principles of trauma surgery

principles of

trauma surgery

edited by

Joseph A. Moylan, M.D.
Professor of Surgery and Chief of Trauma Service
Duke University Medical Center
Durham, North Carolina

Gower Medical Publishing
New York • London

Distributed in the USA and Canada by:
J B Lippincott Company
East Washington Square
Philadelphia, PA 19105
USA

Distributed in the UK and
Continental Europe by:
Gower Medical Publishing
Middlesex House
34-42 Cleveland Street
London W1P 5FB
UK

Distributed Australia and New Zealand by:
HarperEducational (Australia) Pty Ltd.
P.O. Box 226
Artarmon
NSW 2064
AUSTRALIA

Distributed in Southeast Asia, Hong Kong,
India and Pakistan by:
APAC Publishers Service
30 Jalan Bahasa
SINGAPORE 1129

Distributed in Japan by:
Nankodo Co. Ltd.
42-6, Hongo 3-chome
Bunkyo-ku
Tokyo 113
JAPAN

Distributed in South America by:
HarperCollins Publishers Latin America
701 Brickell Avenue - Suite 1750
Miami, FL 33131
USA

Library of Congress Cataloging-in-Publication Data
Principles of trauma surgery / edited by Joseph A. Moylan:
with 30 contributors. — 2nd ed.
p. cm.
Rev. ed. of: Trauma surgery. c1988.
Includes bibliographical references and index.
ISBN 1-56375-013-9
1. Wounds and injuries—Surgery. 2. Traumatology.
3. Emergency medicine. I. Moylan, Joseph A.
II. Trauma surgery.
[DNLM: 1. Critical care—methods. 2. Emergencies.
3. Wounds and Injuries—surgery. WO 700 P9578]
RD93.T6965 1991
617.1—dc20
DNLM/DLC
for Library of Congress 91-25073
CIP

British Library Cataloguing in Publication Data

Principles of trauma surgery. - 2nd ed.
I. Moylan, Joseph A.
617.21

ISBN: 1-56375-013-9

Editor: Jane Hunter
Art Director: Jill Feltham
Designer: Nava Anav
Illustration Supervisor: Alan Landau
Illustrators: Iris J. Nichols,
Catherine Chapin (inking),
Vantage Art, Inc. (charts)

Printed in Singapore by Imago Productions (FE) Pte Ltd.

10 9 8 7 6 5 4 3 2 1

To my wife, Ann Carole; and to my children, Sean, Michael, Brendan, Maura, Kiernan, and Katie. Their zeal for life and deep concern for the well-being of others motivate my every endeavor.

CONTRIBUTORS

ERLE H. AUSTIN, M.D.
Chief of Pediatric Cardiac Surgery
Department of Surgery
University of Louisville
Louisville, Kentucky

WILLIAM H. CHAMBERLIN, M.D.
Director, Intensive Care Unit
Michael Reese Hospital and Medical Center
Associate Professor of Clinical Medicine
Pritzker School of Medicine
University of Chicago
Chicago, Illinois

W. RANDOLPH CHITWOOD, JR., M.D.
Professor and Chief
Division of Cardiothoracic Surgery
Department of Surgery
East Carolina University School of Medicine
Pitt Memorial Hospital
Greenville, North Carolina

CHARLES T. CLOUTIER, M.D.
Assistant Professor of Surgery
College of Medicine
The Ohio State University
The Ohio State University Hospitals
Director, The Ohio State University-Mercy
Hospital Affiliated Surgical Residency
Program
Columbus, Ohio

P. WILLIAM CURRERI, M.D.
Professor and Chairman
Department of Surgery
College of Medicine
University of South Alabama
University of South Alabama Medical Center
Mobile, Alabama

FRANCIS G. DUHAYLONGSOD, M.D.
Research Fellow
Department of Surgery
Duke University Medical Center
Durham, North Carolina

JOHN J. FERRARA, M.D.
Associate Professor of Surgery
Department of Surgery
Tulane University Medical Center
New Orleans, Louisiana

HOWARD C. FILSTON, M.D.
Professor and Chief of Pediatric Surgery
University of Tennessee Medical Center at Knoxville
Knoxville, Tennessee

W. PETER GEIS, M.D.
Vice Chairman, Department of Surgery
Lutheran General Hospital
Associate Professor of Surgery
Abraham Lincoln School of Medicine
University of Illinois at Chicago
Chicago, Illinois

GREGORY S. GEORGIADE, M.D.
Associate Professor of General Surgery and of
Plastic, Maxillofacial and Reconstructive Surgery
Duke University Medical Center
Durham, North Carolina

JOHN L. GLOVER, M.D.
Chief, Surgical Services
William Beaumont Hospital
Royal Oak, Michigan

CLEON W. GOODWIN, M.D.
Associate Professor
Director, Burn Center
Department of Surgery
Cornell University Medical College
Director, Burn Center
Associate Attending Physician
New York Hospital
New York, New York

JOHN P. GRANT, M.D.
Associate Professor of Surgery
Duke University Medical Center
Durham, North Carolina

RAYMOND G. MAKHOUL, M.D.
Vascular Fellow
UCLA Medical Center
Los Angeles, California

MARK E. MANSTEIN, M.D.
Attending Plastic Surgeon
Albert Einstein Hospital
Philadelphia
Holy Redeemer Hospital and
Medical Center
Meadowbrook, Pennsylvania

Richard L. McCann, M.D.
Associate Professor of Surgery
Duke University Medical Center
Durham, North Carolina

Mary C. McCarthy, M.D.
Associate Professor of Surgery
Wright State University
Dayton, Ohio

Norman E. McSwain, Jr., M.D.
Professor of Surgery
School of Medicine
Tulane University Medical Center
New Orleans, Louisiana

Anthony A. Meyer, M.D., Ph.D.
Professor of Surgery
Medical Director of Critical Care
Director, Surgical Intensive Care Unit
University of North Carolina
Chapel Hill, North Carolina

Gerald S. Moss, M.D.
Dean, College of Medicine
University of Illinois
Chicago, Illinois

Joseph A. Moylan, M.D.
Professor of Surgery and Chief of Trauma Service
Duke University Medical Center
Durham, North Carolina

Thomas L. Novick, M.D.
Trauma Service, Carolinas Medical Center
Charlotte Surgical Group, P.A.
Charlotte, North Carolina

David F. Paulson, M.D.
Professor and Chief
Division of Urologic Surgery
Duke University Medical Center
Durham, North Carolina

William C. Pederson, M.D.
Assistant Professor and Division Head
Division of Plastic and Reconstructive Surgery
University of Texas
Health Science Center
San Antonio, Texas

Basil A. Pruitt, Jr., M.D.
Colonel, MC
Commander and Director
U.S. Army Institute of Surgical Research
Department of the Army
Fort Sam Houston
San Antonio, Texas

Jeffrey R. Saffle, M.D.
Assistant Professor of Surgery
University of Utah School of Medicine
Salt Lake City, Utah

John D. Saletta, M.D.
Vice Chairman, Department of Surgery
Lutheran General Hospital
Clinical Professor of Surgery
University of Chicago
Chicago, Illinois

Worthington G. Schenk III, M.D.
Associate Professor of Surgery
Director, Trauma Service
Department of Surgery
University of Virginia Medical Center
Charlottesville, Virginia

Donald Serafin, M.D.
Professor and Chief
Division of Plastic, Maxillofacial and Reconstructive Surgery
Duke University Medical Center
Durham, North Carolina

Glenn D. Warden, M.D.
Shrine Professor of Surgery
University of Cincinnati College of Medicine
Cincinnati, Ohio

Walter G. Wolfe, M.D.
Professor of Surgery
Duke University Medical Center
Durham, North Carolina

PREFACE

Trauma continues to be the major cause of death in the young and productive members of our society. In addition, it is a significant contributing cause of death in the retired and elderly population, who have become very mobile with more leisure time. Increased mechanization, in industry, at home, and in recreation, has resulted in an upsurge in industrial and recreational trauma. The number of admissions to emergency departments secondary to major injuries is increasing each year, making trauma surgery (ie, surgical practice focusing on multisystem, life-threatening, and other injuries resulting in significant morbidity) an increasing portion of the daily practice of general and other specialty surgeons.

Significant progress in trauma surgery during World War II, the Korean War, and the Vietnam conflict was secondary to attention to surgical practice. Improved techniques in managing life-threatening injuries resulted in better survival and decreased morbidity rates. Surgeons providing care for traumatized military personnel acquired much experience in efficient triage, effective resuscitation, and aggressive surgical interventions, and they educated their colleagues during the postwar periods.

During the past two decades, public and governmental demands on improving the organization and delivery of emergency care have resulted in categorization of emergency departments; improved prehospital care delivered by basic-, intermediate-, and advanced-level emergency medical technicians; rapid access to emergency care through region-wide controlled and dispatched communications; better-equipped ground and air ambulances; and the designation and commitment of trauma centers. These improvements have resulted in better field stabilization, accurate triage, and the establishment of resuscitative protocols in emergency departments, which result in the early salvage of more critically injured patients, placing increased demands on surgeons for skilled operative and nonoperative management and care of multisystem-injured patients.

Current attention of trauma care has returned to surgical practice and techniques. The purpose of this volume is to focus on modern-day management of civilian injuries in the environment of sophisticated high technology used in diagnosis and treatment, while sharing practical approaches to the management of both common and complex injuries. Each author brings extensive personal experience in the daily management of trauma patients. The authors were urged to integrate basic pathophysiology with practical technical information on current techniques, diagnosis, and treatment. The practicing general surgeon and specialty surgeon dealing with trauma, as well as the surgeon in training, will benefit from this practical approach to these universal problems.

Joseph A. Moylan, M.D.

Acknowledgments

I am deeply appreciative of the efforts of each of the authors in sharing their extensive expertise in practical and succinct chapters.

I am also indebted to Mary Ann Pickard and Kevin Fitzpatrick for their hard work and careful attention to detail. Eunice Wright's cheerful perseverance during the rewriting and editing of chapters made it possible to complete the task efficiently.

Finally, I am indebted to Duke Hospital; to the Chairman of Surgery, David C. Sabiston, M.D.; and especially to the surgical residents who provided the environment that makes the practice of trauma surgery exciting and whose encouragement and questioning minds have challenged me to seek better solutions to difficult surgical problems.

CONTENTS

initial assessment of trauma

1
2 6
3 7 11
4 8 12 16
5 9 13 17
10 14 18
15 19
20

John D. Saletta
W. Peter Geis

PREHOSPITAL PHASE

Time: The Crucial Factor

Initial assessment of the trauma victim must begin at the scene of the injury. In most large urban areas, trauma victims are initially cared for by emergency medical technicians (EMTs) or paramedics who possess a variety of resuscitation skills depending on their level of training.

EMT-Ambulance (EMT-A) Personnel at the EMT-A level have been trained to provide cardiopulmonary resuscitation; to obtain and maintain an airway using bag-valve mask, valve-to-mouth, mouth-to-mask, and mouth-to-mouth techniques; to control bleeding and to splint fractures using traction splints, spine boards, and bandaging techniques; to employ extrication techniques; and to be familiar with the use of heavy rescue equipment. Mountain, over-water, and special weather training may be included, depending on locale.

EMT-Intermediate (EMT-I) In addition to the basic training outlined above, EMT-I personnel are trained in patient assessment, including the detection and treatment of shock; intravenous fluid therapy and venous access techniques; advanced airway management using endotracheal intubation; defibrillation; and elementary ECG interpretation.

EMT-Paramedic (EMT-P) In addition to the skills taught at the EMT-A and the EMT-I levels, EMT-P training covers the total prehospital management of the patient, which includes pharmacologic therapy of cardiovascular emergencies and decompression of pneumothorax.[22]

Considerable controversy exists regarding which of these EMT skills should be utilized in the trauma victim. Numerous studies have shown the positive benefits of extended cardiopulmonary resuscitation in patients suffering from acute myocardial infarction. In trauma victims, however, the major determinant of survival, other than the injury itself, is clearly the time from injury to definitive treatment.[10,21]

Trauma deaths have been characterized as immediate, early, and late. Approximately 50% of all trauma deaths are classified as immediate, whereby the patient dies instantly or within a few minutes of the injury. In these instances death is usually caused by massive destruction of vital organs and therefore all attempts to salvage this group of patients are hopeless.

Early deaths are those that occur within 2 to 3 hours of injury, and they constitute approximately 30% of all trauma deaths. It is this group of patients whose outcome will be determined largely by the quality of their initial assessment and resuscitation as well as by the rapidity with which they can be transported to a trauma center. Deaths in this group of patients are usually caused by major internal bleeding within the head, chest, or abdomen. A study of traumatic acute subdural hematomas by Seelig and colleagues demonstrated that if surgical intervention was delayed for more than 4 hours after injury, there was a 90% mortality rate and only a 10% functional recovery rate in those who survived. If, on the other hand, definitive surgical care was provided within 4 hours, the mortality rate was 30% with a 60% to 70% functional recovery rate among the survivors.[20] Similarly, massive intra-abdominal or intrathoracic hemorrhage will lead to certain death unless definitive operative intervention can be provided within the first 1 to 2 hours.

During World War I, the time delay between injury and surgery ranged between 12 and 18 hours, resulting in an overall mortality rate of 8.5%. The time interval in World War II was 6 to 12 hours, and the mortality rate was 5.8%. During the Korean War, the time lag was reduced to 2 to 4 hours, with a mortality rate of 2.4%, falling further during the Vietnam War to approximately 1 hour, with a mortality rate of 1.7%. These figures highlight the importance of rapid transport of the trauma victim, and they are all the more impressive when one considers the increased sophistication of military weapons and the resultant increased severity of injury during the Korean and Vietnam wars.

The third mortality group, the so-called late deaths, account for approximately 20% of all trauma deaths; 80% of these patients die of sepsis or multiple organ failure or both. Some of these deaths might be preventable with more appropriate initial surgical treatment and intensive postoperative care.

Medical Control

It is clear from the foregoing discussion that in order to decrease the numbers of early deaths, a system must be in place to give optimum care at the scene of injury and to provide safe and rapid transportation to a sophisticated trauma center. The best system involves the use of EMTs and paramedics whose actions are coordinated by a skilled trauma specialist. EMTs and paramedics must have protocols at the scene of the accident for the management of trauma patients, as well as two-way radio communication with the trauma center personnel who are responsible for directing the resuscitation efforts and ensuring that the patient is transferred to the hospital as rapidly as possible.

Assessment of Injury Severity

Since severity of injury is most closely correlated with mortality, several methods have been developed for its objective assessment. The methods used most frequently are the Injury Severity Score, the Trauma Score, and the Crams Scale.

The Injury Severity Score An anatomical measure of injury severity based on the Abbreviated Injury Scale (a scale for grading injury severity by organ with increasing scores for increased severity), the Injury Severity Score is a reliable index for predicting patient outcome. However, its data base requires identification of anatomical injury, which usually is accurately determined only retrospectively, after definitive management has occurred.[1]

The Trauma Score This is a composite that includes measurements of the status of the cardiovascular, respiratory, and central nervous systems. It measures the physiological state of the patient and can be determined at the scene of injury; it is, therefore, most useful in assessment and trauma triage. It incorporates the Glasgow Coma Scale as its CNS component and grades the three vital organ systems that are likely to fail and result in death shortly after injury (Fig. 1.1). Figure 1.2 shows the correlation between the Trauma Score and patient survival.[2]

It has been estimated that the Trauma Score can be measured in the prehospital phase with 98% accuracy.[3] Experience has demonstrated that patients likely to benefit from prompt diagnosis and timely definitive care at a level I trauma center are those with a Trauma Score of 12 or less.

The CRAMS Scale Developed by S. P. Gormican in 1982, the CRAMS Scale was recently modified by Clemmer and coworkers (Fig. 1.3). CRAMS, which stands for Circulation, Respirations, Abdomen, Motor, and Speech, is an easy scale to remember and simple to apply in the field. In the study by Clemmer and colleagues 94.5% of the patients had field scores of 7 or greater, and in this group there was one emergency room death and two late in-hospital deaths, for a mortality rate of 0.15%. Patients with field scores of 6 or less accounted for 5.5%, and in this group 37% died in the emergency department, for an overall mortality of 62%. Utilizing a CRAMS score of 8 or less as a criterion for transporting patients to a level I trauma center would result in approximately 18% of trauma patients being transported and would encompass all the patients with potentially lethal injuries. It remains for each community to make its own decision with regard to what CRAMS score it will utilize in determining when to transport a patient to a level I trauma center.[4,12]

In addition to utilizing the Trauma Score for triage decisions, "mechanism-of-injury" factors and anatomical factors are also important. Those mechanism-of-injury factors that have a high correlation with life-threatening injuries include evidence of collisions involving high energy dissipation or rapid deceleration; a fall of 15 feet or more; evidence that the patient was in a dangerous environment when injured (e.g., a burning building or icy water); or an automobile accident involving an extrication time longer than 20 minutes, passenger space invaded by 1 foot or more, ejection from the vehicle, death of other passengers, or the striking of a child less than 12 years of age. Anatomical factors that correlate with mortality include a penetrating trauma to the head, neck, torso, groin, or thigh; major amputations above the ankle or wrist; major burns in association with trauma (second- or third-degree over more than 20% of the body); or paralysis.[3]

Triage and Trauma Care Systems

During the past several years, numerous studies have demonstrated that patients with injuries resulting from motor vehicle accidents who were treated in hospitals which were not trauma centers had a significantly greater mortality than those who were taken to a trauma center.[8,23] The American College of Surgeons has defined and published guidelines for levels I, II, and III trauma centers.[7] The major difference in the various levels lies in the 24-hour availability of trauma care specialists, that is, surgeons and anesthesiologists (Fig. 1.4).

By using two-way radio communication with the trauma center, emergency rescue teams in the field can determine which patients require transfer to a level I trauma center. In most trauma systems only 5% to 10% of trauma victims are directed to level I trauma centers.

A model trauma system has been established in West Germany, with designated trauma centers strategically located along major thoroughfares so that 90% of the population is within 15 minutes of one. The government has provided a helicopter system with ground ambulance backup for a response time of approximately 8 to 12 minutes. As a consequence of this regionalized system, West Germany has accomplished a 25% reduction in mortality following motor vehicle accidents. It is imperative that surgeons in our own country work to develop local trauma care systems and participate in the education of EMTs and paramedics.

Lifesaving Measures in the Field

AIRWAY CONTROL AND VENTILATION

The most common form of death in patients with head injuries is airway obstruction or aspiration causing acute hypoxia. The establishment of an adequate airway is the first priority in the management of the injured patient and initially requires the clearing of secretions, broken teeth, dentures, and other obstructions from the airway. Occasionally, an adequate airway may be provided with a jaw-thrust maneuver and use of an oropharyngeal airway, but more often endotracheal intubation is required. Undoubtedly no other skill is more valuable to the emergency medical technician than the ability to perform a successful intubation.

In the past it had been thought that the esophageal obturator airway (EOA) was an effective alternative to endotracheal intubation, but several studies have now demonstrated that the EOA does not function as well as was originally anticipated and that the incidence of inadequate ventilation is unacceptably high.[9] In patients with suspected cervical fractures, hyperextension of the neck in preparation for oral endotracheal intubation may pose a risk of injury to the cervical spinal cord. However, if death from hypoxia is imminent, nasotracheal or orotracheal intubation should be attempted. Nasotracheal intubation is preferable since it can be performed without hyperextending the neck; however, the technique is a blind one which is often more difficult to perform successfully and should not be attempted if the patient has experienced respiratory arrest. The insertion of chest tubes in the field is inappropriate; however, if a tension pneumothorax is strongly suspected, needle aspiration of the pleural space may be lifesaving.

CIRCULATORY SUPPORT

The second most common cause of death in the field is exsanguination. External bleeding is usually best controlled with direct pressure, although occasionally pressure dressings with Ace-type wraps will suffice. The use of tourniquets should be discouraged. Internal bleeding cannot be controlled at the scene of the accident, and therefore rapid transfer to the hospital for operative control of bleeding is essential.

FIGURE 1.1
THE TRAUMA SCORE

TRAUMA SCORE	VALUE	POINTS	SCORE
A. Respiratory rate	10–24	4	
Number of respiration in 15 sec, times 4	25–35	3	
	>35	2	
	<10	1	
	0	0	A. ______
B. Respiratory effort			
Normal	Normal	1	
Shallow—markedly decreased chest movement or air exhange	Shallow or	0	
Reactive—use of accessory muscles or intercostal retraction	Reactive	0	B. ______
C. Systolic blood pressure			
Systolic cuff presssure, either arm, auscultate or palpate	>90	4	
	70–90	3	
	50–69	2	
	<50	1	
No cartoid pulse	0	0	C. ______
D. Capillary refill			
Normal—forehead, lip mucosa, opr nail bed color refills in 2 sec	Normal	2	
Delayed—more than 2 sec of capillary refill	Delayed	1	
None—no capillary refill	None	0	D. ______

E. Glasgow coma scale		Total Points	Score	
1. Eye opening				
Spontaneous	4	14–15	5	
To Voice	3	11–13	4	
To Pain	2	8–10	3	
None	1	5–7	2	E. ______
2. Verbal response				
Orientated	5			
Confused	4			
Inappropriate words	3			
Incomprehensible words	2			
None	1			
3. Motor response				
Obeys commands	6			
Purposeful movement (pain)	5			
Withdraw (pain)	4			
Flexion (pain)	3			
Extension (pain)	2			
None	1			

Trauma Score ______

Total points (1 + 2 + 3) ______

Total Points (A + B + C+ D + E) ______

Champion HR, Sacco WJ, Carnazzo AJ et al: Trauma score. Crit Care Med 9(9):673, 1987.

FIGURE 1.2
PROBABILITIES OF SURVIVAL (P_S) FOR AND PERCENTAGE OF PATIENTS WITH EACH VALUE OF TS

TS	P_S	PERCENTAGE
16	0.99	66.0
15	0.98	14.0
14	0.95	6.3
13	0.91	3.4
12	0.83	2.8
11	0.71	1.3
10	0.55	1.6
9	0.37	0.49
8	0.22	0.24
7	0.12	0.24
6	0.07	0.49
5	0.04	0.00
4	0.02	0.12
3	0.01	0
2	0	3.2
1	0	0

FIGURE 1.3
MODIFIED CRAMS SCALE

Circulation	2—Normal cap. refill and BP greater than 100 mm Hg systolic 1—Delayed cap. refill or BP 85-99 mm Hg systolic 0—No cap. refill or BP less than 85 mm Hg systolic
Respiration	2—Normal 1—Abnormal (labored, shallow, or rate greater than 35) O—Absent
Abdomen	2—Abdomen and thorax not tender 1—Abdomen or thorax tender 0—Abdomen rigid, thorax flail, or deep penetrating injury to either chest or abdomen
Motor	2—Normal (obeys commands) 1—Responds only to pain, no posturing 0—Postures or no response
Speech	2—Normal (oriented) 1—Confused or inappropriate 0—Unintelligible or no sounds
	_____ Total CRAMS score

Clemmer TP, Orme JF, Thomas F, Brooks KA: Prospective evaluation of the CRAMS scale for triaging major trauma. J Trauma 25[3]:188–191, 1985.

FIGURE 1.4
LEVELS OF CATEGORIZATION OF TRAUMA CENTERS AND THEIR ESSENTIAL (E) OR DESIRABLE (D) CHARACTERISTICS

CHARACTERISTIC	LEVEL I	LEVEL II	LEVEL III
HOSPITAL ORGANIZATION			
Trauma service	E	E	D
Surgery departments/divisions/services/sections (each staffed by qualified specialists)			
Cardiothoracic surgery	E	D	
General surgery	E	E	E
Neurologic surgery	E	E	
Obstetrics-gynecologic surgery	D	D	
Opthalmic surgery	E	D	
Oral surgery-dental	D	D	
Orthopedic surgery	E	E	
Otorhinolaryngologic surgery	E	D	
Pediatric surgery	E	D	
Plastic and maxillofacial surgery	E	D	
Urologic surgery	E	D	
Emergency department/division/service/section (staffed by qualified specialists)*	E	E	E
Surgical specialties availability†			
In house 24 hours a day			
General surgery	E	E‡	
Neurologic surgery	E§	E§	
On call and promptly available from inside or outside hospital			
Cardiac surgery	E	D	
General surgery			E
Neurologic surgery			D
Microsurgery capabilities	E	D	
Gynecologic surgery	E	D	
Hand surgery	E	D	
Ophthalmic surgery	E	E	D
Oral surgery (dental)	E	D	
Orthopedic surgery	E	E	D
Otorhinolaryngologic surgery	E	E	D
Pediatric surgery	E	D	
Plastic and maxillofacial surgery	E	E	D
Thoracic surgery	E	E	D
Urologic surgery	E	E	D

FIGURE 1.4
LEVELS OF CATEGORIZATION OF TRAUMA CENTERS AND THEIR ESSENTIAL (E) OR DESIRABLE (D) CHARACTERISTICS (CONTINUED)

CHARACTERISTIC	LEVEL I	LEVEL II	LEVEL III
Nonsurgical specialities availability			
In hospital 24 hours a day			
Emergency medicine	E[‖]	E[‖]	E
Anesthesiology	E[#]	E[**]	E[††]
On call and promptly available from inside or outside hospital			
Cardiology	E	E	D
Thoracic medicine	E	D	
Gastroenterology	E	D	
Hematology	E	E	D
Infectious diseases	E	D	
Internal medicine	E	E	E
Nephrology	E	E	D
Neuroradiology	D		
Pathology	E	E	E
Pediatrics	E	E	E
Psychiatry	E	D	
Radiology	E	E	E

* The emergency department staffing should ensure immediate and appropriate care for the trauma patient. The emergency department physician should function as a designated member of the trauma team, and the relationship between emergency department physician and other members of the trauma team must be established on a local level, consistent with resources but adhering to established standards and ensuring optimal care.

† Requirements may be fulfilled by senior residents capable of assessing emergency situations in their respective specialities. They must be capable of providing surgical treatment immediately and of providing the control and surgical leadership for the care of the trauma patient. When residents are used to fulfill availability requirements, staff specialists must be on call and promptly available.

‡ The established trauma system should ideally ensure that the trauma surgeon will be present in the emergency department at the time of the patient's arrival. When sufficient prior notification has not been possible, a designated member of the trauma team will immediately initiate the evaluation and resuscitation. Definitive surgical care must be instituted by the trauma surgeon in a timely manner consistent with established standards.

§ An attending neurosurgeon must be promptly available and dedicated to the hospital's trauma service. The in-house requirement may be fulfilled by an in-house neurosurgeon or surgeon (or physician in level II facilities) who has special competence, as judged by the Chief of Neurosurgery, in the care of patients with neural trauma and who is capable of initiating measures directed toward stabilizing the patient and initiating diagnostic procedures.

‖ In level I and level II institutions, requirement may be fulfilled by senior-level emergency medicine residents capable of assessing emergency situations in trauma patients and providing an indicated treatment. When residents are used to fulfill availability requirements, the staff specialist on call will be advised and be promptly available.

\# Requirements may be fulfilled by residents capable of assessing emergent situations in trauma patients and of providing any indicated treatment. When residents are used to fulfill availability requirements, the staff anesthesiologist on call will be advised and be available promptly.

** May be fulfilled when local conditions ensure that the staff anesthesiologist will be in the hospital at the time of or shortly after the patient's arrival in the hospital. During the interim, prior to the arrival of the staff anesthesiologist, a certified nurse anesthetist (CRNA) capable of assessing emergency situations in the trauma patients and of initiating and providing any indicated treatment will be available.

†† Requirements may be fulfilled by certified registered nurse anesthetists (CRNAs) capable of assessing emergency requirements, the staff anesthesiologist on call will be advised immediately and will attend promptly.

Modified from the Committee on Trauma of the American College of Surgeons: Hospital and pre-hospital resources for optimal care of the injured patient. ACS Bulletin 68(10):13–18, 1983.

Two schools of thought exist with regard to the establishment of an intravenous line (IV). One school advocates rapid transfer to the hospital with avoidance of any attempts in the field to insert an IV. Once en route to the hospital, an attempt may be made to start an IV, but this is often found to be quite difficult in a hypovolemic patient with collapsed veins in a moving ambulance. In a study of 100 patients who experienced prehospital cardiac arrest, the average time for starting an IV in the field was 11 minutes.[16] For the patient with exsanguinating internal hemorrhage, this time is better spent in reaching a trauma center where multiple large-bore intravenous catheters can be rapidly inserted, intravenous cutdowns performed, and the patient transported to the operating room for definitive hemorrhage control. On the other hand, Jacobs and associates have demonstrated improved Trauma Scores between the scene of the accident and the hospital when patients have received advanced life-support techniques, including the placement of intravenous lines.[13] The present data suggest that for those patients requiring short transit times to the hospital, the placement of IVs should be deferred, whereas in those patients requiring a travel time greater than 30 minutes, placement of IVs should be attempted.

Additional controversy exists regarding the use of the pneumatic antishock garment (PASG), which has been widely employed in civilian trauma systems since its first introduction in Vietnam. The pneumatic antishock garment primarily increases peripheral vascular resistance because of its tourniquet effect below the waist. The garment is especially useful in patients with internal bleeding from sources covered by the garment itself, such as a fractured bony pelvis. Some of the negative effects of the use of this garment include progressive metabolic acidosis, compromise of ventilation due to restriction of rib cage expansion and elevation of the diaphragm, and ischemic damage to the lower extremities when the garment is left inflated for long periods. Additionally, a profound hypotensive effect is noted when the pneumatic antishock garment is deflated prior to the replacement of circulating volume losses. Several recent studies have failed to show any differences in survival among patients with exsanguinating hemorrhage treated with or without a pneumatic antishock garment.[14] The use of a PASG should probably be reserved for patients with major lower extremity and pelvic fractures associated with massive hemorrhage.[5]

EXTRICATION, SPINAL PROTECTION, AND IMMOBILIZATION

For those patients who are trapped in vehicles following an accident, extrication is an additional important lifesaving maneuver. The basic principles are to allow as little extraneous movement as possible, to protect the spine, and to immobilize fractured extremities.

Spinal cord protection is extremely important in any patient who is at risk for a spinal fracture. This is especially true in the unconscious patient or the patient with injuries above the clavicle. The head is usually secured in a neutral position against a spine board and supported with sandbags as well as tape across the forehead. Cervical collars are less reliable in stabilizing the neck. Impaled objects should never be removed unless they are obstructing the airway.

All suspected extremity fractures should be immobilized in order to prevent damage to vessels, nerves, and soft tissue; to control pain, and to prevent further hemorrhage. Fractures may be immobilized with inflatable tubular splints or gauze wrapped against a rigid support.

HOSPITAL PHASE

Trauma Resuscitation Area and the Trauma Team

Hospitals that manage trauma victims should have a designated trauma resuscitation area and a defined trauma team. The trauma resuscitation area should be spacious and well lighted. Essential equipment within the area should include oxygen, suction, focus lighting, oropharyngeal airways, laryngoscopes, endotracheal tubes, nasotracheal tubes, IV catheters and fluids, nasogastric tubes, urinary catheters, thoracostomy tubes, cutdown trays, peritoneal lavage sets, open thoracotomy trays, and monitoring equipment. The trauma resuscitation team should consist of one and preferably two highly skilled physicians who are thoroughly familiar with the techniques required to resuscitate the acutely injured patient. One of these physicians should be designated as the team leader and should direct all of the resuscitation efforts. In addition to the physicians, two nurses, a recorder, a respiratory technician, and a laboratory technician are desirable members of the trauma resuscitation team.

Primary Survey

The ensuing discussion will outline the assessment of the organ systems whose derangements may be immediately life-threatening. The discussion will further describe emergency lifesaving maneuvers that are simple and readily available to provide lifesaving support for approximately 85% of seriously injured patients. It must be emphasized, however, that the first step is identifying the life-threatening injury. The description of the primary survey will, therefore, outline an organized and structured assessment of each of the vital organ systems and will identify derangements that are both immediately life-threatening and detectable on physical examination.

For purposes of organization, assessment is often considered separate from emergency treatment modalities. However, the trauma physician should recognize that the primary survey involves a versatile shifting back and forth between assessment and lifesaving intervention. Clearly, when assessment of the airway reveals the need to intervene and reverse hypoxic state, it is appropriate to do so immediately. Once the lifesaving procedure has been performed, the physician then returns to assessment of breathing mechanics, circulatory status, and so on. The following description of the primary survey is an intermingling of primary assessment and lifesaving intervention.

AIRWAY

The first priority in the management of the trauma patient is the establishment of an adequate airway. Frequently this will require the clearing of broken teeth, secretions, and blood from the mouth, and this can be most readily accomplished by inserting a finger into the pharynx, as well as suctioning the mouth and pharynx. In the unconscious patient, the tongue frequently falls back against the posterior pharynx and obstructs the airway. The chin-lift and jaw-thrust maneuvers can pull the tongue away from the posterior pharynx and allow for the insertion of an oropharyngeal airway. The chin-lift maneuver consists of placing the fingers of one hand beneath the mandible and the thumb behind the lower lip or incisor teeth and pulling the chin anteriorly. The jaw-thrust maneuver is performed by grasping the angles of the mandible bilaterally and pulling them forward.

In the unconscious patient, especially one with head and neck injuries, a cervical spine fracture must be strongly suspected. Consequently, all maneuvers that might either hyperextend or hyperflex the neck must be avoided. Flexion of the neck is disadvantageous for two reasons. Cervical flexion allows the base of the tongue to approximate the posterior wall of the pharynx, thus exaggerating, rather than relieving, a partial airway obstruction. Further, cervical spine injuries most commonly occur in the flexed position. By reproducing the mechanism of injury, flexion, the cervical spinal cord is most apt to be injured. Statistically, therefore, the least desirable manipulation of the cervical spine is flexion. If time permits, a cross-table lateral cervical spine radiograph should be obtained prior to introducing an oral endotracheal tube, which usually requires hyperextension of the neck.

In those patients in whom nasal or oral endotracheal intubation is unsuccessful, either because of technical failure, glottic edema, or severe facial injuries, an immediate cricothyroidotomy should be performed. The procedure is best accomplished by making a transverse incision through skin and cricothyroid membrane utilizing a number 11 blade scalpel. The handle of the scalpel or a curved hemostat may be used to enlarge the opening for insertion of a pediatric tracheostomy tube or a 4-mm to 6-mm endotracheal tube. If long-term endotracheal intubation is required, a formal tracheostomy may be performed as a semi-elective procedure.

Many authors recommend that cricothyroidotomy be avoided in children under the age of 12. The rationale is to avoid damage to the pediatric cricoid cartilage—the only circumferential structure supporting the larynx and upper trachea. However, our experience has indicated that surgical cricothyroidotomy is safe and effective in children as young as 4 to 5 years of age in immediately life-threatening circumstances. Glottic anatomy and size are adequate for emergency surgical cricothyroidotomy in the 4- to 12-year age group when needle cricothyroidotomy is deemed to be less effective. The alternative method of needle cricothyroidotomy is performed by inserting a 12- to 14-gauge needle through the cricothyroid membrane. The needle is then connected to an oxygen outlet at 15 liters per minute. Utilizing a Y connector or a side hole cut in the tubing, an intermittent ventilation pattern of 1 second on, 4 seconds off can be achieved by placing a thumb over the Y connector or the side hole. The technique is usually adequate for a maximum of 30 to 45 minutes, providing a lifesaving approach and allowing time for a semi-urgent intubation or tracheostomy.

Once any tube has been inserted into the trachea, its functional position should be established by auscultating both lung fields, as well as by confirming the tube's position using a radiograph. It is essential to be sure that the tube has not extended into the right main bronchus, thereby partially occluding the left bronchus. Inadvertent intubation of the esophagus must also be immediately recognized and corrected. A well-positioned, cuffed endotracheal tube provides optimum control of the mechanics of ventilation as well as protection against potential aspiration.

The esophageal obturator airway (EOA) or the modified version with a nasogastric tube, the esophageal gastric tube airway (EGTA), has little or no place in the management of the hospitalized trauma patient. The trauma physician should, however, be familiar with these airways, since they are often in place when the patient arrives at the hospital. The EOA and EGTA are utilized by the paramedics to maintain an airway and ventilatory support in unconscious patients only. When the unconscious trauma patient arrives at the hospital, the EOA should be maintained inflated and in place until intubation of the trachea is performed with a cuffed endotracheal tube. The EOA cuff is then deflated, the tube removed, and oral suction made readily available. These steps are aimed at avoiding aspiration of gastric contents in the unconscious patient. Occasionally, an unconscious patient with an EOA inserted will become conscious while the EOA is still in place. In this circumstance, careful decompression of the EOA cuff followed by removal of the tube is safe and effective. In both instances, the EGTA is preferable, since the in-line nasogastric tube decompresses and empties the stomach prior to removal of the esophageal airway tube.

NECK

Inspection of the neck is crucial to the proper assessment of the airway, respiratory, and circulatory systems. Further, the neck must be readily accessible for the performance of lifesaving interventions; a spinal immobilization collar should never stand between the physician and proper assessment of the neck. Immediately after assessment of the airway and prior to assessment of the thorax, the neck should be examined for the following three factors, since each provides data regarding derangements of the airway, respiratory, and circulatory systems: the degree of distention (fullness) of the jugular veins, color and temperature of the skin, and anatomical location of the trachea at the suprasternal location. Nontraumatized patients will have pink, warm skin; barely visible external jugular vein fullness; and a midline trachea. The most common variance in these findings is seen in the hypovolemic patient, where the trachea is midline, the skin is pale and cool, and the external jugular veins are flat in the supine position. In contrast, a blue discoloration of the skin suggests cyanosis, implicating a life-threatening mechanical injury to the chest or airway. Distended jugular veins raise suspicion of cardiac tamponade, tension pneumothorax, or, rarely, flail chest. Petechiae (traumatic cyanosis) suggests a profound compression injury of the upper torso, raising the suspicion of life-threatening intrathoracic injuries (e.g., aortic rupture, myocardial contusion, and diaphragmatic rupture). Shift of the trachea laterally suggests a tension pneumothorax or, infrequently, a massive hemothorax.

The neck is also exposed to determine the presence or absence of direct signs of injury. It is helpful to recall that patients with blunt torso trauma may have experienced a penetrating injury as a component of their traumatic event. Direct inspection of the neck is made for penetrating injuries, direct injury to the larynx, or the presence of an expanding hematoma. As a rule, foreign objects impaled in the neck should be maintained in place and removed only in the operating room. An exception is the foreign object that is both impaled and obstructing the airway; this is the single circumstance in which the risk of removal of the object is outweighed by the benefit.

Systematic assessment of the neck also provides additional evidence regarding the risk of cervical spine injury. Swelling, contusions, or tenderness along the vertebral spinous processes increases the suspicion of cervical spine injury. Occasionally, palpation of the spinous processes reveals a "step-off" deformity, suggesting bony fracture. An additional clue that raises the specter of cervical spine injury is given by the patient who insists on holding his head and neck inappropriately rigid and immobile.

The final rationale for exposure of the neck early in the primary assessment is to accomplish access to the cricothyroid membrane. In the rare circumstance in which a cricothyroidotomy must be performed immediately, the cervical collar must not stand in the way. In our center we emphasize that the best use of the cervical collar is during extrication, during transit in the ambulance or helicopter, and as a message to the trauma physician that there is risk of cervical spine injury based on prehospital information available to the paramedics. The collar is, however, not necessary to accomplish cervical spine immobilization in the controlled emergency department or trauma unit setting.

THORAX

There are a finite number of derangements within the thorax that are life-threatening. Five of these injuries are diagnosed during the primary assessment and thereby treated without the need for diagnostic studies. They are described here in the order in which they are diagnosed during physical examination. Each of these disease processes should have suggested themselves to the examining trauma physician by findings observable during examination of the neck. The remaining intrathoracic injuries are not easily diagnosed during the primary survey and require diagnostic studies to provide direct or indirect evidence of injury, the single best being the chest radiograph.

An *open pneumothorax* is immediately life-threatening and is diagnosed readily upon visual inspection of the chest wall. Appropriately, all garments must be removed for thorough inspection. A defect in the chest wall must be large enough to allow air to pass to and fro during respiration. Thus the "sucking chest wound" pulls air into the pleural space during inspiration and blows air out during expiration. The pathophysiological result is a to-and-fro movement of the mediastinum with respiration. The contralateral lung does not expand appropriately during inspiration and does not deflate appropriately during expiration. This combination of events causes a decreasing cardiac output due to kinking of the great veins accompanied by a combination of hypoxia and hypercarbia (asphyxia). Emergency treatment consists of conversion of the open pneumothorax to a closed pneumothorax by application of a petroleum jelly occlusive dressing over the wound. The urgent use of a tube thoracostomy helps to resolve the pneumothorax and avoid the incipient development of a tension pneumothorax. Definitive surgical closure of the chest wound is deferred until the patient's other life-threatening injuries have been managed.

Flail chest occurs when two or more contiguous ribs are fractured in several locations along each of the ribs, creating a segment of free-floating chest wall. The life-endangering mechanism is similar to that of an open pneumothorax. During inspiration the flail segment is "sucked in," resulting in loss of the negative pleural pressure. During expiration, bulging of the segment dissipates intrapleural pressure; the result is a to-and-fro movement of the mediastinum, kinking the great veins, as well as a lack of expansion of the contralateral lung, causing asphyxia. Flail chest is diagnosed most effectively by palpation. Placing the hands symmetrically along the chest wall provides palpable evidence of the injury, and the position of the examiner's hands provides a yardstick to observe chest wall motion. Emergency treatment consists of external pressure to the unstable segment. Definitive emergency care often requires endotracheal intubation. However, some patients without severe hypoxia or excessively rapid respiratory rate are managed with intercostal nerve blocks and vigorous respiratory care. These patients must be observed closely since many of those who initially are not significantly hypoxic will later demonstrate hypoxia due to respiratory muscle fatigue and the development of an underlying pulmonary contusion. The key element in differentiating a progressive pulmonary contusion from a flail chest is intermittent monitoring of the $PC0_2$, since hypercarbia occurs with flail chest and not with pulmonary contusion.

Tension pneumothorax results from an injury to the lung or to the chest wall which creates a one-way valve effect. The resultant defect allows air to enter the pleural space without being able to escape. Consequently, the accumulation of air within the pleural cavity causes the lung on the injured side to collapse and the mediastinum to shift to the opposite side because of positive pressure. This shift of the mediastinum decreases venous return by kinking of the great veins and results in compression of the contralateral lung, resulting in asphyxia. This combination of pathophysiologic events is immediately life-threatening, and the definitive diagnosis is suggested by deviation of the trachea away from the side of injury, cyanosis, distended neck veins, increased tympany to percussion on the side of injury, absent breath sounds on the side of injury, and a labored breathing pattern. Final corroboration of the diagnosis is made during auscultation when maximum auscultatory heart sounds are shifted from their normal location to a new location away from the side of injury. Treatment should not be delayed to document the diagnosis by chest radiograph. Treatment consists of insertion of a large-gauge needle through the second intercostal space in the midclavicular line. A rush of air through the needle confirms the diagnosis and provides immediate relief. Subsequently, a large-bore chest tube is inserted, usually in the fifth intercostal space midaxillary line and adapted to water seal drainage.

*Massive hemothorax*is recognized in patients with chest injuries who are in shock and have labored respirations. Occasionally, physical findings may mimic tension pneumothorax since the trachea may be deviated along with the mediastinum by the large volume of blood, and the contralateral lung may be compressed, resulting in cyanosis along with absent breath sounds on the affected side. Dullness to percussion, however, suggests massive hemothorax rather than pneumothorax. Emergency treatment consists of decompression of the chest using a large-bore chest tube in the fifth intercostal space, midaxillary line, along with fluid resuscitation of the associated hemorrhagic shock. In patients with an initial chest tube drainage greater than 1500 ml, or continued bleeding at a rate greater than 100 ml per hour, urgent thoracotomy is indicated.

Cardiac tamponade is immediately life-threatening and is suspected when primary assessment reveals jugular venous distention in the absence of a tracheal shift or cyanosis. Auscultation of the chest reveals normal breath sounds; cardiac sounds, although in their normal location, are muffled because of depressed cardiac output as well as blood in the pericardial sac. Tamponade is most often associated with stab wounds of the anterior torso and less commonly with gunshot wounds; blunt torso trauma is rarely implicated. These combinations of findings along with hypotension and tachycardia define the diagnosis. Lifesaving intervention consists of needle aspiration of blood from the pericardial sac using the subxiphoid approach. A large-bore cardiac needle is inserted and directed at a 45° angle toward the left shoulder; if the physician aims the needle tip toward the inferior angle of the left scapula posteriorly and laterally, the needle will always enter the pericardial sac directly through the central tendon of the diaphragm. A rule of thumb regarding needle depth is 10 cm; in the average adult, the distance between the subxiphoid skin and the pericardial sac will be within 10 cm. The necessity to introduce the needle deeper may result in aspiration of blood from the left ventricular chamber. The astute physician will, however, note cardiac pulsations transmitted through the needle if its tip is within the myocardium. We recommend a 50-ml syringe with 3-way stopcock for aspiration of pericardial blood. Many authors advise connecting the hub of the cardiac needle to the V-lead of an electrocardiogram during pericardial aspiration for pericardial effusion; however, because pericardial tamponade in the trauma patient is immediately life-threatening, it should be relieved without delaying to connect cardiac monitoring devices.

The removal of as little as 10 ml of blood from the pericardial sac may result in a dramatic improvement in the patient's cardiac output and will confirm the diagnosis. The blood removed from the pericardial sac decreases the pericardial pressure to less than right atrial filling pressure. This relief of pressure allows improved filling of the right atrium and abrupt improvement in cardiac output. Pericardial blood may be clotting or nonclotting in the presence of an active transmural myocardial injury. Rarely, repeated aspirations will fail to result in improved cardiac output. In these circumstances, clotted blood may be compressing the left atrial inflow in a plombage-like fashion; this mandates that the trauma physician consider emergency thoracotomy. Definitive care of all cardiac wounds which result in pericardial tamponade requires operative exploration of the chest, pericardium, and heart.

CIRCULATION AND SHOCK RESUSCITATION

The next priority in the primary survey is the assessment of the circulatory status. Profound hypovolemic shock, if present, is recognized by signs of decreased organ perfusion, such as prolonged capillary filling time, decreased mentation, or diminished urinary output, as well as diaphoresis, tachycardia, diminished pulse pressure, and hypotension. Quantitation of blood loss is essential in order to estimate the extent of the injury and to define the urgency as well as magnitude of volume replacement. Figure 1.5 delineates physical findings associated with four classes of hypovolemia and illustrates that the physical findings associated with class I hemorrhage (15% or 750 ml blood loss) are very subtle. The most sensitive indicators on a moment-to-moment basis are skin perfusion and an increase in the pulse

FIGURE 1.5
INDICES OF HYPOVOLEMIA

CLASSIFICATION OF HEMORRHAGE	0	I	II	III	IV
Skin perfusion (capillary blanch test)	0 (2 sec)	± (2–3 sec)	+ (>3 sec)	++	+++
Pulse rate	0 (48–100/min)	± (72–100/min)	+ (100/min)	++ (120/min)	+++ (140/min)
Respiratory rate	12–16	12–20	20–32	32–40	>40
Pulse pressure	0	0	±	+	++
Mentation	Normal	Slightly anxious	Mildly anxious	Confused	Lethargic
Urine output (ml/hr)	30	30	20–30	5–15	Negligible
Blood pressure	Normal	0 (>100 mm Hg)	± (±100 mm Hg)	+ (<100 mm Hg)	(<80 mm Hg)
Quantitative blood loss in milliliters	0	750	740–1500	1500–2000	>2000
Percentage blood volume deficit	0	15	15–30	30–40	>40

+, abnormal; ±, equivocal; 0, normal.

rate. In class I hemorrhage the pulse rate increases, but rarely to 100 beats per minute, and the capillary blanch test (skin perfusion) is normal or equivocal. Even class II hemorrhage (750 ml to 1500 ml blood loss) is associated with less than dramatic alterations in physical findings. The capillary blanch test is mildly prolonged (from 2 to 3 seconds) and the pulse rate reaches 100 beats per minute or slightly more. The trauma physician must avoid concluding that the less than dramatic physical findings associated with class II hemorrhage are due to anxiety surrounding the circumstances of the patient's traumatic experience. A triad of symptoms—a mildly anxious patient, pulse rate of 100 per minute, and mildly elevated respiratory rate should be treated aggressively as class II hemorrhage (30% or 1500 ml blood loss) until proven otherwise. In contrast, findings associated with class III or class IV hemorrhages are clearly evident and must be treated as immediately life-threatening.

The physician must consider several modalities as lifesaving procedures to combat the progression and metabolic and ischemic consequences of hypovolemia. The first and simplest emergency treatment is to prevent further external blood loss by applying direct pressure or compression dressings to appropriate areas. Blind clamping into open wounds, especially in areas adjacent to major neurovascular structures, should be avoided since this may lead to irreparable nerve damage or may compromise subsequent vascular repair. Tourniquets should be avoided except in amputations. Bleeding from penetrating neck injuries should be controlled with direct finger pressure; circumferential neck dressings should be avoided.

All patients with signs of class I hemorrhage or greater should have intravenous volume replacement. Estimation of the percentage of total blood loss by the indices described provides an initial basis for determining the magnitude of volume replacement, as well as the choice of fluids. However, because the patient will continue to bleed during the resuscitation phase of the primary survey, the estimate should be in excess of the scale. The initial intravenous fluid replacement is a balanced salt solution delivered through large-bore intravenous catheters. An estimate of the volume of balanced salt solution required to replace blood lost is determined by the three to-one rule: 3 ml of salt solution will be required to replace every 1 ml of blood lost. Therefore, the patient who exhibits class II hemorrhage (1500 ml blood loss) should have a minimum of 4500 ml of balanced salt solution. With regard to blood replacement, most patients with class II hemorrhage and all patients with class III or class IV hemorrhage will require blood as a volume expander. The majority of these patients will continue to bleed during the resuscitation phase and during diagnostic assessment, and the great majority will require operative intervention for control of further blood loss.

Intravenous volume expansion will define three subgroups of patients: the first group will respond by marked improvements in their indices of hypovolemia, the second group will demonstrate a transient improvement in their volume status with dubious stabilization, and the third group will continue to deteriorate. The second and third subgroups are candidates for immediate blood replacement with type-specific blood. Type-specific blood is preferred to low-titer O-negative blood, since the latter may be associated with subsequent type and crossmatch difficulties, besides being more expensive and currently less readily available.[18] The second and third subgroups should be directed to the operating room for further assessment, resuscitation, and possible operative exploration without the benefit of a definitive diagnosis if the physical findings continue to demonstrate deterioration in the cardiovascular status. It is imperative, however, to reassess other possible mechanical causes for the deterioration in cardiac output, such as cardiac tamponade, before proceeding with surgical exploration.

Autotransfusion is occasionally used as a beneficial source of immediately available blood for volume expansion in patients with massive bleeding from thoracic injuries. Blood collected by way of tube thoracostomies is anticoagulated and reinfused. Blood obtained from the abdominal cavity is frequently contaminated and contains large amounts of fat and is therefore inappropriate for autotransfusion. Large amounts of autotransfused blood may precipitate coagulopathies; therefore, autotransfusions should be considered only part of the early resuscitation efforts in the massively hemorrhaging patient in the third subgroup.

The pneumatic antishock garment is frequently already in place in patients arriving in the hospital following severe trauma. The garment should be left in place until the patient is fully resuscitated by aggressive intravenous volume expansion, and then its compartments slowly released with careful monitoring of the patient's vital signs, especially blood pressure. The abdominal compartment should be released initially, then the extremity compartments sequentially. The antishock trousers are clearly beneficial in compressing sites of external blood loss in the pelvis and lower extremities and in immobilizing and stabilizing fractures of the lower extremities and the bony pelvis. Immobilization of these bony structures minimizes continued blood loss from adjacent sources. With the exception of the patient who has a shattered bony pelvis, or the patient with massive internal bleeding (in subgroup III), there is very little indication for applying the pneumatic antishock garment in the hospital setting. It is, however, occasionally beneficial to place the pneumatic antishock garment under the subgroup III patient en route to the operating room.

Venous access for intravenous volume replacement is preferably obtained by percutaneous catheters inserted into upper extremity veins. These catheters should be 16 gauge or larger and be placed as centrally to the torso as possible, recognizing that the rate of flow is directly related to the diameter of the catheter and inversely related to its length.[11] If upper extremity veins are not easily cannulated, intravenous cutdowns should be performed over the long saphenous vein in the area of the medial malleolus or at the femoral triangle. Occasionally, the external jugular vein may be cannulated percutaneously with ease. Any attempt to catheterize the internal jugular vein or the subclavian vein in an agitated patient in shock with collapsed veins is extremely difficult and fraught with a high incidence of complications. Therefore, these latter venous access routes are initially avoided in this category of patient. Blood replacement should be accompanied by in-line filters and blood pumps when needed. Warming of solutions is essential, especially when volume is being replaced rapidly.

Approximately 90% of all trauma victims who arrive at the emergency department with hypotension will be experiencing hemorrhagic hypovolemic shock. It is important to differentiate the various types of shock during the primary assessment. Patients with compromised cardiac output due to mechanical intrathoracic injuries, such as tension pneumothorax, open pneumothorax, and flail chest, will have been diagnosed during assessment of the neck and chest. While this group of patients will have hypotension and tachycardia, they will exhibit cyanosis and occasionally distended neck veins in contrast to flat neck veins and the cool, pale skin of hemorrhagic shock. The patient with cardiac tamponade will also exhibit distended jugular veins and distant heart sounds, differentiating this restrictive process from pure hypovolemia. Spinal shock (neurogenic) is differentiated from hemorrhagic shock by the warm, pink skin of vasodilatation, along with bradycardia in the presence of hypotension. This combination suggests an injury to the spinal cord. Bradycardia also occurs after closed head injuries as part of the Cushing response. The head-injured patient with increased intracranial pressure will exhibit hypertension and should not be confused with the spinal-injured patient. Nontamponade, cardiogenic shock rarely occurs in the early phase after injury, but is most frequently associated with profound myocardial contusion, injuries involving coronary arteries, or ascending aortic injuries with aortic dissection retrograde to the coronary ostia. Cardiogenic shock is most often suspected by failure of therapeutic volume resuscitation and not determined definitively until the secondary survey has been completed. Septic shock almost never appears during the initial assessment unless there has been a combination of injury to the gastrointestinal tract with gross contamination associated with a long delay from injury to initial assessment in the hospital setting. The rare occurrence of septic shock will most often be diagnosed after completion of the secondary survey, which includes diagnostic assessment of each organ system injury. While each of the categories of shock have their own unique definitive therapeutic requirements, it is sufficiently important to recall that all types of shock will initially respond beneficially to aggressive intravenous volume expansion of the vascular space.

In rare circumstances, the trauma patient's vital signs will continue to deteriorate in spite of appropriate and aggressive lifesaving resuscitative procedures. If cardiac arrest (absence of blood pressure and respiratory effort) occurs, a lifesaving emergency thoracotomy should be performed. All comprehensive emergency departments that treat multiple trauma victims should be equipped with an emergency thoracotomy surgical tray. A left anterolateral thoracotomy provides the best exposure to the organs most often injured. Absence of severe injury in the chest along with an empty heart reaffirms massive blood loss from multiple sources other than the chest as the cause of cardiac arrest. Continued volume expansion, cardiac massage, compression of the descending thoracic aorta, and cardiac resuscitation, followed by preparation for emergency abdominal exploration, is indicated. Occasionally, the patient will exhibit marked improvement shortly after the performance of an emergency thoracotomy. This subgroup of patients is likely to have experienced either an undiagnosed tension pneumothorax or flail chest which contributed to cardiac arrest. Equilibration of pressures by thoracotomy, combined with control of respiratory mechanics with positive pressure ventilation, inadvertently reverses the dilatorious effects of these life-threatening injuries. Occasionally, entry into the left hemithorax demonstrates direct evidence of a severe injury. The two most common observations are pericardial tamponade and massive left hemothorax. Decompression of the bluish, tense, distended pericardium using a longitudinal incision anterior to and parallel to the phrenic nerve provides an abrupt increase in cardiac output. If after opening the pericardium and evacuating pericardial blood the cardiac status is either ventricular fibrillation or cardiac standstill, then cardiac massage and cardiac resuscitation must be performed immediately. Definitive treatment of the cardiac injury should be performed in the operating room. The majority of penetrating injuries to the heart will not bleed excessively and are most often controlled by gentle application of a sterile gauze to the surface of the heart. There is generally no need to place balloon catheters through the hole in the myocardium, nor is hurried suturing of the injury indicated. Uncommonly, a large atrial laceration will require occlusion by a balloon catheter, a vascular clamp under direct vision, or moderate pressure. When thoracotomy reveals massive hemothorax, the trauma physician should assume that bleeding is most likely to be from the left pulmonary hilum or from a decelerating aortic injury. A useful technique is to cross-clamp the pulmonary hilum with finger pressure, retract the left lung inferiorly, and compress the descending portion of the aortic arch between the fingers while compressing the descending aorta onto the vertebral bodies with the handle of a retractor or a stick sponge. Definitive control will require the skill of a trauma surgeon and/or a thoracic surgeon, as well as excellent suction.

BRIEF NEUROLOGIC EXAMINATION

The final segment of the primary survey is the brief neurologic examination, which evaluates the patient's level of consciousness, the pupillary size and reactivity, and extremity movement in response to pain or command. The purpose of a concise assessment of the neurologic status of the trauma victim is to raise an early index of suspicion of central nervous system injury. Suspicion of neurologic injury provides the opportunity to perform early diagnostic studies during the secondary survey. Thus, as mentioned earlier, the trauma physician has the opportunity to control the single most important factor for reducing mortality following a central nervous system injury: the time interval from injury to definitive treatment.

The primary indicator of central nervous system injury is the patient's level of consciousness. In the brief exam, level of consciousness is placed in one of four categories by the AVPU method: *A*=alert; *V*=response to vocal stimuli; *P*=response to painful stimuli only; and *U*=unresponsive to any stimulus. Secondary findings appropriate to the brief neurologic exam include the vital signs; hypertension and bradycardia suggest increased intracranial pressure while hypotension and bradycardia indicate a spinal cord injury. Mildly dilated pupils that are sluggishly reactive to light also suggest increased intracranial pressure. Finally, the posture of the patient may indicate intracranial injury (decerebrate vs. decorticate rigidity). Each of these factors implicates central nervous system injury suggests urgent performance of a CT examination of the head.

Additional considerations are important in the assessment of the level of consciousness, since other less obvious factors may adversely influence the patient's level of mentation. Common factors include suppressed cardiac output and resultant decreased cerebral perfusion; persistent, unresolved hypoxia or asphyxia; endogenous metabolic derangements, such as hyperglycemia or hypoglycemia in a patient with diabetes mellitus; and exogenous toxic effects, including drugs and alcohol.

The more detailed neurologic evaluation is reserved for the secondary survey. However, initial documentation of the brief neurologic examination provides objective data for assessing improvement or worsening of the neurologic status during the secondary survey neurologic examination.

Secondary Survey

HISTORY

The secondary survey begins with a brief history, which may be obtained from the patient, the relatives or friends of the patient, a bystander witnessing the accident, or the EMTs who transported the patient to the hospital. A useful mnemonic for remembering the important aspects of the history is AMPLE: *A*=allergies, *M*=medications, *P*=past illnesses, *L*=last meal, and *E*= events preceding the injury. In addition, an attempt should be made to ascertain the mechanism of injury and its magnitude. In instances of blunt vehicular trauma it is important to ascertain the position of the patient in the vehicle, the degree of damage to the vehicle, the condition of other passengers involved in the accident, the use of a seatbelt by the patient, and whether or not the patient was thrown from the vehicle. If the patient was a pedestrian, it is important to know how fast the vehicle was traveling, where the patient was struck, whether the patient was initially conscious or unconscious, and whether the patient regained or lost consciousness on route to the hospital. In patients sustaining penetrating injuries, it is important to ascertain the weapon used and the distance and direction from which the injury was inflicted.

PHYSICAL EXAMINATION

The patient must be completely undressed in order to conduct a complete physical examination.

Head and Neck The physical examination begins with a careful inspection of the face and scalp for lacerations; matted hair should be meticulously parted. Actively bleeding lacerations should be tamponaded with pressure dressings and a head wrap, or closed with monofilament suture, to be repaired with more careful plastic skin closure at a later time. Active bleeding from the nasopharynx may often be controlled by inserting a Foley catheter into the nose, filling the balloon, and applying traction to the catheter.

The skull and all bony facial prominences are carefully palpated for the presence of crepitation or tenderness, suggesting an underlying fracture which may be confirmed with subsequent x-rays. The presence of a "battle sign," "raccoon eyes," blood behind the tympanic membrane, or serous or bloody drainage from the nose or external auditory canal suggests the presence of a basilar skull fracture. The diagnosis of a basilar skull fracture with leaking cerebrospinal fluid may be confirmed by analyzing the glucose level of the nasal or otic drainage, which in the case of cerebrospinal fluid will approximate blood glucose levels.

The pupils are checked for size, reactivity, and other evidence of injury, such as hyphema. Funduscopic examination may reveal injury to the lens, papilledema, retinal hemorrhages, or absence of retinal pulsations. Eye movements should also be checked. Disconjugate gaze suggests brainstem injury, whereas impairment of upward gaze suggests a blowout fracture of the orbit. Binocular vision is assessed by having the patient identify the number of fingers which are being demonstrated, and visual acuity is assessed by asking the patient to read the label on his intravenous fluid bottle.

The nasal canals are examined for patency, and the mouth and pharynx are reevaluated for the presence of broken teeth, lacerations, or hematomas, which may lead to delayed airway obstruction.

The neck is carefully inspected for hematomas or bruits, and the cervical spinous processes are palpated for evidence of crepitus, tenderness, or step-off deformity. Cervical spine fractures cannot be excluded until an adequate cervical spine film is obtained which demonstrates all seven cervical vertebrae. This x-ray and the chest x-ray should be obtained as soon as possible, when suspicion for cervical spine injury exists. Cervical wounds that penetrate the platysma muscle should not be probed. They represent an indication for additional diagnostic testing and surgical exploration. The neck should be further palpated for any evidence of crepitus, suggesting an injury to the tracheobronchial tree, as well as for evidence of a tracheal shift, suggesting a tension pneumothorax. Distended neck veins raise the specter of a possible cardiac tamponade. Sports helmets should not be removed until adequate cervical spine radiographs are obtained. If cervical fractures are demonstrated, the helmet must be carefully removed, preferably utilizing a two-person technique (Fig. 1.6). A one-person technique is acceptable in the conscious, cooperative patient[18] (Fig. 1.7).

Chest The initial chest examination is repeated for evidence of life-threatening mechanical injuries in the thorax. Many of the signs, such as shift of the trachea, distended neck veins, muffled heart tones, or decreased breath sounds, may not have been evident at the time of the initial primary survey. The clavicles, sternum, and all ribs should be individually palpated for evidence of tenderness or crepitus suggesting fractures. Manual compression of the sternum frequently causes pain at the site of a rib fracture.

Abdomen The abdomen is inspected for evidence of abdominal distention, suggesting an ileus or hemoperitoneum. The presence of contusions or abrasions of the abdominal wall increases the suspicion of an underlying injury. Percussion of the abdomen may further help to differentiate between ileus and hemoperitoneum, as well as demonstrate peritoneal irritation. Abdominal tenderness to palpation suggests the presence of muscular contusion or peritoneal irritation, and involuntary guarding confirms the presence of peritoneal irritation. Auscultation of the abdomen is unreliable since bowel sounds

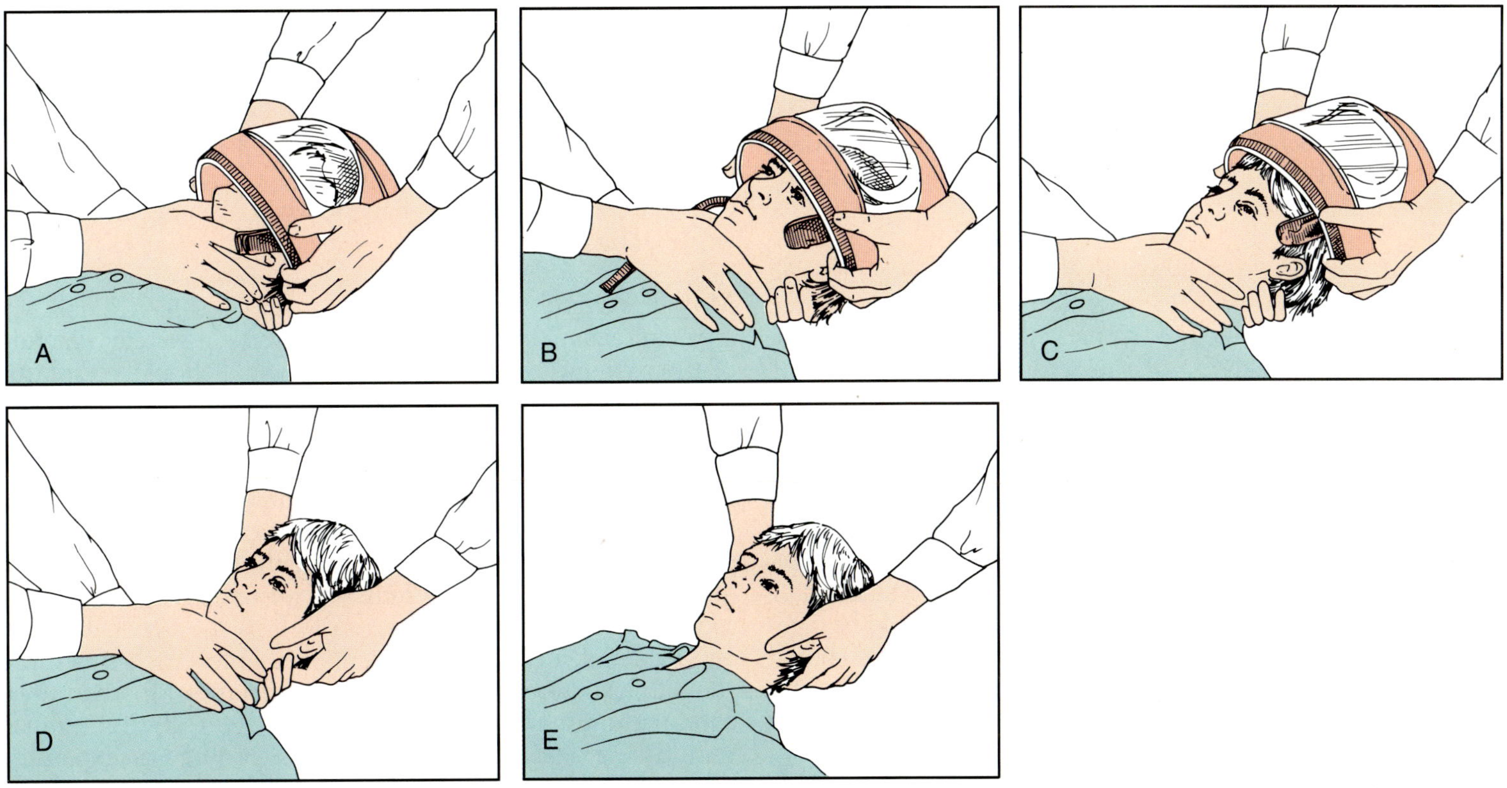

FIGURE 1.6 A One rescuer stabilizes the head while the second spreads the helmen. **B** Traction is applied to the spread helmet. **C** The helmet is removed with continued stabilization and traction from below. **D** Traction is reapplied from above. **E** Traction is maintained until the backboard is placed. (Meyer RD, Daniel WW: The biomehanics of helmets and helmet removal. J Trauma 25[4]:329–332, 1985.)

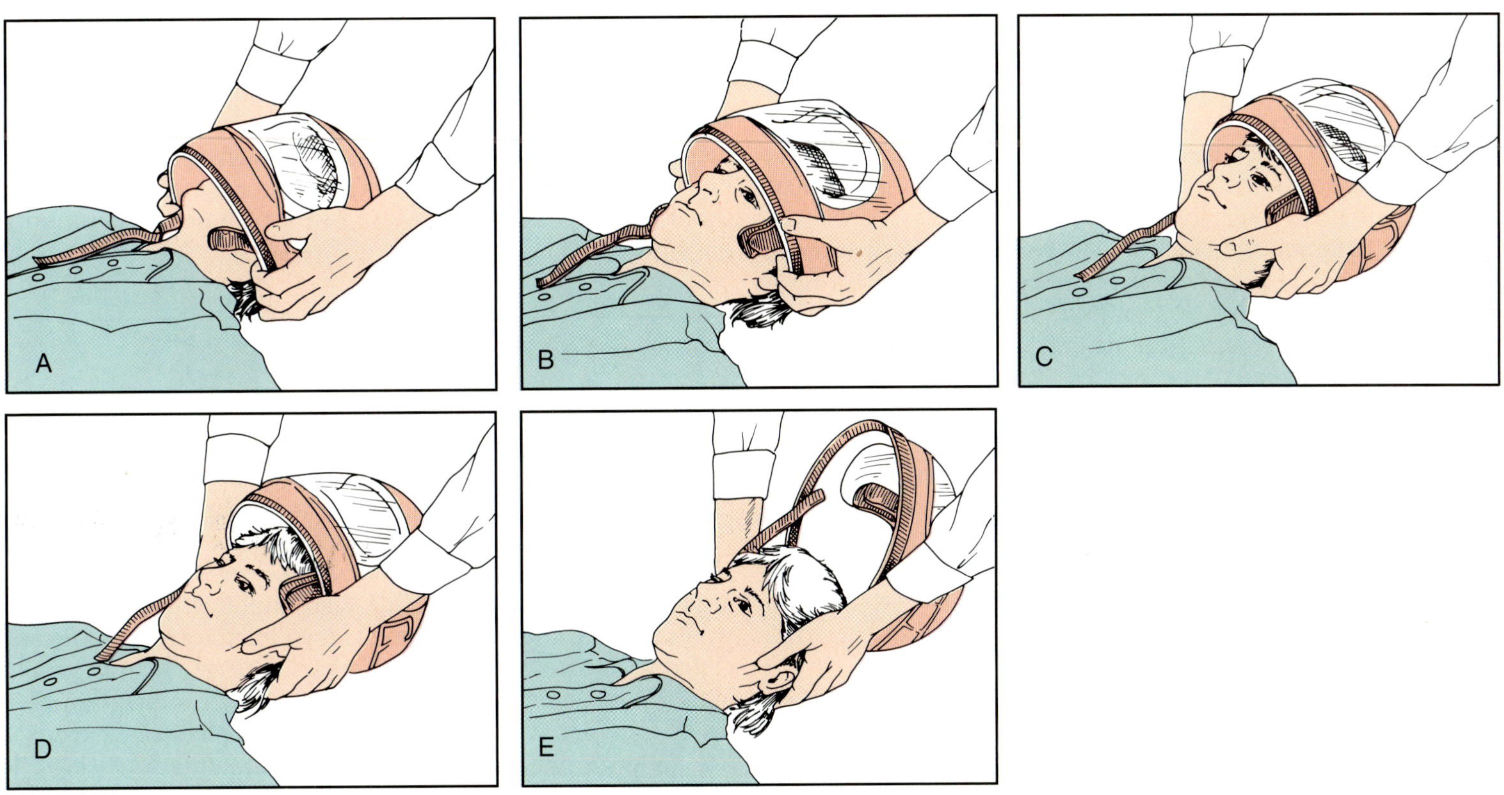

FIGURE 1.7 A Helmet spread. **B** Cephalad traction. **C** Hands "walked" to occiput, maintaining traction. **D** Hands push helmet off while maintaining traction on head. **E** Helmet clears, head lowered onto appropriate backboard. (Meyer RD, Daniel WW: The biomechanics of helmets and helmet removal. J Trauma 25[4]:329–332, 1985.)

may be heard even in the presence of significant intra-abdominal injuries; conversely, bowel sounds may be absent without significant underlying injury. Obvious signs of peritoneal irritation dictate the need for exploratory laparotomy, whereas equivocal signs or an inconclusive examination in the obtunded patient dictate the need for further diagnostic testing, usually including peritoneal lavage.

Pelvis and Rectum Ordinarily, the pelvis and rectum will have been examined prior to insertion of the Foley catheter. Special note must be taken of the presence of blood at the urethral meatus, a hematoma of the scrotum, or a high-riding prostate gland on rectal examination. Any of these findings suggests the possibility of urethral transection and dictates that the tip of the Foley catheter be inserted just into the urethral meatus and then a retrograde urethrogram performed. If the urethra is intact, the Foley catheter may then be inserted into the bladder. If it has been transected, then the patient should have a suprapubic cystostomy performed and a further urologic evaluation by way of a cystogram. The genitalia and perineum should be carefully inspected for lacerations. The vagina and rectum should also be evaluated for lacerations, palpable pelvic bone fragments, or blood on the examining finger. Rectal tone should also be assessed; a lax rectal sphincter usually implies spinal cord injury. Indirect findings which suggest pelvic fractures include tenderness to pressure on the anterior superior iliac spines or pubic symphysis, bony crepitus, urethral blood, grossly bloody urine, distended scrotum, high-riding prostate gland, vaginal or rectal lacerations, a dislocated hip, or internal leg rotation.

Vascular Vascular injury should be suspected in the presence of penetrating injuries or fractures involving the neck or the extremities. Expanding hematomas, bruits, or diminished or absent distal pulses all suggest the presence of an underlying vascular injury. The evaluation of pulses, skin temperature, and capillary refill in the extremities may be difficult in the patient in shock, but an attempt should be made to palpate the carotid, superficial temporal, brachial, radial, ulnar, femoral, popliteal, anterior tibial, and posterior tibial pulses, and the initial findings should be recorded. When asymmetry of pulses or skin temperature exists, vascular injury should be suspected. Comparison of upper extremity blood pressures may give a clue to an underlying subclavian or aortic arch injury. Whenever vascular injury is suspected, appropriate arteriographic studies should be obtained following the secondary survey, provided the patient is stable enough for transfer to the angiographic suite. In the unstable patient, surgical exploration should proceed without the benefit of preoperative arteriography. Whenever the mechanism of injury is a gunshot wound and there is an abrupt loss of pulses in another region of the body, bullet embolus should be considered.

Neurologic The secondary neurologic examination should begin with a repeat of the AVPU examination, which was performed during the primary survey. Gross alterations in the level of consciousness in an otherwise well-oxygenated patient dictate the need for prompt diagnostic evaluation. In the otherwise stable patient an immediate CT scan of the brain is usually obtained at this point. The neurological examination should also include the rating of the patient according to the Glasgow coma scale (Fig. 1.1). Moreover, each of the cranial and spinal nerves should be assessed for motor and sensory function.

Neurosurgical consultation is indicated in patients who are unconscious or have deteriorating levels of consciousness, whose Glasgow coma score is less than 14, who have unequal pupils, or who exhibit focal weakness.

Musculoskeletal The secondary survey is concluded with a careful examination of the musculoskeletal system. Fractures of the extremities are usually obvious and should be splinted and the fractures aligned if possible, especially if the fracture is associated with a diminished or absent distal pulse. The basic principle to remember is that realignment of a fracture usually improves peripheral blood flow, and immobilization reduces further blood loss. When manual compression on the symphysis pubis or bimanual compression on the iliac wings results in pain or tenderness, this usually indicates an underlying pelvic fracture. Fractures of the clavicles as well as the cervical, dorsal, and lumbar spines are often overlooked unless each structure is carefully examined for crepitus and tenderness. In addition to careful examination of the skeletal system, the extremities should be examined for the presence of large or expanding hematomas, as well as for tense fascial compartments. The development of a compartment syndrome is a surgical emergency and should be recognized early before vascular or neurologic compromise develops.

Re-evaluation and Recordkeeping

The trauma patient once stabilized requires frequent re-evaluation in order to detect subtle changes suggesting organ system deterioration. Vital signs, urine output, hematocrit, and arterial blood gases should be monitored frequently. A careful record should be kept of the patient's history, physical examination, diagnostic findings, treatment, and progress.

Medications

In general, trauma patients require a minimum of medications. Narcotics are ordinarily contraindicated in the initial resuscitation period because they may alter the level of consciousness, depress the respiratory center, and mask important symptoms. Steroids and mannitol may be useful in the patient with head injuries and associated cerebral edema. Prophylactic antibiotics are indicated in patients with basilar skull fractures, penetrating wounds of the chest or abdomen, open fractures, or injuries associated with extensive musculoskeletal damage. Tetanus prophylaxis should be provided to all patients with a wound that penetrates the skin. The extent of tetanus prophylaxis depends on the patient's prior history of tetanus immunization[6] (Figs. 1.8 and 1.9). In no instance will antibiotics or tetanus prophylaxis substitute for the need for aggressive debridement of devitalized tissue or grossly contaminated wounds.

Diagnostic Testing

LABORATORY TESTS

Baseline laboratory tests are obtained in all major trauma victims and include CBC, type and crossmatch, urinalysis, arterial blood gases, SMA-12, ECG, and serum amylase. Additional testing, such as cardiac enzymes, echocardiograms or toxicology studies, are obtained as indicated. The ordering of repeat laboratory tests is dictated by the patient's condition.

PERITONEAL LAVAGE

Peritoneal lavage is indicated in most patients with blunt trauma who have equivocal abdominal findings, unexplained fall in

FIGURE 1.8
CLINICAL FEATURES OF TETANUS-PRONE AND NON-PRONE WOUNDS

CLINICAL FEATURES	TETANUS-PRONE WOUNDS	NON-TETANUS PRONE WOUNDS
Age of wound	>6 hours	<6 hours
Configuration	Stellate wound, avulsion, abrasion	Linear wound
Depth	>1 cm	<1 cm
Mechanism of injury	Missile, crush, burn, frostbite	Sharp surface (e.g.,knife, glass)
Signs of infection	Present	Absent
Devitalized tissue	Present	Absent
Contaminants (dirt, feces, soil, saliva, etc.)	Present	Absent
Denervated or ischemic tissue	Present	Absent

Committee on Trauma of the American College of Surgeons: A Guide to Propylaxus Against Tetanus in Wound Management, 1984 Revision. Chicago, ACS Bulletin, 1984.

FIGURE 1.9
SUMMARY GUIDE TO TETANUS PROPHYLAXIS

HISTORY OF TETANUS IMMUNIZATION (DOSES)	TETANUS-PRONE WOUNDS		NON-TETANUS-PRONE WOUNDS	
	TD*	TIG†	TD*	TIG‡
Uncertain	Yes	Yes	Yes	No
0–1	Yes	Yes	Yes	No
2	Yes	No§	Yes	No
3 or more	No‖	No	No#	No

* For children less than 7 years old, Diphtheria and Tetanus Toxoids and Pertussis Vaccine Adsorbed (DPT), (Diphtheria and Tetanus Toxoids Adsorbed [DT], if pertussis vaccine is contraindicated) are preferred to tetanus toxoid alone. For patients 7 years old and older, Td is preferred to tetanus toxoid alone.
† TIG, human tetanus immune globulin
‡ When TIG and Td are given concurrently, separate syringes and separate sites should be used.
§ Yes, if wound is more than 24 hours old.
‖ Yes, if more than 5 years since last dose. (More frequent boosters are not needed and can accentuate side-effects.)
Yes, if more than 10 years since last dose.
Committee on Trauma of the American College of Surgeons: A Guide to Prophylaxis Against Tetanus in Wound Management, 1984 Revision. Chicago, American College of Surgeons, 1984.

hematocrits, or an abdominal examination that is compromised because the patient is obtunded or has spinal cord injury. The bladder is emptied with a Foley catheter, and a nasogastric tube is inserted prior to introducing the peritoneal lavage catheter. The catheter is usually inserted in the midline 2 cm to 3 cm below the umbilicus and directed toward the pelvis. Peritoneal lavage may be performed by an open method in which the peritoneum is opened under direct vision, or by a closed method in which the fasciae and peritoneum are perforated with a trocar. If on insertion of the peritoneal lavage catheter gross blood or bile-stained fluid is obtained, then there is no need for formal lavage. If lavage is performed, approximately 1000 ml of Ringer's lactate solution are infused, and the patient is gently rolled from side to side to allow for adequate mixing of the fluid. The fluid is then allowed to drain into an infusion bottle, which is lowered to the floor. A positive lavage is one in which there is greater than 100,000 red cells per cubic millimeter, a white blood count of greater than 500 per cubic millimeter, or the presence of bile, feces, vegetable matter, or bacteria seen on a Gram stain. Based on these criteria, positive findings are demonstrated in an exploratory laparotomy in 96% to 98% of patients. Others have used figures as low as 20,000 red cells per cubic millimeter in order to avoid missing significant injuries.[15] When this latter criteria is used, higher negative exploratory laparotomy rates can be expected. Regardless of the criteria used, if equivocal results are obtained, the catheter may be left in place and repeat lavage may be performed at frequent intervals. In patients sustaining complex pelvic fractures with suspected pelvic hematomas, the peritoneal lavage catheter is inserted above the umbilicus in order to avoid inserting the catheter into the hematoma. A positive lavage in a patient with a pelvic hematoma presents a dilemma: is the bloody return from an intraperitoneal injury or from a communication with the pelvic hematoma? Additional tests, such as CT scans, are ordinarily used to attempt to differentiate the sources of the bleeding.

Peritoneal lavage is ordinarily not used in patients with gunshot wounds of the abdomen, since most centers routinely explore these patients surgically. However, in patients with tangential gunshot wounds or penetrating injuries of the lower chest, peritoneal lavage is of definite benefit in determining peritoneal penetration. In these patients, a red cell count of $10,000/mm^3$ is considered an indication for surgical exploration.[17]

The use of peritoneal lavage in stab wounds of the abdomen is controversial. Some centers surgically explore all patients with stab wounds of the abdomen; others observe all patients and surgically explore only those who develop peritoneal signs or a falling hematocrit; and a third group uses peritoneal lavage selectively. Peritoneal lavage is ordinarily contraindicated in a patient with a gravid uterus or history of previous abdominal operations.

X-RAYS

Virtually every trauma patient except one who has undergone an emergency room thoracotomy should have a chest x-ray performed as soon as possible and certainly before any operative procedures are initiated. A chest x-ray will often demonstrate findings suggestive of the presence of intrathoracic life-threatening injuries that may have been missed on physical examination, such as a widened mediastinum, fractured first or second rib, pleural cap, blunting of the aortic or pulmonary shadows, shift of the bronchus or esophagus, mediastinal or subcutaneous emphysema, pulmonary contusion, pneumothorax, hemothorax, or ruptured diaphragm—all of which require urgent attention. Patients who have sustained significant blunt trauma, especially those who are unconscious or who have sustained obvious head and neck trauma, should have a lateral x-ray of the cervical spine. The seventh cervical vertebra is frequently injured and often difficult to see on routine cervical x-rays, so that additional views, for example Swimmer's view with the beam directed obliquely through the axilla, may be necessary. If the lateral view is normal, an anteroposterior and open-mouth odontoid x-ray are obtained. If physical examination suggests cervical spine injury and plain x-rays are negative, tomograms should be obtained.

Abdominal x-rays are primarily useful for evaluating retroperitoneal injuries in patients who have sustained blunt trauma. Subtle signs, such as scoliosis, fractures of lumbar transverse processes, obliteration of the psoas shadow and retroperitoneal air, suggest pancreatic or duodenal injuries. In addition, an abdominal x-ray provides evidence for occult bony pelvic fracture, hip dislocation, and separation of the symphysis pubis. Each of these severe injuries requires early assessment. Gunshot and shotgun fragments seen in patients with penetrating trauma may give a clue to potential organs injured.

In patients requiring exploratory laparotomy, as well as those with microscopic hematuria or injuries in the region of the kidneys or ureters, an intravenous pyelogram (IVP) is indicated. One hundred milliliters of contrast material given intravenously prior to transferring the patient to the x-ray suite will ordinarily allow for the demonstration of adequate detail of the kidneys and ureters. Patients with pelvic fractures, gross hematuria, penetrating injuries near the pelvis, or evidence of pelvic hematomas should have a cystogram performed by inserting 150 ml of dye into the Foley catheter and obtaining anteroposterior, oblique, and postvoid views of the bladder. As previously mentioned, a urethrogram is indicated in patients with blood at the urethral meatus, scrotal hematomas, or a high-riding prostate gland on physical examination.

Arteriography is indicated in patients with penetrating neck and thoracic inlet injuries, a widened mediastinum and suspected injuries of the thoracic aorta, nonvisualization of the kidney on IVP, and signs of suspected vascular injuries of the extremities. Arteriography may also be helpful in detecting and sometimes embolizing arterial bleeding sites in the pelvis associated with pelvic fractures.

CT scans of the head are indicated in all patients with depressed skull fractures, as well as in patients with head injuries who are comatose or have worsening neurologic findings. CT scans of the abdomen are helpful in detecting intraperitoneal solid organ injuries as well as retroperitoneal injuries in patients who have sustained blunt trauma. Neither the CT scan or peritoneal lavage are reliable in detecting all intra-abdominal injuries. One study does not necessarily replace the other, and both may be complimentary in some patients. The advantages of peritoneal lavage are that it can be performed in the trauma resuscitation area without the need to transfer the patient to a radiologic suite, and that it does not require a trained specialist to interpret the results.

Unstable patients should never leave the resuscitation area to undergo diagnostic investigation in the radiology department. Under ideal circumstances, a radiology unit complete with CT equipment should be present in the resuscitation area.

REFERENCES

1. Baker SP, O'Neill B, Haddon W, Long WB: The injury severity score: A method for describing patients with multiple injuries and evaluating emergency care. J Trauma 14(3):187–196, 1974.
2. Champion HR, Sacco WJ, Carnazzo AJ et al: Trauma score. Crit Care Med 9(9):672–676, 1981.
3. Champion HR, Sacco WJ: Measurement of injury severity and its practical application. Trauma Quarterly, pp 25–36, November 1984.
4. Clemmer TP, Orme JF, Thomas F, Brooks KA: Prospective evaluation of the CRAMS scale for triaging major trauma. J Trauma 25(3):188–191, 1985.
5. Committee on Trauma: Advanced Trauma Life Support for Physicians. Chicago, American College of Surgeons, 1984
6. Committee on Trauma: A guide to prophylaxis against tetanus in wound management. Chicago, American College of Surgeons, 1984.
7. Committee on Trauma of the American College of Surgeons: Hospital and prehospital resources for optimal care of the injured patient. ACS Bulletin 68(10) 11–18, 1983.
8. Detmer DE, Moylan JA, Rose J et al: Regional categorization and quality of care in major trauma. J Trauma 17(8):592–599, 1977.
9. Gertler JP, Cameron DE, Shea K, Baker CC: The esophageal obturator airway: Obturator or obtundator? J Trauma 25(5):424–426, 1985.
10. Gervin AS, Fischer RP: The importance of prompt transport in salvage of patients with penetrating heart wounds. J Trauma 22(6): 443–448, 1982.
11. Gervin AS, Fischer RP: Resuscitation of trauma patients with type–specific uncrossmatched blood. J Trauma 24(4):327–331, 1984.
12. Gormican SP: CRAMS Scale: Field triage of trauma victims. Ann Emerg Med 11(3):132–135, 1982.
13. Jacobs LM, Sinclair A, Beiser A, D'Agostino RB: Prehospital advanced life support: Benefits in trauma. J Trauma 24(1):8–13, 1984.
14. Mackersie RC, Christensen JM, Lewis FR The prehospital use of external counterpressure: Does MAST make a difference? J Trauma 24(10):882–888, 1984.
15. McLellan BA, Hanna SS, Montoya DR et al: Analysis of peritoneal lavage parameters in blunt abdominal trauma. J Trauma 25(5): 393–399, 1985.
16. McSwain NR, Garrison WB, Artz CP: Evaluation of resuscitation from cardiopulmonary arrest by paramedics. Ann Emerg Med 9:341–345, 1980.
17. Merlotti GJ, Marcet E, Sheaff CM et al: Use of peritoneal lavage to evaluate abdominal penetration. J Trauma 25(3):228–231, 1985.
18. Meyer RD, Daniel WW: The biomechanics of helmets and helmet removal. J Trauma 25(4):329–332, 1985.
19. Millikan JS, Cain TL, Hansbrough J: Rapid volume replacement for hypovolemic shock: A comparison of techniques and equipment. J Trauma 24(5):428–431, 1984.
20. Seelig JM, Becker DP, Miller JD et al: Traumatic acute subdural hematoma. N Engl J Med 304:1511–1518, 1981.
21. Smith JP, Bodai BI, Hill AS, Frey CF: Prehospital stabilization of critically injured patients: A failed concept. J Trauma 25(1):65–70, 1985.
22. Subcommittee on Emergency Services–Prehospital of the Committee on Trauma of the American College of Surgeons: Medical control in trauma care. ACS Bulletin 70(10):1920, 1985.
23. West JG, Trunkey DD, Lim RC: Systems of trauma care: A study of two counties. Arch Surg 114:455–460, 1979.

Suggested Reading

1. Lewis FR: Prehospital Trauma Care: Current Therapy of Trauma, Philadelphia, Brian C. Dekker, 1984–1985.
2. Trunkey DD: Trauma. Scientific American 249:28–35, 1983.
3. Trunkey DD, Halcroft JW: Trauma: General survey and synopsis of management of specific injuries. In Hardy JD (ed): Hardy's Textbook of Surgery, Philadelphia, JB Lippincott, 1983.

pathophysiology and treatment of shock

2

Charles T. Cloutier

Shock is a complex clinical syndrome as old as man. Despite its antiquity, the pathophysiology and effective treatment of various forms of shock were not clearly understood until the middle of the 20th century. For a long time, trauma and shock were thought to be synonymous. In 1859 Samuel D. Gross[24] described different forms of shock and attributed the signs and symptoms of the shock state to a loss of neural innervation. Mitchell and colleagues[33] believed that shock was the result of vasomotor collapse at the level of the medulla. Their theory gained support from the experimental work of Crile,[18] who attributed the shock state to vasomotor exhaustion. With such a poor understanding of the pathophysiology of shock, it is little wonder that treatment was at best symptomatic and at times bordered on witchcraft. Phlebotomy, cold-water applications, turpentine rubs, and sips of brandy and water were once accepted treatments for patients in shock.

What accounted for this lack of understanding? For one thing, shock resulting from trauma was not a major civilian problem. Clearly it was a problem of wartime, and observations of casualties, left to battlefield surgeons, were anecdotal at best. Trauma centers were nonexistent and no animal models were yet available for study.

WARTIME CONTRIBUTIONS TO SHOCK

It is hardly possible to write a chapter on shock without acknowledging the many contributions to our understanding of shock that have come from surgeons caring for battlefield casualties (Fig. 2.1). War and medicine are strange bedfellows: one philosophy is totally committed to death and destruction; the other to the saving of lives.

Mitchell[33] observed during the Civil War the loss of central nervous system control in patients in shock and hypothesized that this was due to vasomotor paralysis. Crile[18] in 1903 and Lockhart-Mummery[31] in 1905 gave additional support to this concept by concluding from experiments in animals that shock was the result of vasomotor exhaustion of the medulla. This remained the dominant thinking concerning shock until World War I.

From wartime experiences came observations that challenged the existing theories of shock. Fracture immobilization significantly lowered morbidity and led to further investigation into the pathophysiology of shock. Cannon[6–8,10] and Bayliss,[4] in addition to providing detailed clinical descriptions of casualties in shock, measured and reported physiologic and biochemical changes in patients and in animals. Cannon[7] concluded that shock was cardiac decompensation caused by loss of vasomotor tone resulting from tissue toxins. His was the first description of the metabolic acidosis of shock and the use of bicarbonate to improve performance.

In World War I an organized effort was made to study battle casualties in the field and was spearheaded by English and French surgeons already on the battlefields of Europe. At their suggestion, they were joined by American physiologists and pharmacologists, and their early observations provided a base of knowledge and uncovered a variety of problems that occupied investigators of shock for the next 20 years. While these studies raised more questions than they answered, they did effectively set the stage for the future investigation of shock.

Despite a body of convincing evidence that accumulated between the two world wars demonstrating that blood loss into injured tissue accounted for the oligemia of shock, so deeply engrained was the concept of liberated tissue toxins and resulting hemoconcentration as the cause of shock that this theory persisted well into World War II. Medical personnel caring for American forces fighting in the European–African campaign early in World War II had to rely on dried plasma and saline solution for shock resuscitation. Logistically, plasma and saline were easier to procure and transport and blood banks were not required. Later in the war, due to the efforts of British surgeons and the observations of Churchill,[13] the use of whole blood was recognized as necessary to effectively treat patients in shock.

In 1943, at the persistence of Colonels Churchill and Stone, the Theater Surgeon-in-Chief General Stayer established the "Board for the Study of the Severely Wounded."[42] For the first time, an organized clinical research unit was present in a battle zone. This unit made many notable observations: (1) Patients exhibited a deficiency in circulating blood volume, except crush injury victims; (2) hemodilution and not hemoconcentration was a characteristic finding in shock; (3) battle casualties had depressed liver function, especially those who received large

FIGURE 2.1
WARTIME CONTRIBUTIONS TO PATHOPHYSIOLOGY AND TREATMENT OF SHOCK

WAR	DATE	CONTRIBUTION
Civil War	1860	Vasomotor paralysis Early amputation Wound debridement
W.W. I	1914	Fracture immobilization Metabolic acidosis
W.W. II	1940	Medical board to study shock Blood banks Biochemical changes
Korean War	1950	Field research Renal failure Asanguinous resuscitation
Vietnam War	1960	Electrolyte resuscitation Respiratory distress Helicopter evacuation

amounts of plasma; and (4) a new clinical syndrome carrying a high mortality (post-traumatic renal failure) was becoming increasingly apparent in patients in shock who were successfully resuscitated.

It was obvious that clinical research could be accomplished in a war zone and that the data could be used in a timely manner to initiate new treatments. Extension of studies on post-traumatic renal failure in the Korean War led to a reduction in mortality.[28] Extremity amputations were significantly reduced because of improved techniques in repairing vascular injuries.[28] Further advances were made in blood and fluid resuscitation and the effectiveness of the helicopter as a medical evacuation vehicle was established. The importance of clinical research in the field was again demonstrated in the Vietnam conflict.

CLASSIFICATION OF SHOCK

Shock is a pathophysiologic condition that results from inadequate perfusion at the cellular level. For normal function of the body, fluid must circulate within certain limits of flow and pressure. Regardless of the cause, the failure of blood to circulate within these limits results in physiologic changes that, if not promptly recognized and corrected, can lead to cellular death. There are four major classes of shock: hypovolemic, cardiogenic, septic, and neurogenic. Each of these will be discussed in detail.

Hypovolemic Shock

Hypovolemic shock is characterized by a critical loss of blood volume as well as other body fluids. It can be corrected by quickly identifying the source of the fluid loss and restoring intravascular volume with the appropriate fluid.

ETIOLOGY

Hemorrhage resulting from trauma remains the single most common cause of hypovolemic shock. Another cause is the loss of circulating plasma or other body fluids, as occurs in burns, peritonitis, protracted vomiting or diarrhea, and acute pancreatitis. The incidence of trauma and hypovolemic shock will probably not decrease in the near future, as long as our society continues to drive faster and is reluctant to use seat belts and helmets.

DIAGNOSIS

In response to inadequate perfusion at the cellular level, the body activates a series of hemodynamic and metabolic compensatory mechanisms. Many of these responses can be readily observed clinically to establish the diagnosis of shock. Although excellent progress has been made in developing sophisticated laboratory tests and accurate monitoring devices, there is no specific laboratory determination or physiologic measurement for shock. Shock remains a clinical diagnosis, with tests and monitoring equipment useful only for observation and management of the patient.

The classic variable used to diagnose shock has been blood pressure, although blood pressure alone may be inaccurate and at times misleading. In the normal steady state, blood pressure is merely a reflection of the balance between cardiac output and peripheral resistance. A loss of intravascular volume will result in reduction of cardiac output, but if this reduction in cardiac output occurs at a slow enough rate, the body's compensatory homeostatic mechanisms are able to increase peripheral vascular resistance and prevent a drop in blood pressure. This compensatory effect will continue until it is overwhelmed by the decreases in blood volume and cardiac output.

A study of severely injured Marines in Vietnam[15] showed that many arrived at the hospital with no significant change in pulse or blood pressure. Of 66 patients, 23 (35%) had no measurable blood pressure on admission, 20 (30%) had a systolic pressure of 80 mm Hg or less, and 23 (35%) had a systolic pressure higher than 80 mm Hg (Fig. 2.2). In 7 patients (11%), the peripheral pulse rate was undetectable on admission. 46 (70%) had a pulse rate between 120 and 180 per minute, 8 (12%) between 100 and 119 per minute, and 2 (3%) less than 100 per minute. No admission pulse rate was recorded in 3 (4%) of the patients. It seemed logical to expect that in patients as severely wounded as

FIGURE 2.2
BLOOD PRESSURE LEVELS AND PULSE RATES OF PATIENTS IN SHOCK

BP SYSTOLIC (MM HG)			PERIPHERAL PR (BEATS/MINUTE)		
VALUES	NO. OF PATIENTS	%	VALUES	NO. OF PATIENTS	%
0	23	35	Unobtainable	7	11
1–80	20	30	120–180	46	70
81–100	8	12	100–119	8	12
Over 100	15	23	80–100	2	3
Totals	66	100	Totals	63	96

these young Marines, longer evacuation time would result in more severe shock characterized by lower systolic blood pressure. However, this assumption was not confirmed, because some of the patients with the lowest blood pressure had the shortest evacuation times. Conversely, several of the patients with evacuation times longer than the mean had adequate perfusion pressures.

The American College of Surgeons Committee on Trauma[2a] has stated that at least a 30% intravascular hemorrhage is required before significant changes can be detected in blood pressure. Therefore, reliance on pulse rate or blood pressure to establish a diagnosis of hypovolemic shock can be and often is misleading.

In arriving at a diagnosis of hypovolemic shock, the following factors should be considered singly or in combination:

- General status of the patient
- Magnitude and site of trauma
- Skin temperature
- Level of consciousness
- Presence of air hunger
- Cuff blood pressure
- Quality and rate of the pulse as an indication of intravascular volume

The capillary blanch test is quite reliable, requires no equipment, and gives an adequate initial reflection of the state of cellular perfusion.

The typical patient in hypovolemic shock is hypotensive, exhibits tachycardia and tachypnea, and has a high level of anxiety. The patients may be oliguric. The degree of fatigue depends upon the degree of shock; patients can be extremely restless or at times frankly comatose. The skin is pale and cool, and there will be a delay in capillary refill because of decreased capillary flow. The patient in shock may have a decreased core body temperature and may exhibit nausea and vomiting.

Unfortunately, there are no laboratory determinations that can confirm optimum care for patients in shock. Ideally, a laboratory test for these patients would be one that accurately depicts the adequacy of cellular perfusion and resuscitation.

PATHOPHYSIOLOGY

The physiologic response to hemorrhage is related to not only the amount of fluid loss, but also to the rate of fluid loss. The human organism, in an attempt to maintain cellular perfusion, initiates homeostatic defense mechanisms at the hemodynamic and metabolic levels. While this homeostatic response is often effective in maintaining perfusion, it is by no means inexhaustible, and appropriate intervention must be prompt for the person to survive.

A low systemic arterial blood pressure stimulates sympathetic receptors in the arterial wall of the carotid sinus. These receptors send diminished afferent impulses to the central nervous system. The stimulated receptors release catecholamines, which bring about arterial and venous constriction. Concomitant with the sympathetic response, venous return to the heart is diminished. As a result, cardiac output decreases, systemic arterial pressure drops, and tachycardia develops with an increase in myocardial contractility.

The body's response is to maintain blood flow to vital organs such as the heart and the brain at all costs. To accomplish this, cardiac output is redistributed, with decreased flow to the skin, kidneys, and skeletal muscles. The fall in renal blood flow is marked by redistribution of flow within the kidney favoring the medulla at the expense of cortical ischemia. If allowed to continue, oliguria and frank anuria will follow. The body also compensates by increasing the respiratory rate in an attempt to improve blood oxygenation and promote increased filling of the right ventricle.

An almost immediate response to hemorrhage is the beginning of a shift of plasma from the interstitial space into the intravascular space. While this attempt at plasma refill is a homeostatic defense mechanism, if allowed to continue uncorrected it can further contribute to the cellular perfusion deficit.

Plasma Refill The endogenous expansion of plasma volume in response to hemorrhage is a well known phenomenon. Moore[34] observed in volunteers who were bled 10% to 20% of their blood volume that plasma refill began in minutes and proceeded at the rate of 50 to 90 ml/min during the first 2 hours, and then averaged 40 to 60 ml/hr for 6 to 10 hours. He reported that the volume added to the vascular space equaled the total volume bled, and complete refill was accomplished in 30 to 40 hours. In patients evaluated in Vietnam, Carey[11] reported rates that exceeded this amount. He observed young patients with a hematocrit of 30% or less and albumin levels of 3% on admission. Thus, it was obvious that plasma volume refill occurred at a much faster rate than previously reported; retrospective calculations suggested a refill rate of several hundred milliliters per hour. For example, in a 70-kg man with a preinjury blood volume of 5000 ml, a hematocrit of 40% represents 2000 ml of red blood cells and 3000 ml of plasma. Following a 40% hemorrhage, the red cell mass would be 1200 ml, plasma volume 1800 ml, and total blood volume 3000 ml. If a hematocrit is 30% on admission, plasma volume would be calculated as follows:

$$1200 \text{ ml red cell mass} = 30\%,$$
$$X \text{ ml plasma volume} = 70\%$$
$$30X = 8400, X = 2800 \text{ ml plasma volume}$$

Where does the fluid come from that refills the vascular space after hemorrhage? The return of interstitial volume to the vascular compartment (transcapillary refill) is governed primarily by Starling forces and is biphasic. Initially, the decrease in blood volume and venous pressure and the accompanying arteriolar vasoconstriction results in a fall in capillary hydrostatic pressure. There then follows a shift of protein-free fluid from the interstitial space into the capillaries. Concomitant with this fluid shift is a return of protein to increase plasma or oncotic pressure. Cope and Litwin[16] found a rapid increase in thoracic duct lymph flow following hemorrhage. It is known that the fluid added to the plasma volume following hemorrhage contains albumin, which comes from the hepatic and mesenteric circulation by way of the lymphatics and enters the circulation rapidly, at a rate as fast as 4 g/hr. The rate of protein breakdown slows and protein synthesis increases.

Still, the cause of transcapillary refill remains unclear. Pirkle and Garan[36] believed it was brought about by an increase in solute load. Friedman, Pearce, and Drucker[23] reported that the transcapillary refill process was dependent upon hyperglycemia. Work in our laboratory with adrenalectomized rats did not produce the typical hyperglycemic response to hemorrhage; rather, we found the same degree of plasma refill as that evidenced by decreased hematocrit and dilution of total protein, albumin, and globulin levels.[14] Thus, the entire process seems to be dependent on many factors acting in synchrony rather than on a single mediating factor.

Endogenous Hemodilution If transcapillary refill occurs at the rate and to the extent described, then it is logical to expect an effect on some of the circulating elements in the blood. This is indeed the case. Total protein, albumin, and globulin are diluted, as observed in 1896 by Stanberg and later confirmed in a study of Korean battle casualties by Frawley and co-workers.[22] Hoch-Ligeti, Irvine, and Sprinkle[27] documented similar changes in civilian surgical patients.

As with plasma refill, serum protein dilution is dependent somewhat on the rate and the extent of the hemorrhage. When volunteers were slowly bled of 10% to 20% of their circulating blood volume, serum albumin levels did not change; however, globulin levels were reduced at the end of several hours. In patients sustaining more severe hemorrhage, total protein, albumin, and globulin levels were all depressed.[38] Evaluating serum protein, globulin, and albumin levels in 66 patients in severe shock, Cloutier, Lowery, and Carey[15] compared these values to a control population and found that total protein was reduced 27%, albumin 20%, and globulin 35% (Fig. 2.3). Thus, it appears that the human organism has the capacity to mobilize albumin in response to hemorrhage, but globulin cannot be mobilized to the same extent.

Assuming no significant preexisting illness, what are the changes in serum electrolytes in patients in shock from trauma prior to the initiation of treatment? Patients in shock from trauma were classically thought to have low sodium, low chloride, and elevated potassium levels. The fall in serum sodium was investigated by Fox and Keston[21] using isotope techniques. They found sodium at the site of the injury to be increased and considered the increase to far exceed what could be expected from edema formation alone. Thus, they concluded that the sodium space of injured tissue was increased as a result of a disruption in the integrity of cell membranes to effectively keep sodium out of the cells. Adding to this hypothesis was the observation that intracellular potassium was decreased. In studying hemorrhagic shock in dogs that had not suffered trauma, Dillon and co-workers[19] found a large functional sodium deficit; because the increase in serum potassium was not significant, the concept that alterations in sodium and potassium were the result of cell membrane exchange of these ions was not an acceptable hypothesis. Crenshaw and associates[17] measured sodium space in tissue following injury by using radioactive sodium sulfate and reported an increase in interstitial space. However, this finding has not been substantiated by others.

In the Vietnamese casualties reported by Cloutier, Lowery, and Carey,[15] serum sodium levels were remarkably similar to baseline controls. Twelve of the 66 casualties had hypocalcemia on admission; the mean potassium level was 2.75 mEq/liter. These findings were obviously unexpected and are contrary to the hypothesis that intracellular water is a source of fluid that refills plasma space. The only possible explanation is that the cells had lost solute-free water, and that is quite unlikely.

Blood Sugar/Insulin Changes For many years, the elevation in the blood sugar level secondary to shock has been accepted and proven at both the clinical and the experimental

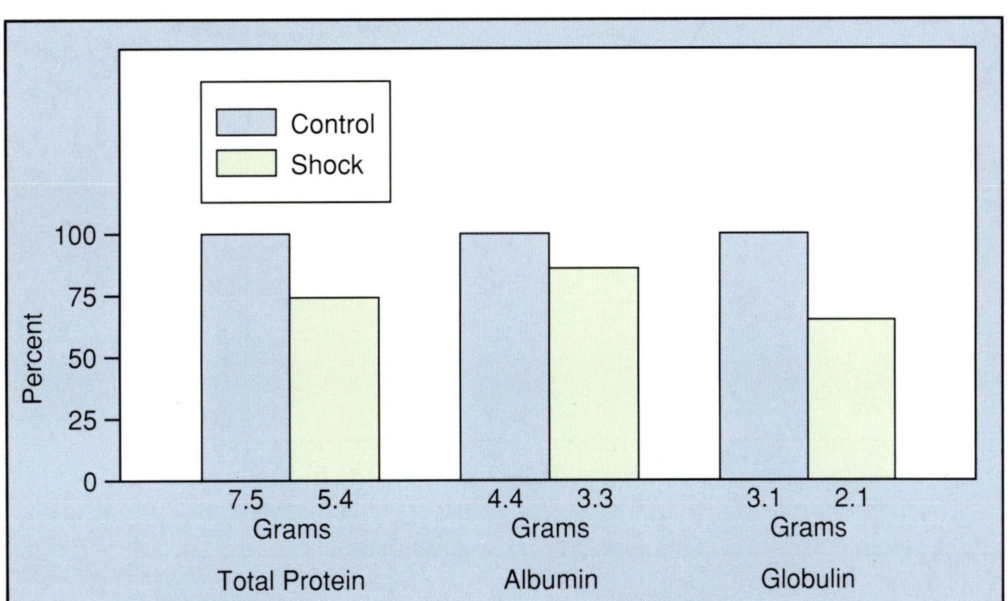

FIGURE 2.3 Serum protein changes following acute hemorrhage and prior to resuscitation. From the time of injury to admission (83 min), total protein was reduced by 25%. Albumin was reduced 15% less than globulin and is added to the plasma space.

levels. In response to shock secondary to trauma there is an outpouring of the sympathoadrenal catecholamines resulting in increased glycogenolysis. At the same time, inadequate cellular perfusion leading to cellular hypoxia contributes to a decreased use of glucose.

While blood sugar elevation is well documented (as occurred in the patients in Vietnam whose mean blood sugar level was 264 mg/dl), opinions concerning insulin conflict. Hyperglycemia is a potent stimulus to insulin release. Several investigators have reported that insulin changes parallel blood sugar changes, rising with hyperglycemia and falling in the late stages of shock.[10,21,33] Others have thought that the catecholamines have a suppressive effect on insulin release. In studies by Carey, Lowery, and Cloutier,[12] on admission of patients in shock, their blood sugar was high and their insulin levels were low. As effective resuscitation was accomplished, the blood sugar level fell and was followed by a rise in circulating insulin (Fig. 2.4). These findings were later confirmed by Moss and colleagues[35] in his studies of baboons in shock. Thus, it is suggested that serum insulin release is more responsive to the suppressive effect of catecholamines than to the stimulating effect of blood sugar. Other studies suggest that the insulin block occurs at the cellular level and is not related to catecholamines.

METABOLIC ALTERATIONS

Lactate Production Shock has been defined as inadequate perfusion at the cellular level. A laboratory test that would accurately reflect the adequacy of resuscitation would be extremely helpful.

In the late 1950s, Huckabee[29] reported a series of experiments that have become classic. He concluded that lactate levels did not correlate well with tissue oxygen deprivation and that the calculation of excess lactate was a more accurate index of tissue oxygen depth. This concept was challenged by Alpert,[1] who questioned the usefulness of excess lactate in judging oxygen depth.

There is no doubt that blood lactate and pyruvate levels increase with shock. In a normal steady state, glucose is converted by the Embden-Meyerhof pathway to pyruvate and lactic acid. In the presence of oxygen, the pyruvate is able to enter the Krebs cycle and is converted to oxaloacetic acid at a high level of energy production efficiency. While in the anaerobic state, the body's attempt to produce energy yields only a fraction of that produced by aerobic metabolism; it is a sufficient amount to allow cellular survival if conversion back to aerobic metabolism is achieved in a relatively short period of time.

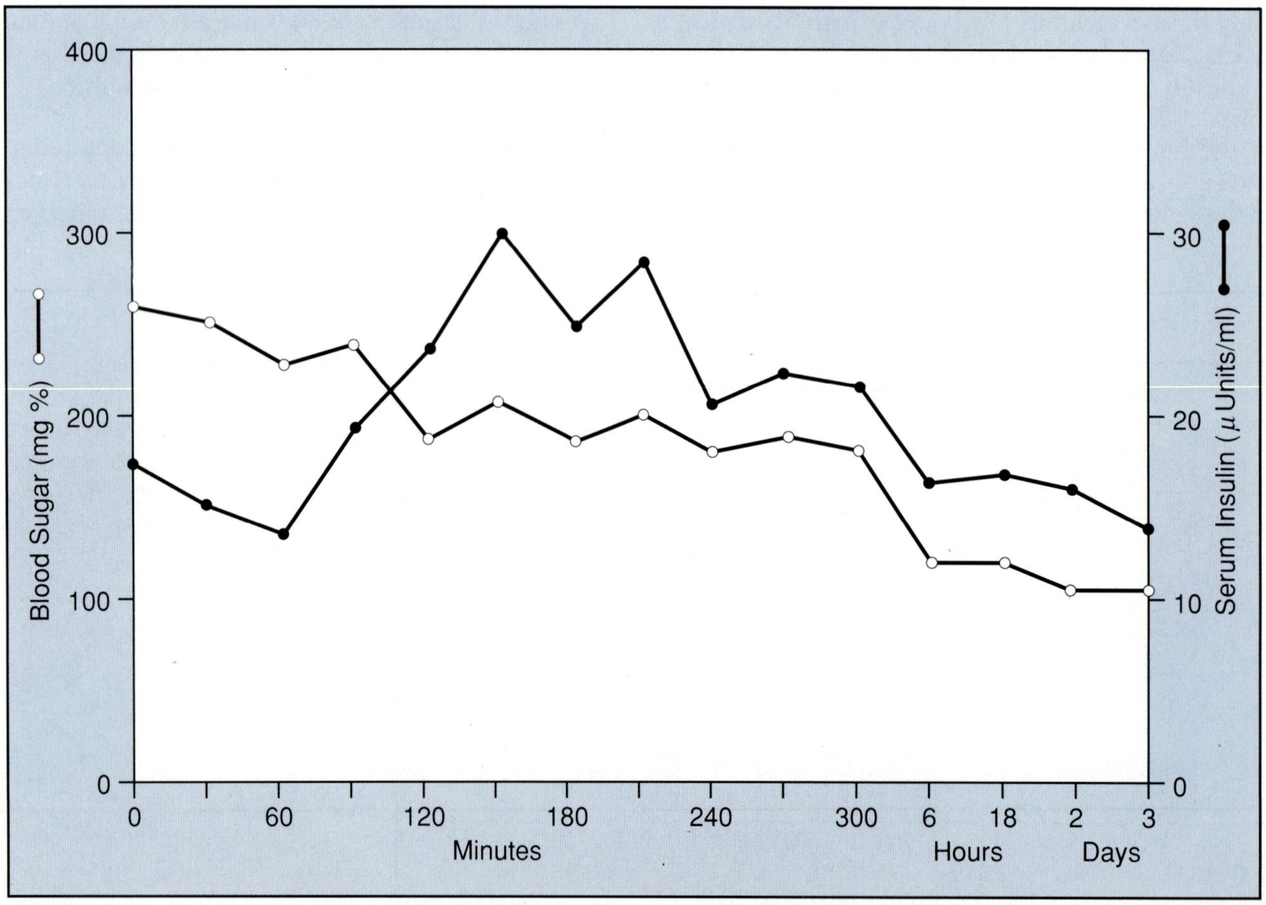

FIGURE 2.4 Blood sugar and insulin changes in 66 men in hemorrhagic shock. Serum insulin does not respond to the hyperglycemia of shock in humans as it does in animals.

Can blood lactate be used to accurately reflect the efficacy of resuscitation from shock? In the 66 patients in shock followed by Carey[11] from admission through resuscitation, it was noted that the blood lactate level was elevated four to five times normal on admission. Immediately following surgery, the blood lactate level rose again, although only slightly, but then fell sharply over the course of the next 6 to 12 hours after resuscitation (Fig. 2.5). In three patients, levels did not return to normal. Retrospectively, it was thought that these patients fell into the category of irreversible shock, since their *p*H levels remained below 7.2, they were all anuric, and they all died within 12 hours of admission to the hospital. It is obvious that the usual clinical signs of adequacy of resuscitation did not apply in these three patients. While their blood pressures did rise with volume replacement and there was other clinical evidence of improvement, such as increased levels of consciousness, their overall status was not consistent with adequate resuscitation.

Retrospectively, the magnitude of lactate elevation was not considered to be a reliable indicator of survival; however, there did seem to be a relationship between the severity of the shock state and the degree of lactate elevation. No specific level of arterial lactate elevation that was incompatible with survival could be determined. In patients admitted without detectable blood pressure, mean lactate levels were 50% higher than in those with detectable blood pressure. Lactate levels appear to be a good indication of the state of resuscitation and the adequacy of restoration of perfusion at the cellular level. A further observation by these investigators was that in several patients who suffered recurrent shock owing to postoperative bleeding, lactate levels again promptly rose. This rise was never seen unless a shock syndrome recurred.

The question arises whether the lactate elevations can be related to the level of arterial oxygen partial pressures. One investigation noted that arterial lactate levels did not rise until the arterial PO_2 reached 36 mm Hg, and in all instances cardiovascular collapse occurred within minutes of the rise in lactate.[29] Haller, Ward, and Cahill[25] used extracorporeal circulation as a means of controlling PO_2, and kept the PO_2 constant while gradually lowering perfusion pressure. They noted that lactate levels rose with lowered perfusion, even though PO_2 levels were maintained at a high level. This was corroborative evidence that arterial lactate levels are useful as an index of the adequacy of cellular perfusion, and that they are not dependent upon PO_2 levels *per se*. In the patients reported by Carey,[11] calculation of excess lactate offered no information beyond that obtained by arterial lactate determination alone.

The use of the arterial lactate level can be offered as a good index of the severity of shock from hemorrhage resulting from trauma. No immediate advantage is gained by measuring excess lactate or deriving lactate/pyruvate ratios. In patients whose lac-

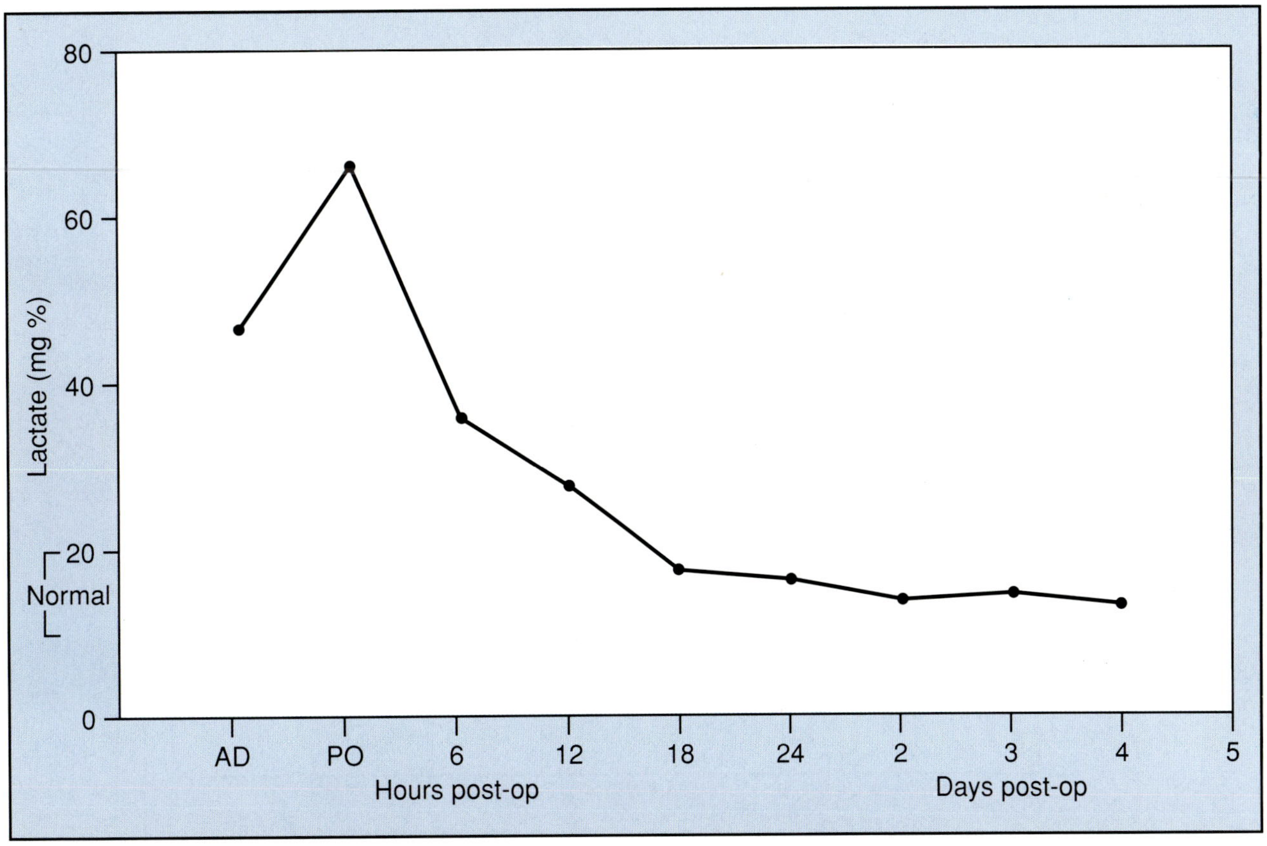

FIGURE 2.5 Arterial lactate levels in 66 men in shock at admission were 4 to 5 times normal. Levels rose in the immediate postoperative period and then fell sharply over the next 6 to 12 hours.

tate levels do not fall promptly with volume restoration, the prognosis remains poor. Inadequate cellular perfusion is reflected well by arterial lactic acidemia.

Acid–Base Balance In 1923, Cannon[9] described a group of soldiers who were acidotic owing to shock and infection. He described these patients as having low *p*H, low PCO_2, increased respiratory rates, and low serum bicarbonate. Hardaway[26] suggested that the acidosis was more severe in hemorrhagic than in endotoxic shock and postulated that this was because of the depressed ability to compensate by respiration.

Acidosis certainly is expected to occur in shock. It is thought that several factors contribute to acidosis. When perfusion at the cellular level is decreased because of low flow, then metabolic responses follow, that is, in carbohydrate, protein, and lipid metabolism. In the normal aerobic pathway, glucose is converted to pyruvate and then to lactic acid, with the major part of the pyruvate entering the Krebs cycle, which converts it to oxaloacetic acid. When anaerobic conditions prevail, the pyruvate is converted to lactate, which readily diffuses out of the cell, producing a rise in blood lactate levels. As the body attempts to compensate for the acidosis with its buffer base, a base deficit ensues as the buffer is consumed.

Under normal conditions, amino acids contribute to the formation of adenosine triphosphate (ATP) in the Krebs cycle. Both amino acids and nitrogen are shown to be increased in urine following shock, suggesting active catabolism. If the catabolism continues, there is a rise in circulating amino nitrogen and a concomitant decrease in the ability of the liver to metabolize amino acids. Catecholamines are stimulated by shock and in turn affect tissue lipids in their conversion of triglycerides to free fatty acids. Fatty acids, when used for ATP production, produce acidosis in much the same way as they do in diabetic ketoacidosis.

In the analysis of 66 men in severe shock in the Vietnam war,[15] it was not surprising that they appeared to be acidotic. However, in order to arrive at a proper evaluation of their acid–base status, we could not rely on a low *p*H alone. Approximately 31% of the patients arrived at the hospital with a *p*H of 7.3 or less; 8 had a *p*H of 7.5 or higher. The majority (40) of the patients arrived with *p*H well within the normal range of 7.31 to 7.45 (Fig. 2.6). The compensatory hallmark for metabolic acidosis is respiratory alkalosis. In patients with no preexisting pulmonary disease, a wide range of compensation is apparently possible. When all acid–base determinants were measured or calculated, 71% of the patients studied showed an element of metabolic acidosis.

Could the time from injury to admission account for the severity of acidosis in these patients? There was no correlation between the severity of acidosis and either the time elapsed from injury to admission or the severity of shock determined by cuff blood pressure measurements. There was a relationship, however, with the degree of lactic acidemia. Perhaps most significant was the definite increase in mortality associated with worsening

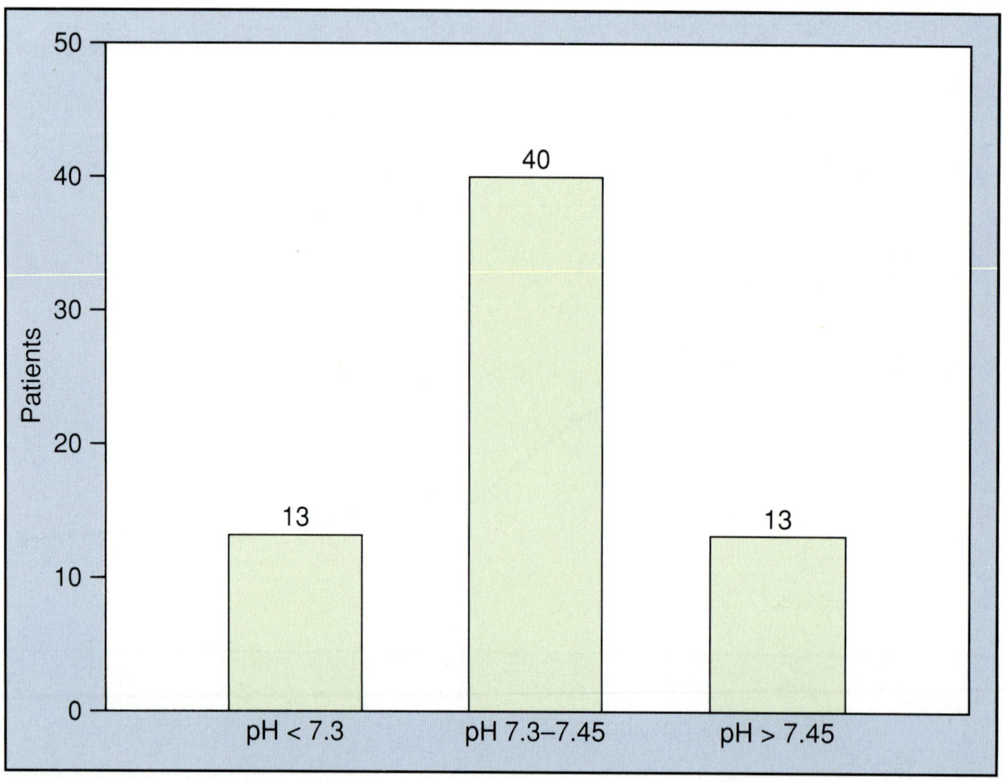

FIGURE 2.6 pH distributions in 66 patients in shock on admission and before treatment. Note that 53 patients had normal or elevated pH on admission.

acidosis. Of 13 (31%) patients with a *p*H of 7.3 or less on admission, 4 died; of these, 3 had been thought to be irreversible and could not be resuscitated. Of the 53 patients with a *p*H above 7.3, only 2 died. Thus, patients suffering from hemorrhage, while they may be expected to be in metabolic acidosis, must be evaluated by measuring or calculating not only the *p*H but also the PCO_2, bicarbonate, and base deficit. The acidosis often can be masked by compensatory mechanisms. In this population of patients, severe metabolic acidosis was a bad prognostic sign.

My colleagues and I have encountered patients with a *p*H of less than 7.1 on admission who were resuscitated. Four of these patients have returned to an active, productive existence. This raises the question of why these patients could be resuscitated when the patients previously described could not. The answer is undoubtedly related to the speed of transportation to a definitive care facility, coupled with vigorous efforts at resuscitation and promptness in getting the patients to definitive surgery.

TREATMENT

To be effective, treatment of hypovolemic shock must be directed toward restoring cellular perfusion.

The patients must be diagnosed quickly and treatment initiated promptly if mortality and morbidity are to be kept at a minimum. The Committee on Trauma of the American College of Surgeons has established excellent procedural guidelines for the initial evaluation of the trauma victim,[2b] which follow the ABCs (airway, breathing, circulation). Once the airway is patent and immediate life-threatening problems have been ruled out or treated, attention is turned to the circulation.

Patients in hypovolemic shock have lost fluid; thus, the goals of treatment are to stop further volume loss and to restore fluid. Obvious external bleeding wounds should receive compression dressings. The use of tourniquets or clamps should be avoided, with the possible exception of a patient who has sustained a traumatic extremity amputation.

Rapid venous access to the vascular system must be established. At least two large-bore (14-gauge) intravascular catheters should be inserted into the peripheral veins. Depending on the severity of injury and degree of shock, three access lines may be needed. The preferred routes of venous access are percutaneous insertion into the forearm or antecubital veins, or saphenous or forearm vein cutdowns. The subclavian and internal jugular veins should be reserved for the judicious insertion of monitoring lines and should not be used as primary access routes for fluid administration. Most catheters used for central vein access are too long and too narrow for rapid fluid administration.

There is no question that the patient who is in hypovolemic shock secondary to blood loss will require blood sometime during the course of treatment. Blood has to be typed and crossmatched and may not always be readily available. However, there are three classes of asanguineous solutions commercially available that may be given to patients in shock to support the circulation: colloids, crystalloids, and electrolytes.

Colloids Colloids are suspensions of particles of varying molecular weight, such as plasma, dextran, hydroxyethyl starch, albumin, and Plasmanate. During World War II and the Korean War, plasma was considered the resuscitative fluid of choice in treating patients in hemorrhagic shock. Plasma's short half-life and the high risk of hepatitis led investigators to search for plasma substitutes. It was believed that substances with a molecular weight similar to albumin (70,000) would be beneficial in restoring oncotic pressure and correcting hypoproteinemia. Thus, great enthusiasm attended the arrival of dextran, a long-chain polymer produced by the action of *Leuconostoc mesenteroides* on sucrose. Two forms of dextran exist: clinical dextran with a molecular weight of 70,000 and low-molecular weight dextran with an average molecular weight of 40,000. Both forms have been used extensively in clinical trials[46] and are still popular in Europe, although they are not widely used in the United States. Aside from being expensive compared to other resuscitative fluids, dextran has inherent disadvantages that preclude its use as a resuscitative fluid. Most patients in shock secondary to trauma require more than 2000 ml of solution for resuscitation, and that amount of dextran can create a bleeding diathesis by diluting clotting factors and increasing capillary flow.

Hydroxyethyl starch, while it is an effective plasma expander[3,44] and is less expensive than dextran, has been shown to prolong prothrombin time and partial thromboplastin time.[30]

Albumin, Plasmanate, and fresh-frozen plasma are not only costly, but also ineffective in treating shock, according to a substantial body of evidence. Carey[11] reported that battle casualties resuscitated with albumin required twice as much blood during and after surgery than did comparable patients treated with electrolyte solution. Furthermore, the patients receiving albumin had lower urine outputs and their total protein and albumin levels were not significantly higher than the patients who did not receive albumin. Thus, the theoretical concept that administering protein solutions restores plasma oncotic pressure in patients in shock was not substantiated in that study. Subsequent studies by Moss and co-workers[35] and Virgilio and associates[45] confirmed that albumin was not needed to resuscitate patients in shock and that it did little to protect the lung from pulmonary edema.

Fresh-frozen plasma does have a place in treating patients who develop a coagulopathy either during resuscitation or while undergoing surgery.

Crystalloids Crystalloids are solutions that contain nonionizing particles such as glucose. Five percent dextrose in water is the most common of the crystalloids. Despite being readily available and inexpensive, they have little value in treating patients in hypovolemic shock. Patients in hemorrhagic shock are hyperglycemic and have impaired utilization of glucose; to add an exogenous glucose load to an already overtaxed metabolic system has no scientific basis.

Because of decreased renal perfusion, patients in shock are often anuric or oliguric. As resuscitation proceeds, the hyperglycemia can cause glucosuria and an obligatory osmotic diuresis, which can, in turn, further compromise vascular volume and deplete sodium and water. Since a functional sodium deficit already exists, further sodium loss is undesirable.

Mannitol is a crystalloid solution that is often used as an osmotic diuretic; however, it has no role early on in the resuscitation of a patient in shock. Once resuscitation is completed and blood loss is arrested, there may be some benefit in administering mannitol to the oliguric patient.

Electrolyte Solution The use of salt-containing solutions in shock resuscitation is not new. Cannon, Fraser, and Hooper[10] in 1918 reported beneficial results in treating battle casualties in shock as long as the volumes used were not so excessive as to worsen hemodilution. Blalock[5] warned that electrolyte solutions diluted serum proteins. Rosenthal[40] in 1942, Fox and Keston[21] in 1945, and Reynolds[39] in 1949 showed in a variety of experimental animals in shock the benefits of saline resuscitation. Subsequent work by Dillon and colleagues[19,20] solidified the rationale for the use of electrolyte solutions in shock resuscitation. In 1966, Dillon and co-workers compared lactated Ringer's solution with colloids and blood in treating dogs in hemorrhagic shock. The importance of their work was not only in the discovery that saline solutions were beneficial in treating a lethal 50% to 75% hemorrhage, but also in the knowledge that these solutions were as good as colloid solutions. They further demonstrated the indisputable need for blood in shock resuscitation. Later, Trudnowski[41] reported that buffered salt solution lowered intraoperative blood requirements in a civilian setting.

As a result of the excellent work cited above, enthusiasm was great for "salt water" resuscitation as the United States entered the Vietnam conflict. Lowery, Cloutier, and Carey[32] compared lactated Ringer's and normal saline solution in 56 battle casualties in severe shock. Twenty-nine received saline and blood, and 27 received lactated Ringer's and blood. The severity of the wounds in both groups was similar, and no formula was used to calculate fluid or blood requirements. From these studies the following observations were reported:

Humans in hemorrhagic shock could be adequately resuscitated with either lactated Ringer's or normal saline solution plus blood.

The fluid and blood requirements to resuscitate and maintain these patients are quite large, averaging 11,700 ml of salt solution and 8,500 ml of blood in the first 24 hours.

Solutions containing lactate do not negate the value of blood lactate measurements, nor do they affect arterial lactate levels any differently than nonlactate-containing solutions.

Despite the infusion of large sodium loads, hypernatremia does not occur, and while the chloride levels are indeed higher in the patients receiving sodium chloride, at no time are they of clinical significance.

A year later, Proctor and colleagues,[37] serving in the same hospital in Vietnam, studied a similar group of casualities. Because of their concern with the volume of salt-containing solutions used in the previous study, they deliberately reduced the amount of salt given. Whereas their patients received an average of 6,300 ml of saline (versus 11,700 ml), their blood requirements averaged 11,000 ml (versus 8,500 ml). These data strongly confirmed the observations of Trudnowski[41] and Pruitt, Moncrief, and Mason[38] that saline solutions can significantly lessen blood transfusion requirements.

It is now widely recognized that salt-containing solutions either in the form of lactated Ringer's or normal saline are the preferred solutions to be used in resuscitating patients in hemorrhagic shock.

Blood and Blood Products Patients who have lost more than 1500 ml of their circulating blood volume will require blood in addition to electrolyte solution as part of the resuscitation regimen. Fresh whole blood, 12 to 24 hours old, while ideal, is rarely available. Properly typed and cross-matched packed red blood cells should be administered as soon as available. The goal of red cell replacement is to maintain the hematocrit at between 30% and 35% (hemoglobin 10–12 g). Hematocrits greater than this may increase viscosity and interfere with the normal rheology of blood flow. Hematocrits below 30% limit the oxygen-carrying capacity of arterial blood.

Patients who require massive transfusions (more than 10 units) may exhibit coagulopathy. A general rule of thumb is to give 1 unit of fresh-frozen plasma for every 4 to 5 units of packed red cells, and 10 units of platelets for every 8 to 10 units of packed red cells. The prothrombin time, partial thromboplastin time, platelet count, and fibrinogen level should be measured when a coagulopathy is suspected, and these values should be monitored serially until coagulation factors return to normal.

Initial Fluid Therapy Once the large-bore intravenous lines are inserted, blood samples should be obtained for laboratory determinations, typing, and crossmatching. Lactated Ringer's is administered as rapidly as possible in an initial bolus of 1000 ml to 2000 ml for an adult. It is absolutely essential that a physician be present who is experienced in treating patients in shock because additional therapeutic decisions will, in large measure, be directed by the patient's response to this fluid challenge.

It is difficult to predict the amount of fluid and blood that will be required to successfully resuscitate a given patient in shock. The American College of Surgeons offers as a guideline the "three-for-one" rule.[2b] This rule is based on retrospective observations that most patients in shock require 300 ml of electrolyte solutions for each 100 ml of blood lost.

My personal preference is not to rely on this or any other rule or formula when managing a patient in shock. Rather, close, careful attention to the same clinical factors that are used in diagnosing shock will determine whether resuscitation is proceeding in the right direction: stabilization of the blood pressure, slowed rate and improved quality of the pulse, cessation of air hunger, improved level of consciousness, return toward normal of the capillary blanch test, and a urine output of 50 ml per hour. If a central venous pressure line was deemed necessary and was inserted after resuscitation was begun, then a central venous pressure of 5 cm H_2O or more is indicative of moving toward an adequate right atrial pressure.

Drugs and Other Measures As a general rule, the patient in hypovolemic shock has lost effective circulating volume and needs volume replacement, not drugs. Occasionally, however, a patient is encountered whose volume is adequately replaced and who has no further volume loss, yet has not responded hemodynamically. In this patient, the use of pharmacologic agents directed at improving cardiac and vascular performance may be indicated.

Dopamine is a sympathomimetic agent, to which the response is directly related to the dose administered. When low dosages (0.5 mg/kg/min) are given, cardiac output is increased, vascular resistance decreased, and mesenteric and renal blood flow increased, thus improving urine output. Used in moderate dosage (2–10 mg/kg/min), there is an increase in cardiac contractility. Large dosages (10 mg/min or more) may lead to increased vasoconstriction, decreased tissue perfusion, and worsening of injury at the cellular level.

Dobutamine in dosages of 2 to 10 mg/kg/min, like Isuprel, increases heart rate and cardiac contractility by stimulating beta-adrenergic receptors. Side effects are many, however, and must be carefully watched for; these include tachycardia, ventricular arrhythmias, vasodilatation, and myocardial ischemia.

Epinephrine is one of the two alpha- and beta-mixed adrenergic agonists commonly employed in treating patients in refractory shock. Epinephrine (1 to 15 mg/min) improves myocardial contractility and increases the heart rate. It is highly arrhythmic and can lead to tissue ischemia secondary to vasoconstriction. Its use should be reserved for those patients who need inotropic support and who do not respond to dopamine or dobutamine.

Norepinephrine (1 to 4 mg/min), the other alpha- and beta-mixed adrenergic agonist, affects primarily the alpha-adrenergic receptors and results in profound vasoconstriction. In a maximally constricted patient this can lead to further tissue ischemia and cellular death. It should be used judiciously only in those patients unresponsive to volume replacement and other pharmacologic manipulations.

Rarely, a patient will be adequately volume resuscitated but does not respond to the usual inotropic agents. The patient may be maximally vasoconstricted and may require an agent to reduce systemic vascular resistance (afterload). Two commonly employed agents to reduce peripheral vasoconstriction are *nitroprusside* (0.5–10 mg/kg/min) and *nitroglycerin* (10–400 mg/min). Nitroprusside has the ability to affect both the arterial and venous end of the microcirculation, thus directly affecting the resistance (arterial) and capacitance (venous) vessels. Nitroglycerin, a venodilator, improves cardiac output in patients with severe vasoconstriction and may be beneficial in patients with known coronary artery disease.

Monitoring Devices While it is always helpful to gather as much relevant information as possible in the treatment of a patient in hypovolemic shock, treatment should never be delayed as a result. A patient who urgently needs a laparotomy to arrest further blood loss cannot possibly benefit from an additional 30-minute delay while central venous pressure, Swan-Ganz catheters, and arterial lines are inserted. Patients in profound shock secondary to trauma most often need urgent, if not emergency, surgery. In these patients it is best to insert intravenous lines as previously described, perform the indicated surgery, and insert monitoring lines in the postoperative period. It is in this period that the information derived from monitoring lines can be of the most value in directing the future course of therapy.

Cardiogenic Shock

Cardiogenic shock occurs when the heart is unable to pump blood in sufficient amounts to maintain adequate cellular perfusion. Myocardial infarction is the major cause of cardiogenic shock. Approximately 20% of patients with myocardial infarction develop cardiogenic shock, and approximately 80% of these patients die. Cardiogenic shock can also occur following rupture of a papillary muscle, rupture of the intraventricular septum, rupture of the myocardium, pericardial tamponade, air embolism, pulmonary embolism, vena cava compression, and end-stage valvular disease.

Occasionally, cardiogenic and hypovolemic shock occur simultaneously, as in a driver of a motor vehicle who has a myocardial infarction that results in an accident in which multiple life-threatening injuries are sustained. The first priority in treating this patient is restoration of volume and arrest of further hemorrhage.

PATHOPHYSIOLOGY

The pathophysiologic responses to cardiogenic and hemorrhagic shock are quite similar, especially at the neurovascular and neuroendocrine levels. A notable difference is the increased venous pressure in cardiogenic shock. Clinically, this is seen as distended neck veins. This important differential sign may be absent in the patient with coexisting hypovolemic and cardiogenic shock. With the rapid infusion of fluids necessary to treat hypovolemic shock, venous pressure may rise quickly, leading to pulmonary congestion.

Thus, it is important in the patient with suspected cardiac dysfunction to monitor venous pressures by the right atrial and pulmonary capillary wedge pressures. This is best accomplished by insertion of a Swan-Ganz catheter, which, in addition to the above measurements, allows other important data (cardiac output, pulmonary and systemic vascular resistance, venous oxygen content, and pulmonary artery pressure) to be measured or calculated. Again, while these data are important in evaluating patients suspected of having concomitant shock problems, its true value is in monitoring the response to therapy. Delays in resuscitation or definitive surgery should not occur because of insertion of monitoring lines.

TREATMENT

Proper treatment of the patient in cardiogenic shock depends on the identification of the reason why the heart is malfunctioning as a pump. Basically, there are four possible causes: reduced diastolic filling pressure of the ventricles (preload), loss of effective myocardial contractility, alterations in vascular resistance, and extremes in the cardiac rate.

If insufficient preload is the problem, treatment consists of volume expansion coupled with a diligent search for a mechanical cause (such as pericardial tamponade, excessive PEEP). Inadequate contractility is managed by pharmacologic agents such as dopamine, dobutamine, Isuprel, and digitalis. Afterload problems are treated initially with drugs such as diuretics and sodium nitroprusside; some patients may require intra-aortic balloon assistance to achieve diastolic augmentation in addition to reduction in afterload. Extremes in cardiac rate (bradycardia below 60 beats/min and tachycardia greater than 180 beats/min) are treated by drugs (digitalis, lidocaine, Isuprel) and sometimes electroversion or external pacing.

Septic Shock

Septic shock occurs when infection produces a decrease in peripheral vascular resistance, resulting in a hyperdynamic circulatory state. In addition to volume restoration, the origin of the sepsis must be identified and often surgically drained, and cultures and sensitivity studies performed so that the discriminate use of antibiotics can be initiated.

Unless an unusual delay in transportation has occurred, septic shock will not be a problem in the initial resuscitation of a trauma victim. However, patients who survive their initial injuries but die weeks later usually do so as a result of sepsis. This is particularly true in patients with major intra-abdominal injuries and peritoneal contamination.

Septic shock can be caused by gram-negative or gram-positive organisms. The gram-negative organisms most frequently implicated are *Escherichia coli*, *Pseudomonas aeruginosa*, *Aerobacter aerogenes*, *Klebsiella pneumoniae*, and, less frequently, *Proteus* and *Bacteroides*. *Streptococcus*, *Staphylococcus*, *Pneumococcus*, and *Candida albicans* are gram-positive organisms that can cause septic shock.

Patients most prone to developing septic shock are the elderly who are often debilitated by preexisting illnesses, such as malignancy, diabetes, or other systemic diseases. Organ systems most frequently implicated as the site of origin of bloodstream bacterial invasion are the genitourinary, respiratory, and gastrointestinal tracts, and the skin in burn patients.

CLINICAL PROFILE

The clinical picture in septic shock often is quite indistinguishable from that seen in hypovolemic shock. Patients may be cold and clammy with poor peripheral perfusion, diminished urinary output, tachycardia, and hypotension. Endotoxins released by gram-negative organisms enter the bloodstream and are carried to cells, where destruction of the cell wall occurs. With cellular destruction comes capillary dilatation, leading to a relative hypovolemia, thus setting in motion the vicious life-threatening cycle of shock. In response to the hypovolemia, cardiac output and cellular perfusion decrease; an increased outpouring of catecholamines leads to vasoconstriction at the arteriolar level and the creation of arteriovenous shunts. Hypoxia results, triggering metabolic acidosis and further destruction at the cellular level.

Occasionally, patients in septic shock may have a condition called "warm shock." In contrast to the appearance of hypovolemic shock and gram-negative sepsis, the patient's skin is warm, dry, and has good color. Urinary output may be adequate. There may or may not be hypotension. Peripheral pooling of blood occurs with loss of regulation of the microcirculation.

Regardless of etiology, septic shock results in impaired tissue perfusion and progressive death at the cellular level. In addition, endotoxins from gram-negative organisms have been incriminated in the production of disseminated intravascular coagulation, believed to result from platelet and vascular endothelial damage. The latter condition produces further impairment of cellular perfusion with worsening cellular hypoxia. Endotoxins apparently impair cellular function by interfering with mitochondrial function. The aerobic metabolic capacity of the cells is further impaired, contributing to the release of destructive lysosomal enzymes.

TREATMENT

Physicians caring for trauma victims recognize that it is easier to prevent septic shock than to treat it. A thorough understanding of the portals of entry of bacteria, awareness of predisposing factors (such as malnutrition, prolonged steroid use), judicious use of antibiotics, and early recognition of the signs and symptoms of septicemia are key ingredients in preventing and treating sepsis.

Patients who have sustained major, life-threatening traumatic injuries and hypovolemic shock have a high potential to develop sepsis. These patients must be monitored very closely for impending signs and symptoms of sepsis. Aseptic technique must be meticulously adhered to, cultures obtained frequently so antibiotics can be used judiciously, and every effort expended to identify the site of pus collections that need prompt surgical drainage. Volume expansion, when needed, must be prompt if tissue perfusion is to be maintained.

Drugs to improve the circulation are sometimes needed and have been previously discussed. Considerable controversy has existed over the use of steroids in treating septic shock. Except for the occasional patient who exhibits adrenal exhaustion, evidence does not support the use of steroids in treating septic shock.[43]

Neurogenic Shock

Neurogenic shock results when there is impairment of central nervous system–mediated vascular control because of an injury or medications. With the exception of nitrous oxide, most general anesthetic agents decrease myocardial contractility and diminish peripheral vascular resistance. These physiologic changes can result in diminished cellular perfusion and may precipitate a dramatic drop in blood pressure in patients who are hypovolemic at the time of induction of anesthesia.

The rapid intravenous administration of barbiturates has also been reported to produce a sharp decrease in peripheral vascular tone, particularly in the venous capillary bed. Once again, the net result is impairment of cardiac filling and reduced cardiac output.

Spinal and epidural anesthesia may cause severe blocking of the autonomic nervous system and a sharp fall in peripheral resistance, which leads to impaired cardiac filling and reduced cardiac output. Acute trauma high in the spinal cord may also result in a loss of peripheral vascular tone and the so-called "spinal shock" syndrome. Central nervous system injuries alone rarely produce a shocklike picture. It behooves the physician to search carefully for other causes of shock in any patient with a primary head injury who suffers clinical shock.

REFERENCES

1. Alpert NP: Lactate production and removal and the regulation of metabolism. Ann NY Acad Sci 119:995, 1964.
2. American College of Surgeons Committee on Trauma: (a) Shock. Chapter III, pp 179–191. (b) Initial assessment of management. Chapter I, pp 139–148. Advanced Trauma Life Support Course Instructors Manual. Chicago, American College of Surgeons, 1984.
3. Ballinger WF II, Solanke TF, Thompson WL: The effect of hydroxyethyl starch upon survival of dogs subjected to hemorrhagic shock. Surg Gynecol Obstet 122:33, 1966.
4. Bayliss WM: Intravenous injections to replace blood. In Wound Shock and Haemorrhage: Their Treatment by Intravenous Infusions, Reports of the Special Committee for the Investigation of Surgical Shock and Allied Conditions, nos. I–VII, pp 11–41. London, Medical Research Committee, National Health Insurance, 1919.
5. Blalock A: Shock. In Military Surgical Manuals. Philadelphia, WB Saunders, 1943.
6. Cannon WB: Acidosis in cases of shock, hemorrhage and gas infection. JAMA 70:531, 1918.
7. Cannon WB: Acidosis and shock. In Wound Shock and Haemorrhage: Their Treatment by Intravenous Infusions. Reports of the Special Committee for the Investigation of Surgical Shock and Allied Conditions, nos. I–VII, pp 245–285. London, Medical Research Committee, National Health Insurance, 1919.
8. Cannon WB: Acidosis in cases of shock, haemorrhage, and gas infection. In Wound Shock and Haemorrhage: Their Treatment by Intravenous Infusions. Reports of the Special Committee for the Investigation of Surgical Shock and Allied Conditions, nos. 1–VII, pp 85–98. London, Medical Research Committee, National Health Insurance, 1919.
9. Cannon WB: Traumatic Shock. New York, D Appleton, 1923.
10. Cannon WB, Fraser J, Hooper AN: Some alterations in distribution and characters of blood in shock and hemorrhage. JAMA 70:526, 1918.
11. Carey LC: Hemorrhagic Shock. Chicago, Year Book Medical Publishers
12. Carey LC, Lowery BD, Cloutier CT: Blood sugar and insulin response of humans in shock. Ann Surg 172:342, 1970.
13. Churchill ED: Introduction. In Beecher HK (ed): Surgery in World War II: The Physiologic Effects of Wounds, pp 1–20. US Army, Board for the Study of the Severely Wounded, Medical Department. Washington DC, US Government Printing Office, 1952.
14. Cloutier CT, Kopolovic R, Thrailkill K et al: Effect of bilateral adrenalectomy on blood sugar level and plasma refill in a rat hemorrhagic shock model. J Trauma 24:586–589, 1984.
15. Cloutier CT, Lowery BD, Carey LC: Acid–base disturbances in hemorrhagic shock. Arch Surg 98:551, 1969.
16. Cope O, Litwin SB: Contribution of the lymphatic system to the replenishment of plasma volume following hemorrhage. Ann Surg 156:655, 1962.
17. Crenshaw CA, Canizaro PC, Shires GT, Allsman A: Changes in extracellular fluid during acute hemorrhagic shock in man. Surg Forum 13:6, 1962.
18. Crile GW: Blood Pressure in Surgery. Philadelphia, JB Lippincott, 1903.
19. Dillon J, Lynch LJ, Myers R, Butcher HR Jr: The treatment of hemorrhagic shock. Surg Gynecol Obstet 122:967, 1966.
20. Dillon J, Lynch LJ, Myers R et al: A bioassay treatment of hemorrhagic shock. Arch Surg 93:537, 1966.
21. Fox CL Jr, Keston AS: The mechanism of shock from burns and trauma traced with radiosodium. Surg Gynecol Obstet 80:561, 1945.
22. Frawley JP, Howard JM, Artz CP, Anderson P: Investigations of serum protein changes in combat casualities. Arch Surg 71:605, 1955.
23. Friedman SG, Pearce FJ, Drucker WR: The role of blood glucose in defense of plasma volume during hemorrhage. J Trauma 22:86–91, 1982.
24. Gross SD: A System of Surgery: Pathological Diagnostic Therapeutique and Operative. Philadelphia, Blanchard & Lea, 1862.
25. Haller JA, Ward MJ, Cahill JL: Metabolic alterations in shock: The effect of controlled reduction of blood flow on oxidative metabolism and catecholamine response. J Trauma 7:727, 1967.
26. Hardaway RM: Studies on [cf2]pH changes in endotoxin and hemorrhagic shock. J Surg Res 1:278, 1961.
27. Hoch-Ligeti C, Irvine R, Sprinkle EP: Investigation of serum protein patterns in patients undergoing operation. Proc Soc Exp Biol Med 84:707, 1953.
28. Howard JM (ed): Battle Casualities in Korea (Surgical Research Team in Korea), vols I–IV. Washington, DC, Army Medical Service Graduate School, Walter Reed Army Medical Center, 1954.
29. Huckabee WE: Relationships of pyruvate and lactate during anaerobic metabolism: Effects of infusion of puruvate or glucose and of hyperventilation. J Clin Invest 37:244, 1958.
30. Lee WH Jr, Cooper N, Weidner MG, Murner ES: Clinical evaluation of a new plasma expander hydroxyethyl starch. J Trauma 8:381, 1968.
31. Lockhart-Mummery JP: The physiology and treatment of surgical shock and collapse. Lancet 1:696–703, 1905.
32. Lowery BD, Cloutier CT, Carey LC: Lactated Ringer's solution versus unbuffered saline in resuscitation of severely wounded humans in shock. Surg Gynecol Obstet 133:273, 1971.
33. Mitchell SW, Morehouse GR, Keen WW: Gunshot Wounds and Other Injuries to Nerves. Philadelphia, JB Lippincott, 1864.
34. Moore FD: The effects of hemorrhage on body composition. New Engl J Med 273:567, 1965.
35. Moss GS, Proctor JH, Herman CM et al: Hemorrhagic shock in the baboon. I. Circulatory and metabolic effects of dilutional therapy: Preliminary report. J Trauma 8:837, 1968.
36. Pirkle JC Jr, Garan DS: Restitution of blood volume after hemorrhage: Role of the adrenal cortex. Am J Physiol 230:1683–1687, 1976.
37. Proctor HJ, Moss GS, Homer LD, Litt BD: Hemorrhagic shock in the baboon. II. Changes in lung compliance associated with hemorrhagic shock and resuscitation. J Trauma 8:842, 1968.
38. Pruitt BA, Moncrief JA, Mason AD: Efficacy of buffered saline as the sole replacement fluid following acute measured hemorrhage in man. J Trauma 7:767, 1967.
39. Reynolds M: Cardiovascular effects of large volumes of isotonic saline infused intravenously into dogs following severe hemorrhage. Am J Physiol 158:418, 1949.
40. Rosenthal SM: Experimental chemotherapy of burns and shock. Public Health Rep 57:1923, 1942.
41. Trudnowski RJ: Hydration with Ringer's lactate solution. JAMA 195:137, 1966.
42. U.S. Army, Board for the Study of the Severely Wounded, Medical Department. In Beecher HK (ed): Surgery in World War II: The Physiologic Effects of Wounds. Washington, DC, US Government Printing Office, 1952.
43. Upjohn Company, Kalamazoo, Michigan. Personal communication.
44. Vineyard GC, Osborne DP: Simultaneous determinations of extracellular water b35-sulfate and 82-bromide in dogs with a note on acute effects of hypotensive shock. Surg Forum 18:37, 1967.
45. Virgilio RW, Rice CL, Smith DE et al: Crystalloid vs. colloid resuscitation: Is one better? A randomized clinical study. Surgery 85:129–139, 1979.
46. Yao ST, Shoemaker WC: Plasma and whole blood viscosity changes in shock and after dextran infusion. Ann Surg 164:973, 1966.

respiratory support following injury

William H. Chamberlin
Gerald S. Moss

Traditionally, ventilatory support for the trauma patient has followed two principles: (1) to support elimination of carbon dioxide and (2) to promote adequate oxygenation of the hemoglobin. Although key, the lungs must be understood as only part of the oxygen delivery system. To that end, this chapter will review the components of that system, beginning with delivery under normal circumstances and focusing on the physiology of the pulmonary circuit as it relates to gas exchange, and concluding with the effects of various injuries on the lungs and the support techniques available.

PHYSIOLOGY OF VENTILATION

Elimination of Carbon Dioxide

The elimination of carbon dioxide (CO_2) is a reasonably straightforward process. That metabolic poison is produced at a basal rate of 200 cc/min and failure to eliminate it results in progressive CO_2 retention, acidosis, and death. Neural centers in the body's medulla sense small decreases in *p*H due to increases in the partial pressure of carbon dioxide (PCO_2) and they respond by increasing the body's ventilatory effort. Air moves in and out of the lung in tidal waves: 400 cc of air breathed 12 times per minute yields a minute ventilation of 4800 cc. Some of that air moves through "dead space" where no gas exchange with the blood occurs, so that only 75% to 80% of the air is exposed to blood in the alveolar exchange units. Thus the minute alveolar ventilation is actually more on the order of 3600 cc for a 75-kg individual. Given that the measured level of any substance in the body is a function of two processes—production and elimination—the balance between normal production (200 cc CO_2/min) and elimination (3600 cc of minute ventilation),

$$\frac{200 \text{ cc } CO_2}{3600 \text{ cc air}} = \frac{1}{8}$$

results in a normal arterial carbon dioxide tension ($PaCO_2$) of 40 torr. According to Dalton's law of partial pressures:

$$PaCO_2 = \text{fraction exhaled } CO_2 \times (\text{Atm. pressure} - H_2O \text{ pressure})$$

$$40 = \frac{1}{18} \times (760-47)$$

Thus, $PaCO_2$ is dependent upon production and elimination. A rise in CO_2 production without a rise in ventilation provokes a rise in $PaCO_2$. A fall in ventilation without a change in CO_2 production will promote a rise in $PaCO_2$. The former occurs rarely because the lungs have an excellent capacity to increase minute ventilation, while the latter may occur in a patient with flail chest. Disease processes in the lung often decrease the efficiency of ventilation. The three most common causes for hypercapnia in trauma patients are related to increases in dead space, decreases in minute ventilation, and marked increases in metabolic demands. Pulmonary embolus, for instance, obstructs blood flow to an area of the lung where ventilation is maintained. The body continues to work to move air in and out of the affected portion of lung, but no gas exchange occurs. The patient becomes tachypneic in an attempt to maintain normal alveolar ventilation.

Hypoventilation is identified by the failure to maintain a $PaCO_2$ below 45 torr. This is a dynamic definition: as carbon dioxide production rises, so should alveolar ventilation. If the rise in alveolar ventilation fails to meet the rise in production, CO_2 retention and acidosis occur. Tachypnea can result from rises in CO_2 production alone. Burn patients may have metabolic rates four to five times normal. Ventilatory rates of 30 breaths/min with tidal volumes of 500 cc are common. Yet measured dead space and $PaCO_2$ may be normal because CO_2 production is over 600 cc/min, or roughly three times normal.

Providing Oxygen to the Tissues

Providing oxygen to the mitochondria at adequate oxygen tensions (PO_2) is necessary to avoid anaerobic metabolism, lactic acidosis, and death. Oxygen delivery is the product of cardiac output and oxygen content, which is dependent upon the concentration of hemoglobin in the blood, the efficiency of the lungs, and the oxyhemoglobin relationship. Oxygen content can be stated thus:

$$\text{Hgb (g/dl)} \times 1.37 \text{ cc } O_2/\text{g Hgb} \times \text{saturation} + PO_2 \times 0.0031$$

Oxygen is carried to the periphery in two compartments of the blood: dissolved in serum and on hemoglobin. These two compartments are in an equilibrium favoring the hemoglobin. The compartment most commonly measured in the clinical environment is the dissolved serum component. However, the arterial oxygen tension (PaO_2) is important only as it reflects hemoglobin saturation. It is not a direct measure of the oxygen content of the blood. Each gram of hemoglobin, when fully saturated, carries 1.37 cc O_2. A patient with 15 g of Hgb/dl of blood when fully saturated with oxygen has 20 cc O_2/dl. A patient with 10 g Hgb/dl at 100% saturation has only 13.7 cc O_2.

Reference to the oxyhemoglobin saturation curve (Fig. 3.1) reveals that when PaO_2 falls below 60 torr, there is a rapid loss of oxygen from the hemoglobin. A rise above 60 torr adds little additional oxygen to the system. If a patient has 15 g Hgb/dl and a PaO_2 of 60, the hemoglobin is nearly 90% saturated and will contain about 18 cc O_2/dl of blood while only an additional 0.18 cc of oxygen is contained in the serum ($0.0031 \times PaO_2$). (However, the dissolved serum component is immaterial to transport when adequate hemoglobin is available; consequently, it will not be considered in calculations concerning the lungs and gas exchange.) If PaO_2 rises 34 torr from 60 to 94 torr, saturation rises to nearly 100%, but only 2 cc of additional oxygen are added to the system. Once the hemoglobin is fully saturated, little additional oxygen is added. A further rise to a PaO_2 of 200 torr results in no significant addition of oxygen to the hemoglobin and only about 0.3 cc of oxygen to the serum. On the other hand, a fall of 34 torr in PaO_2 from 60 to 26 torr results in a loss of 8 cc or nearly 45% of the total oxygen content. Thus, the sigmoid shape of this relationship explains the body's capacity to deliver enormous amounts of oxygen to the tissues over a narrow range of oxygen tension changes from arterial to venous blood. These estimates reveal two important principles of blood oxygenation: (1) Once the hemoglobin is fully saturated, no significant oxygen is added to the system; and (2) with a PaO_2 less than 60 torr, oxygen content is lost rapidly. More simply stated, a PaO_2 greater than 60 torr is seldom needed to satisfy physiologic demand, but less than 60 torr must be supplemented quickly to avoid hypoxic hypoxemia.

The oxyhemoglobin relationship is well established. Oxygen equilibrium between serum and hemoglobin is very rapidly achieved in the blood, and the measure of PaO_2 can suffice for estimates of saturation. This relationship can change, depending on shifts of the curve due to acid-base disturbances, changes in CO_2 tensions, body temperature, and the levels of 2,3 diphosphoglycerate (DPG) in red cells. However, these changes are well established and can easily be taken into account when estimating hemoglobin saturation from the serum PO_2. The Kelman equation (see bibliography) is perhaps the best known calculation used.

Carbon monoxide alters the relationship between saturation and PO_2. Since it competes with oxygen for hemoglobin binding, it can be thought of as shifting the oxyhemoglobin curve far to the right. A saturation estimated from the serum PO_2 will be falsely elevated. Any patient suspected of having smoke inhalation should have blood oxygen analyzed on a co-oximeter which measures saturation directly.

Delivery of oxygen from the capillary to the mitochondria occurs down an oxygen tension gradient. Tissues with a high ratio of utilization to delivery, such as the heart, operate at lower tissue oxygen tensions, while tissues such as skeletal muscle normally operate at a high PO_2 until metabolism is increased; in the case of skeletal muscle, this would occur with exercise. Under most circumstances, the oxygen tension in venous effluent (PvO_2) from the capillary bed is in equilibrium with the tissues and, therefore, can be considered a measure of tissue PO_2. Shifts in the oxyhemoglobin relationship greatly alter tissue oxygen tensions. Shifts to the left lower the oxygen tension associated with any given saturation. Thus alkalosis tends to decrease tissue reserves of oxygen.

Since mixed venous blood obtained from the pulmonary artery is pooled, the mixed venous oxygen tension (PvO_2) is not an index for any one tissue, but rather can be used as a marker for perturbations of the system. It also has profound influence on the ability of diseased lungs to provide adequate arterial oxygenation.

The determinants of PvO_2 saturations are as follows:
Arterial saturation
Cardiac output
Hemoglobin concentration
Rate of oxygen consumption
Oxyhemoglobin relationship

Under normal circumstances, the following occurs in a 75-kg

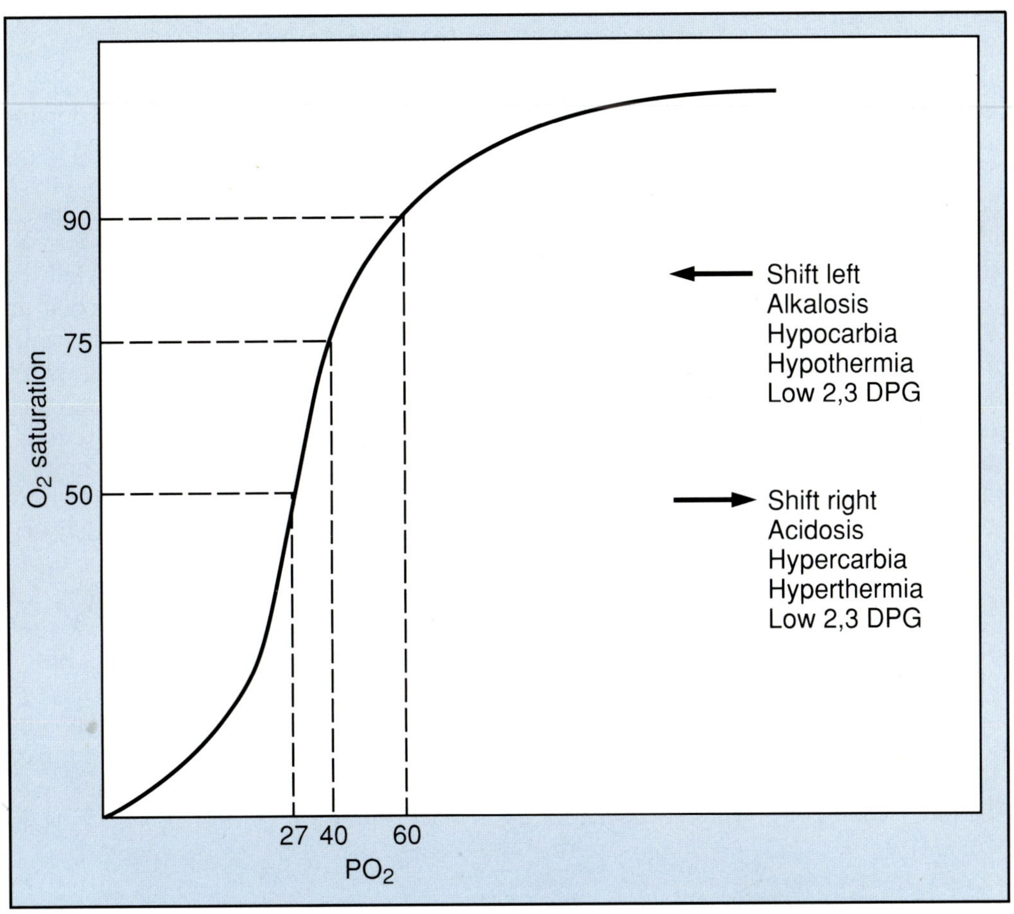

FIGURE 3.1 Shifts in the oxyhemoglobin saturation greatly alter tissue oxygen tensions.

individual. (See the Appendix for calculations.) When 15 g Hgb/dl is 100% saturated, a cardiac output of 50 dl/min delivers 20 cc O_2/dl or 1000 cc O_2/min to peripheral tissues. An oxygen consumption of 250 cc/min leaves 750 cc oxygen to be returned to the lungs. That hemoglobin is 75% saturated. Using the Kelman equation or the oxyhemoglobin saturation curve, the PO_2 of blood with a saturation of 75% and normal *p*H, PCO_2, and temperature is determined to be 40 torr. The Fick principle states: Oxygen consumption equals cardiac output times arterial-venous oxygen-content difference ($AVdO_2$), so that 50 dl/min equals 250 cc O_2/min/$AVdO_2$. The $AVdO_2$ is 5 cc/dl, so the venous content must equal 15 cc O_2/dl. Substituting these values into our original equation for oxygen content,

$$15 \text{ cc } O_2/\text{dl} = 15 \text{g/dl} \times 1.37 \text{ cc } O_2/\text{dl} \times \text{saturation}$$

Saturation is again demonstrated to be 75%. These, then, constitute the numbers one might expect in the normal physiologic state for a 75-kg individual:

Cardiac output = 5.0 liters/min or 50 dl/min
Hemoglobin = 15 g/dl
Oxygen consumption = 250 cc/min
Arterial saturation = 100% and PaO_2 = 95 torr
Venous saturation = 75% and PvO_2 = 40 torr
$AVdO_2$ = 5 cc/dl

The Lungs and Gas Exchange

The lungs are responsible for exposing adequate volumes of blood to air with good PO_2 to assure saturation of hemoglobin. The customary measurement of lung efficiency is the PaO_2. Since a PaO_2 of 60 torr usually ensures hemoglobin saturation of 90%, a PaO_2 below this level defines hypoxia. This is not synonymous with hypoxemia, a condition of inadequate oxygen content, which is difficult to define precisely because its cause is usually anemia, for which the body has good compensatory mechanisms. Hemoglobin levels of 5 to 7 g/dl are not unusual in patients with end-stage renal disease, yet these patients can maintain adequate oxygen delivery even during periods of heavy exercise despite subnormal oxygen content.

Hypoxia has three physiological causes with respect to lung function: ventilation-perfusion mismatch (V/Q), venous admixture, and hypoventilation. These defects account for all problems encountered in the clinical arena. The most devastating of these is severe V/Q mismatch because of the unremitting hypoxemia and high mortality with which it can be associated.

VENTILATION-PERFUSION MISMATCH

For gas to be exchanged, air (ventilation or V) must be exposed to blood (flow or Q) across the thin alveolar surface. The ratio of V to Q determines the oxygen tension that can be achieved in the alveolus and hence in the blood. Each alveolus maintains a V/Q ratio that depends upon the compliance of the alveolus. In the upright position, gravity increases blood flow to the dependent portions of the lung. This stiffens the lung, leading to smaller alveolar volume changes in the bases and lower V/Q ratio than in the apices.

As with CO_2, the level or concentration of oxygen in the body or a compartment of the body, such as the alveolus, is determined by the forces of production and those of excretion acting on that compartment. PO_2 in the alveolus depends on the movement of air into the alveolus through the airway (V) and the consumption of oxygen from the alveolus (Q). A common cause of V/Q inequality is a reduction in ventilation by constriction of the small airways as happens in asthma. For any given alveolus, as ventilation is reduced the partial pressure of alveolar oxygen (PAO_2) must fall, since absorption continues onto the hemoglobin. Blood will be exposed to progressively lower PAO_2, and hypoxia becomes more severe. If the ventilation defect is severe enough, hypoxia can become extreme, and steps must be taken to improve the hypoxic condition in the alveolus. This can be done by increasing the fraction of inspired oxygen (F_IO_2) the patient is breathing. By raising the F_IO_2 to (100% O_2), the production of oxygen to that alveolus will be nearly five times greater than if the patient breathed only room air (F_IO_2 of 0.21). PAO_2 and PaO_2 will also rise. Patients with asthma and pulmonary embolus commonly respond to oxygen therapy. Rarely do these patients need ventilatory support.

A reduction of ventilation to zero results in the clinical condition commonly referred to as shunt, that is, blood flow through an unventilated lung. This most commonly occurs when pus, blood, or water fills the alveoli or the alveoli and smaller airways collapse such that air cannot come into contact with blood. Response to oxygen therapy alone is poor, because blood passing through the shunt is never exposed to oxygen, and blood exposed to open alveoli is 100% saturated on room air.

VENOUS ADMIXTURE PHENOMENON

Arterial hypoxia results when the number of mismatched alveolar units is great. The amount of well oxygenated blood flowing by functioning alveoli and mixing with poorly oxygenated blood flowing through the diseased lung determines the PaO_2. Consider the following model of this principle in gas exchange (Fig. 3.2). Blood arrives in the lung with a PvO_2 of 40 torr. By the oxyhemoglobin curve, this blood is 75% saturated. Half the blood passes through a good lung and is exposed to alveolar air with an oxygen tension of 100 torr and becomes essentially 100% saturated. The other half will be exposed to a lung with a V/Q ratio of zero, that is, unventilated or a shunt. Thus, equal volumes of blood with respective saturations of 75% and 100% will mix. The resulting mixture is 87.5% saturated. Assuming a cardiac output of 5 liters/min and an oxygen consumption of 250 cc O_2/min, as in our example of normal oxygen delivery, this desaturation would result in a delivery of only 875 cc O_2 to the periphery. Following the extraction of 250 cc oxygen, the mixed venous hemoglobin would now be 63% saturated. (See the Appendix for detailed calculations.) Passing this blood through our 50% shunt model once again, equal volumes of arterialized blood with a PaO_2 of 33 torr (63% saturation) and 100 torr (100% saturation), respectively, would result in a mixed arterial saturation of 82% and a PaO_2 of 47 torr. The next pass would account for an arterial saturation of 79% and PaO_2 of 43 torr. By the time equilibrium is reached after five passes through the shunt, the PaO_2 will be about 41 torr and the PvO_2 will be 28 torr. This obviously is severe hypoxia with a resultant compromise of the system.

While these calculations demonstrate how equilibrium is achieved in the system and why shunt disease results in hypoxia, another important principle must be recognized. The patient with this 50% shunt is in desperate need of more oxygen in the bloodstream. Our first response should be to increase the F_IO_2, from, say, 0.21 to 1, causing the PAO_2 to rise above 500 torr, but having no effect on arterial oxygen content. The blood flowing through the shunt is not exposed to an increased PO_2, and the blood flowing through the open lung is already fully saturated. The amount of oxygen dissolved in serum will account for no more than 1.2 cc O_2/dl (400 torr x 0.0031). This will not significantly affect oxygen content and tension; a quick calculation reveals a change from 76% to 79% saturation or a new PO_2 of 43 torr at equilibrium.

Two important principles emerge: (1) Shunt disease is unresponsive to an increasing F_IO_2, and (2) falls in venous oxygen content produce falls in arterial oxygen content in compromised lungs. A common problem in the critically ill patient, shunt disease occurs with pulmonary edema, pneumonia, and parenchymal contusion. Patients with pneumococcal pneumonia in three lobes can present with a PaO_2 of 50 torr on room air and show no response to breathing 100% oxygen. Other supports are required for these patients and will be considered in following sections.

HYPOVENTILATION

There are two variables involved in assuring adequate PAO_2. The first is the F_IO_2. Room air is 21% oxygen and 79% nitrogen. By the gas laws, the fraction of the gas and its partial pressure are proportional. The only other significant gas in the air is evaporated water. Atmospheric pressure at sea level is 760 torr, so room air PO_2 must be 21% of 760 minus water vapor pressure, or $0.21 \times (760 - 47) = 150$ torr. This is the pressure of inspired oxygen (P_IO_2).

The second variable is adequate elimination of carbon dioxide. Oxygen and CO_2 enjoy a reciprocal arrangement. As oxygen leaves the alveolus, CO_2 enters. This ratio is governed by the substrate being burned. That is, the respiratory quotient (RQ) varies with the fuel:

$$RQ = CO_2 \text{ produced}/O_2 \text{ consumed}$$

For instance, the oxidation of glucose is governed by this reaction:

$$C_6H_{12}O_6 + 6O_2 = 6H_2O + 6CO_2$$

Six CO_2 molecules are produced for 6 of oxygen consumed, and

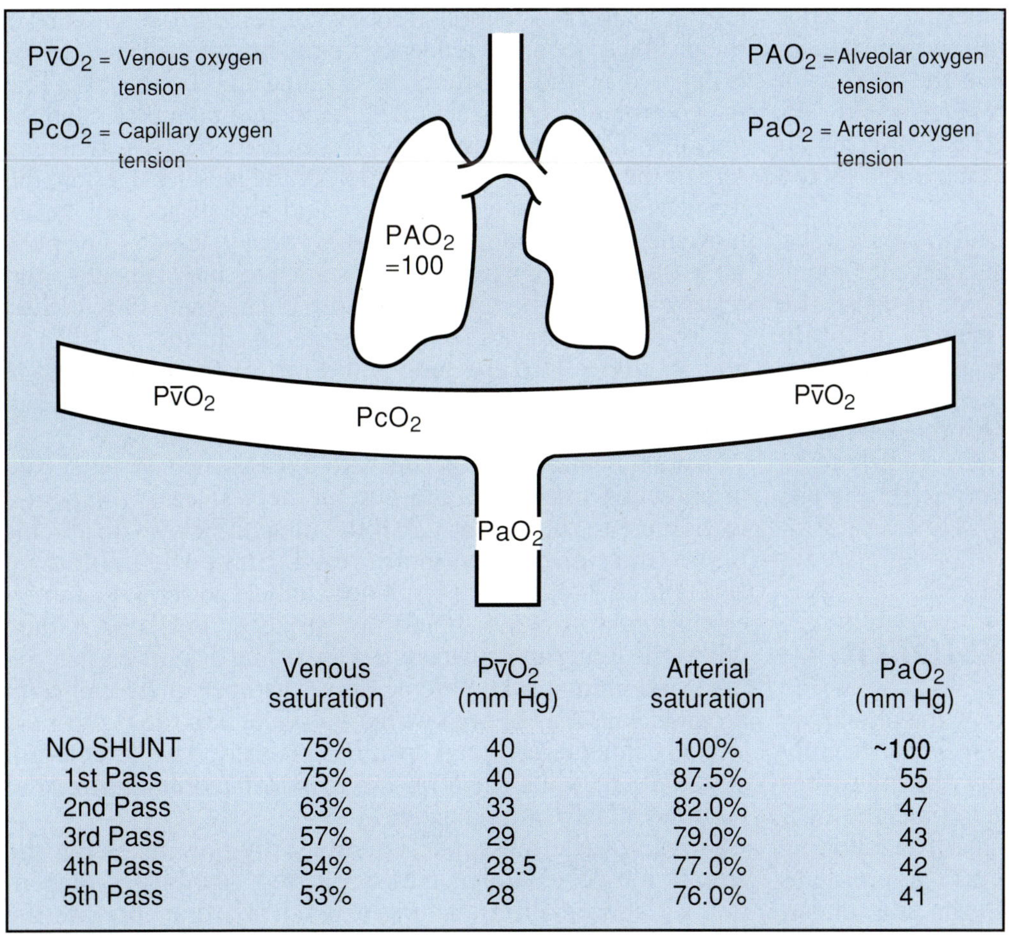

	Venous saturation	$P\bar{v}O_2$ (mm Hg)	Arterial saturation	PaO_2 (mm Hg)
NO SHUNT	75%	40	100%	~100
1st Pass	75%	40	87.5%	55
2nd Pass	63%	33	82.0%	47
3rd Pass	57%	29	79.0%	43
4th Pass	54%	28.5	77.0%	42
5th Pass	53%	28	76.0%	41

FIGURE 3.2 Arterial PO_2 is a function of the amount of blood flowing through the shunt (50% in this model) and the oxygen content of the venous blood going into the shunt.

the RQ is 6:6 or 1. Since the oxidations of fat and protein have different RQs and diet is a mixture of all three substrates, the average RQ for the body is 0.8. The alveolar gas equation is stated thus:

$$PAO_2 = P_IO_2 - [PCO_2/0.8]$$

Under normal circumstances breathing room air,

$$PAO_2 = 150 - 40/0.8 = 100 \text{ torr}$$

Hypoxia can result from a decrease in F_IO_2 or from a rise in PCO_2. $PaCO_2$ rises when alveolar ventilation falls. In the discussion of steady state, it was apparent that a PCO_2 of 40 torr is determined by a CO_2 production of 200 cc/min exhaled in 3600 cc of alveolar air. If minute alveolar ventilation falls to 1800 cc, then $PaCO_2$ must rise to 80 torr.

CO_2 retention commonly occurs in the trauma patient for two reasons: an inability to move air, as with a high cervical spine injury that severs the spinal cord above the phrenic nerves; or a marked increase in dead space, as in a patient unable to compensate. Dead space is defined as ventilation of underperfused areas of the lung (those with very high V/Q ratios). For instance, in our normal example, 1200 cc of 4800 cc total volume of ventilation move in and out of large areas such as the trachea where no gas exchange occurs. In these areas CO_2 cannot be eliminated, even though the lung works to move the gas. Dead space disease increases the work of breathing by decreasing the efficiency of the system. However, when a patient has a thrombotic embolus blocking the perfusion of one entire lung, normal $PaCO_2$ will be maintained. Overall ventilation will be doubled to achieve the 3600 cc of minute alveolar ventilation still needed. Fifty percent of the air is moved in and out of the unperfused lung. The most common clinical sign with thrombotic embolus is tachypnea as the patient increases alveolar ventilation.

However, that reserve can be compromised in other ways. When a patient with flail chest arrives in the emergency room, an elevated PCO_2 might account for hypoxia because the patient cannot move adequate tidal volumes to maintain minute alveolar ventilation. According to the alveolar gas equation, a measured PCO_2 of 80 torr could not be associated with a PaO_2 higher than 50 torr. Given that the lungs normally have a 3% to 5% shunt and mild V/Q inequality, PaO_2 is likely to be closer to 40 torr. With ventilation alone and no oxygen supplementation, this patient's PaO_2 will improve.

MECHANICAL PATHOPHYSIOLOGY

In studying gas exchange abnormalities, not only the physiology but also the pathologic disorders leading to such exchange problems must be considered. Problems develop within the three integrated systems involved in respiratory function: the neurosensory, musculoskeletal, and lung parenchyma. The following is meant only as a simple review relative to the problems encountered in clinical medicine. For a more exhaustive understanding of the physiology of the respiratory system, please see the list of sources at the end of this chapter.

The Neurosensory Centers and Drive

Control of ventilation is accomplished both peripherally and centrally. Brain stem chemo- receptors respond to small changes in the *p*H of the cerebrospinal fluid (CSF). The blood–brain barrier effectively bars hydrogen or bicarbonate ions from passing from the blood to CSF. On the other hand, CO_2 moves readily between the two spaces. For each 1-torr increase in PCO_2, the hydrogen ion concentration is increased by 0.8 nmol/ml. This acidosis stimulates the central chemoreceptors with a consequent increase in minute alveolar ventilation and restoration of normal $PaCO_2$. Narcotics can suppress this drive.

Peripheral chemoreceptors are located in the carotid bodies at the bifurcation of the common carotids and aortic bodies, above and below the arch. These bodies respond to decreases in PaO_2 and *p*H, and increases in PCO_2. In humans, the carotid bodies appear to be the primary sensing site for arterial hypoxia. They have much less responsibility for maintenance of $PaCO_2$ and blood *p*H than does the central chemoreceptor. Bilateral carotid body resection abolishes hypoxic drive but not CO_2 sensitivity.

The Musculoskeletal System

The lung parenchyma is elastic; that is, it tends to assume its resting shape. This elastic property creates negative pressure in the pleural space and a tendency for the lungs to collapse, which is opposed by the stiff thoracic space created by the ribs. This space is enlarged by the action of the intercostal muscles and the muscular diaphragm. Inspiration is the creation of negative pressure in the alveoli by active motion of the muscles. Pressure differences between the atmosphere and alveoli account for air movement in and out of the lungs in "tidal volumes." The pleural space maintains a resting hydrostatic pressure of about –7 torr relative to atmospheric pressure. With enlargement of that chest cavity during inhalation, the pressure falls further to –10 torr and air rushes into the lung and down to the alveoli for gas exchange. Abnormalities of parenchyma, muscles, skeletal system, or drive can each contribute to ventilatory failure.

Neuromuscular failure occurs with diseases such as spinal cord injury when intercostal and phrenic nerves cease to function with injury to the cord at C2. If the injury is below C6, phrenic nerve function will be maintained. Since the diaphragm accounts for two thirds of respiratory muscle power, loss of intercostal function alone should not produce ventilatory failure unless the lung parenchyma is diseased. The diaphragm may fail following injury to the phrenic nerves without intercostal compromise. This may be seen with a stab wound to the neck or use of cold cardioplegia during open heart surgery. The latter is usually transient while the former is most commonly unilateral so both should have a good prognosis.

Fatigue of the muscular system is only now receiving the attention it deserves. The muscular system can usually compensate for abnormalities of lung parenchyma that increase the work of breathing. Respiratory muscles can become fatigued under load and be compromised by other factors affecting strength, such as malnutrition, which leads not only to reduction of skeletal muscle mass, but diaphragm mass as well. Furthermore, some studies indicate that the diaphragm loses more power than would be suggested by the mere loss of mass with starvation. Sick lungs increase the work of breathing by affecting mechanics. As lungs stiffen, for instance, the elasticity increases. This increased tendency to collapse creates more negative pleural pressures and demands more muscular work to expand the lungs for normal tidal volumes. The body usually compensates for this by reducing tidal volume and increasing the respiratory rate. Respiratory rates in excess of 50/min quickly lead to fatigue and failure. Weakness and fatigue of the diaphragm can be evaluated clinically by watching the abdomen during inhalation. Normally expansion of the abdomen precedes expansion of the chest during quiet inhalation. At the point of diaphragm failure, expansion of the intercostal muscles will pull the diaphragm into the chest and "abdominal paradox" occurs, that is, the abdomen collapses during inhalation. A laboratory correlate of this is obtained if tubes are passed into the stomach and esophagus for measurement of pressure during the breathing cycle. Normally abdominal pressure during inhalation is positive as the diaphragm moves caudad. As diaphragm muscles fatigue and abdominal pressure becomes negative, respiratory failure becomes likely. Certain groups of patients are more prone to diaphragm problems. It is estimated that morbidly obese patients lose use of their diaphragm muscles for 24 to 48 hours following an abdominal procedure.

The skeletal frame may also fail. That is, normal inhalation causes enlargement of the chest cavity. With a flail chest, the chest cavity collapses on inhalation, a maneuver that may result in inadequate tidal volumes. This condition usually means that the same rib has been broken in two places on the same side. Without the stiffness of the ribs to oppose them, negative intrapleural pressures cause collapse of the rib cage, rather than expansion of the lung.

Air can enter the pleural space, causing loss of negative pressure. As a result, pneumothorax prohibits adequate expansion, atelectasis occurs, and the lung ceases to ventilate appropriately. These mechanics can be returned to normal by evacuation of the air from the pleural space with a chest tube to water seal. During exhalation, positive pressure in the chest will expel air from the pleura so that the lung can reexpand. Simple pneumothoraces do not require continuous suction, only a simple one-way valve to permit air to leave the cavity but not be sucked in with inhalation.

The Lung Parenchyma, Oxygenation, and Work of Breathing

It is most important to consider two parameters of lung function: compliance and airway resistance. Alterations of either or both can increase the work of breathing and lead to respiratory failure. Both of these factors also markedly affect airway pressures and the complications attendant to positive pressure ventilation.

For clinical purposes, compliance is the relationship between airway pressure and lung volume. The lung can be thought of as a balloon. Such a balloon can be inflated to 1000 cc in 100 cc increments. At each volume increment the pressure in the balloon can be measured to construct a compliance curve (Fig. 3.3). The balloon is considered very compliant if small pressure changes result in large volume changes. The less compliant the balloon, the more pressure would be required to inflate it to the same volume as a more compliant balloon. Lungs are normally very compliant. Airway pressures are measured in spontaneously breathing patients most commonly during pulmonary function testing. The patient interrupts breathing at various points during tidal breathing and mouth pressure is read through a mouthpiece. The pressure in the mouth with glottis open reflects the volume of air in the chest and the compliance of the total system, that is, the lungs, muscles, and skeletal cavity. A lung with 1000 cc of air at a pressure of 10 cm H_2O has a compliance of 100 ml/cm H_2O. However, a patient with pulmonary edema may generate pleural pressures of 40 torr with 600 cc of tidal air, a compliance of 600/40 or 15 ml/cm. These lungs are stiff compared to the compliant lungs of the normal individual. In Fig. 3.3, the curve on the left illustrates compliant lungs. As lungs stiffen the curve moves down and to the right.

Air flow through a tube is met by resistance to that flow. This resistance can be quantified by the relationship described by Poiseuille:

$$R = \frac{8nl}{r4}$$

where R is the flow resistance, r is the radius of the tube, n is the viscosity of the gas, and l is the length of the tube. The smaller the radius of the airway, the greater the resistance to flow. Asthma is a disease that acutely reduces airway diameter with bronchial muscle constriction and markedly increases airway resistance.

Pressure and resistance form another important relationship. Pressure is the product of flow and resistance. Mean airway pressure equals air flow times resistance, or AWP = AF × R. Greater airway resistance increases the pressure differences needed to generate flow. A corollary is that when flow falls to zero, the pressure attributable to resistance also falls to zero.

Work of breathing is done against these two forces. The less compliant the lung, the more work must be done to move tidal air. As airway resistance increases, pleural pressures must become more negative to move air into the alveoli. Abnormalities of either increase the work of breathing. Breathing pattern and rate change according to the pathophysiologic event. When resistance increases, the usual response is to breath more slowly. The lower flow reduces the pressure differences and hence the work of breathing for any given resistance. However, when the lung stiffens, as in a patient with pulmonary edema, expanding to normal volume takes enormous work. The patient attempts to reduce the high energy consumption by limiting the tidal volume. To maintain normal alveolar ventilation, the respiratory rate must be increased. An increased respiratory rate is a good indication that the lung may be stiffening and respiratory work increasing, that is, that there is dysfunction.

Dyspnea is the clinical correlate of work. The sense of an increased work of breathing is reported by the patient as "shortness of breath," and interpreted by physicians as dyspnea. Dyspnea cannot be measured, since its definition is much debated. One thing is clear: patients complaining of dyspnea can have nearly normal blood gases. Changes in compliance and airway resistance increase work of breathing before significant gas exchange abnormalities occur. Blood gases in most patients complaining of dyspnea will generally show a respiratory alkalosis and only mild hypoxia. Therefore, a normal blood gas does not correlate with the absence of disease; it merely suggests that disease is not severe enough to interfere with exchange. In the case of mild pulmonary edema, if the clinician waits until gas exchange is disordered to treat, treatment will be too late.

Support of oxygenation can often be accomplished with an enhancement of F_IO_2. The V/Q mismatch of most diseases responds to an increase in delivered oxygen, and the same is true with hypoxia. Several delivery systems are available. Nasal cannulae are the least obtrusive, but also deliver the lowest flow rates. The Venti-mask tightly controls the F_IO_2 that is delivered to the patient and thus prevents the patient working on hypoxic drive from achieving too high a PaO_2. But for most purposes with the trauma patient, standard 40% or 60% oxygen masks can be used. Up to 80% F_IO_2 can be delivered with a non-rebreathing mask and oxygen reservoir. With continued hypoxia on 80% F_IO_2, more aggressive support must be initiated.

Short of endotracheal intubation, continuous positive airway pressure (C-PAP) masks can be used to deliver up to 10 cm positive end expiratory pressure (PEEP). While the physiology and efficacy of PEEP will be discussed below, it must be noted that techniques for its use are available to improve oxygenation without intubating a patient's trachea and they may be especially useful for conscious patients with fat embolism, smoke inhalation, or cardiogenic pulmonary edema, in whom self-limited deficits are anticipated. PEEP has also been used for therapy of pulmonary contusion and postoperative atelectasis. Several contraindications to its use include unstable facial fractures, extensive facial lacerations, laryngeal trauma, or recent tracheal or esophageal anastomoses.

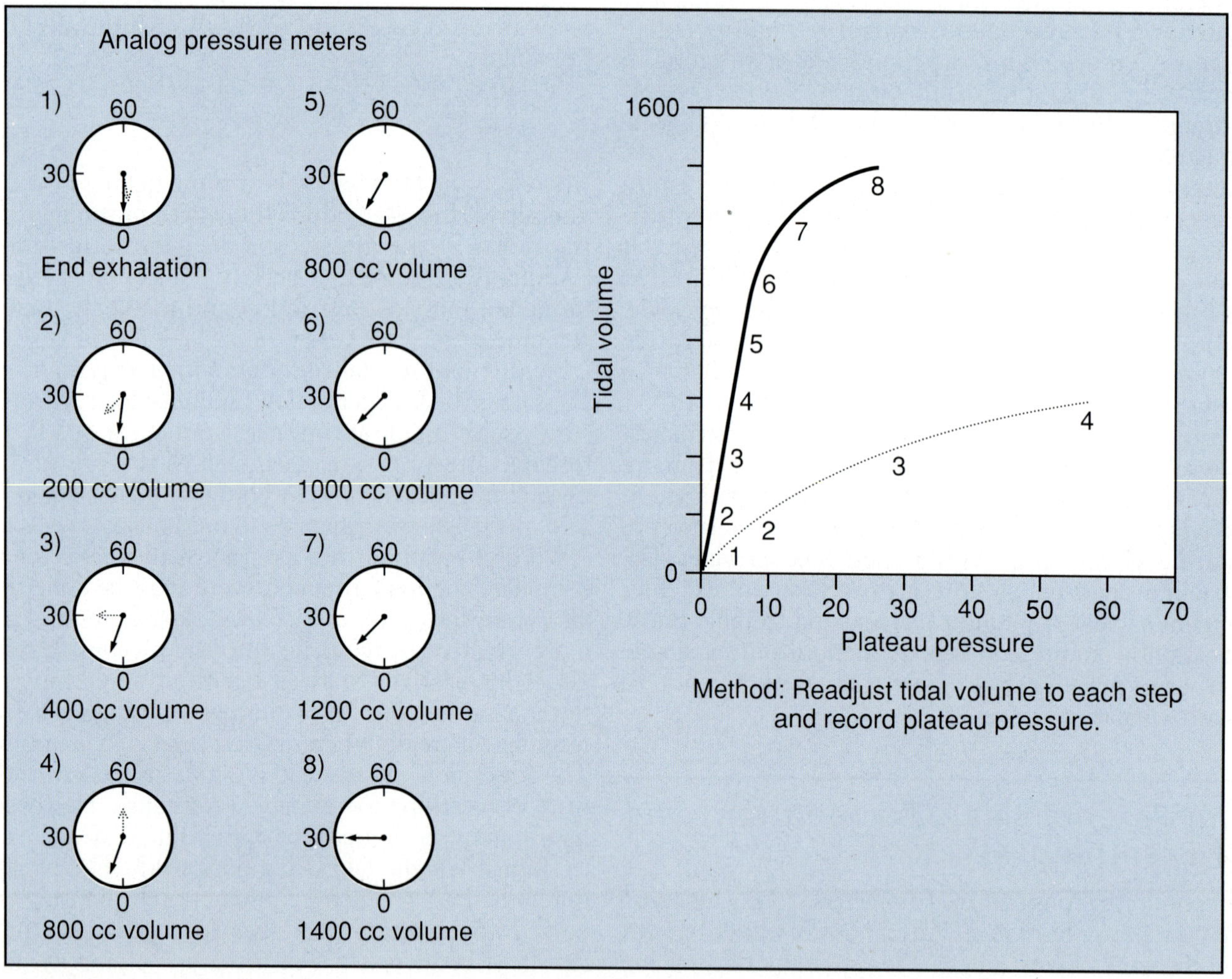

FIGURE 3.3 The dotted arrows represent the plateau pressures for the dotted curve. The shift down and to the right of the compliance curve indicates stiffer lungs.

Improvement of oxygenation does not usually reduce the work of breathing. Hypoxic drive begins significantly at a PaO_2 of less than 50 torr.

Measuring Dysfunction

Several indices exist to grade the severity of disease and follow a patient's progress. The two most popular are the shunt equation and the A-a gradient. (See the appendix for calculations.)

Shunt, as has already been defined, is blood flow by unventilated areas. Blood flow through the shunt, then, is proportional to oxygenation that does not occur, and the shunt becomes an estimate of the efficiency of the lungs. Measurement is only possible when the patient has a pulmonary artery catheter in place for sampling of the mixed venous oxygen content. Less than 10% of blood should normally move through the shunt. Shunts of greater than 20% to 25% are frequently associated with ventilatory failure. Disease with shunt greater than 40% is frequently fatal.

The A-a gradient is the difference between the measured PaO_2 and the PAO_2 estimated from the alveolar gas equation. For example, if a 21-year-old patient has an arterial blood gas drawn, the PaO_2 would likely be 94 torr. Since the PIO_2 is 150 torr on room air, the estimated PAO_2 would be 100 torr. The A-a gradient would be $100 - 94 = 6$ torr. The normal gradient varies as a factor of 0.3 times the age of the patient on room air. The patient's gradient should be 0.3×21 years $= 7$ torr. Since measured and age-estimated values are the same, the lungs are normal. On 100% oxygen, the A-a gradient is normally 25 to 65 torr. Respiratory failure is frequent when values are greater than 450 torr.

We do not always find these values helpful. The concepts are important, and the clinician learning to care for patients in ventilatory failure should become familiar with their use. But each has its limitation. Enormous errors occur when masks are used because the poor seal around most masks makes estimation of alveolar PO_2—dependent upon accurate PIO_2—dubious at best. The ability to maintain adequate gas exchange and a clinical estimate of work remain the most useful measures of dysfunction.

RESPIRATORY FAILURE AND VENTILATORY SUPPORT

Three criteria can be applied to identifying patients with respiratory failure.

RESPIRATORY FAILURE	
Respiratory rate	>50/min
$PaCO_2$	>50 torr
PaO_2	<50torr

Two of the criteria are measurements of gas exchange, but the third, a respiratory rate greater than 50/min, is significant because it correlates with an enormous work of breathing. If allowed to continue, the patient is likely to fail from fatigue. Ventilatory support is designed primarily to support gas exchange when failure occurs.

Endotracheal Intubation

Endotracheal intubation (ET tubes) should not be the first recourse once respiratory failure has been diagnosed. Some causes of failure are readily reversible. Moreover, emergency intubations are not for the uninitiated. They are difficult at best and at worst are a real hazard for the patient. Once the decision to intubate has been made, however, several steps should be followed. An adequate airway should be established with an oral mouthpiece. A suction device should be set up to clear the oropharynx and trachea once intubation is successful. The patient should be bag-ventilated by mask with 100% oxygen. This is a very important step for two reasons. Every attempt should be made to achieve a reasonable PaO_2 for the patient. Putting a tube through the vocal cords initiates a strong vagal response and hypoxemia heightens that response causing many arrests to occur during the intubation process. Additionally, most patients can be supported adequately with bag ventilation by mask until experienced help arrives. In the hospital setting, two individuals are better than one for bagging by mask. One should keep the neck extended and hold the bag firmly over the nose and mouth while the other compresses the bag. Chest movement can be checked to assure adequate ventilation until experienced help arrives. For the nonanesthesiologist, we believe the visualized oral route to be the best for intubation. Blind nasotracheal intubations require more practice and skill. Gentle pressure on the cricoid will close off the esophagus and help prevent aspiration. The endotracheal tube cuff should be tested for leakage. The cords should always be visualized before the tube is advanced between them. The cuff is then inflated just to the point when air leak stops with positive pressure breaths. Overinflation of the cuff damages the tracheal mucosa and leads to stenosis. Several signs can signify the trachea was properly intubated: chest movement with bag compression, full bilateral breath sounds at auscultation, and the presence of humidified air in the ET tube. Proper position should be checked by feeling the cuff in the suprasternal notch, and a chest x-ray should always be obtained to reveal the tip of the tube at least 2 cm above the carina. Patients may become hypotensive after intubation and the initiation of positive pressure. This usually indicates volume depletion and should be evaluated and treated with saline infusion.

Ventilatory Support

With control of the airway accomplished, ventilatory assistance must often be established. Its advantages and limitations will be made clearer by first examining the background physiology.

In considering issues and techniques of support, it is important to remember that improvement in gas exchange does not necessarily reflect an improving patient—merely improved oxygen delivery to the tissues and increased elimination of CO_2. This should not be confused with therapeutic intervention.

Moreover, while the principles concerning the effects of these various parameters are sound, the practice is not always clean. Some evidence suggests that efforts to increase cardiac output frequently increase shunt. The use of dopamine for its inotropic effect also abolishes hypoxic pulmonary vasoconstriction (HPV) thereby increasing pulmonary shunt. Diuresis and aggressive reduction of wedge reduces vascular volume and may precipitate renal dysfunction. Use of vasodilators to reduce afterload and increase cardiac output has even more profound effect on HPV and, in the presence of significant hypoxemia, can be extremely dangerous. Assessment and reassessment of the patient and chosen therapy are most important. Today's high-tech environment permits careful monitoring of cardiac output, oxygen delivery, and gas exchange. The patient and his response to therapy must remain the center of attention.

POSITIVE PRESSURE VENTILATION

Consider again the balloon. Inflation is accomplished and maintained not by the absolute pressure of gas within the balloon, but by the difference in pressures inside and outside the balloon. Hence, the balloon will inflate when enough air is forced into it (positive pressure), or, if the pressure is decreased around it (negative pressure or normal ventilation).

Early ventilators were negative pressure machines. With the iron lung, for instance, the patient was placed inside the large cylinder while his head remained outside. As a bellows decreased the pressure inside the iron lung (and outside the body), air was pulled into the patient's lungs by virtue of the vacuum created in the chest relative to atmospheric pressure. With this mode of ventilation, the pharynx continued to function in the ventilatory circuit to humidify and clean the air on its way into the lungs. This method had two major disadvantages: nursing care was difficult with patients in such an iron encumbrance, and it could not be used to advantage in patients with sick lungs.

Traumatic events tend to make the lungs stiff and difficult to ventilate with negative pressure devices. The early positive pressure devices had a similar disadvantage. They were little more than pressure-cycled valves attached to a high pressure source. As the lungs stiffen, more pressure must be generated to move air in and out of the lung. With the pressure-cycled machines, air flow was cut off when a set pressure was achieved. In the face of decreasing lung compliance, the pressure set point needed

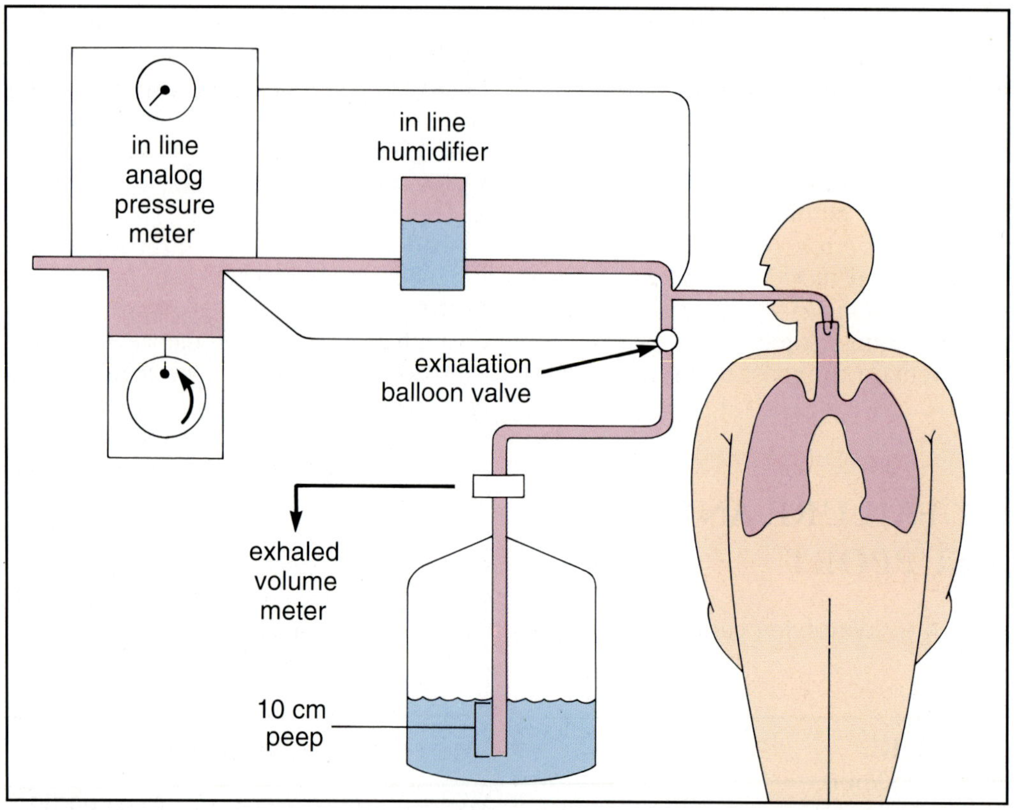

FIGURE 3.4 Typical positive-pressure ventilator. Typical volume ventilators are piston-driven machines with end-expiratory pressure controlled by a threshold resistor valve. The illustration here represents an early technique available for administration of PEEP; immersion of the hose beneath the requisite amount of water maintains the appropriate end-expiratory pressure.

constant adjustment to assure adequate ventilation volumes. The exchange of gases depends upon minute ventilation—not the pressure necessary to transport that volume. Accordingly, the biggest advance in ventilatory support for the critically ill patient came with the introduction of volume-cycled ventilators—those in which the volume of air to be delivered to the patient is preset and delivered despite stiff lungs and high airway pressures. Any technique employing positive pressure to move air in tidal volumes is referred to as intermittent positive-pressure ventilation (IPPV).

THE VENTILATOR

A standard configuration for the volume-cycled ventilator is shown in Fig. 3.4. Valves ensure that the airflow is in one direction as the piston develops pressure in the cylinder. The humidifier is generally a cascade-type system with air picking up moisture as it passes through heated water. This is necessary to prevent the airways from desiccating—a condition that weakens resistance to infection. An exhalation valve inflates as the ventilator develops pressure and a diaphragm closes the exhalation port forcing the set volume to be delivered into the patient's lungs. During exhalation, this port opens and the valves in the inhalation lines close so that air is forced out through the exhalation valve and a spirometer. The excursion of the piston can be set to regulate tidal volume. The frequency of the cycles can also be set to ensure adequate minute alveolar ventilation.

Nearly all ventilators have an analog pressure device for recording the internal pressure the machine must develop to deliver the set volume. This pressure and the airway pressure are identical. Each ventilator also has a control for the maximum or peak inspired pressure (PIP) the machine can be permitted to develop. Without this, the machine could easily cause barotrauma by driving air into stiff lungs at enormous pressure. This cutoff valve is set at 50 cm H_2O pressure, though normal lungs will require only 15 cm to 20 cm H_2O pressure to ventilate properly. As the ventilator delivers volume, pressure develops in the system. If that pressure hits the peak permitted before the entire volume is delivered, the remainder will be vented to the outside. This prevents higher pressures from developing, but at the expense of lost tidal volume. If the ventilator is persistently dumping tidal volume because the peak airway pressure permitted is exceeded, the patient will be underventilated.

The ventilator has several alarms. The peak pressure alarm marks the upper limit of permissible pressures. The apnea alarm identifies prolonged periods without ventilation. The volume alarms can be set to sound when the patient's exhaled volumes fall 200 cc below tidal volume, suggesting a leak in the system. These are the alarms of primary importance. Other features will vary by manufacturer.

All ventilators also control the F_IO_2 by blending oxygen with air. This is accomplished to permit enhancing the oxygen from its value at room air of 21% to the highest possible concentration of 100%. The flow rate of gas is also controlled. While this is normally set at 40 liters/min to start, it may be adjusted according to the physiologic state and the airway pressures encountered.

Most ventilators also have a control which suspends air flow at end inspiration. This ostensibly increases alveolar volumes and improves oxygenation in patients with sick lungs. This feature is only occasionally used to test airway resistance and compliance.

PHYSIOLOGY OF POSITIVE PRESSURE

Positive pressure works to the detriment of V/Q relationships. When the lungs work properly, most gas exchange occurs at the bases and midportions of the lungs. Perfusion to the lung at the low vascular pressures generated by the right side of the heart is very gravity-dependent, causing most blood to flow through the bases. In the presence of the raised airway pressures of positive pressure, flow is diverted away from ventilated areas. This is particularly true in the independent segments of the lung where perfusion pressures may fall below alveolar pressures and capillaries collapse. While this increases dead space, the increased perfusion to the dependent portions of the lung decreases the V/Q ratios of alveoli at the bases and contributes to hypoxia.

IPPV results in increases in intrathoracic pressure, which may decrease venous return to the heart and thereby decrease cardiac output and blood pressure. Additionally, increased pressure in the inferior vena cava, and consequently the renal veins, is associated with intense salt retention and oliguria. The syndrome of inappropriate antidiuretic hormone secretion can also result. Barotrauma in the form of pneumothorax or mediastinal emphysema is encountered most frequently in instances of high peak pressures. However, potential barotrauma does not justify the use of prophylactic chest tubes in patients on positive-pressure ventilation. This has never been satisfactorily demonstrated to reduce morbidity. Chest tubes are indicated primarily for the treatment of pneumothoraces and hemothoraces.

OPERATION OF THE VENTILATOR

The principle of the volume ventilator is the same as normal tidal ventilation: Move enough alveolar air to maintain appropriate $PaCO_2$.

INITIAL VENTILATOR SETTINGS

Tidal volume	10–15 ml/kg
Frequency	10 breaths per minute
F_IO_2	0.60
PEEP	5 cm H_2O
Peak pressure alarm	50 cm H_2O
Flow rate	40 liters/min

A patient with normal lungs, following surgery for example, may require about twice the normal spontaneous tidal volume because of the increase in dead space by a factor of 1.5 to 2 times. The rate should be in the range of 8 to 12 per minute.

There are several modes of ventilation available for patients today. Traditionally, when respiratory support was indicated, the machine entirely controlled the patient's ventilation by discharging at the set rate. The patient could not override the system and would frequently fight the ventilator, trying to exhale as the ventilator was pushing air in. Consequently, the patient had to be heavily sedated. Physicians began to use an assist/control mode, allowing the patient to trigger the machine as many times per minute as his neurocontrol centers would drive him to breath. However, patients tended to overdrive and develop marked respiratory alkalosis. This is not to be encouraged. Low $PaCO_2$ shifts the oxyhemoglobin curve to the left, increases cerebral oxygen consumption, and decreases cerebral blood flow—undesirable in critically ill patients.

A more recent innovation has been the widespread acceptance of intermittent mandatory ventilation (IMV). IMV permits the setting of a minimum respiratory rate while the patient breathes spontaneously through the ventilator circuit. In this mode, the ventilator may deliver a breath as the patient tries to exhale, causing high peak airway pressure. The remainder of the tidal volume is lost and may result in hypoventilation. The most frequently used augmented mode of ventilation in our intensive care unit is synchronized IMV (SIMV). With this method, the ventilator senses each negative inspiratory breath and initiates its cycle at a set frequency but only when the patient inhales. It is synchronized to the patient's efforts. If the patient makes no effort, this mode is identical to total control. With the various modes of IMV, the patient need not be overventilated. Since the patient does not control the ventilator, the amount of minute ventilation can be set to assure appropriate CO_2 tensions and *p*H, yet the patient can continue to draw spontaneous breaths.

In some ventilators popularized in Europe and now making inroads into U.S. markets, the minute ventilation can be set. This allows the patient to breath as on an IMV circuit, but it adds sufficient ventilation to maintain a set minimum minute alveolar ventilation. Thus the machine adjusts to the patient's needs.

Airway pressure plays an important role in adjusting the ventilator for appropriate control. Hence measuring that pressure is important. Once the trachea is intubated, and positive pressure is initiated from a pistonregulated machine (as shown in Fig. 3.4), the ventilator tubing and airway become part of the same circuit. Pressure measured anywhere in the tubing should reflect the pressure throughout the circuit. Most commonly, this is measured in the machine and displayed by an analog dial (Fig. 3.5). At end exhalation, no pressure is recorded in the circuit. As the patient initiates a breath, a small negative deflection will be seen on the dial, as in example 2 of Fig. 3.5. In assist/control mode, the ventilator will sense this negative pressure and deliver its volume. The sensitivity of the ventilator to the detection of that breath can be adjusted. Most commonly, only 2 cm to 3 cm of negative pressure should be required from the patient to trigger the machine.

As inhalation is initiated by the machine and volume delivered to the patient, the needle begins to move clockwise, indicating that pressure is rising as volume is delivered. PIP is achieved at the end of inhalation. This pressure is a function of airway resistance, air flow, and compliance of the lung. High PIPs indicate high airway resistance, stiff lungs, or high tidal volumes; therapy will be adjusted accordingly. Starting tidal volume is usually about 10 ml/kg of body weight, or roughly 700 cc. When tidal volume is normal, continued high PIPs should then be attributable to compliance or airways resistance. One way to

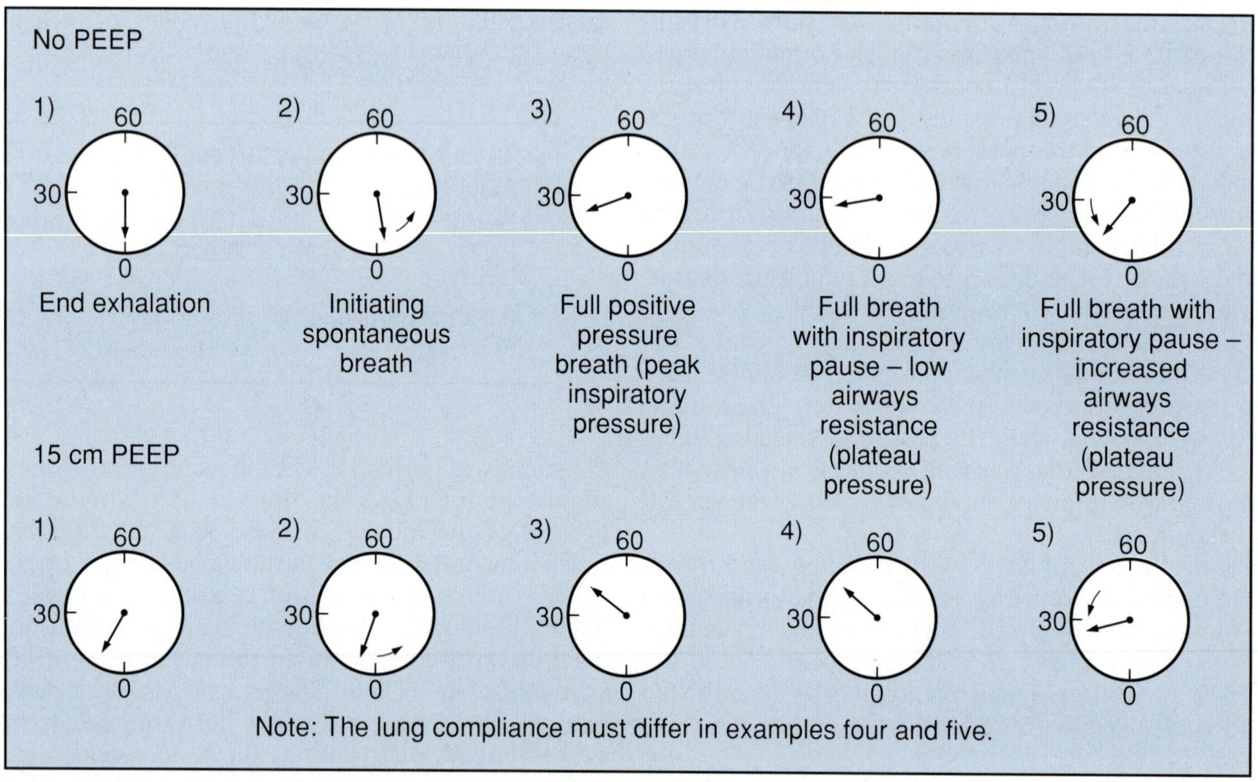

FIGURE 3.5 Ventilator analog dials display airway pressures.

differentiate the two is to estimate the static lung compliance. At the end of inspiration, an adjustment to the ventilator can be made to stop all air flow (an end-inspiratory pause). As gas flow falls to zero, the pressure change attributable to resistance must also fall to zero (AWP = AF × R). The remaining pressure will be a function of the system's compliance. Examples 3, 4 and 5 of Fig. 3.5 illustrate this phenomenon. The bottom row of examples differ from the top row only by the addition of 10 cm PEEP. Example 3 shows the dial at end exhalation. Example 4 shows the dial has not moved during an end-inspiratory pause. Example 5 indicates a fall in pressure with the end-inspiratory pause. It is from this "plateau" pressure that static compliance can be calculated. The difference between PIP and the plateau pressure is a function of the gas-flow rate and airway resistance.

Two examples should suffice. A young asthmatic develops respiratory failure and requires intubation. Peak airway pressures on a tidal volume of 700 cc are noted to be 70 cm H_2O. If an inspiratory pause is given, this analog pressure may fall to 20 cm H_2O indicating tremendous airflow resistance. Compliance would be 700 cc/20 cm H_2O or 35 cc/cm H_2O, hardly normal but certainly not life-threatening.

Another patient with ARDS may also reach PIPs of 70 cm H_2O. With an inspiratory pause of one to two seconds, the plateau pressure remains within 5 cm H_2O of the peak. This indicates the PIP is attributable to poor parenchymal compliance. The measured static compliance would be 700/70 or 10 cc/cm H_2O—a devasting value indicating severely compromised parenchyma.

Many different ventilators can be used to good effect. As support devices, each has certain assets and champions. Each can be used to adequately ventilate patients. The following discussion, however, will deal with the volume-cycled ventilator in SIMV mode.

VENTILATOR ADJUSTMENTS

Two rapid observations must be made with the initiation of positive pressure ventilation: PIP and returned volumes must be checked.

A rapid assessment of the adequacy of tidal volume and hence presumptive alveolar ventilation is usually made first. Intubation of the patient creates a closed system; that is, gas enters and leaves the patient only through the ventilator tubing. Although a small amount of air should leak around the endotracheal tube at end exhalation, virtually the entire exhaled volume passes out through the spirometer. The volume recorded on this spirometer and the volume set on the ventilator should be identical. If they are not, then either the ventilator is not working properly or a leak exists in the system. The most common leak occurs around the endotracheal tube cuff, which may require additional volume. If the ET tube is not leaking, the ventilator tubing should be checked carefully. Leakage most commonly occurs around the cascade or humidifier. This should be checked and tightened. We routinely band all joints of the tubing for the patient. Finally, a disease process like bronchopleurocutaneous fistula will open the system, allowing tidal air to escape through the chest wall or chest tube and not through the spirometer.

Once assured of adequate tidal volumes, attention should be turned to PIP. Pressures above 60 cm H_2O have several undesirable effects. They may reduce cardiac filling and drop cardiac output. Barotrauma—notably pneumothorax and mediastinal emphysema—is seen more frequently in patients with diseased lungs ventilated at high airway pressures and frequent positive-pressure breaths. Pressures should be kept below 50 cm H_2O; pressures in excess of 60 cm H_2O should be reduced.

With tidal volumes of 10 ml/kg and flow rates of 40 liters/min, high PIP is usually due to poor parenchymal compliance, high airway resistance, or the patient fighting the ventilator. The latter is generally obvious from the patient's demeanor, usually restless and coughing. This frequently sets off the peak pressure alarm set at 50 cm H_2O, and exhaled volume through the spirometer will be less than set tidal volume as inhaled air is vented at peak pressure. Sedation is usually effective; in extreme cases, paralysis may be needed.

If the patient is not fighting the ventilator, then high PIP can be attributed to noncompliant lungs or high airway resistance. Knowledge of the underlying process is important. With a diffuse infiltrate on x-ray and no wheezing audible to auscultation, compliance problems should be expected. However, resistance may still be a problem. Observation of the plateau pressure and calculation of static compliance is useful in these circumstances. If PIP does not fall with inspiratory pause, compliance is the problem. Under these circumstances, the usual maneuver is to decrease the tidal volume until PIP falls below 50 cm H_2O. This may necessitate increasing the respiratory frequency to maintain minute alveolar ventilation. Respiratory rates greater than 20 to 25/min are difficult to maintain with conventional ventilation. As mechanical tidal volumes are decreased, the Vd/Vt increases and efficiency of the lung is reduced. Again, support is the issue, and the provision of adequate alveolar ventilation is readily assessed by checking and rechecking $PaCO_2$ after any change of the ventilator. The clinician must balance adequate CO_2 elimination against the bad physiologic effects of positive pressure.

If the plateau pressure is well below the PIP, airway resistance is probably at fault. When no wheezing is heard in the chest, and the ET tube diameter is less than 7.5 mm, the tube may be at fault. With wheezing, small airway disease is likely. Inhaled beta agonists or theophylline may help to diminish the bronchospasm. Inhaled agents are quicker to act and more effective and as such should always be considered superior to theophylline in the acute setting. Paralysis of such patients may also have to be considered. Pulmonary edema as a cause of cardiac asthma will usually respond to diuretic therapy or nitroglycerin. We have a low threshold for initiation of bronchodilator therapy in ventilated patients. Positive pressure often irritates airways and produces bronchospasm. Theophylline is reported to have good effects on mucociliary clearance in the trachea and muscle function for the failing diaphragm. When serum theophylline levels are in the therapeutic range, the toxicity is low, and the therapy is potentially beneficial.

Normal ventilation may be difficult to achieve in some patients with severe bronchospasm. Some physicians drop tidal volumes low enough to keep PIP at less than 40 cm H_2O and underventilate the patient. The resultant acidosis is treated with sodium bicarbonate to maintain normal *p*H. This results in even higher $PaCO_2$, since bicarbonate degrades to CO_2 and water. In the case of the asthmatic, paralysis is preferable, although potentially dangerous.

Once assured that the tidal volumes are being returned and PIP is in a reasonable range, the patient's F_IO_2 should be set to 60% and the arterial blood gases checked within 15 to 20 minutes. This is a most important principle to keep in mind. Ventilator changes are presumptive and do not assure adequate gas exchange. Therefore within 15 minutes after each ventilator change, the patient's blood gases should be checked. This ensures that appropriate readjustments can be made to the ventilator to attain acceptable blood gas parameters. If the patient is overventilated (low $PaCO_2$), then the respiratory rate should be reduced. This is generally preferable to reducing the tidal volume.

Discrepancies between the spirometer value and that set on the ventilator must be assumed to reflect poor delivery, for the spirometer is always right. Where this discrepancy is great and the leak cannot be quickly identified, the patient should be disconnected from the ventilator and ventilated with an ambu bag until the source of problem has been identified. Then, the spirometer or the ventilator can be changed. Until satisfied that the patient is receiving appropriate tidal volumes, the physician should not leave the patient.

OXYGENATION AND POSITIVE END-EXPIRATORY PRESSURE (PEEP)

Intubation, adequate ventilation, and a higher F_IO_2 may be enough to improve oxygenation. However, patients with pulmonary edema, adult respiratory distress syndrome (ARDS), cardiac failure, or pneumonia may have shunt disease unresponsive to these measures. In such circumstances, two abnormalities are responsible. First, many alveoli are flooded with fluid, blocking gas from coming into contact with blood. Second, loss of surfactant and increasing interstitial pressures from water cause alveoli and respiratory bronchioles to collapse. Blood flow will be diminished to these areas by autoregulatory responses, but some flow will continue, and shunt inevitably results. A support technique described by Ashbaugh and colleagues (1967), however, can be used to reopen such closed areas to ventilation and maintain them in the ventilatory circuit. This is the purpose of PEEP.

Positive End-Expiratory Pressure The balloon, given its elasticity, will collapse if pressures are allowed to equalize inside and outside the balloon. The lungs reside in a noncollapsible cavity; that is, pressures inside and outside the chest are not permitted to equalize. Some amount of residual air is always maintained in the lungs at end exhalation; this is the functional residual capacity (FRC). One can keep a balloon inflated by maintaining positive pressure between each "ventilatory" cycle. By the same token, keeping pressure in the airways between breaths will maintain a higher FRC in the lung. This becomes more important as the lungs become sicker. As lungs stiffen from edema, increased pressure is exerted on the alveoli and the smaller airways and eventually causes their collapse, which, in turn, decreases the functional residual capacity and creates shunt. As long as the respiratory muscles are able, enormous pressure can be generated to keep airways open, but ultimately fatigue will occur and airway collapse becomes inevitable. The ventilator can restore balance to these pressures and reopen collapsed airways. More importantly, the airways can be kept open if positive pressure is maintained at the end of exhalation.

FRC increases, shunt decreases, and gas exchange is improved as PEEP is added to the ventilator control of patients with decreased FRC. This can be simply and reliably achieved by placing the end of the exhalation tubing under water, as in Fig. 3.4. If the end is 10 cm under water, the patient is on 10 cm of PEEP. The amount of PEEP can be adjusted by pouring more water into the graduated cylinder, which should be open to air. Or, on modern ventilators, a threshold resistor valve can be adjusted. The analog dial is observed and the dial adjusted until the desired pressure is achieved at end exhalation.

Some confusion exists between the terms C-PAP and PEEP. C-PAP is appropriate for patients who are breathing spontaneously, while PEEP applies to patients who are on an augmented or controlled mode of breathing receiving IPPV. The physiology is the same, differing only in degree. That is, IPPV in the face of end-expiratory pressure further increases positive intrathoracic pressure, exacerbating the complications mentioned before. From here on the term PEEP will be used to refer to any mode of positive end-expiratory pressure.

PEEP is used to best advantage in patients with diffuse disease. Volume always tends to distribute in areas that are most compliant. In patients with contusion, only one area of the lung may be damaged. As that portion stiffens and alveoli fill with hemorrhage, shunt disease will occur. However, the addition of PEEP may not help and can worsen the situation. The stiff areas do not expand as well as the normal compliant areas, so that the largest volume changes occur in normal lung. If these overdistend and alveolar pressure exceeds vascular pressure, capillaries will collapse and blood may be rerouted into the contusion. This increases shunt and causes deterioration of gas exchange. If both lungs are equally stiff, PEEP has a better effect.

Management of Patients With PEEP PEEP is used to good advantage for patients with diffuse parenchymal disease and shunt when an F_IO_2 of 0.6 to 1 is required to keep PaO_2 above 60 torr. Adequate oxygenation at the expense of an F_IO_2 above 0.6 is not an appropriate goal. Normally, alveoli are filled with 79% nitrogen. Since this gas is already at equilibrium with the body, it is not significantly absorbed and is responsible for maintenance of alveolar volumes. Oxygen, however, is continually taken up from the alveolus. In alveoli with low V/Q relationships, ventilation with greater than 80% oxygen can lead to atelectasis as all available oxygen is absorbed, leading to collapse. This is referred to as oxygen atelectasis and is a major reason clinicians have abandoned shunt calculations at 100% oxygen atmospheres.

Additionally, F_IO_2 above 0.6 is associated with oxygen toxicity. The oxygen-rich environment facilitates the production of oxygen radicals which damage alveolar and endothelial cells, leading to marked metabolic and structural changes in the lung. For these reasons, patients should be maintained on an F_IO_2 above 0.6 for only the shortest period of time possible. Some authorities use a F_IO_2 of 0.4 or less as the target. Damage from oxygen toxicity is a function of F_IO_2 and time. Increasing experimental evidence suggests any F_IO_2 above that of room air aggravates the situation in the presence of inflammatory disease. However, a target F_IO_2 of 0.4 to 0.6 remains the clinical standard.

Most authorities begin PEEP at levels of about 5 cm H_2O pressure. Blood gases must be checked within 15 minutes. If the PaO_2 is greater than 80 torr but the F_IO_2 is greater than 0.6, the F_IO_2 should be reduced. If the patient is still inadequately oxygenated at an F_IO_2 of 0.6, the PEEP should be increased to 10 cm H_2O and blood gases again checked. This regimen can be followed until the goal of adequate arterial oxygenation is achieved at an F_IO_2 of 0.6 or less, or the complications of PEEP are encountered. It is most convenient to increase the PEEP in increments of 5 cm H_2O until the desired change in oxygenation is achieved. The blood gases should be checked within 15 minutes each time and readjustments made. Hypotension with an increase in PEEP should prompt a volume challenge on the assumption that cardiac output has fallen from inadequate return to the heart.

Response to PEEP can be dramatic. Just as a balloon pops open at a critical pressure, so do alveoli. This critical opening pressure is not predictable, but it can be identified by patient response. In a patient not responding with an improvement in PaO_2 at 15 cm H_2O, PEEP may suddenly shoot to 170 torr at 20 cm H_2O. This is referred to as recruitment of alveoli. The alveoli require less PEEP to remain open than to pop open, that is, critical closing pressure is less than opening pressure. As a result, PEEP can be reduced slightly once marked improvement has occurred. We usually reduce the level more slowly, however, in increments of 2 cm to 2.5 cm H_2O. Once the PaO_2 is above 80 torr and F_IO_2 is less than 0.6, PEEP can often be reduced without decrement in gas exchange.

We routinely manage all patients except asthmatics on 5 cm of PEEP. No untoward hemodynamic effects are seen, and some evidence exists that fewer problems with atelectasis are encountered in the intubated patient. Keep in mind that intubation abolishes the ability to cough effectively because the patient cannot close the glottis. Lack of cough can lead to microatelectasis and major atelectasis that may be attenuated on small amounts of PEEP. When the time comes, patients are extubated without previously stopping the PEEP.

Controversy does exist about the other effects of PEEP. Some authors suggest that prophylactic PEEP prevents development of ARDS in patients at risk. Others suggest that PEEP decreases the amount of extravascular lung water by pushing it back across the vascular membrane. We are not convinced by current evidence that PEEP has any role other than a supportive one and should be employed only enough to ensure adequate gas exchange. For the majority of patients, even the 5 cm we routinely employ probably does not make a clinical difference in morbidities.

Complications of Increasing PEEP PEEP increases intrathoracic pressure and has the same hemodynamic consequences as IPPV, but is more predictable. That is, PEEP of 10 cm H_2O or above can be associated with significant falls in cardiac output. Since the prime motivation for PEEP is an ultimate improvement in oxygen delivery to the tissues, this fall in cardiac output can have devastating consequences. As practiced in most institutions, patients requiring 10 cm to 15 cm H_2O PEEP for adequate oxygenation have thermodilution pulmonary artery catheters placed to monitor hemodynamic status. Continuous monitoring of mixed venous hemoglobin saturations with a fiberoptic catheter has become routine in some institutions as an aid to adjusting the PEEP. Increases in PEEP that cause a significant fall in cardiac output will cause a fall in mixed venous saturation, which the catheter measures. Other clinicians prefer a constant monitoring of compliance changes as the PEEP is adjusted. Overexpansion of the lung diminishes compliance and is a physiological point at which cardiac output diminishes. This "optimal PEEP" is the level used to achieve the best compliance. Any of these methods can be used to adjust PEEP appropriately. Since this is only a method of support, the minimal level necessary to achieve appropriate and adequate oxygen delivery is best for the patient.

A pulmonary artery wedge pressure (PAWP) is read with the pulmonary catheter in the wedge position. It correlates well with the left ventricular end-diastolic pressure (LVEDP) under most circumstances and is used as an indicator of vascular volume. When cardiac output falls because of vascular volume loss, the PAWP should also have fallen. Patients with PAWP greater than 15 torr may be volume overloaded; those with PAWP greater than 20 torr are at risk of cardiogenic pulmonary edema. However, just as the lungs have a volume-pressure relationship, the phenomenon of compliance pertains to the left ventricle as well. A stiff ventricle will have higher LVEDP readings and therefore higher PAWP for any given left ventricular end diastolic volume than a compliant ventricle at the same volume. Additionally, if the catheter wedges in an area of the lung where alveolar pressures are high enough to collapse the capillaries, the PAWP may more closely approximate airway pressures than capillary pressures. High positive intrathoracic pressure may be transmitted to the PAWP. For all these reasons, the number obtained for PAWP should always be regarded as relative to the end-diastolic volume, not as an absolute value. Hence a PAWP of 20 torr with low cardiac output and a patient on 20 cm H_2O PEEP may prompt more volume challenge to further increase LVEDP. The key to using the catheter to assess volume status lies in the capacity of the clinician to reassess cardiac output after therapy has increased or decreased the PAWP, not in the absolute value of the vascular pressure. Cardiac outputs should be measured and remeasured as necessary. In any event, PEEP should never be stopped to measure PAWP in patients with shunt because that would rapidly decrease oxygenation by permitting closure of airways, loss of functional residual capacity, and increased shunt. Devices are available to permit suctioning of the endotracheal tube while maintaining PEEP. Patients in need of PEEP are better served by remaining on the positive pressure at all times. Hemodynamic alterations caused by the positive pressure must not be overlooked or regarded as measurement artifact.

Levels of PEEP greater than 10 cm H_2O are associated with increased inferior vena caval pressures that have the disadvantage of producing venous congestion of the organs of the abdomen. While PEEP may be necessary to maintain oxygen delivery, it can lead to dysfunction of liver, kidneys, and gastrointestinal tract.

The Nonventilator Issues

Despite all the appropriate maneuvers to reduce shunt and improve oxygenation, patients may remain hypoxic. For any fixed shunt, however, there remain some possibilities for improving oxygenation. In the example of venous admixture, a model for shunt was introduced that emphasized the effect of mixed venous oxygen saturation (SvO_2) on the arterial oxygen content and tension. The higher the oxygen content of the venous blood going into the shunt, the higher the resultant arterial content. Therefore to improve arterial oxygen content, one can effect an improvement in mixed venous oxygen content. There are five factors that affect the SvO_2:

- Arterial saturation
- Hemoglobin
- Cardiac output
- A shift of the oxyhemoglobin saturation curve
- Oxygen consumption

The principle is simple. For any given amount of oxygen delivery, a percentage of that oxygen must be consumed by metabolic processes. The oxygen returned from each organ will mix and determine the mixed venous oxygen content. For instance, in a 75-kg individual with 15 g Hgb/dl, a cardiac output of 5 liters/min will deliver 1000 cc oxygen per minute to the periphery. Such hemoglobin, fully saturated, would contain 20 cc O_2. Normal oxygen consumption is 250 cc or 25% of the delivered load. This leaves 750 cc of oxygen returned to the lungs in 50 dl of blood (15 cc O_2/dl). That blood is 75% saturated, creating a serum PvO_2 of 40 torr. (Details of these and following calculations are in the Appendix.)

If a patient's cardiac output falls to 2.5 liters/min, the corresponding fall in SvO_2 can be readily seen. Only 500 cc would be delivered to the periphery, 250 cc consumed, and only 250 cc returned, with a saturation of 50% and a PvO_2 of 27 torr. Conversely, a rise in cardiac output should improve PvO_2 if the improvement is not at the expense of an increased oxygen consumption.

If a patient experiences a fall in hemoglobin to 10 g/dl, the oxygen delivered at a cardiac output of 5 liters/min falls. Such a fall would result in a decrease of oxygen content and tension in the venous blood. At 10 g, PvO_2 might fall to 32 torr. These calculations are made on the assumption that no physiologic compensation occurs to maintain homeostasis when a perturbation occurs. Under normal circumstances, a fall in hemoglobin occasions a rise in cardiac output to compensate for the diminished red cell mass and to meet oxygen demand. These changes have opposite effects on SvO_2 and PvO_2. For whatever the reason, however, SvO_2 is maintained in the range of 33 to 40 torr. Values outside this range reflect failure of compensatory systems and must be viewed with alarm. Mortality rates of nearly 100% are associated with values below 30 torr in patients with ARDS.

Oxygen delivery may be maintained or increased, but PvO_2 will fall if oxygen consumptions markedly increase. There are not many ways the clinician can alter this process. Oxygen consumptions may double in patients with sepsis, yet respond only to therapy for the infection. Steroids may effect an increase in oxygen consumption, but this is not desirable relative to gas exchange. Hypothermia has been tried in some circumstances, but the dysfunction created by dropping body temperatures below normal and the difficulty accomplishing this anywhere other than in the operating room make it impractical. Fever raises oxygen consumption and to the extent that we reduce fever, we may help gas exchange.

Finally, a shift in the oxyhemoglobin saturation curve can also change venous oxygen tensions at any given venous saturation (see Fig. 3.1). Shifts to the left are accounted for by alkalosis, hypothermia, hypocarbia, and reductions in 2,3 DPG levels. Shift of the relationship to the right is caused by acidosis, hyperthermia, hypercarbia and increases in the 2,3 DPG levels. Thus, while alkalosis produces better saturation of hemoglobin in arterial blood, for any given PO_2, the venous corollary is that at any given saturation of venous blood, the venous and hence tissue PO_2 will be lower. Experimental evidence suggests that animals bled to shock and resuscitated with blood whose oxyhemoglobin was shifted to the right evidence lower cardiac output and cardiac work than those resuscitated with 21-day-old blood.

THE DISEASES

Flail Chest

Normal ventilatory movement expands the rib cage. A fracture of a rib in two places on the same side creates instability and paradoxical motion of that portion of the cage. Negative pressure in the pleural space during inspiration causes the affected portion to move inward. While not always apparent at initial evaluation, parenchymal injury that causes the lung to stiffen can bring out the paradoxical motion. This causes a loss of vital capacity and would characteristically be measured as restrictive disease on lung volume testing. For the injured patient, flail chest can be an important cause of hypoventilation and hypoxia when inadequate volumes of tidal air are moved. Chest pain exacerbates the problem by increasing the restrictive defect and further reducing tidal volumes.

Treatment of flail chest may not be necessary if little interference with ventilatory function is noted. Pain relief may add enough reserve to the circuit for patients to continue to ventilate on their own. Use of epidural morphine has been helpful in the management of selected patients. For the patient with respiratory insufficiency, positive-pressure ventilation is the treatment of choice. The flail usually stabilizes within five days, permitting rapid weaning from the ventilator.

Hemothorax

Hemothorax is rarely a cause of respiratory insufficiency. Blood loss into the chest would cause significant hemodynamic problems long before respiratory failure occurred from loss of lung volume. Treatment of hemothorax depends upon the rate of bleeding.

Pneumothorax

The most common cause of pneumothorax is puncture of the parenchyma by fractured ribs or penetration by knife or bullet. Most young trauma victims will tolerate a simple pneumothorax without difficulty. The collapse of the lung is associated with loss of blood flow to that side, and ventilation and blood are quickly rerouted to the good lung. Thus V/Q ratios are tolerably maintained and gas exchange abnormalities are minimal. However, at the site of the pleural injury a ball valve effect can occur. During inspiration air will be sucked into the pleural space. This air can be forced into the chest wall, resulting in subcutaneous emphysema. During exhalation, the injured lung tissue can flap shut. Continued breathing sucks more air into the pleural space creating the same hemodynamic problems seen with positive pressure ventilation. Neck veins fill as pressure in the chest rises, the trachea and PMI (point of maximal impulse of the heart) shift away from the side of injury and breath sounds may markedly diminish. The chest on the injured side can become quite resonant to percussion. Hypotension results from loss of ventricular filling. Tension pneumothorax is a life-threatening problem that should be clinically diagnosed based on circumstances and physical findings. Without benefit of x-ray, a needle should be placed into the pleural space on the suspected side. By equalizing pleural pressure with atmospheric pressure the tension becomes a simple pneumothorax. Clinical improvement is immediate and a chest tube can then be placed expediently to permit expansion of the lung.

Contusion

Contusion amounts to little more than a parenchymal bruise caused by concussion from blunt injury or bullet. The interstitial and parenchymal blood and water that result can severely affect gas exchange, however. Early PEEP, steroids, and antibiotics have all been reported to reduce the severity of injury and associated morbidity, but most studies do not support their routine use. Therapy should be considered supportive. Contusion of the lung may create significant shunt disease and consequent hypoxia. For most patients, however, supplemental oxygen suffices. In the event of respiratory insufficiency, C-PAP should be instituted. In our experience, the extent of injury in patients with sufficient shunt to require C-PAP usually requires endotracheal intubation and cannot be treated with C-PAP mask alone. Weaning occurs as indicated by improvement in the patient's ventilatory parameters.

Fat Embolus

Long-bone fracture is frequently associated with embolus of marrow fat to the lung. This usually occurs within 12 to 48 hours of injury. However, the syndrome leading to respiratory insufficiency occurs in fewer than 5% of long-bone fracture patients. Fever, petechial rash on the conjunctiva and over the shoulders, confusion, and coagulopathy occur in a substantial portion of the affected patients. The pulmonary insult manifests as diffuse interstitial edema on x-ray and arterial desaturation by blood gas analysis. Prophylaxis with steroids has been beneficial according to one report, though therapy with insulin or heparin has not been demonstrated to be effective. Supportive therapy for this form of ARDS is frequently successful. C-PAP masks used for alert patients often reduce the need for endotracheal intubation.

Smoke Inhalation

Several problems can be identified in patients exposed to fire. Carbon monoxide poisoning will occur frequently and should always be suspected in smoke-inhalation victims. Carbon monoxide competes with oxygen for binding sites on the hemoglobin and effectively shifts the oxyhemoglobin curve far to the right. Thus while oxygen is available in the atmosphere and the PO_2 in the blood is adequate, oxyhemoglobin saturation is quite poor at excellent PaO_2. This is noted in the differences between estimated saturation by PaO_2 from the standard nomograms and the saturation measured directly on a co-oximeter. Oxyhemoglobin saturations of less than 50% are associated with significant morbidity and mortality. Treatment with administration of 100% oxygen usually suffices and is the only therapy available to most victims. Hyperbaric chambers have been used with some efficacy. Steroids, barbiturates, hypothermia, and exchange transfusions are of unproven value.

Singed oral and nasal mucosa from the fire may indicate large airway disease as well. Respiratory distress can be immediate or delayed for as long as 24 to 36 hours. Injury results more commonly from toxic gases than the heat. Clinically the patients may develop tachypnea, stridor, and wheezes. Stridor is an indication for intubation to maintain a patent airway. Fiberoptic bronchoscopy and scintillation lung scanning are frequently used to assess the extent of injury. Therapy is largely supportive. Steroids are contraindicated as the frequency of secondary infection appears to rise significantly and there are no reported benefits. Antibiotics should not be employed prophylactically but rather to treat infection as it occurs.

Aspiration Pneumonitis

Aspiration of material from the oropharynx into the lung is very common. However, in patients with altered mental status or impaired mechanisms of upper airway protection, there is risk of developing secondary infection because they cannot clear this aspiration adequately. Gastric aspiration often causes acid injury initially. Steroids given prophylactically to animals result in attenuation of the subsequent injury, but this is impractical for the treatment of patients and is no longer recommended.

Infection as a result of aspiration of nonacidic oropharyngeal contents evolves slowly. Since mouth anaerobes play a large role, penicillin alone can suffice for therapy of out-of-hospital aspiration. However, in-hospital patients are frequently colonized by staphylococci, gram-negative bacteria, and anaerobes. Clindamycin and an aminoglycoside or a second-generation cephalosporin suffice for most infections as the initial regimen. Therapy should be guided by Gram stain of the sputum and culture results. Chest percussion and postural drainage do not appear to be effective alone or in combination with antibiotics for treating or draining the pneumonia. Positive pressure ventilation is indicated for respiratory failure.

Adult Respiratory Distress Syndrome (ARDS)

Adult respiratory distress syndrome goes by many names: shock lung, wet lung, Da Nang lung. It is best described as a complex collection of clinical events resulting in stiff lungs, a hypoxemic patient, and a diffusely infiltrated chest x-ray. It is seen in a variety of patients, all with an end result of lung injury from capillary leak.

The neutrophil is a key component to any theory about lung damage. Most authorities believe that an inflammatory response accounts for most of the damage to pulmonary capillaries. Lipopolysaccharide from gram-negative organisms enhances neutrophil binding to endothelium, with the subsequent release of lysozymes responsible for the production of oxygen radicals. Oxygen radicals damage cell membranes, which leads to capillary leak. However, capillary leak can occur in the absence of white cells. Complement activation is postulated to cause capillary leakage particularly in the activation of C3a and C5a anaphylatoxins, but the decrease in complement levels may be the result of injury and not its cause. Prostaglandins are frequently invoked for their role in modulating the inflammatory response and may play some therapeutic role, but probably do not represent the final common pathway.

The syndrome will be seen most commonly in the surgical patient as a consequence of undrained pus. Unexplained respiratory failure may be a primary manifestation of subphrenic abscess or infarcted bowel and suspicion must be high for these diseases in the postoperative patient. Drainage and correction of the problem is currently the only effective form of therapy. Early reports attributing the syndrome to the type of resuscitation fluid have been largely discounted, and most emphasis for treatment is placed on demonstrating and correcting the underlying cause.

Support for ARDS patients is based on the degree of dysfunction and understanding of the physiology of the leak. Starling demonstrated and refined his laws of capillary action in the 19th century, and his laws still form the cornerstone of therapy. Under normal circumstances, water is pushed across the capillary membrane by hydrostatic pressure. This most closely correlates with the pulmonary capillary wedge pressure or left-ventricular end diastolic pressure. Flow is impeded by the size of the pores in the capillary and the colloid osmotic pressure (COP) of the serum. The lung is kept dry (less than 100 cc H_2O per lung) by virtue of the relationship between such production and the ability of the lymphatics to drain the interstitium. As wedge pressure rises, flow across the capillary increases, but the total amount of water in the lung does not increase until the capacity of the lymphatics is overcome. If the patient has normal COP, the threshold for the development of cardiogenic pulmonary edema is a PAWP of about 20 to 25 torr. Lower COP results in a lower threshold for pulmonary edema, but even a COP of near zero is not associated with pulmonary edema in the absence of an elevated PAWP, so long as the capillaries are intact. Damage to capillaries has two effects: COP is no longer an effective buffer against rises in PAWP, and the larger holes in the membrane that permit protein to leak across do not impede the movement of water. Therefore, rises in PAWP at any wedge pressure are likely associated with increased amounts of pulmonary edema.

Volume loading such patients often results in worsening pulmonary edema. The dictum for treating these patients is to permit them to function at the lowest wedge pressure consistent with adequate cardiac outputs. Patients operating with good hearts at low wedge pressures are better suited to survival. A failing ventricle with need for high end diastolic volume and consequently high PAWP has high mortality as well. This does not, however, mean that aggressive diuresis benefits these patients. Reduction in PAWP at the expense of reductions of cardiac output may be associated with a higher incidence of renal failure. The coexistence of renal and respiratory failure harbors an 80% mortality.

Hypoxia is much more frequent than hypoventilation in ARDS patients. Supplemental oxygen may suffice, but frequently PEEP is necessary to treat the reduced functional residual capacity resulting from early closure of airways. Most patients will respond in the range of 10 torr to 15 torr, but more may be required. While permanent lung injury for most patients surviving the septic episode is unlikely, some develop chronic ventilator dependency. In this event, nutrition plays a key role in weaning patients from the ventilator.

Malnutrition

Muscular function in respiratory failure has become increasingly important. Loss of diaphragm mass is proportional to lost body mass, and to a greater extent, to loss of strength. With sepsis or trauma, the rate of protein loss is markedly increased and the loss of diaphragm strength, as measured by negative inspiratory force or maximal ventilatory flows, is diminished. Certainly weaning patients from ventilators demands correction of the underlying problem, but it can be enhanced with appropriate nutritional support. Refeeding patients will result in increased ventilatory drive, increased metabolic rate, and, if the respiratory quotient rises from glucose infusions, marked increases in CO_2 production. This alone can lead to ventilatory failure in the poorly compensated patient with chronic obstructive pulmonary disease. Since trauma is a disease of the young, however, this is of less concern; what is important is ensuring adequate nutrition.

Bronchopleurocutaneous Fistula

Injury, pleural space infection, and parenchymal lung infection may lead to difficulties in ventilatory support of the patient due to fistula. An open system, with communication from trachea to pleura and through the chest wall, vents a large portion of the positive-pressure tidal volume administered to patients. This may lead to hypoventilation. It cannot easily be treated by increasing the tidal volume because the associated higher airway pressures magnify volume loss through the fistula.

Support has been enhanced with the use of the JET ventilator. This is a device that defies common logic and traditional thought of tidal volume ventilator support. The JET is a simple device that utilizes a high-pressure gas source separated from the patient by a solenoid valve. This valve opens and closes 60 to 150 times per minute, staying open for about three tenths of its cycle. This permits about 100 cc of air to escape into the trachea, but not enough to fill anatomic dead space. Yet two observations are apparent: airway pressures markedly decrease and carbon dioxide excretion is enhanced. Patients in respiratory failure with a fistula can be supported for prolonged periods to permit recovery from infection and healing of lung parenchyma.

The JET ventilator is also used to support patients with severe parenchymal injury and compliance of less than 10 cc/cm H_2O. We have had several patients fail conventional positive pressure ventilation and retain carbon dioxide at airway pressures in excess of 70 cm H_2O. Instituting the use of the JET ventilator reduced airway pressures and permitted normalization of $PaCO_2$ in every patient. Oxygenation was not affected. This technique may become increasingly used when conventional ventilation fails.

WEANING FROM VENTILATORY SUPPORT

"Weaning begins after intubation." Patients require support for varying periods. Some may be extubated within several hours. Others, suffering the ravages of ARDS, may take weeks to recover. The time for weaning is determined by the reversal of factors that necessitated support. Gas exchange and breathing mechanics should improve. Many parameters may correlate with the successful attempts to discontinue therapy. A negative inspiratory force (NIF) is measured as the patient inhales against a closed valve. NIF is favored by anesthesiologists as a measure of muscle strength in the postoperative period; an NIF of at least –20 cm H_2O is considered adequate. It is not, of course, a measure of endurance or fatigue.

Weaning is unlikely with a Vd/Vt of greater than 0.6 or the appearance of abdominal paradox. The figures for shunt vary according to technique. Assessing muscle fatigue and diaphragm function is becoming more popular with the measurement of transdiaphragmatic pressures. We have found the respiratory rate to be as reliable as any other index. If patients breath without positive pressure support at rates of less than 25 to 30/min, they are likely to succeed off the ventilator. The rate is a good indicator of dysfunction, with higher rates suggesting stiff lungs or weak muscles. The forced vital capacity (FVC) is also useful. Patients are instructed to take as deep a breath as possible and exhale as much as possible. Volumes approaching 1 liter indicate enough reserve for extubation.

The patient should be able to maintain reasonable gas exchange at a rate of less than 30/min. $PaCO_2$ should be normal and PaO_2 should be above 60 torr with a F_IO_2 of less than 0.5 (a level that is easily maintained by mask). PEEP should be 5 cm H_2O or less.

The method of weaning varies by institution and physician, but the techniques all have one thing in common: patients come off support when they have improved sufficiently to sustain their own ventilation. A number of techniques exist for "loading" the respiratory muscles and improving endurance. Placing the patient on a T-piece for hourly intervals is the time-tested method. Some authorities increase the work of breathing by decreasing the sensitivity of the ventilator to the negative inspiratory force of the patient. The ventilator delivers its support only by being driven harder by the patient. The popularity of IMV has focused attention on progressively reducing the ventilator frequency until no support is given. However, in the postoperative patient, in whom ventilatory insufficiency is short-lived, decreasing the ventilator two breaths at a time, sometimes hours apart, prolongs the weaning process. Once awake with paralysis reversed, the patient should be ready to breathe. Once the patient no longer requires support, and no indication for continued endotracheal intubation exists, the trachea should be extubated.

Continued intubation may be indicated if the patient has more tracheal secretions than he may be able to handle or cannot protect his airway sufficiently to prevent major aspiration. IPPV and intubation have their price. Within 24 hours of intubation, most tracheas have been colonized with gram-negative organisms. Intubation abolishes effective cough, since the patient cannot close his glottis to build high positive airway pressures. The patient is susceptible to nosocomial pneumonias, which carry a high mortality.

OTHER SUPPORT TECHNIQUES

Respiratory Therapy

In an era of changing patterns of reimbursement, acceptance of therapeutic dogmatism has changed rapidly. Ten years ago, intermittent positive pressure breathing (IPPB) was used commonly to prevent ateclectasis, to promote the general welfare, and to provide for the common defense. It has virtually disappeared under the weight of studies failing to demonstrate efficacy. Percussion and postural drainage (PPD), except for a few disorders, is rapidly disappearing from use. Even the delivery systems for medication have changed from being therapist-intensive to encouraging inpatients to administer their own.

Among practices that will affect respiratory morbidity in the unit is control of secretions. Secretions in the large airways cause two problems: increased risk of infection when permitted to pool and worsening arterial hypoxia from V/Q disease. Ordering suctioning every 2 hours, however, is irrelevant. The patient must be suctioned as secretions build up, perhaps once a shift or every 15 minutes. Preoxygenation of the patient before suctioning and use of enhanced F_IO_2 by bag will prevent some of the fall in arterial oxygenation observed with suctioning. Venous saturations can be demonstrated to fall more than arterial saturations but the risk to this is unknown. These effects can be attenuated with the use of suction ports on the ventilator tubing that permit maintenance of PEEP during the procedure.

Ventilator tubing should be changed every 48 hours to reduce contamination. The air must be humidified and heated to avoid drying the airways and thus creating breaks in the mucosal barrier, permitting easier entry for infectious agents.

Drugs

BRONCHODILATORS

Therapy of an asthmatic or bronchospastic attack in the trauma patient should be aggressive. Beta agonists are more effective than theophylline for dilation of small airways and are the preferable agent during an attack. Patients who are not intubated may take the drug efficiently through a mistameter available from several manufacturers. Two puffs every 4 to 6 hours should be adequate. Once the technique is learned, the patient can self-administer the drug. Ventilator patients are best given the agonist through a nebulizer hooked up in-line with the ventilator tubing. The same interval can be used. With severe bronchospastic attacks, the drug can be given every hour for prolonged periods. Tachycardia and sympathetic stimulation constitute reasons to cut back on this dose.

Theophylline has several beneficial effects. Recent evidence shows that it enhances diaphragm function in patients with ventilatory failure and improves mucociliary function. Serum levels of 10 to 20 µg/ml are optimal.

Steroids are now used commonly to treat the asthmatic patient in severe exacerbation. Hydrocortisone in dosages of 100 mg every 6 hours should be a sufficient. Methylprednisolone is also used. Dosages of more than 200 mg per day are probably not needed, although we have not hesitated to administer one or two doses of one gram for effect on the recommendation of one pulmonary physician.

VASODILATORS

Use of vasodilators to treat acute or chronic right-sided heart disease caused by marked pulmonary hypertension is of questionable benefit. Most agents, like nitroprusside, interfere with hypoxic vasoconstriction and may prove disastrous by further decreasing arterial saturation. Hydralazine may decrease vascular resistance and has less effect on hypoxic vasoconstriction, as does nifedipine. However, treatment of the underlying process is more important.

INOTROPES

Treatment of right-sided heart failure with inotropes in the presence of ventilatory failure and pulmonary hypertension is not helpful. Any improvement in contractility is usually offset by the increase of pulmonary artery pressures in a system with a fixed resistance. Treatment of left-sided heart disease is accomplished with dobutamine, which has less effect on hypoxic vasoconstriction. The usual starting dosage is 5 µg/kg/min, increased in 5-µg increments until a total dose of 20 µg/kg/min is achieved. Digoxin is used primarily for treatment of arrhythmias, especially atrial fibrillation.

DIURETICS

Diuretics are most useful when cardiac dysfunction accompanies or is the cause of respiratory dysfunction. PAWP in excess of 20 torr is invariably associated with pulmonary edema and should be reduced with a loop diuretic.

COLLOIDS

There is no evidence that the type of fluid used for resuscitation of trauma victims influences the development of pulmonary dysfunction. Colloid administration has more impact on the vascular volume of the patient than on the colloid osmotic pressure, and rapid rises in PAWP associated with colloid administration can precipitate pulmonary edema. Proponents of the use of colloids often advocate diuretic therapy to keep PAWP in the range of 10 to 15 torr. Patients with good hearts operating at low PAWP have no difficulty with administered saline loads. The primary advantage to hetastarch over albumen is cost.

BIBLIOGRAPHY

Physiology

Berger AJ, Mitchell RA, Severinghaus JW: Regulation of respiration. N Engl J Med 297:92–97; 138–143; 194–201, 1977
Demling RH, Staub NC, Edmunds LH: Effect of end-expiratory pressure on accumulation of extravascular lung water. J Appl Physiol 38:907–912, 1975.
Derenne J, Macklem PT, Roussos CH: The respiratory muscles: Mechanics, control, and pathophysiology. Am Rev Respir Dis 118:119–133; 373–390, 1978.
Goldberg HS, Rabson J: Control of cardiac output by systemic vessels: Circulatory adjustments to acute and chronic respiratory failure and the effect of therapeutic interventions. Am J Cardiol 47:696–702, 1981.
Prewitt RM, Oppenheimer L, Sutherland JB, Wood LDH: Effect of positive end-expiratory pressure on left ventricular mechanics in patients with hypoxemic respiratory failure. Anesthesiology 55:409–415, 1981.
Sagawa K: The ventricular pressure-volume diagram revisited. Circ Res 43(5):677–687, 1978.
West J: Pulmonary Pathophysiology. Baltimore, Williams & Wilkins, 1978.
West J: Respiratory Physiology. Baltimore, Williams & Wilkins, 1979.

Ventilatory Support

Ashbaugh D, Bigelow D, Petty TL, Levine B: Acute respiratory distress in adults. Lancet 7511:320, 1967.
Beel J (ed): Respiratory Problems in Critical Care for Surgical Patients. New York, Macmillan, 1982.
Boyd AD: Tracheostomy and cricothroidotomy. In Worth M (ed): Principles and Practices of Trauma Care, pp 23–29. Baltimore, Williams & Wilkins, 1982.
Branson RD, Hurst JM, DeHaven CB: Mask CPAP: State of the art. Respiratory Care 30(10):846–857, 1985.
Craig KC, Pierson DJ, Carrico J: The clinical application of positive end-expiratory pressure (PEEP) in the adult respiratory distress syndrome (ARDS). Respiratory Care 30(3):184–201, 1985.
Kacmarek RM, Dimas S, Reynolds J, Shapiro B: Technical aspects of positive end-expiratory pressure (PEEP): Part I. Physics of PEEP devices. Respiratory Care 27:1478–1489, 1982.

Kacmarek RM, Dimas S, Reynolds J, Shapiro B: Technical aspects of positive end-expiratory pressure (PEEP): Part II. PEEP with posi- tive pressure ventilation. Respiratory Care 27:1490–1503, 1982.
Kacmarek RM, Dimas S, Reynolds J, Shapiro B: Technical aspects of positive end-expiratory pressure (PEEP): Part III. PEEP with spontaneous ventilation. Respiratory Care 27:1505–1518, 1982.
Lavietes MH: Ventilatory control in asthma. Clin Chest Med 5(4):607–617, 1984.
Pepe PE, Hudson LD, Carrico CJ: Early application of positive end-expiratory pressure in patients at risk for the adult respiratory distress syndrome. N Engl J Med 311:281–286, 1984.
Pierson DJ, Hudson LD: Monitoring hemodynamics in the critically ill. Med Clin North Am 67(6):1343–1360, 1983.
Suter PM, Fairley HB, Isenberg MD: Optimum end-expiratory pressure in patients with acute pulmonary failure. N Engl J Med 292:284–289, 1975.
Trunkey D: Thoracic Trauma in Current Therapy of Trauma, pp 85–91. St. Louis, CV Mosby, 1984.
VogelHart NM, Downs JB: Prolonged endotracheal intubation. Chest 76:110, 1979.

Oxygen Delivery

Bishop MJ, Kennard S, Artman LD, Cheney FW: Hydralazine does not inhibit hypoxic pulmonary vasoconstriction. Am Rev Respir Dis 128:998–1001, 1983.
Dantzker DR, Lynch JP, Weg JG: Depression of cardiac output is a mechanism of shunt reduction in the therapy of acute respiratory failure. Chest 77:636–642, 1980.
Dobson K, Greenberg ID, Nolloy W, Prewitt RM: Acute cardiopulmonary effects of dopamine and dobutamine in patients with ARDS. Am Rev Repir Dis (Suppl) 129:A96, 1984.
Kelman GR: Digital computer subroutine for conversion of oxygen tension into saturation. J Appl Physiol 21(4):1375–1376, 1966.
Lynch JP, Mhyre JG, Dantzker DR: Influence of cardiac output on intrapulmonary shunt. J Appl Physiol 46:315–321, 1979.
Murray JF, Gold P, Johnson BL: The circulatory effects of hematocrit variations in normovolemic and hypervolemic dogs. J Clin Invest 42:1150–1159, 1963.
Pinilla JC. Acute respiratory failure in severe chest trauma. J Trauma 22(3):221, 1982.
Prewitt RM, Matthay MA, Ghignone M. Hemodynamic management in the adult respiratory distress syndrome. Clin Chest Med 4:251–268, 1983.
Rice CL, Herman CM, Kiesow LA et al: Benefits from improved oxygen delivery of blood in shock therapy. J Surg Res 19:193–198, 1975.

Diseases

Askanazi J, Rosenbaum S et al: Respiratory changes induced by large glucose loads of total parenteral nutrition. JAMA 243:1444–1447, 1980.
Bassili VE, Wilson EJ, Goldberg AL: Effects of nutritional support on weaning patients off mechanical ventilation. JPEN 5:161–163, 1981.
Burgher LW: Fat embolism syndrome. Chest 79:131, 1981.
Driver AG, LeBrun M: Iatrogenic malnutrition in patients receiving ventilator support. JAMA 244:2195–2196, 1980.
Holcroft JW, Vassar MJ, Weber CJ: Prostaglandin E_1 and survival in patients with the adult respiratory distress syndrome. Ann Surg 203(4):371–378, 1986.
Kelly SM, Rosa A, Feld S et al: Inspiratory muscle strength and body composition in patients receiving total parenteral nutrition therapy. Am Rev Respir Dis 130:33–37, 1984.
Landerscaper J, Cogpill T, Lindesmith L: Long term disability after flail chest injury. J Trauma 24(5):410, 1984.
Larca L, Greenbaum DM: Effectiveness of intensive nutritional regimens in patients who fail to wean from mechanical ventilators. Crit Care Med 10:297–300, 1982.
Lucas CE et al: Pulmonary response to massive steroids in seriously injured patients. Ann Surg 194:256, 1981.
Mattar JA, Velasco IT, Esgail AS: Parenteral nutrition (PN) as a useful method for weaning patients from mechanical ventilation. JPEN 2:50, 1978.
Meyers RAM, Snyder SK et al: Value of hyperbaric oxygen in suspected carbon monoxide poisoning. JAMA 246:2478, 1981
Rochester DF: Malnutrition and the respiratory muscles. Clin Chest Med 7(1):91–100, 1986.
Schonfied SA, Ploysongsang Y, DiLisio R et al: Fat embolism prophylaxis with corticosteroids: A prospective study in high risk patients. Ann Intern Med: 99:438, 1983.
Shim C: Adrenergic agonists and bronchodilator aerosol therapy. Clin Chest Med 5(4):659–668, 1984.
Virgilio RW, Rice CL, Smith DL: Crystalloid vs colloid resuscitation. Is one better? A randomized clinical study. Surgery 85:129, 1979.

APPENDIX

Normal Determinants of Mixed Venous Oxygen Tensions

For a 75-kg patient with
5 liters/min (50 dl/min) cardiac output
250 cc O_2/min oxygen consumption
15 Hgb/dl
100% arterial saturation
Normal *p*H, PCO_2, temperature

O_2 delivery = Cardiac output × O_2 content
= 50 dl/min × 20 cc O_2/dl
= 1000 cc O_2/min

DETERMINANTS OF MIXED VENOUS OXYGEN TENSIONS

O_2 returned = O_2 delivered – oxygen consumption
= 1000 cc O_2/min – 250 cc O_2/min
= 750 cc O_2/min

Venous content = 750 cc O_2/min/50 dl/min = 15 cc O_2/dl
If content = sat. × 1.37 cc O_2/g Hgb × g Hgb/dl,
Then sat. = 15 cc O_2/15 g × 1.37 = 0.75 or 75% sat.
From the saturation curve, PO_2 at 75% sat. is 40 torr.

For Anemia

For a 75-kg patient with
5 liters/min (50 dl/min) cardiac output
250 cc O_2/min oxygen consumption
100% arterial saturation
Normal *p*H, PCO_2, temperature
But 10 g Hgb/dl

O_2 content = Hgb × sat. × 1.37 cc O_2/g Hgb
= 10 g/dl × 1 × 1.37 = 13.7 cc O_2/dl blood

O_2 delivery = cardiac output × 0_2 content
= 50 dl/min × 13.7 cc O_2/dl
= 685 cc O_2/min

DETERMINANTS OF MIXED VENOUS OXYGEN TENSIONS

O_2 returned = O_2 delivered − oxygen consumption
= 685 cc O_2/min − 250 cc O_2/min
= 435 cc O_2/min

Venous content = 435 cc O_2/min/50 dl/min = 8.7 cc O_2/dl
If content = sat. × 1.37 cc O_2/g Hgb × g Hgb/dl,
Then sat. = 8.7 cc O_2/10 g Hgb/dl × 1.37
= 0.63 or 63% saturation
From the saturation curve, PO_2 at 63% sat. is 32 torr.

For Cardiac Output

For a 75-kg patient with
50 cc O_2/min oxygen consumption
100% arterial saturation
15 g Hgb/dl
Normal *p*H, PCO_2, temperature
But 2.5 liters/min (25 dl/min) cardiac output
O_2 content = Hgb × sat. × 1.37 cc O_2/g Hgb
= 15 g/dl × 1 × 1.37 = 20 cc O_2/dl blood
O_2 delivery = Cardiac output × O_2 content
= 25 dl/min × 20 cc O_2/dl
= 500 cc O_2/min

DETERMINANTS OF MIXED VENOUS OXYGEN TENSIONS

O_2 returned = O_2 delivered – oxygen consumption
= 500 cc O_2/min – 250 cc O_2/min
= 250 cc O_2/min
Venous content = 250 cc O_2/min/25 dl/min = 10 ccO_2/dl
If content = Sat. × 1.37 cc O_2/g Hgb × g Hgb/dl,
Then sat. = 10 cc O_2/15 g Hgb/dl × 1.37 = 0.50 or 50% sat.
From the saturation curve, PO_2 at 50% sat. is 26 torr.

For Oxygen Consumption

For a 75-kg patient with
100% arterial saturation
15 g Hgb/dl
2.5 liters/min (25 dl/min) cardial output
Normal *p*H, PCO_2, temperature
But 500 cc O_2/min oxygen consumption
O_2 content = Hgb × sat. × 1.37 cc O_2/g Hgb
= 15 g/dl × 1 × 1.37 = 20 cc O_2/dl blood
O_2 delivery = cardiac output × O_2 content
= 50 dl/min × 20 cc O_2/dl
= 1000 cc O_2/min

DETERMINANTS OF MIXED VENOUS OXYGEN TENSIONS

O_2 returned = O_2 Delivered – oxygen consumption
= 1000 cc O_2/min – 500 cc O_2/min
= 500 cc O_2/min
Venous content = 500 cc O_2/min/50 dl/min = 10 cc O_2/dl
If content = sat. × 1.37 cc O_2/g Hgb × g Hgb/dl,
Then sat. = 10 cc O_2/15 Hgb/dl × 1.37 = 0.50 or 50% sat.
From the saturation curve, PO_2 at 50% sat. is 26 torr.

A Shift in the Oxyhemoglobin Curve

For a 75-kg patient with
5 liters/min (50 dl/min) cardiac output
250 cc O_2/min oxygen consumption
15 g Hgb/dl
250 cc O_2 consumption
Normal temperature, PCO_2
But a change in the P50 due to *p*H change to 7.4
O_2 Delivery = Cardiac output × O_2 content
= 50 dl/min × 20 cc O_2/dl
= 1000 cc O_2/min

DETERMINANTS OF MIXED VENOUS OXYGEN TENSIONS

O_2 returned = O_2 delivered – oxygen consumption
= 1000 cc O_2/min – 250 cc O_2/min
= 750 cc O_2/min
Venous content = 750 cc O_2/min/50 dl/min = 15 cc O_2/dl
If content = sat. × 1.37 cc O_2/g Hgb × g Hgb/dl,
Then sat. = 15 cc O_2/15 g Hgb/dl × 1.37 = 0.75 or 75% sat.
From the saturation curve, PO_2 at 75% sat. is 36 torr.

Dead Space Calculations

(Vd/Vt)
Exhaled air is collected in a Douglas bag for five minutes.

$$Vd/Vt = \frac{PaCO_2 - PeCO_2}{PaCO_2} \times 100\ PaCO_2$$

Where $PaCO_2$ = measured arterial CO_2
(assumed to be alveolar pCO_2)
$PeCO_2$ = measured exhaled CO_2
(from the Douglas bag)
Normal values = 20%
On a ventilator = 40%–60%
Difficult to wean = >60%

Shunt Calculations (Qs/Qt)

$$Qs/Qt = \frac{ccO_2 - CaO_2}{ccCO_2 - CvO_2} \times 100$$

Where Qs = blood flow through the shunt
Qt = total blood flow through the lung
CcO_2 = Calculated oxygen content at the capillary
CaO_2 = Measured arterial oxygen content
CvO_2 = Measured mixed venous oxygen content

pulmonary chest trauma

Norman E. McSwain, Jr.

The earliest written history of the management of trauma of the chest was made six thousand years ago in the Egyptian papyrus discovered by Edwin Smith.[55] In this treatise, which is only partial, there are 47 cases in which the complete treatment of the condition is described and a 48th that is an incomplete analysis of a "sprain in a spinal vertebra."

Eight cases dealt with the thorax and its structures; included were abscesses of the chest wall, dislocations of the sternocostal articulations, and fractured ribs. A spear wound of the heart "perforating the manubrium" was apparently a common injury of war. This wound "was bound with fresh meat for one day then with grease, honey and lint afterward." Vaseline gauze is used today in the same manner to stop the flow of air in a pneumothorax. In a case of abscess, "wound is inflammed . . . whirl of inflammation . . . issues from the mouth of the wound . . . lips . . . are ruddy . . . man continues to be feverish . . . granulation . . . surface is hot and secretions drop in an oily state." An accurate description of an empyema even in today's terms. The history also records a case of fractured ribs with an infection overlying the fractures, still not easily treatable today. Osteomyelitis is a chronic condition that is difficult to manage.

In biblical times there are numerous references to possible thoracic injuries. On the field of Naboth, King Joram, while fleeing from Jehu, was "shot . . . between the shoulders; and the arrow pierced his heart, and he sank down dead in his chariot." The arrow came from the bow of Jehu "drawn with his full strength."[26] Saul, after having been badly wounded by the Philistines, "took his own sword and fell upon the point of the blade and it pierced him through" to produce immediate death and prevent "capture" and "torture" by his enemies.[50] Joab "took three daggers and plunged them into the heart of Absalom."[51] King Ahab was struck with an arrow below the breastplate of his armor to produce a fatal penetrating injury.[11] "On the cross a spear was thrust into the side of Christ, both to validate his death and to assure that he would die, if not already dead."[22]

Peter Lowe wrote a good description of chest tube drainage and the problems of open pneumothorax in 1597:

> Touching those that penetrate (the chest), there is a great difference of opinion in the cure, some are of the opinion that two consolide the wound as soone as may bee to hinder the external ayre to hurt the partes vitall, others give counsell to hold them open, and in case the issue not be large enough, to dilate it, and make it larger, that if there be any bloud or other thing in the cavity . . . the judgement of the expert chirurgian is to bee required: knowing first if it doth penetrate, which shall bee done in closing his mouth and nose, and holding a candle to the wound, if the ayre cometh forth, it is sure, that it penetrates.[31]

He also identified the difficulties of a hemothorax in respiration: "Sometime the bloud cannot evacuate by the wound, it being higher than the diaphragme, which causeth difficulty of respiring." He goes on to describe the complications of, "empiema," to evacuate the "humor contayned, if the putrefaction be great."

A late sixth- or early seventh-century description of the respiratory reaction associated with a hemothorax was translated and printed in 1843 by the Sydenham Society.[2] In it Paulus Aegineta wrote that fractured ribs were easily identified: "The diagnosis is not difficult for an inequity presents itself to the fingers of the examiner and there is crepitus with the arrangement of the fractured part." The physical examination for a fractured rib is the same today and is still the most accurate method of identifying a broken rib. The diagnosis was easy but the management uncertain.

> Hypocrates has advocated that when the broken ends of the ribs are not pushed inward, it seldom happens that a fever or any unpleasant symptoms supervene. In this case a slight bandage will be sufficient, the ribs he said, "become united in twenty days." Soranus on the other hand, described, "And let anything be done as in pleurisy according to the degree of the accident. But if any great necessity compel us owing to the pleura being irritated, we must divide the skin, lay bare the broken part of the rib and then putting the instrument for protecting the membranes under to prevent the pleura from being wounded, cut off properly and remove the irritating pieces of bone. . . .
>
> "When the fractured part incline inwards, there is a violent pungent pain more severe than that in pleurisy from the pleura being wounded, as with a sharp instrument; there is difficulty of breathing, cough and often vomiting of blood. The other modes of displacement then be rectified by the finger, but in that inwards this cannot be done owing to the difficulty of applying distension. Wherefore some direct us to give much flatulent food in order that inflation and distension occasioned by it, the fracture may be propelled outward. But this is not necessary for there is no communication between the chest and the organs of attrition."[2]

Hippocrates put chest wounds in perspective in his lifetime by noting that "penetrating wounds of the bladder, brain, heart, diaphragm, small intestine, stomach or liver are fatal."[2]

John Batiste Morgagni, who was the chief professor of anatomy and president of the University at Tadua, discussed disorders of the respiration in "Letter the 15th" of the *Seats and Causes of Diseases Investigated by Anatomy*.[38] This was first published in Latin in 1761 and translated into English by Benjamin Alexander in 1769. Morgagni described the relationship between injury and respiration by saying, "yet among these few parts there is so great a connection, either by reason of their vicinity, connexions or offices that if one is injur'd or affected, the others are also injur'd or affected by consent."

It was left, however, to John Hunter, perhaps the father of modern trauma surgery, to accurately discuss penetrating trauma. In his *Treatise on the Blood, Inflammation and Gunshot Wounds*, published in 1794 after his death, he noted that wounds that were not opened widely healed better than those that were fully explored.[21] Surgeons prior to his time felt that all bullets should be removed. Hunter stated that "no wound, let it be ever so small, should be made larger, excepting when preparatory to something else, which will imply a complicated wound, and which is to be treated accordingly; it should not be opened because it is a wound, but because there is something else to be done which cannot be executed until the wound is enlarged." In his conservative approach, Hunter was perhaps the first surgeon to advise that one learn the mechanism of injury, the possible anatomy involved, and the differences between the various types of penetrations before attempting exploration.

> It has been hereto recommended in universal practice by almost every surgeon to open immediately upon it being received or as soon as possible the external orifice of all gunshot wounds made by musket balls; so much has this practice been recommended, that they have made no discrimination between one gunshot wound and another.[21]

In the latter part of the 20th century, we readily recognize that 85% of penetrating wounds to the thoracic cavity can be managed without a thoracotomy, basing our decision in part on the mechanism of injury, as Hunter admonished. At about the same time, Larrey described the need to rapidly reach severely injured patients and to begin early treatment.[28] He initiated his "flying ambulance" program in Napoleon's army, a method of getting to the patient in the field early and starting resuscitation and wound care.

Trauma is like any other disease affecting the human body. Although the initial insult is physical, the condition follows the same pathophysiological progression of any other disease process, from hemorrhage and associated hypoperfusion to anoxia, anaerobic metabolism, and cellular death. This secondary metabolic acidosis results in the patient's death. Inappropriately early or delayed management of anaerobic metabolism leads to interstitial edema, cellular failure, or leaky capillaries, to compromise of the immune system, and to other organ system failure with sepsis, acute tubular necrosis, hepatic, and pulmonary or cardiac failure. Anaerobic metabolism itself is probably the precursor of all multiple organ system failure. This has been identified as the culprit in acute tubular necrosis, adult respiratory distress syndrome, and cardiac failure in the trauma patient. There is no reason to believe that hepatic failure, failure of the immune system, or failure of the coagulation system is of other etiology. This then being true, there is a linear, even logarithmic, relationship between cellular anoxia and patient death. Based on the Fick principle of adequate on-loading of oxygen into the red cell tissue, perfusion by these oxygenated red cells, and adequate off-loading of oxygen, the thoracic cavity can be described as one of the major sources of early patient compromise.

Pulmonary ventilation must be initiated early by the emergency medicine technician (EMT) and maintained with adequate oxygen to enable the patient to survive and reach the hospital, pass rapidly through the emergency department (while resuscitation is continued and quick diagnostic steps are taken), and continue into the operating room for definitive management of the problem. All providers of emergency health care must be adequately experienced in airway management and ventilation. They must be able to respond to a patient with decreased expansion, air in the pleural cavity, or decreased ventilatory effect because of compromise of the thoracic cage if they are to keep the patient from succumbing to this "neglected disease of modern society."[42]

An understanding of the pathophysiology of trauma begins with an understanding of the mechanisms of injury, especially since 25% of traumatic deaths result from thoracic injury.

MECHANISMS OF INJURY

The Halstedian philosophy that 90% of an accurate diagnosis is in the obtaining of a correct and complete history applies to the disease of trauma. However, history of the injury of the trauma patient is an often overlooked aspect of the care. The physician in the emergency department and the EMT in the field begin to take the patient's history immediately to determine the cause of injury. An accurate history will, in most instances, identify the specific organs injured and the severity of the organ injury before the examiner's hand is ever laid on the patient.

The Physical Laws of Energy Exchange

An understanding of organ injury begins with the physical laws of energy exchange. Trauma is defined as an absorption of energy into the human body and the resultant tissue deformations produced by this energy exchange.[40]

Energy Can be Neither Created nor Destroyed Energy is never created or lost. It can, however, be changed in form. The energy of a moving bullet can be exchanged for a hole in body tissues. The energy of a moving automobile can be partially exchanged by the bending of the ribs to the point of fracture in the thoracic cage of a pedestrian.

Kinetic Energy is Equal to One Half the Mass Times the Velocity Squared ($KE = 1/2 \times V^2$) Energy contained in any moving object (knife, automobile, bullet, or fist) is determined in part by the weight of the object, but more importantly, by its velocity.

Force Is Equal to Mass Times Acceleration (Deceleration) ($F = M \times A$) A stationary object requires force to set it in motion. The amount of force necessary is determined by the weight of the object times the rate at which it is accelerated to its terminal velocity. Once the object reaches that speed, in order to slow that object an equal force is required to decelerate it back to zero (since energy can be neither created nor destroyed). The body is injured as energy is transferred from the moving missile to the body and the missile decelerates.

A Body in Motion or Body at Rest Will Remain in That State and Travel a Straight Line Until Acted Upon by an Outside Force Newton's First Law of Motion is the principle used to determine the injury inflicted upon a body by a moving object.

If each of these laws is understood and the energy of the moving object before it hits the patient approximated, the force required to slow the object and the structures and organs involved in this slowing process (transfer of energy) can be more accurately assessed. The specific diagnosis in a traumatic incident is then easy to determine.

The Traumatic Incident

Although they all involve similar energy laws, traumatic incidents can be broken down into three categories: penetrating, blunt, and blast.

Any object moving through time and space must impact the particles of the medium through which it moves. As each particle is impacted, it is pushed away from the pathway of the moving object. The energy required for this transition removes energy from that moving object based on the force formula. The mass of the particle hit and the speed that was given to the particle determine the amount of energy exchanged and the subsequent slowing of the original moving body. The denser the medium, the more particles that are likely to be impacted. In a vacuum, or near-vacuum, the moving body will hit very few particles and therefore lose very little energy. It may continue forever, like the Pioneer II in its fly-by of Uranus and out into space. As the medium becomes denser, more particles are hit by the moving body and more energy exchange occurs. For purposes of medical discussions, the density of the medium can be divided into air, liquid (soft tissue), and solid.

It is apparent that the faster the moving body is traveling, the more potential it has for giving the hit particle a higher energy level in exchange and, therefore, the greater distance these particles will travel away from the pathway of the moving body. As already noted, the denser the medium the more likely that the moving object will run into particles and the more likely that energy exchange will occur. By the same token, the greater the frontal surface area of the moving body, the more likely it is to hit particles whatever the medium. The frontal presentation of a sharp-pointed ice pick and that of the radiator of a semi-trailer tractor truck (Fig. 4.1) illustrates the difference between penetrating and blunt trauma.

PENETRATING TRAUMA

In penetrating trauma, three factors determine the area of the frontal presentation of the penetrating object.[14] A narrow, sharp-pointed moving body will obviously hit fewer particles than will a broad, flat object. Considering ballistics, it is important for a missile to penetrate air easily, to be streamlined, and not to lose energy, but this all changes as soon as the missile hits its intended target. In order to hit many particles so that energy exchange occurs rapidly, missiles fired from weapons employ profile change, tumbling, and fragmentation.

Profile Profile modification is classically illustrated by the hollow-pointed missile that mushrooms and changes from a sharp-pointed, streamlined object to a blunted one with a large frontal surface (Fig. 4.2). The increase in frontal projection increases the number of particles affected.

Tumbling A pointed-nose missile has more of its mass in back than in front and, therefore, the center of gravity is more toward the back (Fig. 4.3). The missile spins to maintain its nose-first orientation and the flow of particles tends to be around the missile and not directly onto it. However, when the point suddenly encounters a denser medium (tissue), the tail end of the missile is still in a less dense medium (air), causing the nose to slow while the end portion continues to move with little energy loss. The center of gravity continues forward and, if it is in any way off-center, it pulls the base of the missile into the lead position. As this rotation, or tumble, occurs, the missile will be turned at right angles to its forward pathway (Fig. 4.4), creating a large frontal area capable of impacting many particles.

Fragmentation If the missile breaks up into many pieces, each piece becomes an individual missile, thus enlarging the frontal projection and increasing the number of moving particles (Fig. 4.5). The ultimate in fragmentation is the shotgun

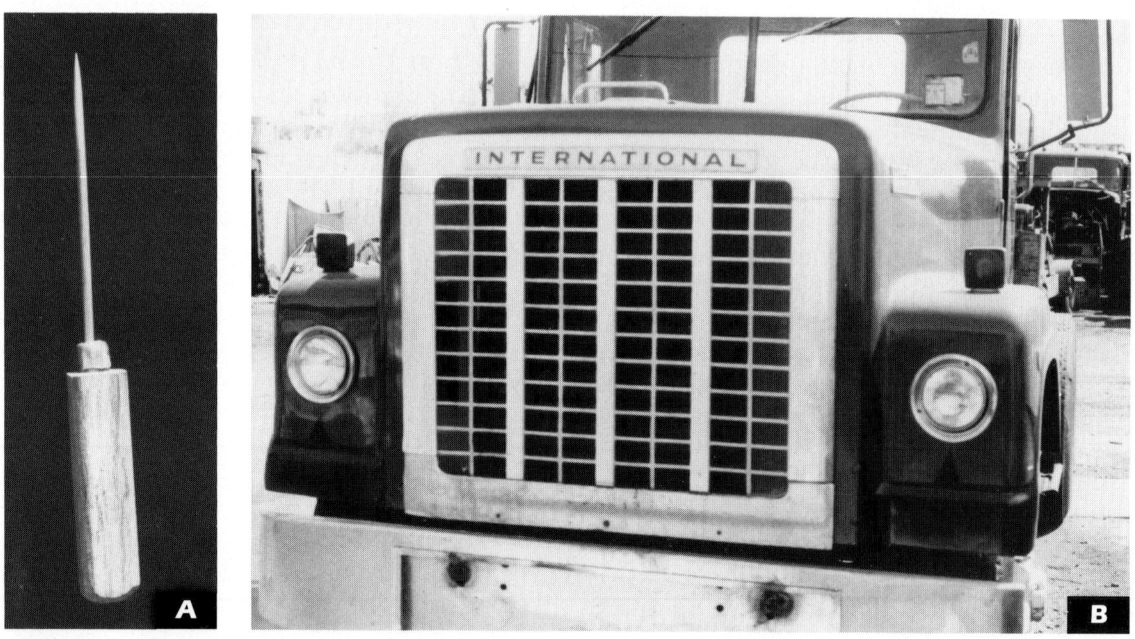

FIGURE 4.1 The energy forces of penetrating trauma produce similar energy waves. In penetrating trauma, such as that caused by an ice pick **A**, the energy wave is laterally away from the penetrating object, while in blunt trauma, such as that caused by a truck **B**, the force is in the same direction as the impact.

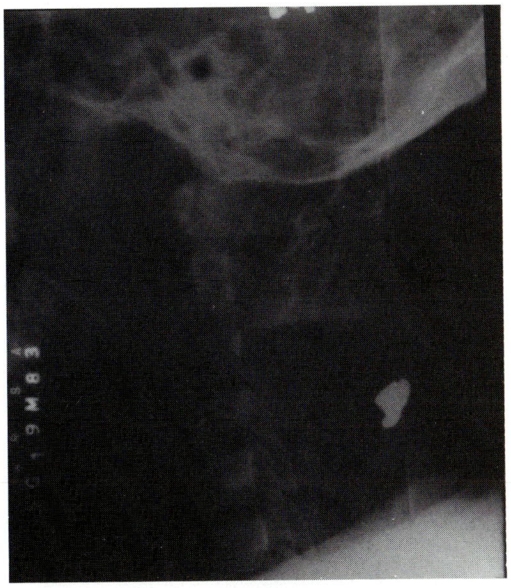

FIGURE 4.2 Changes in the profile or trauma projection increase the particles hit and therefore the amount of energy dispersal.

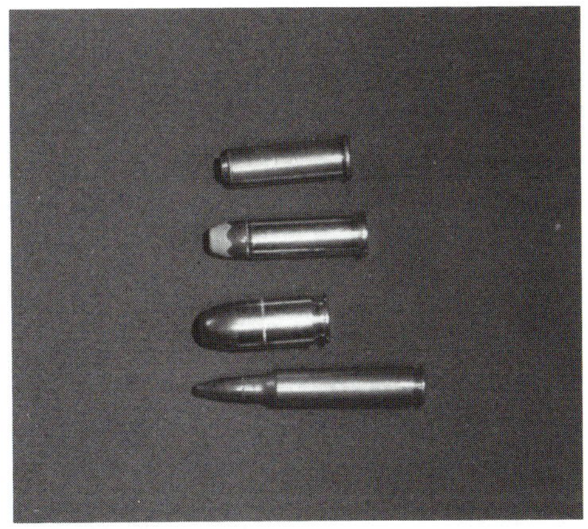

FIGURE 4.3 The center of gravity of a projectile is more toward its aft end, since the fore end is much smaller. This center of gravity tends toward the lead point as the front of the missile stops, producing tumble.

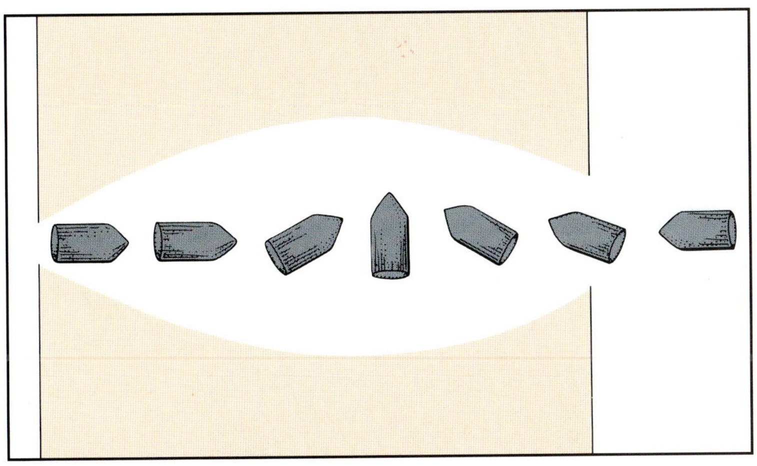

FIGURE 4.4 As the missile tumbles when it reaches a 90° point, its frontal area impacts more tissue particles than when its lead point is small and narrow. This produces a larger temporary cavity.

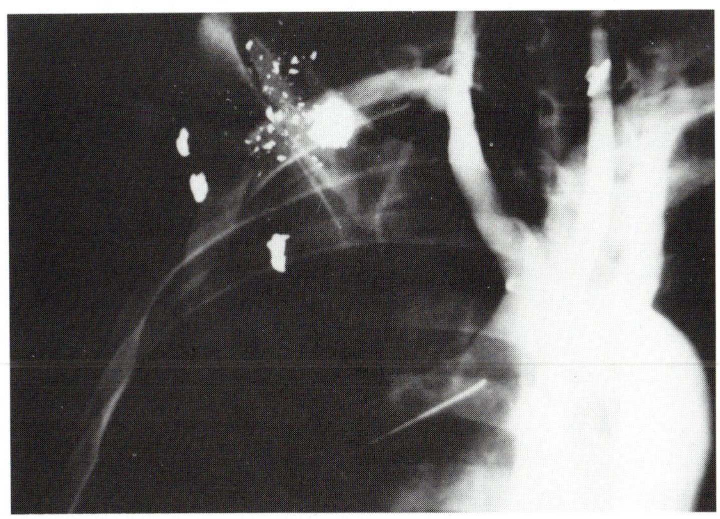

FIGURE 4.5 When the missile breaks up into smaller particles, this fragmentation increases its frontal area and increases the energy distribution.

missile (Fig. 4.6). The deficit in the shotgun, however, is that fragmentation occurs as the missile leaves the muzzle of the weapon, and although it carries with it great wounding potential, because of its energy early on, each of the shots hits air particles and slows down rapidly. A shotgun blast, for example, is extremely devastating within 3 yards, but after 7 yards, so much energy has been spent on air particles that the individual shots seldom penetrate deeper than into the subcutaneous tissue or muscle.

Cavitation On the break in a game of pool, the cue ball is the moving body and the other 15 balls are stationary (Fig. 4.7). The cue ball hits the ball at the apex of the triangle, and that

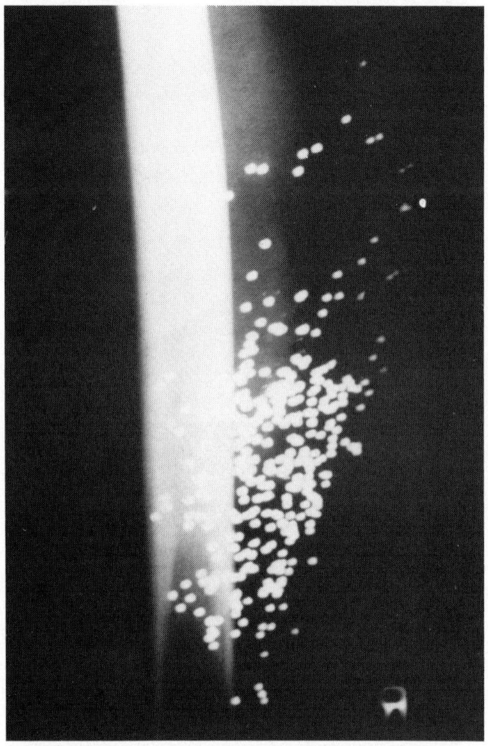

FIGURE 4.6 The ultimate in fragmentation are the missiles from a shotgun.

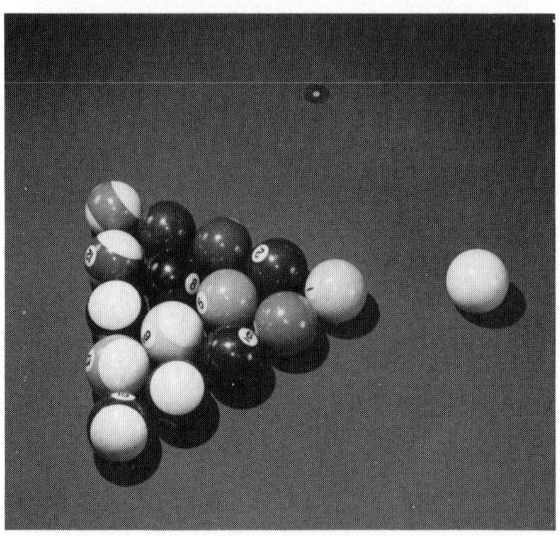

FIGURE 4.7 The cue ball is like a penetrating missile. The tissue particles (the racked balls) have no energy and are stationary.

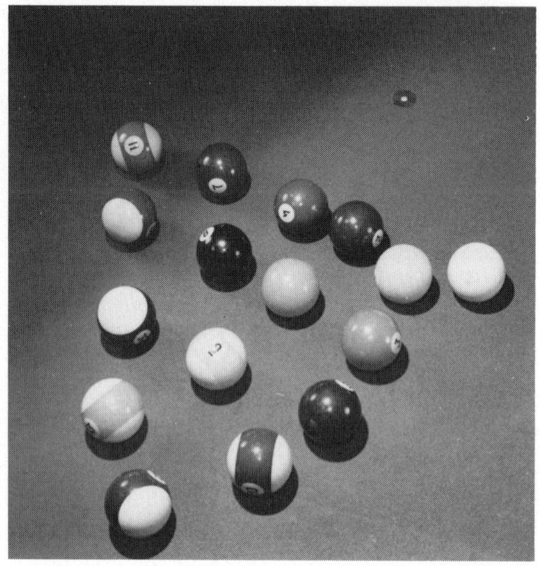

FIGURE 4.8 As the cue ball impacts the object ball, energy is exchanged from the cue ball to the object ball to the balls behind it. In progression, all balls receive some of the energy (motion) of the cue ball.

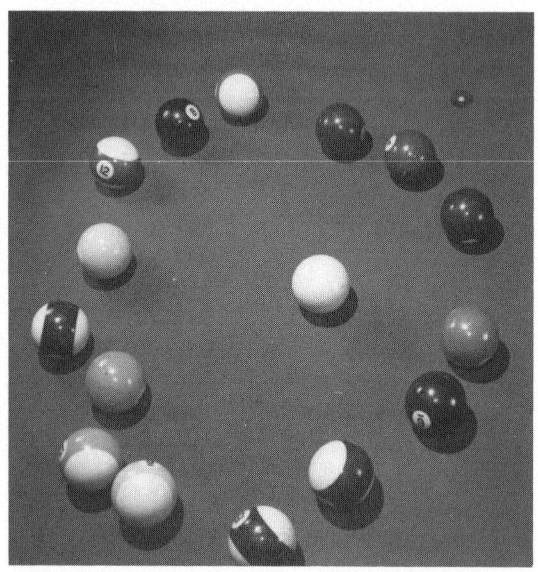

FIGURE 4.9 Since the pool balls now have energy, they move away from the point of impact. The size of the cavity depends on the amount of energy exchanged from the cue ball to the racked balls.

ball in turn hits the two balls behind it, which hit the three behind it (Fig. 4.8). This progressional distribution of energy from the cue ball knocks all of the balls from their racked position, creating an empty space (Fig. 4.9). So it is when a moving object penetrates the body tissues. They are knocked away from the pathway of the missile, creating a *temporary cavity* (Fig. 4.10). The size of the cavity depends upon the amount of energy distributed from the moving body to the tissue particles. These tissue particles compress the adjacent tissue and stretch surrounding tissue out of its normal position.[10] As the missile continues, an area of decreased pressure is created in the original cavity and the stretched tissue surrounding the cavity rebounds the particles back toward their original position. This is not unlike the pool balls hitting the rubber bumper on the sides or ends of the pool table and being returned toward the center (Fig. 4.11). The *permanent cavity* in the tissue is much smaller

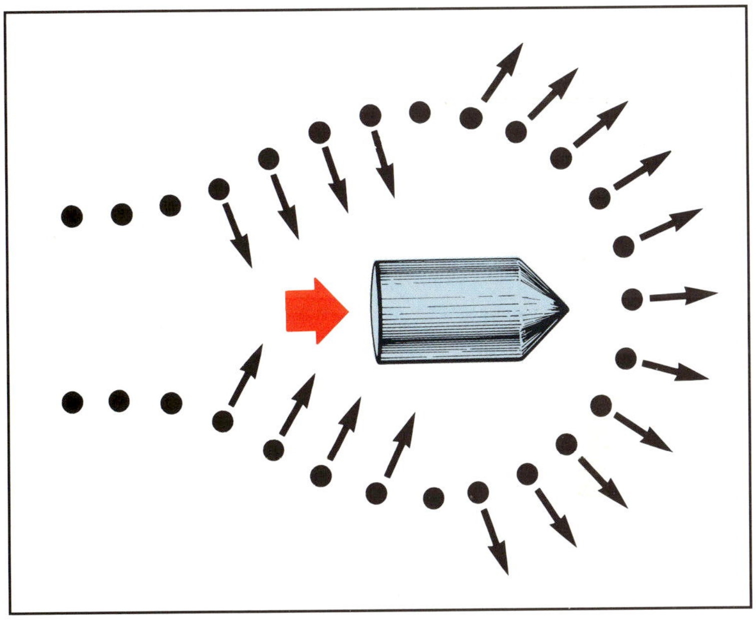

FIGURE 4.10 The pool balls move away from the point of impact, creating a temporary cavity, just as the tissue particles move away from a penetrating missile traversing the body.

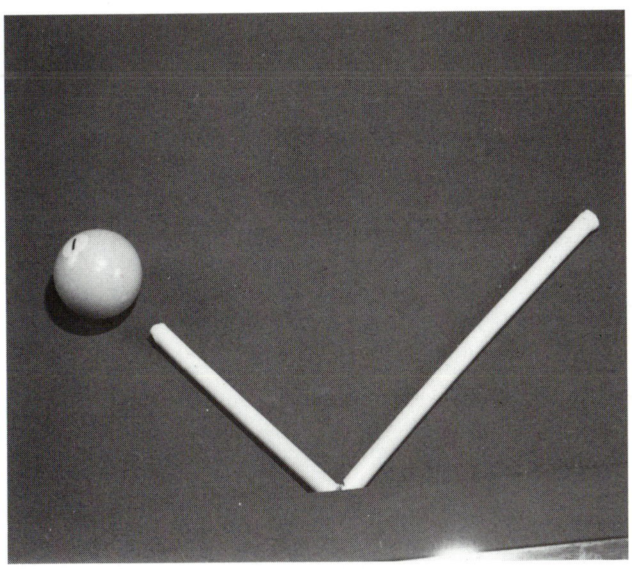

FIGURE 4.11 In the body the elastic fibers in the tissue stretch and then force tissue particles back toward their original positions. The rubber bumpers on the pool table are similar. The amount of elastic tissue present determines the size of the permanent cavity. The size of the temporary cavity is determined by the amount of energy imparted from the penetrating object to the tissue.

than the temporary cavity at its apogee. In the evaluation of any energy, penetrating or blunt, it is important to consider where the body tissues were when furthest from the pathway of trauma, in order to identify organs which may have been injured, but are not in direct contact with the missile pathway.

The amount of injury distributed to organ tissue by a moving body is determined by two factors. One is the energy of the missile at the moment of penetration and the other is the density of particles in the organ struck. The energy of penetration can vary from that of an extremely low-energy missile, such as a small needle used for thoracentesis, to that of a large high-energy missile used in elephant hunting. For practical purposes in the management of trauma, the range can be divided into three general categories: *low-energy*, penetrating objects of a hand-driven device such as a thoracentesis needle, a knife, or an ice pick, wherein the amount of damage is directly proportional to the individual organs struck and the size and direction of the sharp object; *medium-energy* missiles, which are fired from handguns and most rifles, producing a permanent cavity two to three times the diameter of the missile with only a minimal temporary cavitation; and *high-energy* missiles, such as many hunting rifles and most military rifles, which produce not only a permanent cavity, but a temporary cavity that may be 30 times the diameter of the missile itself (Fig. 4.12).

This range is a continuum, however. A .22 shot may create little or no cavitation, while a .44-magnum semi-jacket, hollow-point bullet will create a large one and a .223 M16 rifle a larger one still. The density of the tissue struck determines the number of particles hit which in turn determines the amount of energy transferred. The less energy transferred, the smaller the temporary cavity and the less tissue damage or destruction. The individual tissue particles can become missiles themselves, especially in extremely dense tissue, such as bone. Bone fragments continue to spread the amount of energy in other directions, damaging other particles (Fig. 4.13).

Much of the thoracic cavity is filled with air-containing tissue of relatively low density. There will be much less energy absorbed from a penetrating object if it passes through the lung than if it penetrates a denser organ, such as the liver. For this reason, when a bullet penetrates the thoracic cavity, unlike in the abdominal cavity where exploration is almost mandatory, approximately 85% of cases can be managed by observation and a chest tube.

Shotgun wounds are treated as any other wound as long as it is recognized that close-range injuries distribute a lot of energy into the victim. This is because the shot wadding—also a missile at close range—discharges a blast of expanding gases, which can do tremendous soft tissue damage, particularly to the outer thoracic

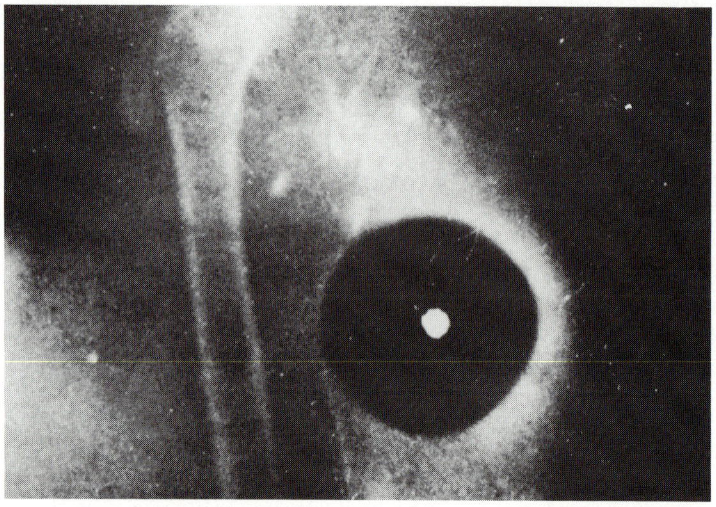

FIGURE 4.12 The more energy that the penetrating object has, the greater the exchange and therefore the greater the size of the temporary cavity.

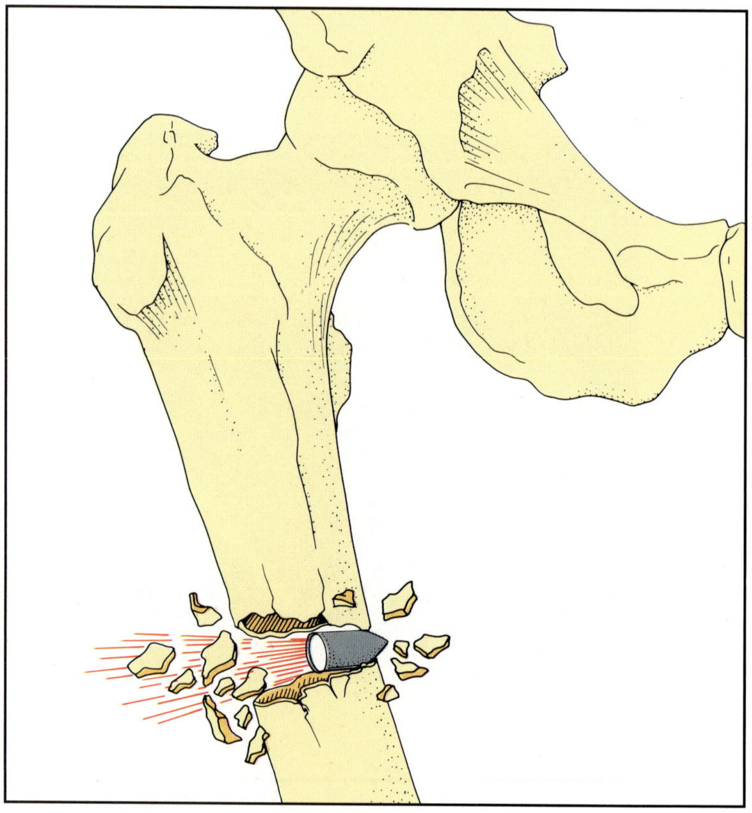

FIGURE 4.13 Bone fragments become secondary missiles themselves, producing damage by the same mechanism as the original penetrating object.

wall. In longer-range shotgun injuries, the chest film will show multiple pellets, frequently just through the skin and into the subcutaneous tissue (Fig. 4.14). (It takes approximately 137 foot-pounds of energy to penetrate the skin.) The diagnostic question arises, however, as to when one of the pellets has penetrated deep enough to produce injury of clinical significance.

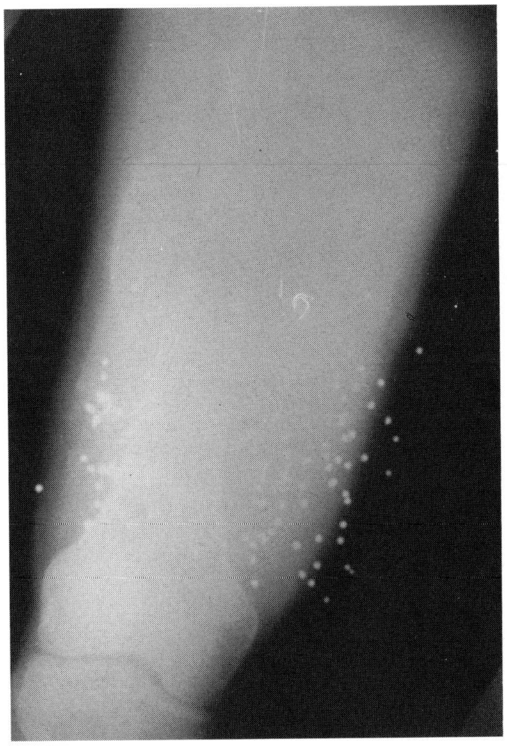

FIGURE 4.14 The greater the distance from the shotgun, the less energy the missiles have to travel through the body. A significant amount of energy is absorbed by the skin, so the depth of penetration may be extremely shallow.

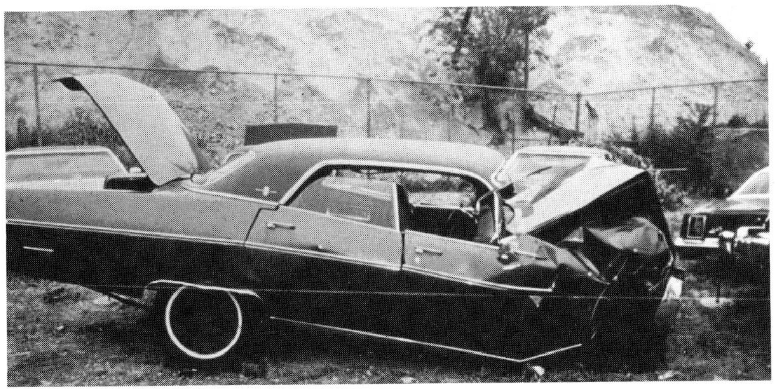

FIGURE 4.15 Very little elastic tissue exists in an automobile body; therefore, the deformation of an impact is the same as that seen later. This is in contrast to the human body, which, because of its elastic tissue, conceals the extent of deformation. It must be estimated based on the mechanism of injury.

BLUNT TRAUMA

The physical principles of blunt trauma differ from those of penetrating trauma in two respects. First, the object that strikes the body is much larger and is not able to penetrate; all the energy is dissipated without an obvious point of internal damage. Diagnosis is thus much more difficult unless the examining physician understands the forces involved. Second, with the exception of pedestrian accidents, the body is the missile that strikes a stationary object. For example, in a head-on collision the car and occupant are traveling through time and space together when the car hits another car or something that suddenly stops the car's motion. The occupant if unrestrained continues forward until striking some part of the car. If this should be the steering wheel, the forward motion of the anterior chest is stopped, but the organs inside the thoracic cavity as well as the thoracic spine continue forward. The broken ribs, contused heart, and pneumothorax that are produced are a result of the occupant being in motion, rather than the object struck.

Greater than 90% of the automobile accidents that produce thoracic trauma involve either head-on or side-impact collisions. The history of blunt trauma as obtained by the physician, either from the patient, a bystander, or perhaps more importantly, the EMTs, is a description of the accident itself. What was the type of impact (frontal or lateral)? How fast were the cars going? What was the amount of damage to each car (inches of deformation, if possible)? What parts of the car were damaged? This last item is particularly important, for if the physician knows the part of the car that is damaged, he can usually surmise the part of the occupant that is also damaged. Finally, was the occupant restrained? If there was another occupant involved who was killed immediately, the physician knows that the energy exchange involved was great.

Frontal Impact Collisions Newton's first law of motion identifies that a body at rest or a body in motion will remain in that state until acted upon by some outside force. All parts of the car, following the tenets described by Newton, continue in motion until this energy can be absorbed. Since energy can be neither created nor destroyed, it is dissipated by changing form from motion itself to bent parts of the car. The front of a car stops against an object, but the back part continues forward. It only ceases its forward motion when the frame is bent to absorb this energy.

It is the same with the occupant in the car. When the car ceases its forward motion, the occupant continues at the same speed as at the time of impact. This forward motion of the occupant is absorbed by the dashboard or steering column, which the occupant hits unless restrained by a life-belt (seat and diagonal strap). Approximately 40% of the population used life-belts in 1990. Life-belt laws will most probably improve these statistics, as they have when enacted in many states and in other countries. The United States is one of the few major countries left that has not taken this step as a nation, although all states have some form of legislation for infants. At the end of 1990 only 25 states had passed life-belt legislation.

When the front of an automobile impacts an immovable object, the auto parts are pushed in but in general do not rebound (Fig. 4.15). It is easy to look at the car and see what damage it sustained. Steel, aluminum, and other metals in general do not have the elastic characteristics of the human body, which has enough resiliency and memory in its tissues to return nearly or exactly to the same configuration as before the impact. This temporary cavitation is similar to what occurs with penetrating trauma. As the sternum or chest wall stops its forward motion, the organs in the posterior thoracic wall continue forward; one can envision the bending of the thoracic cage. If the tensile strength of the ribs is exceeded, the ribs will break (Fig. 4.16). The organs (heart and lung) get trapped between the stationary sternum and the moving thoracic cage and are compressed. Cellular structures are ruptured, vessels are broken, and interstitial hemorrhage occurs. The resulting compression injuries that one can expect are cardiac contusion or chamber rupture, pulmonary contusion or lung rupture (leading to pneumothorax), and a flail chest. If the tensile strength is exceeded in two or more ribs and they are broken in two or more places, a loose segment of chest wall is created (a flail chest). When the lungs are compressed between the anterior and posterior thoracic wall, the lung parenchyma is bruised. In many instances the occupant, seeing the accident impending, takes a deep breath and closes the glottis. This is similar to blowing up a paper bag, holding the end closed with one hand, and hitting the bag with the other—the paper bag pops (Fig. 4.17). So it is with the lungs: compression of a distended lung against a closed glottis can rupture the alveoli and result in a pneumothorax. This is probably more common than a rib actually penetrating the pleura and lacerating the lung itself. Continued leakage of air from the damaged lung can convert a simple pneumothorax into a tension pneumothorax.

Compression of the myocardium produces much the same tissue damage as compression of the lung. The myocardial muscle itself can be bruised and contused, or the myocardium can actually be ruptured. The anterior wall of the right ventricle is just beneath the sternum, the posterior wall of the left ventricle overlays the vertebra, and the septum is between. Any of these structures are vulnerable to compression.

Some of the contents of the thoracic cavity, most notably the aorta, may be between two compressive forces not directly in line and can sustain distraction damage. The heart and arch of the aorta are fairly mobile, in contrast to the descending aorta, which is tightly attached to the vertebral column by strong fasciae. If the heart and arch of the aorta continue in their forward motion, there will be shear forces created at the junction of the stable and unstable portions and distraction of the arch from the descending thoracic aorta, at about the point of the ligamentum arteriosum (Fig. 4.18). This deceleration injury is fairly characteristic and in 80% of patients leads to exsanguination within the first hour. However, 20% of the patients will survive from several hours to several days. Unless the managing physician has taken a close history of the incident, understands the mechanisms of injuries, and has a high index of suspicion, such injuries may not be identified. The subtlety of the associated physical findings is such that they must be suspected to be found.

Lateral Impact Collisions As one car proceeds through an intersection and is struck in the side by another, its direction changes from forward to sideways. Unfortunately, no change in direction of the unrestrained occupant occurs until the occupant is hit from the side. The door of the car is pushed in (Fig. 4.19), and so is the vulnerable, lateral part of the occupant. As in a head-on collision, the resilience and memory of the chest wall frequently does not retain this deformation, but returns to its precrash position.

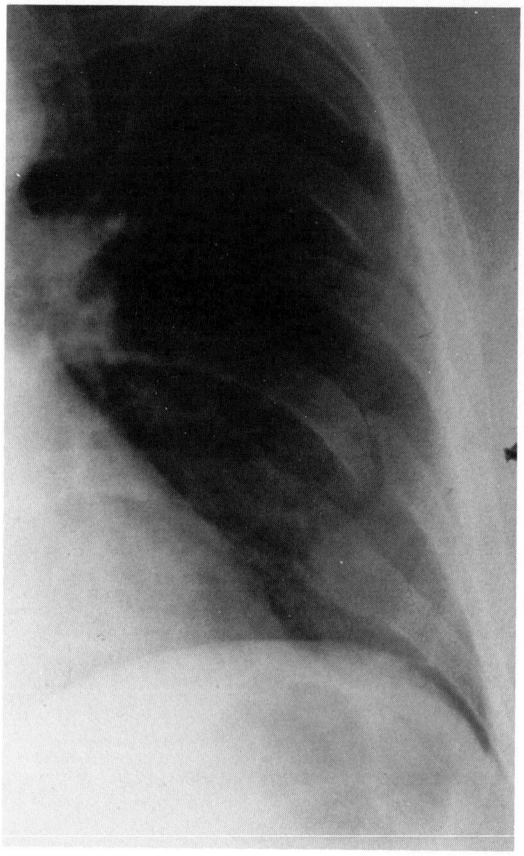

FIGURE 4.16 When the tensile strength of ribs is exceeded, they will suddenly give way, no longer protecting the soft intrathoracic organs from impact.

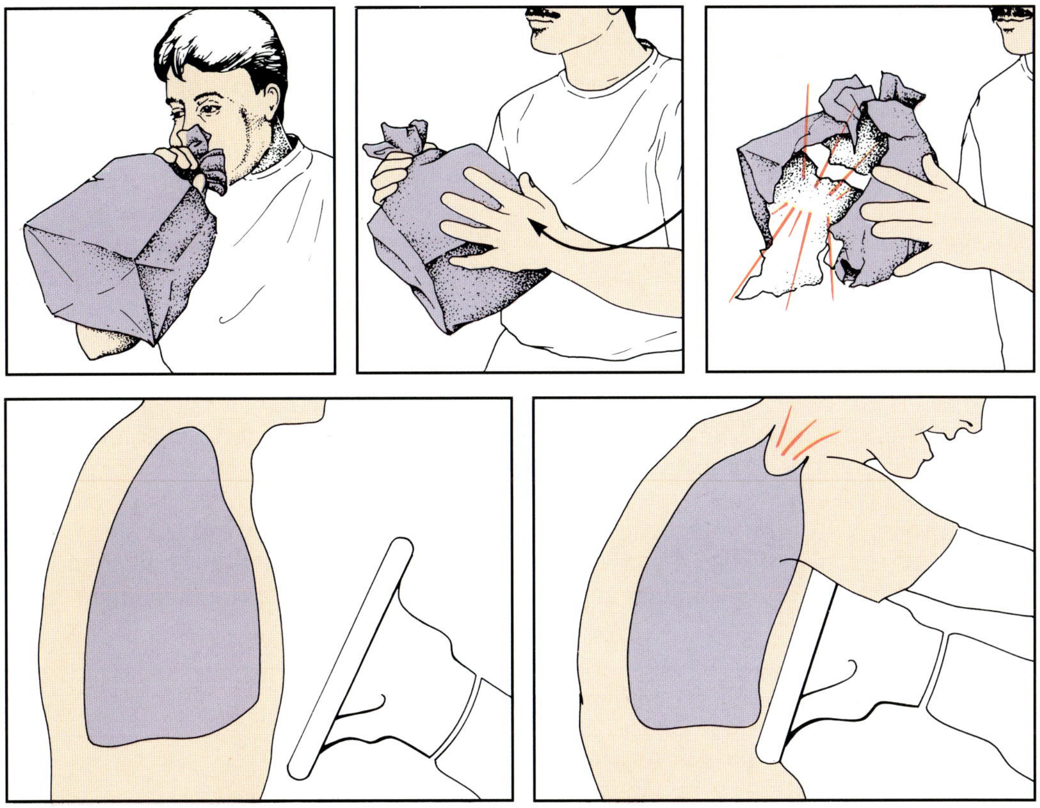

FIGURE 4.17 The lungs in an accident are similar to a paper bag held tightly at the neck and compressed with the other hand. Thoracic compression against the closed glottis causes the lungs to pop—just like the paper bag.

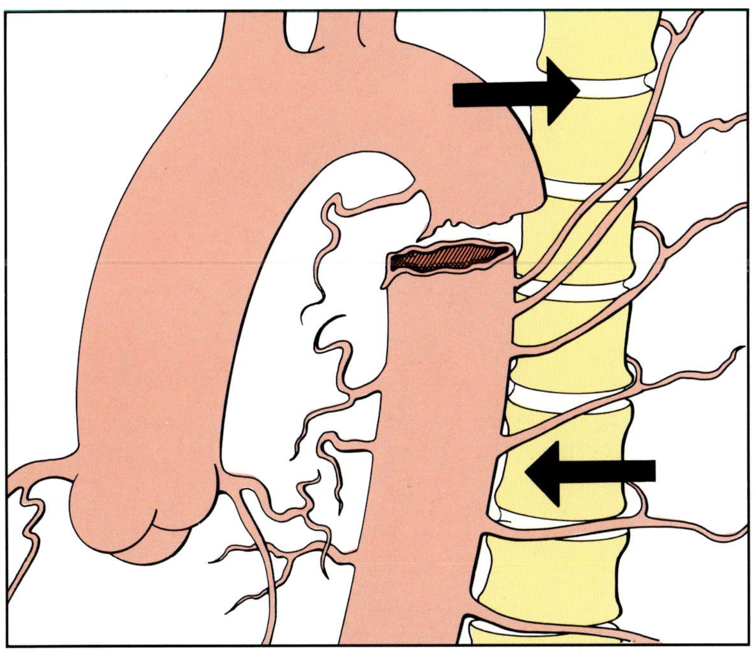

FIGURE 4.18 The descending aorta is tightly attached to the vertebral column, while the arch and heart are unattached. Sudden deceleration of the thoracic wall in a frontal impact or acceleration in a lateral impact makes the arch and heart a pendulum, with shear forces at the junction of the arch and the descending aorta.

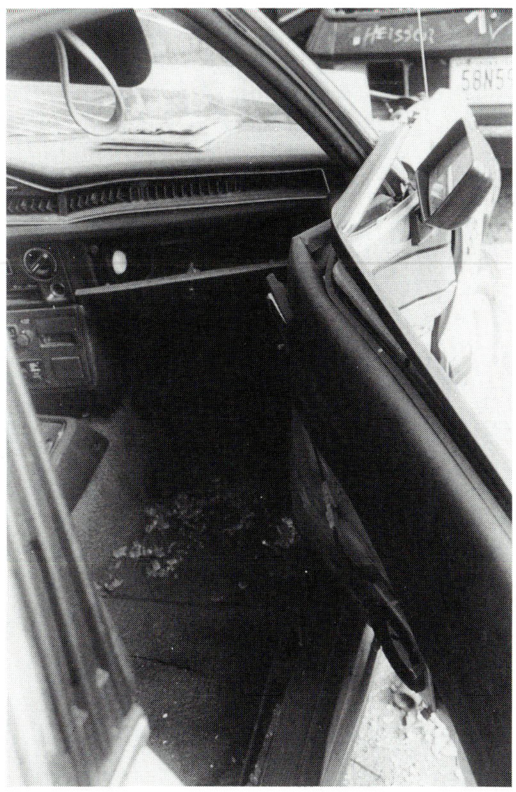

FIGURE 4.19 A lateral automobile impact pushes the door into the passenger compartment. The same mechanism pushes the chest wall into the thoracic and abdominal compartments.

There are three major points of impact in a lateral collision: the femur at the greater trochanter, the lateral chest wall, and the shoulder. Injuries are to the neck (lateral impact collisions produce more spinal fractures than do rear impact collisions), the thoracic and abdominal cavities as ribs are pushed in (Fig. 4.20), and the pelvis as the head of the femur is driven through the acetabulum.

The thoracic injuries that result from this compression are a flail chest from the multiply fractured ribs and a pulmonary contusion. The deceleration injuries to the aorta described for frontal impact collisions can also occur, although they occur as results of acceleration.

Complications can arise from associated injuries of retroperitoneal hemorrhage from a fractured pelvis, splenic injuries (when the occupant is on the driver's side), hepatic injuries (when the occupant is on the passenger's side), and cervical spine fractures. The trauma surgeon cannot be a thoracic surgeon alone, but must be able to appropriately identify and manage injuries in the abdomen as well as chest.

Abdominal compression can produce injuries to the thoracic cavity itself. Compression of the lungs against the closed glottis produces rupture of the lungs. Similarly, compression of the abdominal cavity (by definition a closed sac) can cause rupture of a weak portion of the abdominal wall. The abdominal cavity is strengthened anteriorly by the rectus abdominis and its supporting fascia, laterally by three muscles and their supporting fasciae, posteriorly by the paraspinal muscles, and inferiorly by the muscles of the perineum. Superiorly, however, there is only the 5-mm-thick muscle of the diaphragm, which has minimal associated fascia. It is extremely weak and vulnerable to increased intra-abdominal pressure.

When the abdomen is the major focus of pressure from a lateral impact, the diaphragm can rupture and force abdominal contents into the chest (Fig. 4.21). On the left, bowel sounds upon auscultation of the chest, or air- and fluid-filled loops of bowel on the chest film make this a relatively easy diagnosis to make (Fig. 4.22). On the right, the water density of the liver and the diaphragm are so similar that a rupture of the diaphragm when

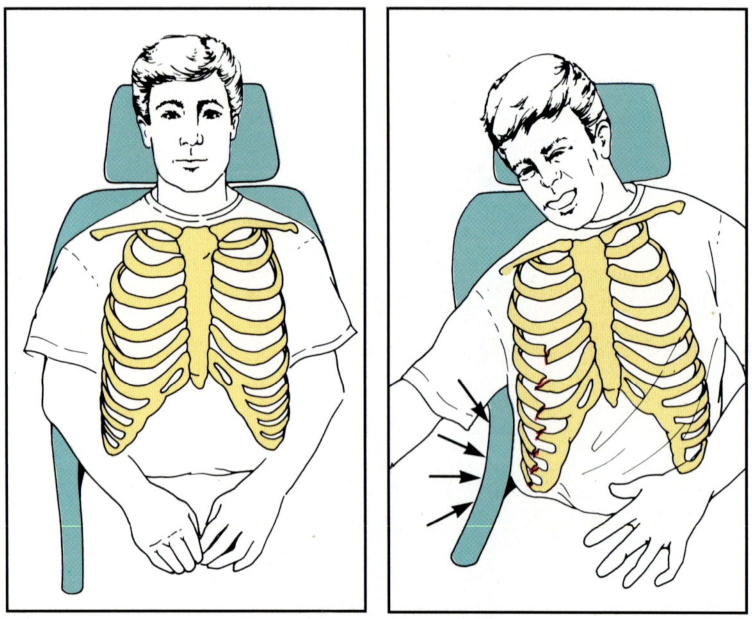

FIGURE 4.20 Compression of the lateral aspect of the thoracic cage fractures the ribs, contuses the lung, and injures the liver (driver) or spleen (other front seat occupant).

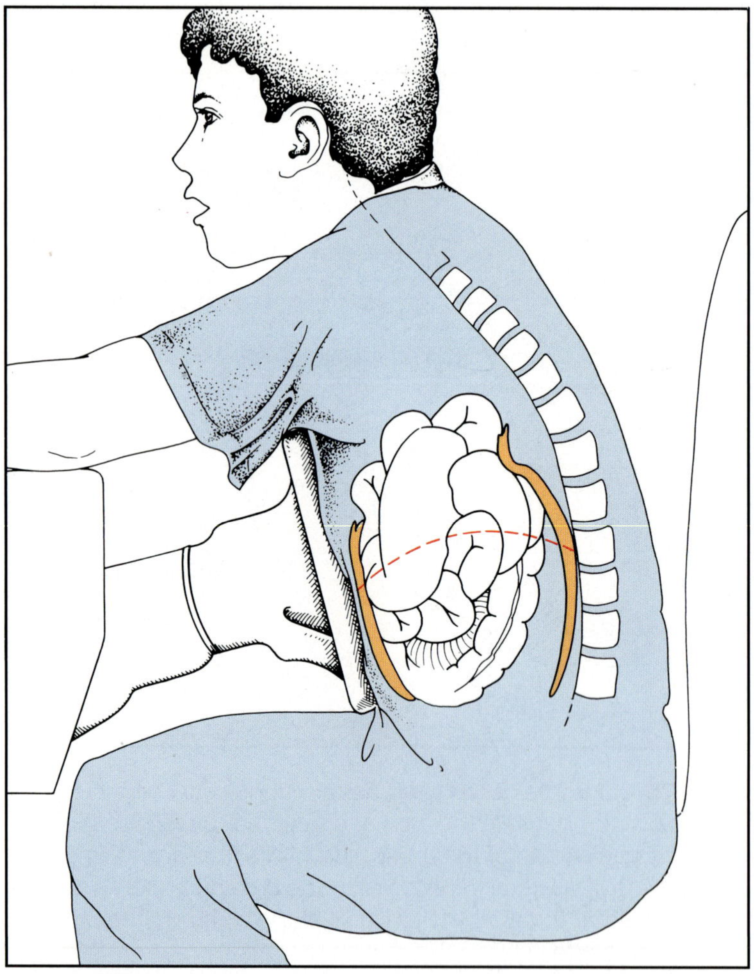

FIGURE 4.21 Just as lungs rupture at their weakest point with thoracic compression, the abdomen will rupture at its weakest point with abdominal compression. The weakest wall is the superior one, the diaphragm.

the liver is protruding into the chest cavity is very difficult to discern (Fig. 4.23). If the examining physician does not understand the kinematics that have been discussed, an injury may be overlooked and produce complications several years later.

Increased intra-abdominal pressure may also force blood back up the aorta to rupture the aortic valve, mitral valve, sinus of Valsalva, or ventricle. Antegrade blood flowing up the vena cava may be of sufficient force to rupture the right side of the heart.

Pedestrian Collisions Unlike the occupant in the automobile, the pedestrian is relatively stationary when struck by a vehicle. The injury patterns of acceleration and compression produce the same outcome as deceleration does, except the direction of impact is changed. There are three separate impacts that occur in pedestrian trauma: first, the vehicle hits the victim on the lower half of the body with the pelvis and legs receiving the most force; second, the body rotates into the hood or fender, the thoracic cage receiving the major thrust of the force; and finally, the victim strikes the pavement with the head receiving intracranial and cervical spine trauma.

There are two differences in adult and pediatric pedestrian injuries. First, the height of the child is lower, making the impact relatively higher on the body. Second, a child will usually turn toward the vehicle out of curiosity; the adult will turn away and try to escape. The result is that pediatric injuries tend to be anterior while adult injuries are lateral or posterior.

BLAST TRAUMA

A *blast* is a rapid burning (3000 ft/sec) of a substance that burns in 0.00001 seconds. The pressures created by such rapid burning can vary tremendously from a firecracker to a hydrogen bomb, but most "civilian" explosions, which would be found in terrorist-type situations, create pressures in the range of 1.4×10^6 pounds per square inch.

There are three components to such a blast that must be considered by the physicians and other health care personnel managing the patient.

First phase (primary) The shock wave itself is formed by the rapid expansion of gases and movement away from the point of the explosion. The recipient of this shock wave is knocked from his feet, possibly hitting some other object such as the ground, and may be forced into unusual positions that may produce lacerations, avulsions, fractures, or severing of body parts.

Softer, more compressible body parts such as the eye may be ruptured. Organs that have an air/tissue/air interface, such as the tympanic membrane, are subject to implosion in any overpressure event. The lungs are especially vulnerable to this overpressure condition as the blast forces air at sudden high pressures against the chest wall. This pressure transmitted through thoracic cage compression to the parenchma and eventually to the bronchi and alveoli. Rupture of the alveolus, pneumothorax, and air embolus can be expected as pulmonary contusion occurs

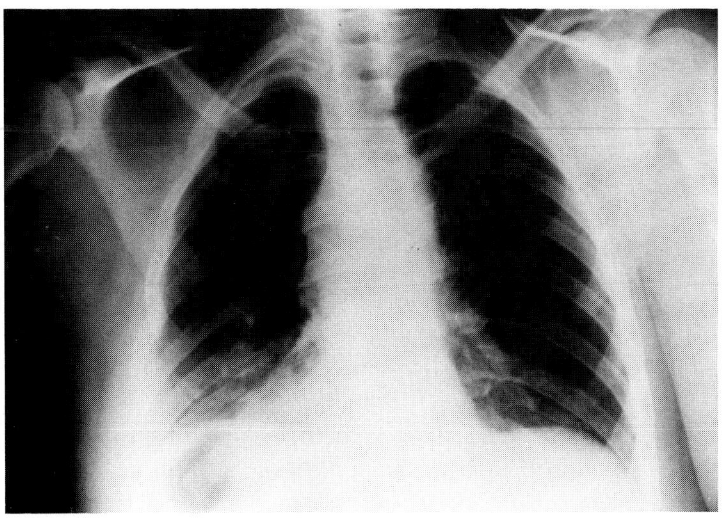

FIGURE 4.22 Disparity of the x-ray density of the lung and the abdominal contents on the right make diagnosis of a diaphragmatic hernia on the left relatively easy.

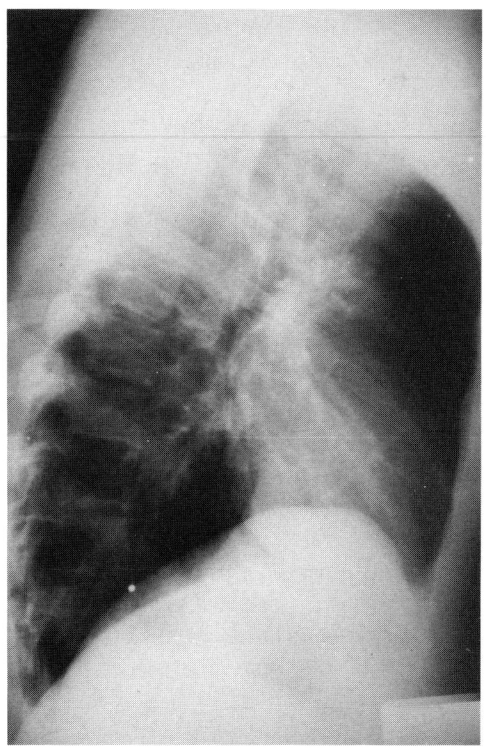

FIGURE 4.23 On the right, similarity between the density of the diaphragm and that of the liver make diagnosis of such a diaphragmatic hernia much more difficult.

from the outside. The pulmonary complications associated with rupture of the tissue, compression hemorrhage, and later edema are the same as occur with a flail chest, except the entire lung is involved.

Second phase The heat from the blast can cause thermal damage on the side facing the explosion at close range. Clothing provides some protection and causes a spotty burn pattern. The clothing can also ignite, causing secondary burns.

Third phase A blast may also result in flying debris. Pieces of metal, glass, wood, stone, and other loose material in the area can become missiles with enough force to penetrate deeply.

The major thoracic problem to be produced by such a blast is the so-called blast or shock lung. This overpressure event can produce a severe pulmonary contusion-type pattern, penetrating injuries to the thoracic wall, burns to the skin overlying the ribs, and fractured ribs in a victim who has been forced into a solid structure or hit in the chest by a large flying object.

RESUSCITATION AND INITIAL EVALUATION

Primary Assessment

The resuscitation of the trauma patient starts with the initial identification of immediate life-threatening problems, then total evaluation of the patient for all injuries and establishing priorities for management. The American College of Surgeons Committee on Trauma in the Advanced Trauma Life-Support Course has established an outstanding procedure to accomplish these priorities.[12] Because the acutely traumatized patient requires action so quickly, the examining physician frequently does not have time to think, but must react according to a previously memorized protocol in order to ensure that the priorities are recognized in order and appropriate steps taken to solve the complications from the specific injuries involved. The primary survey assesses the airway (with attention to probable cervical spine injury); breathing, with initiation of adequate ventilation and addressing the three critical thoracic problems that compromise respiration: tension pneumothorax, open pneumothorax, and flail chest; the cardiac system, identifying output problems by evaluating peripheral perfusion (capillary refilling, temperature and color of the extremity, and presence or absence of radial or carotid pulses), identifying hypovolemia or decreased myocardial contractibility, and attending immediately to cardiac tamponade and dysrhythmias produced by myocardial contusion; and disability, evaluating total body perfusion and oxygenation by surveying one of the most sensitive tissues to ischemia, the brain. Identification of the level of consciousness based on the simplistic but extremely definitive system of AVPU (*A*, *a*lert; *V*, responsive to *v*ocal stimuli; *P*, responsive to *p*ainful stimuli; *U*, *u*nresponsive) carries the examining physician through the primary survey to recognize these critical, life-threatening injuries and begin their management.

The specifics of initial assessment and airway management are well covered in the other chapters of this text. These will not be addressed here; however, the techniques for the initial evaluation of the patient, and specifically those that relate to the thoracic cavity, will be discussed.

Depending on the number of physicians available in the resuscitation room, one physician can evaluate and manage the airway while another evaluates and manages the thoracic injuries, or a single physician can evaluate both. The nurses should evaluate other vital signs and start large-bore (14-gauge) peripheral, not central, intravenous access lines.

When a single physician is accomplishing the entire primary survey, the physician should position himself at the head of the patient, and as the EMTs roll the patient into the room, ask them for a history of the incident and patient's condition. He should ask the patient what happened while simultaneously checking the patient's carotid pulse. A description of the entire accident by the patient identifies that the patient's airway is open, he is ventilating moderately well, and that his level of consciousness is not depressed. The follow-up question of "Where do you hurt?" will point out specific areas that the patient is aware of that received trauma. Following the identification of the presence of a carotid pulse, the physician should immediately examine the patient's hand, checking for a radial pulse and capillary refill and noting the color, temperature, and moisture of the hands. A radial pulse identifies a systolic pressure above 80 mm Hg. Good capillary refill in the thumb indicates adequate peripheral perfusion; lack of capillary refill identifies decreased extremity perfusion and possible hypovolemia. Pink skin denotes oxygenated periphery; pale skin reinforces the lack of peripheral perfusion, and blue skin identifies a cyanotic patient with lack of appropriate ventilation or stagnated blood flow in the capillary beds.

Absence of correct and appropriate patient response to the initial questions alerts the examiner to decreased cerebral activity with three prominent possible etiologies: (1) overdose on alcohol or drugs, (2) cerebral injury, or (3) decreased cerebral oxygenation. Since neither (1) nor (2) can be specifically managed in the acute situation and (3) can, the examiner must assume that decreased cerebral oxygenation is the cause. With no response from the patient, the airway must be immediately addressed. The three critical thoracic conditions which compromise ventilation—open pneumothorax, tension pneumothorax, and flail chest—must be accessed. The major concern at this point of patient evaluation is oxygenation.

Ventilation

The presence of anaerobic metabolism is the definition of shock. Its prevention and early reversal is the goal of resuscitation. Inadequate reversal leads to cellular death. When cellular death extends to the whole organ it produces failure of that organ, and ultimately of the patient. Organ failure, although it occurs late, is frequently due to inadequate resuscitation early on, and failure to reverse or prevent anaerobic metabolism in the first hour following the injury.

The Fick principle states that the oxygenation of any tissue and, therefore, its aerobic metabolism is based on three conditions: (1) on-loading of oxygen into the red cells in the lungs, (2) delivery of oxygenated red cells to the peripheral tissue, and (3) off-loading of oxygen from the red cells into the cells lining the capillaries. Violation of these principles produces operative or early postoperative cardiac failure, pulmonary failure 2 to 3 days post-trauma, renal failure 4 to 5 days after trauma, hepatic failure 7 to 10 days after trauma, and cerebral failure 5 to 10 minutes after trauma. Sepsis is probably of a similar etiology and is a failure of the immune system secondary to anaerobic metabolism, and various coagulopathies are probably a failure of platelets in the reticuloendothelial system due to such anaerobic metabolism, in the same manner. Other components of multiple organ system failure probably begin with anaerobic metabolism that compromises these systems' ability to perform. The long-term results may be a compromise of these specialized cells plus additional insult when other organ system failure has occurred also. The best solution to these problems at the present time seems to be early reversal and prevention of organ and cellular anaerobic metabolism. According to the Fick principle, there are two major problems that must be immediately addressed and solved: adequate red cell oxygenation and adequate red cell delivery. These are best accomplished by rapid, effective good prehospital care and delivery of the patient by adequate general and specialized staff to a trauma center operating room within an hour after the accident. During this hour adequate restoration of oxygenation and perfusion should have been accomplished or at least started. Of all the problems that produce inadequate tissue oxygenation, hypovolemia from blood loss and inadequate early management of the airway, and of pathology within the thoracic cavity, are most often to blame.

As the physician prepares to evaluate the patient being brought into the resuscitation room, the airway is a prime concern. If it is compromised, bag-valve-mask ventilation with 100% oxygen is used to quickly reverse as much hypoxia and acidosis as possible. After about 1 minute of such reestablishment of adequate oxygenation, an endotracheal tube is placed with direct laryngoscopy via the mouth (or nose, if the patient is breathing) while another member of the patient-care team maintains in-line stability of the cervical spine, preventing its hyperextension or hyperflexion. Auscultation of the chest and abdomen assures correct placement of the endotracheal tube, if such is required.

Visual inspection of the thoracic cage is made by opening the clothing down the midline of the chest to expose the anterior and lateral thoracic walls. The chest is auscultated with particular attention to the lungs for adequacy of ventilation; the supraclavicular and infraclavicular areas are listened to first for decreased breath sounds, indicating a tension pneumothorax, then laterally on both chest walls to reassess the depth of ventilation (either spontaneous or mechanical). The thoracic cage is palpated anteriorly, laterally, and posteriorly for major rib fractures, flail segments, or penetrations that cannot be visualized. Heart sounds are assessed next. Last, the stethoscope is placed in the epigastrium to check that the endotracheal tube is in the correct position, or that the patient is adequately ventilated by the bag-valve-mask. Visual inspection of the neck to identify the status of the neck veins completes the primary assessment.

Unless the examining physician specifically questions all seven diagnostic traumatic processes, their signs and symptoms are so subtle that the delay in identifying their presence may significantly compromise the survival of the patient. These are as follows:

- Airway obstruction
- Inadequate ventilation
  - Auscultation
  - Pulmonary retraction
  - Decreased thoracic cage movement
- Tension pneumothorax
  - Cyanosis
  - Unilateral absent breath sounds
  - Distended neck veins
  - Deviation of the trachea
  - Subcutaneous emphysema
- Cardiac tamponade
  - Distended neck veins
  - Muffled heart sounds
  - Narrowed pulse pressure
  - Paradoxical pulse
- Open pneumothorax
  - Decreased breath sounds
  - Penetration of thoracic wall
- Myocardial contusion
  - Dysrhythmia
- Flail chest
  - Loose segment
  - Multiple palpable fractured ribs
  - Decreased or moist breath sounds
  - Hemoptysis

Many of the signs and symptoms of the above-listed conditions are very subtle and extremely difficult to detect upon initial physical examination and may require other diagnostic techniques. Until they can be specifically ruled out, however, the resuscitating physician cannot disregard their possible contributions to the current status of the patient.

Venous Access

There are three reasons for accessing the vascular system in any patient: administration of intravenous fluid, administration of drugs, and measurement and monitoring of cardiac parameters.

In a trauma patient the major need is to administer IV fluids, preferably whole blood. According to Poiseuille's law, the rate of fluid flow is inversely proportional to the length of the catheter and directly proportional to its internal diameter. It says nothing of the vein in which the catheter is placed. A 14-gauge, 5-cm catheter in a peripheral vein will pass fluid twice as fast as a 16-gauge, 20-cm catheter placed centrally. No drugs are required for the resuscitation of a trauma patient, and since most patients are young and healthy, measurement of cardiac parameters is significant only when there is a question of cardiac tamponade. Therefore, the central placement of a catheter is an intensive care unit or operating room technique, one that in general should not be accomplished in the emergency department until after the patient has been stabilized, unless no other routes of venous access are available. It has been shown that a saphenous cutdown is still an excellent venous access, even when the pneumatic antishock garment (PASG)[69] is inflated; this device does not slow fluid flow through the legs.

The complications of central venous catheter placement are all potentially dangerous to the trauma patient. The addition of a pneumothorax further complicates ventilation. Hemorrhage into the thoracic cavity may go unnoticed for several hours unless a chest tube is in place. Blood, Ringer's lactate, platelets, fresh-frozen plasma, and other fluid placed in the thoracic cavity by intrathoracic location of the central venous catheter not only compromises ventilation, but gives a false impression of intravascularly administered fluids and clotting factors. Finally, cold or even room temperature fluids administered by central venous catheter will significantly lower the patient's body temperature, increasing susceptibility to other complications.

Chest Tube Insertion

There are three reasons to insert a chest tube. The first is to rapidly decompress a tension pneumothorax; the second, to prevent a simple or potential pneumothorax from developing into a tension pneumothorax when positive-pressure ventilation is required; and the third is to evacuate and assess the severity of intrathoracic hemorrhage. Due to its rapidly deleterious effects, a tension pneumothorax is best managed by either a quick stab wound into the pleural cavity through the lateral thoracic wall or insertion of a needle into the second intercostal space at the midclavicular line. A stab wound can result in complications because of injury to the lung beneath if the diagnosis is incorrect. The second technique is safer and almost as rapid. Formal tube thoracostomy, which requires much more time, can then proceed safely while continued resuscitation is accomplished.

PROCEDURE

Insert a large-bore needle through the second intercostal space at the mid-clavicular line. This provides not only immediate relief, but also early management of the condition via a one-way valve that allows continued evacuation of the air under pressure but prevents to-and-fro air flow. The midclavicular line is chosen because the internal mammary artery lies 1 cm lateral to the sternum and posterior to the anterior rib cage. Injury to this vessel produces rapid blood loss and, because it lies inside the thoracic wall, direct pressure to control hemorrhage is extremely difficult to apply.

The second intercostal space is chosen because with a pneumothorax, the air tends to rise to the upper chest and periphery, while the lung falls toward the mediastinum. The lateral high chest wall can also provide easy access to the pleural cavity, but it is not ideal when movement of the patient is required, for the device may interfere with the patient's arm motion.

THORACOSTOMY

Chest tube thoracostomy in a severely injured trauma patient is most frequently initiated in the resuscitation room based on history and physical diagnosis criteria. There is no time for confirmation of hemothorax or pneumothorax by x-ray.

After preparing the lateral chest wall and identifying the landmarks of the seventh intercostal space, the following steps should be taken:

1. Lidocaine is injected into the skin if the patient's condition permits.
2. A 2-cm transverse incision is made overlying the fifth intercostal space at the midaxillary line. The skin incision is continued into the subcutaneous tissue (Fig. 4.24).
3. With a Kelly clamp, the dissection is carried over the fifth rib into the fourth intercostal space through the intercostal muscles, and with a sharp, thrusting motion the pleura is penetrated (Fig. 4.25).
4. The hole is widened by expansion of the clamp.
5. A gloved finger is inserted to ensure that (a) the pleural cavity has been entered (not the abdominal cavity), (b) no intra-abdominal organs that would be injured by the tube are in the way of the chest tube, and (c) that the lung has not adhered to the lateral pleural walls (Fig. 4.26).
6. Gloved fingers are withdrawn, and the chest tube is guided into the thoracic cavity with a Kelly clamp and then directed upward toward the apex of the thoracic cavity.
7. The chest tube is immediately connected to suction to evacuate the pleural cavity and reexpand the lung.
8. Shed blood is collected in a sterile container to be reinfused into the patient after anticoagulation and filtration, using a Sorenson autotransfuser.

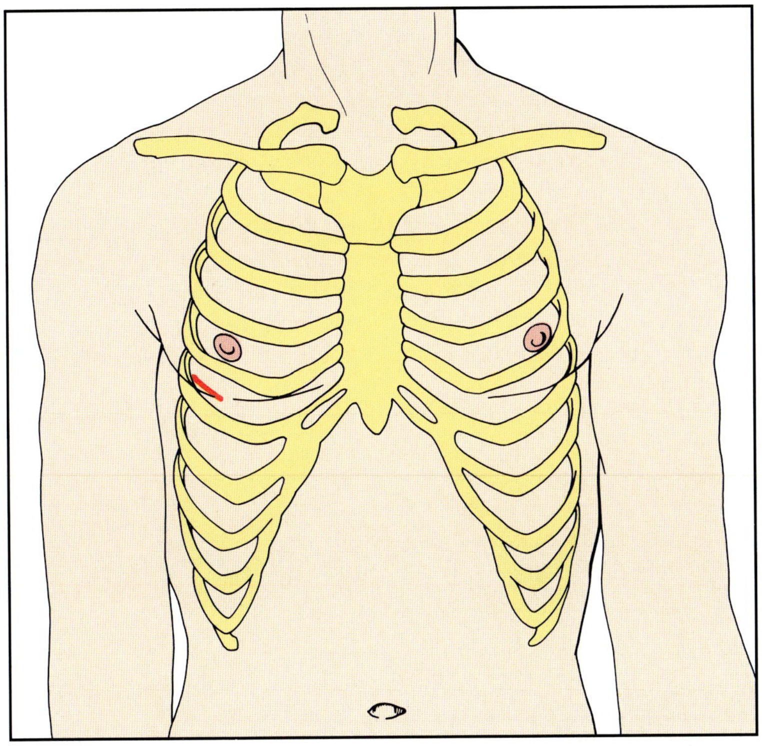

FIGURE 4.24 The skin incision over the fifth intercostal space is continued through the skin and into the subcutaneous tissue.

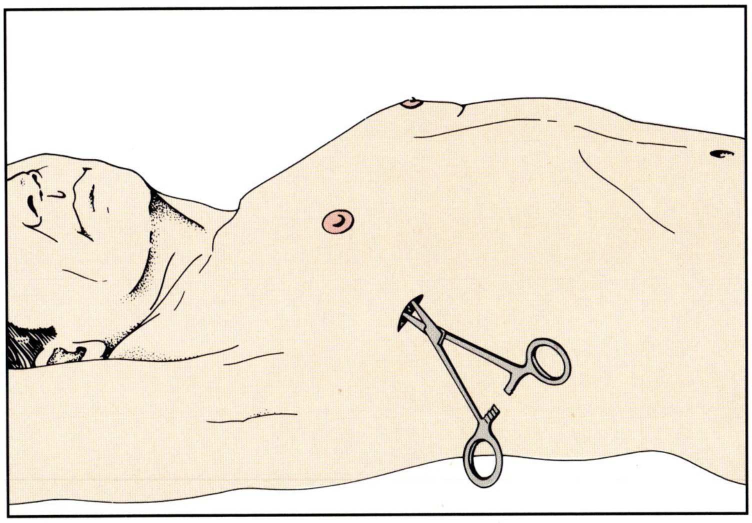

FIGURE 4.25 Utilization of a Kelly clamp to dissect through the intercostal muscles bluntly at the fourth intercostal space allows full penetration.

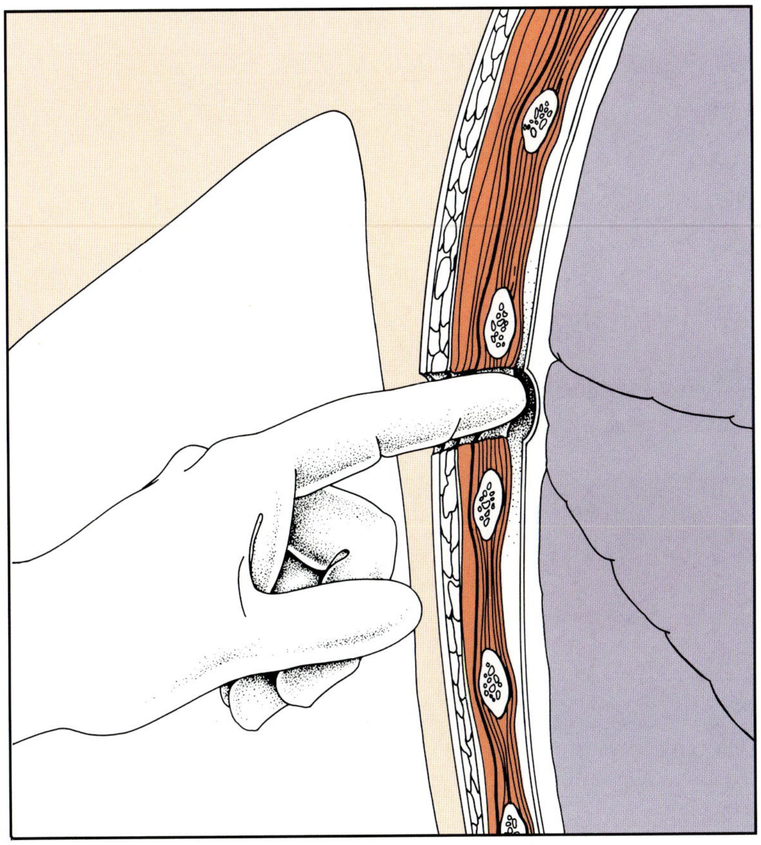

FIGURE 4.26 The gloved finger must be inserted into the full cavity to ensure that the correct cavity has been entered and that no adhesions of the lung or intra-abdominal organs that would be injured by the tube are present.

Resuscitative Thoracotomy

There are three basic reasons for doing a thoracotomy on an immediate basis either in the emergency department or in the operating room:

1. To control exsanguinating intrathoracic hemorrhage
2. To manage a cardiac tamponade that cannot be decompressed via needle aspiration
3. To cross-clamp the thoracic aorta to control intra-abdominal exsanguinating hemorrhage

In the second instance, when a patient's blood pressure decreases below 60 mm Hg, it is probable that one of the above conditions exists and the patient is not going to survive without such a procedure. Figure 4.27 is an algorithm developed at Tulane University Medical Center for assessing an emergency situation.

A thoracotomy should be performed by a surgeon adequately trained in its techniques, one who knows how to evacuate a cardiac tamponade, to cross-clamp the aorta, and to control intrathoracic hemorrhage by cross-clamping the hilum of the lung.[67] The surgeon should have done several thoracotomies in

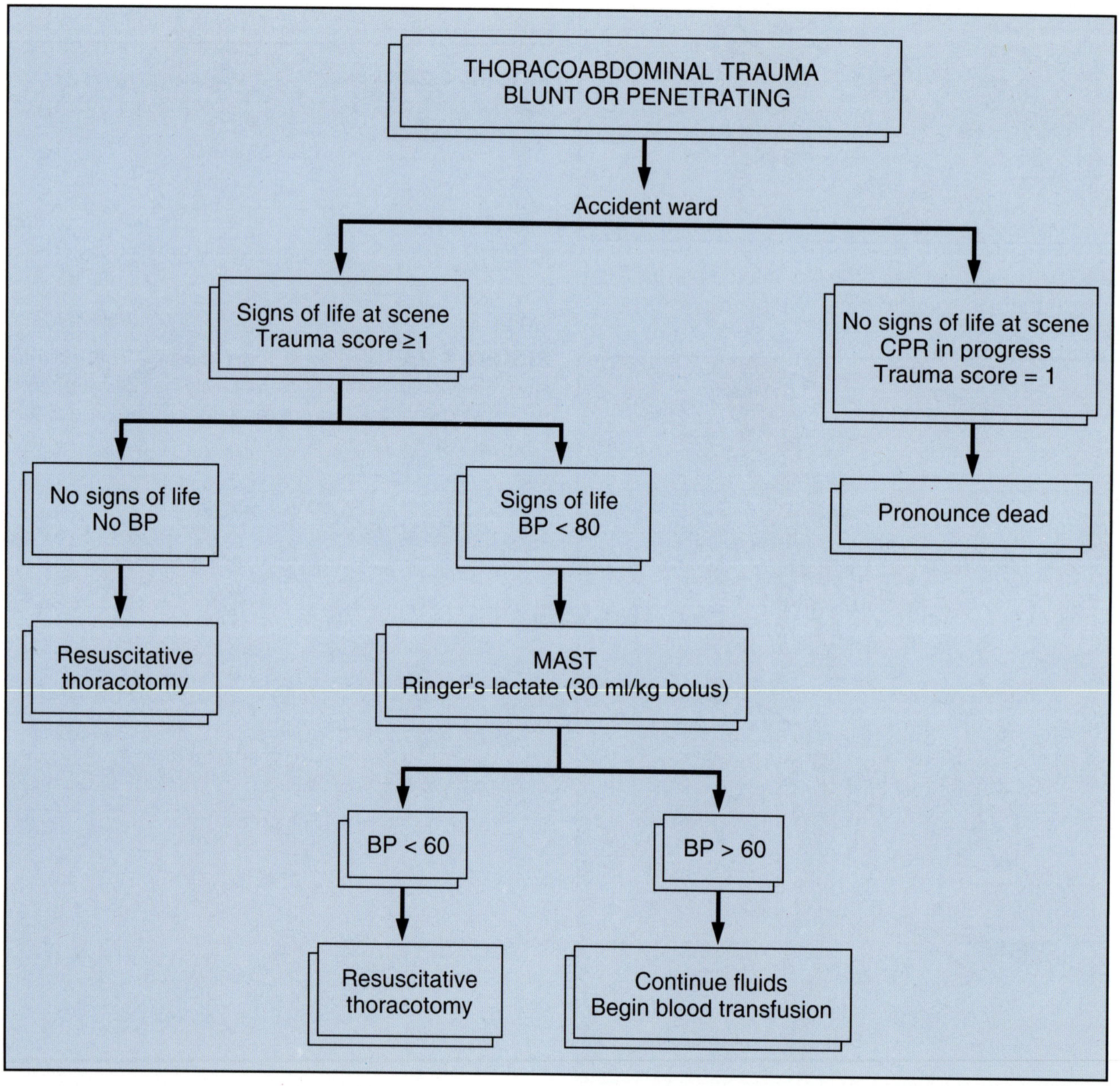

FIGURE 4.27 The decision to accomplish a resuscitative thoracotomy is frequently delayed until it is of no benefit to the patient, or it is attempted in the emergency department when it could be better accomplished in the operating room. This flowchart describes the correct evaluative steps to determine when the technique should be attempted.

the operating room under controlled conditions, supervised by a thoracic or trauma surgeon, and have accomplished the same procedure in the emergency department with the above-described supervision. The operation is best performed in the operating room. If a patient cannot survive to reach the operating room, it must be done in the emergency department.

There is another major factor that must be understood before attempting such a procedure, however. The opening of the chest and the opening of the pericardium, cross-clamping the aorta, or cross-clamping the pulmonary hilum represent only one fourth of the procedure. The intrathoracic lesions must be repaired, the condition producing the pericardial tamponade must be fixed, the lung removed if necessary or the abdomen opened, and the source of exsanguinating hemorrhage controlled and repaired. The final task is closure of the thoracic wound. If an operating room, anesthesiology staff, and trauma surgeon are not immediately available to complete the procedure it should not have been started. Just because one has the ability to open a chest with a knife does not mean that one has the ability, equipment, or staff available to complete the procedure.

The cost of resuscitative thoracotomy can be high. With signs of life in the field but not in the emergency department, the salvage rate is almost zero. There is a greater survival rate when there are signs of life in the emergency department and the procedure is initiated promptly. A delay in the procedure reduces salvage again to zero.[67] There is some chance for survival if there are signs of life in the field that subsequently disappear en route to the hospital. Rapid transportation and immediate resuscitative thoracotomy on arrival in the emergency department are absolute necessities if this latter group is to be recovered.

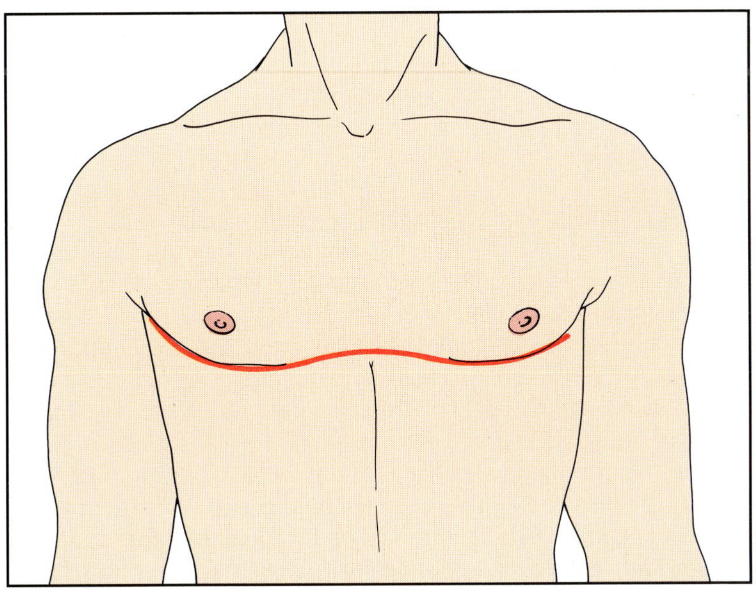

FIGURE 4.28 The "butterfly" incision extends a thoracotomy on one side of the chest to the other side, allowing access to both hemithoraces as well as the heart and other structures in the mediastinum.

PROCEDURE

1. The patient is intubated and prep solution is poured on the thoracic wall. Drapes are applied if time permits.
2. A fourth intercostal anterolateral incision is made from just medial to the nipple to the posterior axillary line. In the trauma patient the incision is under the breast, and the breast is not transected.
3. The operator's left hand is inserted through the incision and to the aorta.
4. A large self-retaining, rib-spreading retractor is inserted by an assistant and the wound opened wide.
5. After the operator's left hand has mobilized the aorta, it is cross-clamped just superior to the diaphragm.
6. The pericardium is inspected and if blood is visualized inside the distended sac, it is opened parallel and anterior to the vagus nerve.
7. The lung is inspected for exsanguinating hemorrhage. If any is found, a vascular clamp is placed proximal to the bleeding. The hilum of the lung may be the only such location. Other procedures cease while blood volume is restored. After the patient is stabilized, a definitive repair can be accomplished.
8. A hole in the heart is immediately sutured with 2-0 cardiovascular suture with Teflon pledgets, while the operator's finger is kept in the hole to prevent further blood loss.
9. The patient is immediately removed to the operating room where the abdomen can be opened, or definitive repair of thoracic pathology can be completed.

Pitfalls

A tension pneumothorax on the right side that goes unrecognized by the operating surgeon can cause severe injury to the heart and lung, which may both be forced against the lateral thoracic wall. If care is not taken with the incision through the pleura, one or both organs can be lacerated. A lung which bulges through the incision is indicative of a right tension pneumothorax. Immediate steps must be taken to decompress it.

The internal mammary artery lies 1 cm lateral to the sternum. Extending the incision too far medially will cut this vessel and rapid, large-volume blood loss can result. If the patient is already severely hypotensive, or if perfusion is reduced for other reasons, injury to the vessel may not be immediately apparent. When significant hemorrhage occurs as the blood pressure increases and perfusion improves, internal mammary artery laceration should be immediately investigated.

After opening the left chest, if it becomes apparent that the right side of the chest is also a source of pathology, the incision is extended across the sternum to "butterfly" the whole chest open (Fig. 4.28). This provides access to the right hemithorax and also the mediastinum. Such an incision, however, will transect both internal mammary arteries; they must be ligated.

These arteries derive blood from two sources, the subclavian arteries above, and the superior epigastric arteries below (through the inferior epigastric and femoral arteries). The cephalad and caudad portions must both be ligated, and because the internal mammary artery is inside the thoracic cage, control must be made under the ribs, not on the anterior surface (Fig. 4.29).

SECONDARY SURVEY AND DIAGNOSTIC TECHNIQUES

Before the patient is moved for anything other than an AP film, a lateral cervical spine x-ray visualizing all seven cervical vertebrae and the top of T1 should be done to rule out a cervical-spine fracture (blunt trauma). Insertion of a Foley catheter, nasogastric tube, and other techniques required for adequate total patient management should also be done, including an electrocardiogram, blood gas studies, blood transfusion if indicated, and other resuscitative techniques as required. Immediately after the patient is stabilized, chest films should be obtained (upright, PA, and 6 feet if the patient's condition permits; if not, AP supine and lateral x-rays) to identify correct placement of the chest tube, evacuation of possible pneumo- or hemothorax, correct placement of the central venous catheter if cardiac monitoring was required, and evaluation of the lung field for pulmonary contusion.

The patient's total condition at this point must be assessed to identify what other diagnostic techniques are needed to complete the evaluation of the thoracic cavity. Based on the patient's overall condition, these procedures are to be considered: arteriography, bronchoscopy, computed tomography, hemodynamic cardiac parameters, and thoracoscopy. All of these procedures have been adequately described in the literature except thoracoscopy, which is of great value in trauma.

Thoracoscopy

Many intrathoracic injuries are inadequately evaluated by indirect methods. Thoracoscopy, which allows a direct look at the pathology, can prevent unnecessary surgery or hasten intervention. In fact, one series identified that in 39% of patients receiving a thoracoscopy, the operative management of the patient was changed.[24]

INDICATIONS

The indication for a thoracoscopy is a penetrating thoracic injury in which a real question exists as to whether operative intervention is required. Thoracoscopy can, for example, identify the presence or absence of diaphragmatic penetration in any patient with an abdominal gunshot wound. At maximal expiration the dome of the diaphragm is on a plane with the fourth intercostal space anteriorly, the sixth intercostal space laterally, and the eighth intercostal space posteriorly. Any penetration in a lateral or downward direction below this line (one half of the true thoracic cavity, two thirds of the rib cage) would otherwise necessitate a laparotomy. A thoracoscopic evaluation can identify such a perforation or, perhaps more importantly, its absence.

The indication for a thoracotomy is continued intrathoracic hemorrhage, regardless the rate of blood loss. Very frequently clots or an incorrectly placed chest tube prevent the adequate assessment of hemorrhage. The etiology may be an intercostal vessel that is continually bleeding, but can be controlled by electrical coagulation. The thoracoscope can assess whether the blood loss is continuing or has stopped. Continuing, significant blood loss would most likely require a thoracotomy. The thoracoscope can also be used to evacuate clotted blood from the thoracic cavity, which might otherwise require a later thoracotomy to prevent development of a peel; and to evaluate for pericardial tamponade, mediastinal penetration, or expanding mediastinal hematoma.

PROCEDURE

Thoracoscopy is best performed under general anesthesia. The previously inserted chest tube is removed and the thoracoscope inserted through the site. A pediatric rigid sigmoido scope can serve the function of a thoracoscope even more accurately and conveniently. Through a separate, small stab wound, a long rigid suction catheter is inserted in order to move the lung out of the way, to allow inspection of the entire thoracic cavity, and to aspirate blood clots or continued hemorrhage. The anesthesiologist controls expansion of the lung to facilitate visualization of the entire cavity. If a formal thoracotomy is not indicated, the chest tube can be reinserted.[24]

Antibiotics

The use of antibiotics has remained controversial. The conservative approach in all thoracic trauma that would require a chest tube or a thoracotomy is to start every patient on a general broad spectrum antibiotics regimen. LeBlanc and Tucker identified no statistical difference in using prophylactic cephapirin and using no treatment (the actual percentages were 2.6% treated and 10.8% untreated).[30] Stone, Symbas, and Hooper reported a decrease in infections when antibiotics were used.[57] Mandal, Montano, and Thadepalli reported "no appreciable difference between the two groups in duration of chest tube drainage, length of hospital stay or incidence of infection."[33] Grover and co-workers reported from a prospective blind study that clindamycin-treated patients had less pneumonia, less-elevated temperatures, lower incidences of positive cultures, less empyema, and required fewer operations and fewer days of hospitalization. With the literature still mixed at present, the conservative approach is to use antibiotics in penetrating thoracic trauma or when a chest tube is required.

Autotransfusion

During the late 1960s at Grady Hospital in Atlanta, Peter Symbas investigated and revived the use of autotransfusion for patients with acute thoracic blood loss. While his initial studies were in thoracic trauma, the procedure was adapted for use for blood loss anywhere in the body. Blood from the acutely traumatized chest is reinfused in the emergency department after being anticoagulated by one of the many commercially available devices. In the operating room an autotransfusion device washes the blood cells with saline to remove debris, clots, and other material. With bowel injury there is reinfusion of bacteria, but as long as the patient is placed on antibiotics this does not seem to be of clinical significance.[8,16,68]

CHEST INJURIES AND MANAGEMENT

Pneumothorax

Pneumothorax in penetrating trauma can be a result of injury of the thoracic wall or the lung or both, resulting in air leaking into the pleural space. In more than half of the pneumothoracotomies that occur in blunt trauma, the accident victim has instinctively taken a deep breath and closed the glottis, causing the lung to burst. A smaller number are due to the fractured rib actually penetrating the pleural space and lacerating the lung.[41]

PATHOPHYSIOLOGY

A ball or flap valve is created in either the injured thoracic wall or the lung in most penetrating thoracic injuries. As the thoracic cage expands, intrathoracic pressure becomes negative and air is sucked in from the outside through the thoracic wall defect, or out of the bronchus through the pulmonary parenchyma defect. When intrathoracic pressure becomes positive, air is usually retained in the pleural space as the flap-type valve is forced closed in either the lung or thoracic wall. If the defect does not seal readily with subsequent breaths, the air in the intrapleural space continues to increase. As the volume builds, the lung on the affected side is compressed. As more compression occurs, the mediastinum is shifted and a tension pneumothorax develops. As the mediastinum is pushed farther, the lung on the unaffected side is compressed, reducing its ventilatory capacity, the vena cava is kinked, and the intrapleural pressure is increased—a combination that decreases cardiac filling, increases central venous pressure, and distends the neck vein.

In blunt trauma, a tension pneumothorax develops by the same mechanism, except that there is no hole in the thoracic wall, only in the lung itself.

DIAGNOSIS

With time of the essence, the initial evaluating physician must depend on his physical examination techniques and ability to identify a tension pneumothorax without the use of x-ray films. He or she must correct the hypoxia before the brain and heart develop terminal ischemic damage.

The classic signs of a tension pneumothorax are unilateral absent breath sounds, cyanosis, distended neck veins, deviated trachea, and subcutaneous emphysema. Unfortunately, subcutaneous emphysema is not always apparent, a deviated trachea is extremely difficult to identify on physical examination, and cyanosis is not as apparent on persons with dark skin or patients with decreased cardiac output. For distended neck veins to be visible, cardiovascular volume must be close to normal. An extremely hypovolemic patient does not have enough preload to cause distended neck veins. Further, when a PASG is applied, preload may be increased to the point that neck veins are distended without an increase in intrathoracic pressure. Only unilateral absent breath sounds can be consistently relied upon to identify a tension pneumothorax. However, the physician must listen at the apex of the lung—not the base—in the supraclavicular or infraclavicular area. The physician should be experienced enough to differentiate between bronchial and parenchymal breath sounds and, perhaps most importantly, to detect the subtlety of a unilateral decrease in breath sounds.

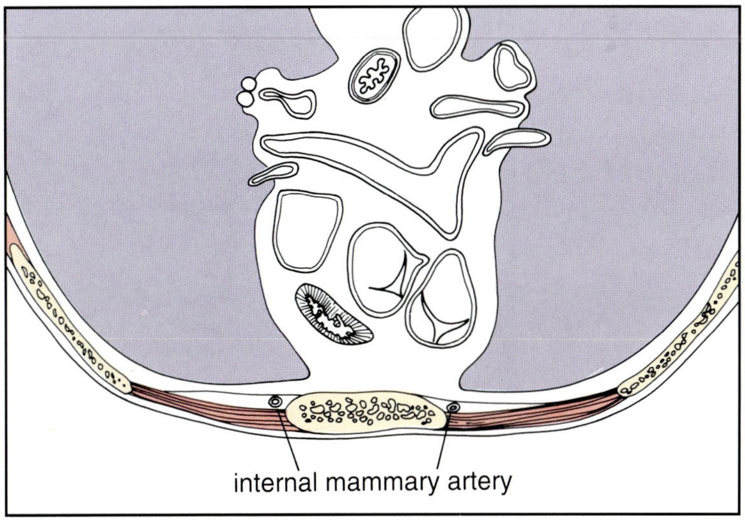

FIGURE 4.29 The "butterfly" incision cuts across the internal mammary artery, which must be ligated. External compression will not provide hemostasis, since the artery is under the rib cage and not between the skin and ribs.

A chest film provides a definitive diagnosis of a pneumothorax. The early or small pneumothorax may be difficult to identify on the inspiratory chest film because the pleural line may be extremely close to the lateral or superior chest wall (Fig. 4.30). An expiratory chest film may be required to make this identification (Fig. 4.31). Identifying a small pneumothorax by expiratory chest film is critically important to the patient who is going to be intubated, either for anesthesia or to manage a flail chest. Positive-pressure ventilation will convert a small pneumothorax to a tension pneumothorax in extremely short order, and in an ICU or operating room setting it can go undetected until too late. Frequently, too, a tension pneumothorax is missed when the signs of decreased cardiac output and increased central venous pressure are mistaken for myocardial failure.

The subtleties of a tension pneumothorax can be confusing. For example, Werne and Sands reported a left tension pneumothorax that was actually misdiagnosed as an anterior myocardial infarction.[78] Slay, Slay, and Luehrs have reported a transient ST elevation associated with tension pneumothorax, which could be misleading.[54]

Air from a pneumothorax and more specifically from a bronchus defect can produce a pneumomediastinum or a pneumopericardium. The subtleties of these are such that both chest and neck films can be read as normal unless specific attention is directed toward the soft tissues of the neck and the pericardium itself. Associated with these conditions is a "bruit demoulin" first described in 1844 by Drichteau.[13]

With a penetrating injury across the mediastinum, a patient with an injured esophagus must also be suspected of having air either in the mediastinum or the pericardial sac.

MANAGEMENT

Management of a tension pneumothorax consists of urgent decompression, either with a needle or a stab wound in the chest. By performing a quick decompression, the clinician will then have the time to carefully insert a chest tube without risk of injuring the heart, lung, or diaphragm and the organs below it.

Flail Chest

Flail chest, as described earlier, is created when two or more ribs break in two or more places, and can be the result of a frontal impact collision or pedestrian trauma.

PATHOPHYSIOLOGY

Three clinical conditions produce the ventilatory compromise characteristic of flail chest: paradoxical movement, pain, and pulmonary contusion. Early in the management of a multiply injured patient (1 to 3 hours), these conditions may be overshadowed. Even in the patient with an isolated flail chest, the psychological shock of the incident suppresses pain, and muscle spasms suppress paradoxical movement, so that it may be several hours before the clinical condition is recognized.

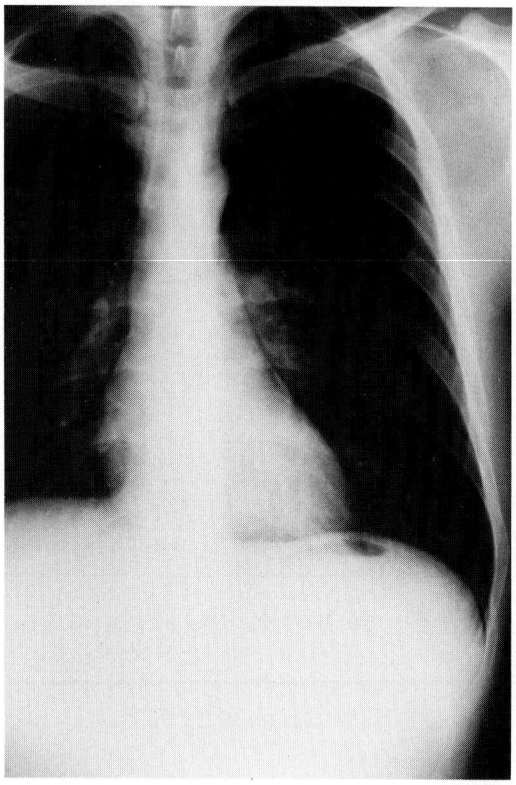

FIGURE 4.30 A small pneumothorax is difficult to identify on an inspiratory chest film.

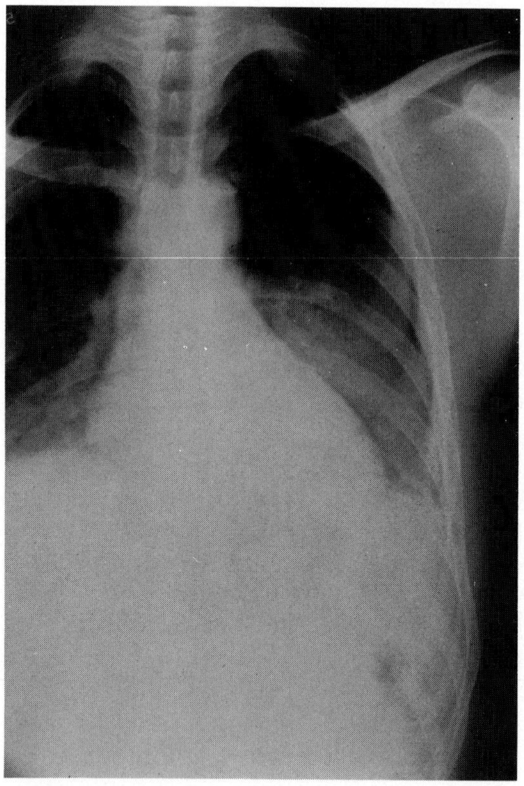

FIGURE 4.31 An expiratory chest film makes such identification far easier.

Paradoxical movement is defined as movement of the flail segment of the chest wall opposite to normal respiration. The larger the involved segment, the more clinical significance the process has in decreasing the volume of ventilation. In the first few hours after the traumatic incident, spasms of the intercostal muscles may reduce the pathological effect of this loosened segment. On visual inspection of the thoracic cavity, no apparent paradoxical motion is visible. It is only after the patient begins to tire, and the spasms in these muscles relax, that the condition develops to a point of reducing the volume of air moved on inspiration and expiration.

Any fractured bone produces pain. The patient usually holds a fractured arm tightly to the side or with the opposite hand so as not to move it and produce pain. The self-splinting of multiple rib fractures, however, is of far greater consequence than the self-splinting of a forearm fracture. Decreased rib movement translates into decreased thoracic cage expansion, which in turn translates into decreased pulmonary expansion and decreased ventilation. Prolonged over 8 to 12 hours, this produces atelectasis and subsequent pneumonia.

Both the delayed development of clinically apparent atelectasis and clinically apparent paradoxical motion are factors in the delayed recognition, decreased ventilation, and compromised respiration of flail chest.

By far the most significant and serious consequence of flail chest is a pulmonary contusion. Hemorrhage into the interstitium, the alveolar-capillary membrane, and the alveolar space itself immediately decreases oxygen transport to the red cells. The edema that develops around the injured cells over a period of several hours further compromises this decreased oxygen transport and is another factor in the delayed onset of the clinical problems of flail chest.

The "pendleluft," or pendulum-like movement of the mediastinum from one chest cavity to the other classically described in the older textbooks of surgery and trauma probably does not exist, as was originally thought in 1960.[77]

DIAGNOSIS

Visual examination of the patient on arrival in the emergency department may not identify flail chest, nor will blood gases, pulmonary pressures, or cardiac pressures. Initially only a chest film may identify multiple rib fractures and the early radiopaque density of the contused lung. Bruising and pulmonary hemorrhage are usually apparent on the admission chest film, with edema worsening in the next 6 to 12 hours.

Blood gas determination is a significant factor in the diagnosis of the severity of pulmonary contusion. A blood gas below 60 mm Hg on room air or 80 mm Hg with an F_1O_2 of 40 identifies a significant decrease in oxygen exchange produced by the damaged segments of lungs.

Increasing pulmonary compliance and pulmonary artery pressure, indicating increased pulmonary vascular resistance, are also indicators that the pulmonary contusion present is significant enough to compromise a patient's clinical condition.

MANAGEMENT

Until the early 1950s flail chest was managed by external fixation. Towel clips were placed around each fractured rib and the chest was suspended with weighted rope. Tracheostomies and pulmonary ventilation for 8 to 14 days replaced this method of management until recently.[77] Moore and co-workers attempted placement of pins to stabilize these fractures, but increased morbidity and mortality resulted.[37] In Europe and in some centers in the United States there is a renewed interest in operative stabilization, especially for a patient undergoing a thoracotomy for other reasons. Better understanding of pulmonary physiology, positive end-expiratory pressure, and intermittent mandatory ventilation in the 1980s have led to shorter stays on ventilators in the ICU.

Patients with flail chest who show up in the accident room can be classified into three groups:

1. Patients with associated injuries that require laparotomy and thoracotomy
2. Patients with obvious pulmonary compromise on admission
3. Patients with no apparent pulmonary compromise on admission

The patients in the first two categories are noncontroversial as to their method of management. Those in the first category require intubation and positive-pressure ventilation at least through the operation. Such patients should stay on positive-pressure ventilation, intermittent mandatory ventilation (IMV) and positive end-expiratory pressure (PEEP) until arterial blood gas, pulmonary compliance, and cardiac pressures indicate that extubation can be safely accomplished. Patients with obvious pulmonary compromise on admission are similarly treated with intubation, IMV, and PEEP. Initial PaO_2 below 60 mm Hg on room air or below 80 mm Hg with oxygen supplementation, and decreased pulmonary compliance, are indicators on admission that pulmonary assistance will be required and should be started immediately in the resuscitation room.

Treatment of the third category of patients, whose initial pulmonary parameters are within normal limits and whose chest film does not identify severe pulmonary contusion, is controversial. Trinkle and Shackford introduced symptomatic management of flail chest.[51,71] Unless and until the parameters deteriorate requiring intubation and positive-pressure ventilation, the patient is managed with pain medication alone.[47] Others feel that if a patient is initially intubated and placed on IMV and PEEP, that the time on the ventilator and in the ICU can be shortened to 2 to 3 days, whereas waiting until the patient's clinical condition deteriorates can increase that time to 10 to 14 days. At present no prospective study has been completed to evaluate these two methods of treatment. I favor the latter, unless the patient has an extremely mild pulmonary contusion.

Following the selective method of management, the patient's pain is suppressed by systemic analgesics given either orally or by injection. Intercostal blocks are performed on a frequent basis to suppress pain and allow adequate ventilation. However, they must be done as often as every 6 hours, and the patient's discomfort associated with this and the possibility of complications (intercostal hematomas, sterile abscess, and pneumothorax) are overriding factors against this type of management. Thoracic epidural anesthesia with lidocaine or morphine has produced analgesia with fewer complications, and is probably the best initial management of the pain of multiple rib fractures.

Methylprednisolone will reduce the pulmonary vascular resistance and prevent and reduce complications of pulmonary contusion. However, glycerol produces similar results.[3,25] Steroids will have a deleterious effect on the ability of the contused and noncontused lungs to clear bacteria.[3,48] The contused lung is not more susceptible to bacterial infection, unless it is associated with acute blood loss, making it less able to clear bacteria. Crystalloid infusion will also markedly depress lung bacteria clearance.

Cardiac Tamponade

Larrey performed the first successful periocardiocentesis in 1849.[28] Billroth decried it in 1883,[6] but in 1943 Baylock and Roberts[4] identified pericardiocentesis as the treatment of choice for pericardial tamponade. This was the standard treatment until 1968 when Sugg analyzed 459 cases and set the stage for the change toward using pericardiocentesis as a temporizing measure and thoracotomy as the treatment for pericardial tamponade.[60]

The most prominent cause of cardiac tamponade is secondary to penetrating trauma. This can come either from a coronary artery laceration (most commonly, left anterior descending) or a myocardial penetration itself. Victims of close-range shotgun injuries frequently show up in the emergency department with not enough vital signs to be resuscitated. Some medium-high gunshot wounds, however, will develop a pericardial tamponade despite the missile penetration of the pericardium. If a patient with this type of injury does not exsanguinate from the myocardial injury, the hole in the pericardium will decompress itself enough that the patient is able to reach the hospital alive.

Stab wounds, however, are a far more frequent cause of pericardial tamponade in the emergency department. The blood loss is frequently less and the patient can be more easily managed.

PATHOPHYSIOLOGY

In an acute tamponade, the pericardial sac is rigid and does not dilate. It fills during systole, as blood leaks from either the myocardium itself or a lacerated coronary artery. Blood is forced out from a ventricular defect during systole, and the contracting myocardium gives it space to accumulate. As more and more blood accumulates, there is less space for the myocardium to distend during diastole, compromising the amount of interventricular volume available for ejection into

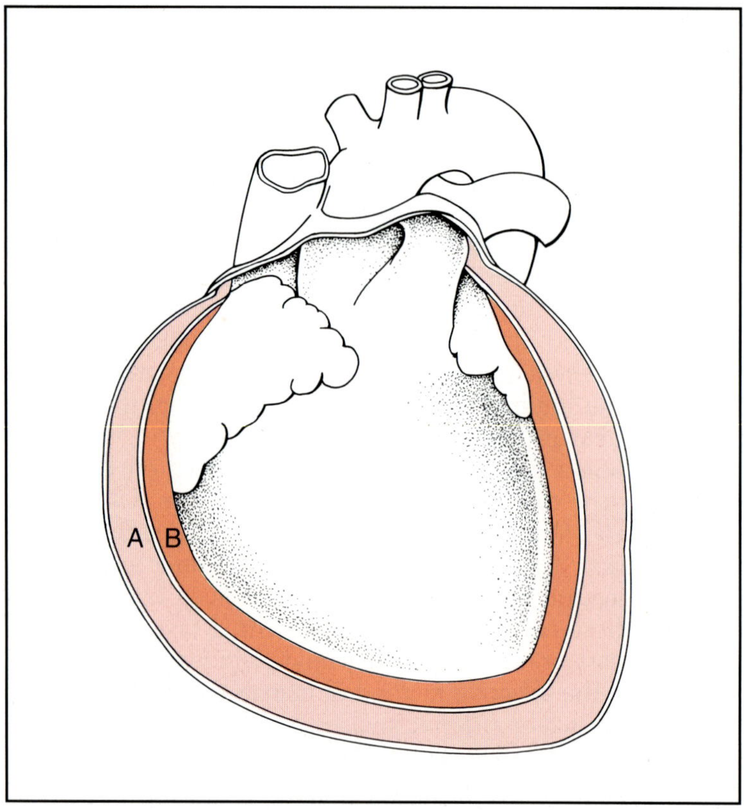

FIGURE 4.32 Pericardial fluid prevents expansion of the heart during diastole, limiting its filling volume. This reduces the blood volume available for ejection.

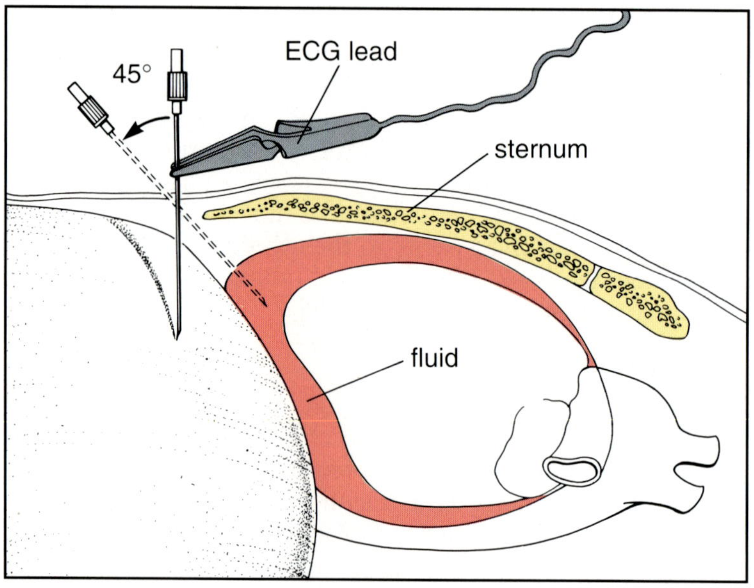

FIGURE 4.33 The needle is directed at a 45° angle downward beneath the sternum toward the apex of the heart. "V" ECG leads can be used to identify contact with the myocardium.

the aorta (Fig. 4.32). This decreased cardiac filling and subsequent cardiac ejection leads to decreased cardiac output and narrowing of the pulse pressure. There is only so much space in the pericardial sac. Acutely the pericardial sac does not dilate; chronically it can.

DIAGNOSIS

The signs and symptoms of a patient with a tension pneumothorax and a patient with a cardiac tamponade are so similar as to present a very confusing picture for the clinician. In addition, it is not unusual for a patient to have both a tension pneumothorax and a cardiac tamponade because the penetrating object has traversed first the lung and then the pericardium, into the heart itself. As in other trauma, the history of the event, direction of penetration, length of the penetrating object, and caliber of weapon are all extremely important when the physician initially assesses a patient. Beck's triad has long been used as the diagnostic criterion, although in actuality the onset is much more subtle than Beck's triad implies.

Although all signs and symptoms are not uniformly present, the following are hallmarks of cardiac tamponade: muffled heart sounds due to both fluid in the pericardial sac and decreased strength of contractions, distended neck veins secondary to decreased cardiac filling, paradoxical pulse-enhanced cardiac filling due to increased intrathoracic pressure during expiration, and decreased systolic pulse pressure while diastolic pressure remains stable. A diagnostic central venous pressure measurement is one of the few procedures in which a central catheter placement is highly beneficial to the trauma patient. When the index of suspicion is high, pericardial aspiration should be attempted both to confirm the diagnosis and to relieve the tamponade while a patient is moved to the operating room.

Once in the operating room, a subxiphoid incision is made under local anesthesia. Dissection is carried above the diaphragm to visualize the pericardial sac. The sac is grasped with two Allis clamps and opened to relieve the tamponade. General anesthesia is then induced.

The vasodilatory effects of general anesthesia can produce such a profound decrease in afterload that cardiac arrest (decreased coronary perfusion during diastole) may ensue if the tamponade has not been decompressed. Especially in gunshot wounds, but also in stab wounds and blunt trauma, the possibility exists that the etiology of the cardiac tamponade is a large hole in the myocardium. Relieving the pressure by the creation of a subxiphoid window may result in acute, profound blood loss. The surgical team should be ready and the patient prepared and draped so that anesthesia can be rapidly induced, the sternum opened to access the myocardium, and any exsanguinating hemorrhage following the opening of the pericardial sac checked by a finger in place.

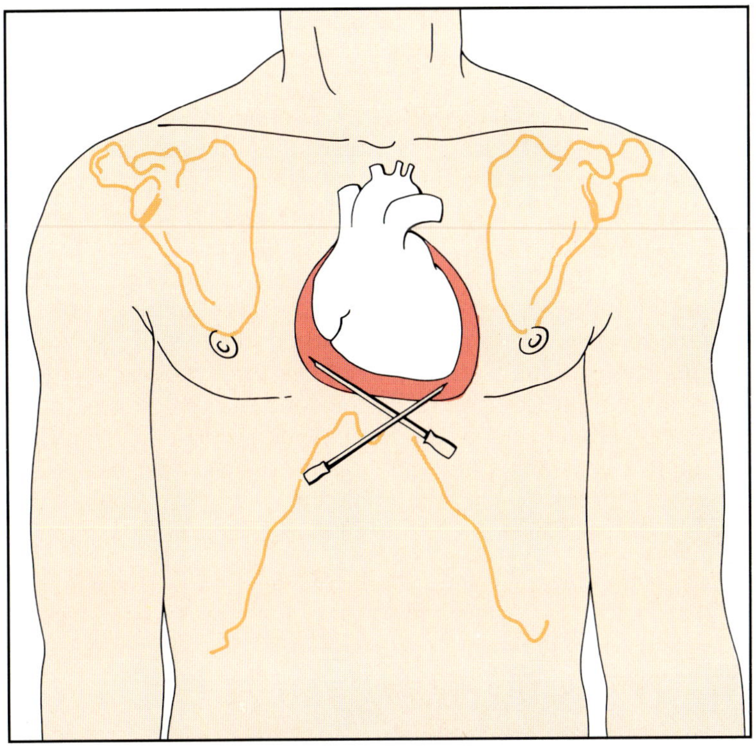

FIGURE 4.34 The needle can be directed toward the left scapular tip to encounter the pericardial sac where the fluid should be the thickest or toward the right scapula to skim between the sac and the myocardium.

BECK'S TRIAD

- Distended neck veins
- Muffled heart sounds
- Hypotension

PROCEDURE FOR PERICARDIOCENTESIS

After preparing the subxiphoid and epigastric areas and anesthetizing the skin with local anesthesia (if time permits), a long spinal needle with the "V-lead" attached with an alligator clip is connected to a 10-ml syringe and advanced at 90° to the patient until the tip of the needle is posterior to the sternum (Fig. 4.33). At this point, the needle is advanced at a 45° angle to the patient cephalad and posteriorly, either toward the tip of the right scapula or to the tip of the left scapula (Fig. 4.34). Proponents of the right scapular approach feel that the pericardium will be entered and the point of the needle will traverse parallel to the myocardium for a greater distance than if aimed directly at the apex. Proponents of the left scapular approach believe that there is less chance of missing the pericardial sac, and that with the pericardium distended with blood the distance between the myocardium and pericardial sac will be great enough to allow aspiration of the fluid without damage to the heart itself.

When the tip of the needle is advanced into the myocardium, an ischemic ST segment change on the ECG identifies that the myocardium has been touched (Fig. 4.35). Backing the needle out until the current of injury reverses itself (1 mm to 2 mm) will ensure that the tip of the needle is within the pericardial sac and not inside the ventricle. Aspiration of blood at this point will decompress the pericardial tamponade. Some feel the use of ECG is unnecessary, since once the pericardium is perforated, the rush of blood and positive response of the blood pressure and pulse are adequate signs of the needle's proper position. Preferably, a sheath-over-stylette-type needle is used so that the sheath can be left in place and aspiration can be repeated if necessary, through a three-way stopcock while en route to the operating room. This procedure is relatively innocuous and should be used early when the diagnosis of pericardial tamponade is suspected.

It is not a technique which is 100% accurate, however. Trinkle and associates found false-negative or false-positive results in 12 of 47 patients in which the technique was attempted.[72] A clot within the pericardial sac was to blame for up to 50% of the false-negative results.

A markedly distended abdomen is an obvious sign of intra-abdominal injury in an otherwise stable patient. The pericardium can be accessed transdiaphragmatically for a diagnostic tap.[16] After the abdomen is evaluated and the hemorrhage controlled, the triangular ligament of the liver is taken down through the tendinous portion of the diaphragm in the midline, and the pericardial sac is exposed and opened. Retraction downward on the tendinous portion with Allis clamps protects the heart as this area is sharply incised. If pathology is present after evacuation, the midline abdominal incision can be extended upward in a mediastinotomy to access the heart and make appropriate repairs.

Myocardial Compression

Borch reported in 1676 a child with a suspected myocardial contusion. In 1859 a similar patient was autopsied and found to have multiple epicardial hemorrhages.[7]

ETIOLOGY

In a frontal impact collision the heart can be compressed, caught between the sternum and steering wheel in front, and the continued motion of the vertebral column and posterior thoracic wall behind. Forces in the range of 5000 foot-pounds have been recorded (only 40 to 50 pounds of force are required to compress the sternum 1 1/2 to 2 inches in standard CPR). In actuality it is amazing that the heart is not damaged more often than it is. In 10% to 15% of motor vehicle accident deaths, the myocardium is contused.

The points of contact on the anterior myocardium are the right ventricle, the septum, and the left anterior descending coronary artery. Posteriorly there is the left ventricle. All of these components are vulnerable to injury. Although the left anterior descending artery is in the direct pathway of myocardial compression, direct damage to the vessel does not seem to produce enough spasm to cause dysrhythmias.[5,36]

PATHOPHYSIOLOGY

Two conditions have been described.[64] In cardiac concussion, dysrhythmias are the only indication of cardiac injury. Actual myocardial damage practically does not exist, since there is no CK-MB isoenzyme evaluation indicating muscular injury. Myocardial contusion is actual contusion, intercellular and intracellular hemorrhage, myofibril disruption, and other pathophysiology of compressive damage. Depending on the energy absorbed, the damaged area can be partial thickness or full thickness, and involve a small or large segment of the myocardial wall. Since the damage is usually limited to extravasation of blood and myofibril damage, rather than interruption of major vascular supply, the myocardium can repair itself. It does not carry the long-term disability of a myocardial infarction, when this section of the heart would actually be devascularized and ischemic.

Stein and co-workers reported that animals that survived the ordinarily fatal arrhythmia of experimentally induced cardiac contusion immediately after impact showed functional impairment that was only moderate.[56] The exact pathophysiology of myocardial compression is not well known. The majority of patients with this syndrome neither die nor have thoracotomies, and its seriousness generally corresponds to the size and depth of muscular damage. As in any traumatized body tissue, however, scarring can develop to the point of causing paradoxical movement of the injured segment. As the condition progresses, interstitial and cellular edema can develop and produce a progression of symptoms. As with pulmonary contusion, the damage present in the first hour following the trauma may only be the tip of the iceberg. Cellular swelling, leaky capillaries, and fluid accumula-

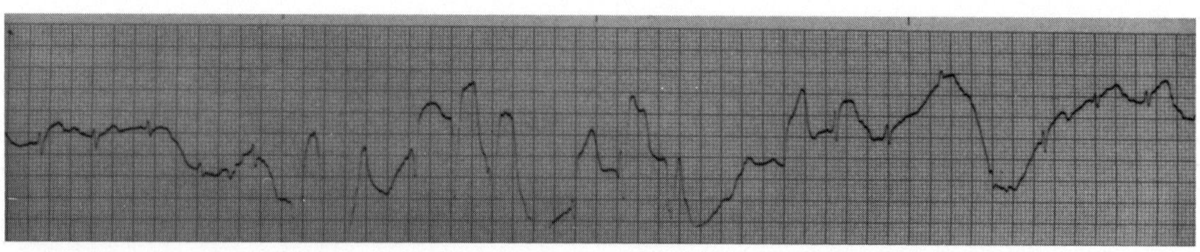

FIGURE 4.35 With the "V" electrode of the ECG attached to the needle, a normal sinus pattern is seen until the myocardium is touched with the needle. A sudden and immediate ST segment change is apparent.

tion can compromise oxygen influx into the tissue and produce delayed localized anaerobic metabolism and cellular failure.

A seldom-reported complication is pulmonary emboli secondary to ventricle wall thrombus; two recent patients have been reported at Charity Hospital in New Orleans.[65] Many mural thrombi go undiagnosed because they do not produce emboli. Emboli have not been associated with this problem in the literature. When a post-trauma patient develops post-embolus, the contused myocardium should be investigated as a possible source.

DIAGNOSIS

Because symptoms may develop late as edema further compromises the initial contused area, the examining physician should suspect that myocardial compression has occurred. Prompting this suspicion is a moderate- to high-speed frontal impact; a bent steering wheel; bull's-eye fracture of the windshield over the steering column (Fig. 4.36), indicating the point of impact of the head and the vulnerable position of the chest; central circular sternal contusion, identifying the impact of the steering column; or a knee impact area on the dash. The patient should be hospitalized for 48 to 72 hours for continuous ECG monitoring, serial enzyme studies every 6 to 8 hours, and two-dimensional echocardiography.

Dysrhythmias Ventricular fibrillation is the most frequent dysrhthymia that occurs at the scene of the accident, and it causes death in many patients before they reach the hospital. Although speculation and animal research bear this out, the exact statistics are almost impossible to attain, since very few patients are wearing Holter monitors at the time of impact.[32,45,47,61] Tachycardia that is inappropriate, unrelated to blood loss, and does not resolve once the initial "fright" of the situation is over, is probably the most common dysrhythmia seen. Premature ventricular contractions, both multifocal and frequent, are extremely common, along with atrial fibrillation. ST segment change and bundle branch block, usually on the right, are other ECG changes that are frequently seen in myocardial compression injuries.[23,35,74]

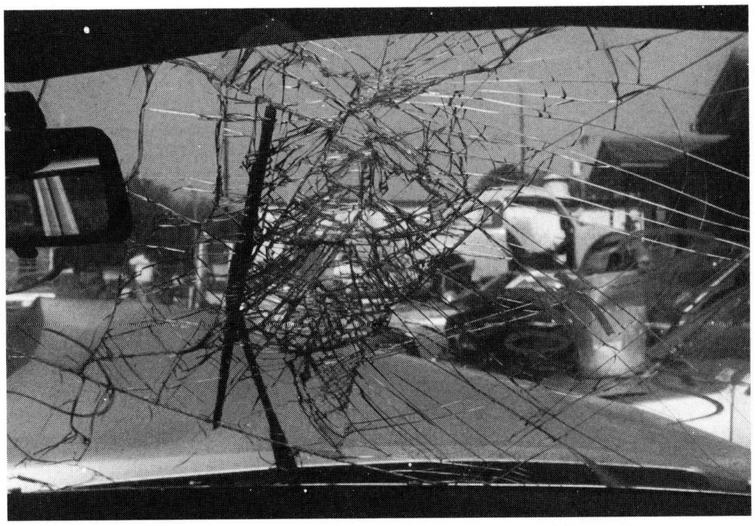

FIGURE 4.36 Bull's-eye fracture of the windshield indicates the point of head contact. If this is located directly above the steering wheel, chest impact into the steering column should be expected.

Enzymes The extensive muscular damage that occurs in blunt trauma will elevate creatine kinase (CK) enzymes. Fractionation of the MB bands in which these are elevated, or represent greater than 5% of the total CK elevation, signifies damage to the muscle itself.

Two-dimensional echocardiography obtained 24 hours after the injury can be an extremely important diagnostic tool in evaluating abnormal ventricular and septal-wall patterns. The diagnostic parameters with two-dimensional echocardiography that are helpful in identifying cardiac contusion are generalized or segmental right ventricle dilatation, localized myocardial thinning, generalized or segmental wall motion abnormalities, fibrinous pericardial effusion, ruptured chordae tendineae and flail leaflet, and aneurysm of sinus of Valsalva.[35] It is also an important tool for identifying mural thrombi and thereby the need for anticoagulant therapy. Miller and co-workers found mural thrombi in five of seven patients with myocardial contusion.[61]

Nuclear scans and other tests have been advocated as helpful in identifying myocardial contusion. Potkin and colleagues felt that "non-invasive abnormalities were nonspecific and did not reflect myocardial contusion which led to clinically important cardiac complications." However, their reliability is such that the three major tests, ECG, CK-MB, and two-dimensional echocardiography, can pick up most of the injuries in patients with significant myocardial damage without relying on other studies.[45]

MANAGEMENT

Patients who are suspected of having myocardial compression damage on initial presentation to the emergency department should be hospitalized and monitored for 48 to 72 hours while diagnostic studies are obtained. Dysrhythmias are managed with the usually cardiac regimes, as the specific rhythm dictates. Maintenance of a high F_1O_2 protects cells with decreased profusion and decreased oxygen exchange secondary to edema. Patients with mural thrombi should be under prophylactic anticoagulation therapy unless contraindicated by some other traumatic injury.

Hemothorax

ETIOLOGY

Penetrating injuries into any major blood vessel including the pulmonary artery, pulmonary vein, intercostal artery, aorta, or heart are associated with hemorrhage into the thoracic cavity. A missile that has penetrated the diaphragm or a neck vessel such as the subclavian artery or vein, carotid or innominate artery, vena cava, or jugular vein can produce minimal to massive amounts of hemorrhaging into the pleural cavity.

Blunt compression injuries to the ribs can lacerate intercostal arteries or pulmonary vessels and produce an accumulation of blood in the thoracic cavity. Deceleration injuries to the aorta frequently exsanguinate into the pleural cavity; these patients, however, do not reach the hospital. Hemorrhage into the mediastinum and above the lung, creating a pleural cavity, are considerations when evaluating patients with a hemothorax. Blunt abdominal trauma can rupture the diaphragm while producing intra-abdominal hemorrhage, from which blood can seep into the chest to produce a hemothorax.

PATHOPHYSIOLOGY

Hemorrhage into the chest produces not only hemodynamic compromise (hypovolemia), but also ventilatory compromise as the lung on the affected side is compressed. However, blood loss, even up to 3 to 4 liters within one thoracic cavity, is of much greater clinical significance in the healthy trauma patient than is the loss of effectively ventilated lung tissue.

DIAGNOSIS

Physical diagnosis with percussion and auscultation can demonstrate a large hemothorax, but is ineffective in identifying a smaller one. Usually, clinical suspicion of pulmonary pathology and insertion of a chest tube is the method of identifying hemothorax in the severely injured trauma patient. In a patient with minor injuries, a chest film is often obtained before the chest tube is inserted. Differentiation between pulmonary contusion and a hemothorax is usually difficult in the supine AP film, but becomes apparent as the fluid layers out either in the upright or the lateral decubitus x-ray. Previous pulmonary injury and adhesions of the parietal to visceral pleura can make the identification of a hemothorax difficult at times (Fig. 4.37), since the blood does not layer out against the diaphragm as one would expect.

MANAGEMENT

A hemothorax is most often self-limiting and requires nothing more than the insertion of a chest tube and replacement of lost blood. However, if blood loss continues at a rate greater than 200 ml/hr up to a total of 1500 ml, or if blood loss is more than 1000 ml when the chest tube is initially inserted, operative intervention is indicated. A thoracoscopy is an excellent diagnostic and therapeutic step for checking hemorrhage status, locating its source, and possibly controlling it with electrocoagulation, without the increased morbidity associated with a thoracotomy.[24]

Once a decision has been made to open the chest, appropriate steps to control hemorrhage, from the ligation of intercostal arteries to a pulmonary resection, may be required.

Before starting a thoracotomy in the multiply traumatized patient, the clinician should ascertain whether the hemothorax is being produced by intra-abdominal hemorrhage associated with a diaphragmatic rupture. In a patient with a markedly distended abdomen, a grossly positive peritoneal tap, or other signs of major intra-abdominal hemorrhage, the abdomen should be opened unless cross-clamping the aorta is required. The indication for a thoracotomy before laparotomy is intra-abdominal hemorrhage, blood pressure of less than 70 mm Hg, and tachycardia in the operating room.[79] In this instance the chest should be opened first, the aorta cross-clamped, aggressive resuscitation with whole blood begun, and the abdomen then opened. A patient with hemothorax is ideal for autotransfusion, as demonstrated by Peter Symbas in his initial work in the late 1960s at Grady Hospital in Atlanta, in which he reintroduced autotransfusion in the care of the trauma patient.[61]

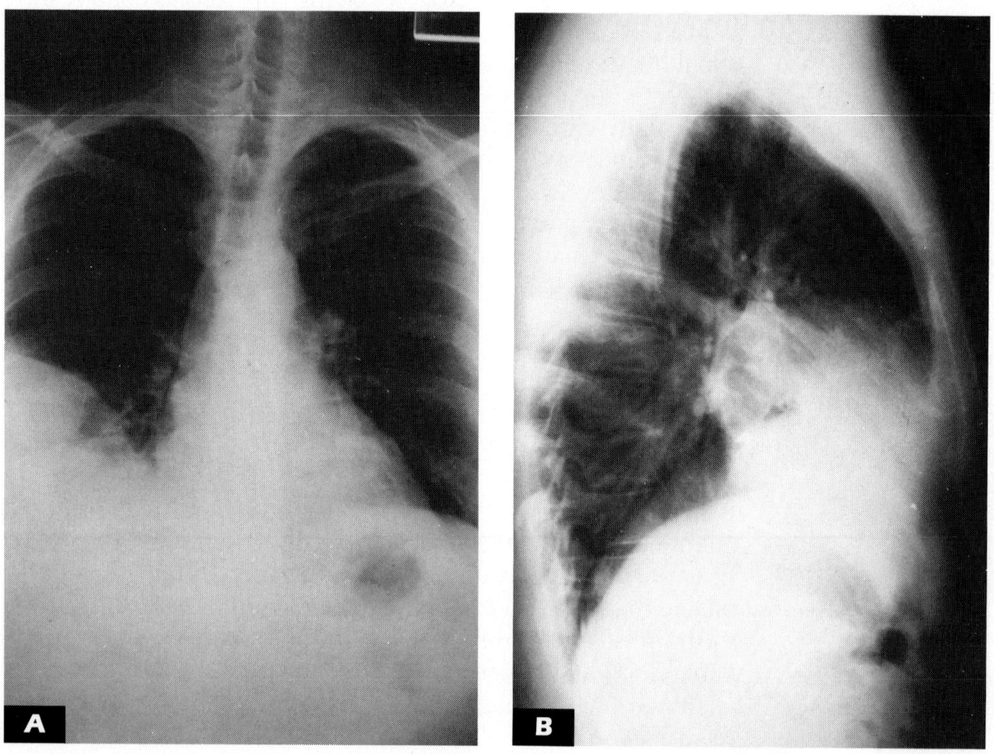

FIGURE 4.37 Hemorrhage into a loculated space can produce a hemothorax that does not layer out, is difficult to aspirate, and resolves very slowly.

Aortic Shearing Injury

ETIOLOGY

The descending aorta is tightly attached to the posterior abdominal wall just distal to the arch through the diaphragm. Proximal to this point, including the arch, the ascending aorta and the heart, there is only a tenuous attachment. Any situation that produces an acute change in motion or direction of the thoracic cavity can produce shear forces on the aorta. With rapid deceleration during a frontal impact collision, or rapid acceleration during a lateral impact collision, the descending aorta moves with the body while the arch, ascending aorta, and heart do not. These components move only when dragged along by the descending aorta or when stopped by it. Shear forces create tremendous stress on the areas of the ligamentum arteriosum, just distal to the arch, or between the left subclavian and left carotid arteries. A tearing of the aorta results.

PATHOPHYSIOLOGY

Exsanguination into the thoracic cavity because of a total loss of continuity of the thoracic aorta occurs, according to Parmley, in approximately 80% of the cases, with these patients dying within the first hour after impact.[43] Twenty percent of the patients will survive the first hour because the hemorrhage is contained within the adventitia, avoiding immediate exsanguination. Of these, approximately one third will exsanguinate within the first 6 hours, another one third within 24 hours, and the final one third may survive for 3 days or longer.

DIAGNOSIS

A high index of suspicion is necessary when such forces are involved in automotive trauma. Definitive diagnosis can be made only with aortography. Some centers advocate aortography on every patient in whom the mechanism of injury is sufficient to produce such trauma. Others rely on a high index of suspicion produced by the mechanism of injury, and use aortography whenever any of the eight major signs of possible injury are visible on the chest film (Fig. 4.38).[10,34,58,59] These signs are extremely subtle and must be specifically kept in mind when the chest film is examined. The most reliable of these signs is the first one, widening of the mediastinum.[34]

CHEST X-RAY FINDINGS INDICATING POSSIBLE AORTIC TEAR

- Widening of the mediastinum
- Blurring of the aortic knob
- Left pulmonary cap
- Deviation of the trachea to the right
- Deviation of the esophagus to the right (NG tube)
- Angle of the left main-stem bronchus greater than 140°
- Obliteration of the pulmonary aortic window
- Fracture of the first and second ribs

MANAGEMENT

Repair of the thoracic aorta with an interposition prosthetic graft should be instituted as soon as possible. A cardiopulmonary bypass is in general not required. Controversy exists as to whether repair should be accomplished by cross-clamping the aorta and rapidly replacing the damaged segment, or by a Gott shunt. The major institutions report an approximate 1% chance of paraplegia resulting with either approach.[75] Since paraplegia is a major complication in a patient with a successful repair, the experienced trauma surgeon should use the technique with which he is most familiar and deems most appropriate.

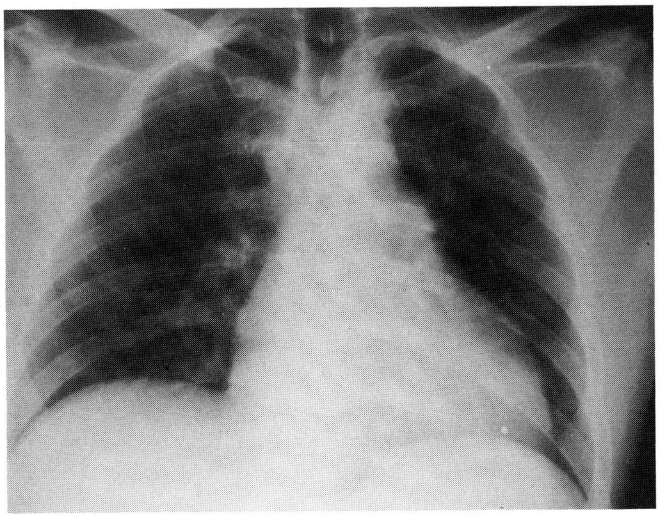

FIGURE 4.38 Five of the classic eight findings that identify a thoracic aortic tear are visible on this film. They were missed when the patient was initially seen in the emergency department.

Pulmonary Contusion

ETIOLOGY

Contusion injury to the lung is produced by an intrusion into the thoracic cavity as ribs are pushed in by frontal or lateral impact. Pulmonary contusion can also be produced by a sudden overpressure through the nose and mouth in a blast situation, when the body does not have an opportunity to equalize and compensate. A scuba diver, commercial diver, or a patient undergoing hyperbaric oxygen therapy may sustain tremendous pulmonary pressures, but slow enough equalization inside the vascular compartment and pleural space does not cause injuries to the lung. Sudden decompression in such a situation, however, can produce an acute underpressure that has similar pathophysiologic consequences.

PATHOPHYSIOLOGY

Initial injuries to the alveolar linings, pulmonary capillaries, and parenchyma of the lung are localized hemorrhage and cellular disruption. They are the results of the compression and stretching associated with a penetrating injury, blast, or motor vehicle accident. Edema develops both within the cell and within the interstitial space over the next 6 to 12 hours. This edema additionally compromises the oxygenation of the cells, both from decreased perfusion and decreased ability of the oxygen molecules to cross through the edema to red cells, leading to anaerobic metabolism within the cells. (See also discussion on flail chest.)

DIAGNOSIS

On the initial chest film increased opacification will be seen around the bruised lung from automotive trauma, surrounding the point of penetration from gunshot, or bilaterally with blast injury (Figs. 4.39 and 4.40). As edema increases over several hours following trauma, this pulmonary opacification will become more dense and more widespread.

Moist rales on auscultation and bloody nasotracheal secretions alert the physician on initial physical examination that pulmonary contusion is a significant possibility.

MANAGEMENT

A patient with initially compromised pulmonary functions has increased pulmonary compliance and arterial blood gas of less than 60 mm Hg on room air or less than 80 mm Hg on an F_1O_2 of 0.04 intubation. PEEP and IMV are the treatment of choice. Weaning should occur as the patient's pulmonary compliance and blood gas return toward normal, between 3 to 10 days on the ventilator. If a patient's initial pulmonary values are not compromised, it is debatable whether the patient should be put on prophylactic IMV and PEEP, or only observed and ventilated if conditions warrant. Proponents of prophylactic IMV and PEEP argue that although not all patients require it, those that do will have their hospitalization and their time on the ventilator significantly shortened if managed early. If, on the other hand, the situation is allowed to deteriorate first, time on the ventilator will be increased from 48 to 72 hours to 10 to 14 days.

Proponents of observational management contend that the unnecessary costs incurred by the use of ventilatory support in patients who do not require it offsets the savings for those who do. Until prospective random studies are available to answer these questions, the trauma surgeon must follow his or her own best clinical judgment. In one study on animals, 1 hour of mechanical ventilation, beginning 1 hour after injury, reduced the rate of mortality to 20%, while in animals that did not receive the treatment it was 80%.[49] Rutherford and Velenta felt that mechanical ventilation impeded and reversed the pulmonary edema and thereby prevented a diffuse consolidation of the lung tissue.

Traumatic Diaphragmatic Herniations

ETIOLOGY

The abdominal cavity is a closed container, well protected anteriorly by the rectus abdominis and the posterior and anterior rectus sheaths, laterally by the external and internal obliques and the transversus abdominis and its associated investing fascia, posteriorly by vertebral column and psoas, and inferiorly by the pelvis and muscles of the pelvic floor and perineum. Superiorly,

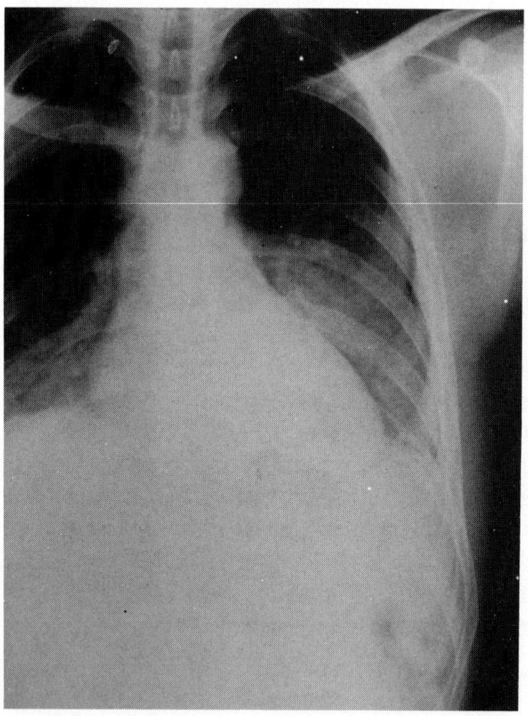

FIGURE 4.39 Pulmonary contusion resulting from blunt trauma can be seen on the initial chest film.

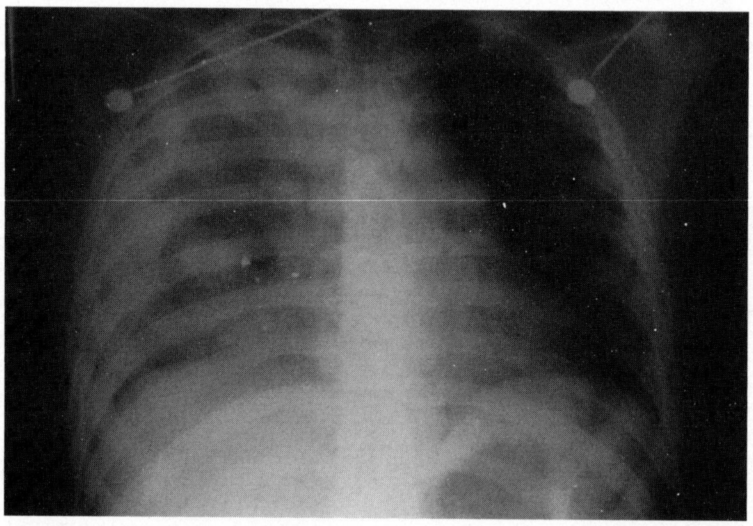

FIGURE 4.40 Pulmonary contusion from penetrating trauma surrounds the point of penetration and represents the extent of cavitation injury.

protection is provided only by the 5-mm diaphragm, which has a supporting fascia only on its periphery.

Increased intra-abdominal pressure produced by compression in a frontal or lateral impact collision suddenly forces the abdominal contents against the walls of the abdomen. Because of its comparative weakness, the diaphragm is most likely to rupture. Early studies into this problem reported most ruptures (in excess of 80%) occurred on the left. This was thought to be due to the protective influence of the liver on the right.[39] However, Waldschmidt and Laws identified that an equal number occurred on the left and the right.[76] The apparent disparity in these two reports probably relates to the difficulty in making the diagnosis on the right from the chest film alone. Proper identification needs to be done in the operating room or on the autopsy table.

PATHOPHYSIOLOGY

Acute symptoms, when they occur, are produced when a large amount of the contents of the abdominal cavity is forced into the thoracic cavity and compromises ventilation. A delayed presentation of strangulated bowel or intestinal obstruction can occur from months to years after the initial trauma because it went unrecognized and produced no symptoms during the latent period.

The problem of diaphragmatic herniation in penetrating trauma has been infrequently highlighted. A recent animal study has shown that a small laceration of the diaphragm left untreated produces almost 100% diaphragmatic herniation with a mortality rate in excess of 50%.[66] These lacerations usually go undetected when associated with a stab wound of the chest, which produces no early interabdominal symptomatology. However, the long-term effect in the human has not been identified in the literature.

Contrasted with the 1-cm to 2-cm laceration in penetrating trauma, a 10-cm tear in blunt trauma allows abdominal contents immediate entry into the thoracic cavity. Then more of the gastrointestinal (GI) tract will be drawn into the cavity by negative intrathoracic pressure and a continued pressure differential between the abdominal and thoracic cavities.

On the right, the liver is large enough to prevent herniation of the small or large intestines through the defect in the diaphragm. Only the liver protrudes through, and unless the liver tissue is injured and bleeds, or the rent is large enough to appear on x-ray film, such an injury will only be apparent at the time of autopsy, thoracotomy, or thoracostomy.

DIAGNOSIS

The acutely injured patient is seen in the emergency department. Abdominal contents producing unusual gas patterns from the small or large intestines, or an unusually dense profile of the spleen in the chest film will identify the presence of a diaphragmatic injury (Fig. 4.41). If the stomach is in the defect, the nasogastric tube present in the thoracic cavity may provide a clue. Definitive diagnosis, short of emergency surgery for other reasons, can be made from a barium contrast study of the GI tract (Fig. 4.42). Comparison views of earlier chest films (if available) may identify a change in the contour of the diaphragm on the right. Otherwise, the diagnosis is extremely difficult to make in the asymptomatic patient.

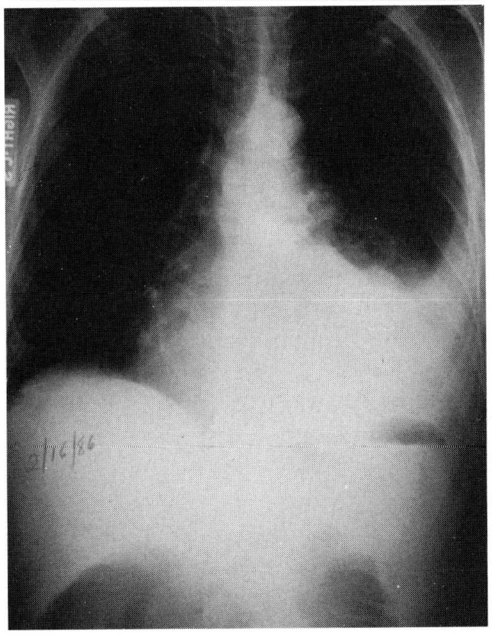

FIGURE 4.41 A diaphragmatic hernia on the left is much easier to identify than on the right because of the small volume of contents present above the diaphragm.

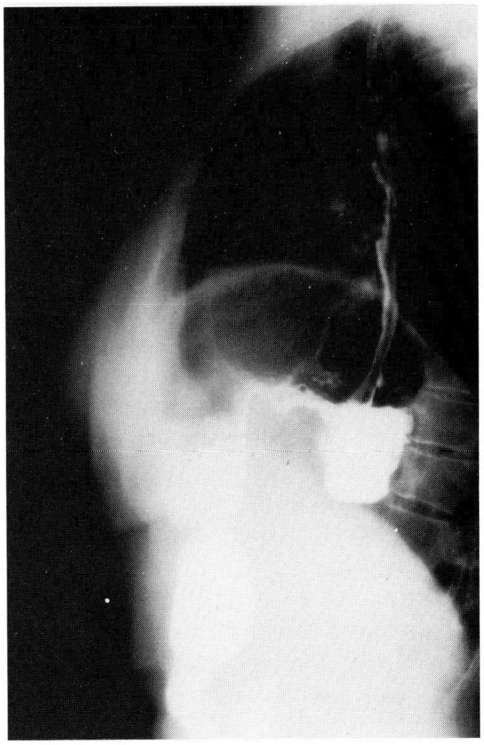

FIGURE 4.42 Barium in the GI tract may be required to differentiate a diaphragmatic hernia from an acutely contused lung.

MANAGEMENT

The diaphragmatic hernia is best repaired from the abdominal approach. Repairs of the frequently associated injuries of abdominal organs are much easier from below, as is investigation of the entire abdominal cavity for other pathology. Exploratory laparotomy for blunt trauma of the abdomen obviously includes evaluation of such retroperitoneal structures as the pancreas and duodenum, which are virtually impossible to reach effectively through the thorax. Repair of the diaphragm done with interrupted nonabsorbable sutures can be accomplished as easily from below as above.

If a thoracic incision has already been made, the repair can be accomplished transthoracically. However, because of the tremendous force that is required to rupture the diaphragm and the real possibility of injuring intra-abdominal organs, an exploratory laparotomy should also be performed. Moreover, it is extremely difficult to explore the pancreas, duodenum, liver, and kidneys through the diaphragm from the thoracic approach.

Rib Fracture

Compression of the rib beyond its tensile strength produces an isolated fracture. It can occur in automotive trauma, contact sports, martial arts, street fights, or even spontaneously with severe coughing.

PATHOPHYSIOLOGY

The fractured rib produces pain on respiration and in response, the patient spontaneously decreases ventilation in this section of the thoracic wall. The alveolar bronchial stasis produces an accumulation of secretions that will lead to atelectasis and pneumonia if not cleared.

DIAGNOSIS

The multiple rib fractures of the flail chest are frequently difficult to identify. A singular nondisplaced rib fracture is even more difficult. In order to identify a fracture on film, the x-rays themselves must pass through the fracture parallel to its fissure. If the film is not aligned exactly right, the fracture will not be identified (Fig. 4.43). Multiple views are required, and even then are frequently unreliable. Obtaining rib views to identify a fractured rib is generally a waste of time and money. The identification of the fractured rib is a clinical one based on physical examination. The point of maximal tenderness of the rib is identified by palpation. The body of the rib is then followed proximal and distal to the fracture and pressure applied at least 5 cm away. If this pressure produces pain at the site of the suspected rib fracture, then a fractured rib is presumed to be present.

MANAGEMENT

The principle of fracture management is bone immobilization. However, taping a fractured rib to provide this immobilization is one of the worst things that can be done, as this promotes pulmonary stasis, atelectasis, and the development of pneumonia. The management of a fractured rib is pain suppression, usually a codeine-containing compound will suffice.

Esophageal Laceration/Penetration

ETIOLOGY

Penetrating injuries that cross the midline can damage the esophagus.[44] Such injuries are likely to be through-and-through lacerations, but they can also pass between the trachea and the esophagus to produce a tracheoesophageal fistula.

Blunt trauma is rare because the esophagus is relatively soft and pliable and is protected in the lower half of the chest by the heart, and in the upper half by the trachea and other mediastinal structures. However, in 1980 Layton, DiMarco, and Pellegrini found 34 cases of tracheoesophageal fistulae in the literature since the first reported case in 1936.[29] The mechanism of injury, as they described it, is compression of the trachea onto the esophagus by the sternum in front and the vertebral column in back. Laceration of the membranous trachea should seal rapidly. However, the contusion of the anterior wall of the esophagus may develop an infection, with a fistula becoming apparent 4 to 5 days later. The anterior wall, because of the compromised blood supply, will probably rupture. Fistulas not identified until many years after the blunt trauma have been reported.

PATHOPHYSIOLOGY

Rupture of the esophagus into the mediastinum, if unrepaired and undrained, produces marked inflammation which will indurate the entire mediastinum if identified early, or develop into mediastinitis and gross abscess if overlooked.

The injury usually becomes clinically apparent 3 to 5 days after the initial trauma, as the infection produces a persistent elevated temperature and an abnormal chest film.

DIAGNOSIS

Physical findings are pneumothorax, pneumomediastinum (visualized on the chest film), subcutaneous emphysema, leucocytosis, hydrothorax, and elevated temperature. If the injury is high in the chest, neck tenderness and inflammation in the lower neck may be palpable.

Any patient with a gunshot wound or other penetrating injury crossing the midline should have either an immediate thoracotomy or detailed evaluation with a rigid esophagoscope, esophagogram, bronchoscopy, and perhaps even bronchogram. Thorascopic evaluation may also be helpful in delineating the pathway of the missile. Negative bronchoscopy and esophagography, however, do not completely rule out this lesion. A rigid esophagoscope better visualizes the mucosa, and is more effective in identifying a small laceration or hemorrhagic area, which might otherwise be missed.

MANAGEMENT

An early minimal perforation without inflammation and contamination may be treated with primary repair, an esophageal tube proximally and a gastrostomy distally for the diversion of GI contents along with adequate mediastinal drainage. The lack of serosa surrounding the esophagus, which is extremely protective in abdominal GI wounds, creates a greater propensity for leaking. If possible a surrogate serosa can be made by creating a parietal pleural flap (Fig. 4.44).

If there is any question about the viability of the esophagus due to contamination, late exploration, or presence of much devitalized tissue, the recommended procedure is a cervical esophagoscopy and gastrostomy with ligation of the distal esophagus, using two absorbable ligatures around the lower esophagus.[62]

Tracheal Laceration/Penetration

ETIOLOGY

Both the trachea and esophagus are well protected from blunt trauma on their anterior and lateral surfaces. However, the membranous portion is extremely susceptible to overpressure injuries, as well as compression. Penetrating trauma can produce either through-and-through lacerations or tangential ones, depending on the pathway of the missile. The pathway of the missile and the possibility of bronchial injuries must be considered when repairing pulmonary parenchyma.

PATHOPHYSIOLOGY

Positive-pressure ventilation will continue to force air into the free pleural cavity. A continuous pneumothorax may result from such a large leak that cannot be controlled even with two chest tubes.

DIAGNOSIS

Bronchoscopy is a useful technique to diagnosis tracheal injuries. However, unless the bronchial injuries are in the main-stem bronchus, it is difficult to visualize them even with the flexible bronchoscope. The diagnosis of a pneumothorax that does not resolve with a continuous large volume of air flow in both tubes is usually made by exclusion and with a high index of suspicion. A bronchogram may be helpful in establishing its exact location.

MANAGEMENT

Large tears of the distal bronchi may not be repairable without segmental or low resection of the involved portion of the bronchus. Proximal injuries to the trachea are repaired primarily with an endotracheal tube placed distal to the repair while it

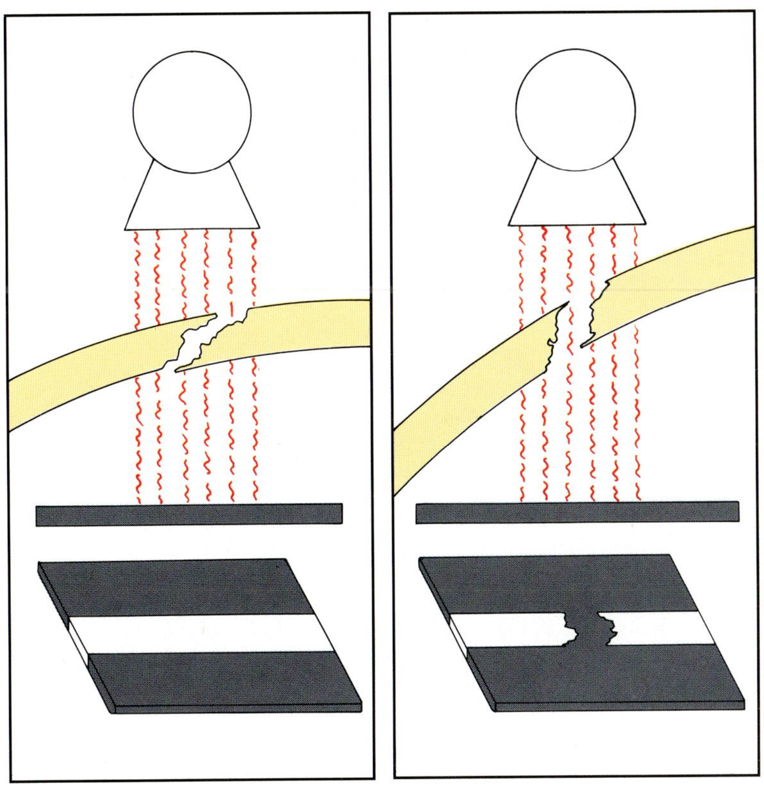

FIGURE 4.43 The standard AP or PA x-ray is a poor film with which to try to identify fractures of the rib. Rib detail films are most often a waste of time and money, since a rib fracture is a clinical diagnosis. Confirmatory films are not necessary. To identify a fracture in a well-aligned bone (as ribs often are), the rays from the tube must proceed parallel through the fracture line; otherwise, the fracture will probably not be visible.

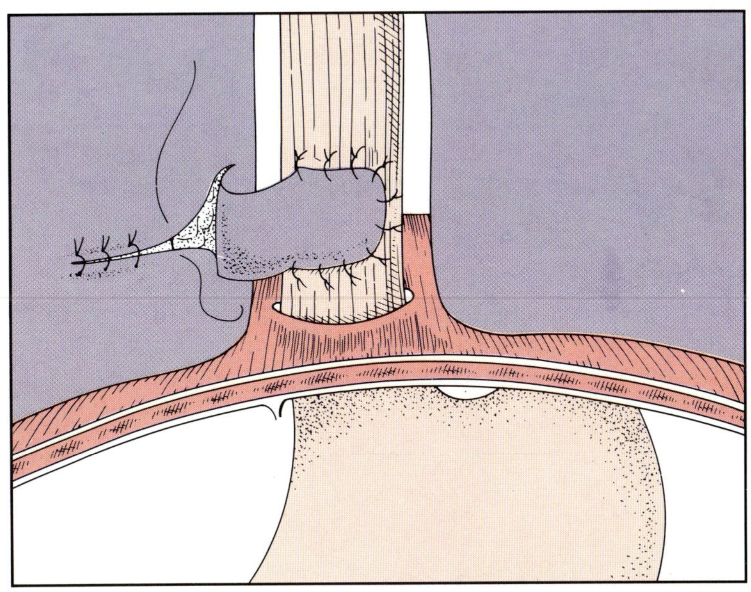

FIGURE 4.44 To provide serosa-like coverage of an esophageal injury, a pleural flap can be developed and sewn into place to assist in covering the defect.

heals. Injuries to the proximal main-stem bronchi produce the most difficulty, since positive-pressure breathing, coughing, other necessary techniques, or pulmonary toilet can produce overpressure and blow-up in these areas, with a high recurrence of bronchopleurocutaneous fistulas.

Air Embolism

ETIOLOGY

Simultaneous rupture of the trachea and an adjacent vessel, or laceration of the pulmonary parenchyma with a moderate-sized vessel and bronchus adjacent will allow air into the pulmonary venous system. Positive-pressure ventilation increases this possibility. None of the literature reports a very high incidence of such air emboli, perhaps due to a lack of sophistication in diagnosis. The close proximity to pulmonary veins and bronchi would make this condition seem extremely likely.

PATHOPHYSIOLOGY

A return to the heart through the pulmonary veins will block capillaries and small to moderate-sized vessels. If the blocked vessels lead to critical organs such as the brain or heart, ischemic pathology of these organs results.

DIAGNOSIS

Hemoptysis following trauma indicates that there is hemorrhage into the air-containing pleural tree. Visualization of air in a coronary artery or an arteriographic demonstration of a block is the only definitive diagnostic method at present. Central nervous system or cardiac abnormalities without other possible pathology are indicative, but not diagnostic.

MANAGEMENT

Management of such conditions is only possible through acute compression to 2 atmospheres with 100% oxygen as is available in the hyperbaric oxygen chamber unit.

REFERENCES

1. Abouhatem R, Hendrickx P, Titeca M: Thoracic epidural analgesia in the treatment of rib fractures. Acta Anaesthesiol Belg 35(Suppl): 271–275, 1984
2. Aegineta P: On Surgery, book VI, sec. xcvi. London Sydenham Society, 1843
3. Appenheimer L, Craven KD, Forkert L et al: Pathophysiology of pulmonary contusion in dogs. J Appl Psychol 47(4):718–728, 1979
4. Baylock A, Roberts NM: A consideration of the non-operative treatment of cardiac tamponade resulting from wounds of the heart. Surgery 14:157–163, 1943
5. Beckman DL, Friedman BA: Mechanics of cardiothoracic injury in primates. J Trauma 12(7):620–629, 1972
6. Billroth, Diechirurgieda, Bluntgefoss: Des Herenus, 295. Berlin, Hishwala, 1913
7. Borch A, in Halter BL: Nonpenetrating trauma to the heart. Am J Surg 70:237, 1955
8. Boudreaux JP, Bornside GH, Cohn I: Emergency autotransfusion: Partial cleansing of bacteria-laden blood by cell washing. J Trauma 23(1):31–35, 1983
9. Bugge-Asperheim B, Svennevig JL, Birkeland S: Haemodynamic and metabolic consequences of lung contusion following blunt chest trauma. Scand J Thorac Cardiovasc Surg 14(3)295–299, 1980
10. Burney RE, Gundry SR, Mackenzie JR et al: Comparison of mediastinal width mediastinal-thoracic and -cardiac ratios, and "mediastinal widening" in detection of traumatic aortic rupture. Ann Emerg Med 12(11):668–671, 1983
11. 2 Chron 18:33 (RSV)
12. Committee on Trauma, American College of Surgeons: Advanced Trauma Life Support Course, Chicago, 1985
13. Drichteau: J Arch Gen Med, series 4(4):334, 1844
14. Fackler ML: Physics of missile injury. In Kerstein MD, McSwain NE Jr (ed): The Evaluation and Management of Trauma. East Norwalk, CT, Appleton-Century-Crofts, 1986
15. Franbaugh RF, Elings VB, Christensen J: Determinants of pulmonary interstitial fluid accumulation after trauma. J Trauma 22(10): 820–826, 1982
16. Garrison RN, Richardson JD, Fry DE: Diagnostic transdiaphragmatic pericardiotomy in thoracoabdominal trauma. J Trauma 22(2): 147–149, 1982
17. Glover JL, Smith R, Yaw PB: Autotransfusion of blood contaminated by intestinal contents. JACEP 7:142–144, 1978
18. Grover FL, Richardson JD, Fewil JA et al: Prophylactic antibiotics in the treatment of penetrating chest wounds. J Thorac Cardiovasc Surg 74(4):528–536, 1977
19. Hankins, JR, Baekhyo S, McAslan C: Management of flail chest: An analysis of 99 cases. Am Surg 45:176–181, 1979
20. Hippocrates: The Aphorisms of Hippocrates, sec VI, XVIII. Coar T (trans): London, AJ Valpy, 1822
21. Hunter J: A Treatise on the Blood, Inflammation and Gunshot Wounds, 529–532. London, Richardson, 1794
22. John 19:35 (RSV)
23. Jones JW, Hewitt RL, Drapanas T: Cardiac contusion: A capricious syndrome. Ann Surg 181(5):567–574, 1975
24. Jones JW, Kitahama AK, Webb WR et al: A logical approach to chest trauma management. J Trauma 21:280–284, 1981
25. Just-Viera JO, Gonzalez A, Santiago-Delphin E: Glycerol and methlprendisolone in lung contusion. Am Surg 46(1):33–37, 1980
26. 2 Kings 9:21–24 (RSV)
27. Kouwenhoven WB, Jude JR, Knickerbocker GG: Closed-chest cardiac message. JAMA 173:1064–1067, 1960
28. Larrey DJ: Memoirs of Military Surgery. Willmott R (trans): Special edition by Classics of Surgery Library. Birmingham, AL, Joseph Cushing, 1985
29. Layton TR, DiMarco RF, Pellegrini RV: Tracheoesophageal fistual from nonpenetrating trauma. J Trauma 20(9):802–805, 1980
30. LeBlanc KA, Tucker WY: Prophylactic antibiotics and closed tube thoracostomy. Surg Gynecol Obstet 160:259–263, 1985
31. Lowe P: The whole course of chirurgerie. In Purfott T: Wounds of the Thorax, chap XI. London, 1597
32. Louhimo I: Heart Injury after Blunt Thoracic Trauma: An Experimental Study of Rabbits. Helsinki, Oy Weilin & Goos Ab, Tapiola, 1967
33. Mandal AK, Montano J, Thadepalli H: Prophylactic antibiotics and no antibiotics compared in penetrating chest trauma. J Trauma 25:639–643, 1985
34. Marnocha KE, Maglinte DD, Woods J et al: Blunt chest trauma and suspected aortic rupture: Reliability of chest radiograph findings. Ann Emerg Med 14(7):644–649, 1985
35. Miller FA Jr, Seward JB, Gersh BJ et al: Two-dimensional echocardiographic findings in cardiac trauma. Am J of Cardiol 50(5):1022–1027, 1982
36. Miller MS, Scott FC: Cardiac contusion and right bundle branch block. JACEP 6(11):504–505, 1977
37. Moore BP: Operative stabilization of nonpenetrating chest injuries. J Thorac Cardiovasc Surg 70(4):619–630, 1975
38. Morgagni JB: The Seats and Causes of Diseases Investigated by

Anatomy, book II:Letter the fifteenth. Alexanderus B (trans): London, Millar and Cadell, 1769
39. Morley JE: Traumatic diaphragmatic rupture. S Afr Med J 48:325, 1974
40. McSwain NE Jr: Motor vehicle occupant kinematics and injury patterns. American Association for Automotive Medicine Quarterly 3:31–33, 1981
41. McSwain NE Jr: Resuscitation. In Kerstein MD, McSwain NE Jr (eds): The Evaluation and Management of Trauma. East Norwalk, CT, Appleton-Century-Crofts, 1987
42. National Council, National Academy of Sciences: Accidental Death and Disability: The Neglected Disease of Modern Society. Rockville, MD, US Dept of Health, Education, and Welfare, 1966
43. Parmley LF, Mattingly TW, Manion WC et al: Nonpenetrating trauma of the aorta. Circulation 17:1086–1101, 1958
44. Popovsky J: Perforations of the esophagus from gunshot wounds. J Trauma 24(4):337–339, 1984
45. Potkin RT, Werner JA, Trobaugh GB et al: Evaluation on noninvasive tests of cardiac damage in suspected cardiac contusion. Circulation 66(3):627–631, 1982
46. Reynolds M, Jones JW: CPK-MB isoenzyme determinations in blunt chest trauma. JACEP 8(8):304–306, 1979
47. Richardson JD, Adams L, Flint LM: Selective management of flail chest and pulmonary contusion. Ann Surg 196(4):481–487, 1982
48. Richardson JD, Woods D, Johnson WG Jr et al: Lung bacterial clearance following pulmonary contusion. Surgery 86(5):730–735, 1979
49. Rutherford RD, Velenta J: An experimental study of trauma wet lung. J Trauma 11:146, 1971
50. 1 Sam 31:3–5 (RSV)
51. 2 Sam 18:14 (RSV)
52. Shackford SR, Smith DE, Azrins CK et al: The management of flail chest: A comparison of ventilatory and nonventilatory treatment. Am J Surg 132:759–762, 1976
53. Shackford SR, Virgilio RW, Peters RM: Selective use of ventilator therapy in flail chest injury. J Thorac Cardiovasc Surg 81(2):194–201, 1981
54. Slay D, Slay E, Luehrs JG: Transient ST elevation associated with tension pneumothorax. JACEP 8(1):16–18, 1979
55. Smith E: The Edwin Smith Papyrus. Special Edition of Classics of Surgery Library. Birmingham, AL, Joseph Cushing, 1985
56. Stein PD, Sabbah HN, Viano DC et al: Response of the heart in nonpenetrating cardiac trauma. J Trauma 22(5):364–73, 1982
57. Stone HH, Symbas PN, Hooper CA: Cefamandole for prophylaxis against infection in closed tube thoracotomy. J Trauma 21:957–977, 1981
58. Strum JT, Olson FR, Cicero JJ: Chest roentgenographic findings in twenty-six patients with traumatic rupture of the thoracic aorta. Ann Emerg Med 12(10):598–600, 1983
59. Strum JT, Perry JF, Olson FR: Significance of symptoms and signs in patients with traumatic aortic rupture. Ann Emerg Med 13(10):876–878, 1984
60. Sugg WL, REA WJ, Ecker RR et al: Penetrating wounds of the heart: Analysis of 459 cases. J Thorac Cardiovasc Surg 56:531–543, 1968
61. Symbas PN: Fundamentals of clinical cardiology. Am Heart J 92(3):387–396, 1976
62. Symbas PN, Hatcher CR Jr, Vlasis SE: Esophageal gunshot injuries. Ann Surg 191(6):703–707, 1980
63. Taylor GA, Miller HA, Shulman HS et al: Controversies in the management of pulmonary contusion. Can J Surg 25(2):167–170, 1982
64. Tenzer ML: The spectrum of myocardial contusion: A review. J Trauma 25(7):620–627, 1985
65. Timberlake GA, McSwain NE Jr: Thromboembolism as a complication of myocardial contusion: A new capricious syndrome. J Trauma 25(40):535–540, 1988
66. Timberlake GA, Crumlin LE, McSwain NE Jr et al: Penetrating Diaphragmatic Injuries: Is herniation inevitable? American College of Surgeons Forum 1986(A)
67. Timberlake G, McSwain NE Jr, Martinez G: Resuscitation thoracotomy factors critical to failure. American Association for the Surgery of Trauma, 1986(A)
68. Timberlake G, McSwain NE: Immediate autotransfusion of washed red cells contaminated by abdominal trauma. Unpublished data.
69. Tucker JF, Danzl DF, Teague E et al: Infusion of intravenous fluids distal to pneumatic antishock trousers. J Emerg Med 2(2):79–83, 1884
70. Treasure RL: Management of flail chest. Milit Med 144(9):588–589, 1979
71. Trinkle JK, Richardson D, Franz JL: Management of flail chest without mechanical ventilation. Ann Thorac Surg 19(4):355–363, 1975
72. Trinkle JK, Toon RS, Franz JL et al: Affairs of the wounded heart: Penetrating cardiac wounds. J Trauma 19(6):467–472, 1979
73. Trunkey D: Operative stabilization at flail chest. Presented at Trauma '86, Las Vegas, March 14, 1986
74. Viano DC, Artinian CG: Myocardial conducting system dysfunction from thoracic impact. J Trauma 18(6):452–459, 1978
75. Verdant A, Cossette R, Dontigny L: Acute and chronic traumatic aneurysms of the descending thoracic aorta: A ten year experience with a single method of aortic shunting. J Trauma 25(7):601–606, 1985
76. Waldschmidt ML, Laws HL: Injuries to the diaphragm. J Trauma 20(7):587–592, 1980
77. Webb WR: Thoracic trauma. Surg Clin North Am 54:(5):1179–1192, 1974
78. Werne S, Sands M: Left tension pneumothorax masquerading as anterior myocardial infarction. Ann Emerg Med 14(2):164–170, 1985
79. Wilson RF, Murray C, Antonenko DR: Nonpenetrating thoracic injuries. Surg Clin North Am 57(1):17–36, 1977

cardiac trauma: penetrating and blunt

W. Randolph Chitwood, Jr.
Erle H. Austin

Cardiac trauma has been categorized classically as being either penetrating or blunt. The chest wall offers little protection from penetration, often making these wounds lethal, with 60% to 80% of patients dying before arrival at an emergency center.[126,205,245] Usually, mortality results from bleeding, tamponade, valvular injury, or coronary artery involvement. Also, delayed complications, including coronary artery fistulas and retained intramyocardial foreign bodies, can become problematic. Imbedded bullets and shrapnel can either embolize or become infective and are often removed electively. With most patients sustaining penetrating cardiac trauma, immediate management is needed to optimize survival. Individuals sustaining blunt trauma may decompensate acutely from chamber, valvular, or septal disruption. Presently, survival from blunt cardiac rupture is infrequent. However, blunt injuries may remain subtle, presenting as myocardial contusions with the potential for hemodynamic compromise. Although rare, delayed ventricular rupture can occur, with few patients salvaged. Pericardial, valvular, and coronary injuries are uncommon blunt cardiac injuries but important consequences of blunt trauma.

Iatrogenic catheter retention as well as ventricular perforations from cardiac catheterization and pacemaker insertion are occurring with increasing frequency. Also, therapeutic pericardiocentesis can cause ventricular or coronary lacerations resulting in tamponade. Myocardial and coronary injuries may result from standard radiation therapy for malignancies as well as electrical countershock for life-threatening arrhythmias. Devastating cardiac injury may develop during both prosthetic valve insertion and forceful cardiac resuscitation. The latter injuries are difficult to manage and may occur at a most inopportune time.

HISTORICAL ASPECTS

Throughout recorded medical history, mystery and intrigue have surrounded observations and treatment of cardiac injuries. For centuries all heart wounds were considered mortal, and only in the last century was this tenet disproved.[31] Claude Beck titled the era prior to 1700 "the period of mysticism," extending from Homer to Paré.[22] Pessimism surrounded the potential of recovery, and Aristotle, Ovid, Celsus, Pliny, and Galen were prophets of doom regarding cardiac injuries. Although early reports by Cabriolanus (1604) and Wolf (1642) suggested that heart wounds were capable of healing, most authorities were doubtful until Senac provided encouragement (1749).[13,22,31]

Morgagni first described the treacheries of pericardial tamponade in *De Sedibus* (1761), and Jobert proposed that cardiac compression must be the cause of related hemodynamic decompensation (1839).[122,168] Although Riolan suggested pericardiocentesis in 1649, Dupuytren first performed a successful pericardial decompression using a transthoracic probe.[13,22] Subsequently, Napoleon's surgeon, Larrey, introduced a catheter into the pericardium for drainage with four survivors (1829).[13] Larrey is credited with being the first to consider these injuries not uniformly lethal. In 1866 Allbutt and Wheelhouse performed the first successful pericardiocentesis in England with the news spreading rapidly to Bowditch in Boston, who apparently was the first to do the procedure in America.[13] Rose termed cardiac compression "Herztamponade" in 1884.[211] Cohnheim discovered experimentally in 1889 that with a rising intrapericardial pressure, a concomitant elevation in venous pressure and fall in arterial blood pressure occurred.[56] Later, Beck confirmed these studies and documented the restorative physiologic effects of pericardial drainage.[22]

During the 19th century, European surgical education and opinion was flavored by Billroth, who is said to have stated that "the surgeon who should attempt to suture a wound of the heart would lose the respect of his colleagues."[31,121] Few clinicians would rebel in the cautionary atmosphere of that era. By 1868 no repairs of a cardiac injury had been reported, and only 10% of patients were found to have recovered by all known modes of therapy including pericardiocentesis.[86] In 1882, Block of Danzig showed experimentally in rabbits that closure of heart wounds was possible and suggested this modality in humans.[32] Two years later, Del Vechio demonstrated healed wounds in dog hearts to the eleventh International Medical Congress in Rome.[65]

In 1896, Stephen Paget wrote prophetically in his well-known text, "no new method and no new discovery, can overcome the natural difficulties that attend a wound of the heart. It is true that heart suture has been vaguely proposed but I cannot find that it has ever been attempted in practice."[179] It is interesting that earlier, on September 4, 1895, Cappelen of Norway had

IX.

Ueber penetrirende Herzwunden und Herznaht.

Von

Professor Dr. L. Rehn

in Frankfurt a. M.[1])

In einem verzweifelten Fall von Stichverletzung des rechten Ventrikel wurde ich durch die andauernde Blutung zum Eingreifen gezwungen. Ich wollte das Möglichste thun, um den Kranken zu retten und so kam ich im Lauf der Operation in die Nothwendigkeit, eine Herznaht auszuführen. Es blieb mir kein anderer Weg, so schwer er war, denn der Patient hätte sich unter meinen Augen verblutet.

FIGURE 5.1 Ludwig Rehn's report of the first successful closure of a penetrating cardiac injury performed on September 9, 1896, in Frankfurt. (Rehn L: Ueber penetrirende Herzwunden und Herznaht. Arch Klin Chir 55:315, 1897.)

sutured a 2-cm left ventricular stab wound with chromic catgut in a 24-year-old man. Unfortunately, the youth died 2–4 days later of "anemia and pericarditis."[47] Subsequently, in March 1896, Farina closed a ventricular dagger injury with silk. The patient died 8 days later of bronchopneumonia.[13,84] After two prior attempts, Ludwig Rehn performed the first successful repair of a cardiac stab wound on September 9, 1896, in Frankfurt (Fig. 5.1). He closed a 1.5-cm right ventricular injury with three silk sutures and reported his triumph to the German Surgical Society.[13,201] The first successful atrial repair was done by Gentil of Lisbon in 1901.[13] Despite the skeptical climate, by 1907 Rehn had compiled 124 cases of cardiac suture with a 40% recovery rate.[202] Fischer and Rehn independently established that the right ventricle was the most common chamber injured.[13,86,202]

In America, H. C. Dalton of St. Louis sutured a pericardial wound on September 6, 1891, as did Daniel H. Williams in 1893 at Providence Hospital in Chicago.[61,123,278] Roberts had suggested this procedure earlier.[207] The first successful repair of a true cardiac injury in this country is illustrated in Figures 5.2 through 5.4.[213] On the evening of September 14, 1902, Luther L. Hill sutured the left ventricular stab wound of 13-year-old Henry Myrick in a dim, backwoods cabin near Montgomery, Alabama. Myrick's pulse improved immediately and many years later the patient was found to be quite healthy.[110,213]

In 1903, Ricketts of Cincinnati reported 20 out of 56 cardiac wounds repaired successfully, and in 1906 described 12 successful cases of open chest cardiac resuscitation.[13,206] Although many times unhelpful, the "Saurbruch grip" was introduced in 1907 as a method of simultaneous compression of the venae cavae, right atrium, and pulmonary veins, limiting cardiac preload and reducing hemorrhage until suture closure could be effected (Fig. 5.5).[22,218] By 1920, Rehn, Pool, Vaughan, and Tuffier had independently reported over 300 cases of cardiac suture with an optimistic 40% to 65% rate of survival.[13,191,202,263] In the now famous 1919 Bradshaw Lecture to the Royal College of Surgeons, Sir Charles Ballance stated, "the operations now practised on the pericardium and heart are: pericardiotomy, paracentesis of the right auricle and ventricle, operation for embolism of the heart [Trendelenburg], cardiac stimulation for arrest, cardiolysis, and cardiorraphy."[13] He detailed the "chondroplastic Kocher flap," "intercostal Spangaro incisions," and the "Duval-Barasty median sternotomy" for exposure of cardiac injuries. Moreover, he advocated removal of intracardiac foreign bodies under fluoroscopy as, "a bullet may perforate the heart or aorta [and] may be ejected from the right ventricle into the pulmonary artery or from the left ventricle into the aorta." In the 1920 Hunterian Lecture, Moynihan reported successful removal of foreign bodies from the heart or pericardium in five patients.[172]

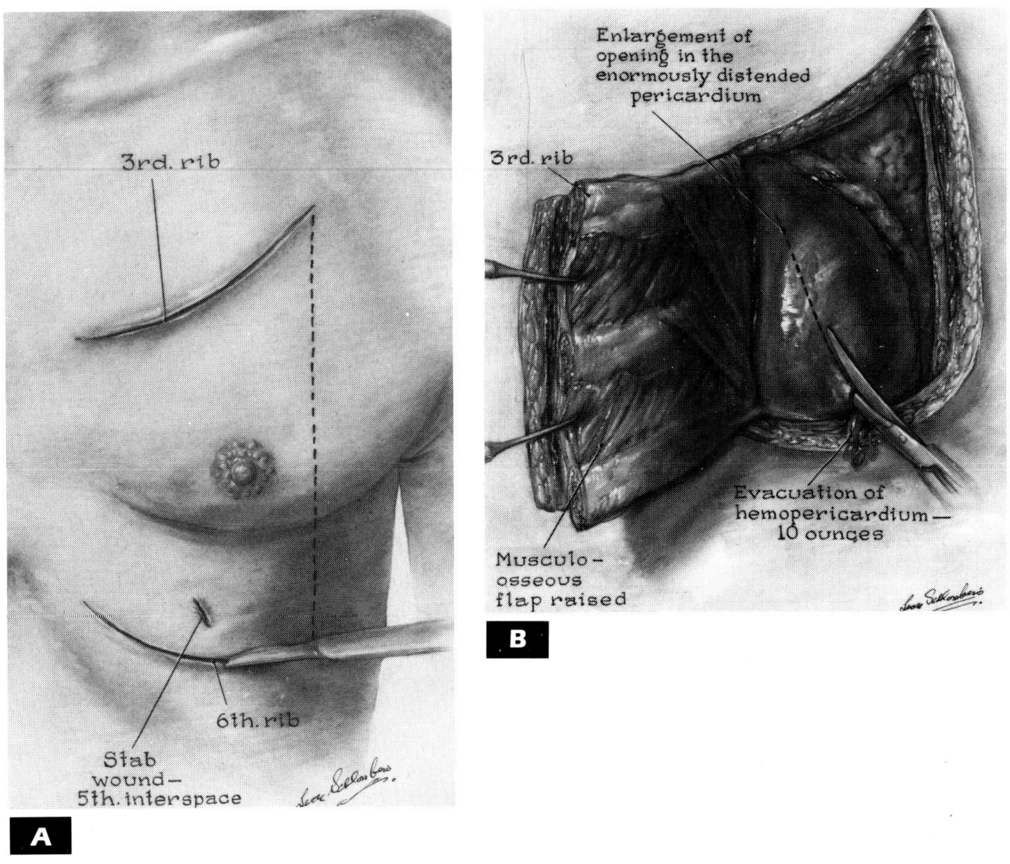

FIGURE 5.2 The first successful repair of a cardiac injury in the United States by Luther L. Hill in 1902. **A** To provide adequate cardiac exposure, a "trapdoor" incision was made along the third and sixth ribs. **B** After retraction of the chest wall flap, a tense pericardium was found and evacuated. (Sabiston DC: Major contributions to surgery from the south. Ann Surg 181:487–507, 1975.)

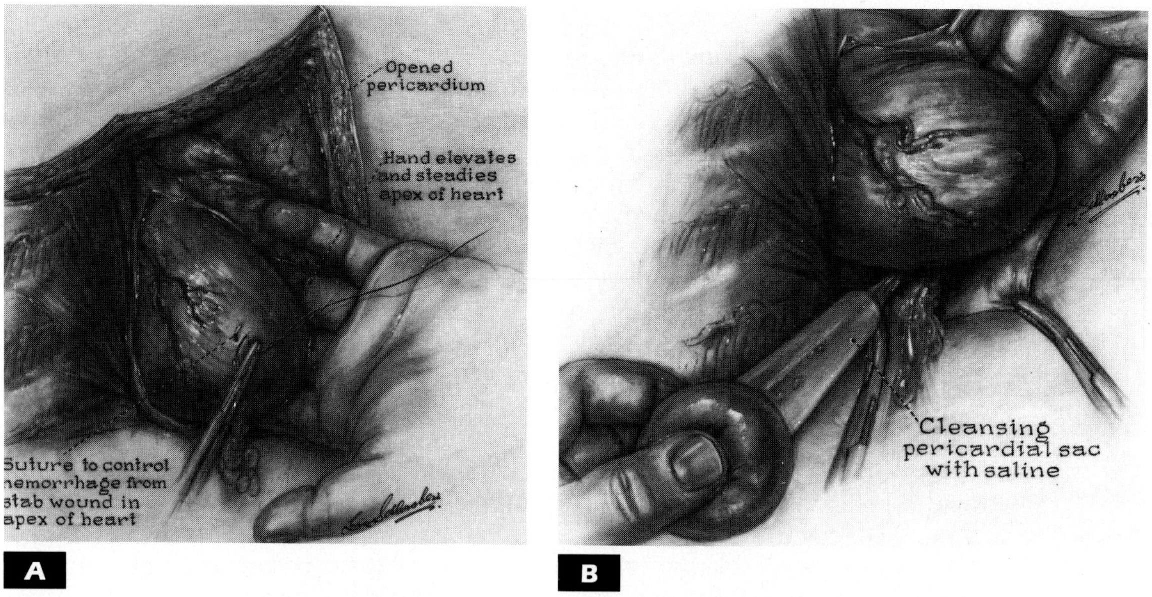

FIGURE 5.3 A Control of hemorrhage was established by digital compression. Subsequently, catgut suture material was used to close the ventricular injury. **B** The pericardium was irrigated with saline. (Sabiston DC: Major contributions to surgery from the south. Ann Surg 181:487–507, 1975.)

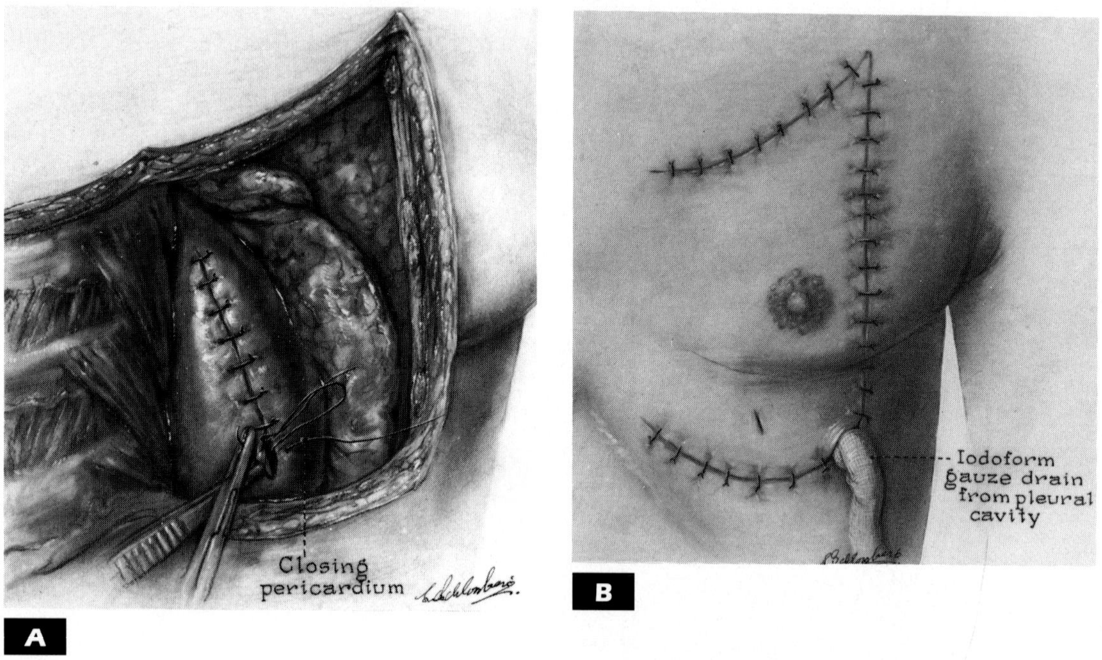

FIGURE 5.4 A The pericardial incision was closed after ventricular repair. **B** After chest wall closure the cavity was drained by a gauze wick without the benefit of lung re-expansion. (Sabiston DC: Major contributions to surgery from the south. Ann Surg 181:487–507, 1975.)

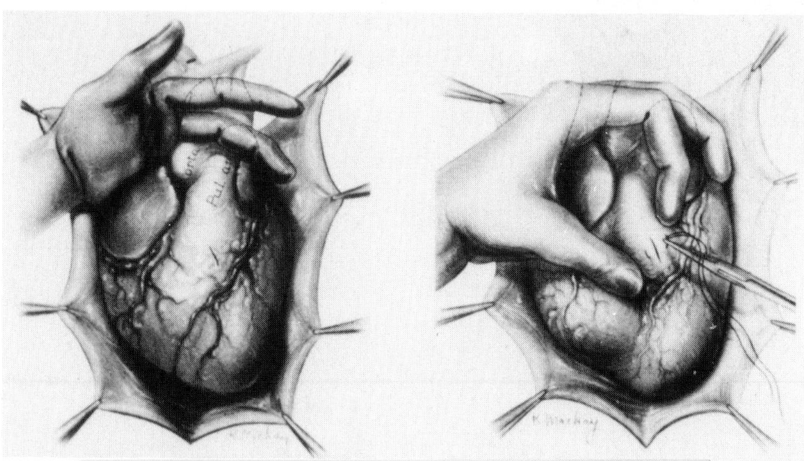

FIGURE 5.5 The Saurbruch grip was used to decrease cardiac preload during emergency repair of heart wounds (Elkin DC: Diagnosis and treatment of cardiac trauma. Ann Surg 114:169–180, 1941.)

In 1926 Claude Beck described a new method of cardiac wound closure applying crossed sutures to control bleeding, minimize coronary inclusion, and relieve myocardial tension (Fig. 5.6).[22] Subsequently, permanent sutures were made to close the wound safely. Today similar methods are commonly used when pledgeted sutures are unavailable. Beck and Bright's 1935 article "Contusions of the Heart" should be noted as another classic work that was early in relating concomitant myocardial ischemic changes.[23] By 1934 Ramsdell of New York found that 55 stab wounds had been operated on in the United States with only a 47% mortality rate.[197]

Bigger (1939) and Elkin (1941) reaffirmed independently the most common locations of civilian cardiac injuries and advocated operative intervention.[28,78] Blalock and Ravitch (1943) were concerned over the operative mortality and emphasized that pericardiocentesis was a safer form of therapy. If repeat drainage became ineffective then surgery was advocated.[30] This later conservative approach was the therapeutic posture for U.S. military surgeons during World War II.[31] In the 1943 course "War Surgery of the Chest," given to British surgical officers, Grey-Turner advocated operative therapy, stating, "Open wounds over the heart area require emergency operation to arrest hemorrhage and anticipated infection."[98] Also he suggested that selected cardiac foreign bodies should be removed. Harken and Samson were responsible for many advances in cardiac repair during World War II (Fig. 5.7).[104,214] In the 10 months following D-

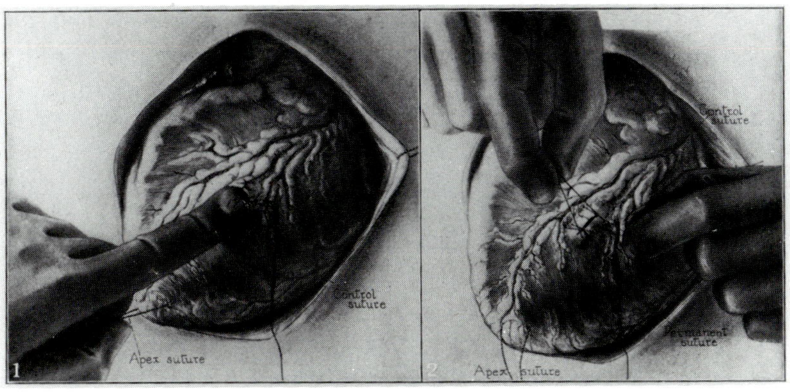

FIGURE 5.6 "Crossed suture technique" developed by Claude Beck for closure of penetrating cardiac wounds. (Beck CS: Wounds of the heart: The technique of suture. *JAMA* 13:205–227, 1926. Copyright 1926, American Medical Association.)

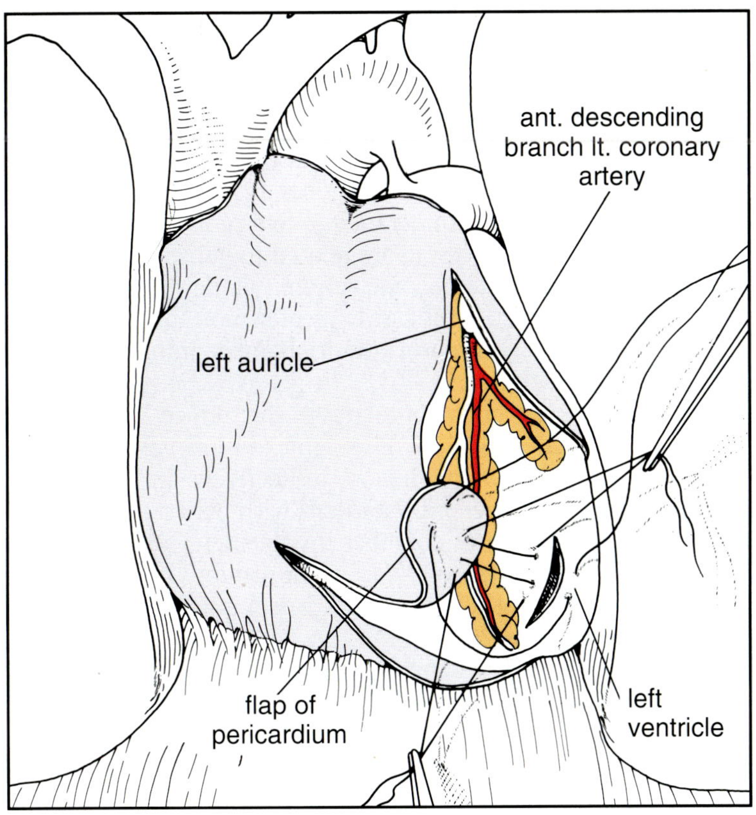

FIGURE 5.7 Closure of a left ventricular penetrating injury during World War II using a pericardial pledget. This method was used by Dr. Paul C. Samson at the Eleventh Evacuation Hospital in Italy. (Adapted from Samson PC: Two unusual cases of war wounds of the heart. *Surgery* 20:373–381, 1946.)

Day, Captain Dwight Harken and his team performed 134 operations at Cirencester, England, for either thoracic aortic or intracardiac missiles, remarkably without a death.[104] He considered such injuries at a high risk for embolism and infection, and this opinion generally remains today. Controversy between conservative and operative management of cardiac wounds persisted well into the 1960s when Sugg and Beall among others showed that early surgery provided a significantly lower mortality.[19,238]

PENETRATING CARDIAC INJURIES

Etiology

Among the civilian population, penetrating cardiac wounds have resulted primarily from knives and other sharp objects (70%–90%). However, the number of gunshot wounds has been increasing, especially in the United States.[49,245,251,280] Recently, Evans of Louisville and Taveres of Baltimore reported that 60% to 66% of all cardiac wounds were from guns.[81,252] Despite these trends, in less-developed civilian populations stab wounds still constitute nearly all (96%) of these injuries.[66] Although gunshot wounds account for only 30% of penetrating cardiac injuries in many civilian studies, they occur in over 50% of patients dead on arrival, reflecting their lethal potential.[124,251] Shotgun wounds of the heart are often irreparable and have an exceedingly high mortality.[81] In the Vietnam War cardiac injuries resulted primarily from shell fragments (71%), gunshots (11.5%), flechettes (3%), and knives (3%).[205] Moreover, in the recent Lebanon war, 56% of military cardiac injuries were incurred from shrapnel fragments and 42% of these were from high-velocity Kalashnikov, M15, and M16 weapons, all of which cause severe internal cavitation defects.[282] Unusual injuries from high-velocity nail and staple guns, ice picks, and projectiles from lawnmowers and other mechanical devices occur infrequently, but may be lethal.[24,146,157,219]

Incidence and Mortality

In a classic autopsy study Parmley concluded that the overall incidence of penetrating cardiac injuries was difficult to establish.[182] In World War I, chest wounds in general had a mortality of nearly 60%, with 8% of such patients dying of cardiac injuries of all types.[42] During World War II, 3.3% of all thoracoabdominal wounds involved the heart, and Brewer reported a 40% mortality in these soldiers.[42] The incidence of cardiac injuries had not changed appreciably by either the Korean (4.8%) or Vietnam wars (2.8%).[90,205,266] However, these wounds had increased to 14% during the Lebanon military conflict between 1969 and 1982.[282] Prior to 1955, the overall hospital mortality from cardiac injuries was approximately 30% in patients arriving alive for care.[114] Prehospital mortality was highest with gunshot patients (80%).[114,238] During this period, Griswold and others emphasized that without exploration, the site and extent of injury often remained ill-defined and that pericardial aspiration alone may be insufficient.[34,99,100,238] A mixture of conservative pericardiocentesis and definitive surgical exploration was reflected by several early studies.[20,34] At many major trauma centers, a gradual transition to early thoracotomy occurred in the mid-1960s.[260] In 1968, Sugg analyzed 459 patients with penetrating heart injuries and found that prehospital mortality was highest among cardiac gunshot and left-ventricular injured patients (90%), but was 61% among those with stab wounds.[238] With immediate exploration, hospital mortality fell from 43% with pericardial aspiration alone to 16% with definitive surgical therapy.

By 1960 to 1970 gunshot wounds still had a 60% mortality rate while only 17% to 20% of patients with stab wounds died.[114,124] In several more modern studies, the overall survival of those arriving for treatment has been better than 70%.[64,153,195,200,260,261] Recently Symbas showed that of patients arriving alive with cardiac stab wounds, 89% survived, compared to 69% of patients with gunshot wounds.[245] Trinkle treated 100 consecutive patients with penetrating cardiac wounds by a combination of pericardiocentesis, subxiphoid pericardial tube insertion, and thoracotomy, with an 11% mortality rate.[261] Although overall survival from penetrating cardiac wounds continues to improve, gunshot injuries still portend a much higher mortality both in military and civilian situations.[150,205,224] Moreover, associated chest injuries in cardiac trauma patients, including hemothorax, pneumothorax, and other visceral injuries, contribute to a substantially higher mortality.

Pathology and Pathophysiology

Most commonly, the right ventricle is injured and chances of survival are better if only this chamber is involved.[78,124,126,205] Some series relate a preponderance of left ventricular penetrating injuries, and usually these are related to gunshot wounds.[150] When the left ventricle becomes injured alone or in combination with the right, a significantly greater mortality exists (Fig. 5.8).[49,205,238,251,260] Fortunately, multichamber injury from stab wounds is relatively rare (7%).[67] In general the potential for injury to a particular chamber relates to the surface area exposed to the anterior chest wall.[245] The right and left ventricles subtend 55% and 20% of this region, respectively. In 20 separate studies representing over 1800 patients with penetrating cardiac injuries, the incidence of chamber involvement was right ventricle (42%), left ventricle (33%), right atrium (15%), and left atrium (6%), with intracardiac great vessel injuries constituting the remainder.[126,205,245,261]

Occasionally, small ventricular injuries may self-seal and not require surgical exploration. More often this occurs with right ventricular catheter and pacing wire perforations. Because of the greater transmural thickness and vigorous myocardial contraction, left ventricular penetrations less than 1 cm have a tendency to close spontaneously.[7] Bullet wounds almost never become self-limiting due to significant tissue destruction.[245] Large ventricular injuries usually promote rapid bleeding, little defibrination, and either early tamponade or exsanguination. Although intracavitary atrial pressures are less than those of the ventricles, injuries to these thin-walled chambers frequently continue to bleed, requiring exploration and repair.[174,244] Right atrial injuries have a slightly higher mortality rate than those of the left atrium.

With chamber penetration, hemorrhage becomes an obvious problem; however, cardiac tamponade is often the presenting malady. The hemodynamic consequences of tamponade are found in up to 65% of patients having significant penetrating cardiac injuries[81]: 90% of patients with stab wounds and 20% of those with gunshot injuries arrive with tamponade.[41] Also, tamponade is discovered more frequently in patients arriving alive for treatment compared with those dead on arrival.[66,67] Generally, right-sided injuries are slower to induce tamponade, and survival has been better with right ventricular stab wounds, as high as 90%.[67]

The pericardium is a relatively noncompliant sac that expands significantly only in the presence of a chronic transmural stress. Rapid cardiac displacement with 150 ml to 250 ml of blood usually

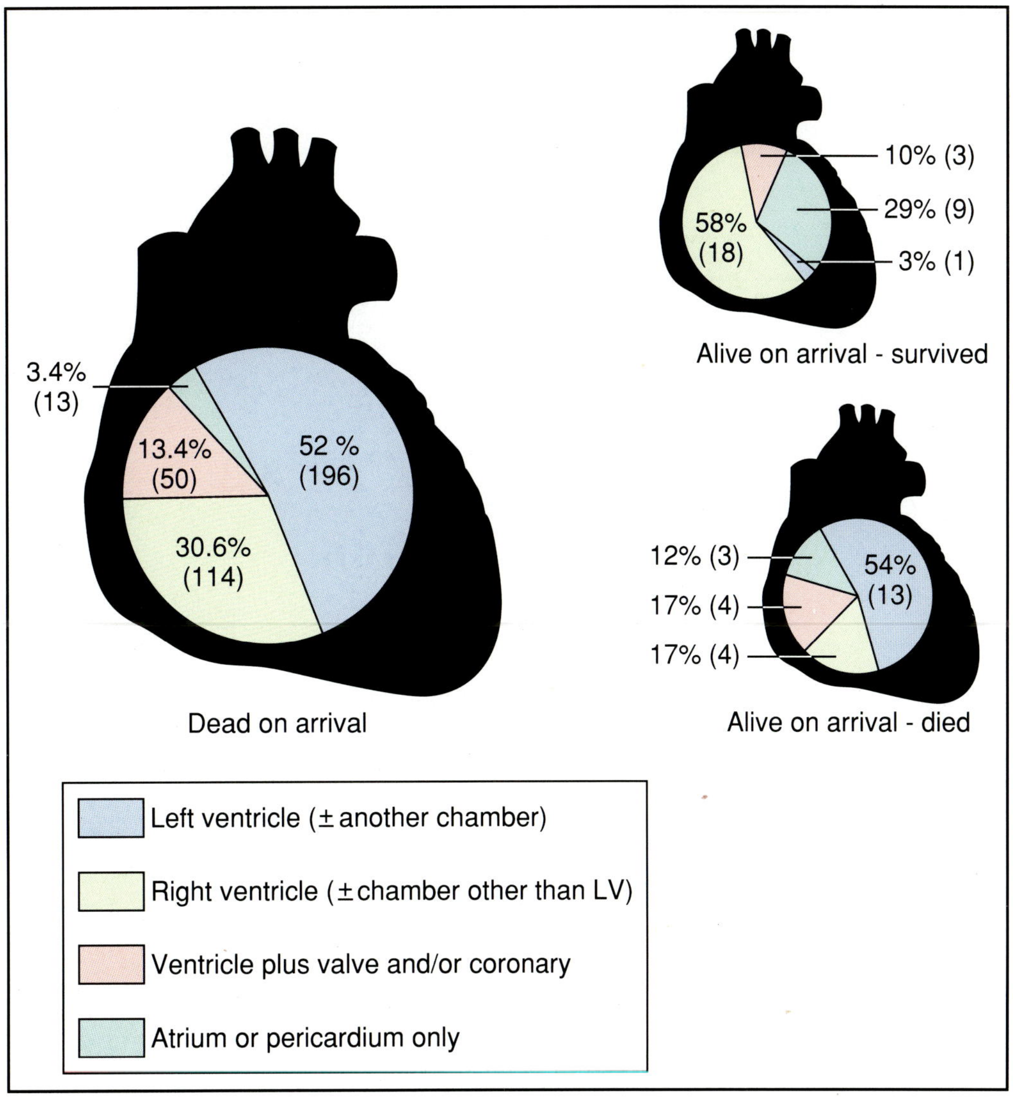

FIGURE 5.8 The overall distribution of cardiac wounds is shown for 459 patients with penetrating cardiac injuries. Comparisons are made for surviving and nonsurviving individuals as well as chamber injured. (Sugg WL, Rea WJ, Ecker RR et al: Penetrating wounds of the heart: An analysis of 459 cases. J Thorac Cardiovasc Surg 56:531–545, 1968.)

results in a significant blood pressure decrement.[245] Acute tamponade eventuates in a combination of unphysiologic events occurring almost simultaneously. During tamponade, as stroke volume becomes diminished, a compensatory tachycardia may enhance the cardiac output initially to maintain homeostasis. Cardiac filling depends on the difference between venous inflow and left ventricular end-diastolic pressures. A progressive intrapericardial pressure rise becomes manifest transmurally as a higher left ventricular end-diastolic pressure. Therefore, as the filling pressure gradient falls, cardiac stroke volume and output decrease concurrently.[192] Although the end-diastolic chamber volume becomes reduced progressively during tamponade, end-systolic dimensions generally remain unaltered, resulting in a lowered ejection fraction. Thus, temporizing therapy should be directed toward optimizing ventricular end-diastolic filling pressures by volume infusion and enhancing ejection by inotropic support.[192,223]

During progressive chamber volume displacement by the extra-cardiac pericardial fluid, both ventricles become less compliant. Subsequently, intravascular volume recruitment occurs by renal and vasoconstrictive mechanisms resulting in higher intracavitary pressures. Therefore, for a while, these diastolic Starling properties help maintain cardiac output and stabilize hemodynamics. Without therapy the ultimate fall in cardiac output is followed by uncompensated hypotension. Although the central venous pressure becomes elevated in many cases of tamponade, in hemorrhaging patients this finding may not be evident until blood volume is restored.[66,244,245] As hypotension develops intrapericardial bleeding may become self-limiting.

Experimental and clinical studies have demonstrated an exponential pericardial pressure-volume relationship during progressive cardiac tamponade (Fig. 5.9, A).[169,264] These characteristics are largely dependent upon pericardial compliance

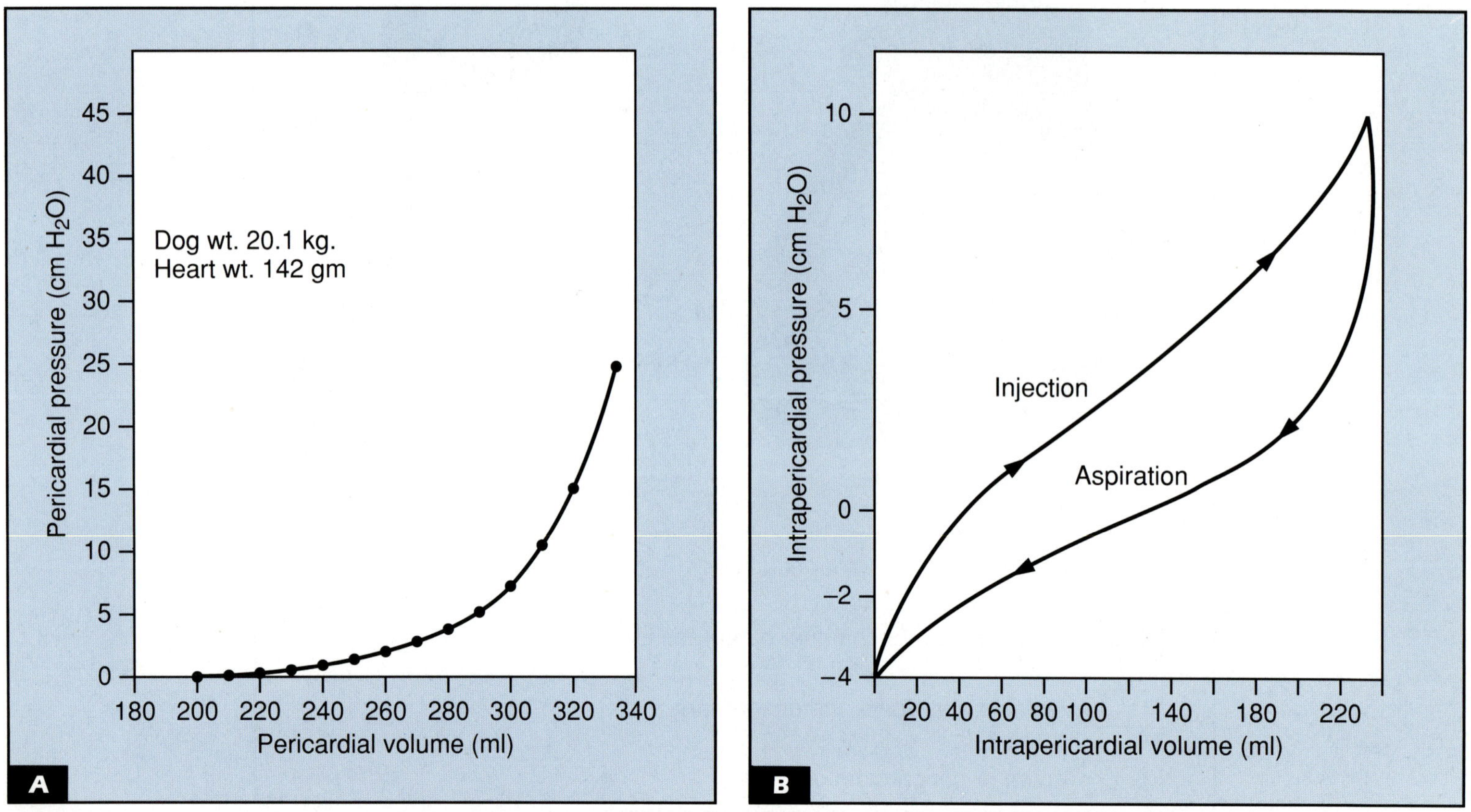

FIGURE 5.9 A Nonlinear experimental pericardial pressure-volume relationship. **B** The pressure volume relationship is shown for both infusion and removal phases, demonstrating hysteresis or noncongruent curves. (Morgan BC, Able FL, Mullins GL: Flow patterns in cavae, pulmonary artery, pulmonary vein, and aorta in intact dogs. Am J Physiol 210:903–909, 1966; Reproduced with permission from Color Atlas of Chest Trauma and Associated Injuries. Copyright ©1983 by A. Besson & F. Saegesser. Published by Medical Economics Company Inc., Oradell, NJ 07649. All rights reserved.)

rather than ventricular properties. Although impaired cardiac filling may develop rather slowly, the latter part of the pericardial volume curve yields higher intracardiac pressures with more rapid tamponade. Moreover, the fluid-withdrawal relationship does not remain congruent with infusion curves, exhibiting a pattern of hysteresis (Fig. 5.9, *B*).[169] Therefore, removal of even a small aliquot is often sufficient to restore hemodynamic stability until bleeding recurs. In the presence of concomitant systemic volume depletion and positive-pressure ventilation, the detrimental effects of tamponade on overall cardiac function become exaggerated.[101] Care should be exercised when anesthetizing and ventilating patients even in very early tamponade.

With acute tamponade, myocardial ischemia may develop in concert with the restrictive filling properties just described. As the left ventricular end-diastolic pressure rises with tamponade, transmural diastolic coronary perfusion pressure diminishes *a priori* even before diastolic hypotension becomes manifest.[54,120,250,275] Coronary blood flow becomes limited almost completely to a diastolic event as intracavitary pressures become more influential.[120] Thus, the transmural myocardial flow gradient decreases with continuing tamponade. Several studies suggest that as tamponade progresses myocardial ischemia develops and becomes greatest at the endocardium. A reactive hyperemic response has been shown to occur following rapid withdrawal of tamponading fluid, indicating a metabolic debt repayment. The compensatory tachycardia aggravates developing ventricular ischemia. Thus, during late tamponade, the effects of ischemia appear to be combined with unfavorable ventricular geometric alterations eventuating collectively in irreversible hemodynamic decompensation.[264] In trauma patients the early removal of tamponading blood, before irreversible tissue damage and arrhythmias develop, remains optimal. This is especially true for those with preexisting coronary lesions. Acute cardiac tamponade commonly occurs following elective cardiac surgical procedures. This problem may develop in a subtle fashion at a time when myocardial reserve has been compromised and patients are being ventilated with positive pressure. In this and other tamponade situations, rapid recognition, clear analysis, and efficient decompression remain the touchstone to hemodynamic stability.

Pulsus paradoxus is a normal physiologic occurrence and is defined as an inspiratory decline in systolic blood pressure of 8 to 10 mm Hg.[222] As it occurs, aortic flow decreases slightly. In pericardial tamponade this fall in inspiratory pressure is accentuated. These changes may be exaggerated also by hypovolemia, pulmonary disease, and ventilator support. With eupneic inspiration an increase in caval blood flow occurs, concurrent with an increase in right ventricular output. Generally, a two-to-three-beat phase shift occurs in the pulmonary arterial circuit resulting in an inspiratory decline in systemic pressure. Figure 5.10 shows these exaggerated pressure-flow effects developing during tamponade. Other physiologic mechanisms probably contribute to the notable pulsus paradoxus of cardiac tamponade.[222] In late tamponade, peripheral arterial pulses may vanish completely with inspiration. When this occurs, vascular decompensation is near, and pericardial drainage must be established immediately. The magnitude of pulsus paradoxus during tamponade may be determined as the difference in cuff pressure measured between the first systolic Korotkoff sound, heard only in expiration, and those audible during both respiratory phases.[192]

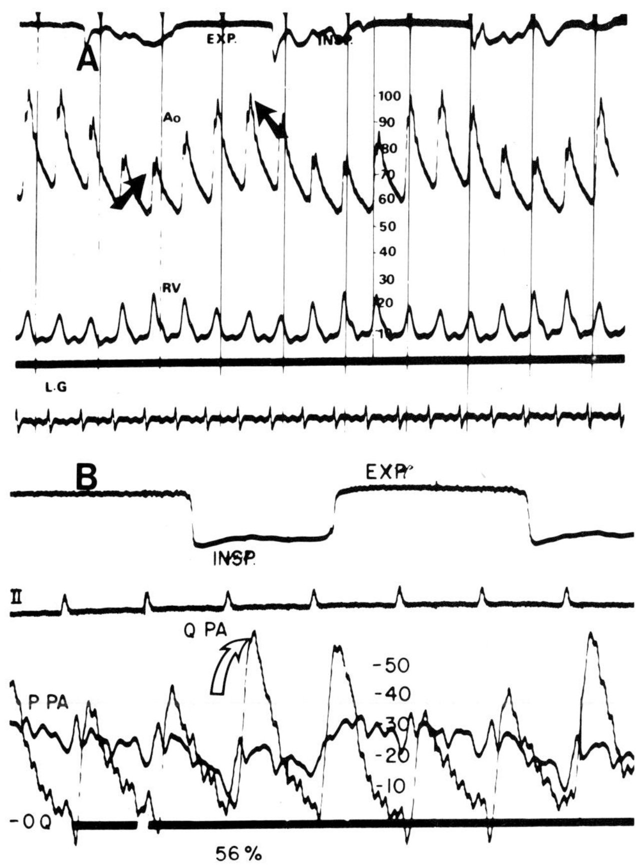

FIGURE 5.10 A Aortic and right ventricular pressures in a hypovolemic patient with concomitant pericardial tamponade. Note the 25.mm Hg paradox with inspiration (arrows). A two-to three-beat phase shift exists between right ventricular and aortic pressure. (EXP, expiration; INSP, inspiration; Ao, aortic pressure; RV, right ventricular pressure) **B** Pulmonary arterial pressure and flow in a patient with cardiac tamponade. During inspiration the systemic pressure falls despite simultaneous increased pulmonary flow (arrow). **C** PA, pulmonary arterial blood flow; P Pa, pulmonary artery pressure; 0 Q, zero flow) (Shabetai R, Fowler N, Guntheroth WG: The hemodynamics of cardiac tamponade and constrictive pericarditis. Am J Cardiol 26:480–489, 1970.)

Evaluation and Treatment

As 60% to 80% of patients with penetrating cardiac injuries die either from bleeding or tamponade before arrival, proximity to the treatment facility and rapid transport have been shown to influence patient survival markedly.[156,157,252,259] Transport to larger facilities just for the availability of facilities for cardiopulmonary bypass may be detrimental in very unstable patients as this procedure is needed for only 4% to 5% of cardiac trauma victims.[252,261] The initial evaluation and therapy must be carried out in an organized expedient fashion to provide optimal recovery. In most patients treatment of penetrating cardiac wounds takes precedence over associated injuries, although cardiac injuries may be difficult to differentiate from other causes of intrathoracic bleeding.

Penetrating wounds that enter the anterior left part of the chest or traverse the mediastinum are highly suspect for a cardiac injury.[81] The "danger zone for injury" includes the entire anterior and posterior mediastinum as well as supraclavicular and epigastric areas.[217,245] DeGennaro found cardiac injuries in 62% of patients having penetrating wounds within the cardiac silhouette.[64] In general, suspected injuries should be explored early even in the presence of hemodynamic stability. With thoracic gunshot wounds, entrance and exit sites should be identified in an effort to determine the pathway of injury and predict organ involvement.

In cases of penetrating cardiac trauma, isolated and serial chest radiographs are usually unhelpful for diagnosing pericardial tamponade or the extent of myocardial injury. Enlargement of the cardiac silhouette, which often occurs with chronic pericardial effusions, is not obvious in most acute situations. However, routine x-ray studies will help establish the diagnosis of a concurrent hemopneumothorax or congestive heart failure resulting from valve injury or an intracardiac shunt. X-ray studies should help identify projectiles entering the abdomen from the chest. In stable patients echocardiography may help identify pericardial bleeding, but to do so means delay and often fails to correlate with the degree of therapeutic concern. Radionuclide scanning techniques, which may be efficacious for diagnosing blunt cardiac injuries, offer little help in evaluating acute penetrating cardiac injuries. Early fluoroscopy and echocardiography may be helpful in stable patients to localize retained intramyocardial fragments.[112]

In unstable individuals algorithmic thinking may help provide optimal triage, evaluation, and care under suboptimal conditions (Fig. 5.11). With real or potential penetrating cardiac trauma, aggressive care must be instituted on arrival at the emergency facility. Patients with thoracic penetrating wounds presenting *in extremis* need little evaluation: immediate therapy offers the only chance for recovery. In comparison, the stable individual can be evaluated more extensively. In most cases, stab and low-velocity gunshot injuries occurring more than an hour before arrival can be evaluated thoroughly prior to definitive therapy. Patients occupying the middle ground are of greatest concern, since instability may develop rapidly. In trauma patients, delays in diagnosis and appropriate fluid therapy have been shown to be the most common errors in early management.[76]

Because of unresponsiveness, cardiac arrest, or other thoracic injuries, many patients require immediate intubation and ventilation. Ventilation must be done with utmost caution, since positive intrathoracic pressure aggravates hemodynamic instability in patients with tamponade. When possible, many allow these patients to breathe spontaneously until the surgeon is fully prepared for exploration. Immediate intravascular volume expansion should be initiated through several large-bore catheters (16–14 gauge) and escalated rapidly. Usually, at least 3 to 4 liters of fluid are necessary to achieve any hemodynamic stability.[268] One large intravenous line should be placed centrally for venous pressure assessment. Crystalloid volume expanders and type specific O-negative blood should be available, as should infusion pumps and warmers. Several liters of fluid can be administered per minute with aggressive management through large catheters. A chest tube should be placed on the side of injury to identify and treat a large hemothorax or tension pneumothorax.

Patients who can be stabilized rapidly should be transported to the operating room for definitive therapy. When either massive chest-tube blood loss or hemorrhagic shock is evident, rapid transport and an immediate operating room thoracotomy are preferred, with little additional therapy. If excessive bleeding from the chest tube occurs, the tube should be clamped to help prevent exsanguination during transport to surgery. In the presence of a large parenchymal air leak, the decision to clamp the tube becomes more difficult.

Beck's classic triad of distended neck veins, muffled heart sounds, and hypotension may be present in only 35% of patients with traumatic pericardial tamponade. However, one or more signs, including those of Beck's triad, tachycardia, confusion, a paradoxical pulse, Kussmaul's sign, and the skin changes of shock will be present in up to 87% of tamponading patients.[7,174,192,225] The central venous pressure remains the best indicator of tamponade but, as mentioned earlier, elevated right-sided pressures may not be evident in the hypovolemic patient.[7,174]

The emergency room pericardiocentesis has fallen into disfavor at most centers because clotted blood in either the needle or the pericardium may render the technique ineffectual in a dire emergency.[238, 260] It may occasionally be the only recourse, however, and should be mastered by physicians involved in emer-

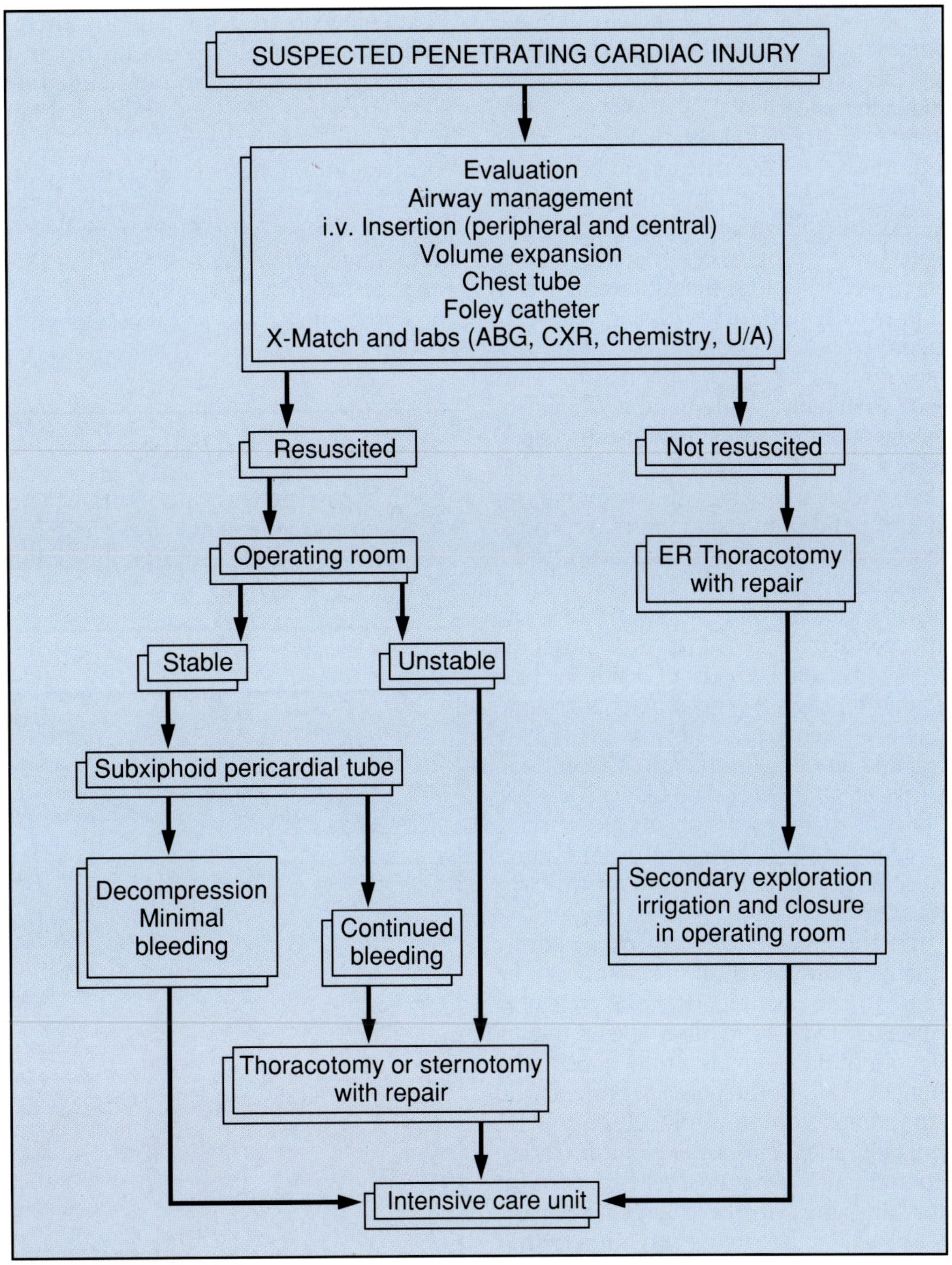

FIGURE 5.11 Algorithm for the early evaluation and treatment of patients with suspected acute cardiac injuries.

gency care (Fig. 5.12).[205] Withdrawal of unclotted blood usually indicates pericardial aspiration, since heart motion causes defibrination. However, rapid bleeding often prevents clot liquefaction, making the technique less effective.

In most trauma centers a subxiphoid pericardial tube can be inserted almost as expeditiously.[7,260] The subxiphoid pericardial tube has been helpful for diagnosis and treatment of stable patients in whom a question of cardiac injury exists.[7,81,261] Moreover, in patients who develop tamponade following catheterization and pacemaker insertion, these tubes may provide the definitive therapy. In patients with large cardiac defects, care must be taken to prevent exsanguination following tube placement and some authors have not supported the early use of pericardial tubes.[66] Preferably, stable patients should be transported to the operating room for pericardial tube drainage.

Recently, the emergency room thoracotomy has been popularized as saving lives.[156] The pulseless patient with a potential cardiac injury who does not respond immediately to massive fluid resuscitation should be considered for emergency room exploration and attempted cardiac repair. Although mortality in patients undergoing these procedures ranges between 28% and 100%, some centers report a 70% to 85% success rate.[11,64,126,156,166,245, 252,272] The major causes of death in these patients include exsanguination (33%), central nervous complications (18%), shock (17%), ventricular fibrillation (13%), myocardial injury (12%), and air embolism (7%). A recent collective review suggests that up to 35% of patients with cardiac gunshot wounds and 45% of those with stab injuries survive emerLgency room thoracotomies.[126] This and other studies have shown a much worse prognosis (85%–100%) for this type of exploration for blunt cardiac lacerations.[39,126]

Trinkle emphasized that the emergency room thoracotomy should be reserved for the most dire situation. If stability can be obtained rapidly, transport to the operating room is preferable and has an improved survival. Even in modern level I trauma centers, the emergency room thoracotomy is always done under less than ideal circumstances. Still, in the pulseless patient who fails to respond to immediate volume replacement, little recourse exists.[39,252] Generally, an emergency exploratory thoracotomy in the trauma room should be reserved for patients with an isolated cardiac injury and arrest in the emergency department, patients with an isolated cardiac injury and arrest within 4 minutes of arrival, rapidly deteriorating patients who would not survive transport to the operating suite, and moribund patients who fail to respond to rapid volume infusion, chest tube insertion, and simultaneous pericardiocentesis, and definitely cannot be transported.[11,126,156]

Supporting the *selective* use of the emergency room thoracotomy, Baker concluded that patients without vital signs and who cannot be resuscitated at the accident scene should not be transported for this procedure.[115] Other authors also have considered the procedure not efficacious in moribund patients and have advised against indiscriminate usage.[53,166] Vij suggested that the absence of pupillary responses and spontaneous respirations predicts an unsuccessful emergency room thoracotomy.[268] However, he found that the ability to resuscitate these patients did not correlate with a presence or absence of hypotension or a palpable pulse.

Patients who are resuscitated in the emergency room by this method should be explored further in the standard operating room, irrigated copiously, and closed under sterile conditions. Also, attendant chest and abdominal injuries should be assessed and repaired at that time.[153] Most authors suggest that associated intracardiac defects be repaired in a subsequent operation.[198,245,255] The objectives of both the emergency room and operating suite exploration remain the same: to release cardiac tamponade, to perform internal massage, to control hemorrhage, to repair cardiac injuries, and occasionally to cross-clamp the descending aorta to raise cerebral and coronary perfusion pressures.

Surgical Techniques

When a patient with a potential penetrating cardiac injury arrives in the emergency area the algorithm shown in Figure 5.11 can be applied. After stabilization and transport to the

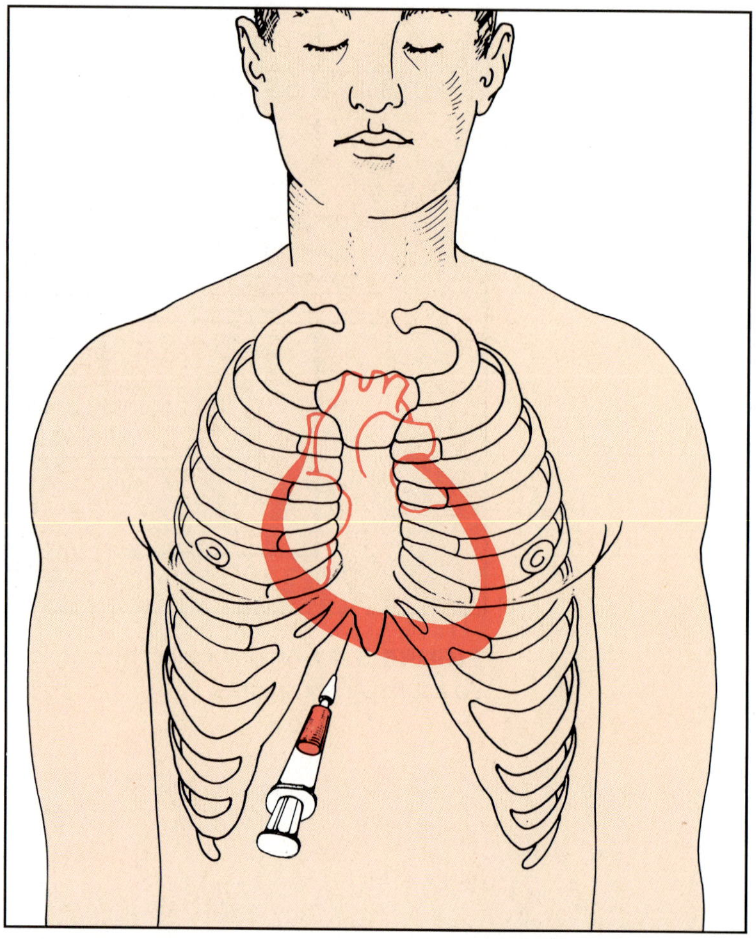

FIGURE 5.12 The appropriate technique for pericardiocentesis in the cardiac trauma patient. Electrocardiographic control often is not possible with traumatic tamponade. (Adapted from Rich NM, Spencer FC: Wounds of the Heart in Vascular Trauma. Philadelphia, WB Saunders, 1978.)

operating room, many surgeons proceed directly with an operating room thoracotomy for bullet and stab injuries, believing this the most conservative management. Often hemodynamically stable patients will tolerate pericardial tube insertion without difficulty. In these individuals the entire chest and upper abdomen should be prepared either for a thoracotomy or sternotomy before placing the drainage tube through a subxiphoid pericardial window. To insert a pericardial drainage tube, a vertical 10-cm midline incision is made over the lower sternum, xiphoid, and upper abdomen. The xiphoid process can be grasped with a Kocher's clamp or elevated using a retractor and mobilized completely with the electrocautery. After xiphoid detachment from rectus and diaphragmatic fibers, the pericardium can be identified by blunt dissection (Fig. 5.13).[5,199] After opening the pericardial sac, thrombus extraction and decompression are facilitated by suction. Adding a Silastic tube may be enough to control bleeding from small penetrating injuries from catheters and pacing wires, as bleeding often is self-limiting. At our university, pericardial tubes are left in place until drainage ceases completely.

When pericardial hemorrhage persists after initial tube decompression and hemodynamic restoration, either an exploratory thoracotomy or median sternotomy should be performed. Superb access to both right and left ventricles, right atrium, and great vessel origins can be obtained by extending the subxiphoid incision into a median sternotomy. Although cardiopulmonary bypass is required infrequently, cannulation is easier by a sternotomy. However, the descending aorta and proximal pulmonary artery can be used for perfusion when bypass becomes necessary through a left thoracotomy. Exploration and repair of associated tracheal, esophageal, and descending aortic injuries are difficult through the sternotomy approach.

In unstable patients the exploration must be performed in a precise, expedient manner. At East Carolina University, a cardiopulmonary perfusionist is notified during patient transport and is available to maintain blood-conserving equipment and potential bypass perfusion. Autotransfusion has been helpful for patients with these and other chest injuries both in the operating room and postoperative Lunit. To perform an exploratory thoracotomy, the left side of the chest is elevated 30° and the anterolateral fourth intercostal space opened (Fig. 5.14).[119] With this approach the chest can be entered rapidly and a retractor inserted for wide exposure. When the entire mediastinum and right side of the chest must be entered, this incision can be extended across the sternum with a Lebsche knife or Gigli's saw. The pericardium should be opened 2 cm to 3 cm

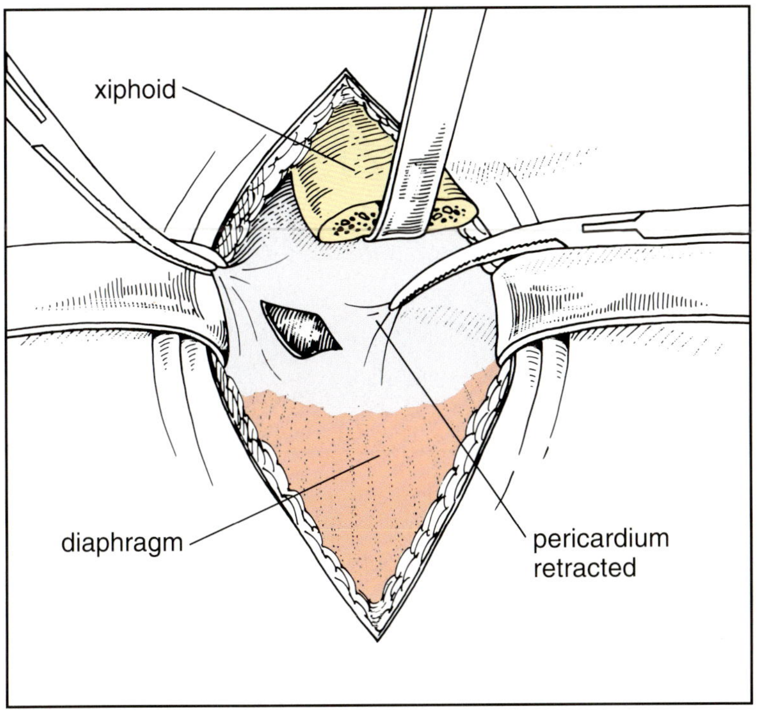

FIGURE 5.13 The subxiphoid approach for emergency pericardial tube insertion and decompression. (Adapted from Arom KV, Richardson JD, Webb G et al: Subxiphoid pericardial window in patients with suspected traumatic pericardial tamponade. Ann Thorac Surg 23:545–549, 1977.)

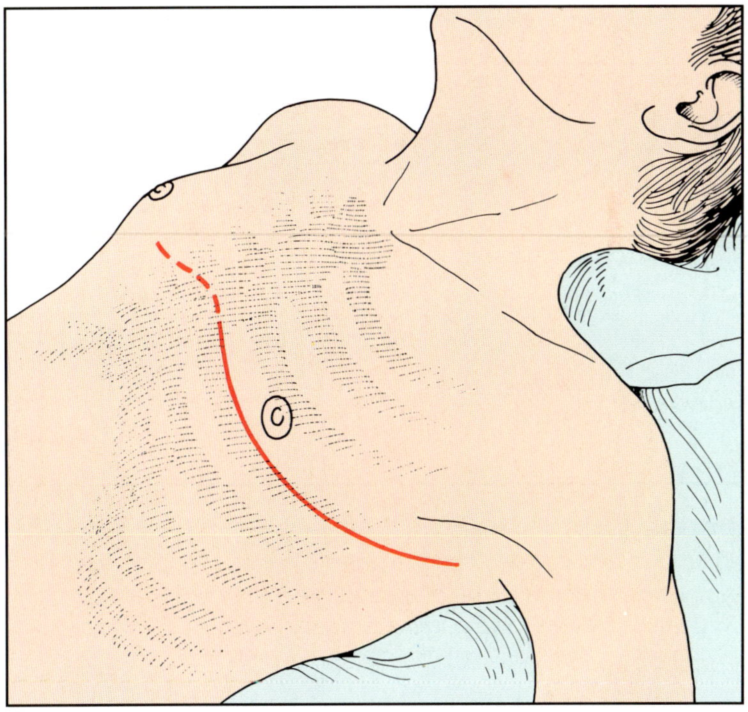

FIGURE 5.14 The appropriate incision for an emergency thoracotomy. The same incision can be used in either the operating room or emergency department for rapid cardiac access. (Adapted from Symbas PN: Trauma to the heart and great vessels. In Jamieson SW [ed]: Rob & Smith's Operative Surgery. St. Louis, CV Mosby, 1986.)

anterior and parallel to the phrenic nerve, avoiding transection and crush injury (Fig. 5.15). Pericardial thrombus removal, injury identification, and hemorrhage control should be done in rapid sequence. In many cases digital compression will stop the bleeding and allow careful inspection. For small wounds pressure may be held until arrhythmias quieten and cardiac hemodynamics are restored.[245] Subsequently, suture closure can be effected by one of several methods, depending on the site and nature of injury. Care should be taken to prevent myocardial tearing and extension into a greater injury. Sutures tied during cardiac contraction may lacerate the ventricular wall even more. Either the crossed stitch technique or Teflon-felt-pledgeted sutures are best for closing most cardiac injuries (Figs. 5.16 and 5.17). We believe the latter method to be preferable. Mattress sutures and Teflon strips are helpful to buttress larger ventricular lacerations (Fig. 5.18). Extensive ventricular injuries may require cardiopulmonary bypass, chamber decompression, and patch closure.[138,245] Prior to chest closure, the heart should be palpated for thrills, which may indicate either a residual intracardiac shunt or valvular disruption.[138] No attempt should be made to repair these defects unless hemodynamic instability would persist without additional surgery.[245] Postoperative echocardiography and catheterization are helpful for detecting residual internal cardiac problems.

Ventricular lacerations near major coronary arteries warrant special consideration to avoid myocardial ischemia, and most can be closed by undersewing the vessel (Fig. 5.19). Most atrial tears can be controlled with a partial occlusion clamp and closed

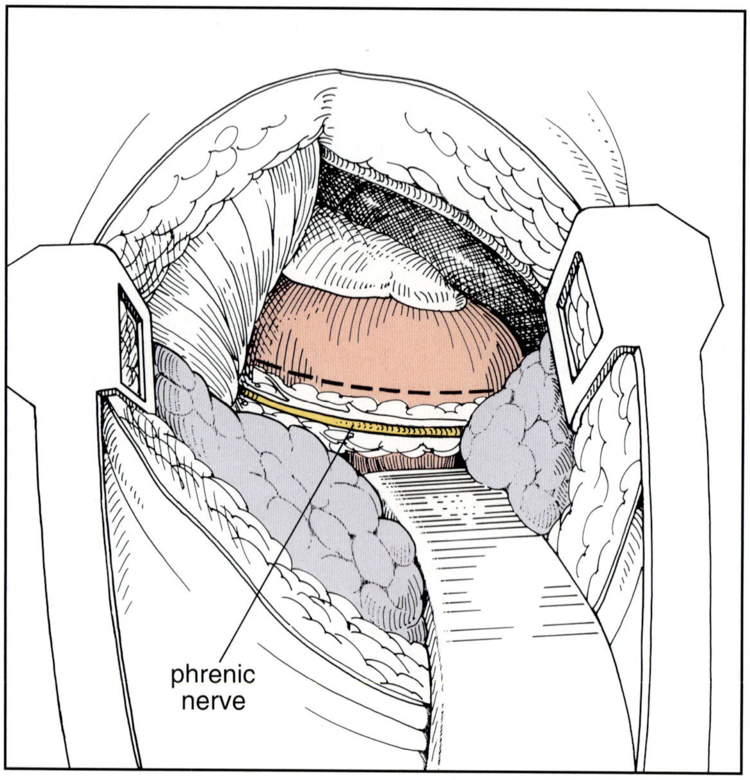

FIGURE 5.15 After the chest is entered, an incision is made anterior to and parallel with the phrenic nerve. (Adapted from Symbas PN: Trauma to the heart and great vessels. In Jamieson SW [ed]: Rob & Smith's Operative Surgery. St. Louis, CV Mosby, 1986.)

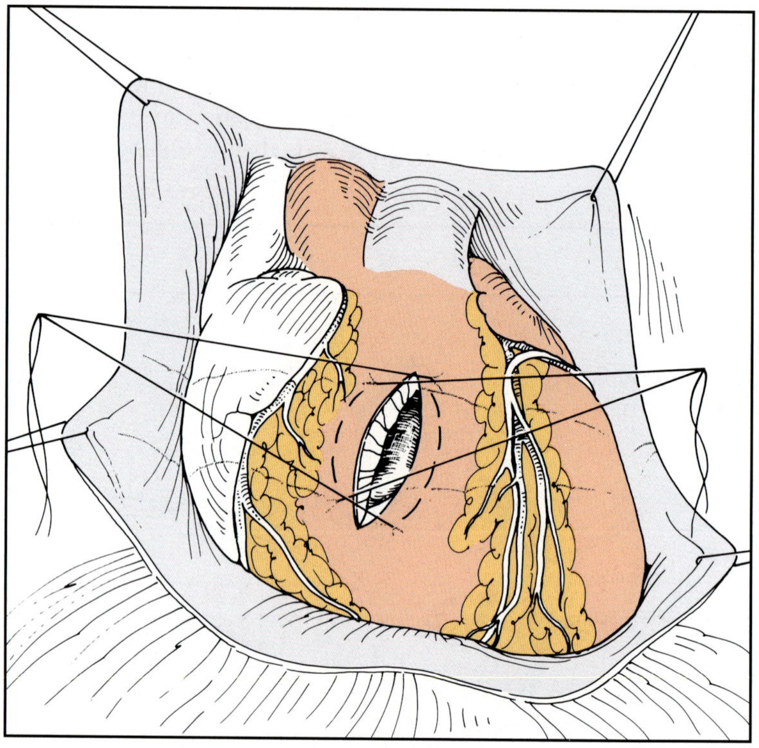

FIGURE 5.16 To relieve wall tension and control bleeding, the crossed suture technique may be applied even for relatively large cardiac wounds. (Adapted from Symbas PN: Trauma to the heart and great vessels. In Jamieson SW [ed]: Rob & Smith's Operative Surgery. St. Louis, CV Mosby, 1986.)

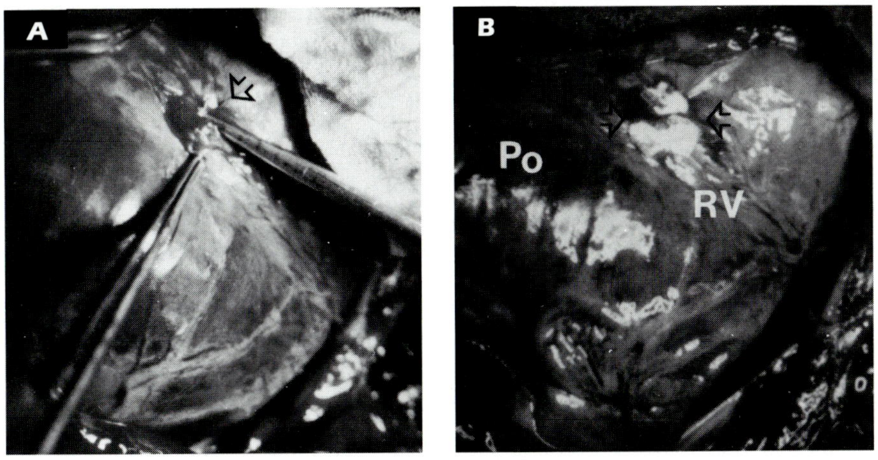

FIGURE 5.17 A Felt pledgeted sutures are being used to close a right ventricular stab wound (arrow). **B** Two pledgets (arrows) buttress the wound closure in the ventricle. (Po, pulmonary artery outflow tract; RV, right ventricle) (Courtesy of Dr. Daniel Rosenthal, Brooke Army Hospital.)

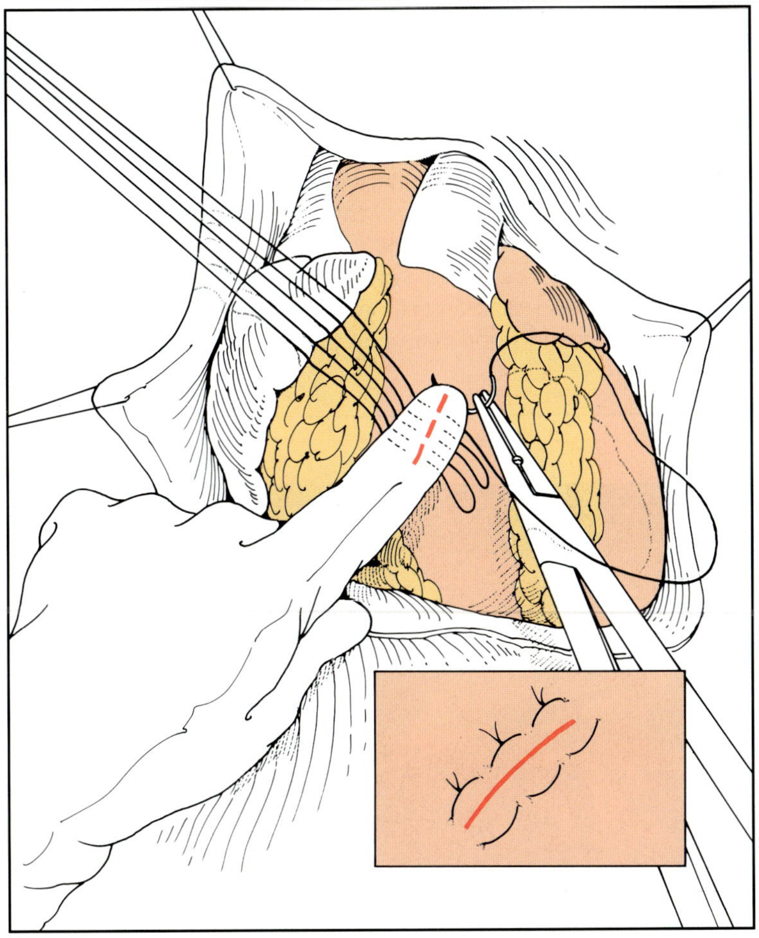

FIGURE 5.18 Multiple mattress sutures are shown to close a relatively long right ventricular injury. (Adapted from Symbas PN: Trauma to the heart and great vessels. In Jamieson SW [ed]: Rob & Smith's Operative Surgery. St. Louis, CV Mosby, 1986.)

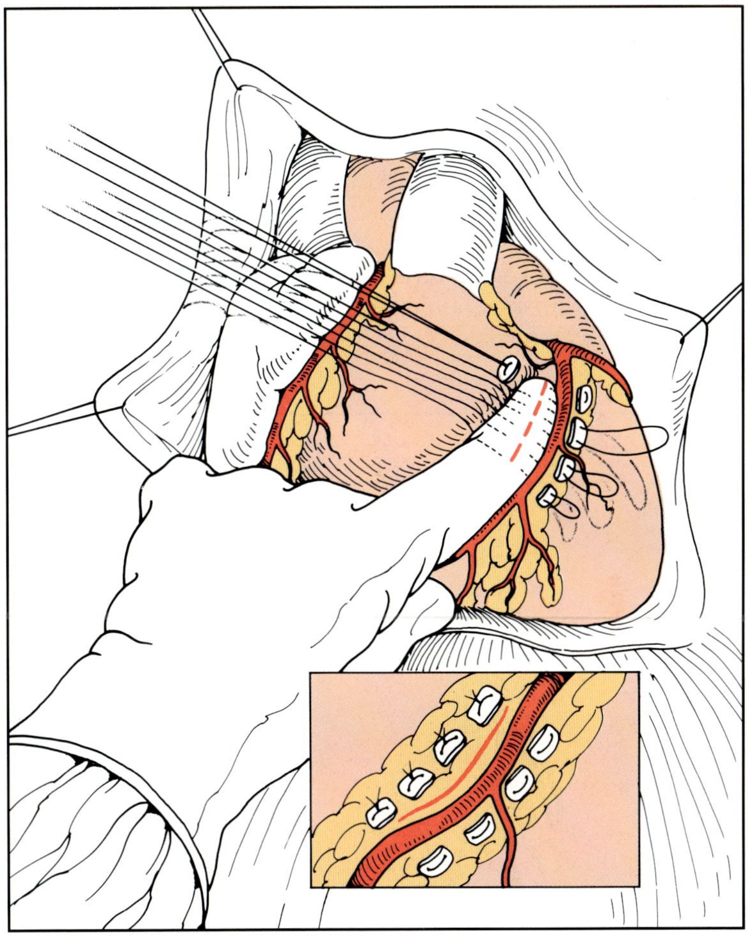

FIGURE 5.19 A ventricular laceration is present close to the left anterior descending coronary artery. Pledgeted sutures are used to undersew the coronary and close the laceration without creating myocardial ischemia. (Adapted from Symbas PN: Trauma to the heart and great vessels. In Jamieson SW [ed]: Rob & Smith's Operative Surgery. St. Louis, CV Mosby, 1986.)

by oversewing the injury (Figs. 5.20 and 5.21). Also, balloon catheters may be inserted to control bleeding temporarily. Atrial injuries can be treacherous, especially with large tears from blunt trauma. Moreover, lacerations in the atrioventricular groove, near the right or circumflex coronary arteries or posterior coronary sinus, often require cardiopulmonary bypass for meticulous repair. Levitsky and Arbulu independently described intra-atrial stenting techniques to repair multiple penetrating superior caval injuLries occurring close to the right atrium (Fig. 5.22).[4,138] The short intrapericardial segment of inferior vena cava may be repaired by Foley catheter obturation and purse-string closure.[7] Prior to chest approximation, the posterior wall of the heart should be inspected, as should mammary and intercostal vessels. The pericardial incision should be approximated in several places to allow continued drainage and avoid cardiac herniation.

The emergency room thoracotomy should be performed in a similar fashion as the procedure just described. Obviously, chest preparation must be abbreviated. Should cardiac arrest be evident on opening the chest, the cardiac wound may be repaired rapidly before defibrillation, which may help avoid additional myocardial tearing. Resuscitation, to the point when defibrillation will be effective, may require intracardiac epinephrine injections (2–3 ml of 1:10,000 epinephrine) and correction of both arterial blood gases and base deficits.[245] All emergency room thoracotomy instruments should be checked after each use and kept available in well marked trays. At our institution monofilament sutures (3-0 and 2-0 polypropylene), Teflon-felt strips, sterile open-chest defibrillator paddles, pacing wires, and intracardiac medications are available in the emergency trauma rooms.

Associated Cardiac Injuries

Secondary cardiac injuries may accompany penetrating wounds in up to 50% of patients. These may include coronary injuries and fistulas, intracardiac shunts, valvular damage, retained intramyocardial foreign bodies and emboli, and pericarditis. Some of these complications should be repaired during the original exploration; however, a number require further evaluation and therapy. Figure 5.23 provides a diagnostic plan for evaluating these patients.

CORONARY ARTERY INJURIES AND FISTULAS

Penetrating cardiac trauma has been compounded with coronary injuries in 4% to 12% of patients.[80,199,205,245] Traumatic coronary lesions include lacerations, arteriovenous and coronary-cameral fistulas, dissections, and secondary aneurysms.[88] The incidence of direct traumatic involvement in the left anterior descending system is 62%; the right, 28%; and circumflex arteries, 10%.[80,83,199] Rea found only 36 cases of coronary lacerations reported until 1969 when he added an additional 22 cases with a 44% mortality overall.[199] Left and right main coronary injuries often resulted in

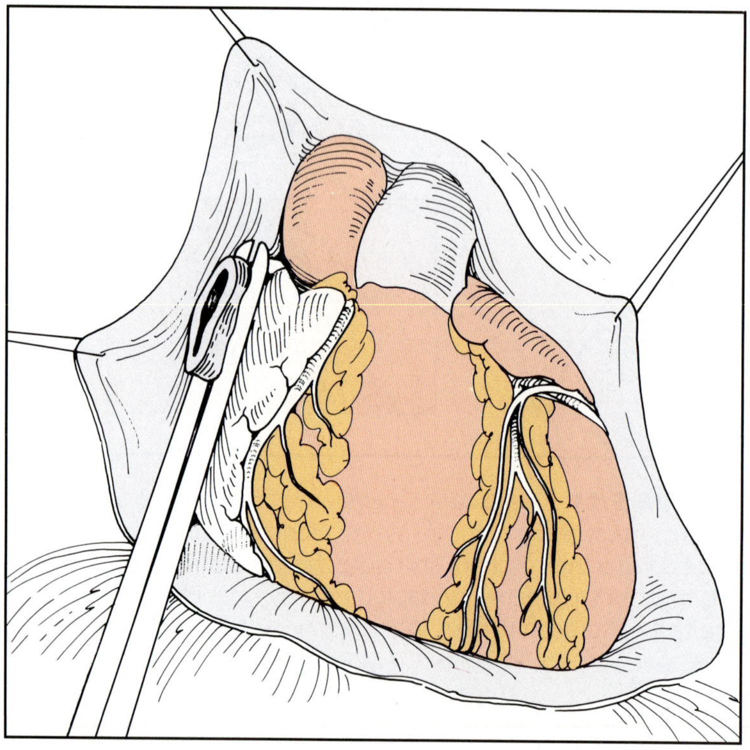

FIGURE 5.20 A partial occlusion clamp is shown to control a penetration atrial laceration. (Adapted from Symbas PN: Trauma to the heart and great vessels. In Jamieson SW [ed]: Rob & Smith's Operative Surgery. St. Louis, CV Mosby, 1986.)

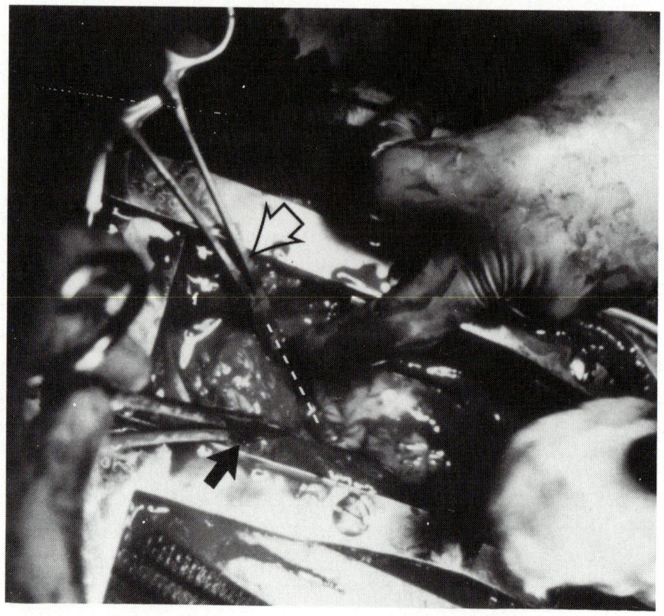

FIGURE 5.21 This patient sustained a gunshot injury of the right atrium (dotted line). Control has been effected by a Satinsky-type clamp (open arrow). The laceration is being oversewn (solid arrow, needle holder). (Courtesy of Dr. Daniel Rosenthal, Brooke Army Hospital.)

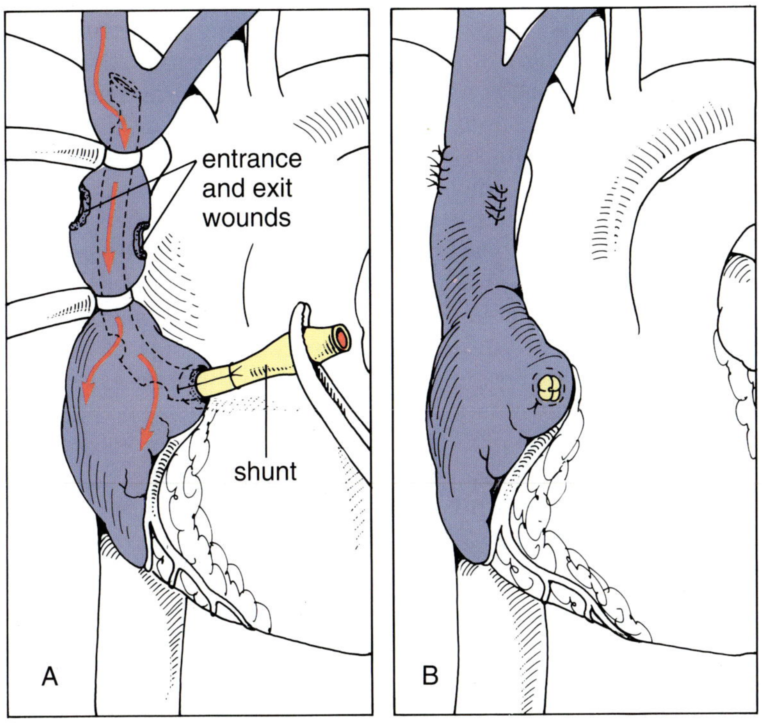

FIGURE 5.22 Two small-caliber gunshot wounds are located near the right atrial-caval junction. **A** A stent has been inserted through the right atrial appendage to control bleeding. Cardiopulmonary bypass was not required using this method. **B** The superior vena cava is shown after repair. (Adapted from Levitsky S: New insights in cardiac trauma. Surg Clin North Am 55:43–55, 1975.)

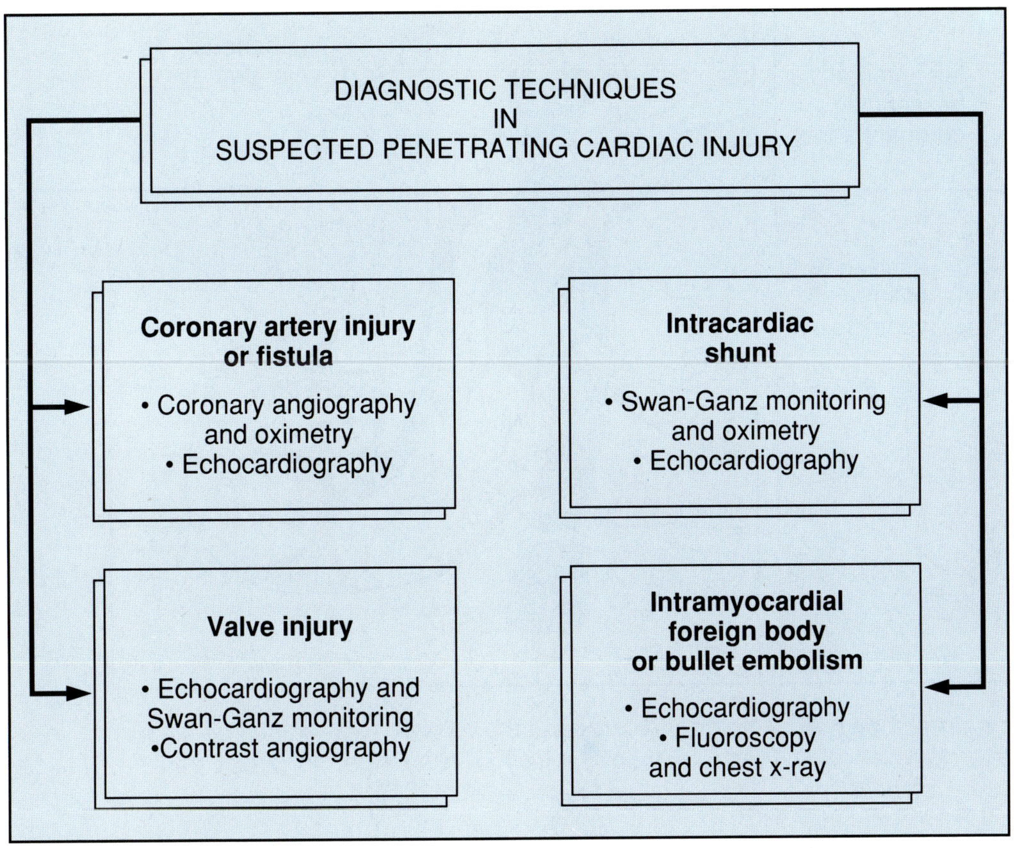

FIGURE 5.23 A diagnostic plan for evaluating penetrating heart trauma patients who are suspected of having other cardiac injuries.

death because these early patients were treated by ligation alone; of those surviving, 90% developed myocardial infarctions. However, Rea did propose that primary coronary repair would be the optimal therapy if possible. The authors concluded that concurrent coronary injuries carried a 20% higher hospital mortality than with chamber wounds alone.[199]

In the presence of a major coronary laceration, patients may die of acute tamponade, intrathoracic bleeding, myocardial ischemia, or attendant arrhythmias. With major coronary injuries, control of hemorrhage and direct suture, patch closure, or coronary grafting remain the repairs of choice. Injuries to smaller vessels may require ligation despite the probability of myocardial infarction and ventricular aneurysms. Literature reports of coronary artery repair following penetrating injuries are relatively sparse. In 1973 Tector treated two patients with direct coronary stab injuries by saphenous bypass grafting during cardiopulmonary bypass.[253] Levitsky repaired a tangential coronary-ventricular gunshot wound by a similar method (Fig. 5.24).[138] Subsequently, Espada reported seven traumatic coronary injuries bypassed successfully.[80] Modern cardiopulmonary bypass techniques should allow precise grafting and repair of major coronary injuries.

Coronary-cameral and coronary-venous fistulas are rare but may develop following penetrating cardiac injuries.[40,203,216] By 1973 only 11 cases had been reported.[139] The 1983 review by Lowe covered this subject most comprehensively and detailed 26 patients treated since 1958.[144] In this study, coronary fistulas were the result of gunshot and shrapnel injuries in 61% of patients and of stab wounds in 15%, while the remainder were due to blunt cardiac trauma. The right coronary artery and ventricle were involved most frequently. Detailed locations of coronary and cavitary involvement are related in Figure 5.25. The majority of patients presented either with angina pectoris (68%) or congestive heart failure (19%). In general, these fistu-

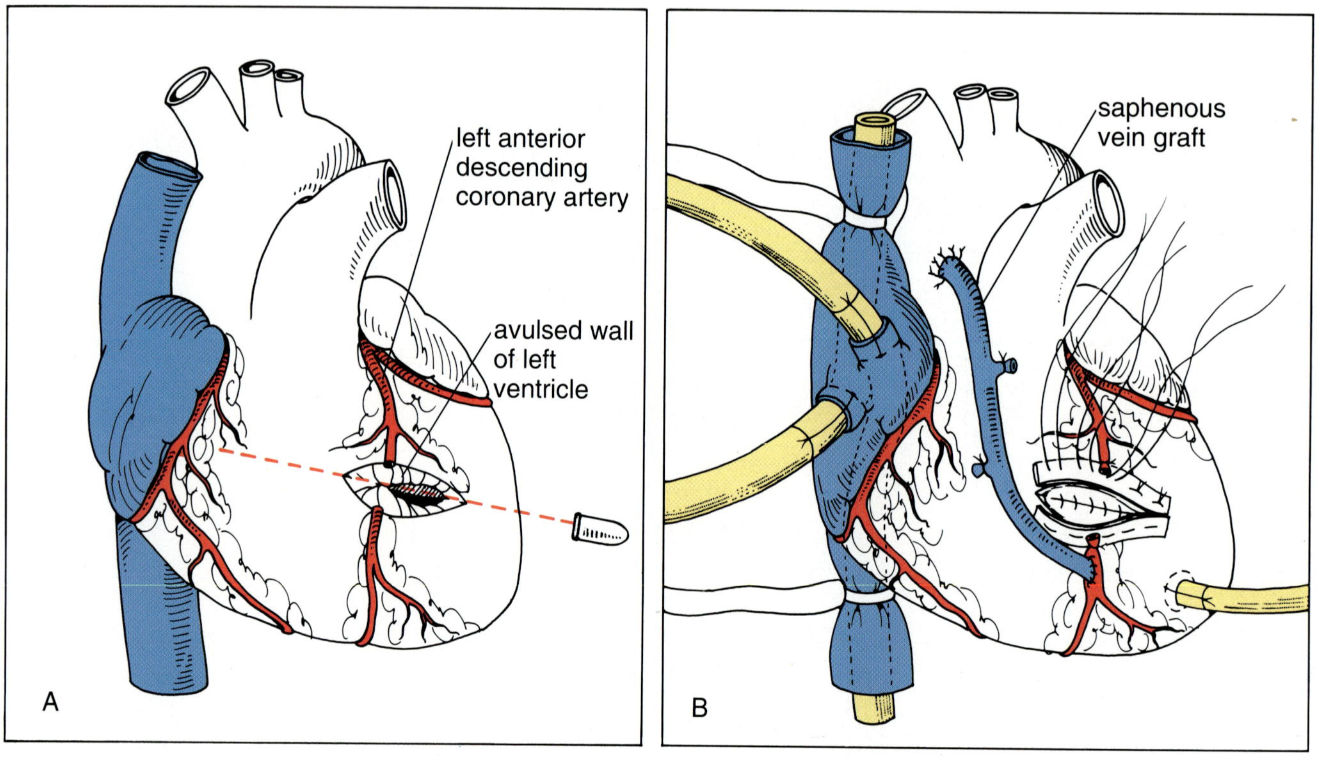

FIGURE 5.24 A tangential gunshot injury is shown **A** to avulse a segment of the left ventricular wall along with the left anterior descending coronary artery. **B** The ventricular laceration was closed with a Teflon strip and mattress sutures and the coronary was grafted distally. Adapted from (Levitsky S: New insights in cardiac trauma. Surg Clin North Am 55:43–55, 1975.)

las mature with time and the involved vessels enlarge markedly.[144] Typical continuous murmurs are often present; however, patients with connections between the left anterior descending coronary artery and left ventricle may have the diastolic component alone.[245]

Right heart and selective coronary angiography provides the diagnosis in most cases.[88] Figure 5.26 shows the angiogram of a right coronary atrial fistula that was repaired when the patient developed symptoms 31 years following a Korean War injury.[144] Recently, contrast echocardiography and computed tomography have been used for diagnosing these fistulas, but angiography remains the definitive test.[59,149] In coronary fistula patients, pulmonary-to-systemic flow ratios have averaged 1.5:1, but little correlation with the magnitude of symptoms has existed.[144]

Collateral arteries often supply vessels distal to coronary fistulas. Angina appears to result from coronary blood flowing preferentially through the low-resistance fistula. Thus, the more proximal left-to-right shunt steals blood flow instead of supplying distal myocardium. Lowe and others have proposed that collaterals develop from the decreasing coronary pressure gradient. Increased retrograde flow through these collaterals from other coronary beds may even result in extension of the ischemic zone.[144,227,242] Only 11.5% of traumatic coronary fistula patients have normal electrocardiograms.

As symptoms develop in most patients, surgical therapy has been recommended for both congenital and traumatic coronary fistulas.[139,144,145] In the majority of patients, fistulas can be closed from within the cardiac chamber on cardiopulmonary bypass, reconstituting distal flow effectively. However, occasionally bypass grafting will become necessary. Other operations that have been used include external fistula obliteration or fistulaorrhaphy, ligation with distal bypass grafting, and simple proximal ligation. However, the internal approach appears

FIGURE 5.25
LOCATIONS OF TRAUMATIC CORONARY ARTERY FISTULAS[144]

LOCATION	PERCENTAGE*
Coronary Artery	
Right	54
Left anterior descending	46
Communicating Chamber	
Right ventricle	50
Right atrium	34
Right atrium and ventricle	4
Left ventricle	4
Pulmonary artery	4
Coronary vein	4

*Of 26 fistulas treated since 1958

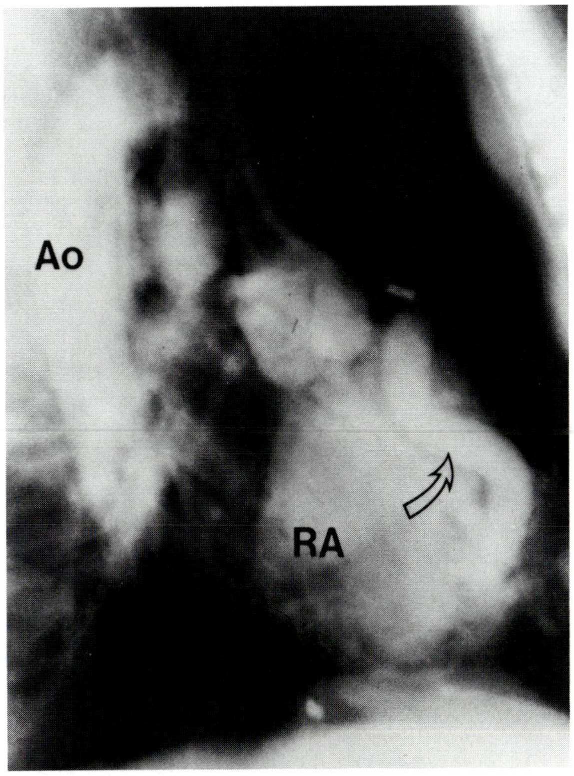

FIGURE 5.26 A large traumatic right coronary artery–atrial fistula (arrow). (Ao, aorta; RA, right atrium) (Lowe JE, Adams DH, Cummings RG et al: The natural history and recommended management of patients with traumatic coronary artery fistulas. Ann Thorac Surg 36:295–305, 1983.)

superior; brief cardiopulmonary bypass, normothermia, and ventricular fibrillation will allow complete identification of shunting connections (Fig. 5.27).[145]

INTRACARDIAC SHUNTS AND VALVE INJURIES

Residual intracardiac shunts result in 4% to 5% of all cardiac injuries.[36,276] Approximately 101 cases had been reported by 1981.[255] Of 15 post-traumatic intracardiac shunts reported from Baylor University, 60% were from stab wounds.[276] Of patients with traumatic intracardiac shunts, ventricular septal defects (VSD) have occurred in 54% to 67% and 20% to 27% have had an ascending aorta–right ventricular fistula (A-RVF).[198,210,255,276] The remainder have included right ventricular–vena caval, aorto–pulmonary artery, and aorto–right atrial fistulas, all of which occur uncommonly but need repair.[198,210,255] Multiple cardiac chamber injuries may result in separate but concurrent intracardiac shunts.[210] Often these shunts are not detected at the time of the initial exploration. A palpable thrill, characteristic murmur, and radiographic stigmata of heart failure may suggest either a residual intracardiac shunt or valve injury (Fig. 5.28). The murmur and thrill may not be evident immediately but may mature with time.[255] In all cases additional diagnostic echocardiography, oximetry, and angiography should be done to confirm the clinical impression and localize the lesion. Generally, these injuries are repaired 4 to 6 weeks later when patients have become more stable, tissues are less friable, and some defects have had the opportunity to close spontaneously.[198,212,245]

In 1951, O'Neill first closed a VSD resulting from a stab wound. Between 1% and 4% of all penetrating cardiac injuries may result in a residual VSD.[18,245] Most patients become symptomatic (88%), with cardiac failure developing several days to weeks later. Although a small traumatic VSD may remain asymptomatic, nearly all patients with an A-RVF develop symptoms requiring relatively early repair. Moreover, traumatic aortic incompetence occurs in almost 50% of A-RVF patients but valvuloplasty or valve replacement is rarely indicated.[198,255] Some authors recommend not repairing the small asymptomatic VSD with a shunt of less than 1.5:1 and a normal heart size.[255] In one study up to 32% of these did not require repair.[8] Usually, a VSD or A-RVF resulting from a penetrating injury can be repaired on cardiopulmonary bypass from within the right ventricle with pledgeted sutures; however, patch closure and a left ventricular approach may be necessary for larger penetrating defects (Figs. 5.29 and 5.30).[8,276] Up to 13% of traumatic VSD patients have residual right-sided conduction defects; however, complete heart block is rare.[198]

Symbas has related that in cardiac gunshot and stab wounds, the true incidence of concurrent *valve injuries* has been difficult to establish because many patients die before evaluation.[245]

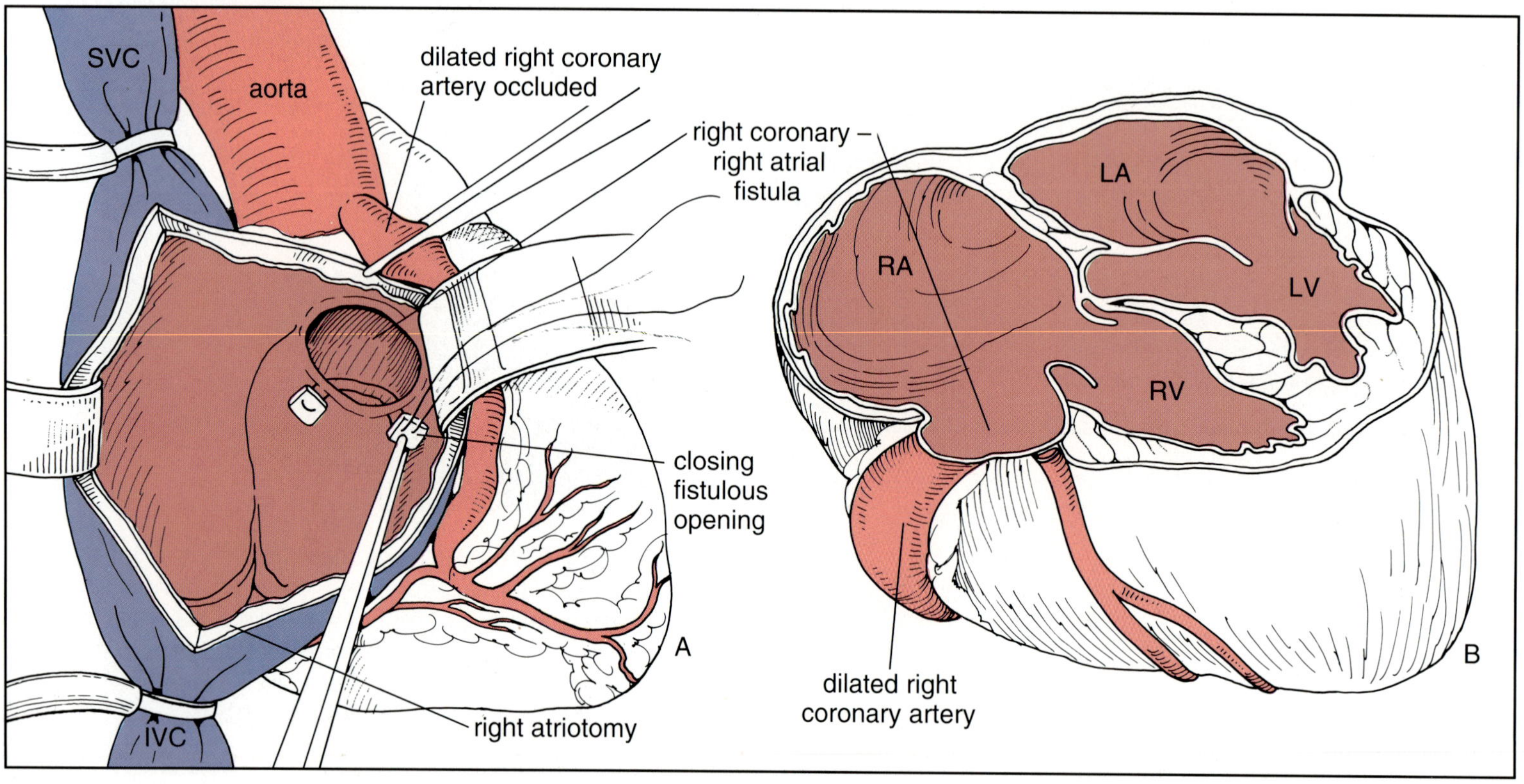

FIGURE 5.27 Closure of a right coronary–atrial fistula on cardiopulmonary bypass. Under normothermic beating and fibrillating conditions, the fistula orifice can be seen easily within the right atrium and closed. This illustrates closure of a congenital fistula; the traumatic variety is repaired by the same technique. (Adapted from Lowe JE, Oldham HN, Sabiston DC: Surgical management of congenital coronary artery fistulas. Ann Surg 194:373–380, 1981.)

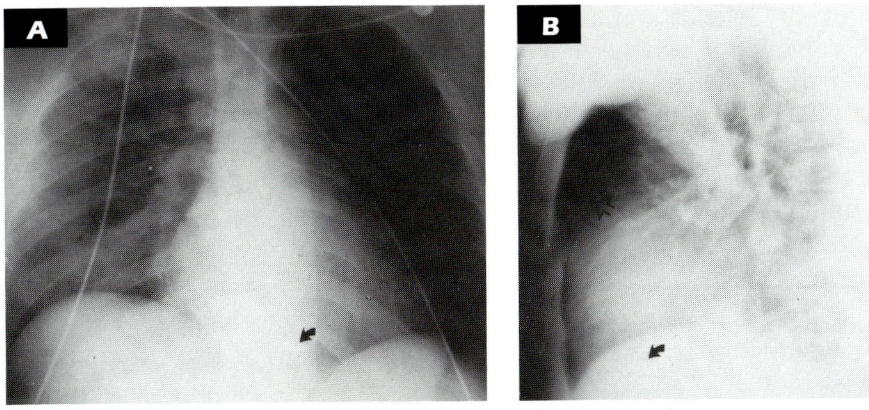

FIGURE 5.28 This patient sustained a .32-caliber gunshot wound (**A**, arrow) resulting in a traumatic ventricular septal defect. Radiographic cardiomegaly and pulmonary vascular congestion suggest an intracardiac shunt. **B** In this lateral view the bullet is marked by the solid arrow. Note the right ventricular prominence (open arrow), suggesting the shunt. (Courtesy of the Department of Radiology, Duke University.)

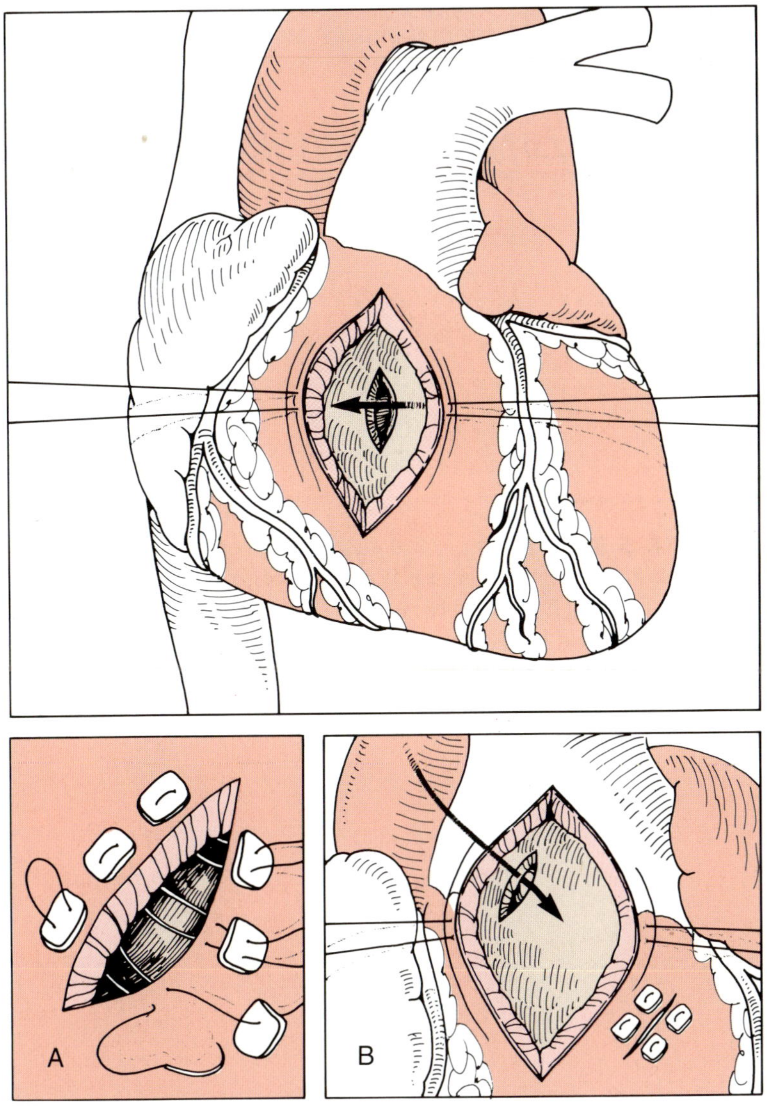

FIGURE 5.29 A ventricular septal defect resulting from a penetrating injury. **(Inset A)** Penetrating communications can often be closed by simple pledgeted mattress sutures. **(Inset B)** An aorto–right ventricular shunt can be closed by a similar technique. (Adapted from Whisennand HH, Van Pelt SA, Beall AC et al: Surgical management of traumatic intracardiac injuries. Ann Thorac Surg 28:530–536, 1979.)

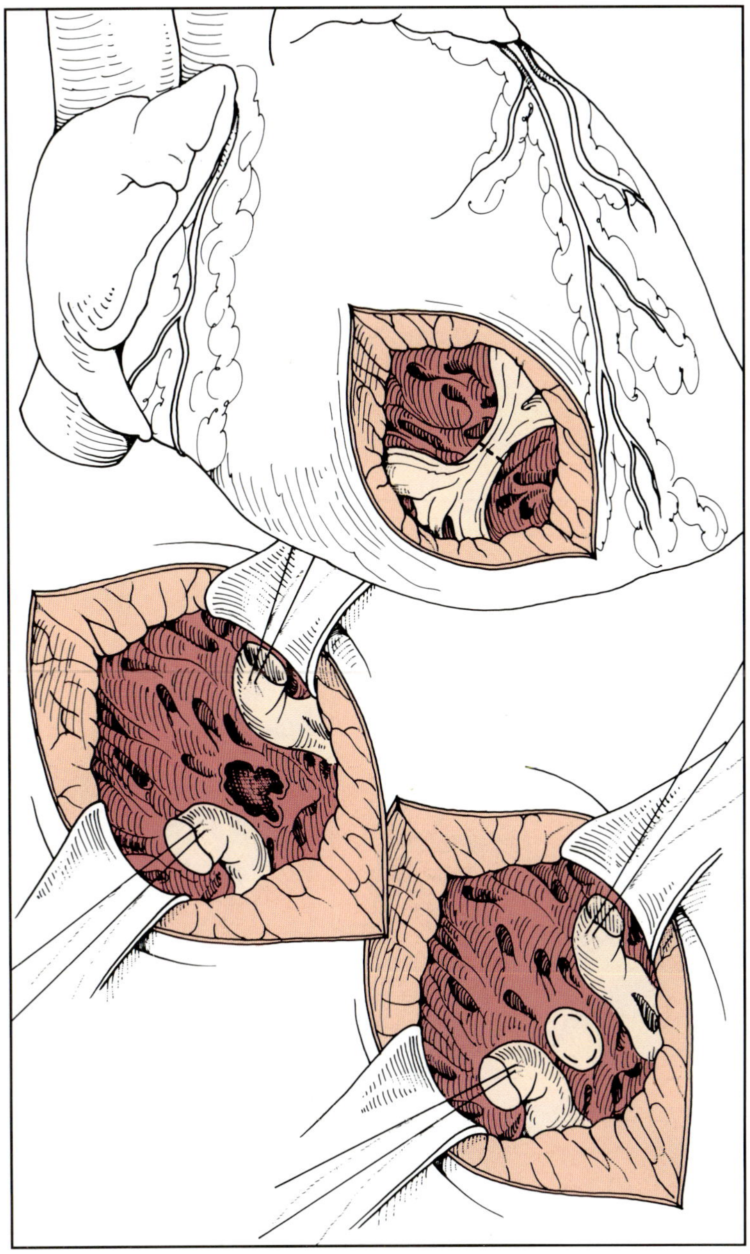

FIGURE 5.30 Closure of ventricular septal defect from penetrating injuries may require a left ventriculotomy and patch closure. (Adapted from Asfaw I, Thoms NW, Arbulu A: Interventricular septal defects from penetrating injuries of the heart. J Thorac Cardiovasc Surg 69:450–457, 1975.)

Roughly 4% of patients with penetrating injuries sustain concomitant valvular involvement; blunt trauma results in valve disruptions even less frequently. Valve injuries occur in the leaflets, annulus, or supporting structures and are most often associated with other cardiac maladies. Penetrating injuries most frequently involve the aortic valve, followed by the tricuspid valve.[111,198] Symptoms usually result from valvular insufficiency and associated cardiac injuries. Although many advocate valve replacement, the aortic, mitral, and tricuspid leaflets have successfully been repaired both primarily and with autologous pericardium (Figs. 5.31 and 5.32).[25,79,111,113, 138,183] Cryopreserved homograft aortic valves may be optimal in young patients requiring elective replacement for penetrating valve injuries.

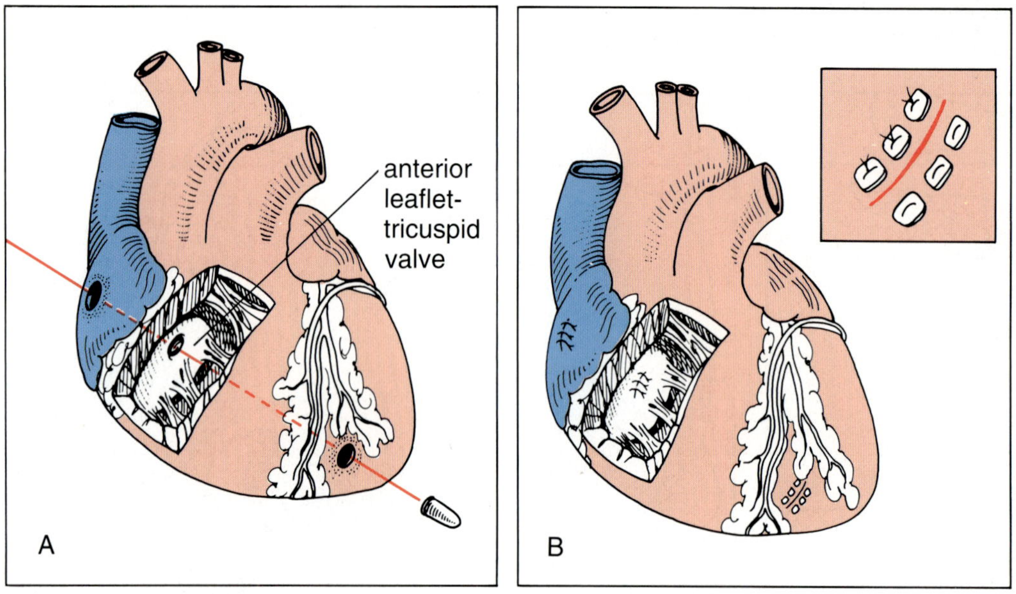

FIGURE 5.31 A A transmural projectile has injured a tricuspid valve leaflet. **B** This leaflet was repaired primarily. (Adapted from Levitsky S: New insights in cardiac trauma. Surg Clin North Am 55:43–55, 1975.)

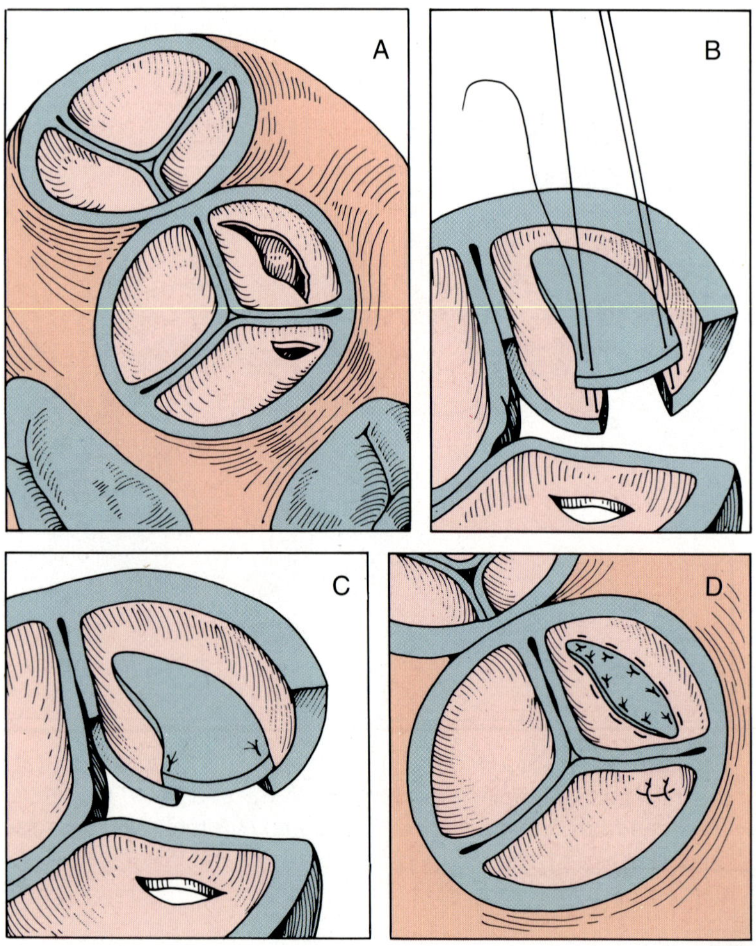

FIGURE 5.32 This aortic valve cusp was lacerated by a knife in an altercation and was repaired using an autologous pericardial patch. (Adapted from Hutchinson JE, Schmidt DM, Cameron A, McCord CW: The surgical management of intracardiac defects due to penetrating trauma. J Thorac Cardiovasc Surg 65:103–107, 1973.)

INTRAMYOCARDIAL FOREIGN BODIES AND EMBOLI

Concern over a retained intramyocardial bullet or foreign body has persisted over the years.[63,172] Harken popularized this concern and showed that bullets and shell fragments could be removed safely.[104] These materials can embolize or become infective or may be the nidus for a cardiac neurosis.[245,247] Projectiles may enter the myocardium at the primary injury site or migrate to the heart from peripheral veins. Body position, bullet size, gravitational forces, and respiratory movements all influence central venous movement of foreign bodies to the right side of the heart. Cardiac contraction influences embolization to pulmonary and peripheral systemic arteries.[109,134,245]

Materials imbedded near the endocardial surface may erode and subsequently embolize. Pulmonary infections and limb ischemia may be the presenting symptoms of a foreign body retained earlier in the left heart wall. Many patients with intramyocardial materials are asymptomatic, but post-traumatic pericarditis may result. Most clinicians believe that ventricular intramyocardial foreign bodies should be removed electively at a time distant from the original injury or cardiac repair. However, easily palpable, intra-atrial, and obvious ventricular projectiles should be extracted at the initial operation. Up to 50% of bullets may have positive pericardial cultures at exploration. For this reason and to prevent erosion, most pericardial bullets should also be removed.[163]

Recent individual reports by Symbas, Harrison, and Hassett have suggested newer techniques for localizing intramyocardial foreign bodies prior to and during surgical removal.[106,107,247] Retained bullets, birdshot, and shell fragments seen within the mediastinal shadow on the emergency room x-ray film are of concern even in stable patients. Blurring of the projectile image suggests motion and either cardiac or great vessel retention (Fig. 5.33). With shotgun wounds numerous small pellets may make the task of identification more difficult (Fig. 5.34). In stable patients flouroscopy is very helpful for identifying possible cardiac retention. In one of our patients, a shotgun pellet was imbedded in the wall of the right atrial appendage, creating an interesting orbital pattern on fluoroscopy.

Recently, portable two-dimensional and M-mode echocardiography have been helpful for identifying location, transmural depth, and surgical accessibility of intramyocardial missiles immediately after injury (Fig. 5.35).[107] On echo studies these fragments may be seen as bright targets with multiple reverberations (Fig. 5.36). Simultaneously, wall motion abnormalities, pericardial bleeding and effusions, residual intracardiac defects, and valve injuries can be assessed with good resolution. Microcavitation bubble studies have allowed early detection of

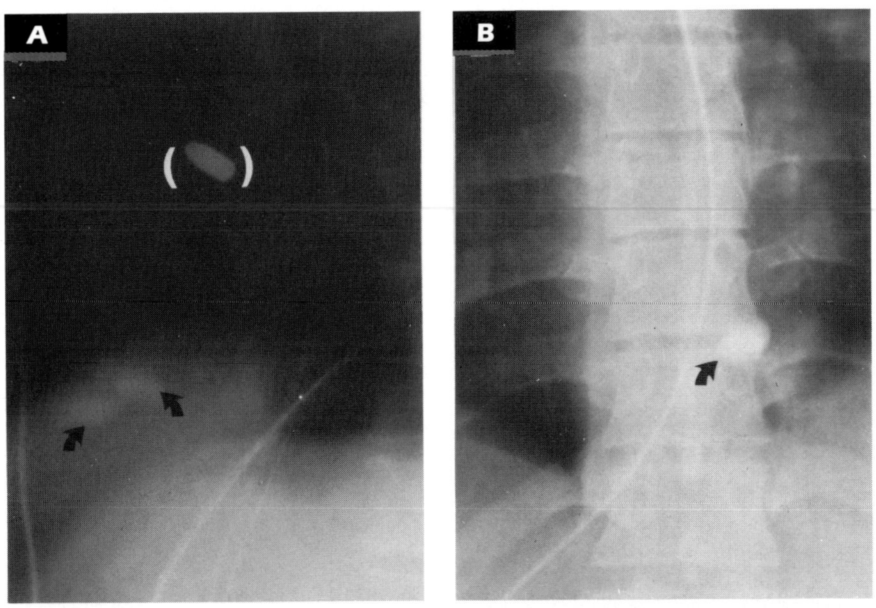

FIGURE 5.33 A Two bullets are seen as blurred shadows on a detailed spot film indicating a probable intramyocardial location (dark arrows). This location was confirmed both by echocardiography and surgical exploration. The clear bullet image (parentheses) indicates localization in either the chest wall or less-mobile lung tissue. **B** Another intramyocardial bullet is demonstrated on a plain spot radiograph. (Courtesy of Dr. Jon Moran, University of Kansas Medical Center.)

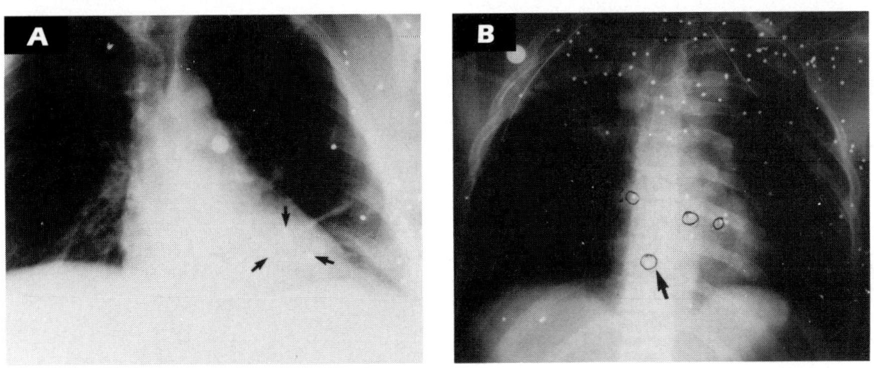

FIGURE 5.34. A Three intramyocardial pellets (arrows) are from a shotgun injury. **B** Four intramyocardial pellets are circled. The upper-and lower-left ones (arrow) demonstrated a peculiar orbital pattern on fluoroscopy suggesting a right atrial location. (Courtesy of Dr. Jon Moran, University of Kansas Medical Center.)

residual septal defects and other shunts.[107] In patients identified as having either metallic fragments close to coronary vessels or intracardiac defects, adjunctive angiography is warranted several days following the initial injury (Figs. 5.37 and 5.38).

Even with standard diagnostic techniques, up to 30% of retained cardiac foreign bodies cannot be localized at surgery despite meticulous searching.[63,182,246] These projectiles may have a subendocardial, intraventricular septal, or intrapapillary muscle location, which makes palpation difficult, even in the asystolic flaccid heart. Harrison and others have facilitated the localization of bullet fragments intraoperatively using a sterile two-dimensional echocardiographic probe (Figs. 5.39 and 5.40).[106,107] Rapid identification and precise intraoperative echo localization usually provide short arrest times and a conservative ventriculotomy.[106] At Duke University, a number of foreign bodies have been retrieved successfully with these echocardio-

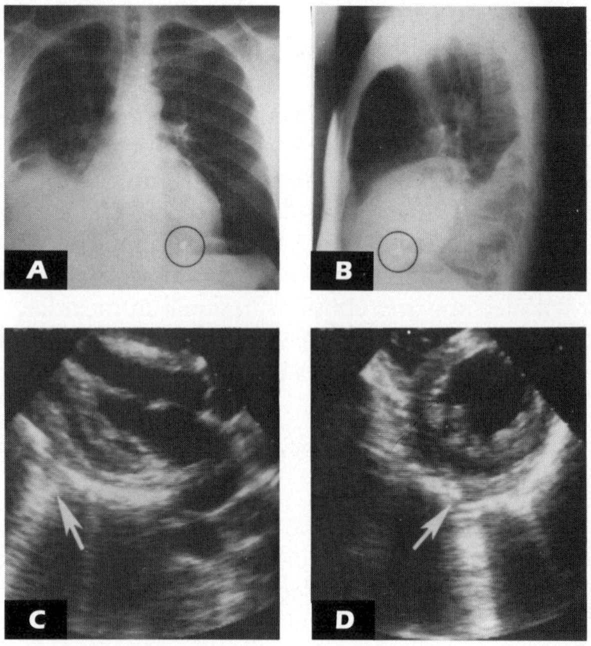

FIGURE 5.35 A,B Chest x-ray from a patient with a single bullet fragment in the cardiac silhouette. **C,D** Left parasternal long and short axis echocardiograms. The missile fragment projects typical diagnostic trailing reverberations (arrows). (Reprinted with permission from the American College of Cardiology ;obJournal of the American College of Cardiology Vol 7, May 1986, pp 1151–1156;cb.)

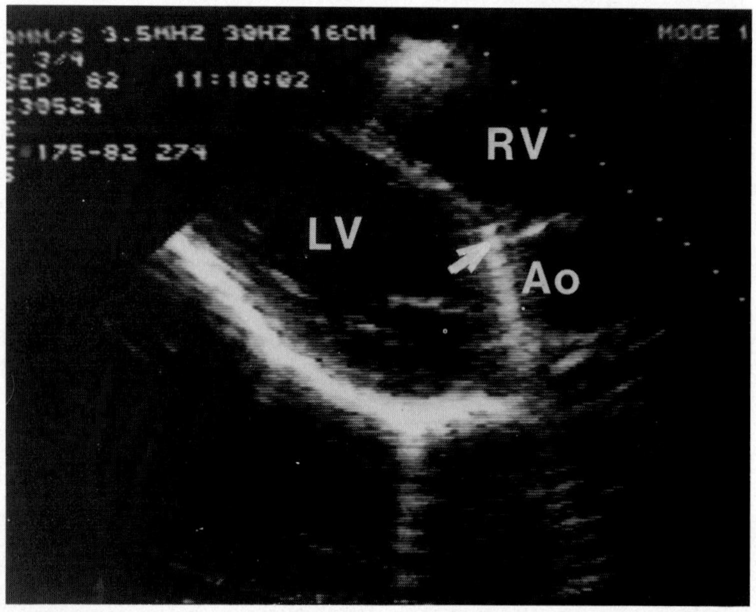

FIGURE 5.36 On this echocardiogram dense trailing reverberations (arrow) suggest location of this pellet high in the interventricular septum. (LV, left ventricle; RV, right ventricle; Ao, aorta.)

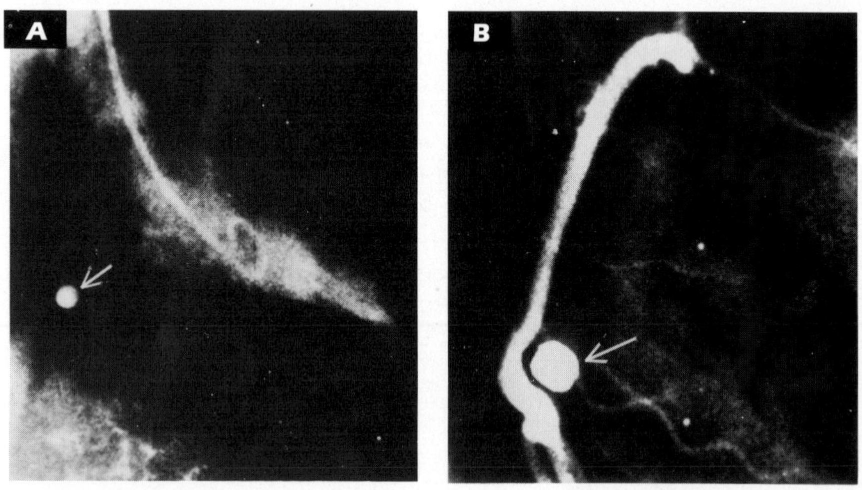

FIGURE 5.37 Ventriculogram **A** and selective coronary angiogram **B** of a patient diagnosed initially as having an intramyocardial .32-caliber bullet wound by echocardiography. Subsequently, the projectile (arrows) was extracted surgically under echocardiographic control. (Courtesy of Dr. Jon Moran, University of Kansas Medical Center.)

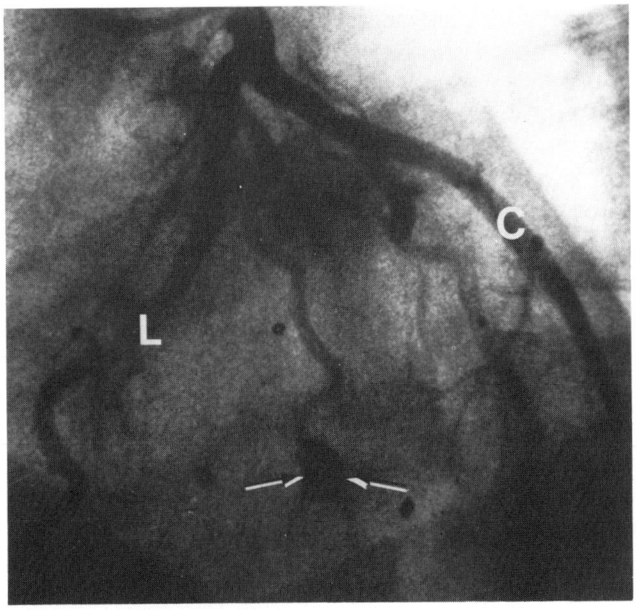

FIGURE 5.38 Coronary arteriogram showing a metallic fragment (arrows) located between the left anterior descending (L) and circumflex coronary arteries (C). (Harrison L, Kisslo JA, Sabiston DC: Extraction of intramyocardial foreign body utilizing operative ultrasonography. J Thorac Cardiovasc Surg 82:345–349, 1982.)

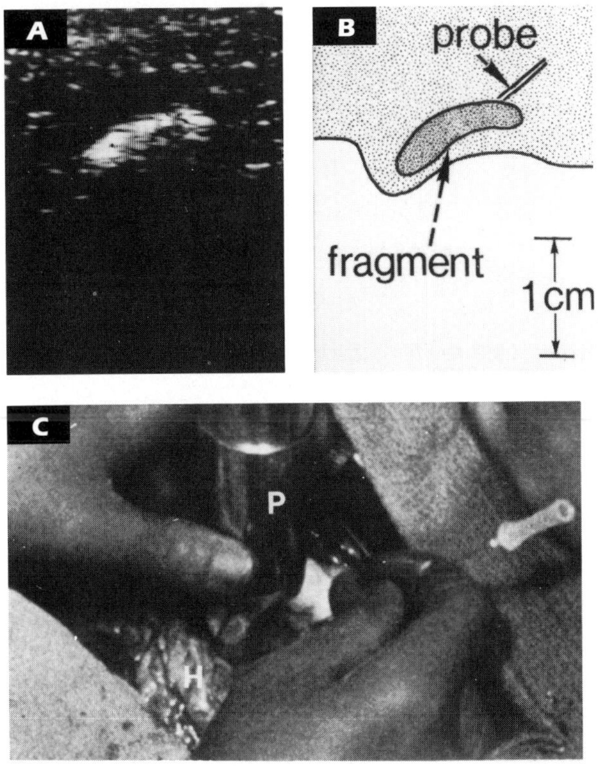

FIGURE 5.39 A An operative echocardiogram of the metallic intramyocardial fragment shown in Figure 5.37. **B** Diagram of the subendocardial location of the fragment. **C** Operative localization of an intramyocardial bullet fragment using a sterile echo probe (P) and needle. (Harrison L, Kisslo JA, Sabiston DC: Extraction of intramyocardial foreign body utilizing operative ultrasonography. J Thorac Cardiovasc Surg 82:345–349, 1981.)

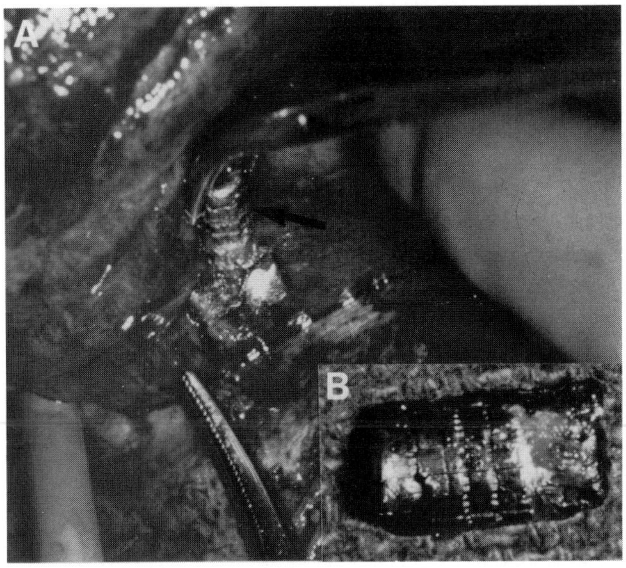

FIGURE 5.40 The bullet shown preoperatively by coronary arteriography in Figure 5.36 is being removed after intraoperative localization with a sterile echo transducer. (Courtesy of Dr. Jon Moran, University of Kansas Medical Center.)

graphic techniques (Fig. 5.41).[107] Intraoperative transesophageal echocardiography seems advantageous for locating these materials and may be applied in the future.

Bullet embolism should be suspected if the projectile is not located on a radiograph of the injured area and no exit wound is found (Fig. 5.42).[245,247] The presence of limb or organ ischemia and projectiles found a distance from the injury also suggest the diagnosis. In 1974 Ward reviewed 36 cases of peripheral arterial bullet emboli and found that ten came from primary cardiac injuries (Figure 5.43).[271] In 12 patients, the aorta was the entrance site. In the remainder, the thorax was penetrated but vascular entrance locations remained undiscovered. Although Ward showed an almost equal incidence of emboli to both legs and a 20% upper extremity involvement, other reports show a predilection for left lower extremity involvement. Most authors have indicated that upper extremity embolization is rare but occurs more often on the right when present. Carotid involvement has been reported.[258] Immediate angiography, exploration, and embolectomy are warranted in patients with limb ischemia and stable cardiac injuries.

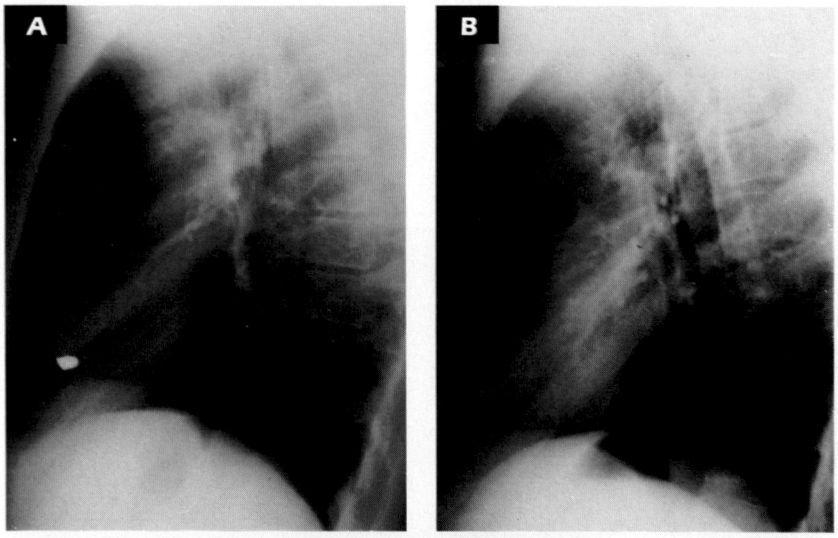

FIGURE 5.41 A Lateral x-ray of a patient having a retained intramyocardial bullet. **B** The same patient following surgical removal. (Courtesy of the Department of Radiology, Duke University Medical Center.)

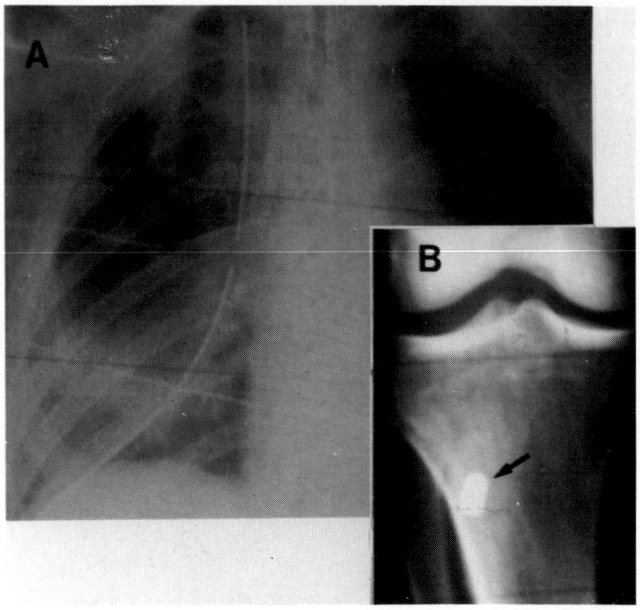

FIGURE 5.42 A Portable chest x-ray film of a patient who sustained a gunshot wound to the left side of the chest resulting in a hemopneumothorax. The bullet was not found on the chest or abdominal x-rays. **B** After searching, the bullet was found to have embolized to the lower extremity (arrow). (Courtesy of Dr. Jon Moran, University of Kansas Medical Center.)

Exploration should be near the site of the missile as manipulation may cause intimal tears.[134] Missiles located in the wall or in close proximity to major vessels should be extirpated to avoid subsequent erosion.[245]

Small fragments, such as birdshot, migrating through the venous system to the right ventricle may be followed in some cases (Fig. 5.44); however, the prophylactic removal of larger bullets has been advocated to avoid further embolization and bacterial endocarditis and to prevent valvular damage. Ledgerwood emphasized the frustration of searching for bullets migrating within the venous system.[134] Stephenson reviewed 18 patients with pulmonary bullet emboli since 1946, with eight undergoing a successful embolectomy.[236] Patients with pulmonary artery bullet emboli either are asymptomatic or may develop chest pain or cough.[247] The diagnosis can often be made by the combination of chest radiography and pulmonary V/Q scanning with arteriography done for confirmation.[134,247] These missiles should be removed electively to prevent continued symptoms as well as pulmonary infection and possible infarction.[236,247]

FIGURE 5.43
LOCATIONS OF SYSTEMIC ARTERIAL BULLET EMBOLI[271]

LOCATION	PERCENTAGE*
Final Arterial Destination	
Lower Extremity	
Femoral	44
Iliac	25
Aorta	8.5
Popliteal	3
Upper Extremity	
Subclavian	5.5
Axillary	5.5
Brachial	5.5
Innominate	2.5
Site of Bullet Origin	
Heart	28
Left ventricle	17
Left atrium	8
Pulmonary vein	3
Thorax (artery unidentified)	32
Thoracic aorta	25
Abdominal aorta	16

*Of 36 patients

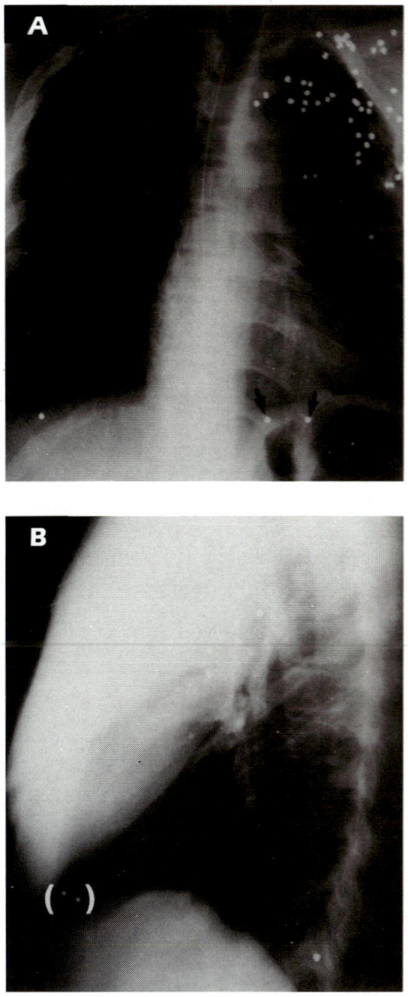

FIGURE 5.44 A PA chest x-ray of a patient following a shotgun assault. The two lower pellets (arrows) were believed to have moved to the right ventricular chamber via the venous system. **B** Lateral chest x-ray of the same patient. (Courtesy of Dr. Jon Moran, University of Kansas Medical Center.)

NONPENETRATING CARDIAC INJURIES

Etiology

With greater reliance on high-speed transportation has come an increase in blunt cardiac injuries. An early review of nonpenetrating cardiac trauma indicated that only 33% of blunt injuries resulted from automobile accidents.[270] That figure is now over 80%.[125,159,193] Blunt cardiac trauma results from several general pathophysiological mechanisms including rapid deceleration, sternal compression of the heart against the thoracic spine, direct precordial blows, and abrupt increases both in intrathoracic and intra-aortic pressures from sudden leg or abdominal compression. Blast exposure is another unusual mechanism of cardiac trauma. The steering wheel injury is the most typical injury, combining mechanisms of deceleration and compression. The type and extent of blunt cardiac injury vary widely (see Types of Cardiac Injury From Blunt Trauma). At one extreme, a mild cardiac contusion may be asymptomatic and resolve spontaneously, never having been detected. At the other end of the spectrum, myocardial rupture may occur, often resulting in instant death. Also, the pericardium, cardiac valves, and coronary arteries may be injured concomitantly, producing varied clinical manifestations with differing levels of severity and acuteness.

Incidence and Mortality

Most autopsy studies emphasize which injuries will result in early mortality. Among 50 nonselected consecutive necropsies following fatal automobile accidents, Leinoff noted 16% with definite cardiac injury.[135] Later, Parmley reviewed 546 autopsies of patients dying of nonpenetrating cardiac injuries, which represented 0.1% of all patients from the Armed Forces Institute of Pathology (Fig. 5.45).[181] The majority were found to have either chamber or septal rupture, but many had myocardial contusions or lacerations. The coexistence of an aortic rupture in 25% indicates the severity of associated injuries in these patients.

TYPES OF CARDIAC INJURY FROM BLUNT TRAUMA

- Myocardium
  - Contusion
  - Laceration
  - Rupture
  - Aneurysm, true or false
  - Ventricular septal defect
- Cardiac valves
  - Aortic insufficiency
  - Mitral insufficiency
  - Tricuspid insufficiency
- Coronary arteries
  - Thrombosis
  - Laceration
  - Fistula
- Pericardium
  - Hemorrhage
  - Effusion
  - Laceration
  - Cardiac herniation

FIGURE 5.45
LESIONS FOUND IN 546 AUTOPSY CASES OF BLUNT CARDIAC TRAUMA

TYPE OR SITE OF INJURY	NUMBER OF CASES	CASES WITH COEXISTENT AORTIC RUPTURE	TOTAL
Chamber rupture	230	68	298
Septal rupture	43	12	55
Contusion/laceration	105	24	129
Pericardial laceration	18	18	36
Hemopericardium	13	12	25
Valvular injury	2	0	2
Coronary artery injury	0	1	1
Total	411	135	546

Parmley LF, Manion WC, Mattingly TW: Nonpenetrating injury to the heart. Circulation 18:371–396, 1958.

Clinical blunt trauma studies have demonstrated wide variations in incidence and mortality (Fig. 5.46), and wide differences in selection criteria for detecting cardiac injury have made comparisons difficult. In these studies the incidence of electrocardiographic abnormalities in patients sustaining blunt thoracic trauma has varied between 14% and 76%. Although life-endangering complications and death occurred in some patients, the majority showed myocardial recovery without residual dysfunction. More recent studies have included determinations of myocardial isoenzymes and radionuclide function measurements.[105,131,193,241] Although the mortality from blunt cardiac injury remains less than 5%, the overall incidence has increased significantly over the past 30 years. In 1958, Parmley estimated that in the United States alone, 150,000 cases of blunt cardiac injury resulted annually.[181] In 1973, Jackson and Murphy escalated this estimate to 900,000.[116] In view of the overall increase in traffic accidents since 1973, it is likely that there are more than 1,000,000 cases of nonpenetrating cardiac trauma annually in the United States.[173] Because of this high incidence, any physician treating traffic accident victims should be familiar with the evaluation and management of the nonpenetrating cardiac injury.

Pathology and Pathophysiology

With blunt injuries, pathologic findings range from no detectable anatomical changes to chamber rupture, valve injury, and coronary artery lacerations. The least severe injury in which no myocardial cellular damage can be demonstrated is referred to as a "cardiac concussion." Parmley described two such cases in which the patients died moments after the accident, presumably from a dysrhythmia.[181] One individual was struck in the chest with a stick, and in the other, the precordium was hit by a pitched ball. The most typical pathologic cardiac injury following blunt trauma is a myocardial contusion, which appears as a dark hemorrhagic area on the wall of the heart (Fig. 5.47). The early lesion consists of erythrocyte extravasation into subepicardial and myocardial tissues. Muscle fibers become separated and often are disrupted. Blood vessels in the region of injury dilate and during the first few days, leukocytes migrate from vessel margins into these hemorrhagic areas. Standard patterns of inflammation and fibroblastic proliferation ensue. These changes resemble those seen in typical myocardial infarctions. However, the transition from normal to abnormal myocardial regions is more abrupt with traumatic lesions.[170]

A classical experimental study of myocardial contusion was reported by Bright and Beck in 1935.[43] After a significant myocardial impact, the majority of animals developed transient Q-and T-wave changes but remained in good health 3 months after injury. Subsequent pathologic examinations showed firm epicardial scar tissue. However, several animals did die within 48 hours following the insult from ventricular arrhythmias. These studies were important in changing the prevailing concept that nonpenetrating cardiac trauma was nearly always lethal. Up to that time, pathologic and clinical studies had demonstrated only 11 survivors among 168 reported cases of blunt cardiac injuries.[43] From these experimental studies Bright and Beck concluded that "the vast majority of nonpenetrating wounds of the heart are not recognized clinically."

Recent experimental studies have examined the effects of myocardial contusion on arrhythmia development, ventricular function, and coronary blood flow.[1,3,74,133,142, 235,265] Using a controlled impact technique, Anderson and Doty produced transient arrhythmias, but no pathologic evidence of acute

FIGURE 5.46
INCIDENCE OF CARDIAC INJURY IN BLUNT CHEST TRAUMA*

AUTHOR	YEAR	CARDIAC INJURY/TOTAL	PERCENTAGE	LIFE-ENDANGERING COMPLICATIONS	DEATH FROM CARDIAC INJURY
Barber	1942	8/33	24.2	0/8	0/8
Sigler	1945	32/42	76.2	2/32	1/32
Watson	1960	17/44	38	0/17	0/17
Dolara	1967	19/98	19	0/19	0/19
Jones	1975	45/210	21	14/45	1/45
Potkin	1982	70/100	70	0/70	0/70
Sutherland	1983	15/77	19	3/15	3/15
Kron	1983	7/50	14	0/7	0/7
Harley	1984	21/74	28	1/21	1/21

*Data derived from electrocardiographic evidence of myocardial damage.

injury at lower velocities (13 m/ sec).[3,133] With impacts at 17 m/sec, significant myocardial injury with attendant hemodynamic consequences developed. In most studies, ventricular fibrillation and death resulted at levels of 24 m/sec. Similarly, Stein found that the propensity for lethal arrhythmias and diminished left ventricular function was related to the severity of the blunt impact.[235] Other studies have confirmed these correlations between quantitative myocardial injury, cardiac function, and the incidence of ventricular fibrillation.[194,265]

Using radioactive microspheres, Utley found coronary blood flow to increase immediately following contusion in both normal and injured areas, returning to control levels in survivors.[265] Also, Doty infused barium gel into coronary arteries of dogs, sacrificed immediately after a myocardial impact. By microscopic evaluation, collections were noted within dilated vascular channels of injured zones, and these were thought to represent arteriovenous communications.[74] More recently, Liedtke noted a significant decrement in distal coronary vascular resistance with concurrent regional myocardial dysfunction following a blunt impact.[140] Although total regional coronary flow increased, elevated epicardial/endocardial flow ratios resulted, along with decreased myocardial oxygen consumption. These later data suggest that impaired cardiac function after myocardial contusion may result from a combination of inadequate oxygen delivery secondary to arteriovenous shunting and altered microcirculatory flow patterns.

Clinical studies relating pathophysiologic characteristics of myocardial contusions have been limited. However, recent noninvasive techniques have provided insight into the hemodynamic effects of myocardial contusions in patients. Both regional and global ventricular changes have been found following blunt injuries. The preponderance of right ventricular blunt injuries parallels the vulnerable position of this chamber immediately beneath the sternum. Two-dimensional echocardiography has shown global right ventricular dilation and regional thinning as the predominant finding following these injuries.[164] Using radionuclide angiography, Sutherland assessed both early and late right and left ventricular function changes in 25 patients.[239] In most, focal ventricular wall motion abnormalities were detected early in the post-trauma period. Moreover, 68% had dysfunction confined to the right ventricle. The left ventricle was involved in 8%, with both ventricles being affected in 12%. In patients available for follow-up, either complete or partial resolution occurred in 85%.

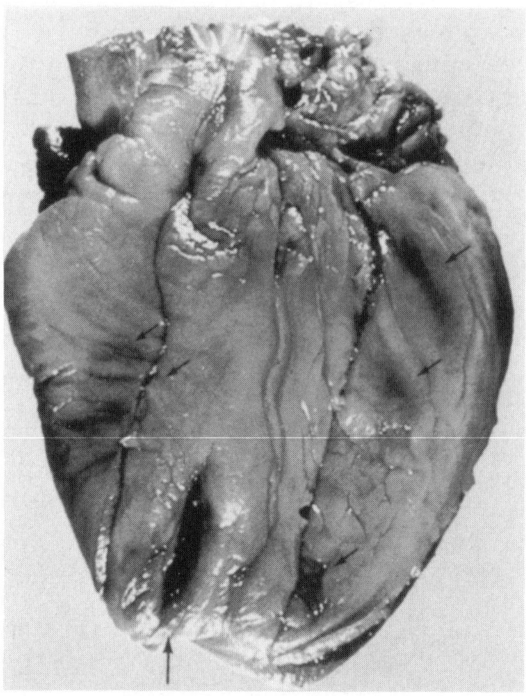

FIGURE 5.47 Autopsy specimen demonstrating multiple myocardial contusions (small arrows) and a large right ventricular rupture. (Reproduced with permission from Color ATLAS of Chest Trauma and Associated Injuries. Copyright © 1983 by A. Besson & F. Saegesser. Published by Medical Economics Company Inc., Oradell, NJ 07649. All rights reserved.)

Diagnostic Studies and Techniques

Although most patients show external evidence of major trauma, cardiac problems may remain unnoticed unless clinical curiosity prompts further diagnostic investigation. No single best technique for determining the presence of myocardial injury has yet been determined, since pathologic verification is impossible except in patients who have died. Diagnostic techniques most often used have included electrocardiography, serum enzyme analysis, radionuclide scanning, radionuclide angiocardiography, and echocardiography. Also, invasive catheter techniques have been helpful for identifying specific cardiac lesions. In addition to detecting serious injuries, by identifying significant myocardial dysfunction, these methods may help plan elective surgery and indicate when advanced monitoring should be used during emergency procedures for other injuries.

ELECTROCARDIOGRAPHY

The most common diagnostic technique used for detecting blunt myocardial injury has been the 12-lead surface electrocardiogram. Early experimental studies demonstrated that ST-segment and T-wave changes following myocardial contusions were similar to those of ischemia or infarction. Arrhythmias, including atrial fibrillation and flutter, ventricular tachycardia and fibrillation, as well as premature ventricular contractions, all may be manifestations of blunt cardiac injury.[3,29,141] Moreover, conduction disturbances, including complete heart block, may indicate the presence of a myocardial contusion.[141] The incidence of electrocardiographic abnormalities in patients sustaining severe blunt chest trauma ranges from 14% to 76% (see Table 5.4). In the past, this easily performed test has been considered relatively sensitive for identifying myocardial contusions.

Despite these notions, several recent studies have questioned both the sensitivity and specificity of the electrocardiogram.

Kumar found electrocardiographic abnormalities in only 25% of those having evidence of a myocardial contusion as determined by enzyme and scanning methods.[132] In a consecutive group of patients who had sustained blunt chest trauma, Harley found significant electrical abnormalities in only 28% of patients compared with abnormal radionuclide angiographic findings in 74%.[105] This relative insensitivity may be related to a high incidence of right ventricular and nontransmural injuries. Moreover, independent studies by Blair and Potkin showed a number of patients whose post-traumatic electrocardiograms suggested definite myocardial contusions to have normal hearts at autopsy.[29,193] Conversely, of five patients with pathologically documented cardiac contusions, Potkin noted previous electrocardiographic changes in only three.[193] Extracardiac factors including pulmonary contusion, hypoxemia, altered serum electrolytes, and acid–base imbalances may produce factitious electrocardiographic patterns suggesting myocardial injury. Thus, an abnormal electrocardiogram is not always indicative of a definite cardiac injury; and conversely, a normal study does not exclude significant myocardial damage.

SERUM ENZYME ANALYSIS

Generally, elevated serum glutamic-oxaloacetic transaminase (SGOT) levels, lactic dehydrogenase (LDH), and creatine kinase (CK) levels result from myocardial damage. However, with injury of other tissues during major trauma, marked increases in these enzymes occur also. Recently, adjunctive measurements of cardiac CK isoenzymes (CK-MB) have added specificity to this analysis. Usually, CK-MB levels peak 24 hours following cardiac trauma and return to normal within 72 hours.[254] Some authors consider CK-MB levels of over 2% as being diagnostic of myocardial injury, while others require levels greater than 6%.[105,127,193] In several series of severe nonpenetrating chest trauma, the incidence of CK-MB positively has ranged between 8% and 27%.[105,193] Recently, several studies have questioned the accuracy of CK-MB determinations for diagnosing blunt myocardial injury. Harley found positive CK isoenzyme studies in only 6 of 74 patients (8%) sustaining severe nonpenetrating chest injuries, compared with abnormal radionuclide studies in 55 (74%).[105]

Although these studies may be insensitive, CK-MB levels probably provide an acceptable overall specificity for cardiac damage: In a recent study of 78 patients who had suffered blunt trauma, Kettunen determined elevated serum CK-MB levels in 19 (24%).[127] In this group the incidence of electrocardiographic abnormalities, cardiac dilation, pulmonary edema, and death was significantly higher than in patients with negative CK-MB levels. However, similar correlations were not evident in patients studied by Potkin, who suggested that CK isoenzyme measurements were of limited usefulness in the diagnosis of blunt cardiac injury.[193] Severe crush injuries, myopathies, and tachyarrhythmias, as well as gas gangrene and Rocky Mountain Spotted Fever, may also cause CK-MB levels to be elevated, impairing the accurate diagnosis of coexisting blunt cardiac injuries. Despite these considerations, the presence of elevated CK-MB isoenzymes may alert clinicians to significant blunt myocardial damage. However, if CK-MB values are not elevated, the clinician *cannot* be assured that myocardial damage has not occurred.

RADIONUCLIDE SCANNING AND ANGIOCARDIOGRAPHY

Recently, technetium-99m pyrophosphate scanning techniques have been employed for diagnosing blunt myocardial injury. However, the successful results seen in experimental animals have not carried through to clinical situations.[93] Brantigan found positive scans in only 6% of patients having probable myocardial injury.[38] Also, Rodriguez and Shatney found normal scans in six patients with significantly elevated CK-MB isoenzymes.[208] In another series only 2% of scans done for blunt myocardial trauma were positive; however, in patients dying of cardiac injuries pyrophosphate scans were never diagnostic.[193] Although these scans have gained significant utility for diagnosing acute myocardial infarctions, they remain of little value for evaluating cardiac trauma patients. Factors that probably contribute to inadequate diagnostic sensitivity include the necessity of a transmural injury, as well as difficulty in separating right ventricular damage from sternal fractures and other chest wall injuries.

Radionuclide angiocardiography (RNA) has been used to measure both global and regional ventricular function noninvasively. Sutherland studied 77 consecutive patients and found focal wall motion abnormalities in 55% on gated equilibrium evaluations.[241] Sudden cardiac deaths occurred in three patients having positive RNA studies, and myocardial contusions were confirmed pathologically in each patient. In a similar study, Harley found 74% of patients evaluated by first-pass RNA to have significant myocardial dysfunction. Follow-up studies performed 3 weeks following injury demonstrated improvement in function in all patients studied.[105] In addition to demonstrating focal wall motion abnormalities, RNA can provide an excellent assessment of global cardiac function. This information may be valuable in the multiply traumatized patient whose injuries may require general anesthesia for surgical treatment. Identification of significant myocardial dysfunction may help plan elective surgery or indicate when advanced cardiovascular monitoring should be used during emergency procedures. The disadvantages of RNA for assessing nonpenetrating cardiac trauma relate to the expense, complexity, and availability. Many hospitals do not have this equipment, and most devices are still not portable. Evaluation and interpretation of RNA studies can be complex and time-consuming. Nevertheless, improvements in technology are making these techniques easier to interpret, more portable, and less expensive.

ECHOCARDIOGRAPHY

Recent developments in echocardiography have provided a portable, noninvasive technique for rapidly assessing the heart and pericardium. Although some experimental and clinical studies have been performed using M-mode techniques, two-dimensional methods appear to provide more information on potential cardiac injuries.[57,128] Experimental studies have shown two-dimensional echocardiography to be both sensitive (97%) and specific (86%) for diagnosing myocardial contusions.[180] This technique was first used in 1981 to diagnose blunt cardiac injury.[171] An isolated right ventricular aneurysm was demonstrated by both RNA and two-dimensional echocardiography. Subsequently, Miller described seven victims of blunt chest trauma in whom two-dimensional echo studies were of diagnostic value.[164] King found two-dimensional echocardiographic abnormalities in 47% of patients with elevated CK-MB levels after chest trauma.[130] In these and other studies, helpful findings have included right ventricular dilation, regional wall thinning and dyskinesia, pericardial effusions, mural thrombi, and intramyocardial hematomas.[152] Also, two-dimensional echocardiography has been of value for assessing valvular and septal abnormalities following blunt trauma.[89,95,130,248] Microcavitation studies are very helpful for detecting flow abnormalities. The recent application of adjunctive doppler techniques has increased the specificity for detecting intracardiac valve lesions and shunts.[95,158]

Thus, two-dimensional echocardiography may offer clinicians more information than any other readily available noninvasive technique. In addition to evaluating focal wall motion abnormalities, it can be used to assess global ventricular function, detect the presence of pericardial fluid with the potential for cardiac tamponade, and help identify traumatic injuries of either intracardiac valves or septa. Specifically, cross-sectional echocardiographic studies may be the only noninvasive diagnostic method that can discriminate between significant right ventricular contusions and restrictive pericardial effusions—a differentiation that is important for appropriate early management. Two-dimensional echocardiography remains relatively inexpensive and is more widely available than RNA and scanning techniques. However, inadequate studies may result from imperfect transducer placement, secondary to either patient discomfort or concomitant chest wall injuries.

INVASIVE HEMODYNAMIC MEASUREMENTS AND ANGIOGRAPHY

Although noninvasive methods may detect specific myocardial injuries, other techniques may be necessary to help identify patients most likely to develop hemodynamic instability. The insertion of a Swan-Ganz thermodilution catheter has become commonplace in critical care units and may be quite helpful. These catheters are inserted through the subclavian, internal jugular, or brachial veins with minimal difficulty and patient risk. After flow-directed distal pulmonary artery positioning, serial central venous, pulmonary artery diastolic, and pulmonary capillary wedge pressures, as well as cardiac output values, can be measured serially. Moreover, from these data, derivations of other hemodynamic parameters including cardiac index, right and left ventricular stroke-work indices, and systemic and pulmonary vascular resistances are possible. Also, Starling function curves can be determined by measuring ventricular output values at different filling pressures obtained by progressive volume infusions. By using direct hemodynamic measurements and determining ventricular function curves in those with enzyme and electrocardiographic changes of myocardial contusion, patients at risk for mortality and significant morbidity may be identified early.[257] These methods may be used in conjunction with RNA and echocardiographic studies for added sensitivity.[240] Thus, patients in whom noninvasive evaluations suggest myocardial injury should be considered for early placement of a pulmonary artery thermodilution catheter. However, when patients are hemodynamically stable and do not have other injuries or the need for general anesthesia, Swan-Ganz catheterization may be unnecessary.

In victims of nonpenetrating cardiac trauma, complete cardiac catheterization with contrast ventriculography is indicated rarely and almost never in the acute period. However, when clinical and noninvasive diagnostic findings suggest the presence of valvular injury or a residual intracardiac shunt, these studies become indicated. Left to right shunts via ventricular septal defects may be quantitated by oximetry obtained during Swan-Ganz catheter positioning.[245] Contrast ventriculography may be preferred to characterize a chronic ventricular aneurysm or septal defect, but often is ill-advised in the acute period. Although more common after penetrating injuries, coronary artery fistulas and aneurysms occur following blunt trauma and, if suspected, must be confirmed by selective coronary angiography.[245]

Specific Nonpenetrating Cardiac Injuries

Specific cardiac abnormalities that result from blunt trauma include myocardial contusions, formation of ventricular aneurysms, cardiac chamber ruptures, ventricular septal defects, valvular injuries, and coronary artery occlusions and fistulas. Pericardial injuries and pericarditis may also occur. Fig. 5.48 relates how various diagnostic tests may be helpful for diagnosing specific blunt cardiac injuries.

MYOCARDIAL CONTUSION

Myocardial contusions are the most common cardiac injury secondary to nonpenetrating trauma.[43] The spectrum of injuries ranges from an asymptomatic and difficult-to-detect lesion to a profound myocardial insult severely compromising cardiac function. Any patient sustaining significant blunt chest trauma should be evaluated thoroughly for this injury. Serial electrocardiograms and serum CK-MB isoenzyme assays should be obtained along with either two-dimensional echocardiography or RNA. The high incidence of arrhythmias following a myocardial contusion warrants continuous electrocardiographic monitoring for up to 48 hours following injury. Although prophylactic antiarrhythmic medications have been administered to patients sustaining contusions, no studies either support or refute this therapy. Most clinicians monitor patients continuously after these injuries and if rhythm disturbances develop, antiarrhythmic medications are begun.

The majority of patients with myocardial contusions have an uneventful recovery. Unfortunately, other injuries may complicate recovery and increase myocardial oxygen demands. Concomitant pulmonary contusions occur frequently and may require prolonged intubation and respiratory support. Moreover, associated orthopaedic, thoracic, and intra-abdominal injuries may require early operative intervention. The presence of a concurrent myocardial contusion increases the risk of anesthesia[68,223] and therefore the adjunctive risk of this injury should be considered carefully in the decision to proceed with an early operation for another surgical problem.

Patients with isolated myocardial contusions may be treated symptomatically and discharged after careful observation. An evaluation 4 to 6 weeks later should be mandatory to identify the development of any late complications. This evaluation should include a physical examination, chest film, and electrocardiogram, and when possible a follow-up two-dimensional echocardiogram or RNA. The latter two tests are helpful for detecting residual wall motion abnormalities. More aggressive management is needed for the more severely injured patients whose myocardial contusion is associated with other serious injuries. The early insertion of a Swan-Ganz thermodilution catheter is appropriate, especially when general anesthesia is unavoidable. Patients having a concomitant pulmonary contusion may also profit from more objective fluid management. Hypotension and decreased cardiac output may be the presenting hemodynamic manifestations of a contusion, and optimal management requires careful adjustment of inotropic medications and intracardiac filling pressures. At times cardiogenic shock occurring secondary to a myocardial contusion may necessitate insertion of an intra-aortic balloon for support.[232]

TRAUMATIC VENTRICULAR ANEURYSM

Occasionally, blunt cardiac trauma can result in the late appearance of a ventricular aneurysm.[6,26,91,97,204,230,234] Although right ventricular myocardial contusions occur most often, left ventricular aneurysms develop more frequently. The development of differential intracavitary pressures between the two chambers is the presumed explanation for this discrepancy. Traumatic left ventricular aneurysms have been associated with occlusions of the left anterior descending coronary artery; however, in the majority of cases, no evidence of coronary injury exists.[229]

Most traumatic aneurysms probably result from a transmural injury as reflected by wall thinning and full-thickness myocardial fibrosis. However, pseudoaneurysms have been described.[129] Patients with aneurysms may remain asymptomatic but often present with congestive heart failure, systemic embolization, and

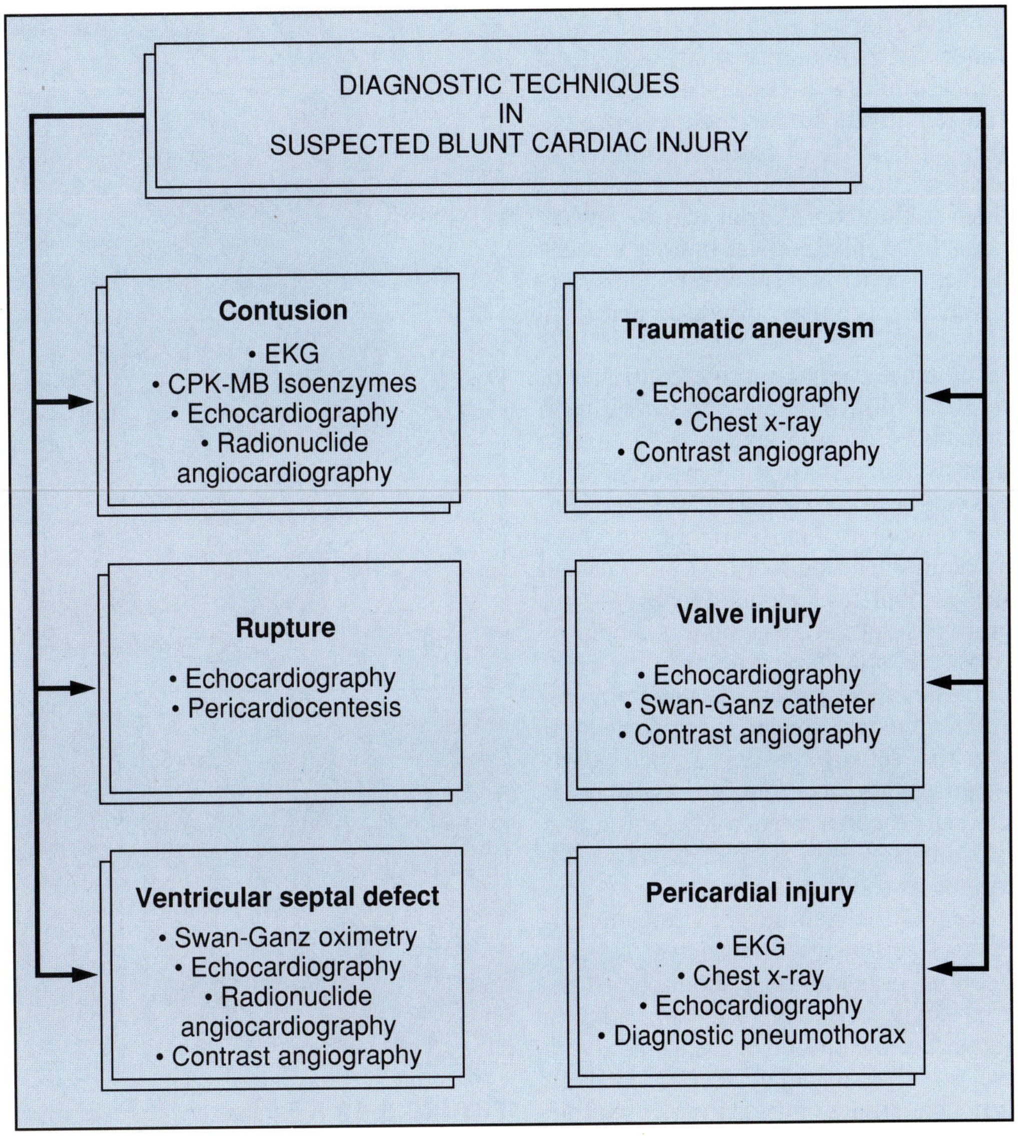

FIGURE 5.48 These diagnostic tests are used currently for evaluating patients suspected of having blunt cardiac injury.

dysrhythmias. Traumatic aneurysm rupture rarely occurs but remains a disastrous complication.[229] Ventricular aneurysms are often detected initially by an abnormal cardiac silhouette on a routine chest film. When the chest film and echocardiogram suggest a traumatic aneurysm, cardiac catheterization should be performed to further delineate the size and position. Moreover, coronary abnormalities, valvular injuries, and residual ventricular septal defects can be detected concurrently by angiography. The advisability of aneurysm resection in asymptomatic patients continues to be controversial. However, in patients who have not undergone resection, a high incidence of complications including aneurysm rupture, fatal dysrhythmias, and systemic embolization have been reported.[129,229] Because of the low risk of operation and excellent prognosis following resection, most clinicians prefer surgical extirpation at present.

CARDIAC RUPTURE

Cardiac rupture from nonpenetrating chest trauma is most often a lethal injury (See Fig. 5.43). In an early review of 152 patients, only 30 patients lived longer than 1 hour following cardiac rupture.[43] In Parmley's 1958 autopsy study, 64% of all deaths resulted from chamber rupture.[181] Because most patients die before evaluation, in most clinical studies the incidence has remained low, representing only 0.5% of patients admitted to the Baylor trauma service between 1977 and 1982.[154] Desforges first identified and repaired a blunt right atrial tear in 1955.[69] Since then, other clinicians have treated these injuries successfully[108,165,226,231,262]; however, the early mortality remains very high, with 50% to 80% of those surviving transport to a medical center dying subsequently.[15,147,154,157,231,262,279]

The accurate diagnosis of acute cardiac rupture continues to be difficult. In patients with blunt trauma presenting with hypotension, engorged neck veins, and an elevated central venous pressure, the diagnosis of cardiac rupture should be considered. Pericardiocentesis can be both diagnostic and therapeutic provided that there is temporary hemodynamic improvement prior to availability of an operating room. Most successful cases have been performed without cardiopulmonary bypass, but when blunt cardiac rupture is suspected, this option should be kept available, and a perfusionist should be present in the operating room.[69,147,184,279] The emergency room thoracotomy has been of little value in the treatment of this injury, and the mortality of the procedure in this setting has approached nearly 100%.[33,156] With acute cardiac tamponade from these injuries, most authors have selected the median sternotomy for the best exposure of all cardiac chambers.[262,245,279] Others have considered an anterior thoracotomy as the incision of choice.[279] This incision can be extended across the sternum for complete cardiac access or laterally to treat a concurrent aortic transection. After exposure, manual control of hemorrhage should be effected immediately. A partial occlusion clamp will approximate most atrial lacerations and either the crossed or pledgeted suture technique should control small ventricular lacerations (Figs. 5.16, 5.20 and 5.21). Although closure of these injuries without extracorporeal circulation is preferable, immediate cardiopulmonary bypass may be necessary for extensive cardiac lacerations. With this technique, the heart can be emptied rapidly, and the lesion repaired with large mattress sutures and Teflon pledgets and strips (Fig. 5.49).[119] When primary closure does not appear possible, a Teflon or Dacron patch can be used.[245] Although fibrillation without bypass may be helpful for rapid suture closure of major chamber lacerations, elective fibrillation should be reserved for only the more dire circumstances. In several reports, cardiac arrest was present before exposure could be obtained. In these patients, the cardiac laceration was repaired just prior to defibrillation and resuscitation.[147,184]

VENTRICULAR SEPTAL DEFECT

Ventricular septal defects resulting from blunt chest trauma are rare[77,85,187,188] but were identified in 5.5% of patients in Parmley's large autopsy series.[181] Moreover, in only 0.9% was a ventricular septal defect the singular cardiac finding. In 1955,

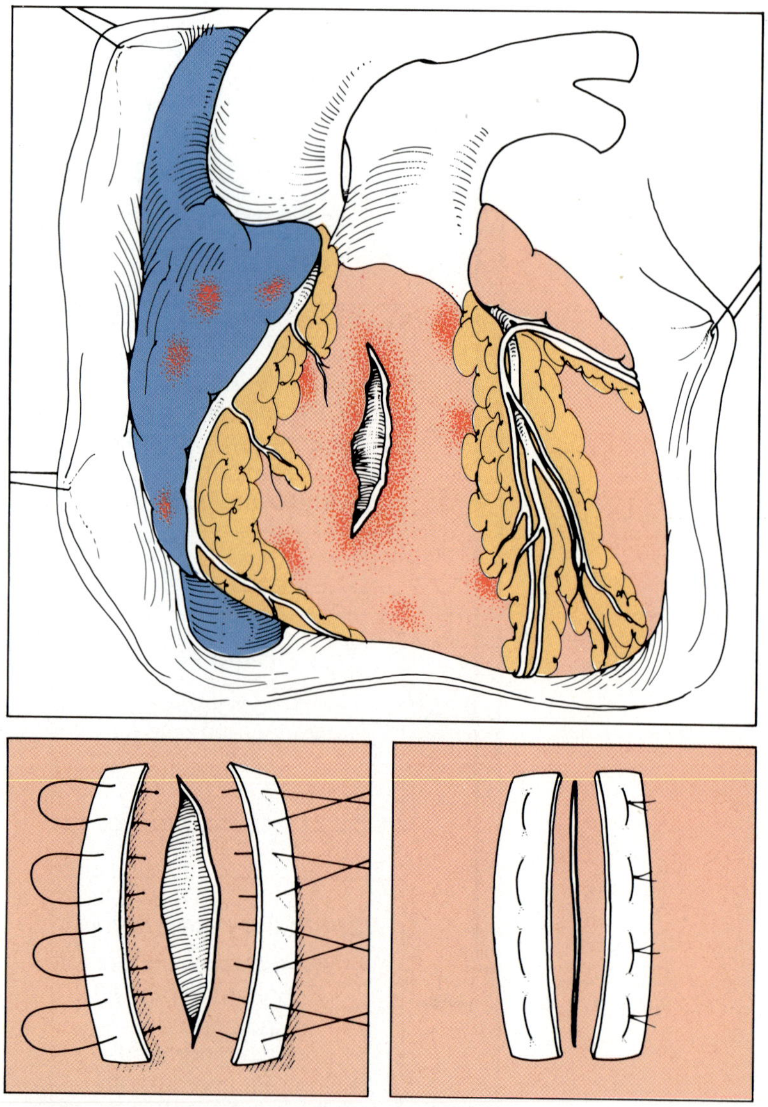

FIGURE 5.49 A right ventricular blunt rupture is shown along with closure using Teflon strip–buttressed mattress sutures. (Adapted from Symbas PN: Trauma to the heart and great vessels. In Jamiesan SW [ed]: Rob & Smith's Operative Surgery. St. Louis, CV Mosby, 1986.)

Lillehei repaired a ventricular septal defect that had resulted from a blunt injury.[46] These defects probably resulted from compression of the heart between the sternum and spine either during late diastole or early systole—a time when both ventricular chambers are full and the atrioventricular valves are closed. Lacerations of the ventricular septum may occur acutely or present several days following the insult. In the latter case, further necrosis of the contused ventricular septum results in subsequent perforation.[82] In some cases, blunt coronary artery damage has affected septal infarction and subsequent rupture.[189] Most commonly these defects are found in the apical muscular septum; however, perimembranous and multiple septal perforations have been described.[181] In some cases, the intraventricular conduction pathways have been injured concomitantly.[46]

A new systolic murmur following closed chest trauma should alert the astute clinician to a new septal defect. To differentiate this lesion from either acute mitral or tricuspid insufficiency, a Swan-Ganz catheter should be passed to detect sequential elevations in oxygen saturation. This step-up is diagnostic, and the magnitude of shunting can be quantitated from oximetry data. First-pass RNA has also been used to demonstrate and calculate the magnitude of ventricular septal defect shunts (Fig. 5.50).[248] With the use of microcavitation techniques, two-dimensional echocardiography, and more recently, Doppler methods, the diagnosis can be made noninvasively with relative ease.[95,158,248] Formal cardiac catheterization is rarely necessary for evaluating acute patients, but may be helpful later (Fig. 5.51).

The prognosis in patients having traumatic ventricular septal defects relates to the defect size and the presence of associated cardiac lesions. As mentioned earlier, those resulting from penetrating injuries tend to be small, while blunt defects are larger and have an additional myocardial contusion, making many of these patients desperately ill. When severe refractory congestive heart failure occurs, immediate repair may be necessary.[51] Unfortunately, the rate of mortality from emergency surgery under these circumstances is very high.[167] Therefore, every effort to control congestive failure by inotropic medications and the intra-aortic balloon pump is warranted. Hopefully, conservative therapy will allow gradual recovery from the concomitant myocardial contusion, decreasing the risks from arrhythmias and ventricular dysfunction. Ideally, patients should be stabilized for four to eight weeks prior to elective closure. In some cases dur-

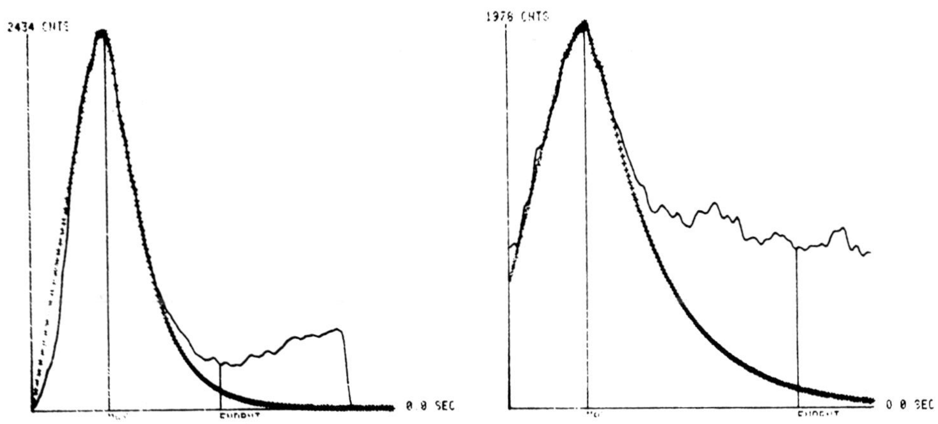

FIGURE 5.50 A time-activity curve obtained from a right-sided injection using first-pass radionuclide angiocardiography. The left curve demonstrates a normal washout pattern. The curve on the right suggests a left-to-right shunt from a ventricular septal defect following a blunt chest injury. (Szabo JR, Chen JT, Putman CE: New murmur following blunt chest trauma. Invest Radiol 19:163–167, 1984.)

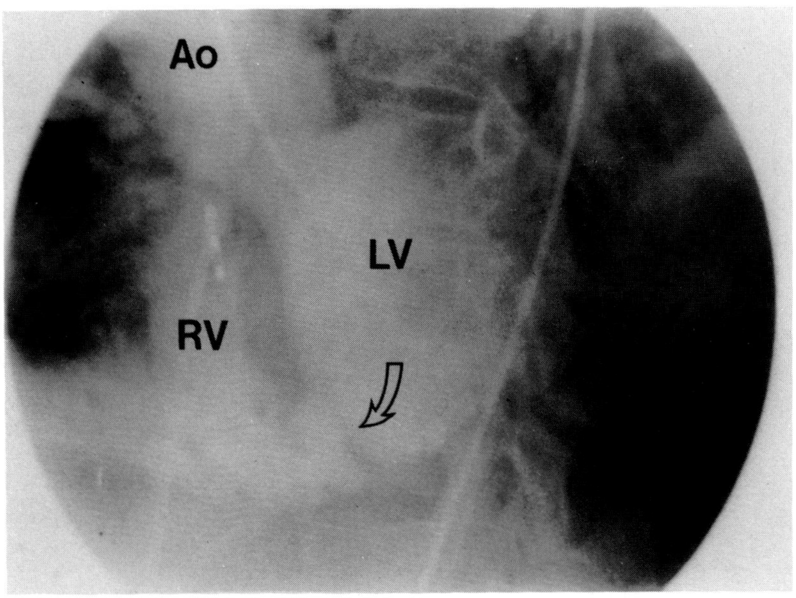

FIGURE 5.51 Left ventriculogram from a patient developing a large ventricular septal defect (arrow) following a baseball bat injury of the anterior chest. (Ao, aorta; RV, right ventricle; LV, left ventricle) (Courtesy of Dr. Norman A. Silverman, University of Illinois.)

ing the recovery period, ventricular septal defects become hemodynamically less significant, with spontaneous closure in a few.[27,212] Patients maintaining continued left-to-right flow values of 2:1 or more should undergo elective surgical correction to prevent chronic pulmonary vascular changes.

For defects requiring early repair, the surgical approach is similar to closure of those developing after a myocardial infarction. The left ventricle should be entered through the most traumatized myocardial zone. Teflon-pledgeted sutures are placed on the opposite side of the septum to anchor the Teflon or Dacron septal patch (Figs. 5.52 and 5.53). Subsequently, the ventriculotomy should be closed with pledgeted sutures and strips. For large contusions, a large Dacron patch will be required to close the ventricle securely. When closure is elective, much of the acute myocardial injury has resolved, with fibrosis present, and the technique should be similar to that for closing a congenital ventricular septal defect.

CARDIAC VALVE INJURY

Injuries to cardiac valves from nonpenetrating trauma are rare, although some reports appear in the literature. Blunt valve injuries have occurred in the aortic, mitral, and tricuspid valves. Symptoms result from acute valvular insufficiency with coexistent myocardial contusions. The severity of the clinical presentation varies with the valve involved, degree of insufficiency, and amount of concomitant ventricular dysfunction caused by the associated contusion. Although these lesions are rare, they should be considered when a new heart murmur occurs following closed chest trauma.

The first report of blunt aortic valve injury was by Bouillaud in 1841, and the first successful surgical repair was in 1954 by Hufnagel, who placed a plastic ball valve in the descending aorta.[35,136] By 1984 a total of 19 patients had been corrected surgically following aortic insufficiency from blunt injuries.[21,71,143,185] Aortic valvular injury is thought to result from a sudden increase in intra-aortic pressure during early diastole. The resultant large aortic valve pressure gradient develops a rupture either at the cusp-free border or base, or detaches the commissures, allowing leaflet prolapse into the ventricle (Fig. 5.54).[137] Similar lesions have been produced by Barie when pressures of approximately 480 mm Hg were applied to the aortas of human cadavers.[16]

Typically, the occurrence of a new diastolic murmur following blunt chest trauma in a patient without previous heart disease

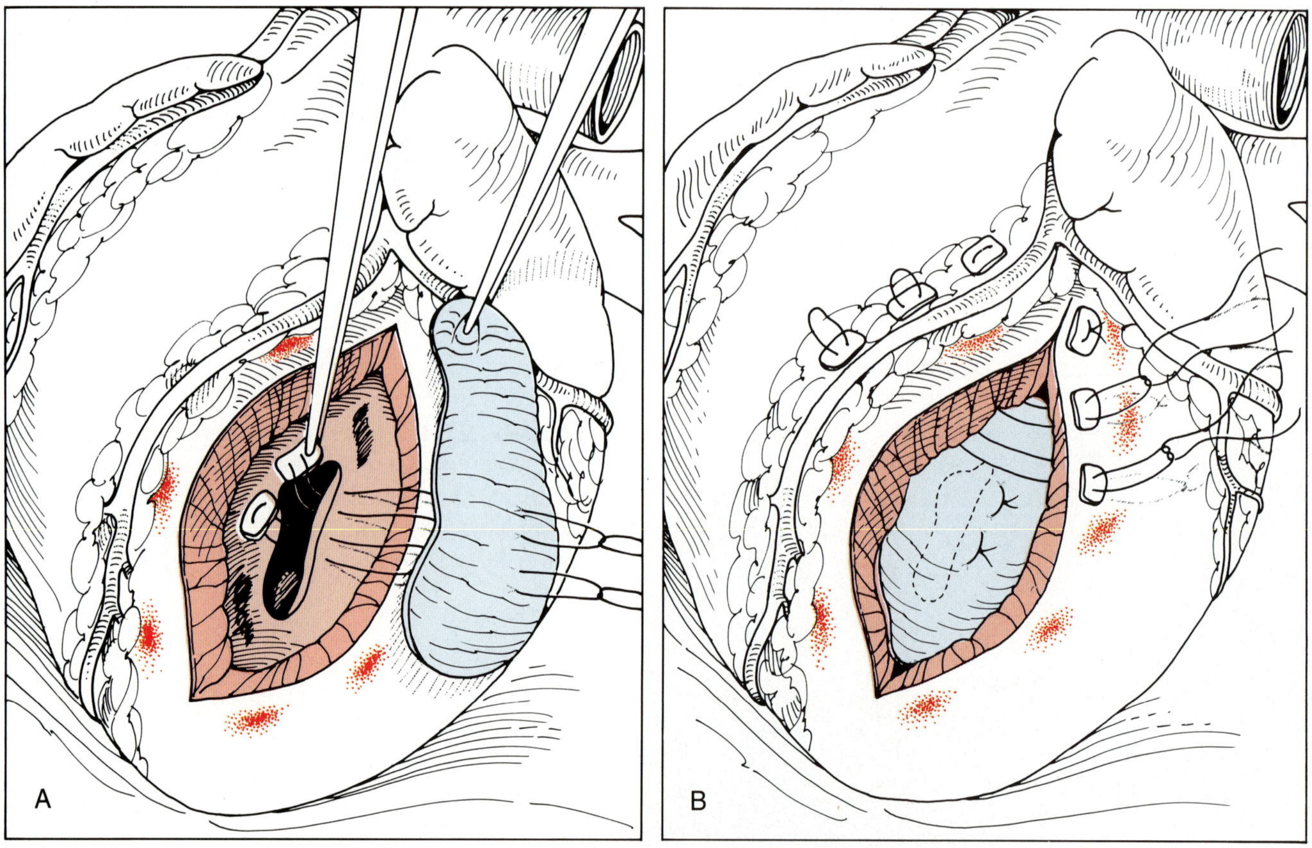

FIGURE 5.52 A Diagrammatic illustration of a traumatic ventricular septal defect closure via the left ventricle. Pledgeted sutures are placed on the right ventricular side of the septum and the patch is secured in the left ventricle. **B** The ventriculotomy is closed with Teflon-buttressed mattress sutures to avoid tearing the contused anterior wall. (Adapted from Symbas PN: Trauma to the heart and great vessels. In Jamieson SW [ed]: Rob & Smith's Operative Surgery. St. Louis, CV Mosby, 1986.)

suggests aortic valve injury. The murmur has been described as being more musical than that in patients with chronic acquired aortic insufficiency. Symptoms may be insignificant; however, refractory congestive heart failure with pulmonary edema may result. The diagnosis can be confirmed by two-dimensional echocardiography, but most clinicians prefer full cardiac catheterization with an aortic root contrast injection to estimate the degree of insufficiency.[89] Swan-Ganz catheters have been helpful for following the hemodynamic response to preoperative medical therapy, which includes diuretics and inotropic medications. As coexistent myocardial contusions increase the operative risk from dysrhythmias and ventricular dysfunction, a 4-to-8-week delay in operative intervention is preferable. In some patients this is not possible, and emergency aortic valve repair or replacement has been performed as early as 14 hours after the injury.[220] At the other extreme, patients with trivial aortic insufficiency may need only close follow-up without surgical therapy.

The choice between repair or replacement of aortic valve injuries depends on the type of lesion as well as experience of the surgeon. Among the cases reported previously, most surgeons have replaced the aortic valve with good success.[71] However, in four cases, aortic valvuloplasties have been reported. Of these patients, one died in the operating room and two others developed recurrent insufficiency.[21] Thus, valve replacement appears to be the procedure of choice with blunt aortic injuries. In instances in which commissural detachment occurs, simple resuspension may be adequate, obviating the potential long-term complications of prosthetic valve replacement.

In 1936, Glendy reported the first case of mitral insufficiency resulting from nonpenetrating trauma. The first successful repair did not occur until 1962.[92,162] By 1984, 13 cases of traumatic mitral insufficiency had been corrected surgically.[10,60,70,160,190] With blunt mitral injuries, chordae tendineae and papillary muscles are involved more frequently than leaflets themselves. Injury is thought to occur from a sudden compression of the distended heart either during late diastole or early systole when the valve is

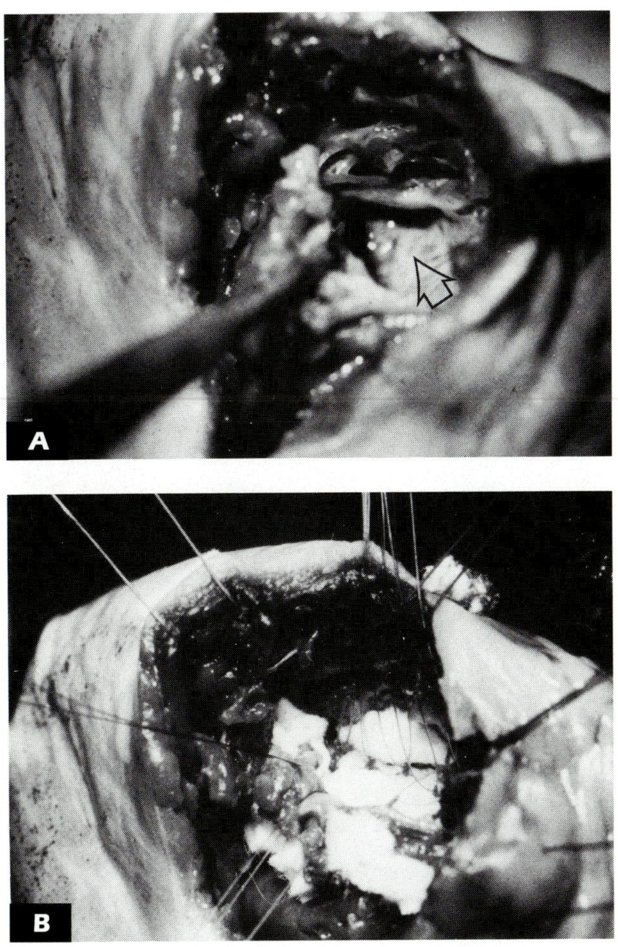

FIGURE 5.53 A A large ventricular septal defect (arrow) shown in Figure 5.46 is demonstrated just prior to surgical closure. This injury resulted from a baseball bat injury. **B** The defect was closed with pledgeted sutures and a Teflon felt patch. (Courtesy of Dr. Norman A. Silverman, University of Illinois.)

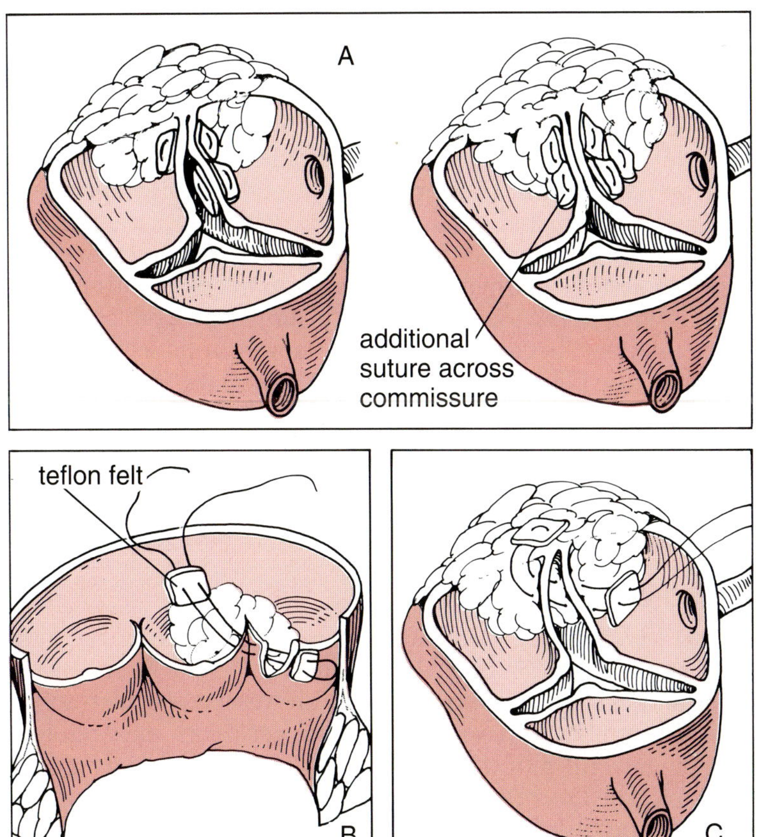

FIGURE 5.54 Aortic valve cusp rupture is shown following a blunt injury. The right coronary cusp was repaired primarily by pledgeted sutures. (Adapted from Levine RJ, Roberts WC, Morrow AG: Traumatic aortic regurgitation. Am J Cardiol 10:752–763, 1962.)

closed. Often patients present with a new holosystolic murmur and signs of congestive heart failure. As mentioned earlier, Swan-Ganz catheter data may help differentiate this lesion from a traumatic ventricular septal defect by the absence of high right ventricular oxygen saturations and the presence of large V waves on wedge tracings. Two-dimensional echocardiography may be diagnostically valuable by imaging a prolapsing leaflet.[60,164]

Management depends on how well patients compensate for their valvular defects. As with aortic valve injuries, supportive therapy with close follow-up is preferred for minor amounts of insufficiency, which can be tolerated for many years without surgery. However, patients with moderate to severe levels of regurgitation should undergo operative treatment, preferably after significant myocardial contusions have resolved. Recent improvements and experience suggest that mitral valve repairs should be attempted when possible, especially when simple chordal rupture or partial papillary muscle injury is present.[48] With complete papillary muscle rupture, prosthetic valve replacement has been preferred.

Fewer than 20 cases of blunt tricuspid valve injuries exist in the literature.[37,45,118, 178,222] The mechanism of disruption appears to be similar to that of mitral valve injury. Jahnke reviewed nine cases, with five having papillary muscle injury, three having chordal ruptures, and only one having a true leaflet injury.[118] Because right-sided cardiac pressures are low, tricuspid problems may be less significant clinically than left-sided valvular injuries.[245] Although tricuspid insufficiency may be tolerated without symptoms, these patients present with symptoms of fatigue, dyspnea, and lower extremity edema. Neck vein distention with prominent systolic regurgitation is characteristic. A soft holosystolic murmur that increases in intensity with inspiration is often noted. As with traumatic mitral valve prolapse, two-dimensional echocardiography may show systolic leaflet excursion into the right atrium.[273] In some patients the increased right atrial pressure has opened the foramen ovale, producing right-to-left shunting and resulting in severe hypoxemia.[117] Most cases of tricuspid injury may be treated medically; however, some patients develop progressive right-sided heart failure or cyanosis and should undergo repair or replacement of the valve.

CORONARY ARTERY INJURY

Until 1982, acute coronary thrombosis from blunt chest trauma had been reported in only 18 patients.[176,177,189,237,269] The mechanism of occlusion is thought to be an intimal tear with subsequent thrombosis. In some cases, these occlusions have resolved within several months, resulting in normal coronary arteriograms. The left anterior descending coronary artery is most frequently involved, and an anteroseptal myocardial infarction usually results. A secondary left ventricular aneurysm or postinfarction ventricular septal defect may develop. Unfortunately, the diagnosis of an acute coronary occlusion in this setting continues to be difficult, and under only the most unusual circumstances would emergency revascularization be possible. Most patients respond to supportive therapy and require surgical treatment only if they develop subsequent angina pectoris, a significant left ventricular aneurysm, or a septal defect.

As mentioned earlier, most traumatic coronary artery fistulas occur as a result of penetrating wounds. However, by 1984, five cases from blunt cardiac trauma had been reported.[9,87,148,186,215] Each developed a fistula between the left anterior descending coronary artery and the right ventricle. In these patients, other coincident cardiac injuries included tricuspid insufficiency, a ventricular septal defect, and a left ventricular aneurysm.[186,215] Four of the five patients underwent surgical correction of the fistula between 1 month and 10 years following the injury, and two required reoperation later. One patient, not undergoing surgery, remained asymptomatic because of a very small residual fistula. This exceedingly rare lesion may become obvious at various times following the traumatic event. The clinical hallmark is development of a new continuous cardiac murmur. Electrocardiographic evidence of either anterior myocardial ischemia or an infarction often occurs. Although two-dimensional echocardiography may suggest a coronary fistula by showing a dilated left anterior descending coronary artery, selective coronary arteriography is necessary to confirm the diagnosis. Large fistulas that produce either congestive heart failure or myocardial ischemia should be closed surgically; small fistulas may be treated by observation.

PERICARDIAL INJURY

Both contusion and rupture of the pericardium may occur with blunt injuries. Most often these are found incidental to other life-threatening cardiac injuries such as a myocardial contusion and rupture. However, isolated pericardial involvement may occur and, if not identified readily, may become life-threatening. Parmley found isolated disruption in only 18 of 546 (3.3%) blunt cardiac trauma autopsies.[181] In a more recent collective review, Clark described 142 reports of blunt pericardial rupture and con-

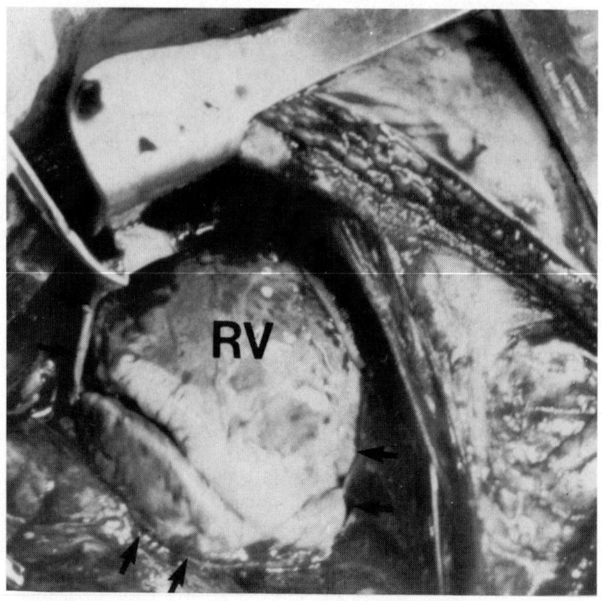

FIGURE 5.55 Blunt pericardial rupture shows the pericardial edges (arrows) with part of the right ventricle (RV) and atrium herniating through the defect. (Courtesy of Dr. Daniel Rosenthal, Brooke Army Hospital.)

sidered survival possible with this lesion.[50] Disruptions occur most frequently at the coronal margins of the heart, involving the left pleuropericardium (50%) (Fig. 5.55). Other prevalent sites include the diaphragmatic pericardium (27%) and the right pleuropericardium (19%). The primary danger of pericardial rupture is potential cardiac herniation or so-called luxation, resulting either in torsion or constriction of the great vessels.[2,52,155,209] Herniation is more likely to occur with intermediate-size defects (8–12 cm). Although this complication presents acutely in most cases, sudden death can result years after the inciting traumatic event. Moreover, herniation of abdominal viscera into the pericardium through a diaphragmatic defect can occur, resulting in findings similar to those of cardiac tamponade.

The diagnosis of pericardial rupture may be difficult. However, when cardiac herniation has occurred and symptoms develop, an urgent thoracotomy is required to reposition the heart and either repair or open wide the pericardial defect to eliminate the possibility of recurrence. In stable patients either displacement of the heart or evidence of intestinal loops in the pericardial sac on the chest film may suggest herniation. Conversely, pericardial tears without herniation may often go unnoticed. When suspected, induction of a pneumothorax or pneumoperitoneum followed by appropriate patient positioning may be helpful diagnostically.

Following blunt trauma, pericardial injuries may become manifest as acute or chronic pericarditis.[96,102,249] Symptoms are similar to those seen occasionally following a myocardial infarction (Dressler's syndrome) or after cardiac surgery (postpericardiotomy syndrome). Pericarditis usually presents 3 to 5 days following the injury. Symptoms include chest pain, fever, a friction rub, and often electrocardiographic changes. Furthermore, pericardial effusions may be quantitated on echocardiography. Although symptoms are usually self-limiting, anti-inflammatory agents may provide symptomatic relief. Should chest discomfort persist or evidence of central venous pressure elevation develop, corticosteroids are indicated.[245] Although unusual, post-traumatic pericarditis can produce cardiac tamponade. Therefore, these patients should be observed closely until resolution occurs. At times pericardiocentesis may be indicated for larger hemodynamically significant collections. Occasionally, either open pericardial drainage or a pericardiectomy must be performed to obtain relief.[151] Moreover, constrictive pericarditis can occur as a late complication of pericardial injury.[161,196] Although a rare complication, symptoms of constriction may develop weeks, months, or years after the trauma. The typical clinical presentation includes dyspnea, lower extremity edema, and hepatomegaly. The diagnosis may be confirmed most reliably by cardiac catheterization. As with pericardial constriction from other etiologies, these cases respond best to complete surgical decortication.

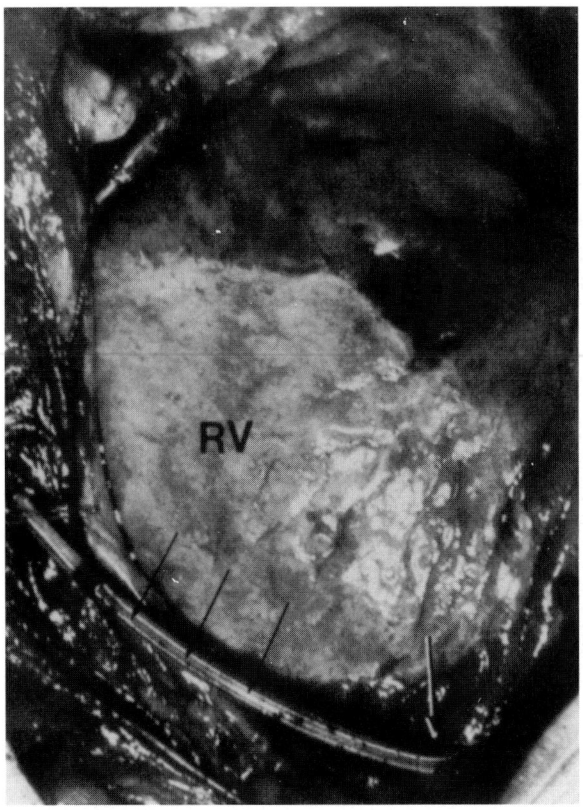

FIGURE 5.56 A right ventricular (RV) perforation by a permanent endocardial pacing lead (black arrows). The lead exits the ventricle near the cardiac apex (black and white arrow). (Reproduced with permission from Color Atlas of Chest Trauma and Associated Injuries. Copyright © 1983 by A. Besson & F. Saegesser. Published by Medical Economics Company Inc., Oradell, NJ 07649. All rights reserved.)

Iatrogenic Cardiac Injuries

In an attempt to render therapy for a number of conditions, physicians may induce reparable and irreparable cardiac damage. These types of trauma injuries include perforations, catheter and pacing wire retention, ventricular tears, and myocardial and coronary injuries from radiation therapy and electrical countershock. Although perforations following diagnostic cardiac catheterization are relatively few today (0.5%), pathologic conditions including valvular and subvalvular aortic stenosis, cardiomyopathies, and older age may predispose to continued bleeding from ventricular injuries.[243] In many cases, perforations fail to cause symptoms, especially in right-sided catheter injuries.

Pericardiocentesis is required in less than half of patients and exploration is rarely necessary.[58] The inadvertent intramyocardial injection of contrast material is particularly dangerous and may cause ventricular fibrillation.[243] Catheter perforation of valve leaflets causing insufficiency is very rare. During selective coronary angiography or angioplasty, dissection may occur, necessitating emergency coronary artery bypass grafting.[75,103] In the recent Coronary Artery Surgery Study only 1.6% of 19,300 patients sustained a diagnostic catheter–related complication.[75]

Cardiac perforations have been reported in 3% to 9% of patients during insertion of both temporary and permanent transvenous pacing wires (Fig. 5.56). After recognition of a perforation, the pacing wire should be withdrawn into the ventricle and repositioned. Echocardiography may be helpful for detecting significant pericardial collections. Certain electrocardiographic patterns or diaphragmatic pacing may indicate a pacing wire perforation.[267] Because the right ventricle is under low pressure, bleeding often becomes self-limiting; however, pericardiocentesis and subxiphoid pericardial tube insertion may be required.[17] Surgical exploration is the exception rather than the rule.

Figure 5.57 shows a Swan-Ganz catheter retained in the right ventricle. This may result from entrapment by a suture during cardiac closure. These should be removed surgically if nonoperative manipulation fails. Swan-Ganz and other tube catheters have been reported to cause fatal hemorrhage from pulmonary artery rupture and ventricular perforations.[62,94] Endocardial pacing wires often cannot be removed without cardiac exploration, especially tine-tipped leads that interdigitate with myocardial trabeculations. These leads can usually be left in place without ill effects after the new one has been positioned (Fig. 5.58). A persistent attempt at extraction of these without surgical exploration may result in a ventricular laceration. Although very rare, removal of temporary epicardial pacing wires following cardiac surgery can result in significant bleeding and tamponade.[12]

Other unusual causes of cardiac trauma can be mentioned. During a therapeutic pericardiocentesis, coronary and ventricular lacerations may occur, especially when performed for a hemopericardium.[281] Both coronary and myocardial damage can result from direct electrical countershock as well as high-voltage injuries.[72,277] Moreover, radiation therapy for malignancies has been reported to cause occasional coronary, valvular, percardial, and myocardial damage.[55] Vigorous cardiac compression has been shown to elevate serum CK-MB isoenzymes; however, direct changes of infarction may not be present.[256] In the presence of a prosthetic cardiac valve, precordial compression against the rigid spine may be responsible for a venticular laceration near the atrioventricular groove or coronary artery rupture (Figs. 5.59 and 5.60).[44] Sethi reported a right venticular outflow tract injury from precordial compression.[221] During mitral valve replacement, the posterior wall is susceptible to perforating injuries and lacerations (0.5%-2.0%), especailly with a difficult native valve removal.[175] These injuries are difficult to repair and the mortality remains very high. Thus, careful removal of the posterior leaflet and delicate positioning of the prosthesis are extermely important.

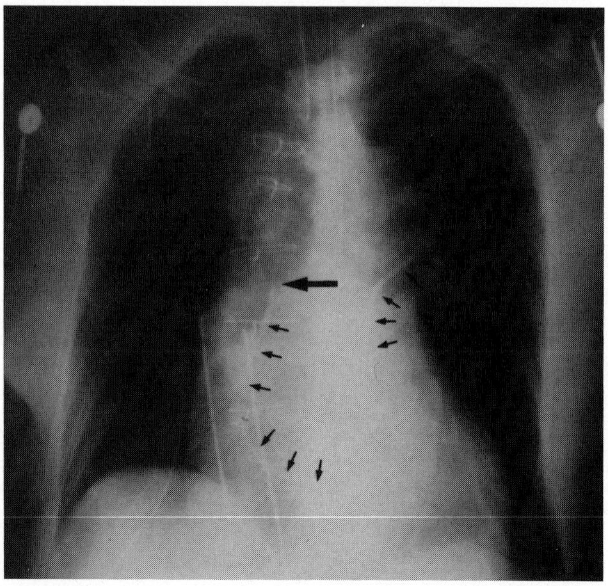

FIGURE 5.57 On a postoperative chest x-ray a broken Swan-Ganz catheter (small arrows) is shown in the right ventricle. The distal end (large arrow) is still located in the pulmonary artery. Removal of the catheter required reexploration. (Courtesy of the Department of Radiology, Duke University Medical Center.)

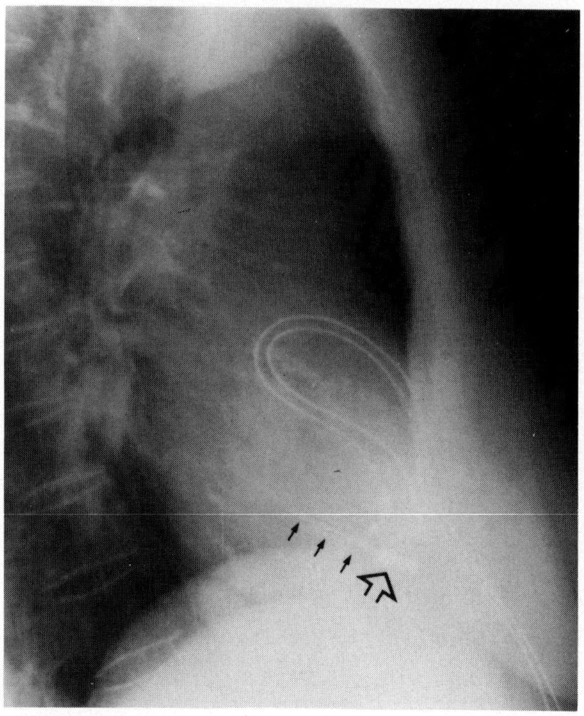

FIGURE 5.58 On this lateral chest x-ray the retained tip of an old endocardial pacing lead is shown. These leads may be difficult to remove without cardiotomy and generally do not cause problems when left in situ. Large arrow shows tip of broken wire; small arrows show wire. (Courtesy of the Department of Radiology, Duke University Medical Center.)

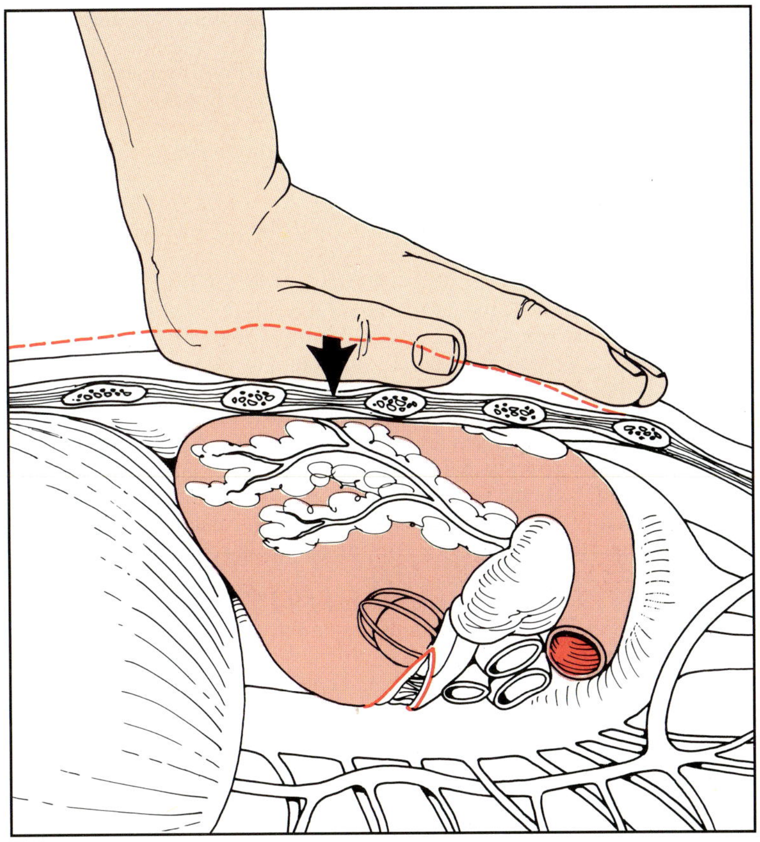

FIGURE 5.59 In the presence of a rigid prosthetic valve, vigorous external cardiac compression may result in cardiac laceration of either the posterior ventricular wall or the great vessels.

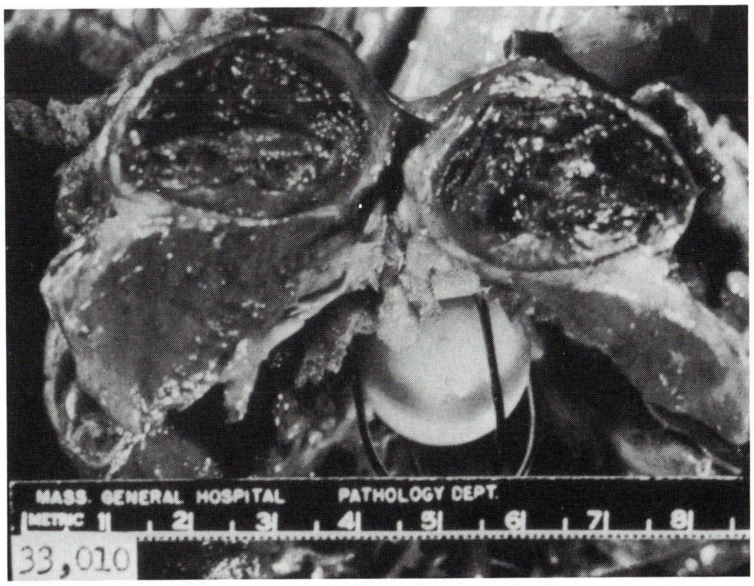

FIGURE 5.60 In this patient external cardiac compression resulted in rupture of the circumflex coronary artery and death. (Burnside J, Daggett WM, Austen WG: Coronary artery rupture by a mitral valve prosthesis after closed chest massage. Ann Thorac Surg 9:267–270, 1970.)

REFERENCES

1. Allen RP, Liedtke AJ: The role of coronary artery injury and perfusion in the development of cardiac contusion secondary to nonpenetrating chest trauma. J Trauma 19:153–156, 1979.
2. Andersen M, Fredens M, Olesen KH: Traumatic rupture of the pericardium. Am J Cardiol 27:566–569, 1971.
3. Anderson AE, Doty DB: Cardiac trauma: An experimental model of isolated myocardial contusion. J Trauma 15:237–244, 1975.
4. Arbulu A, Thoms NW: Control of bleeding from a gunshot wound of the inferior vena cava at its junction with the right atrium by means of a Foley catheter. J Thorac Cardiovasc Surg 63:427–429, 1972.
5. Arom KV, Richardson JD, Webb G et al: Subxiphoid pericardial window in patients with suspected traumatic pericardial tamponade. Ann Thorac Surg 23:545–549, 1977.
6. Aronstam EM, Strader LD, Geiger JP, Gomez AC: Traumatic left ventricular aneurysms. J Thorac Cardiovasc Surg 59:239–242, 1970.
7. Asfaw I, Arbulu A: Penetrating wounds of the pericardium and heart. Surg Clin North Am 57:37–48, 1977.
8. Asfaw I, Thoms NW, Arbulu A: Interventricular septal defects from penetrating injuries of the heart. J Thorac Cardiovasc Surg 69:450–457, 1975.
9. Austin SM, Applefeld MM, Turney SZ, Mech KF Jr: Traumatic left anterior descending coronary artery to right ventricle fistula: Report of two cases. South Med J 70:581–584, 1977.
10. Bailey CP, Vera CA, Hirose T: Mitral regurgitation from rupture of chordae tendineae due to ``steering wheel" compression. Geriatrics 24:90–105, 1969.
11. Baker CC, Thomas AN, Trunkey DD: The role of emergency room thoracotomy in trauma. J Trauma 20:848–855, 1980
12. Baldwin BJ, Dorney ER: Acute cardiac tamponade following the removal of temporary epicardial pacemaker wires after open heart surgery. Am J Med Sci 261:241–243, 1971.
13. Ballance CA: 1919 Bradshaw Lecture: Surgery of the Heart. London, Macmillan 1920.
14. Barber H: Electrocardiographic changes due to trauma. Br Med J 83:241–243, 1942.
15. Barbero-Marcial M, Gregori F Jr, Verginelli G et al: Rupture of the heart due to non-penetrating chest trauma. J Cardiovasc Surg 16:16–20, 1975.
16. Barie E: Recherche sur les ruptures valvulaires due coeur. Revue Medicale 1:132–144, 1881.
17. Bassan MM, Merin G: Pericardial tamponade due to perforation with a permanent endocardial pacing catheter. J Thorac Cardiovasc Surg 74:51–54, 1977.
18. Beall AC, Hamit H, Cooley DN, DeBakey ML: Surgical management of traumatic intracardiac lesions. J Trauma 5:133–141, 1965.
19. Beall AC, Ochsner JL, Morris GC et al: Penetrating wounds of the heart. J Trauma 1:195–210, 1961.
20. Beall AC, Patrick TA, Okies JE et al: Penetrating wounds of the heart: Changing patterns of surgical management. J Trauma 12:468–473, 1972.
21. Beall AC, Shirkey AL: Successful surgical correction of traumatic aortic valve regurgitation. JAMA 187:507–510, 1964.
22. Beck CS: Wounds of the heart: The technique of suture. JAMA 13:205–227, 1926.
23. Beck CS: Contusions of the heart. JAMA 104:109–113, 1935.
24. Ben Hur N, Gemer M, Milwidsky H: Perforating injury of the heart caused by a nail fired from a stud-gun. J Trauma 4:850–853, 1964.
25. Berger RL, Gibson H, Riemer RW, Ramaswamy K: Traumatic aortic regurgitation ventricular septal defect, and fistula of the sinus of Valsalva. N Engl J Med 281:887–888, 1969.

26. Berkoff HA, Rowe GG, Crummy AB, Kahn DR: Asymptomatic left ventricular aneurysm. Circulation 55:545–548, 1977.
27. Berman RW, Rook GD, Bronsther B, Abrams MW: Traumatic nonpenetrating ventricular septal defect: Recovery under conservative management. J Pediatr Surg 1:275–283, 1966.
28. Bigger IA: Diagnosis and treatment of heart wounds with summary of thirty-four cases. J Thorac Surg 8:239–253, 1939.
29. Blair E, Topuzlu C, Davis JH: Delayed or missed diagnosis in blunt chest trauma. J Trauma 11:129–145, 1971.
30. Blalock A, Ravitch M: A consideration of the nonoperative treatment of cardiac tamponade resulting from wounds of the heart. Surgery 14:157–162, 1943.
31. Blatchford JW, Anderson RW: The evolution of the management of penetrating wounds of the heart. Ann Surg 202:615–622, 1985.
32. Block MH: Ueber wunden des herzens und ihre heilung durch die naht unter blutenleere verhandlungen der Deutschen Gesellschaft fur Chirurgie. Elften Congress 11:108–109, 1882.
33. Bodai BI, Smith JP, Blaisdell FW: The role of emergency thoracotomy in blunt trauma. J Trauma 22:487–491, 1982.
34. Borja AR, Lansing AM, Ransdell HT: Immediate operative treatment for stab wounds of the heart. J Thorac Cardiovasc Surg 59:662–667, 1970.
35. Bouillaud T: Trait;aae Clinic des Maladies du Coeur. Paris, Balliere, 1841.
36. Boyd TF, Streider JW: Immediate surgery for traumatic heart disease. J Thorac Cardiovasc Surg 50:305–315, 1965.
37. Brandenburg RO, McGoon DC, Campeau L, Giuliani ER: Traumatic rupture of the chordae tendineae of the tricuspid valve. Am J Cardiol 18:911–915, 1966.
38. Brantigan CO, Burdick D, Hopeman AR, Eiseman B: Evaluation of technetium scanning for myocardial contusion. J Trauma 18:460–463, 1978.
39. Brautigan MW, Tietz G: Emergency thoracotomy in an urban community hospital. Am J Emerg Med 3:311–315, 1985.
40. Bravo AJ, Glancy DL, Epstein SE, Morrow AG: Traumatic coronary arteriovenous fistula. Am J Cardiol 27:673–676, 1971.
41. Breaux EP, Dupont JB, Albert HM et al: Cardiac tamponade following penetrating mediastinal injuries: Improved survival with early pericardiocentesis. J Trauma 19:461–466, 1979.
42. Brewer LA: Wounds of the chest in war and peace, 1943–1968. Ann Thorac Surg 7:387–408, 1969.
43. Bright EF, Beck CS: Nonpenetrating wounds of the heart. Am Heart J 10:293–321, 1935.
44. Burnside J, Daggett WM, Austen WG: Coronary artery rupture by a mitral valve prosthesis after closed chest massage. Ann Thorac Surg 9:267–271, 1970.
45. Cahill NS, Beller BM, Linhart JW, Early RG: Isolated traumatic tricuspid regurgitation: Prolonged survival without operative intervention. Chest 61:689–691, 1972.
46. Campbell GS, Vernier R, Varco RL, Lillehei CW: Traumatic ventricular septal defect. J Thorac Surg 37:496–501, 1959.
47. Cappelen A: Vulnia cordis, sutura af hjertet. Norsk Mag F Laegevidensk 11:285–288, 1896.
48. Carpentier A, Chauvaud S, Fabiani JN et al: Reconstructive surgery of mitral valve incompetence. J Thorac Cardiovasc Surg 79:338–348, 1980.
49. Carrasquilla C, Wilson RF, Walt AJ, Arbulu A: Gunshot wounds of the heart. Ann Thorac Surg 13:208–212, 1972.
50. Clark DE, Wiles CS, Lim MK et al: Traumatic rupture of the pericardium. Surgery 93:495–503, 1983.
51. Clark TA, Corcoran FH, Baker WP, Mills M: Early repair of traumatic ventricular septal defect. J Thorac Cardiovasc Surg 67:121–124, 1974.
52. Clifford RP, Gill KS: Traumatic rupture of the pericardium with dislocation of the heart. Br J Surg 16:123–126, 1984.
53. Cogbill TH, Moore EE, Millikan JS, Cleveland HC: Rationale for selective application of emergency department thoracotomy in trauma. J Trauma 23:453–460, 1983.
54. Cohen MV, Greenberg MA, Grose R, Yipintsoi T: Cardiac tamponade in dogs with normal coronary arteries. II. Myocardial flow and metabolism with moderate and severe hemodynamic impairment. Basic Res Cardiol 79:542–550, 1984.
55. Cohn KE, Stewart JR, Fajardo LF, Hancock EW: Heart disease following radiation. Medicine 46:281–298, 1967.
56. Cohnheim J: Lectures in general pathology. London, New Sydenham Society, 1887.
57. Coleman J, Gonzalez A, Harlafter N, Symbas PN: Myocardial contusion: Diagnostic valve of cardiac scanning and echocardiography. Surg Forum 27:293–294, 1976.
58. Conti CR, Ross RS: The risks of cardiac catheterization. Am Heart J 78:289–291, 1969.
59. Cooper MJ, Bernstein D, Silverman NH: Recognition of left coronary artery fistula to the left and right ventricles by contrast echocardiography. J Am Coll Cardiol 6:923–926, 1985.
60. Cuadros CL, Hutchinson JE III, Mogtader AH: Laceration of a mitral papillary muscle and the aortic root as a result of blunt trauma to the chest. J Thorac Cardiovasc Surg 88:134–140, 1984.
61. Dalton HC: Report of a case of stab wound of the pericardium. Ann Surg 21:147–152, 1895.
62. Dane TEB, King EG: Fatal cardiac tamponade and other mechanical complications of central venous catheters. Br J Surg 62:6–10, 1975.
63. Decker HR: Foreign bodies in the heart and pericardium—should they be removed? J Thorac Surg 9:62–79, 1939.
64. DeGennaro VA, Bonfils-Roberts EA, Ching N, Nealon TF: Aggressive management of potential penetrating cardiac injuries. J Thorac Cardiovasc Surg 79:833–837, 1980.
65. Del Vechio S: Sutura del cuore. Riforma Med 11:38, 1895.
66. Demetriades D: Cardiac wounds: Experience with 70 patients. Ann Surg 203:315–317, 1986.
67. Demetriades D, Van Der Ven BW: Penetrating injuries of the heart: Experience over two years in South Africa. J Trauma 23:1034–1041, 1983.
68. DeMuth WE Jr, Baue AE, Odom JA Jr: Contusions of the heart. J Trauma 7:443–455, 1967.
69. Desforges G, Ridder WP, Lenoci RJ: Successful suture of ruptured myocardium after nonpenetrating injury. N Engl J Med 252:567–569, 1955.
70. Devineni R, McKenzie FN: Acute mitral insufficiency resulting from blunt chest trauma. J Thorac Cardiovasc Surg 85:797–798, 1983.
71. Devineni R, McKenzie FN: Avulsion of a normal aortic valve cusp due to blunt chest injury. J Trauma 24:910–912, 1984.
72. Doherty PW, McLaughlin PR, Billingham M et al: Cardiac damage produced by direct current countershock applied to the heart. Am J Cardiol 43:225–232, 1979.
73. Dolara A, Morando P, Pampaloni M: Electrocardiographic findings in 98 consecutive non-penetrating chest injuries. Dis Chest 52:50–56, 1967.
74. Doty DB, Anderson AE, Rose EF et al: Cardiac trauma: Clinical and experimental correlations of myocardial contusion. Ann Surg 180:452–460, 1974.
75. Douglas JS, King SB: Management of complications. In King SB, Douglas JS (eds): Coronary Arteriography and Angioplasty. New York, McGraw-Hill, 1985.
76. Dove DB, Stahl WM, DelGuercio LRM: A five-year review of deaths following urban trauma. J Trauma 20:760–766, 1980.
77. East T: Traumatic rupture of the interventricular septum. Br Heart J 7:116–118, 1945.
78. Elkin DC: Diagnosis and treatment of cardiac trauma. Ann Surg 114:169–185, 1941.
79. Enders GC, Graeber GM, Poirier RA: Wounds traversing two or more cardiac chambers. J Thorac Cardiovasc Surg 76:83–89, 1978.
80. Espada R, Whisennand HH, Mattox KL, Beall AC: Surgical management of penetrating injuries to the coronary arteries. Surgery 78:755–760, 1975.
81. Evans J, Gray LA, Rayner A, Fulton RL: Principles for the management of penetrating cardiac wounds. Ann Surg 189:777–784, 1979.
82. Evora PRB, Ribeiro PJF, Brasil JCF et al: Late surgical repair of ventricular septal defect due to nonpenetrating chest trauma: Review and report of two contrasting cases. J Trauma 25:1007–1009, 1985.
83. Fallahnejad M, Kutty ACK, Wallace HW: Secondary lesions of penetrating cardiac injuries. Ann Surg 191:228–233, 1980.
84. Farina: Betrag zur Chirurgie der Herzens. Centralblatt fur Chir 23:1224, 1896.

85. Feruglio GA, Bayley A, Greenwood WF: Non-penetrating chest injury resulting in isolated rupture of the ventricular septum and angina pectoris. Can Med Assoc 82:261–269, 1960.
86. Fischer G: Die wunden des herzens und des herzbeutels. Arch Klin Chir 9:571–910, 1868.
87. Forker AD, Morgan JR: Acquired coronary artery fistula from nonpenetrating chest injury. JAMA 215:289–291, 1971.
88. Gaspard P, Clermont A, Villard J, Amiel M: Non-iatrogenic trauma of the coronary arteries and myocardium: Contribution of angiography—report of six cases and literature review. Cardiovasc Intervent Radiol 6:20–29, 1983.
89. Gay JA, Gottdiener JS, Gomes MN et al: Echocardiographic features of traumatic disruption of the aortic valve. Chest 83:150–151, 1983.
90. Gielchinsky I, McNamara JJ: Cardiac wounds at a military evacuation hospital in Vietnam. J Thorac Cardiovasc Surg 60:603–606, 1970.
91. Glancy DL, Yarnell P, Roberts WC: Traumatic left ventricular aneurysm. Am J Cardiol 20:428–433, 1967.
92. Glendy RE, White PD: Nonpenetrating wound of heart-rupture of papillary muscle and contusion of heart resulting from external violence: Case report. Am Heart J 11:366–369, 1936.
93. Go RT, Doty DB, Chiu CL, Christie JH: A new method of diagnosing myocardial contusion in man by radionuclide imaging. 1. Radiology 116:107–110, 1975.
94. Golden MS, Pinder T, Anderson WT, Cheitlin MD: Fatal pulmonary hemorrhage complicating use of a flow-directed balloon-tipped catheter in a patient receiving anticoagulant therapy. Am J Cardiol 32:865–867, 1973.
95. Goldman AP, Kotler MN, Goldberg SE et al: The uses of two-dimensional doppler echocardiographic techniques preoperatively and postoperatively in a ventricular septal defect caused by penetrating trauma. Ann Thorac Surg 40:625–627, 1985.
96. Goodkind MJ, Bloomer WE, Goodyear AVN: Recurrent pericardial effusion after nonpenetrating chest trauma. N Engl J Med 263:874–881, 1960.
97. Green L, Oakley CM, Cleland WP, Davies DM: Successful repair of left ventricular aneurysm and ventricular septal defect after indirect injury. Lancet 984–986:874–881, 1965.
98. Grey-Turner G: Lecture Notes—War Surgery of the Chest. University of London, British Postgraduate Medical School, 1943.
99. Griswold RA, Drye J: Cardiac wounds. Ann Surg 139:783–785, 1954.
100. Griswold RA, Maguire CH: Penetrating wounds of the heart and pericardium. Surg Gynecol Obstet 74:406–418, 1942.
101. Grose R, Greenberg MA, Yipintsoi T, Cohen MV: Cardiac tamponade in dogs with normal coronary arteries. I. Effect of changing intravascular volume on hemodynamics and myocardial blood flow. Basic Res Cardiol 79:531–541, 1984.
102. Guest JL Jr, Hall DP, Yeh TJ, Ellison RG: Late manifestations of trauma to the pericardium. Surg Gynecol Obstet 787–791:531–541, 1965.
103. Haas JM, Peterson CR, Jones RC: Subintimal dissection of the coronary arteries: A complication of selective coronary arteriography and the transfemoral percutaneous approach. Circulation 38:678–683, 1968.
104. Harken DE: Foreign bodies in and in relation to the thoracic blood vessels and heart. Surg Gynecol Obstet 83:117–125, 1946.
105. Harley DP, Mena I, Narahara KA et al: Traumatic myocardial dysfunction. J Thorac Cardiovasc Surg 87:386–393, 1984.
106. Harrison LH, Kisslo JA, Sabiston DC: Extraction of intramyocardial foreign body utilizing operative ultrasonography. J Thorac Cardiovasc Surg 82:345–349, 1981.
107. Hassett A, Moran J, Sabiston DC, Kisslo J: Utility of echocardiography in the management of patients with penetrating missile wounds of the heart. J Am Coll Cardiol 7:1151–1156, 1986.
108. Hendel PN, Grant AF: Blunt traumatic rupture of the heart—successful repair of simultaneous rupture of the right atrium and left ventricle. J Thorac Cardiovasc Surg 81:574–576, 1981.
109. Hiebert CA, Gregory FJ: Bullet embolism from the head to the heart. JAMA 229:442–443, 1974.
110. Hill LL: A report of a case of successful suturing of the heart, and table of 37 other cases of suturing by different operators with various terminations and the conclusions drawn. Med Rec 62:846–848, 1902.
111. Hines GL, Doyle E, Acinapura AJ: Post-traumatic ventricular septal defect, mitral insufficiency, and multiple coronary camera fistulas. J Trauma 17:234–237, 1977.
112. Hipona FA, Paredes S: The radiologic evaluation of patients with chest trauma. Med Clin North Am 59:65–93, 1975.
113. Hutchinson JE, Schmidt DM, Cameron A, McCord CW: The surgical management of intracardiac defects due to penetrating trauma. J Thorac Cardiovasc Surg 65:103–107, 1973.
114. Isaacs JP: Recent advances in surgery: Sixty penetrating wounds of the heart. Surgery 45:696–707, 1959.
115. Ivatury RR, Shah PM, Ito K et al: Emergency room thoracotomy for the resuscitation of patients with "fatal" penetrating injuries of the heart. Ann Thorac Surg 32:377–385, 1981.
116. Jackson DH, Murphy GW: Nonpenetrating cardiac trauma. Mod Concepts Cardiovasc Dis 45:123–128, 1976.
117. Jacob L, Bonnet F, Pavie A et al: Severe hypoxemia revealing traumatic tricuspid regurgitation with right-to-left intracardiac shunt. J Trauma 25:659–661, 1985.
118. Jahnke EJ Jr, FitzGibbon GM, Nelson WP, Aaby GV: Tricuspid insufficiency. Arch Surg 95:880–886, 1967.
119. Jamieson SW: Trauma to the heart and great vessels. In Jamieson SW (ed): Rob & Smith's Operative Surgery. St. Louis, CV Mosby, 1986.
120. Jarmakini JM, McHale PA, Greenfield JC: The effect of cardiac tamponade on coronary haemodynamics in the awake dog. Cardiovasc Res 9:112–117, 1975.
121. Jeger E: Die chirurgie der blutgefasse und des herzens. Berlin, A. Hirschwald, 1913.
122. Jobert JA: Reflexions sur les plaies penetrantes du cour. Arch Gen Med 6:1, 1839.
123. Johnson SL: Heart wounds. In Johnson SL: The History of Cardiac Surgery 1896–1955. Baltimore, Johns Hopkins Press, 1970.
124. Jones EW, Helmsworth J: Penetrating wounds of the heart: Thirty years' experience. Arch Surg 96:671–682, 1968.
125. Jones JW, Hewitt RL, Drapanas T: Cardiac contusion: A capricious syndrome. Ann Surg 181:567–574, 1975.
126. Karrel R, Schaffer MA, Franszek JB: Emergency diagnosis, resuscitation, and treatment of acute penetrating cardiac trauma. Ann Emerg Med 11:504–517, 1982.
127. Kettunen P: Cardiac damage after blunt chest trauma, diagnosed using Ck-Mb enzymes and the electrocardiogram. Int J Cardiol 6:355–371, 1984.
128. Kettunen P, Nieminen M: Creatine kinase Mb and M-mode echocardiographic changes in cardiac contusion. Ann Clin Res 17:292–298, 1985.
129. Killen DA, Gobbel WG Jr, France R, Vix VA: Post-traumatic aneurysm of the left ventricle. Circulation 39:101–108, 1969.
130. King RM, Mucha P Jr, Seward JB et al: Cardiac contusion: A new diagnostic approach utilizing two-dimensional echocardiography. J Trauma 23:610–614, 1983.
131. Kron IL, Cox PM Jr: Cardiac injury after chest trauma. Crit Care Med 11:524–526, 1983.
132. Kumar SA, Puri VK, Mittal VK, Cortez J: Myocardial contusion following nonfatal blunt chest trauma. J Trauma 23:327–331, 1983.
133. Lau V, Viano DC, Doty DB: Experimental cardiac trauma—ballistics of a captive bolt pistol. J Trauma 21:39–41, 1981
134. Ledgerwood AM: The wandering bullet. Surg Clin North Am 57:97–109, 1977.
135. Leinoff HD: Direct nonpenetrating injuries of the heart. Ann Intern Med 653–666:97–109, 1940.
136. Leonard JJ, Harvey WP, Hufnagel CA: Rupture of the aortic valve. N Engl J Med 252:208–212, 1955.
137. Levine RJ, Roberts WC, Morrow AG: Traumatic aortic regurgitation. Am J Cardiol 10:752–763, 1962.
138. Levitsky S: New insights in cardiac trauma. Surg Clin North Am 55:43–55, 1975.
139. Liberthson RR, Barron K, Harthorne JW et al: Traumatic coronary arterial fistula: A case report and review of the literature. Am Heart J 86:817–821, 1973.

140. Liedtke AJ, Allen RP, Nellis SH: Effects of blunt cardiac trauma on coronary vasomotion, perfusion, myocardial mechanics, and metabolism. J Trauma 20:777–785, 1980.
141. Liedtke AJ, DeMuth WE Jr: Nonpentrating cardiac injuries: A collective review. Am Heart J 86:687–697, 1973.
142. Liedtke AJ, Gault JH, DeMuth WE: Electrocardiographic and hemodynamic changes following nonpenetrating chest trauma in the experimental animal. Am J Physiol 226:377–382, 1974.
143. Loop FD, Hofmeier G, Groves LK: Traumatic disruption of the aortic valve. Cleve Clin Q 38:187–194, 1971.
144. Lowe JE, Adams DH, Cummings RG et al: The natural history and recommended management of patients with traumatic coronary artery fistulas. Ann Thorac Surg 36:295–305, 1983.
145. Lowe JE, Oldham HN, Sabiston DC: Surgical management of congenital coronary artery fistulas. Ann Surg 194:373–380, 1981.
146. Lowen HJ, Fink SA, Helpern M: Transfixion of the heart by embedded ice pick blade with eight months' survival. Circulation 11:426–433, 1950.
147. Ludington LG, Boskind AS, Miguel A: Rupture of left ventricle from blunt cardiac trauma. Ann Thorac Surg 18:195–200, 1974.
148. Lynn RB, Fay JE: Post-traumatic cardiocoronary fistula. Can J Surg 14:335–336, 1971.
149. MacMillan RM, Shahriari A, Sumithisena et al: Contrast-enhanced cine computed tomography for diagnosis of right coronary artery to coronary sinus arteriovenous fistula. Am J Cardiol 56:997–998, 1985.
150. Mandal AK, Awariefe SO, Oparah SS: Experience in the management of 50 consecutive penetrating wounds of the heart. Br J Surg 66:565–568, 1979.
151. Mannix EP Jr, Dennis C: The surgical treatment of chronic pericardial effusion and cardiac tamponade. J Thorac Surg 381–397: 565–568, 1954.
152. Markiewicz W, Best LA, Burstein S, Peleg H: Echocardiographic evaluation after blunt trauma of the chest. Int J Cardiol 8:269–274, 1985.
153. Marshall WG, Bell JL, Kouchoukos NT: Penetrating cardiac trauma. J Trauma 24:147–149, 1984.
154. Martin TD, Flynn TC, Rowlands BJ et al: Blunt cardiac rupture. J Trauma 24:287–290, 1984.
155. Mattila S, Silvola H, Ketonen P: Traumatic rupture of the pericardium with luxation of the heart. J Thorac Cardiovasc Surg 70:495–498, 1975.
156. Mattox KL, Beall AC, Jordan GL, DeBakey ME: Cardiography in the emergency center. J Thorac Cardiovasc Surg 68:886–895, 1974.
157. Mattox KL, Koch LV, Beall AC, DeBakey ME: Logistic and technical considerations in the treatment of the wounded heart. Circulation (Suppl) 51–52:210–214, 1975.
158. Mattox KL, Limacher MC, Feliciano DV et al: Cardiac evaluation following heart injury. J Trauma 25:758–765, 1985.
159. Mayfield W, Hurley EJ: Blunt cardiac trauma. Am J Surg 148:162–167, 1984.
160. Mazzucco A, Rizzoli G, Faggian G et al: Acute mitral regurgitation after blunt chest trauma. Arch Intern Med 143:2326–2329, 1983.
161. McKusick VA, Kay JH, Isaacs JP: Constrictive pericarditis following traumatic hemopericardium. Ann Surg 142:97–103, 1955.
162. McLaughlin JS, Cowley RA, Smith G, Matheson NA: Mitral valve disease from blunt trauma. J Thorac Cardiovasc Surg 48:261–271, 1964.
163. McLaughlin JS, Suherlis HR, Yeager G: Sterile pericarditis from foreign body: Acute tamponade one month following gunshot wound. Ann Thorac Surg 3:52–56, 1967.
164. Miller FA Jr, Seward JB, Gersh BJ et al: Two-dimensional echocardiographic findings in cardiac trauma. Am J Cardiol 50:1022–1027, 1982.
165. Miller GE, Rueb AE: Blunt thoracic trauma producing heart laceration. Ann Surg 166:852–853, 1967.
166. Moore EE, Moore JB, Galloway AC, Eiseman B: Postinjury thoracotomy in the emergency department: A critical evaluation. Surgery 86:590–598, 1979.
167. Moraes R, Victor E, Arruda M et al: Ventricular septal defect following nonpenetrating trauma. Angiology 24:222–229, 1973.
168. Morgagni JB: The Seats and Causes of Disease. Alexander B (trans): London, Miller and Cadell, 1769.
169. Morgan BC, Able FL, Mullins GL: Flow patterns in cavae, pulmonary artery, pulmonary vein, and aorta in intact dogs. Am J Physiol 210:903–900, 1966.
170. Moritz AR, Atkins JP: Cardiac contusion an experimental and pathological study. Arch Pathol 25:445–462, 1938.
171. Motro M, Barzilay Z, Schneeweiss A, et al: Isolated right ventricular infarction and aneurysm due to blunt trauma: Valve of two-dimensional echocardiography and radionuclide angiography. Am Heart J 101:679–680, 1981.
172. Moynihan B: The surgery of the chest in relation to retained projectiles. Br J Surg 7:444–486, 1920.
173. National Safety Council: Accidents SATS. Chicago, National Safety Council, 1985.
174. Neville WE, Bolanowski PJP: Cardiac Trauma. In Gay WA (ed): P Goldsmith's Practice of Surgery. Philadelphia, Harper & Row, 1985.
175. Nunez L, Celemin D, Gil-Aguado M, Pinto AG: Left ventricular rupture related to mitral valve replacement. In Roberts AJ (ed): Difficult Problems in Adult Cardiac Surgery, p 151. Chicago, Year Book Medical Publishers, 1985.
176. Oliva PB, Hilgenberg A, McElroy D: Obstruction of the proximal right coronary artery with acute inferior infarction due to blunt chest trauma. Ann Intern Med 91:205–207, 1979.
177. Oren A, Bar-Shlomo B, Stern S: Acute coronary occlusion following blunt injury to the chest in the absence of coronary atherosclerosis. Am Heart J 92:501–505, 1976.
178. Osborn JR, Jones RC, Jahnke EJ Jr: Traumatic tricuspid insufficiency hemodynamic data and surgical treatment. Circulation 30:217–222, 1964.
179. Paget S: The Surgery of the Chest. London, John Wright & Co, 1896.
180. Pandian NG, Skorton DJ, Doty DB, Kerber RE: Immediate diagnosis of acute myocardial contusion by two-dimensional echocardiography: Studies in a canine model of blunt chest trauma. J Am Coll Cardiol 2:488–496, 1983.
181. Parmley LF, Manion WC, Mattingly TW: Nonpenetrating traumatic injury of the heart. Circulation 18:371–396, 1958.
182. Parmley LF, Mattingly TW, Manion WC: Penetrating wounds of the heart and aorta. Circulation 17:953–973, 1958
183. Pate JW, Richardson RL: Penetrating wounds of cardiac valves. JAMA 207:309–311, 1969.
184. Patton AS, Guyton SW, Lawson DW, Shannon JM: Treatment of severe atrial injuries. Am J Surg 141:465–471, 1981.
185. Payne DD, DeWeese JA, Mahoney EB, Murphy GW: Surgical treatment of traumatic rupture of the normal aortic valve. Ann Thorac Surg 17:223–229, 1974.
186. Pellegrini RV, Layton TR, Dimarco RF et al: Multiple cardiac lesions from blunt trauma. J Trauma 20:169–173, 1980.
187. Pickard LR, Mattox KL, Beall AC Jr: Ventricular septal defect from blunt chest injury. J Trauma 20:329–331, 1980.
188. Pierce EC, Dabbs CH, Rawson FL: Isolated rupture of the ventricular septum due to nonpenetrating trauma. Arch Surg 77:87–93, 1958.
189. Pifarre R, Grieco J, Garibaldi A et al: Acute coronary artery occlusion secondary to blunt chest trauma. J Thorac Cardiovasc Surg 83:122–125, 1982.
190. Pillai R, Fountain SW, Qureshi SA et al: Avulsion of the anterior papillary muscle of the mitral valve due to non-penetrating trauma to the chest. Thorax 37:943–944, 1982.
191. Pool EH: Treatment of heart wounds: Report of successful cardiography and tabulation of cases. Ann Surg 4:485–512, 1912.
192. Pories WJ, Gaudiani VA: Cardiac tamponade. Surg Clin North Am 55:573–589, 1975.
193. Potkin RT, Werner JA, Trobaugh GB et al: Evaluation of noninvasive tests of cardiac damage in suspected cardiac contusion. Circulation 66:627–631, 1982.
194. Potter RT, Stefko PL, Bertrand CA et al: Blunt cardiac trauma. Ann Thorac Surg 1:432–443, 1965.
195. Radtke HJH, de Wet Lubbe JJ, Janson PMC, Barnard PM: Penetrating wounds of the heart and pericardium. J Thorac Cardiovasc Surg 27:18–23, 1979.
196. Raker JW, Langfeld SB, Gowens GF: Traumatic hemopericardium producing late constrictive pericarditis. Ann Surg 148:134–138, 1956.

197. Ramsdell J: Stab wounds of the heart. Ann Surg 99:141–151, 1934.
198. Rayner AVS, Fulton RL, Hess PJ, Daicoff GR: Post-traumatic intracardiac shunts: Report of two cases and review of the literature. J Thorac Cardiovasc Surg 73:728–732, 1977.
199. Rea WJ, Sugg WL, Wilson LC et al: Coronary artery lacerations. Ann Thorac Surg 7:518–528, 1969.
200. Reece IJ, Davidson KG: Emergency surgery for stab wounds to the heart. Ann Coll Surg Engl 65:304–307, 1983.
201. Rehn L: Ueber penetrierende herzwunden und henznaht. Arch Klin Chir 55:315–329, 1897.
202. Rehn L: Zur chirurgie des herzens und herzbeutels. Arch Klin Chir 83:723–820, 1907.
203. Reyes LH, Mattox KL, Gaasch WH et al: Traumatic coronary artery–right heart fistula. J Thorac Cardiovasc Surg 70:52–56, 1975.
204. Rheuban KS, Tompkins DG, Nolan SP et al: Myocardial necrosis and ventricular aneurysm following closed chest injury in a child. J Trauma 21:170–173, 1981.
205. Rich NM, Spencer FC: Wounds of the Heart in Vascular Trauma. Philadelphia, WB Saunders, 1978.
206. Ricketts J: Injuries of the heart. NY Med J 77:993, 1903.
207. Roberts JB: The surgery of the pericardium. Ann Anat Surg 4:247, 1881.
208. Rodriguez A, Shatney C: The value of technetium 99m pyrophosphate scanning in the diagnosis of myocardial contusion. Am Surg 48:472–474, 1982.
209. Roebuck EJ, Minford J: Traumatic rupture of the pericardium with herniation of the heart. Br J Radiol 56:585–588, 1983.
210. Rogers MA, Chesler E, Du Plessis L: Surgical management of traumatic cardiac fistulae. Thorax 24:543–546, 1969
211. Rose E: Herztamponade (Ein beitrag zur herzchirurgie). Dtsch Z Chir 20:329–340, 1884.
212. Rosenthal A, Parisi LF, Nadas AS: Isolated interventricular septal defect due to nonpenetrating trauma. N Engl J Med 283:338–341, 1970.
213. Sabiston DC: Major contributions to surgery from the south. Ann Surg 181:487–507, 1975.
214. Samson PC: Two unusual cases of war wounds of the heart. Surgery 20:373–381, 1946.
215. Sareli P, Goldman AP, Pocock WA et al: Coronary artery-right ventricular fistula and organic tricuspid regurgitation due to blunt chest trauma. Am J Cardiol 54:697–699, 1984
216. Sarot IA, Schechter DC, Weber DJ: Post-traumatic coronary arteriovenous fistulas with surgical cure. Ann Thorac Surg 6:172–177, 1968.
217. Sauer PE, Murdock CE: Immediate surgery for cardiac and great vessel wounds. Arch Surg 95:7–11, 1967.
218. Saurbruch F: Die verwendbarkeit des unterdruckverfahrens bei der herzchirurgie. Arch Klin Chir 83:537–545, 1907.
219. Schechter DC, Gilbert L: Injuries of the heart and great vessels due to pins and needles. Thorax 24:246–253, 1969.
220. Schwaitzberg SD, Khalil KG: Isolated traumatic aortic valvular insufficiency with rapid pulmonary deterioration. Arch Surg 120:971–973, 1985.
221. Sethi GK, Scott SM, Takaro T: Complications of external cardiac massage: Report of a case of laceration of the right ventricular outflow tract. J Cardiovasc Surg 18:187–190, 1977.
222. Shabetai R, Aravindakshan V, Danielson G, Bryant L: Traumatic hemopericardium with tricuspid incompetence. J Thorac Cardiovasc Surg 57:294–297, 1969.
223. Shabetai R, Fowler NO, Guntheroth WG: The hemodynamics of cardiac tamponade and constrictive pericarditis. Am J Cardiol 26:480–489, 1970.
224. Sherman MM, Saini VK, Yarnoz MD et al: Management of penetrating heart wounds. Am J Surg 135:553–558, 1978.
225. Shoemaker WC, Carey JS, Yao ST et al: Hemodynamic alterations in acute cardiac tamponade after penetrating injuries of the heart. Surgery 67:754–764, 1970.
226. Siderys H, Strange PS: Rupture of the heart due to blunt trauma. J Thorac Cardiovasc Surg 62:84–86, 1971.
227. Siepser SL, Kaltman AJ, Mills N et al: Coronary collateral flow after traumatic fistula between right coronary artery and right atrium. N Engl J Med 287:754–756, 1972.
228. Sigler LH: Traumatic injury of the heart. Am Heart J 30:459–478, 1945.
229. Silver GM, Spampinato N, Favaloro RG, Groves LK: Ventricular aneurysms and blunt chest trauma. Chest 63:628–631, 1973.
230. Singh R, Nolan SP, Schrank JP: Traumatic left ventricular aneurysm. JAMA 234:412–414, 1975.
231. Smith JM, Grover FL, Marcos JJ et al: Blunt traumatic rupture of the atria. J Thorac Cardiovasc Surg 71:617–620, 1976.
232. Snow N, Lucas AE, Richardson JD: Intra-aortic balloon counterpulsation for cardiogenic shock from cardiac contusion. J Trauma 22:426–429, 1982.
233. Snow N, Richardson JD, Flint LM Jr: Myocardial contusion: Implications for patients with multiple traumatic injuries. Surgery 92:744–750, 1982.
234. Stansel HC Jr, Julian OC, Dye WS: Right ventricular aneurysm. J Thorac Cardiovasc Surg 46:66–76, 1963.
235. Stein PD, Sabbah HN, Viano DC, Vostal JJ: Response of the heart to nonpenetrating cardiac trauma. J Trauma 22:364–373, 1982.
236. Stephenson LW, Workman RB, Aldrete JS, Karp RB: Bullet emboli to the pulmonary artery: A report of 2 patients and review of the literature. Ann Thorac Surg 21:333–336, 1976.
237. Stern T, Wolf RY, Reichart B et al: Coronary artery occlusion resulting from blunt trauma. JAMA 230:1308–1309, 1974.
238. Sugg WL, Rea WJ, Ecker RR, et al: Penetrating wounds of the heart: An analysis of 459 cases. J Thorac Cardiovasc Surg 56:531–542, 1968.
239. Sutherland GR, Calvin JE, Driedger AA et al: Anatomic and cardiopulmonary responses to trauma with associated blunt chest injury. J Trauma 21:1–12, 1981.
240. Sutherland GR, Cheung HW, Holliday RL et al: Hemodynamic adaptation to acute myocardial contusion complicating blunt chest injury. Am J Cardiol 57:291–297, 1986.
241. Sutherland GR, Driedger AA, Holliday RL et al: Frequency of myocardial injury after blunt chest trauma as evaluated by radionuclide angiography. Am J Cardiol 52:1099–1103, 1983.
242. Sutherland RD, Gholston DE, Gulde RE, Martinez HE: Traumatic fistula between left anterior descending coronary artery and right ventricle. J Thorac Cardiovasc Surg 70:692–695, 1975.
243. Swan HJ: Complications associated with angiocardiography. Circulation 37:81–84, 1968.
244. Symbas PN: Cardiac trauma. Am Heart J 92:387–396, 1976.
245. Symbas PN: Trauma to the Heart and Great Vessels. New York, Grune & Stratton, 1978.
246. Symbas PN, DiOrio DA, Tyras DH et al: Penetrating cardiac wounds. J Thorac Cardiovasc Surg 66:526–532, 1973.
247. Symbas PN, Harlaftis N: Bullet emboli in the pulmonary and systemic arteries. Ann Surg 185:318–320, 1977.
248. Szabo JR, Chen JT, Putman CE: New murmur following blunt chest trauma. Invest Radiol 19:163–167, 1984.
249. Tabatznik B, Isaacs JP: Postpericardiotomy syndrome following traumatic hemopericardium. Am J Cardiol 7:83–96, 1961.
250. Taichman GC, Byrne P, Forester GV, Keon WJ: Regional myocardial blood flow during pericardial tamponade. Can J Physiol Pharmacol 62:539–543, 1984.
251. Tate JS, Horan DP: Penetrating injuries of the heart. Surg Gynecol Obstet 157:57–63, 1983.
252. Tavares S, Hankins JR, Moulton AL et al: Management of penetrating cardiac injuries: The role of emergency room thoracotomy. Ann Thorac Surg 38:183–187, 1984.
253. Tector AJ, Reuben CF, Hoffman JF et al: Coronary artery wounds treated with saphenous vein bypass grafts. JAMA 225:282–284, 1973.
254. Tenzer ML: The spectrum of myocardial contusion: A review. J Trauma 25:620–627, 1985.
255. Thandroyen FT, Matisonn RE: Penetrating thoracic trauma producing cardiac shunts. J Thorac Cardiovasc Surg 81:569–573, 1981.
256. Tonkin AM, Lester RM, Guthrow CE et al: Persistence of MB isoenzyme of creatine phosphokinase in the serum after minor iatrogenic cardiac trauma. Circulation 51:627–631, 1975.
257. Torres-Mirabal P, Gruenberg JC, Brown RS, Obeid FN: Spectrum of myocardial contusion. Am Surg 48:383–392, 1982.
258. Trimble C: Arterial bullet embolism following thoracic gunshot wounds. Ann Surg 168:911–916, 1968.

259. Trinkle JK: Penetrating heart wounds: Difficulty in evaluating clinical series. Ann Thorac Surg 38:181–182, 1984.
260. Trinkle JK, Marcos J, Grover FL, Cuello LM: Management of the wounded heart. Ann Thorac Surg 17:230–236, 1974.
261. Trinkle JK, Toon RS, Franz JL et al: Affairs of the wounded heart: Penetrating cardiac wounds. J Trauma 19:467–472, 1979.
262. Trueblood HW, Wuerflein RD, Angell WW: Blunt trauma rupture of the heart. Ann Surg 177:66–69, 1973.
263. Tuffier T: Cinquieme Congres de la Societ;aae Internationale de Chirurgie. Paris, Extrait Hayez, 1920.
264. Tyson G, Maier G, Olsen CO et al: Pericardial influences on ventricular filling in the conscious dog: An analysis based on pericardial pressure. Circ Res 54:173–184, 1984.
265. Utley JR, Doty DB, Collins JC et al: Cardiac output, coronary flow, ventricular fibrillation and survival following varying degrees of myocardial contusion. J Surg Res 20:539–543, 1976.
266. Valle AR. War injuries of the heart and mediastinum. Arch Surg 70:398–404, 1955.
267. Venkataraman K, Bilitch M: Intracardiac electrocardiography during permanent pacemaker implantation: Predictors of cardiac perforation. Am J Cardiol 44:225–231, 1979.
268. Vij D, Simoni E, Smith RF et al: Resuscitative thoracotomy for patients with traumatic injury. Surgery 94:554–561, 1983.
269. Wainwright RJ, Edwards AC, Maisey MN, Sowton E: Early occlusion and late stricture of normal coronary arteries following blunt chest trauma. Chest 78:796–798, 1980.
270. Warburg E: Myocardial and pericardial lesions due to non-penetrating injury. Br Heart J ii:271–280, 1940.
271. Ward PA, Suzuki A: Gunshot wound of the heart with peripheral embolization. J Thorac Cardiovasc Surg 68:440–446, 1974.
272. Washington B, Wilson RF, Steiger Z, Bassett JS: Emergency thoracotomy: A four-year review. Ann Thorac Surg 40:188–191, 1985.
273. Watanabe T, Katsume H, Matsukubo H et al: Ruptured chordae tendineae of the tricuspid valve due to nonpenetrating trauma. Chest 80:751–753, 1981.
274. Watson JH, Bartholomae WM: Cardiac injury due to nonpenetrating chest trauma. Ann Intern Med 52:871–880, 1960.
275. Wechsler AS, Auerbach BJ, Graham TC, Sabiston DC: Distribution of intramyocardial blood flow during pericardial tamponade. J Thorac Cardiovasc Surg 68:847–856, 1974.
276. Whisennand HH, Van Pelt SA, Beall AC et al: Surgical management of traumatic intracardiac injuries. Ann Thorac Surg 28:530–536, 1979.
277. Wilkinson C, Wood M: High voltage electric injury. Am J Surg 136:693–696, 1978.
278. Williams DH: Stab wound of the heart and pericardium—suture of the pericardium—patient alive three years afterwards. Medical Record 51:437, 1897.
279. Williams JB, Silver DG, Laws HL: Successful management of heart rupture from blunt trauma. J Trauma 21:534–537, 1981.
280. Wilson RF, Bassett JS: Penetrating wounds of the pericardium or its contents. JAMA 195:105–110, 1966.
281. Wong B, Murphy J, Chang CJ et al: The risk of pericardiocentesis. Am J Cardiol 44:1110–1114, 1979.
282. Zakharia AT: Cardiovascular and thoracic battle injuries in the Lebanon war. J Thorac Cardiovasc Surg 89:723–733, 1985.

traumatic thoracic aneurysm

Walter G. Wolfe
Francis G. Duhaylongsod

1
2 6
3 7 11
4 8 12 16
5 9 13 17
10 14 18
15 19
20

THORACIC AORTIC RUPTURE

Few traumatic injuries have succeeded in captivating the interest of surgeons as much as the disruption of the thoracic aorta consequent to high-speed deceleration and blunt chest trauma. Although only a minority of trauma centers will manage more than four cases of aortic rupture a year, over two hundred scientific articles on this subject have appeared in the English literature since the first successful repair approximately thirty years ago. Undoubtedly, fascination is borne from the almost unimaginable circumstance that anyone could survive a complete transection of this major artery, yet a considerable number do survive.

Vesalius, in 1557, is credited with the first description of a traumatic aortic rupture in a patient who fell from a horse.[110] Although Dshanelidze successfully repaired a penetrating wound to the thoracic aorta in 1923,[19] the first successful repair of an acute, nonpenetrating, traumatic aortic injury did not occur until 1958, by Klassen,[81] marking the 400th anniversary of Vesalius' original description.

Incidence

Modern automobile transportation ushered in the new age of rapid deceleration injury involving the thoracic aorta. Strassman,[100] from 1936 to 1942, found only 51 motor vehicle-related cases of thoracic aortic rupture among 7000 autopsies (0.7%) performed by the Chief Medical Examiner's Office of New York City. In comparison, Greendyke,[36] from 1961 to 1965, noted 35 traumatic aortic ruptures among 218 autopsies (16%) of motor vehicle-related fatalities in Monroe County, New York, or 1 in every 6 persons dying in a motor vehicle accident. Notably, among 49 driver and passenger fatalities involving ejection from the vehicle, 13 (27%) sustained aortic rupture.[36] In a recent review of the literature, 94% of all traumatic aortic ruptures were related to motor vehicle accidents, involving either drivers, passengers, or pedestrians.[26]

In Parmley's often-cited work,[80] 38 of 275 patients with traumatic aortic rupture, or 13.8%, survived the initial injury. Of these 38, only 3 died within the first hour; thus, most survived long enough to obtain medical treatment. In the United States alone, more than 8000 cases of traumatic aortic rupture are estimated annually.[65] Therefore, well over 1000 accident victims harboring a thoracic aortic rupture may be predicted to survive the initial trauma and present to our nation's medical centers each year.

The prevalence of traumatic aortic rupture is highest during the third and fourth decades of life, with a mean age of 30 years. Few reported cases have involved children below the age of 10 years or adults above the age of 70. The male to female ratio is 3:1.[26] The age and gender distribution among victims of aortic deceleration injury reflect the population at risk for violent vehicular trauma, and therefore, should not be interpreted as indicating inherent risk. The probability of thoracic aortic rupture is equally likely among patients of all age and gender given a sufficient mechanism of injury.

Mechanism of Injury

Deceleration injuries may be either impact or momentum injuries.[85] The mechanism by which an impact or momentum injury results in a thoracic aortic tear has interested numerous investigators during this century. The forces acting upon the thoracic aorta during rapid deceleration include:

1. Acute pressure alteration within a closed compartment
2. Shear stress
3. Bending stress
4. Torsion stress

In studies by Oppenheim[79] and Zehnder,[119] a bursting pressure of 2070 mm Hg and 2500 mm Hg, respectively, was required to rupture a normal human aorta. However, rapid deceleration from 120 m.p.h. in 0.1 to 0.2 seconds will result in an intraluminal pressure of only 1000 mm Hg.[18] This observation, coupled with reports of aortic rupture following mild deceleration from 30 m.p.h.,[88] has cast reasonable doubt that the usual deceleration force encountered in a motor vehicle accident could produce an aortic tear through acute pressure alteration alone.

In 1944, Haas proposed that whenever one part of the body is decelerated at a rate different from another part, the connection between the two is subjected to shearing stress proportional to the difference in the rates of deceleration.[43] Thus, as the body experiences violent deceleration, a shearing force is produced by the mass/inertia of a mobile structure relative to its point(s) of fixation.[76,85] One area of debate has centered upon the extent of movement of the aortic arch relative to the descending thoracic aorta. In 1893, Rindfleisch first advanced the concept of an aortic arch fixed by the brachiocephalic vessels and ligamentum arteriosum, with a relatively mobile descending aorta.[89] During rapid deceleration, the momentum of the mobile descending thoracic aorta leads to a tear at its junction to the fixed aortic arch, in the region of the ligamentum arteriosum (aortic isthmus). Indeed, the fact that the aortic isthmus is the most common site of traumatic aortic rupture has popularized this theory.[5,17,32,48,50,51,53,67,94,95] Others, however, contend that if the descending aorta actually continues to move forward upon abrupt deceleration, avulsion of the intercostal arteries may be expected, but this is not seen.[67,83] Instead, they propose that the aortic arch, great vessels, and isthmus are freely mobile, while the descending thoracic aorta is securely fixed to the posterior chest wall by the intercostal branches and parietal pleura.[31,37,38,67,73,77,82,88,91,119] Similarly, the site of maximal shear stress would also be focused in the region of the aortic isthmus.

Bending stress and torsion stress both involve an impact injury as the patient is thrown violently on the road or against the steering wheel, dashboard, or body of the vehicle. As the AP diameter of the chest is compressed, the heart is displaced further into the left chest resulting in hyperflexion of the aortic arch as it courses over the left mainstem bronchus and torsion of the aortic wall.[31,47,59]

During rapid deceleration, the inner surface of the aortic lumen bears the greatest stress.[18] Therefore, tears usually begin in the intima and extend peripherally. In about 20% of traumatic ruptures, the adventitia remains intact creating a false aneurysm.[16,113] Since the adventitia accounts for 60% of the tensile strength in the healthy aorta, the false aneurysm may remain intact for hours to days depending on the strength of the residual adventitia.[36] The aortic rupture is usually a single, transverse laceration, which may be complete (involving the entire wall) or partial. The extent of rupture may not have a significant bearing on survival. In Parmley's series, 9 of 38 patients who survived the immediate trauma had complete transections of the aorta, and 8 survived beyond 5 days.[80]

Natural History

Eighty to 85% of all victims of thoracic aortic rupture will not survive the immediate trauma.[80,100] Because of the violent mechanism of injury, associated non-cardiovascular injuries are common and may account for over 50% of the prehospital mortality.[80] The 15% to 20% of victims who survive long enough to receive medical attention will usually have an injury at the aortic isthmus with intact adventitia or surrounding mediastinal tissues capable of containing the pulsating hematoma (Fig. 6.1).[13] The mortality rate if left untreated is 20% at 6 hours, 31% at 24 hours, 74% at 8 days, and 83% at 4 months.[80] A subgroup of patients, up to 20%, may be predicted to form a chronic false aneurysm if left untreated.[80]

Clinical Presentation

Central to the successful management of thoracic aortic rupture is a heightened level of suspicion leading to a deliberate and thorough diagnostic workup. Patients with aortic injury often present with multisystem trauma, including head injury, abdominal hemorrhage, severe extremity injury, pelvic fracture, and frequently, absence of external chest injury. In fact, one-third to one-half of patients will have no external evidence of thoracic injury at the time of initial physical examination.[19,23,50,54,55,58,80,90,103] The number and severity of associated injuries often divert the physician's attention away from the chest, resulting in an inordinate delay in recognition of the aortic injury. Constant awareness of the possibility of aortic injury in victims of high-speed deceleration, or blunt chest trauma, and careful inspection of the chest radiograph will reduce the frequency of undetected thoracic aortic rupture.[69,70]

The pathogenesis of traumatic aortic injury underscores the importance of the patient history in assessing the risk for thoracic aortic rupture in any given patient. Although a history of deceleration injury or blunt trauma to the chest remains the most sensitive indicator of aortic rupture, a positive history alone is extremely nonspecific. Nevertheless, certain events obtained from the patient history may increase suspicion, including: ejection from the vehicle,[4] head-on collision, death of a passenger or

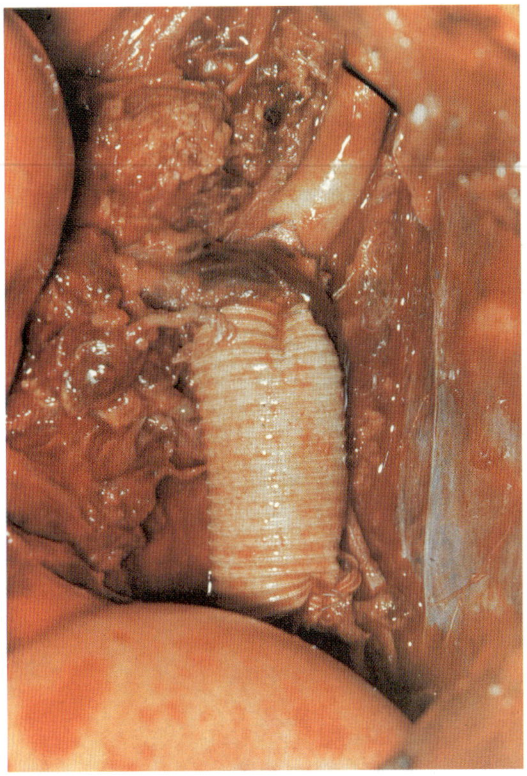

FIGURE 6.1 Operative photograph of a 14-year-old victim of high-speed deceleration injury following graft repair of an acute aortic transection occuring at the most common location, just distal to the origin of the left subclavian artery (aortic isthmus). Note periaortic hematoma and marked distortion of the normal mediastinal tissue planes.

driver within the same vehicle, fall of more than 2 floors,[65] and aircraft crash.[80] Kirsh[53,56] and Redman[86] advocate compulsory contrast angiography in any patient who has sustained a deceleration injury or blunt chest trauma, even without clinical or chest radiographic findings that suggest aortic rupture. However, given the low specificity of the patient history combined with the high negative predictive value of a normal chest radiograph, most workers support a more judicious approach.[69,70]

The spectrum of findings on physical examination in patients with traumatic aortic rupture emphasize the violent nature of the inciting trauma. Based upon the experience at Duke University Medical Center over a 20-year period, in 105 patients sustaining acute thoracic aortic rupture, the distribution of physical findings underscores the frequency of multisystem involvement and the poor sensitivity of any specific sign or symptom (Fig. 6.2). Associated injuries were common (Fig. 6.3). No patient in our experience had a completely negative physical examination. Forty-five percent of our patients had no evidence of rib, sternal, or clavicular fractures.

Although the physical examination remains poorly sensitive for the diagnosis of traumatic aortic rupture, several findings should raise suspicion, including: a difference in pulse amplitude between the upper and lower extremities, hypertension of the upper extremities with hypotension of the lower extremities (pseudocoarctation),[55,57,60,62,66,99,105] paraplegia,[24,45] systolic murmur heard maximally to the left of the spine in the midscapular area,[28,29,48] and midscapular chest pain in the absence of a vertebral fracture.

Chest Radiography

Radiographic manifestations of mediastinal hemorrhage are often invaluable in the diagnosis of traumatic aortic rupture. However, no single radiographic sign or combination of signs provides both the sensitivity to enable identification of all cases of thoracic aortic injury, and the specificity to avoid an appreciable number of negative angiographic studies.[69] Ayella et al. believed the inability to discern the normal anatomy of the superior mediastinum in a true erect chest film is the *raison d'etre* for the diagnosis of thoracic aortic injury.[8] Hence, any irregularity in the normal configuration of the superior mediastinum is an indication for aortography, and a large number of negative aortograms should be accepted as standard practice.[115] Conversely, a normal superior mediastinum makes the likelihood of an aortic isthmus tear remote,[96] excluding the diagnosis of traumatic aortic rupture and eliminating unnecessary aortography in this group of patients.[69]

Chest radiographic findings (Fig. 6.4) associated with mediastinal hemorrhage and traumatic aortic rupture include:

1. Widening of the superior mediastinum greater than 8 cm
2. Mediastinal-width/chest-width ratio greater than 0.25
3. Abnormalities of aortic knob contour
4. Apical capping
5. Opacification of the aorticopulmonary window
6. Widening of the paraspinal lines
7. Widening of the right paratracheal stripe greater than 5 mm
8. First rib and multiple rib fractures

FIGURE 6.2
SIGNS AND SYMPTOMS OF ACUTE TRAUMATIC THORACIC ANEURYSM IN 105 PATIENTS: DUKE UNIVERSITY MEDICAL CENTER 1970–1990

Chest pain	75% (45 of 60)
Loss of consciousness or coma	68% (50 of 74)
Dyspnea	55% (18 of 33)
Shock (SBP <90 mmHg)	49% (51 of 105)
Midscapular backpain	38% (9 of 24)
Paresis or paralegia (includes coma)	31% (33 of 105)
Difference in pulse amplitude	25% (24 of 96)
Systolic murmur	16% (15 of 96)
Hypertension	6% (6 of 99)
Dysphagia	0% (0 of 9)
Cough	0% (0 of 24)
Hoarseness	0% (0 of 42)
	(number of patients)

FIGURE 6.3
ASSOCIATED INJURIES IN 105 PATIENTS WITH ACUTE TRAUMATIC THORACIC ANEURYSM: DUKE UNIVERSITY MEDICAL CENTER 1970–1990

Orthopedic	
Ribs/clavicle/sternum fracture	55% (54 of 99)
Femur/extremity fracture	61% (44 of 72)
Pelvis/hip fracture	26% (27 of 102)
Vertebral fracture	21% (17 of 81)
Cardiopulmonary	
Cardiac contusion	17% (6 of 36)
Pulmonary contusion	46% (18 of 39)
Neurological	
Intracranial hemorrhage	30% (21 of 69)
Cerebral contusion	21% (15 of 72)
Skull fracture	6% (6 of 93)
Gastrointestinal	
Spleen	29% (27 of 93)
Liver	10% (9 of 90)
Diaphragm	10% (9 of 93)
Kidney	13% (12 of 93)
Pancreas	3% (3 of 93)
Small bowel/mesentery	10% (9 of 93)
Maxillofacial	
Facial fracture	13% (12 of 93)
Negative physical examination	0% (0 of 105)
	(number of patients)

9. Displacement of nasogastric tube to the right
10. Depression of the left mainstem bronchus
11. Tracheal deviation to the right
12. Left hemothorax without rib fracture

The table shown in Figure 6.5 summarizes the results from several studies regarding the value of specific radio-graphic findings in the diagnosis of traumatic aortic rupture.[2,6,10,33,40,41,46,53,54,58,63,64,68,86,92,93,96,101,102,106,107,111,116,117]

Radiographic Imaging

Aortography is the only definitive diagnostic technique for establishing the diagnosis of traumatic aortic rupture. The inability to discern the normal anatomy of the superior mediastinum on the screening radiograph remains a highly sensitive indicator of mediastinal hemorrhage, but it is not sufficiently specific to distinguish the patients who possess a traumatic aortic rupture from those who do not. Efforts to improve the specificity of the initial chest radiograph risk diminishing its ability to identify patients with major thoracic arterial injury. This fact, coupled with the extremely low mortality associated with contrast aortography[117] constitutes a strong argument for its liberal use in any patient with one, or more, of the aforementioned radiographic manifestations of mediastinal hemorrhage.

The retrograde femoral approach is the technique of choice. It is relatively quick (average time 30 to 40 minutes), safe, generally more convenient than using the upper extremities, and it allows study of the abdominal, cerebral, or peripheral sites, if indicated.[53,86,91] The most common finding is a pseudoaneurysm without extravasation of contrast material (Figs. 6.6 and 6.7). Radiolucent lines extending into the lumen of the aorta represent aortic wall flaps, which are essential for the diagnosis

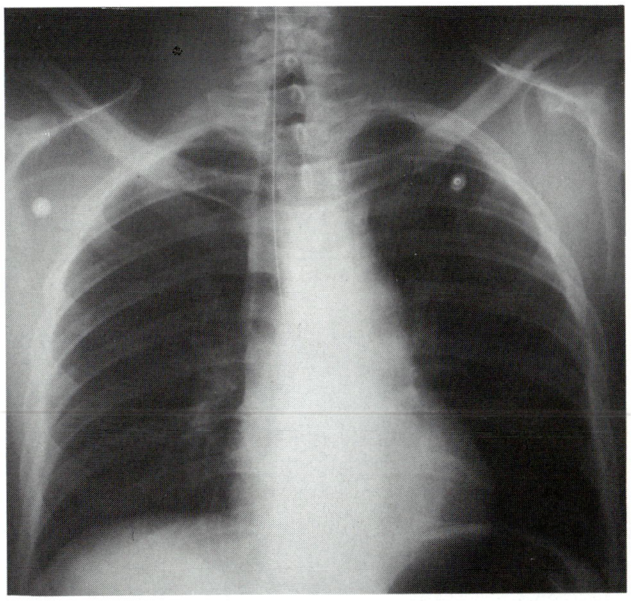

FIGURE 6.4 True erect portable chest radiograph of a 29-year-old male after sustaining high-speed deceleration injury in an automobile accident. The film shows several radiographic findings suggestive of traumatic aortic injury: a subtle left apical cap, wide right paraspinal stripe, wide right paratracheal stripe, loss of sharpness of the aortic contour, deviated nasogastric tube, deviated trachea, and depression of the left mainstem bronchus. The patient underwent an arteriogram, which confirmed the diagnosis of aortic transection, and underwent successful operative repair.

FIGURE 6.5
RADIOGRAPHIC FINDINGS IN ACUTE TRAUMATIC THORACIC ANEURYSM: A LITERATURE REVIEW OF 423 PATIENTS

RADIOGRAPHIC FINDING	SENSITIVITY	SPECIFICITY	ACCURACY
Mediastinal widening	0.87	0.44	0.56
>8cm at aortic arch	0.82	0.43	0.56
M/C <0.25	0.95	0.42	0.54
subjective	0.81	0.52	0.56
Loss aortic contour	0.88	0.46	0.62
Loss aortic knob	0.69	0.76	0.75
Left apical capping	0.48	0.70	0.64
Opacified AP* window	0.74	0.73	0.73
Left paraspinal line widening	0.57	0.74	0.67
Right paraspinal line widening	0.33	0.90	0.62
Right paratracheal stripe	0.67	0.89	0.78
First rib fracture	0.31	0.71	0.58
Any rib fracture	0.35	0.55	0.49
Nasogastric tube deviation	0.42	0.94	0.78
Depressed left main bronchus	0.43	0.94	0.78
Tracheal deviation	0.49	0.89	0.77
Left hemothorax	0.37	0.77	0.65
Pneumothorax	0.27	0.74	0.63

* Aorticopulmonary.

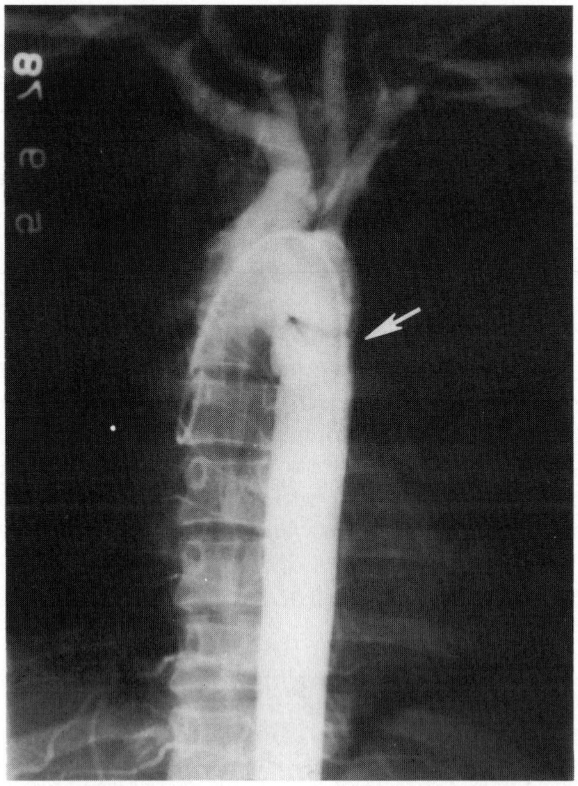

FIGURE 6.6 Retrograde femoral arteriogram demonstrates a pseudoaneurysm (arrow) just distal to the origin of the left subclavian artery (aortic isthmus). An aortic wall tear is visualized as a linear filling defect.

(Fig. 6.8).[6] A localized bulge in the aortic wall without an aortic wall flap may be seen in an atherosclerotic aorta, ductus diverticulum, or vascular ring.[8]

Proponents of intra-arterial digital subtraction angiography (IA-DSA) for the diagnosis of traumatic aortic rupture claim a 50% reduction in study time compared to conventional aortography and 100% accuracy. Mirvis et al. reported on 10 patients diagnosed with aortic rupture by IA-DSA. Induced paralysis and mechanical ventilation, or patient cooperation reduced the artifactual distortion accompanied by patient motion in these studies.[70,71] Although computerized tomography (CT) was first used in the diagnosis of traumatic aortic rupture in 1983,[44] its current role in the management of blunt chest injury remains controversial. Several studies have reported a low sensitivity and specificity for the diagnosis of traumatic aortic rupture based on the presence of a false aneurysm, linear lucency within the opacified aortic lumen, irregularity of the opacified aortic lumen, periaortic or intramural hematoma, or dissection.[34,68,112] Miller et al., reported that CT completely missed 2 of 5 traumatic aortic tears detected by aortography.[68]

Management

Successful management of the accident victim with deceleration aortic injury is dependent on expeditious prehospital transport, rapid resuscitation, thorough assessment of all

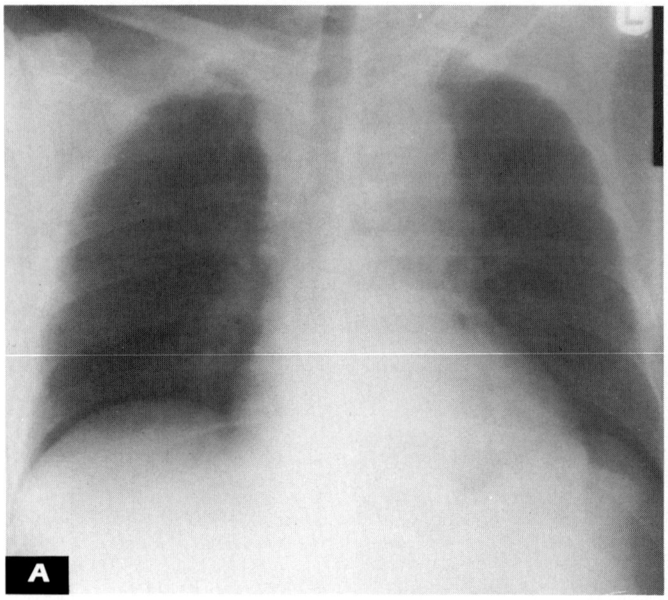

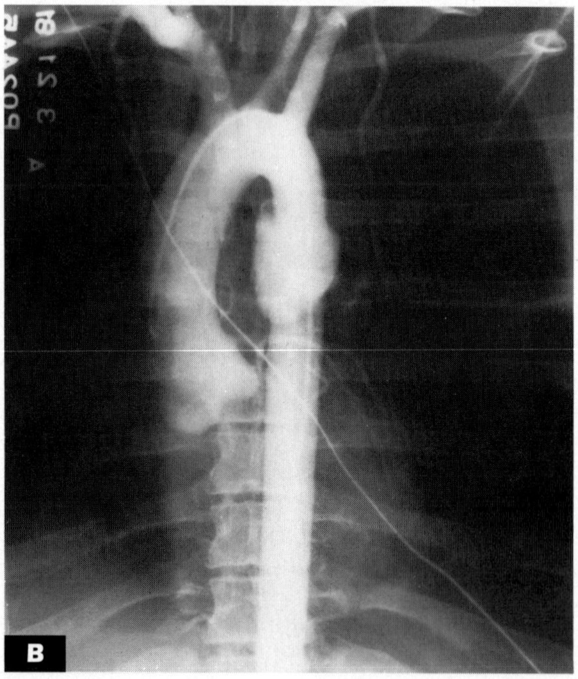

FIGURE 6.7
A Supine portable chest radiograph of a 30-year-old male ejected from an automobile.
B Retrograde femoral arteriogram demonstrates a large pseudoaneurysm at the aortic isthmus.

injuries, prioritizing treatment based on injury severity, and prompt surgical repair. Due to the inherent complexities in treating serious cardiovascular and associated injuries, these patients should be transported to a regional trauma center that is well-prepared for such contingencies.

The resuscitation of the accident victim with multisystem involvement follows firmly established principles and guidelines.[1] Airway maintenance, ventilation, and stabilization of hemodynamics are the first priority in all patients. Shock is present in one-third to one-half of patients with traumatic aortic rupture[26] and vigorous volume replacement with balanced salt solution is often required. The role of emergency room thoracotomy in blunt trauma has been addressed by numerous authors.[9,14,15,72] Survivorship following this procedure is virtually nonexistent. Patients with severe shock caused by traumatic aortic rupture are unlikely to survive with any treatment, thus emergency thoracotomy should not be performed. In patients without shock, and in particular, the 5% to 20% of traumatic aortic rupture patients who present with hypertension,[26] close attention should be given to the unnecessary and potentially harmful administration of intravenous fluids. If traumatic aortic injury is suspected, we recommend keeping the systolic blood pressure between 100 to 120 mm Hg[2] until chest radiography or aortography can exclude the diagnosis, or definitive surgical repair is accomplished. Systemic hypertension may be controlled with the use of short-acting vasodilators, in the absence of closed head injury,[98] calcium-channel blockers, or beta-adrenergic blockers. The use of beta-adrenergic blockade has the added benefit of reducing cardiac contractility and ejection fraction, thereby decreasing the possibility of progressive subadventitial dissection of the aortic tear.[53]

Treatment priorities in patients with deceleration aortic injury is determined by the severity of each associated injury relative to the potential for exsanguinating aortic hemorrhage. In Parmley's autopsy series, among patients surviving beyond 30 minutes of initial trauma, the risk of death from aortic rupture was 20% and 31%, within the first 6 and 24 hours, respectively.[80] However, if only injuries to the aortic isthmus are included, the risk of death within the first 6 hours becomes 12.5%. Thus, nearly 90% will survive beyond the first 6 hours.

In the hemodynamically stable patient, the diagnostic workup should proceed deliberately and methodically. Computerized tomography will reveal most intra-abdominal solid viscera and intracranial injuries if suspected on physical examination. Aortography is then performed, and repair of the aortic rupture assumes first priority. In the hemodynamically unstable patient, a rapidly expanding, tense abdomen or grossly positive peritoneal lavage suggests an abdominal source and demands urgent laparotomy. Following successful eradication of the abdominal hemorrhage, aortography and definitive aortic repair may then proceed. Witnessed neurological deterioration with lateralizing signs or coma are indications for immediate head CT and neurosurgical intervention, if indicated. This is then followed by aortography, and repair of the aortic rupture. Elective

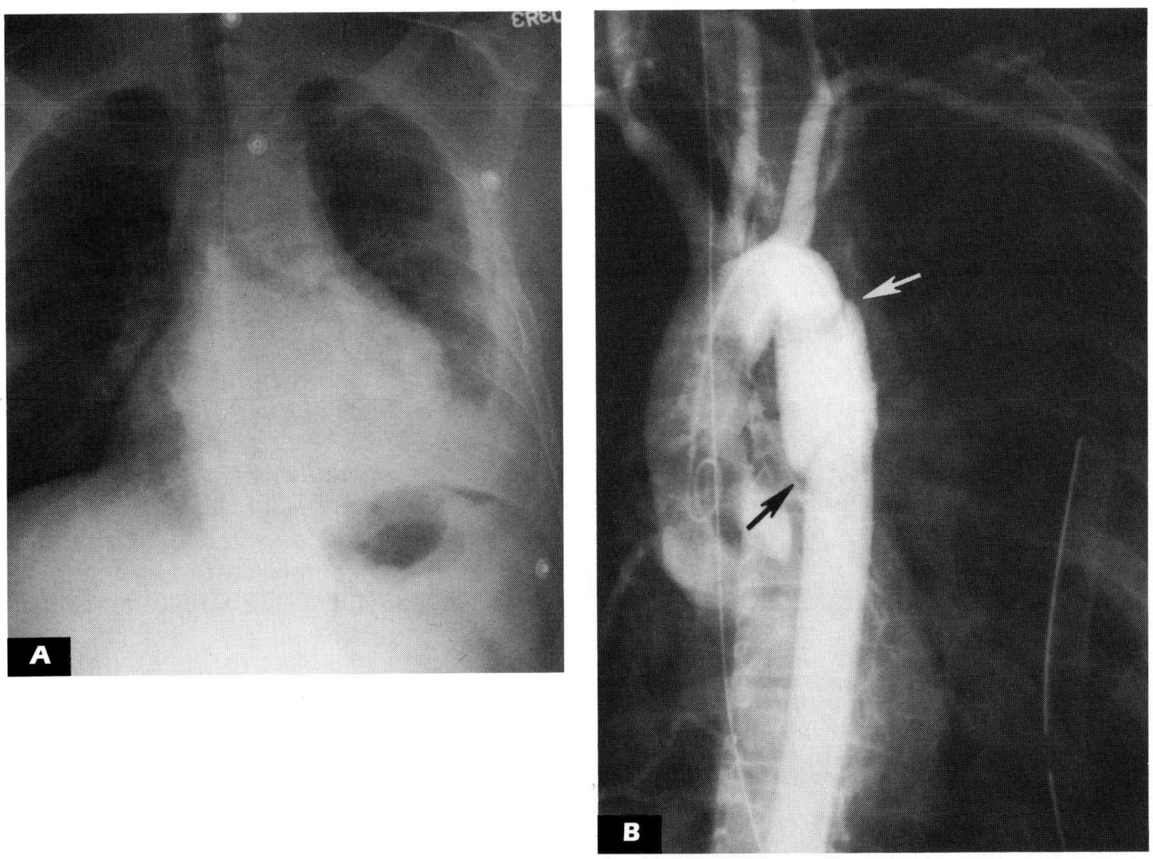

FIGURE 6.8 A Supine portable chest radiograph of a 40-year-old male after blunt chest trauma. **B** Retrograde femoral arteriogram demonstrates a large pseudoaneurysm secondary to complete transection of the aorta, with two transected aortic wall flaps (arrow) visualized within the lumen.

delay of aortic repair has been advocated by some under special circumstances, including:

1. Stabilization of extensive central nervous system trauma
2. Extensive total body surface area burns that have a high risk of sepsis
3. Severe colon injury with abdominal contamination
4. Established sepsis
5. Severe respiratory insufficiency
6. Extensive extremity or pelvic fractures[2,84,104]

However, with the advent of methods to avoid systemic heparinization during aortic surgery and the option of primary repair with avoidance of prosthetic grafts, fewer situations exist to justify delayed repair of a documented aortic rupture.

Early operative experience in the repair of the thoracic aorta utilized adjunctive methods to protect the splanchnic viscera and spinal cord from ischemia when the aorta was cross-clamped.

Cardiopulmonary bypass, left-heart bypass, and femoral venoarterial bypass allowed unhurried repair with preservation of distal flow, however, spinal cord ischemia with resultant paraplegia was not completely eliminated. Furthermore, the need for systemic heparinization drew valid concern over the potential for catastrophic hemorrhage and increased mortality in patients with multiple traumatic injuries.[51,53,97,107,114] Popularized as an effective alternative to previous bypass methods, heparin-bonded (TDMAC) shunts provided adequate distal perfusion without an interposed pump and eliminated the need for systemic heparinization.[7,20,35,74,91,109,118] Disadvantages, however, included uncontrolled bleeding from cannulation sites,[21,25,61,75,107] ventricular tears,[74] prolonged aortic cross-clamp time,[107] and unpredictable and uncontrollable flow.[78, 87] Resurgence of the clamp repair technique, without adjuncts to preserve distal flow, was supported by reports demonstrating no difference in the incidence of paraplegia, and a decrease in the operative blood loss, cross-clamp time, and operative mortality relative to left heart bypass (with systemic heparinization).[3,21,53,108] Although it is clear that aortic repair can be safely performed using this technique, careful consideration must be given to aortic cross-clamp time, proximal hypertension, and left ventricular strain. Recently, Benckart et al. updated their experience with left atrial-femoral artery bypass using the Biomedicus centrifugal pump in 21 patients with traumatic aortic rupture.[12] This approach combines all the advantages of shunt bypass with the ability to regulate distal perfusion by augmenting pump flow.[78] In addition, it is easily inserted and, once in place remains out of the operative field. Currently, it is our method of choice for the repair of acute traumatic aortic rupture.

Technique

The patient is anesthetized with consideration taken to avoid dangerous elevations in blood pressure due to excessive volume loading by the anesthetist, whose main concern is hypotension upon induction.[98] A Carlen's double-lumen endotracheal tube is used to allow selective ventilation of the right lung and collapse of the left lung, permitting easier dissection and exposure. The patient is positioned on the operating table in the right lateral decubitus position with the pelvis rotated 45° backward and the left hip fully extended. This affords full exposure of the left chest and gives access to the left femoral artery for left heart bypass. The posterolateral thoracotomy incision is performed through the fourth or fifth interspace. The mediastinal structures must be dissected with particular attention given to preserving the vagus, recurrent laryngeal, and phrenic nerves (Fig. 6.9). Proximal control is accomplished by carefully encircling the aorta between the left common carotid and left subclavian arteries. Distal control is obtained on the descending thoracic aorta, well outside the area of the hematoma. The left subclavian artery is dissected and encircled with a heavy silk tie. Partial left heart bypass is established from the left atrium to the previously exposed left femoral artery. The pump is adjusted to maintain flow between 2.5 to 3.5 liters per minute.

After the aorta is clamped between the left common carotid and subclavian arteries, and distal to the hematoma, it is opened revealing the full extent of the transection (Fig. 6.10). The aorta may be repaired either primarily or with the use of a Dacron graft (Fig. 6.11). Primary repair will not be acceptable if it creates undue tension at the suture line, despite meticulous dissection around the healthy aorta proximally and distally. If there is any doubt as to the feasibility of a primary repair, a prosthetic graft should be used.

Once repair is completed, the chest is closed and ventilatory support continued as necessary, depending on associated lung, chest wall, and nonthoracic injuries. Immediately following the operation, a full neurologic evaluation should be undertaken to detect the presence of lower extremity paresis or paraplegia.

Mortality and Morbidity

In our experience, traumatic aortic rupture carries an overall mortality of 37%.[26] Severe associated injuries constitute approximately 80% of the overall mortality. The intraoperative mortality for acute aortic repair is 4.8%, or 5 of 105 patients. However, only 3 of the 5 patients succumbed to their aortic injury; severe cardiac contusion and intractable hepatic bleeding each accounted for one death.

The most dreaded complication following surgery for traumatic aortic injury is paraplegia. In our experience, 5 out of 99 patients (5%) developed this complication. The pathogenesis of paraplegia remains unknown. The uncertainties in management of traumatic aortic rupture reflects the confusion prevalent in the literature regarding the technique which best protects the spinal cord from ischemic injury during aortic occlusion. Multivariate analysis reveals that spinal cord injury is6 more likely to occur with long aortic cross-clamp times when no shunt is employed to maintain distal perfusion.[49] Other factors include:

1. Intraoperative periods of hypotension[75,98]
2. The inclusion of intercostal arteries critical to the spinal cord blood flow to the exteriorized segment of the aorta[52]
3. The clamping of important intercostal arteries which are prevented from functioning as an important collateral blood supply to the distal aorta[22]

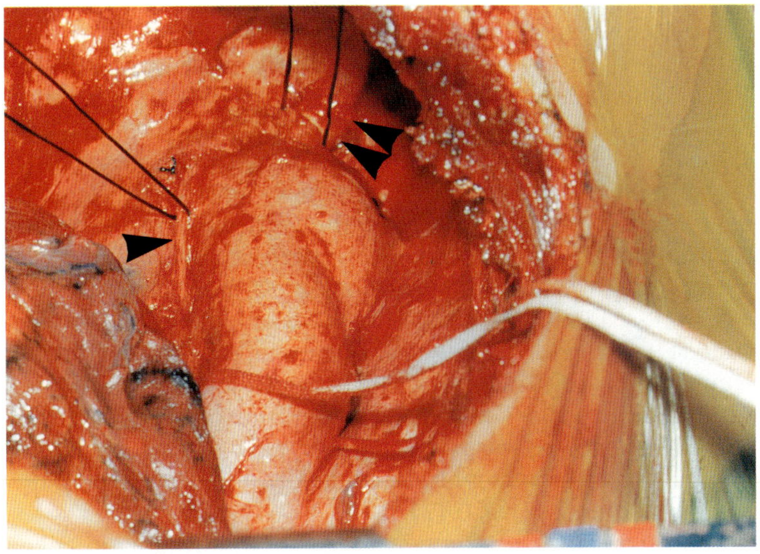

FIGURE 6.9 Operative photograph demonstrating a saccular traumatic aortic aneurysm just distal to the origin of the left subclavian artery. The subclavian artery is encircled with heavy silk suture (double arrows). Care is taken to identify the vagus (single arrow), recurrent laryngeal, and phrenic nerves. Umbilical tape surrounds the normal descending thoracic aorta, beyond the hematoma.

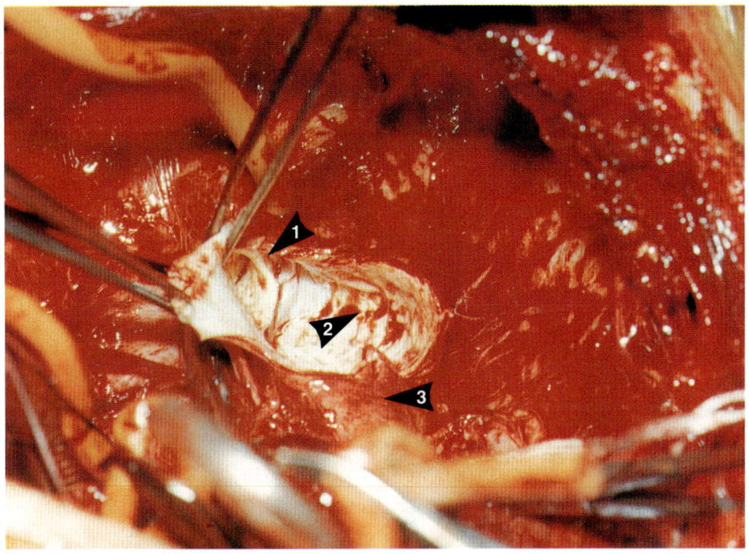

FIGURE 6.10 Operative photograph taken following the placement of proximal (not seen) and distal (bottom) aortic cross-clamps to provide vascular exclusion, and left atrial-distal descending aorta bypass with interposed Biomedicus pump. Keeper (top) is secured around the left subclavian artery. The proximal edge of normal aorta (arrow 1), the cavity of the false aneurysm (arrow 2), and normal distal descending aorta (arrow 3) are shown.

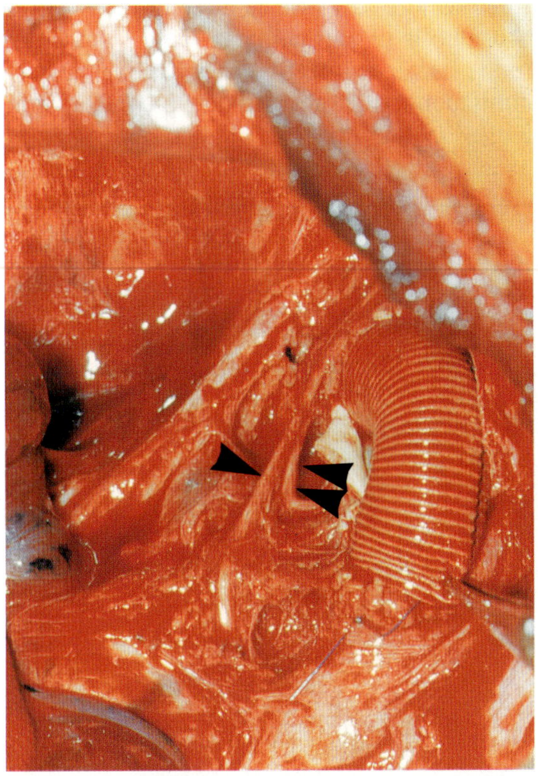

FIGURE 6.11 Operative photograph showing completed repair. An interposed Dacron graft allows restoration of vascular continuity without tension at the suture lines. Preservation of the vagus (single arrow) and recurrent laryngeal (double arrows) nerves are also shown.

4. Compression and occlusion of intercostal arteries by the mediastinal hematoma[11]
5. Unrecognized spinal cord injury
6. A rise in cerebrospinal fluid pressure after aortic cross-clamping
7. The body and spinal cord temperature during the period of cross-clamping[52]
8. Complete cord reperfusion after removal of the cross clamps[52]

Until more information is available regarding the pathogenesis of cord ischemia and paraplegia following repair of traumatic aortic rupture, no definitive statements concerning appropriate management can be made. Thus, the choice of operative procedure and method to preserve distal perfusion, if any, should be based on the individual surgeon's experience and considerations towards minimizing aortic cross-clamp time.

Other complications following acute thoracic aortic repair include phrenic and recurrent laryngeal nerve injury, and persistent bleeding.

CHRONIC TRAUMATIC ANEURSYM OF THE AORTA

Bennett and Cherry defined chronic traumatic aneurysm as an aortic false aneurysm present for at least 3 months after the inciting trauma.[13] Parmley, et al. described 7 out of 35 patients who survived for periods beyond 4 months, a prevalence of 20%.[80] The constellation of signs and symptoms found in chronic traumatic aneurysms are a direct result of progressive enlargement and compression of contiguous structures. Shortness of breath, air trapping, or chronic cough may follow extrinsic compression of the trachea or left main bronchus.[39] Pressure on the main or left pulmonary artery may result in right-sided heart failure, dyspnea on exertion, and shortness of breath.[39] Impingement on the left recurrent laryngeal nerve or the esophagus may manifest as hoarseness or dysphagia. Chest pain is also a common complaint. Radiographic manifestations include direct evidence of a false aneurysm, or manifestations of pulmonary artery, tracheal, bronchial, or esophageal compression, including loss of the left pulmonary artery contour, decreased left-sided vascular markings, right ventricular hypertrophy,[39] tracheal or esophageal deviation, and depression of the left main bronchus (Fig. 6.12).

Appreciation for the propensity of chronic traumatic aneurysms to progressively enlarge, become symptomatic, and rupture, combined with current low operative mortality rates,[31] supports the policy of operative management in all patients; except in cases of extreme medical risk. From a review of the English and French literature, Bennett, determined that 50% of all chronic traumatic aneurysms were symptomatic, while 21% showed definite radiographic evidence of enlargement.[13] Aneurysms have demonstrated enlargement after 43 years,[27] and have ruptured as late as 27 years after injury.[13] Distal embolization and thrombosis of an aneurysm have been reported.[13,42,62] Furthermore, bacterial infection may develop *de novo* or via spread from contiguous structures and may present a formidable surgical challenge.[13,30,42]

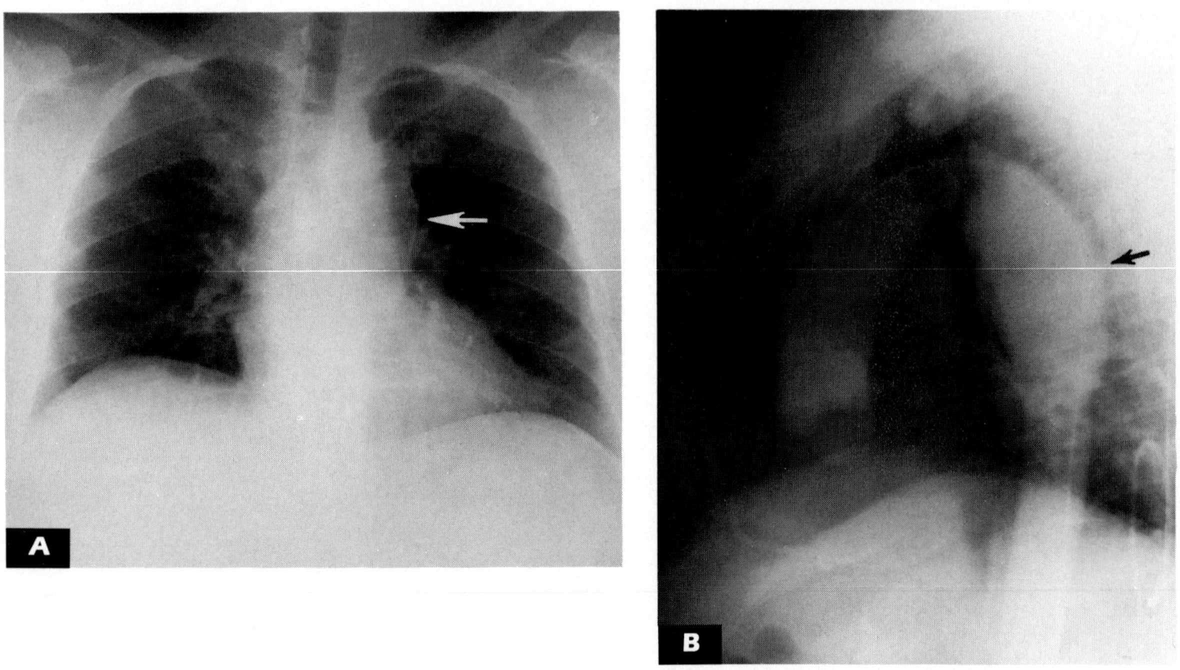

FIGURE 6.12 A An upright PA chest radiograph of a 40-year-old male who sustained violent blunt trauma to the chest five years previously. A calcified pseudoaneurysm of the thoracic aorta (arrow) is demonstrated. **B** Retrograde femoral arteriogram demonstrates a large, chronic traumatic aneurysm of the thoracic aorta (arrow).

REFERENCES

1. Advanced Trauma Life Support Course for Physicians. American College of Surgeons, 1985.
2. Akins CW, Buckley MJ, Daggett W, McIlduff JB, Austen WG: Acute traumatic disruption of the thoracic aorta: a ten-year experience. Ann Thorac Surg 31(4):305–309, 1981.
3. Appelbaum A, Karp RB, Kirklin JW: Surgical treatment for closed thoracic aortic injuries. J Thorac Cardiovasc Surg 71(3):458–460, 1976.
4. Arajarvi E, Santavirta S, Tolonen J: Aortic ruptures in seat belt wearers. J Thorac Cardiovasc Surg 98(3):355–361, 1989.
5. Athey P, Harle TS, Roehm J, Fred HL: Transection of the thoracic aorta: special reference to routine chest roentgenograms. South Med J 63:971–974, 1970.
6. Attar S, Ayella RJ, McLaughlin JS: The widened mediastinum in trauma. Ann Thorac Surg 13(5):435–448, 1972.
7. Avery JE, Hall DP, Adams JE, Headrick JR, Nipp RE: Traumatic rupture of the thoracic aorta. South Med J 72(10):1238–1240, 1979.
8. Ayella RJ, Hankins JR, Turney SZ, Cowley RA: Ruptured thoracic aorta due to blunt trauma. J Trauma 17(3):199–205, 1977.
9. Baker CC, Thomas AN, Trunkey DD: The role of emergency room thoracotomy in trauma. J Trauma 20(10):848–855, 1980.
10. Barcia TC, Livoni JP: Indications for angiography in blunt thoracic trauma. Radiology 147:15–19, 1983.
11. Beall AC Jr, Arbegast NR, Ripepi AC, Bricker DL, Diethrich EB, Hallman GL, Cooley DA, DeBakey ME: Aortic laceration due to rapid deceleration. Arch Surg 98:595–601, 1969.
12. Benckart DH, Magovern GJ, Leibler GA, Park SB, Burkholder JA, Maher TD, Magovern GJ Jr: Traumatic aortic transection: repair using left atrial to femoral bypass. J Cardiac Surg 4(1):43–49, 1989.
13. Bennett DE, Cherry JK: The natural history of traumatic aneurysm of the aorta. Surgery 61(4):516–523, 1967.
14. Bodai BI, Smith JP, Blaisdell FW: The role of emergency thoracotomy in blunt trauma. J Trauma 22(6):487–491, 1982.
15. Bodai BI, Smith JP, Ward RE, O'Neill MB, Auborg R: Emergency thoracotomy in the management of trauma. JAMA 249(14):1891–1895, 1983..
16. Bower DAL, Teare RD: Delayed traumatic rupture of aorta. Thorax 17:150, 1962.
17. Bromley LL, Hobbs JT, Robinson RE: Early repair of traumatic rupture of the thoracic aorta. Br Med J 2:17–19, 1965.
18. Cammack K, Rapport RL, Paul J, Baird WC: Deceleration injuries of the thoracic aorta. Arch Surg 79:90–96, 1959.
19. Clarke CP, Brandt PWT, Cole DS, Barratt-Boyes BG: Traumatic rupture of the thoracic aorta: diagnosis and treatment. Br J Surg 54(5):353–358, 1967.
20. Connors JP, Ferguson TB, Roper CL, Weldon CS: The use of the TDMAC-heparin shunt in replacement of the descending thoracic aorta. Ann Surg 181(5):735–741, 1975.
21. Crawford ES, Rubio PA: Reappraisal of adjuncts to avoid ischemia in the treatment of aneurysms of descending thoracic aorta. J Thorac Cardiovasc Surg 66(5):693–704, 1973.
22. Cunningham LN, Laschinger JC, Merkin HA: Measurement of spinal cord ischemia during operations. Ann Surg 196:285–296, 1982.
23. DeMeules JE, Cramer G, Perry JF Jr: Rupture of aorta and great vessels due to blunt thoracic trauma. J Thorac Cardiovasc Surg 61(3):438–442, 1971
24. DeMuth WE, Roe H, Hobbie W: Immediate repair of traumatic rupture of thoracic aorta. Arch Surg 91:602–603, 1965.
25. Donahoo JS, Brawley RK, Gott VL: The heparin-coated vascular shunt for thoracic aortic and great vessel procedures: a ten-year experience. Ann Thorac Surg 23(6):507–513, 1977.
26. Duhaylongsod FG, Glower DG, Wolfe WG: Acute traumatic disruption of the thoracic aorta: the duke experience from 1960 to 1990: submitted for publication, 1990.
27. Eiseman B, Rainer WG: Clinical management of postraumatic rupture of the thoracic aorta. J Thorac Surg 35:347–358, 1958.
28. Flaherty TT, Wegner GP, Crummy AB, Francyk WP, Hipona FA: Nonpenetrating injuries to the thoracic aorta." Radiology 92:541–546, 1969.
29. Fleischaker RJ, Mazur JH, Baisch BF: Surgical treatment of acute traumatic rupture of the thoracic aorta. J Thorac Cardiovasc Surg 47(3):289–297, 1964.
30. Garamella JJ, Schmidt R, Jensen NK, Lynch MF: Traumatic aneurysms of the thoracic aorta: report of four cases, including one of spontaneous rupture into the esophagus. N Engl J Med 266(26):1341–1348, 1962.
31. Gazzaniga AB, Khuri EI, Mir-Sepasi HM, Bartlett RH: Rupture of the thoracic aorta following blunt trauma. Arch.Surg 110:1119–1123, 1975.
32. Gerbode F, Braimbridge M, Osborn JJ, Hood M, French S: Traumatic thoracic aneurysms: treatment by resection and grafting with the use of an extracorporeal bypass. Surgery 42(6):975–985, 1957.
33. Gerlock AJ Jr, Muhletaler CA, Coulam CM, Hayes PT: Traumatic aortic aneurysm: validity of esophageal tube displacement sign. AJR 13S:713–718, 1980.
34. Goodman PG: Computed tomography in chest trauma. Computed Tomography in the Evaluation of Trauma. Federle and Brant-Zawadzki ed, 1986, Williams and Wilkins, Baltimore.
35. Gott VL: Heparinized shunts for thoracic vascular operations (editorial). Ann Thorac Surg 35:219, 1972.
36. Greendyke RM: Traumatic rupture of aorta. JAMA 195:119–122, 1966.
37. Griffin JS, Ochsner JL, Bower PJ: Posttraumatic coarctation of the aorta. Am J Cardiol 31:391–392, 1973.
38. Groves LK: Traumatic aneurysm of the thoracic aorta. N Engl J Med 270(5):220–224, 1964.
39. Gundry SR, Burney RE, MacKenzie JR, Jafri SZ, Shirazi K, Cho KJ: Traumatic psuedoaneurysms of the thoracic aorta. Arch Surg 119:1055–1060, 1984.
40. Gundry SR, Burney RE, MacKenzie JR, Wilton GP, Whitehouse WM, Wu SC, Kirsh M: Assessment of mediastinal widening associated with traumatic rupture of the aorta. J Trauma 23(4):293–299, 1983.
41. Gundry SR, Williams S, Burney RE, Cho KJ, MacKenzie JR: Indications for aortography in blunt thoracic traumas: a reassessment. J Trauma 22(8):664–671, 1982.
42. Gwathmey O, Byrd CW: Clinical experience with acute traumatic rupture of the thoracic aorta in a general hospital. Ann Surg 159(6):846–857, 1964.
43. Haas GM: Types of internal injuries of personnel involved in aircraft accidents. J Aviation Med 15:77–84, 1944.
44. Heiberg E, Wolberson MK, Sundaram M, Shields JB: CT in aortic trauma. AJR 140:1119–1124, 1983.
45. Herendeen TL, King H: Transient anuria and paraplegia following traumatic rupture of the thoracic aorta. J Thorac Cardiovasc Surg 56(4):599–602, 1968.
46. Heystraten FM, Rosenbusch G, Kingma LM, Lacquet LK, de Boo T, Lemmens, WA: Chest radiography in acute traumatic rupture of the thoracic aorta. Acta Radiol 29:411–417, 1988.
47. Iyengar SRK, Charrette EJP, Lynn RB, McArthur R: Traumatic rupture of the thoracic aorta. Can J Surg 15:350–359, 1972.
48. Jahnke EJ, Fisher GW, Jones RC: Acute traumatic rupture of the thoracic aorta. J Thorac Cardiovasc Surg 48:63–77, 1964.
49. Katz NM, Blackstone EH, Kirklin JW, Karp RB: Incremental risk factors for spinal cord injury following operation for acute traumatic aortic transection. J Thorac Cardiovasc Surg 81(5):669–674, 1981.
50. Keen G, Bradbrook RA, McGinn F: Traumatic rupture of the thoracic aorta. Thorax 24:25–31, 1969.
51. Ketonen P, Jarvinen A, Luosto R, Ketonen L: Traumatic rupture of the thoracic aorta. Scand J Thor Cardiovasc Surg 14:233–239, 1980.
52. Kirklin JW, Barratt-Boyes BG: Cardiac Surgery. Morphology, Diagnostic Criteria, Natural History, Techniques, Results, and Indications. John Wiley & Sons, New York, 1985.
53. Kirsh MM, Behrendt DM, Orringer MB, Gago O, Gray LA, Mills LJ, WalterJF, Sloan H: The treatment of acute traumatic rupture of the aorta: a 10-year experience. Ann Surg 184(3):308–316, 1976.
54. Kirsh MM, Crane JD, Kahn DR: Roentgenographic evaluation of trau-

matic rupture of the aorta. Surg Gynecol Obstet 131:900–904, 1970.
55. Kirsh MM, Kahn DR, Crane JD, Anastasia LF, Lui AH, Moores WY: Repair of acute traumatic rupture of the aorta without extracorporeal circulation. Ann Thorac Surg 10:227–236, 1970.
56. Kirsh MM, Orringer MB, Behrendt DM, Mills LJ, Tashian J, Sloan H: Management of unusual traumatic ruptures of the aorta. Surg Gynecol & Obstet 146:365–370, 1978.
57. Koroxenidis GT, Moschos CB, Landy ED, Poulos PP, Lehan PH: Traumatic rupture of the thoracic aorta simulating coarctation. Am J Card 16:605, 1965.
58. Kram HB, Wohlmuth DA, Appel PL, Shoemaker WC: Clinical and radiographic indications for aortography in blunt chest trauma. J Vasc Surg 6(2):168–176, 1987.
59. Lacquet LK, Kuijpers PJ, Van Lent D, Linssen GH, Sutherland I: Traumatic rupture of the aortic isthmus after blunt chest trauma. J Cardiovas Surg l5:537–546, 1974.
60. Laforet EG: Acute hypertension as a diagnostic clue in traumatic rupture of the thoracic aorta. Am J Surg 110:948–950, 1965.
61. Lawrence GH, Hessell EA, Sauvage LR, Krause AH: Results of the use of the TDMAC-heparin shunt in the surgery of aneurysms of the descending thoracic aorta. J Thorac Cardiovasc Surg 73:393–398, 1977.
62. Malm JR, Deterling RA: Traumatic aneurysm of the thoracic aorta simulating coarctation. J Thorac Cardiovasc Surg 40:271–277, 1960.
63. Marnocha KE, Maglinte DDT: Plain-film criteria for excluding aortic rupture in blunt chest trauma. AJR 144:19–21, 1985.
64. Marsh DG, Sturm JT: Traumatic aortic rupture: roentgenographic indications for angiography. Ann Thorac Surg 21(4):337–340, 1976.
65. Mattox KL: Decelerating aortic injury. Vascular Surgical Emergencies. Bergan and Yao ed 1987 Harcourt Brace Jovanovich, Orlando.
66. McClenathan JE, Brettschneider L: Traumatic thoracic aortic aneurysms. J Thorac Cardiovasc Surg 50:74–82, 1965.
67. McKnight JT, Meyer JA, Neville JF Jr: Nonpenetrating traumatic rupture of the thoracic aorta. Ann Surg 160(6):1069–1072, 1964.
68. Miller FB, Richardson JD, Thomas HA, Cryer HM, Willing SJ: Role of CT in diagnosis of major arterial injury after blunt thoracic trauma. Surgery 106(4):596–603, 1989.
69. Mirvis SE, Bidwell JK, Buddemeyer EU: Value of chest radiography in excluding traumatic aortic rupture. Radiology 163:487–493, 1987.
70. Mirvis SE, Bidwell JK, Buddemeyer EU, Diaconis JN, Pais SO, Whitley JE: Imaging diagnosis of traumatic aortic rupture: a review and experience at a major trauma center. Invest Radiol 22:187–196, 1987.
71. Mirvis SE, Pais SO, Gens DR: Intraarterial digital subtraction angiography (IA-DSA) in the diagnosis of thoracic aortic rupture. AJR 146:987–991, 1986.
72. Moore EE, Moore JB, Galloway AC, Eiseman B: Postinjury thoracotomy in the emergency department: a critical evaluation. Surgery 86(4):590–598, 1979.
73. Mulder DG, Grollman JH Jr:Traumatic disruption of the thoracic aorta: diagnostic and surgical considerations. Am J Surg 118:311–316, 1969
74. Murray GF, Young WG Jr: Thoracic aneurysmectomy utilizing direct left ventriculofemoral shunt (TDMAC-heparin) bypass. Ann Thorac Surg.

hepatic trauma

Thomas L. Novick
Joseph A. Moylan

1 2 3 4 5 6 7 8 9 10 11 12 13 14 15 16 17 18 19 20

Although the prognosis for patients with liver injuries has improved markedly since the time of Hippocrates, hemorrhage and postoperative complications continue to present difficult problems to the trauma surgeon. The liver, although protected by the rib cage, is injured in 5% to 10% of patients with blunt abdominal trauma. In these patients, it is second only to the spleen as the most commonly injured organ. However, approximately 80% of liver injuries in most studies in the United States are secondary to penetrating abdominal trauma and as such the liver is the most frequently injured organ other than the small bowel.[17,67] Although great strides have been made in the treatment of hepatic injuries, particularly because of better physiological support of the patient and more rapid transport of patients to treatment facilities, they still have a 10% to 15% mortality rate.[13,17,46,57] Also, as a result of better preoperative support, the trauma surgeon is now seeing a greater number of complex hepatic injuries.

Since the time of Hippocrates to the late 1800s, liver injuries were considered uniformly fatal and management was generally nonoperative. There were, however, isolated incidences of successful surgical management. Bruns in 1870 successfully resected a portion of liver following a gunshot wound. Buckhart, in 1887, successfully packed a wound to the liver, and in 1896 Kausnetzoff and Penski described several methods of repair of liver wounds still used today.[6] Then, as now, exsanguinating hemorrhage was the leading cause of death. Pringle, in 1908, described occlusion of the porta hepatis as an adjunct to packing, to control bleeding from the injured liver.[58] The Pringle maneuver, as it is now called, has remained a valuable technique in hepatic surgery.

The experience from World War II led to the development of the principles currently in use today. During World War I, an overall mortality of 66% was reported for all wounds of the liver. In the interval between the World Wars and during the early stages of World War II, operative intervention was expectant; it consisted of packing, suturing, and grafting free muscle in order to achieve hemostasis in a damaged liver. Mortality rates remained high, but, with the experience of Madding, Lawrence, and Kennedy, they were lowered from 34% in 1944 to 15% in 1945.[45] These authors stressed that all patients with intra-abdominal injuries should undergo surgery rather than be treated expectantly and that the previous mainstay of the treatment, the gauze pack, should be abandoned and drainage used instead. Now these concepts are being challenged, since the need for drainage of the liver has been questioned, and the use of packing for temporary control of hemostasis has been reinstituted.[11] In addition, selective hepatic artery ligation has established itself as a valuable adjunctive measure in recent years.[23,24] Since sepsis was frequently a major complication of liver injury, debridement and hepatic resection have been used frequently in the past 30 years. Recent data suggest that more conservative treatment may be indicated.[36]

CLASSIFICATION

Hepatic injury varies from a small capsular tear to the complex bursting injury secondary to severe blunt trauma. In most large series of hepatic trauma, penetrating trauma makes up 80% to 90% of the cases; however, other series have indicated a higher mortality rate for patients with blunt trauma.[13,36,55,70] This is probably due to the increase in high-speed motor vehicle accidents and the multisystem injuries that these patients often suffer.

Several classifications of liver injuries have been proposed.[2,23,53] A grade I injury is a superficial parenchymal injury or a capsular tear. This injury is not bleeding at the time of laparotomy, having stopped spontaneously. A grade II injury is a deeper parenchymal injury, smaller than 3 cm to 5 cm, or a through-and-through peripheral injury. This bleeding can be easily controlled. A grade III injury is a deeper bursting parenchymal injury or central penetrating wound. The Pringle maneuver is often necessary to control this hemorrhage. Grade IV injuries are the more complex injuries with lobar tissue destruction and often intraparenchymal damage to major hepatic vessels. Grade V injuries are those with damage to the retrohepatic vena cava or hepatic veins or bilobar tissue destruction. As one would conclude from this classification, grades I, II, and III make up the majority of cases, while grades IV and V carry a higher morbidity and mortality.

CLASSIFICATION OF HEPATIC INJURIES

Grade I
Grade II
Grade III
Grade IV
Grade V
Superficial injury or capsular tear, not bleeding
Deeper laceration (3 cm-5 cm)
Peripheral, through-and-through
Bleeding, easily controlled
Deep parenchymal or bursting injury
Central penetrating injury
Large fracture, lobar destruction
Major interparenchymal vessel injury
Extensive or bilobular injury with injury to hepatic veins or retrohepatic vessels

DIAGNOSIS

The diagnosis of hepatic trauma is often made initially at laparotomy. In fact, the major decision in trauma is not what specific organ is injured, but whether exploratory laparotomy is indicated. The decision regarding laparotomy is made based on physical examination, the condition of the patient, laboratory studies, plain x-ray films, peritoneal lavage, and other special studies such as abdominal CT, ultrasound, radionuclide scans, laparoscopy, and arteriography.

On physical examination, the patient may exhibit abdominal tenderness, guarding, rebound, distention, and hypoactive or absent bowel sounds. A significant percentage of these patients may not have any of these findings initially. The presence of penetrating wounds, upper abdominal bruising or ecchymoses, or lower chest injury may be indications of hepatic trauma.

Hypovolemic shock may be present in up to 50% to 65% of the patients. A falling hematocrit may be indicative of continued intra-abdominal bleeding. Elevated peripheral leukocyte counts are commonly seen in patients with liver or splenic injury.

Abdominal paracentesis has been replaced by peritoneal lavage as a quick, simple, inexpensive method for determining intra-abdominal injury. Lavage can be performed in 10 to 15 minutes and is accurate in over 90% of cases.[34] Lavage fluid should be examined for red blood cell count, white blood cell count, bile, amylase, and bacteria.

Certain findings in plain x-ray films of the abdomen and chest may raise the diagnosis of hepatic trauma: presence of right lower rib fractures, elevated right hemi-diaphragm, pleural effusion or right hemopneumothorax, loss of normal hepatic outline or increased hepatic shadow, gastric dilatation and displacement of the gastric shadow, increased opacification of the right upper quadrant, and duodenal or intestinal paralytic ileus.

There has been considerable controversy lately concerning the use of computed tomography (CT) in the diagnosis of abdominal trauma.[19,51] Abdominal CT has been shown to be very sensitive in revealing free fluid in the peritoneal cavity and inhomogeneity of solid organs, and can detect abnormalities as small as 1 cm in solid organs. Since as many as half of all hepatic injuries are not found to be bleeding at the time of laparotomy and may not require operative intervention, abdominal CT may be useful in the diagnosis and management of these patients (Figs. 7.1 and 7.2).

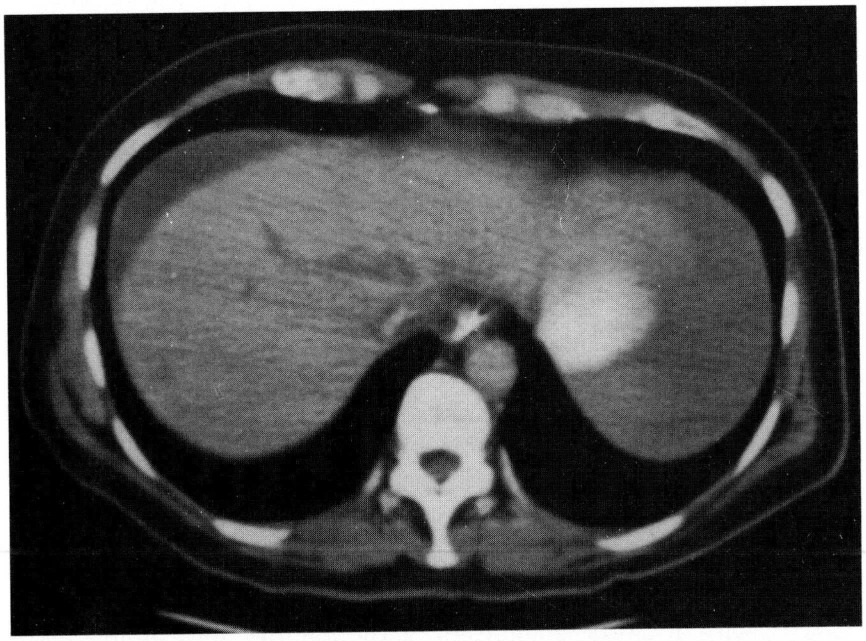

FIGURE 7.1 Subcapsular hematoma of liver treated by observation.

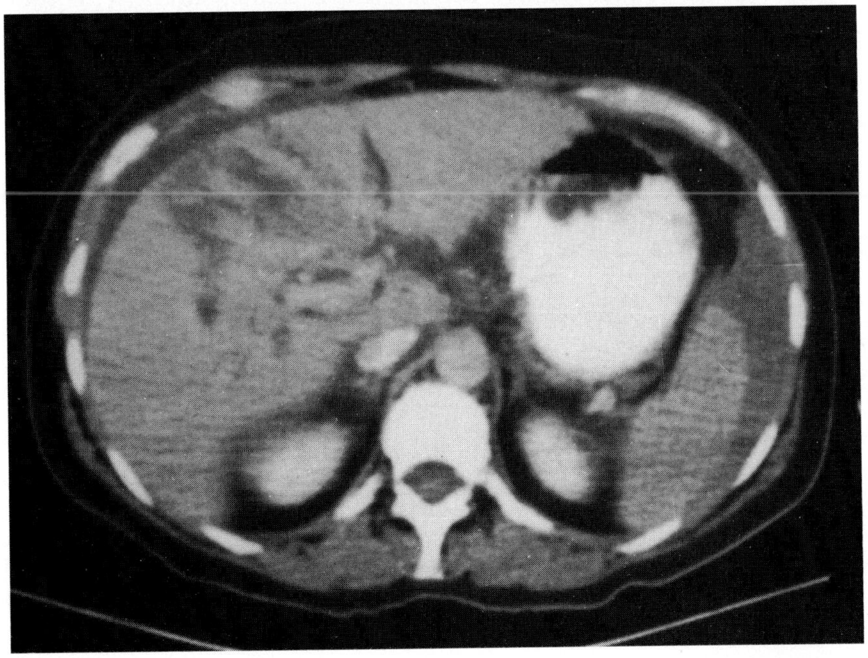

FIGURE 7.2 Major stellate laceration of the right lobe of the liver in a transferred patient.

However, since scanning requires the availability of a skilled radiologist for interpretation and may take 45 minutes or longer, its use should be limited to patients who are hemodynamically stable, who do not have other indications for laparotomy, and who can be followed closely by staff trained in the care of trauma patients. In most cases, CT should not supplant the use of physical examination and peritoneal lavage in the management of trauma patients.

Radionuclide scanning is time-consuming and has no greater accuracy than the other methods in the diagnosis of acute liver trauma. It may be more useful in follow-up, especially in following subcapsular hematoma or identifying liver abscesses. HIDA scan may be useful in the nonemergency or postoperative stages in the detection of biliary leaks or biloma.[27,73] Although ultrasound is inexpensive and less time-consuming than CT, it has been used infrequently in the preoperative diagnosis of hepatic trauma.[29]

Arteriography is accurate in determining the presence of hepatic hemorrhage. However, like CT, its use should be reserved for the stable patient who has no other indication for laparotomy initially, since it is time-consuming and expensive. It does have a definite place in the management and diagnosis of postoperative bleeding and intrahepatic hematoma.[63] Laparoscopy offers no advantage and is of limited usefulness because it cannot be used to rule out other organ injuries. In general, if laparoscopy is considered, the patient, in all likelihood, should undergo laparotomy.

PREOPERATIVE PREPARATION

The patient should be rapidly resuscitated, have appropriate diagnostic studies performed, and be rapidly moved to the operating room. Since more than half of all deaths due to hepatic trauma are secondary to hemorrhage, time should not be wasted by attempting to obtain a specific diagnosis prior to surgery. CT or other tests should not be attempted in the unstable patient; rather, resuscitation may be continued in the operating room, where bleeding may be temporarily arrested while the anesthesia team continues to stabilize the patient. The patient's entire chest and abdomen should be prepared and draped for access to the chest should a median sternotomy or left thoracotomy for cross-clamping of the aorta become necessary.

MANAGEMENT

Incision

Most of the patients with hepatic injury are victims of major trauma undergoing emergency exploration and often have other intra-abdominal injuries. A long midline incision should be made and if there is injury to a major hepatic vein, retrohepatic vena cava, or the dome of the liver, or if major hepatic resection becomes necessary, this incision may be extended to a partial or complete median sternotomy. In the past, a right thoracoabdominal incision was used; however, the median sternotomy is quicker, provides adequate exposure of the vena cava and hepatic veins, causes less diaphragmatic injury, has a lower incidence of postoperative complications, and is easier to close. This should be the incision of choice.[26]

Operative Techniques

The abdomen should be rapidly opened and a quick appraisal of bleeding sites made. All blood clots and debris should be removed rapidly by scooping them out with the hand. Suction drainage is often too slow. Temporary control of bleeding sites may be obtained by the placement of packs and the use of manual compression. Obvious bleeding vessels may be temporarily clamped. A quick exploration should be carried out of the liver, spleen, and major vessels, and attention turned to the area of most obvious bleeding. If major bleeding from the liver is noted, compression of the portal triad between the thumb and index finger to include the hepatic artery and portal vein (Pringle maneuver) may be a useful adjunct to packs and manual compression.[58] Alternatively, an atraumatic clamp may be placed across the hepatoduodenal ligament (Fig. 7.3). If packing and the Pringle maneuver fail to arrest arterial hemorrhage, one should keep in mind the possibility of anomalous vascular supply to the liver, which may occur in 20% to 25% of cases. The Pringle maneuver may not occlude the right and left hepatic arteries, since these may frequently arise from the superior mesenteric and left gastric arteries, respectively. If persistent hemorrhage occurs from the lateral aspect of the liver in spite of the above maneuvers, some authors have advocated the use of a variety of liver compression clamps.[4,66] These, however, are often cumbersome, and a simple hepatic tourniquet may be constructed by using a large DeBakey aortic clamp and a Penrose drain[64] (Fig. 7.4). The aorta may be temporarily occluded just below the diaphragm using manual compression with an aortic compressor or the hand of an assistant. If the patient's preoperative condition is extremely unstable, consideration may be given to cross-clamping the aorta above the diaphragm prior to laparotomy through a left thoracotomy incision.

When persistent hemorrhage is found and continues in spite of the use of packing and the Pringle maneuver, injury to the hepatic vein or retrohepatic vena cava is likely. In this situation, control of the infrahepatic and suprahepatic vena cava must be obtained. The incision should be rapidly extended to a median sternotomy and the inferior vena cava encircled with a vascular tourniquet within the pericardium. The infrahepatic and suprahepatic vena cava may then be temporarily occluded. This is a last-resort temporizing maneuver, since occlusion of the inferior vena cava impedes 60% of the blood return to the right atrium and may lead to rapid further deterioration of the patient.[26] Recently, the use of various intracaval shunts has alleviated this problem. Several shunting methods have been proposed.[62] The simplest method is that described by Yellin, consisting of a number 8 endotracheal tube with multiple sideholes cut into it and inserted through a purse-string suture in the right atrial appendage[75] (Fig. 7.5).

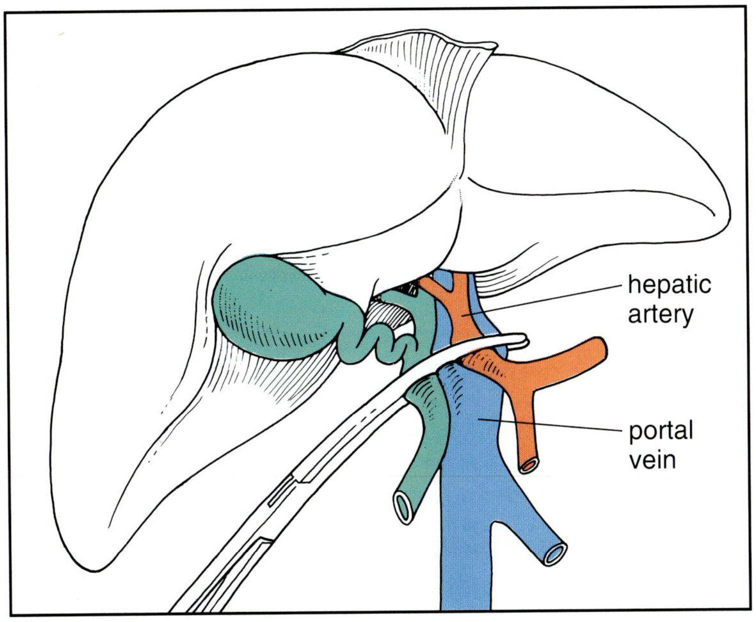

FIGURE 7.3 "Pringle maneuver'"—occlusion of the porta hepatis with an atraumatic vascular clamp.

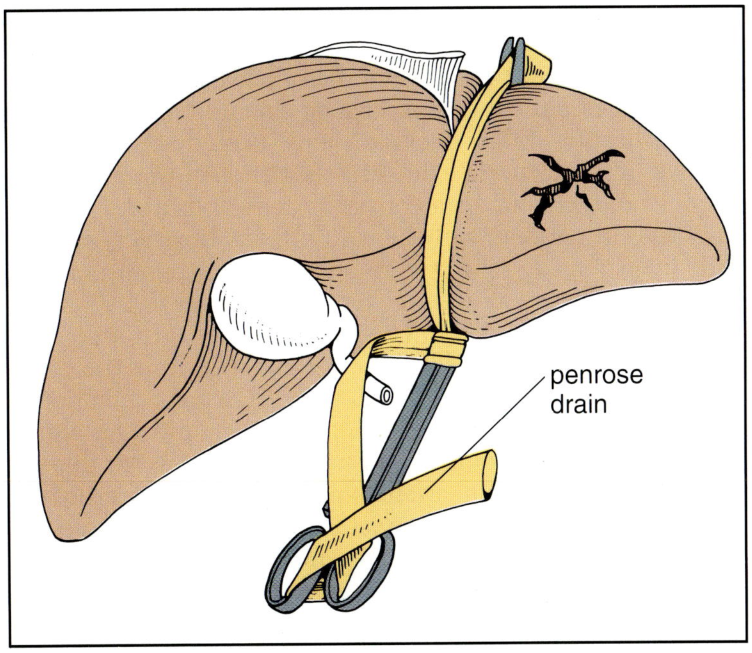

FIGURE 7.4 Simplified hepatic tourniquet utilizing a large DeBakey aneurysm clamp and a Penrose drain.

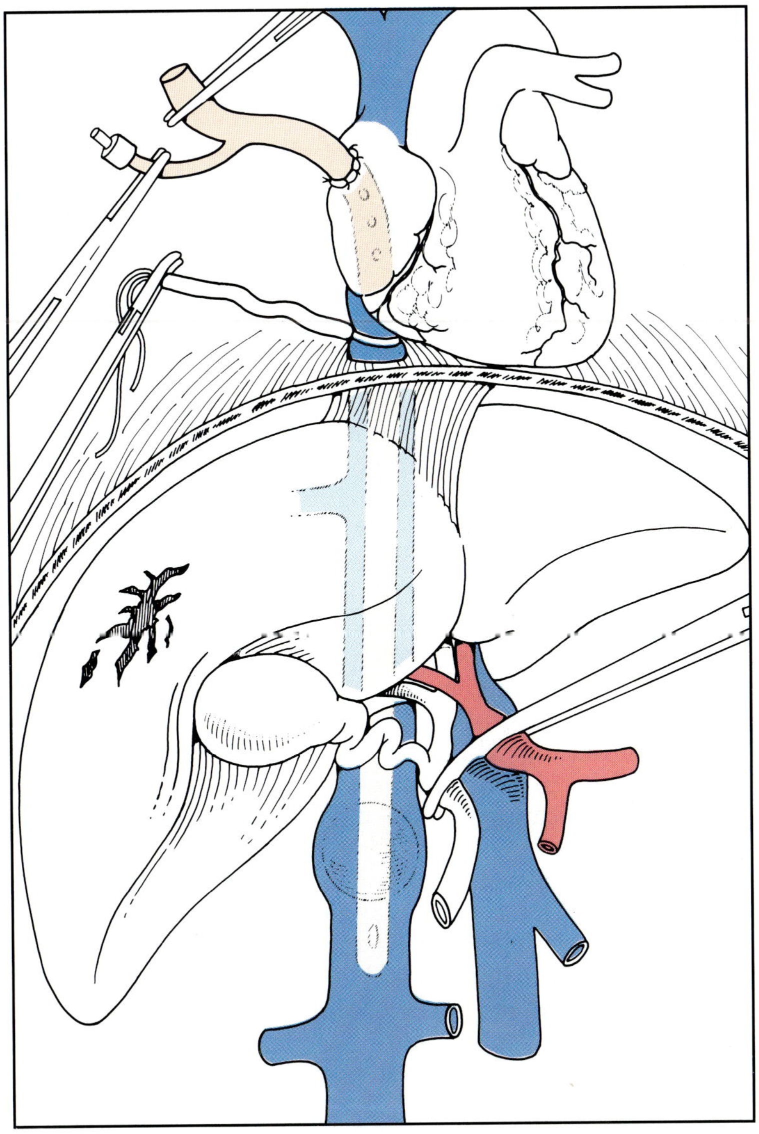

FIGURE 7.5 Atrial-caval shunt using a #8 endotrachial tube as described by Yellin and colleagues.[29]

The sensitivity of the liver to warm ischemia has been a concern to surgeons. It is generally considered safe to completely occlude blood flow to the normothermic liver for periods of up to 20 minutes without causing cellular damage.[49] Longer periods of total hepatic inflow occlusion have been described during elective liver resections, extending the period of warm ischemia up to 1 hour without apparent hepatocellular damage.[32,33] This was done in patients with hepatic tumors, however, and not with livers already subjected to anoxia and hypotension from trauma. The liver receives an average blood flow of 25% of the cardiac output in man.[35,69] The hepatic artery with an oxygen saturation of 95% provides 25% of this flow, while the portal vein provides the remaining 75% with an oxygen saturation of approximately 80%. Thus the hepatic artery provides almost half of the total liver oxygen. For many years it was felt that the hepatic arteries were end-arteries and total occlusion of the hepatic artery flow was uniformly fatal. This was largely based on canine experiments. It has since been shown that as many as 26 collateral channels exist in man and that hepatic survival in man has probably been due to higher venous portal oxygen content and the presence of collaterals.[7]

Adrenal steroids, local hypothermia, and glucagon have also been used to extend the period of warm ischemia. Pachter and Spencer gave patients a 30-mg to 40-mg/kg bolus of methylprednisolone sodium succinate (Solu-Medrol) intravenously prior to inflow occlusion. Inflow occlusion time was greater than 20 minutes in 80% of the 22 patients and greater than 30 minutes in 45% of the patients, with an operative mortality rate of 4.5%. All of these patients had complex hepatic injuries.[55] The authors felt that the steroids prolonged the tolerated rate of warm ischemia. They also used local hypothermia, using a liter of iced Ringer's lactate solution applied topically to the liver, but they state that this method cannot be adequately evaluated, since they did not use an intrahepatic temperature probe to monitor its effects. The dangerous effects of hypothermia on the cardiovascular system and clotting cascade may limit the usefulness of this technique in trauma patients, and the role of steroids in prolonging warm ischemic time will need further study before a universal recommendation for their use can be made.

Glucagon has been advocated to increase splanchnic blood flow in liver trauma. In addition to increasing portal vein flow, glucagon causes glycogenolysis and increases oxygen demand of hepatocytes. If the trauma patient has a limited availability of oxygen, the administration of glucagon may have a deleterious effect on hepatic function despite its theoretical advantage of increasing portal vein flow. The failure of glucagon to improve hepatic function in a hypoxic liver has been demonstrated by several investigators.[25,74] Although glucagon may not cause problems in the patient with adequate oxygen availability to meet the increased demand it causes, glucagon may cause hepatic failure if hypotension, shock, or oxygen desaturation occurs.

DRAINAGE

Grades I and II liver injuries make up nearly 85% of all liver injuries. By definition, grade I injuries are not bleeding at the time of laparotomy. In the past, most surgeons agreed that all liver injuries should be drained; however, this has recently been challenged. In a large retrospective series, Fischer studied the use of drains and the incidence of associated sepsis and concluded that drainage was not indicated for capsular tears, minor liver lacerations, and most major liver lacerations. The effectiveness of drains after major bursting injuries was also questioned.[21] More recently, Mullins and Stone conducted a prospective randomized trial using Penrose drains versus no drainage in 167 patients. They felt that their data supported the use of drains only if a bile leak from the wound was noted at laparotomy; that without bile leak, drainage may not be necessary.[54]

For grades I and II liver injuries with the absence of either bile leak or bleeding, drainage may not be indicated, but selectivity in drainage should be used only by experienced hepatic surgeons. In the presence of contamination from concomitant hollow viscus perforation, drainage should be used. If drainage is elected, the preference is for Silastic closed suction drains left in place for short periods and removed when drainage ceases.

CONTROL OF BLEEDING

Hemorrhage from grade II liver injuries can usually be halted by the placement of heavy mattress sutures (1-0 or 2-0) of an absorbable material (chromic catgut) on a blunt-tipped liver needle. Buttressing of these sutures is almost never necessary if gentle technique is used and if they are placed at least 2 cm away from the defect. If buttressing is necessary, the use of omentum is preferred to Gelfoam or other foreign objects.

It is fortunate that grades III and IV injuries constitute less than 15% of all hepatic injuries, because the management of these is more complex. The previously discussed methods of obtaining initial hemostasis, direct compression with temporary packs, and the Pringle maneuver may be used for temporary control of hemorrhage. If the bleeding continues, the next approach for definite hemostasis should be direct ligature of bleeding points with sutures or surgical clips. Blind mass suture ligature of the liver parenchyma may lead to further bleeding, bile leaks, and devitalized tissue.

If some of these bleeding points are inaccessible to direct ligation, there are several alternatives available. A hot electrocautery may be useful in obtaining hemostasis in the diffuse ooze. Alternatively, the application of one of the topical hemostatic agents may help stem oozing from the raw bed. Oxidized cellulose (Surgicel) has been shown by Dineen to be superior to gelatin sponge (Gelfoam) with respect to infection.[15,16] This is probably due to the acidic *p*H of oxidized cellulose. More recently, Scher demonstrated an increased infection rate in a subcutaneous wound model with use of a microfibrillar collagen (Avitene) compound compared with oxidized cellulose.[60] If a topical hemostatic agent must be left in the wound, these results must be considered. The use of thrombin USP (Thrombostat) may be helpful in controlling the diffuse ooze. However, the potential complications, if it should enter the bloodstream, may limit its use.

If bleeding continues from a deep fissure or cavity despite direct ligation of accessible vessels, tractotomy may be performed using the finger fracture technique in order to provide exposure for direct ligation of bleeding vessels in bile ducts. This method has been used successfully by Pachter and Spencer in 75 consecutive patients with complex hepatic injuries.[55,56] These authors detail several steps necessary for the management of these complex injuries and they also pretreat the patient with methylprednisolone sodium succinate (Solu-Medrol) prior to inflow occlusion. Their steps consist of (1) temporary compression for hemostasis while hypovolemia and acidosis are corrected, (2) occlusion of the portal triad, (3) the use of finger fracture technique to achieve adequate exposure, (4) direct vision ligation of lacerated blood vessels and bile ducts, (5) debridement of nonviable parenchyma, (6) filling the dead space with a viable omental pedicle, and (7) wide dependent drainage. Using this technique, they reported a 5% mortality rate. Care must be taken when performing the tractotomy to avoid causing severe bleeding due to the tractotomy itself. The finger fracture technique is one of gentle dissection. Another important aspect of this method of treatment is the debridement of the nonviable parenchyma. This does not imply a formal resection, but rather it is carried out along the planes of the injury. Other authors have used the finger fracture technique or recommend exposure of the wound and direct ligation of bleeding vessels, and several studies report good success with these methods.[23,39,52,72]

If direct ligation of bleeding points is not possible, the next step should be consideration of selective hepatic artery ligation. If the Pringle maneuver is successful in reducing the hemorrhage and the bleeding appears arterial, the right or left hepatic arteries may be ligated selectively.[1,23,24,37,39,44,47,52] The Pringle maneuver may be used to estimate both the effectiveness of selective hepatic artery ligation and the likelihood of hepatic ischemia. The appropriate lobar artery, right or left, should be ligated distal to the bifurcation of the proper hepatic artery. Although there have been reports of ligation of the proper hepatic artery between the bifurcation and the gastro-duodenal artery without hepatic necrosis, the danger of hepatic ischemia and liver failure is significant. When selective hepatic artery ligation is used, portal venous flow and collateral flow to the liver will prevent cases of hepatic necrosis.

Flint and Polk reported 540 cases of hepatic trauma in which 94 (17%) underwent selective hepatic artery ligation. Selective hepatic artery ligation failed in 15 patients (16%). Eight intraoperative failures occurred secondary to injury to either major hepatic or lobar portal veins. Four patients had early rebleeding and 3 of these 4 had ligation of the incorrect artery. Lobar hepatic necrosis necessitated formal hepatic lobectomy at a later date in 1 patient in whom the viability of the lobe was in doubt at the time of the operation. Seven of the 15 patients died. The authors state that selective hepatic artery ligation should be avoided in patients with cirrhosis or in other patients in whom extensive dissection has interrupted potential collaterals by way of the inferior phrenic or gastroduodenal arteries.[24]

Although the incidence is low, hepatic necrosis may occur after selective hepatic artery ligation.[40] Even though frank necrosis may not occur, relative ischemia of the liver may lead to sepsis or intrahepatic abscess.[3] Selective hepatic artery ligation should not be taken lightly and should not be used as a first-line or prophylactic treatment. If selective hepatic artery ligation fails to control hepatic bleeding, venous injury to either the portal or hepatic systems or the vena cava should be considered, as should the possibility of anomalous origin of the right or left hepatic artery. A search should then be made for anomalous vessels. Several authors report ligation of the associated portal vein branch without apparent complications.[24,47] It is unrealistic to expect that selective hepatic artery ligation will stop portal or retrograde hepatic venous bleeding.

Rebleeding after selective hepatic artery ligation has been reported.[24,39,71] A cholecystectomy should be performed if either the right or common hepatic artery has been ligated, or as Mays recommends, if the left hepatic artery has been ligated due to the possibility of acalculous cholecystitis developing. Many authors, however, do not feel that this is necessary.[1]

Through-and-through gunshot wounds to the liver have been treated by using liver sutures to close the entrance and exit wounds and obtain hemostasis. This treatment remains controversial because of the possible development of intrahepatic abscess, hematoma, or hemobilia. Lucas and Ledgerwood reported several patients in whom this technique was used to avoid hepatic resection. In their follow-up of 5 years, only 1 patient developed an intrahepatic abscess and no patient developed hemobilia.[39] If this technique is used, the liver should be observed for at least 10 minutes for an increase in size and for bleeding through the suture line, which would indicate persisting intrahepatic hemorrhage. If the bleeding continues and the tract is near the periphery of the liver, a wedge resection with individual ligation of bleeding points may be performed. If the tract is longer or more centrally located, a tractotomy may be performed to ligate the bleeding vessels if selective hepatic artery ligation fails to achieve hemostasis. A report by Bluett, Woltering, and Adkins recently described achieving tamponade in through-and-through wounds to the liver by placing a red rubber catheter through the wound and using it to draw several Penrose drains back through the defect. These drains were left in place through the tract and then brought out through the abdominal wall.[8] Using this technique, they were able to preserve hepatic parenchyma without hepatic hematoma or abscess in 15 patients. They felt that the Penrose drains provided a tamponade effect as well as allowing the drainage of bile. Drawbacks to this procedure are the need for the drains to remain in place for long periods, averaging 23 days in their patients, and the possibility of causing more bleeding as the drains are drawn through the defect. Enough experience has not been gained in this procedure to universally recommend it at this time.

In an effort to achieve hemostasis and avoid resection in hepatic injuries, the placement of multiple packs has been used extensively. This was the preferred method of treatment of severe hepatic injuries for many years until Madding and Kennedy reported on problems experienced in World War II.[45] They found an unacceptable incidence of sepsis and delayed hemorrhage, and this technique gradually fell out of use. More recently, there have been several reports of the use of intra-abdominal packs to obtain hemostasis in severe injuries when all other methods have failed.[11] Carmona and co-workers and Feliciano and associates have reported 18 and 10 patients, respectively, in whom all other methods to control bleeding failed.[10,20] The wounds were tamponaded with gauze packs and the patient stabilized while clotting parameters corrected. Once the patients' conditions improved, they were taken back to the operating room for a second-look operation, during which the packs were removed, areas of devitalized tissue debrided, and drains placed. Both groups found this method of treatment very effective in controlling bleeding in the unstable patient with life-threatening hemorrhage uncontrolled by other means. In Feliciano's group, 9 of the 10 patients survived without rebleeding after removal of the packs. Carmona's patients had a 17% (3 patients) mortality rate. One patient died before return to the operating room. Carmona's group planned a second-look operation 12 to 24 hours after the initial surgery in order to decrease the complications of sepsis and abscess formation.

An alternative to the gauze pack has been reported by Stone and colleagues.[18,65] They were able to arrest massive hepatic bleeding in 100 of 104 cases of primary venous bleeding and 105 of 113 cases overall using an omental pedicle pack (Fig. 7.6). Their technique consists of the development of an omental pedicle by dissecting the omentum free from its avascular attachment to the transverse colon while an assistant applies bimanual compression of the liver to achieve hemostasis. If only one pack is needed, the left gastroepiploic vessels are divided and the vascular pedicle developed using the right gastroepiploic vessels. If two packs are needed, the omentum is divided vertically in the midline and each pack is placed on its own gastroepiploic pedicle. The omentum is then packed into the depths of the liver fracture and the edges of the hepatic defect approximated under mild tension with a continuous large polypropylene suture, avoiding deep bites to prevent injuries to main vessels and bile ducts. Sump drains are then placed to avoid accumulation of bile or blood.[18] Their mortality rate was 8% with approximately a 40% complication rate consisting mainly of complications caused by massive hemorrhage, hypotension, or massive transfusion.

Fischer and Gervin recently devised the use of the falciform ligament as an alternative for patients whose omentum is not adequate for use either as a buttress or a pack. They suggest that the abdomen be opened in the midline and the preperitoneal fat bluntly dissected to the right prior to incising the peritoneum. The falciform ligament may then be harvested later by dividing it at the umbilicus and incising its anterior peritoneal reflection along the posterior rectus sheath. If additional length is needed, the umbilical vein is divided at the umbilical notch and the anterior incision extended cephalad along the undersurface of the diaphragm to the triangular ligament. They do not report any experience with this maneuver.[22] The use of packs—omental, falciform or gauze—may gain control of life-threatening venous hemorrhage in grade IV or V injuries, when all other methods have failed. This method is particularly useful in patients with disseminated intravascular coagulation with diffuse oozing or those patients who are extremely unstable or hypotensive and acidotic. The use of the pedicle omental flap has the advantage of not requiring a second-look operation, but good results have been obtained through the use of gauze packs and early second-look procedures. The use of packs may be particularly helpful to the general surgeon in the community hospital who is otherwise unable to obtain hemostasis. Hemostasis can then be obtained using this technique and the patient stabilized and transferred to a trauma center for definitive care.

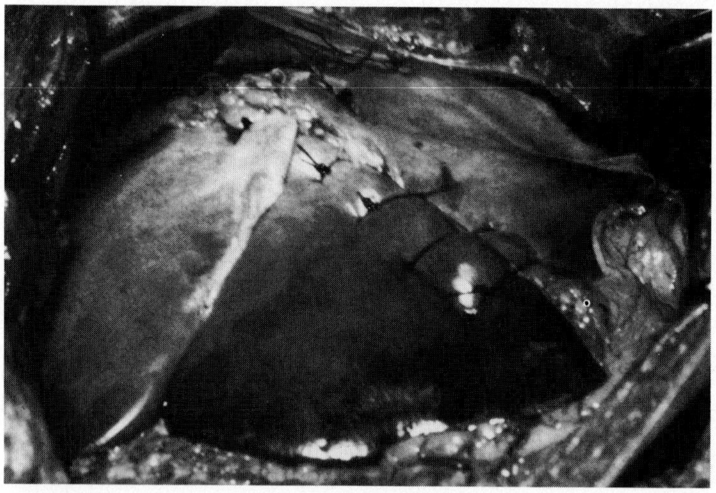

FIGURE 7.6 Pedicle omental pack used in controlling hemorrhage from a laceration to left lobe of the liver.

RESECTION

Resection or debridement may be carried out whenever there is a ragged wound with nonviable tissue present. This is typically found in gunshot wounds or in blunt trauma with stellate fractures. All nonviable tissue should be removed and the individual vessels and bile ducts suture-ligated. Only if this technique fails to control hemorrhage from the raw liver surface should mattress sutures be placed in the hepatic parenchyma. If hemorrhage continues despite the use of finger fracture and direct ligation or selective hepatic artery ligation, mattress sutures may be placed running parallel to the cut edge of the liver. Care should be taken when placing these sutures because if they are placed too far from the liver edge, they may cause further devitalization of tissue and potentially create a contaminated closed space or hematoma within the liver parenchyma. Formal hepatic lobectomy in liver trauma has been advocated extensively in the past.[5] Because of the high mortality rate associated with this procedure when used in the trauma setting, specific guidelines for formal hepatic lobar resection should be followed. If resection or debridement, direct ligation of vessels, selective hepatic artery ligation, or packing fail to control hemorrhage, or if there is extensive damage isolated to one lobe of the liver, or if anatomical location precludes the use of direct control, lobar resection may be considered.[55,71] Several authors report mortality rates as high as 50% when using lobar resection in the trauma setting. Although the formal lobectomy has been used extensively since 1945, indications for this procedure have narrowed, and other treatment modalities have been developed, so that lobectomy is now indicated in less than 5% of all patients with hepatic trauma. The technique for hepatic resection is similar to that used in elective resection and may be found in any number of excellent atlases of surgery and will not be described here. Suffice it to say that the resection should be performed as expediently as possible and techniques to limit blood loss, such as the use of liver clamping or hepatic tourniquets, should be used. The use of the cell-saver device may limit the need for transfusion and the recently developed ultrasonic aspirator (CUSA) described by Hodgson[31] may be helpful. Our experience thus far using this device in hepatic trauma has been limited, but favorable.

Grade V injuries to the liver are rare. This is fortunate because the control of retrohepatic vena caval or hepatic vein injuries may be difficult owing to their location. These injuries can often be managed by primary repair and an intracaval shunt is necessary only in the extreme situation. If the venous injury cannot be repaired, it has been shown that ligation of the vessel may be tolerated.[14]

Intrahepatic Hematoma

In a small group of patients, blunt trauma may cause parenchymal damage and bleeding contained within the liver capsule, resulting in an intrahepatic hematoma. Although the majority of these hematomas will resolve spontaneously, a significant number may expand and rupture or result in other complications including abscess formation and hemobilia. Controversy exists as to the correct treatment of intrahepatic hematoma. It is well known that incision and drainage of these hematomas may result in life-threatening hemorrhage; at the same time it has been demonstrated that a number of these patients may be treated by conservative nonoperative management.[12,28,59]

If one suspects hepatic trauma in a stable patient who has no other indications for urgent laparotomy, an abdominal CT or radionuclide liver/spleen scan should be performed. CT scanning may be more accurate but is much more expensive; a liver/spleen scan may be technically more difficult to obtain in the patient with multisystem trauma. Once the diagnosis is made, the patient may be watched conservatively with bed rest, serial examinations and hematocrits, and the scan repeated in a few days. Any time the patient develops an acutely falling hematocrit, a change in abdominal examination, signs of intra-abdominal sepsis, or evidence of enlarging intrahepatic hematoma by scanning, consideration should be given to immediate operation. If there is evidence of an expanding yet still contained intrahepatic hematoma, arteriography and embolization of the bleeding vessel may be performed.[30,61] In fact, with patients who have evidence of intrahepatic hematoma and who are stable, arteriography may be the initial study of choice, since it will more accurately define the anatomy and may also prove therapeutic if embolization is used. Geis and his co-workers recently followed 16 patients with intrahepatic hematoma. Of these, 6 (37.5%) required emergency surgery after initially being treated nonoperatively. Their complications occurred 1 to 28 days postinjury and included rupture with hemorrhage and abscess formation with sepsis. They also found that 3 of 4 patients with a palpable liver at initial examination and large hematoma on scan developed complications and concluded that the combination of the two is an ominous finding. These authors concluded that arterial bleeding within the hematoma may be more likely to cause surrounding necrosis due to expansion and may also lend itself to arterial embolization.[28]

Patients with intrahepatic hematoma should be followed for a minimum of 28 days and possibly as long as 8 weeks, since delayed rupture has been reported to occur up to 6 weeks after injury.[68] If signs of an expanding hematoma are present, consideration should be given to arteriography with embolization. Signs of a ruptured hematoma or sepsis and abscess formation require immediate operative intervention.

Other Methods

In 1963, Merendino proposed the use of routine biliary tract drainage of patients with major hepatic trauma.[50] In several studies since, it has been shown that placement of a T-tube in the absence of ductal injury does not decompress the biliary tree and prevent bile leakage. Indeed, it has been associated with increased incidence of stress ulcers, sepsis, biliary fistula, and late bile duct stricture.[9,38,41,43,57] The placement of a T-tube does have the advantage of ready access for performance of postoperative cholangiography; however, in the absence of ductal injury, it should not be used routinely.

POSTOPERATIVE COMPLICATIONS

Although hemorrhage remains the most common cause of death in hepatic trauma, pulmonary complications including pneumonia, atelectasis, and effusion are the most common complications, occurring in 20% to 30% of survivors. The high incidence may be due to the high incidence of associated injuries to the thorax in patients with hepatic trauma. Sepsis may occur in 10% to 15% of hepatic trauma patients and may account for 10% of the deaths. Overall, sepsis is associated with intrahepatic abscess formation in 4% to 5% of patients. Patients with concurrent colon injuries are particularly at risk for developing abscess and septic complications. Hemobilia, biliary fistula, liver failure, and delayed bleeding are other relatively uncommon complications.[13,42,48]

REFERENCES

1. Aaron S, Fulton RL, Mays ET: Selective ligation of the hepatic artery for trauma of the liver. Surg Gynecol Obstet 141:187, 1975
2. Aldrete JS, Halpern NB, Ward S, Wright JO: Factors determining the mortality and morbidity in hepatic injuries. Ann Surg 189:466, 1979
3. Aust JB: Discussion of Flint et al, 1977. Ann Surg 185:618, 1977
4. Balasegaram DM: Hepatic resection in trauma. Adv Surg 17:129, 1984
5. Balasegaram M, Joishy SK: Hepatic resection: The logical approach to surgical management of major trauma to the liver. Am Surg 142:580, 1981
6. Beck C: Surgery of the liver. JAMA 38:1063, 1902
7. Bengmark S, Rosengren K: Angiographic study of the collateral circulation of the liver after ligation of the hepatic artery in man. Am J Surg 119:620, 1970
8. Bluett MK, Woltering E, Adkins RB: Management of penetrating hepatic injuries. Am Surg 50:131, 1984
9. Bowen JC, Fleming WH: Upper gastrointestinal bleeding associated with biliary diversion after hepatic injury. Ann Surg 177:402, 1973

10. Carmona RH, Lim RC Jr, Clark GC: Morbidity and mortality in hepatic trauma. Am J Surg 144:88, 1982
11. Carmona RH, Peck DZ, Lim RC Jr: The role of packing and planned reoperation in severe hepatic trauma. J Trauma 24:779, 1984
12. Cheatham JE, Smith EI, Tunell WP, Elkins RC: Nonoperative management of subcapsular hematoma of the liver. Am J Surg 140:852, 1980
13. Defore WW Jr, Mattox KL, Jordan GL Jr, Beall AJ Jr: Management of 1590 consecutive cases of liver trauma. Arch Surg 111:493, 1976
14. Depinto DJ, Muchs SJ, Powers PC: Major hepatic vein ligation necessitated by blunt abdominal trauma. Ann Surg 183:243, 1976
15. Dineen P: The effect of oxidized cellulose on experimental intravascular infections. Surgery 82:575, 1972
16. Dineen P: Antibacterial activity of oxidized, regenerated cellulose. Surg Gynecol Obstet 146:481, 1976
17. Elerding SC, Moore EE Jr: Recent experiences with trauma of the liver. Surg Gynecol Obstet 150:853, 1980
18. Fabian TC, Stone WH: Arrest of severe liver hemorrhage by an omental pack. South Med J 73:1487, 1980
19. Federle MP, Crass RA, Jeffrey RB et al: Computed tomography in blunt abdominal trauma. Arch Surg 117:645, 1982
20. Feliciano DV, Mattox KL, Jordan GL: Intra-abdominal packing for control of hepatic hemorrhage, a reappraisal. J Trauma 21:285, 1981
21. Fischer RP, O'Farrell KA, Perry JF Jr: The value of peritoneal drains in the treatment of liver injuries. J Trauma 18:393, 1978
22. Fischer RP, Gervin AS: The use of falciform ligament in the repair of hepatic injuries. Surg Gynecol Obstet 161:383, 1985
23. Flint LM, Mays ET, Aaron WS et al: Selectivity in the management of hepatic trauma. Ann Surg 185:613, 1977
24. Flint LM, Polk HC: Selective hepatic artery ligation: Limitation and failures. J Trauma 19:319, 1979
25. Fredlund PE, Callum B, Tibblin S: Influence of glucagon on the ischemic liver in the pig. Arch Surg 105:615, 1972
26. Fullen WD, McDonough JT, Popp MJ, Altemeier WA: Sternal splitting approach for major hepatic or retrohepatic vena caval injury. J Trauma 14:903, 1974
27. Gartman DM, Zeman RK, Cahow CE, Baker CC: The value of hepatobiliary scanning in complex liver trauma. J Trauma 25:887, 1985
28. Geis WP, Schulz KA, Gibschin JL, Freeark RJ: The fate of unruptured intrahepatic hematomas. Surgery 90:689, 1981
29. Gregory NV, Ramon G, Kenneth JU et al: Ultrasonic evaluation of hepatic and splenic trauma. Arch Surg 115:320, 1980
30. Heimbach DM, Ferguson GS, Harley JD: Treatment of traumatic hemobilia with angiographic embolization. J Trauma 18:221, 1978
31. Hodgson WJB: Ultrasonic surgery. Ann Coll Surg Engl 62:459, 1980
32. Huguet C, Nordlinger B, Block P, Conard J: Tolerance of the human liver to prolonged normothermic ischemia. Arch Surg 113:1448, 1978
33. Huguet C, Nordlinger B, Galopin JJ et al: Normothermic hepatic vascular exclusion for extensive hepatectomy. Surg Gynecol Obstet 147:189, 1978
34. Jordan GL Jr: Hepatic trauma. Contemp Surg 27:19, 1985
35. Leevy CM: Evaluation of Liver Function in Clinical Practice. Indianapolis, Lilly Research Laboratories, 1965
36. Levin A, Gover P, Nance FL: Surgical restraint in the management of hepatic injury: A review of Charity Hospital experience. J Trauma 18:399, 1978
37. Lewis FR, Lim RC, Blaisdell FW: Hepatic artery ligation adjunct in the management of massive hemorrhage from the liver. J Trauma 14:743, 1978
38. Lucas CE: What is the role of biliary drainage in liver trauma? Am J Surg 120:509, 1970
39. Lucas CE, Ledgerwood AM: Prospective evaluation of hemostatic techniques for liver injuries. J Trauma 16:442, 1976
40. Lucas CE, Ledgerwood AM: Liver necrosis following hepatic artery transection due to trauma. Arch Surg 113:1107, 1978
41. Lucas CE, Ledgerwood AM: Factors influencing morbidity and mortality after liver injury. Ann Surg 44:406, 1978
42. Lucas CE, Walt AJ: Critical decisions in liver trauma. Arch Surg 101:277, 1970
43. Lucas CE, Walt AJ: Analysis of randomized biliary drainage for liver trauma in 189 patients. J Trauma 12:925, 1972
44. Madding CF: Injuries to the liver. AMA Arch Surg 70:748, 1955
45. Madding GF, Lawrence KB, Kennedy PA: Forward surgery of the severely injured. Second Auxiliary Surgical Group 1:307, 1942–1945
46. Martin JR, Roys GD, Bricker DL: The treatment of liver injuries. Surg Gynecol Obstet 134:298, 1972
47. Mays ET: Critical wounds of the liver and the juxtahepatic veins. Ann Surg 43:635, 1977
48. McInnis WD, Richardson JD, Aust JB: Hepatic trauma, pitfalls in management. Arch Surg 112:157, 1977
49. McMaster P, Madd R: Total hepatic ischemia in the rhesus monkey. Br J Surg 64:819, 1977
50. Merendino KA, Dillard DH, Cammoch EE: The concept of surgical biliary decompression in the management of liver trauma. Surg Gynecol Obstet 117:285, 1963
51. Meyer AA, Crass RA, Lim RC Jr et al: Selective nonoperative management of blunt liver injury using computed tomography. Arch Surg 120:550, 1985
52. Moore EE: Critical decisions in the management of hepatic trauma. Am J Surg 148:712, 1984
53. Moore FA, Moore EE, Seagraves A: Nonresectional management of major hepatic trauma, an evolving concept. Am J Surg 150:725, 1985
54. Mullins RJ, Stone H, Dunlop WE, Strom PR: Hepatic trauma: Evaluation of routine drainage. South Med J 78:259, 1985
55. Pachter HL, Spencer FC: Recent concepts in the treatment of hepatic trauma, facts and fallacies. Ann Surg 190:423, 1979
56. Pachter HL, Spencer FC, Hofstetter SR, Coppa GF: Experience with the finger fracture technique to achieve intrahepatic hemostasis in 75 patients with severe injuries to the liver. Ann Surg 197:771, 1983
57. Pinkerton JA, Sawyers JL, Foster JH: A study of the postoperative course after hepatic lobectomy. Ann Surg 173:800, 1971
58. Pringle JH: Notes on the arrest of hepatic hemorrhage due to trauma. Ann Surg 48:541, 1908
59. Richie JP, Fonkalsrud EW: Subcapsular hematoma of the liver. Arch Surg 104:781, 1972
60. Scher KS, Coil JA: Effects of oxidized cellulose and microfibrillar collagen on infection. Surgery 91:301, 1982
61. Schmidt B, Bhatt GM, Abo MN: Management of post-traumatic vascular malformations of the liver by catheter embolization. Am J Surg 140:332, 1980
62. Schrock T, Blaisdell FW, Mathewson C Jr: Management of blunt trauma to the liver and hepatic veins. Arch Surg 96:698, 1968
63. Sclafani SJA, Shaftan GW, McAuley J et al: Interventional radiology in the management of hepatic trauma. J Trauma 24:256, 1984
64. Smith GW: Trauma to the liver. In Shackleford RT, Zuidema GD (eds): Surgery of the Alimentary Tract, vol. 4. Philadelphia, WB Saunders, 1983
65. Stone HH, Lamb JM: Use of pedicled omentum as an autogenous pack for control of hemorrhage in major injuries of the liver. Surg Gynecol Obstet 141:92, 1975
66. Storm FK, Longmire WP Jr: A simplified clamp for hepatic resection. Surg Gynecol Obstet 133:103, 1971
67. Trunkey DD, Shires GT, McClelland R: Management of liver trauma in 811 consecutive patients. Ann Surg 179:722, 1974
68. Turrill FL, Donovan AJ, Facey FL: Traumatic hepatic sequestra. Am J Surg 122:175, 1971
69. Wakim KG: Basic and clinical physiology of the liver, normal and abnormal. Anesth Analg 44:636, 1965
70. Walt AJ: The surgical management of hepatic trauma and its complications. Ann R Coll Surg Engl 45:319, 1969
71. Walt AJ: The mythology of hepatic trauma or Babel revisited. Am J Surg 135:12, 1978
72. Walt AJ: Hepatic injuries, a 1980 overview, p658. South Afr Med J, April 19, 1980
73. Weissman HS, Freeman LM: Role of Tc99m IDA scintigraphy in the evaluation of hepatobiliary trauma. Semin Nucl Med 8:199, 1983
74. Witte CL, Witte MH, Kintner K: Effect of glucagon on hepatic lymph (tissue) PO^2 after ligation of the hepatic artery: An experimental study. J Trauma 18:27, 1978
75. Yellin AE, Chaffee CB, Donovan AJ: Vascular isolation in treatment of juxtahepatic venous injuries. Arch Surg 102:566, 1971

splenic trauma

Mary C. McCarthy
John L. Glover

In the past, trauma to the spleen was considered a simple subject that could be summarized succinctly:

> The spleen is frequently injured by blunt or penetrating trauma, and injury to this organ is usually associated with serious hemorrhage that may be fatal if not treated promptly. Any injury to the spleen should be treated by splenectomy because the spleen apparently has no function, and attempts at repair would be associated with unacceptably high rates of recurrent bleeding.

Three important medical trends in the last decade have produced significant changes in the management of trauma to the spleen. One of these trends is the widespread recognition of the role of the spleen in infection; the second is the more liberal application of noninvasive tests for intraperitoneal bleeding, such as computed tomography (CT). Finally, delineation of the anatomic basis for splenic repair, increasing experience with splenorrhaphy, and confirmation of acceptable rates of morbidity associated with splenic preservation have led to increasing conservatism in operative and even non-operative management. While these trends generally represent significant improvements in care, they have also been a source of some confusion with regard to the management of splenic trauma. This chapter will consider how these trends and the resultant conservative approaches developed in specialized centers affect the management of splenic trauma in practice.

The spleen may be injured by blunt or penetrating trauma, and it is still the organ most commonly injured in blunt trauma. The overall rate of mortality due to splenic injury is approximately 11%; but it is 19% in those with blunt trauma, largely because of concomitant serious injuries such as craniocerebral trauma. In patients with penetrating trauma from gunshot wounds, mortality is 9%; it is 0% in those with stab wounds.[44]

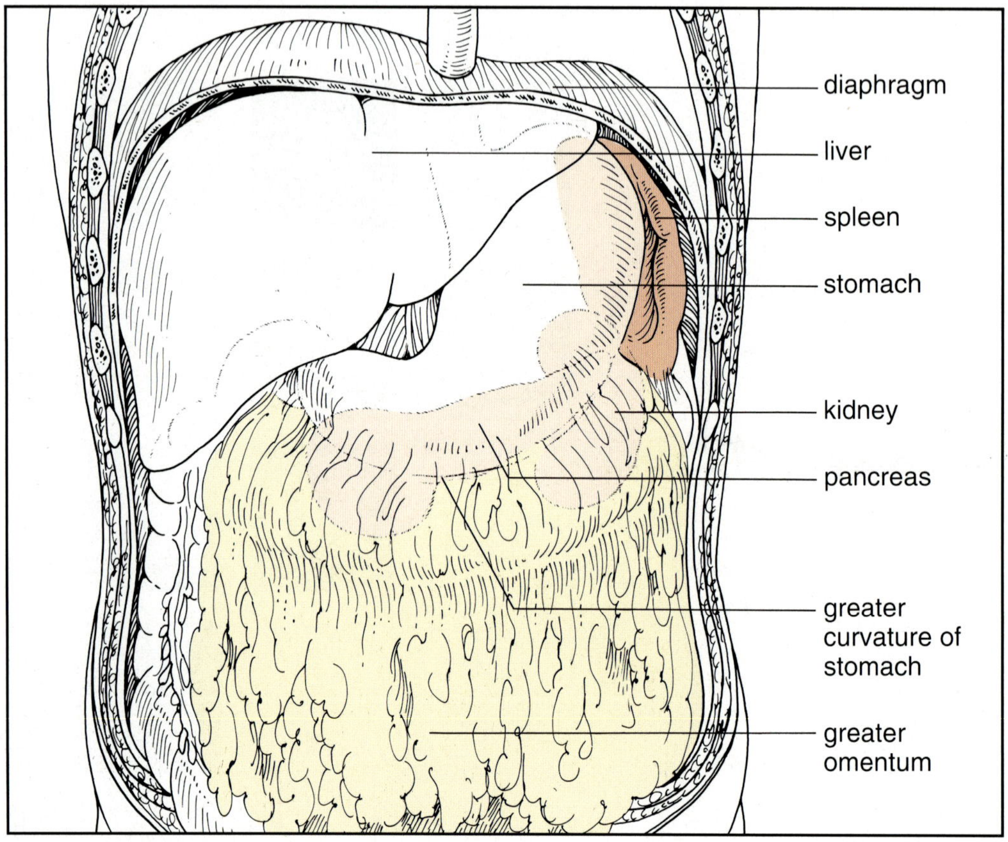

FIGURE 8.1 The spleen is shown in relation to other intra-abdominal organs.

The spleen is also subject to injury from penetrating trauma to the lower portion of the left thorax, and this type of injury may present a problem in diagnosis. Finally, iatrogenic trauma may cause injury to the spleen in a variety of situations: traction on the stomach or colon during laparotomy, inadvertent placement of a chest tube below the left diaphragm, and percutaneous catheter drainage of intra-abdominal abscesses.

ANATOMY

The spleen is located in the left upper quadrant of the abdomen, juxtaposed to the 9th, 10th, and 11th ribs. Normally, it is completely protected by the costal arch. The superior anterior surface of the spleen is closely applied to the greater curvature of the stomach. Inferiorly, the lower pole of the spleen is often attached to the splenic flexure of the colon and the greater omentum. The lateral and posterior surface of the spleen is apposed to the diaphragm, the medial surface to the left kidney (Fig. 8.1).

The peritoneal attachments of the spleen are the gastrosplenic, phrenosplenic, splenorenal, and splenocolic ligaments (Fig. 8.2). The gastrosplenic ligament contains the short gastric and left gastroepiploic vessels, but in the absence of portal hypertension or myeloproliferative disorders, the remainder of the splenic attachments are generally avascular.[55] The layers of the gastrosplenic ligament separate at the hilum of the spleen. The anterior layer invests the outer surface of the spleen, passes posteriorly, and is reflected over the surface of the left kidney. The inner layer covers the splenic vessels and is continuous with the floor of the lesser sac, where it covers the pancreas and forms

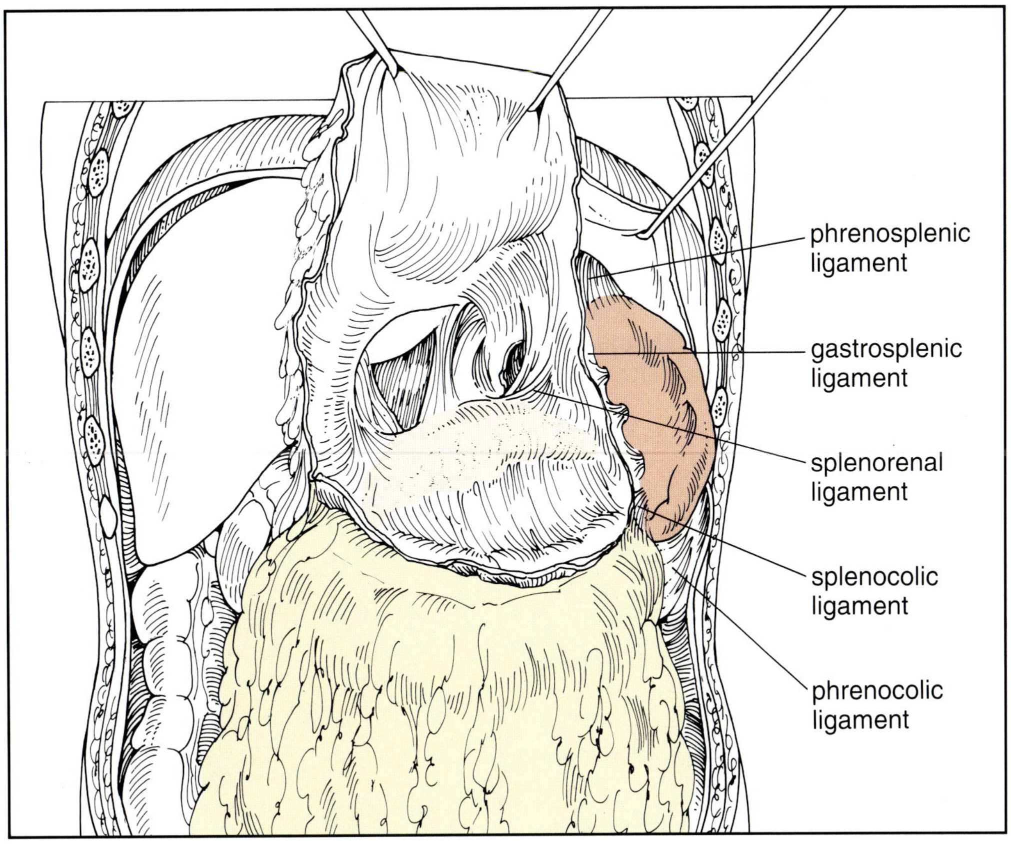

FIGURE 8.2 Ligamentous attachments of the spleen.

the splenorenal ligament (Fig. 8.3). The inferior pole of the spleen lies upon, and is occasionally connected to, the phrenocolic ligament, which attaches the splenic flexure of the colon to the diaphragm.[34]

The arterial blood supply is provided by the splenic artery, which runs transversely from right to left at the superior margin of the pancreas, distributing multiple small branches to the pancreatic substance and occasionally to the posterior aspect of the stomach. At the hilum, this artery divides into numerous branches, the major ones being the left gastroepiploic, superior polar, and superior and inferior terminal arteries (Fig. 8.4). The left gastroepiploic artery passes inferiorly and along the greater curvature, providing branches to the stomach and greater omentum. The superior polar artery, which may arise at some distance from the splenic hilum, gives off short gastric branches to the greater curvature of the stomach and then enters the splenic parenchyma. Additional short gastric arteries may arise from the main splenic arterial trunk before it branches.

The superior and inferior terminal arteries arise and then resolve into several secondary branches before entering the splenic pulp. There may also be an intermediate terminal branch. Inferior polar arteries frequently occur. These may arise from the left gastroepiploic, splenic, or inferior terminal artery.

The vessels within the splenic parenchyma are sequentially distributed and run in a transverse plane, perpendicular to the long axis of the spleen. This distribution is important to the understanding of the anatomical basis for partial splenectomy.

The splenic vein arises in six or more large branches leaving the hilum, and passes from left to right in a much more direct course than the artery. It runs dorsal to the pancreas and joins with the superior mesenteric vein to form the portal vein behind the head of the pancreas.

PATHOLOGY

The normal adult spleen weighs approximately 150 g. It measures about 12 cm in length, 7 cm in breadth, and 3 cm to 4 cm in thickness. The splenic capsule is 1 mm to 2 mm thick and is composed of an external serous coat derived from the peritoneum and a fibroelastic layer that invests the spleen. This layer is continuous with the trabeculae and, together with a fine network of reticulum fibers, supports the splenic pulp.

The complex nature of the splenic microcirculation is responsible in large part for its active role in the reticuloendothelial system. Two major theories about intermediary splenic circulation exist. The *open circulation theory* holds that the arterial capillaries open directly into the cordal meshwork of the red pulp and the blood cells, then pass through the reticular meshwork of the cords and through the pores (interendothelial spaces) of the walls of the venous sinuses. The *closed circulation theory* states that the arterial capillaries connect directly to the venous sinuses. Animal studies reveal that both types of circulation may occur in the spleen, with about 90% of blood passing through the open route. Trabecular arteries give off central arteries that supply arteriolar branches to the splenic pulp. The blood is filtered slowly through the reticular network of the sinuses, then into trabecular veins, and eventually into the main splenic vein and the portal circulation.[8]

The spleen is a friable and highly vascular organ and is therefore often subject to injury. Traumatic injuries to the spleen may consist of splenic capsular avulsions, minor parenchymal disruptions, transverse fractures oriented along the planes of the internal vascular architecture of the spleen, disruption of the hilar vasculature, or massive injuries. A Splenic Injury Scale developed by the Organ Scaling Committee of the American Association for the Surgery of Trauma is depicted in the table displayed in Fig. 8.5.[39]

Changes in the spleen occurring with aging may affect the type of splenic injury, the response to conservative management, and the ease of surgical repair. Morgenstern and Uyeda report that there is more functional smooth muscle and elastica in the spleens of children than in those of adults.[41] Thus the splenic vasculature and the spleen itself are more contractile, possibly enabling easier tamponade of hemorrhage. Also, the splenic capsule increases almost five times in thickness between birth and the sixth year of life, thereafter remaining relatively constant. Splenic weight increases tenfold in the first 6 years of life, then doubles again by adulthood, the capsular thickness decreasing proportionally. This thinning of the capsule makes suture repair much more difficult in adults than in children.[33]

Splenectomy may be followed by hypertrophy of accessory spleens or the development of splenosis, the growth of splenic

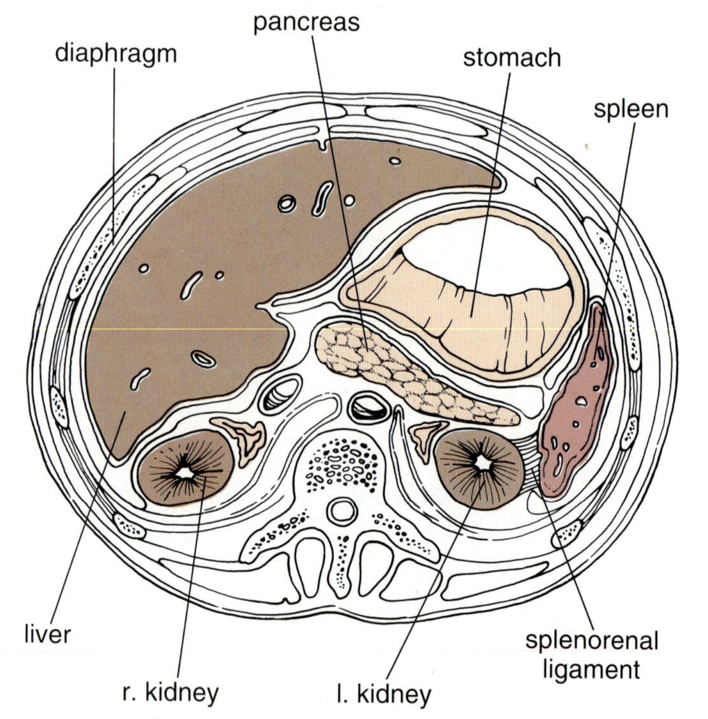

FIGURE 8.3 The spleen and its relations to other organs, shown in a transverse section.

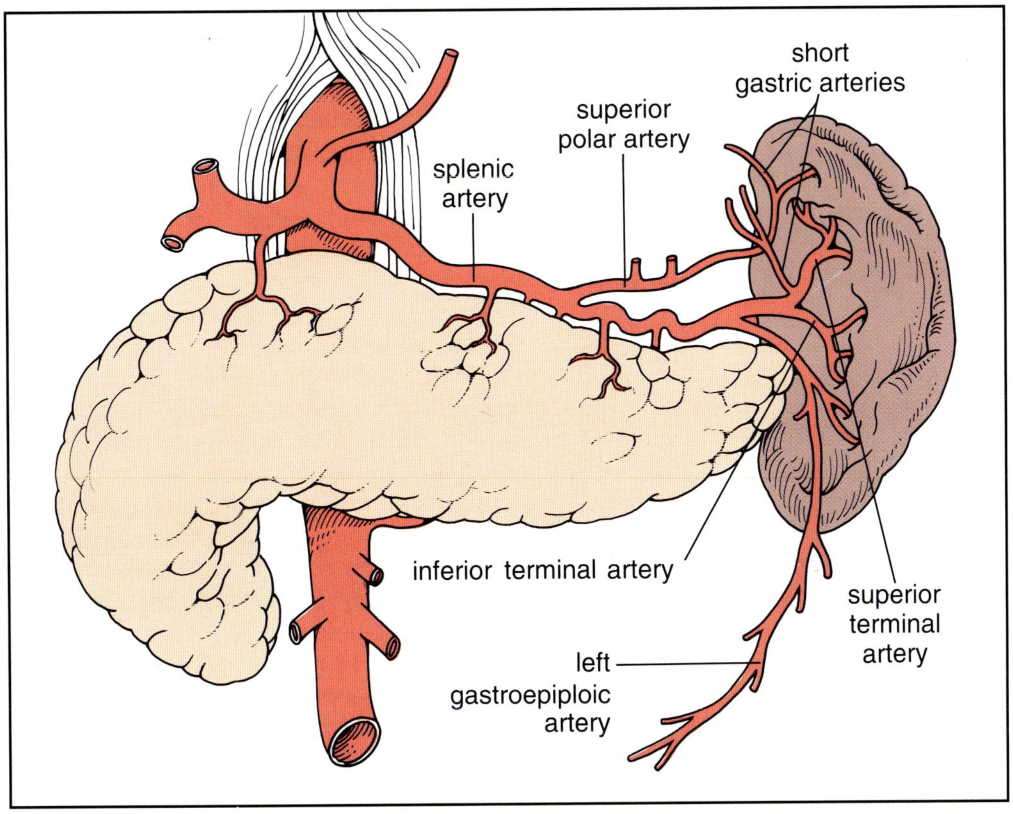

FIGURE 8.4 Blood supply of the spleen.

FIGURE 8.5 SPLENIC INJURY SCALE

GRADE*		INJURY DESCRIPTION†	ICD-9	AIS 85	AIS 90
I.	Hematoma:	Subcapsular, nonexpanding <10% surface area	865.01 865.11	2	2
	Laceration:	Capsular tear, nonbleeding, <1 cm parenchymal depth	865.02 865.12		
II.	Hematoma:	Subcapsular, nonexpanding, 10–50% surface area Intraparenchymal, nonexpanding, <2 cm in diameter	865.01 865.11	2	2
	Laceration:	Capsular tear, active bleeding; 1–3 cm parenchymal depth which does not involve a trabecular vessel	865.02 865.12	2	2
III.	Hematoma:	Subcapsular, >50% surface area or expanding Ruptured subcapsular hematoma with active bleeding Intraparenchymal hematoma >2 cm or expanding		3	3
	Laceration:	>3 cm parenchymal depth or involving trabecular vessels	865.03 865.13	3	3
IV:	Hematoma:	Ruptured intraparenchymal hematoma with active bleeding		3	4
	Laceration	Laceration involving segmental or hilar vessels producing major devascularization (>25% of spleen)	865.04 865.14	3	4
V.	Laceration:	shattered spleen	865.04 865.14	5	5
	Vascular:	Hilar vascular injury which devascularizes spleen		5	5

* Advance one grade for multiple injuries to the same organ.
† Based on most accurate assessment at autopsy, laparotomy, or radiologic study.

tissue implants in the peritoneal cavity. Inflammation around these implants has caused small bowel obstruction in some patients long after surgery.

Accessory spleens may be found in the splenic hilum or along the splenic vessels in the tail of the pancreas, in the splenocolic ligament, in the greater omentum, the perirenal area, the small bowel mesentery, or the presacral, adnexal, or peritesticular regions.

PHYSIOLOGY

The spleen plays an exceedingly active role in the reticuloendothelial system. The splenic microcirculation is the primary site of clearance for blood-borne bacteria and particulate antigens. The spleen responds to systemic infection by increasing phagocytic activity and increasing the numbers of neutrophils in the sinusoids and cords. Splenic macrophages are particularly effective at engulfing blood-borne particles. These particles are then transported to the splenic lymphoid follicle where a reaction center develops and a specific class M immunoglobin (IgM) antibody is formed. In addition, B lymphocyte maturation and the production of class G immoglobin occurs in the spleen. It is also a site for the maturation of T-helper, T-cytotoxic/suppressor, and natural killer cells.[35] The spleen is a major site for the synthesis of opsonic proteins, tuftsin and properdin, which are essential to the processing of antigens. The spleen also has other roles in the modification of reticulocytes and destruction of senescent red blood cells.[12]

Several factors may be responsible for the impaired immune response seen following splenectomy.[2] The anatomical integrity of the spleen, with 90% of its blood flow passing through the red pulp where particles are exposed to phagocytic cells, is crucial. The spleen is an important source of antibody. Following splenectomy, IgM levels fall and remain low for a year or more. There is also a reduction in phagocytic capacity, with a resultant inability to clear encapsulated bacteria from the bloodstream, and an impaired antibody response to blood-borne antigens. These factors may result in overwhelming postsplenectomy sepsis due to meningitis, pneumonia, or septicemia; these diseases may occur days to years following splenectomy. The majority (80%) of the serious infections occur within 2 years, and almost half occur within 12 months. There is a trend, however, toward longer intervals between operation and septic episodes in older children and adults.[62] Repeated episodes of severe infection may occur in some patients.

The onset of postsplenectomy sepsis is usually quite sudden, with nausea, vomiting, headache, and confusion, progressing to coma. Fever as high as 104°F has been noted. Most commonly, the causative organism is *Streptococcus pneumoniae* (50%). Other organisms that have been identified include *Neisseria meningitidis*, *Hemophilus influenzae*, *Escherichia coli*, *Staphylococcus*, *Streptococcus*, and *Pseudomonas*. Viral and protozoal infections have also been described. Encapsulated organisms are most frequently involved, because the presence of a capsule inhibits phagocytosis. Thus, when encapsulated organisms with a rapid doubling time invade the bloodstream, the asplenic person is unable to clear them from the bloodstream. As the bacteria invade, hypoglycemia, electrolyte imbalance, disseminated intravascular coagulation, and shock may ensue. Organisms may be identified on peripheral blood smears, and cultures may grow as many as 10^6 organisms per cubic millimeter. The overall mortality rate is 50% to 80%, and patients may die within 12 to 18 hours. Antibiotic therapy is often futile.[56] At autopsy, the Waterhouse-Friderichsen syndrome (hemorrhagic adrenal necrosis) may be evident.

The syndrome of overwhelming sepsis after splenectomy was noticed in children as early as 1952, when King and Shumacker reported fulminant sepsis in five infants who had undergone splenectomy for congenital spherocytic anemia.[24] Those under 2 years of age were thought to be at greatest risk, probably because they had not developed the "library" of antibodies needed for resistance to systemic infection. Following the reports of Singer in 1973[57] and others, there was increased awareness of the syndrome and, for the first time, appreciation that adults may be susceptible to it, too. Singer reviewed 2,796 patients from the literature and evaluated the incidence of septic morbidity and mortality. The overall incidence of postsplenectomy sepsis was 4.25%, and the rate of ensuing mortality was 2.52%. Commonly used figures currently place the annual risk at 0.5% for post-traumatic splenectomy, as opposed to approximately 2% for other diseases requiring splenectomy. Appreciation of this information developed concomitantly with advances in techniques for monitoring physiological status, availability of methods of imaging organs, and recognition of pediatric surgery as a specialty. It was natural, therefore, that procedures to conserve the spleen would develop in children's hospitals. These techniques, as well as nonoperative care in selected situations, are being widely used today.

DIAGNOSIS

Clinical Manifestations

The ease of diagnosis depends upon the clinical presentation, of which there are three common types: a stable ambulatory patient with abdominal pain after blunt trauma; emergency presentation of patients with penetrating trauma, stable or unstable; and emergency presentation of patients with severe blunt trauma and multiple injuries, such as victims of automobile accidents.

AMBULATORY PATIENTS WITH BLUNT ABDOMINAL TRAUMA

When patients come to the emergency department on an ambulatory basis after isolated blunt abdominal trauma and complain of abdominal pain, rupture of the spleen is usually considered early in the course of the evaluation. The antecedent trauma is usually a direct blow to the abdomen, as may occur in a fight, in contact sports, or in a fall from a bicycle or from heights. If the patient is of high school or college age and has considerable abdominal pain after minor trauma, the possibility of the rupture of a diseased spleen must be considered. For example, symptoms of infectious mononucleosis may be vague and minor enough that a busy student may not have sought medical attention.

Moreover, an enlarged spleen in such patients is more prone to rupture from blunt trauma than a normal one.[53]

These patients are usually hemodynamically stable, but postural hypotension is often present and should be further evaluated and treated before the patient is sent for radiographic studies or left unattended. If the patient complains of pain associated with respiration, suspicion of splenic rupture is heightened. If this sign is present, it may mean peritoneal irritation from blood or pleural irritation from fractured ribs or costal cartilages. A ruptured spleen seems even more likely if the left 10th or 11th rib is fractured, a diagnosis best made during physical examination by gentle, careful palpation along the course of the ribs. However, it is possible for such injuries to be present without underlying visceral trauma, and the pain associated with them makes evaluation of the abdomen more difficult. In such instances, direct tests for intra-abdominal bleeding, such as peritoneal lavage or CT scan, may be needed; these will be discussed in the section on diagnostic tests.

If there is no injury to ribs or costal cartilages and no contusion of the abdominal wall, there may be tenderness in the left upper quadrant or generalized abdominal tenderness. Some patients, however, will have very little, if any, tenderness; they may have a minor injury to the spleen with a small amount of clotted blood contained adjacent to the spleen. Kehr's sign, pain at the top of the shoulder, may be elicited by pressure in the left upper quadrant or by placing the patient in the Trendelenburg position. Ballance's sign, fixed dullness to percussion in the left upper quadrant, and Seagesser's sign, pain in the neck with pressure over the phrenic nerve, are only rarely identified. The presence of associated injuries may, of course, alter these findings.

The majority of patients with splenic rupture present acutely, although some patients may present with delayed rupture, following a period referred to as "the latent period of Baudet."[54] (Increasing use of early CT of the abdomen has cast doubt on the existence of this syndrome.) These patients may present a more difficult diagnostic picture, often presenting only with evidence of occult blood loss, which might be more appropriately called "delayed hemorrhage." In most instances, this presentation is not a delayed rupture of an expanding subcapsular hematoma, but represents the sudden onset of bleeding due to lysis of clot that had sealed tears in the parenchyma immediately after the injury.[46]

PATIENTS WITH PENETRATING TRAUMA

When patients are brought to the emergency department with penetrating trauma to the left upper quadrant, splenic injury must always be considered. If the patient is hemodynamically unstable, laparotomy must be performed as quickly as possible, with the usual preparation but a minimum of time-consuming tests. If the patient is stable, there is a possibility of delayed or missed diagnosis if the patient is merely observed until abdominal tenderness develops. We see no virtue in such a delay; if tenderness develops after observation, either bleeding has recurred or peritonitis has developed. These problems can be avoided if patients with penetrating trauma are properly evaluated.

Stab wounds to the anterior abdominal wall are explored locally, using local anesthesia and sterile technique. A small cutdown over the wound tract should be performed to determine whether penetration of the peritoneal cavity has occurred. If it has, peritoneal lavage is performed to assess the presence of injury. If there is no penetration, the patient may be discharged. However, all patients with gunshot wounds of the abdomen should undergo exploratory laparotomy because of the high incidence of intra-abdominal injuries. Even tangential wounds without peritoneal penetration may cause injuries due to blast effect, and peritoneal lavage is not reliable for determining peritoneal penetration in these injuries.

Penetrating wounds in other areas present more problems, especially wounds in the lower left hemithorax and flank. The diaphragm may be as high as the fifth rib anteriorly when a patient is supine (Fig. 8.6). Externally, this level is identified by the nipples anteriorly and the angle of the scapula posteriorly. If

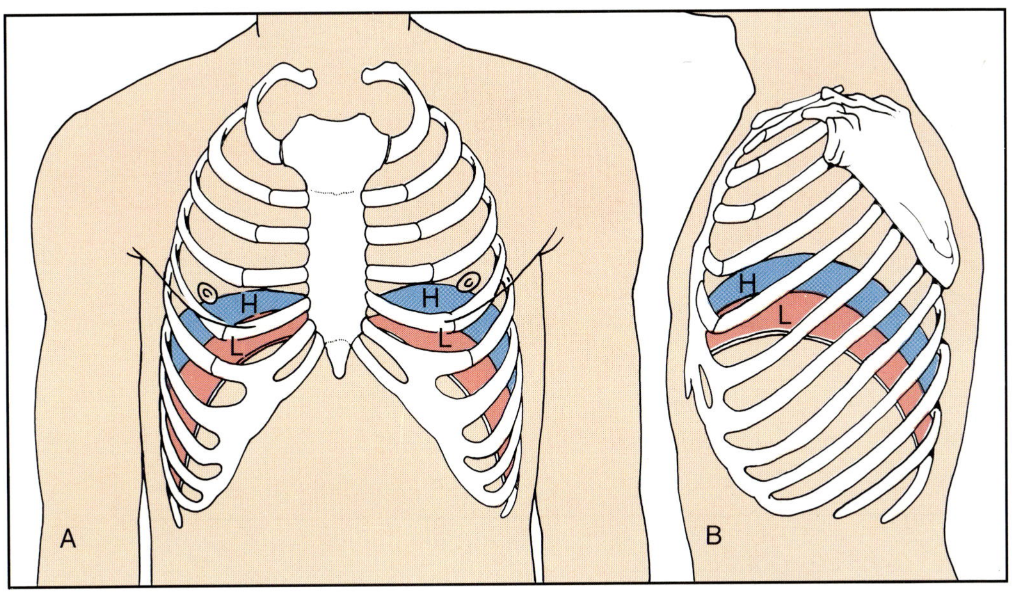

FIGURE 8.6 A Anteroposterior view of the chest showing diaphragmatic respiratory excursion. **B** Lateral view of the chest showing diaphragmatic respiratory excursion.

a patient has a penetrating wound below the nipple and is hypotensive, the greatest immediate concern is whether there is a wound of the heart, and if the patient is unstable, the question affects the initial management profoundly. In most cases, the problem is intra-abdominal bleeding unless there is obvious pericardial tamponade or a large hemothorax. Immediate peritoneal lavage will confirm the presence of intra-abdominal bleeding and the necessity for laparotomy. Chest tubes, if needed, may be inserted in the operating room; these patients should be prepared and draped so that the sternum can be split or a bilateral anterior thoracotomy can be performed if necessary.

If significant suspicion of cardiac injury remains, the pericardium can be opened by a subxiphoid approach during laparotomy (Fig. 8.7). In this technique, the midline laparotomy wound is continued up to the left of the xiphoid process. Blunt dissection is performed, peeling the peritoneum and areolar tissues from the posterior aspect of the xiphoid and staying in the plane just behind it. When the level of the pericardial sac is reached, the movement of the heart within it can be clearly felt. The pericardium is elevated with fine forceps, and a small opening is made with Metzenbaum scissors. If there has been pericardial penetration, the pulsations of the heart will force blood out through the opening. In general, however, patients with penetrating wounds at or below the fifth rib and between the midclavicular lines are more likely to have hypotension from intra-abdominal bleeding or injury to vascular structures in the upper retroperitoneum than from cardiac or pulmonary wounds.

If the patient is stable and has a small hemopneumothorax, there may be a tendency to insert a chest tube and observe the patient's progress, especially if the wounding agent is a knife or if a bullet appears to be in the chest or upper peritoneum away from the midline. Such treatment ignores the fact that the path of a missile, and therefore the damage it has caused, cannot be determined by the locations of the wound of entry and exit or the position of a bullet on a radiograph.

Patients with stab wounds over the left anterior and lateral hemithorax below the nipple level should routinely undergo peritoneal lavage to rule out intra-abdominal injury. Patients with gunshot wounds in this area should be operated upon, since lavage is unreliable. Flank stab wounds below the costal margin may be managed like abdominal wounds, with local exploration followed by lavage if there is peritoneal penetration.

PATIENTS WITH BLUNT TRAUMA AND MULTIPLE INJURIES

In patients with blunt trauma, the problem may be considerably more subtle. As in the situation with penetrating trauma, these patients may be stable or unstable, but the instability may appear to be related to other injuries, such as skeletal trauma or head injuries. In fact, most articles on blunt abdominal trauma comment on the misleading lack of abdominal tenderness and rigidity in these patients despite the presence of visceral injuries.

In dealing with patients with blunt trauma, two principles help clarify the indications for diagnostic tests for abdominal injury. The first principle is that *craniocerebral trauma is not a cause of hypotension*. Quadriplegic patients may be hypotensive because of spinal shock, but their lesions are obvious. Patients with cerebral contusions who have hypotension nearly always have an extracranial source of major blood loss. The absence of hypotension, of course, does not exclude significant injury.

The second principle is that *the severity of the impact determines the extent of the injury*. Any fracture of the hip or femur is associated with significant loss of blood, but a young adult who has sustained a fracture of the femur, several fractured ribs, and a cerebral contusion in an automobile accident has a high likelihood of having an injury to the spleen, liver, pancreas, or small

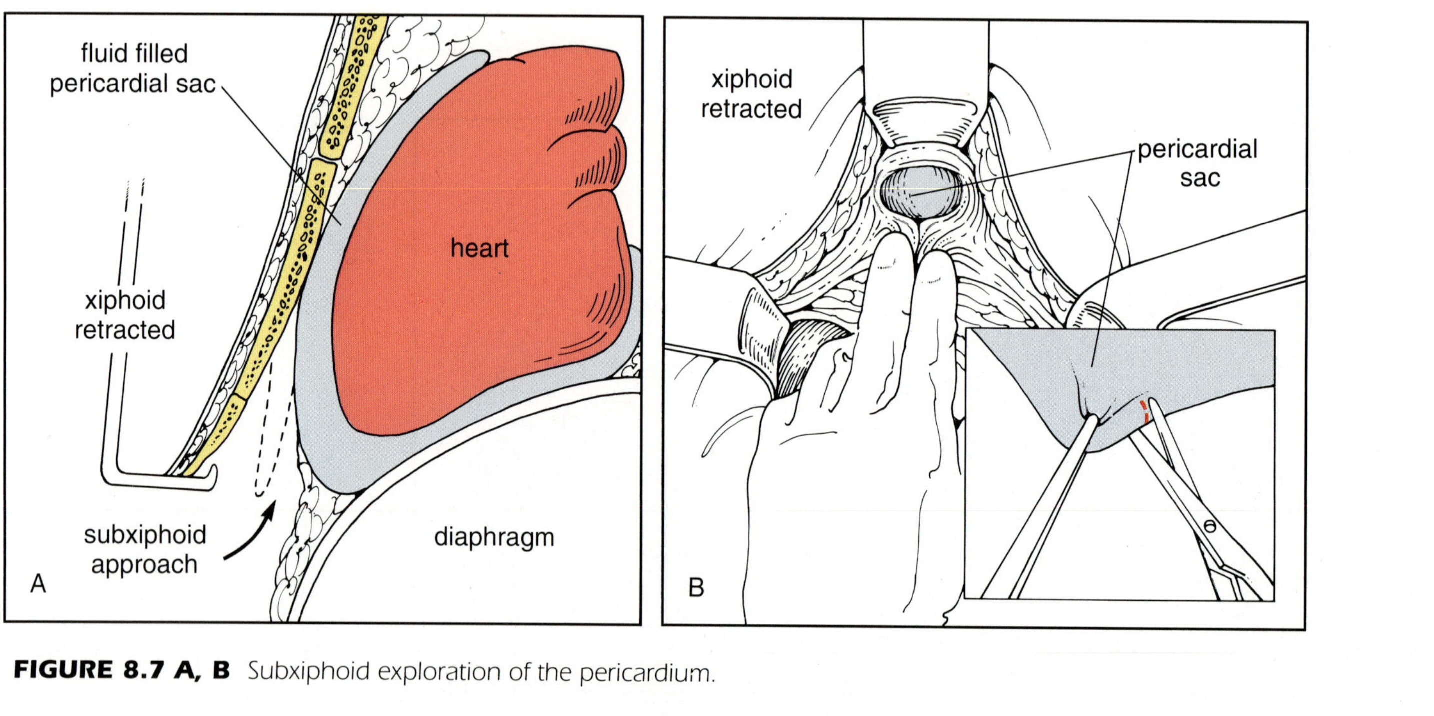

FIGURE 8.7 A, B Subxiphoid exploration of the pericardium.

bowel. In a report on blunt trauma from 1950 to 1960, Fitzgerald and associates[15] found head injuries in 18%, long bone fractures in 29%, and rib fractures in 37% of patients who had arrived alive and were found to have abdominal injuries at laparotomy. The spleen was the most commonly injured organ, and 20% of these patients had multiple intra-abdominal injuries. When the patients with intra-abdominal trauma who were dead on arrival were examined at autopsy, 44% had head injuries, 45% had long bone fractures, and 71% had rib fractures. Again, the spleen was the most commonly injured organ, and 40% of patients had multiple intra-abdominal injuries. In a similar review of patients at Indiana University Medical Center from 1960 to 1970, the statistics were remarkably similar except that more patients had head injuries (40% of those arriving alive and 68% of those dead on arrival), and more had multiple intra-abdominal injuries (57% of those arriving alive and 73% of those dead on arrival). These increases in just one decade were attributed to more high-speed motor vehicle accidents. Recent passage of mandatory seat-belt laws may affect these statistics, but the importance of this type of information cannot be overemphasized to those acting as primary physicians in emergency departments. Patients with multiple injuries from blunt trauma, especially young adults with head injury, rib fractures, and long bone fractures, must be evaluated thoroughly for evidence of trauma to the spleen before care is turned over to a specialist not trained in managing abdominal trauma.

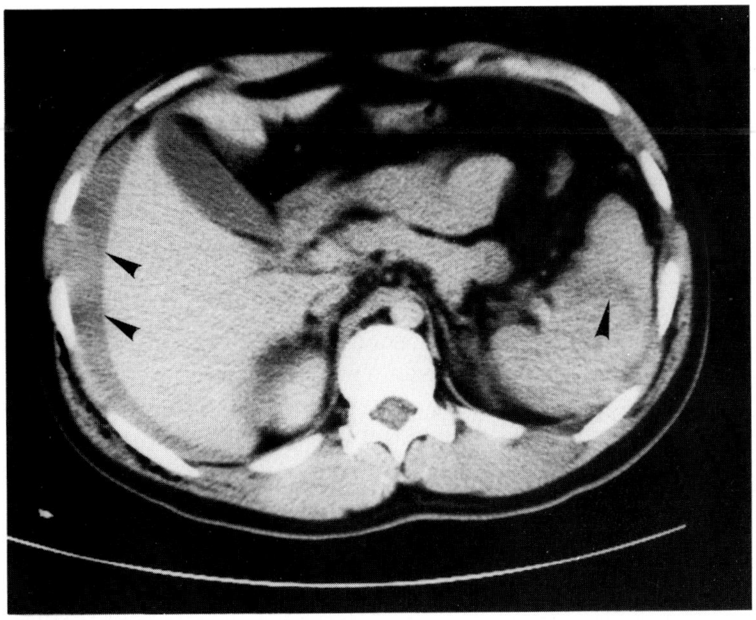

FIGURE 8.8 CT scan of the abdomen shows splenic fracture (single arrowhead) with free intraperitoneal blood (double arrowheads).

Laboratory Values

A complete blood count obtained on admission may show evidence of blood loss. However, if this study is obtained early, the hematocrit may be normal, in which case serial studies should be helpful. The white blood cell count is frequently greater than 15,000 to 20,000/mm[34]. Other studies, such as a serum amylase, which may be elevated in pancreatic trauma, are usually done in consideration of associated injuries. All these patients should have an evaluation of their coagulation system: prothrombin time, partial thromboplastin time, and estimation of adequacy of platelets are usually sufficient. If there is a history of muscosal bleeding after previous surgery, however, a standardized bleeding time should be done to screen for von Willebrand disease.

Radiography

Routine chest and abdominal films may be helpful in diagnosis. The presence of fractures of the left 8th, 9th, and 10th ribs should increase suspicion of splenic injury, and a left pleural effusion or an elevated left hemidiaphragm may be indicative of splenic injury. Abdominal films may demonstrate an increase in the size of the splenic shadow in the left upper quadrant, with displacement of the gastric air bubble medially and the hepatic flexure inferiorly.

A CT scan of the abdomen is becoming an invaluable diagnostic study in the management of patients sustaining blunt trauma and is essential if nonoperative therapy is planned. Iodinated water-soluble contrast material is given orally or by the nasogastric tube 45 minutes prior to examination, in order to opacify the gastrointestinal tract and to facilitate the identification of small bowel loops. Additional doses of contrast material are given every 15 minutes. Contrast material given immediately before the examination will enable visualization of the stomach and duodenum. The nasogastric tube should be pulled back into the esophagus before the study is performed in order to prevent streak artifacts in the left upper quadrant. Intravenous contrast is also imperative because acute hematomas have the same attenuation value as the adjacent parenchymal organs.

Splenic fractures or lacerations appear as irregular intrasplenic low-density regions. The bolus technique is most useful in trauma patients, with occasional supplemental doses required to evaluate subtle injuries more completely. In addition to the area of the spleen itself, the paracolic gutters, subhepatic space, and cul-de-sac should be examined for the presence of free intraperitoneal blood (Fig. 8.8). The CT scan is also valuable in the delineation of other intra-abdominal injuries, lesser sac and retroperitoneal hemorrhage, and in the evaluation of the pelvis. Splenic injuries appear as simple or complex fractures accompanied by either subcapsular hematoma or intraperitoneal blood. Subcapsular hematomas appear as crescentic, low-density fluid collections that flatten or indent the lateral margin of the spleen.

In a recent review of 55 consecutive cases of surgically proven splenic injuries,[13] CT scan permitted correct identification of 54 splenic injuries, with 1 false negative and 3 false positive scans. CT demonstrated hemoperitoneum (98%), perisplenic clot (85%), splenic laceration (71%), and subcapsular hematoma (24%). Recently, CT scanning has been used to develop scoring systems predictive of splenic salvage or successful nonoperative therapy.[5] In other series, however, clinical evaluation was more reliable.[36]

There are some potential pitfalls in using CT scan for evaluation of the spleen. One is that streak artifacts from adjacent ribs may degrade the splenic image. Another is that the normal spleen does not always enhance as homogeneously as the liver and does not have the added enhancement provided by the portal venous system in the liver. Consequently, identification of splenic fractures may be more difficult than identification of hepatic fractures.[51] Also, computerized tomographic imaging may be difficult in the patient who is restless, uncooperative, or has an irregular breathing pattern. However, in patients who are undergoing cerebral CT, performing an abdominal CT adds little time to the exam.

Ultrasonography provides an additional method for noninvasive assessment of the patient with blunt trauma. The spleen may be difficult to visualize, however, because of its location beneath the ribs, and gaseous distension may also make imaging more difficult. The superior anatomical detail provided by CT scanning makes ultrasound less useful, although lower cost and ready availability make it more appealing.

Radionuclide scans may occasionally be helpful in the evaluation of splenic trauma. Radioactive technetium sulfur colloid particles are cleared by the reticuloendothelial system, and images of the liver and spleen are obtained in six different projections: anterior, posterior, right and left lateral, left anterior oblique, and right posterior oblique. The last three are specific for the spleen. Collections of blood within the splenic parenchyma will compress surrounding tissues and produce focal areas of decreased uptake. The area of involvement will appear larger on scan than it actually is because of the hypofunction of compressed tissues.

These scans are most valuable in detecting parenchymal subdiaphragmatic lesions, although some initial confusion may be caused by misinterpretation of morphologic variants, or by the presence of abscesses, tumors, cysts, or infarctions unrelated to the episode of trauma.[31] Although useful for the serial evaluation of the healing of traumatic defects, the lack of significant anatomic abnormalities in the remote post-injury period has led many authors to abandon otherwise unnecessary follow-up scanning.[23]

Arteriography has also been used to delineate the source of intraperitoneal bleeding, but because it is more invasive, expensive, and time consuming, it is seldom used as the primary means of diagnosis in the uncomplicated case. In one study comparing the arteriographic findings with injuries found at operation, selective splenic arteriography was found to be reliable in delineating the extent of injury, although 5% of the angiograms were falsely positive.[3] Angiographic signs of injury are either direct or indirect. Direct signs include extravasation or pooling of contrast material in the parenchyma, arteriovenous shunting, or pseudoaneurysm formation within the spleen. Stretching or dislocation of either intrasplenic channels or vessels adjacent to the spleen due to collections of blood are indirect signs. Other indirect signs include splenic enlargement, widening of the space between the spleen and the diaphragm, indistinct splenic margins, and inhomogenous splenogram during the capillary phase of the examination. These indirect findings are useful only if supported by additional clinical evidence of splenic injury.

Peritoneal Lavage

When hemodynamic instability or multiple injuries are present, hemoperitoneum is a sufficient indication for laparotomy in most circumstances; peritoneal lavage is an excellent method for identifying its presence. It has an accuracy of 95% to 98% in the diagnosis of intra-abdominal injuries due to blunt trauma,[1] and similar sensitivity has been reported for stab wounds.[59] For gunshot wounds, however, some modification of the criteria is required, and the test is not as reliable.[38] The open technique for peritoneal lavage is the safest, and patients with significant pelvic fractures should undergo lavage through a supra-umbilical, open technique.

Previous major laparotomy is a contraindication to lavage because there may be difficulty entering the peritoneal cavity due to adhesions, with a resulting increased risk of bowel injury. In addition, results of lavage may be unreliable because of the walling off of an area of injury by adhesions and, therefore, inadequate mixing of the lavage fluid.

Following placement of a nasogastric tube and Foley catheter to reduce the likelihood of visceral injury, a site for lavage is selected approximately two thirds of the way from the umbilicus to the pubis. The area is infiltrated with 1% lidocaine with epinephrine, and an incision approximately 2.5 cm in length is made. The incision is carried down to the fascia, where a small opening is made. The peritoneum is grasped with clamps and elevated to prevent injury to the underlying bowel. A small nick is made, and the peritoneal dialysis catheter is then threaded inferiorly and posteriorly. If initial aspiration returns greater than 10 ml of gross blood, it is considered positive; otherwise, lavage is performed. A liter of normal saline is allowed to flow into the peritoneal cavity and return by gravity siphon, then a specimen is sent to the laboratory for analysis. The presence of greater than 100,000 red blood cells/mm^3[4] is considered a positive lavage. Some authors have used a gross estimation of red cell count, a spun hematocrit of two, or the inability to read through the intravenous fluid connector tubing as an indication for operation.

TREATMENT

Decision to Operate

The presence of hemodynamic instability in a patient with abdominal trauma is an indication for surgery unless there is another obvious cause such as myocardial contusion, or if there is spinal shock. The liberal use of peritoneal lavage clarifies the decision to operate in such patients, as well as in many others. A suggested algorithm for evaluation and treatment, modified from one presented by Luna and Dellinger,[30] is depicted in the table in Figure 8.9. Noninvasive testing may require significant time, however, and observation of the patients may not be optimal during this interval. Furthermore, there will be a significant number of instances in which the images are less than ideal and the interpretation difficult. If there is question about the accuracy of peritoneal lavage in such cases because of previous surgery or morbid obesity, for example, laparotomy is the safest course in the unstable patient who has sustained severe trauma. Laparoscopy is being studied for its efficacy in trauma, but it would be subject to the same limitations as lavage in cases of obesity or previous surgery. We consider confirmation of intraperitoneal bleeding, hemodynamic instability, and peritoneal signs as indications for operation.

Resuscitation

A nasogastric tube should be placed for the evacuation of gastric contents. If possible, the patient should be hemodynamically stabilized by the administration of crystalloid solutions and blood products as needed. Evaluation of the patient for con-

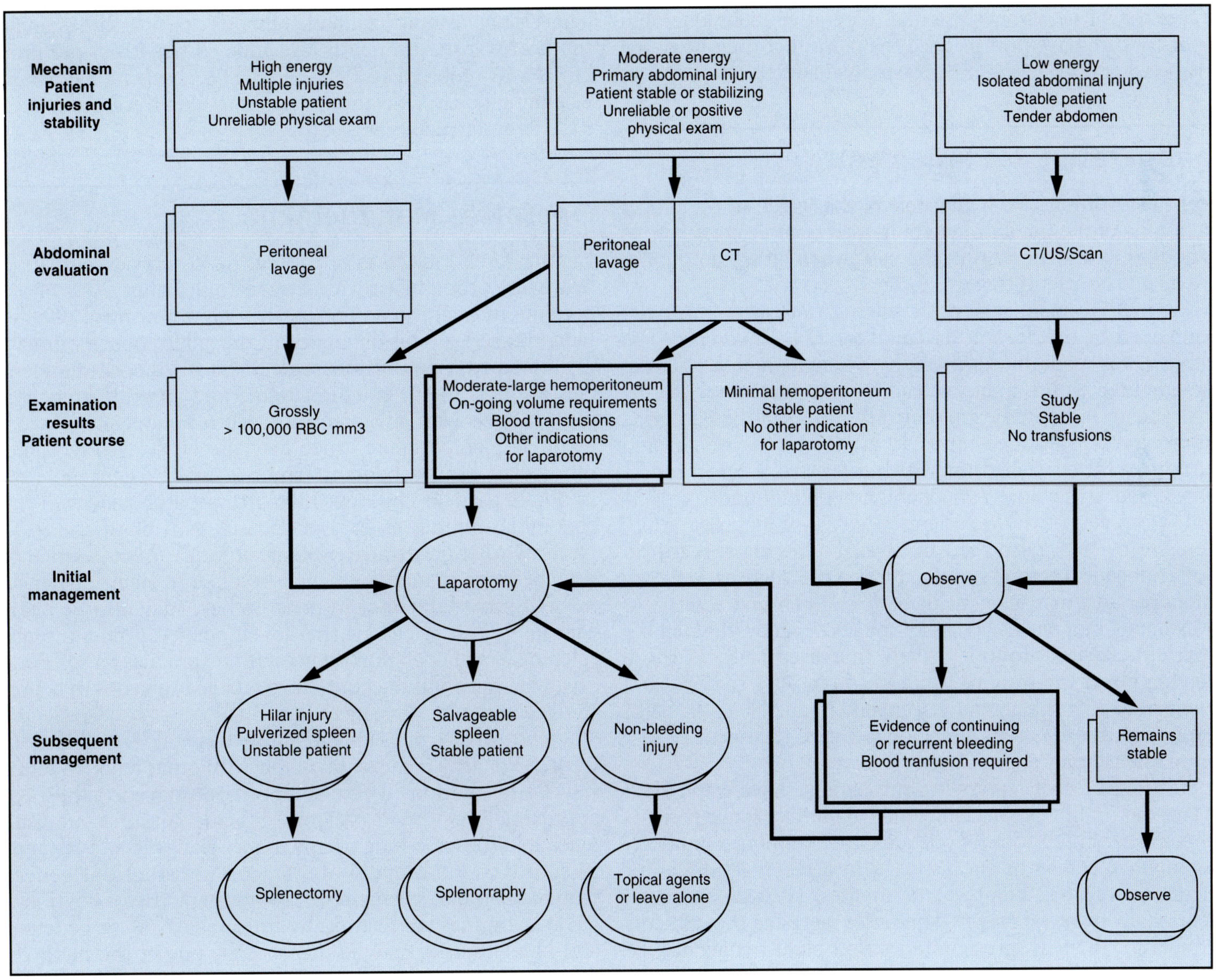

FIGURE 8.9 Flow chart for decisions in the management of splenic injuries.

comitant injuries should be completed if the patient is stable; otherwise, immediate laparotomy should be performed. If the patient is unstable, type-specific blood should be administered rather than waiting for completely crossmatched blood. Patients who have been hypotensive at any time in their course should have at least two large, secure intravenous lines and a Foley catheter in place. If laparotomy is planned, prophylactic antibiotics are administered preoperatively in the event that attendant gastrointestinal tract injury is found.

Renal injury is frequently associated with splenic trauma, and a urinalysis should be obtained to check for hematuria. However, since 20% of patients with renal injuries may not have blood in the urine, an intravenous pyelogram should be performed if there is a strong suspicion of renal injury. If emergency operation precludes obtaining this study before exploration, it may be obtained on the operating table if a large retroperitoneal hematoma is found. Operative techniques and supportive care have now reached the point that the care of the patient (adult or pediatric) must be individualized.

Nonoperative Management

Recent recognition of the vital role of the spleen in the proper functioning of the immune system has led to more conservative methods of treatment than in the past, when all spleen injuries were treated by splenectomy.

Nonoperative management of splenic trauma was initially championed by the Toronto Hospital for Sick Children.[61] The diagnosis was made by scintigraphy or angiography; children were admitted to the intensive care unit for observation using both repeated physical examinations and serial hematocrits. Children were transfused up to 40 ml/kg of body weight and maintained on strict bedrest with nasogastric suction for 72 hours. Under this policy, 70% of children did not undergo operation. However, of those patients who did require operation, splenectomy was performed in 80%. Following this initial report, subsequent studies have confirmed the safety and efficacy of nonoperative management in both children and adults.[22,63] For example, in a recent update of the above study, the number of patients treated nonoperatively increased to 87%, those receiving blood transfusions decreased from 36% to 23%, and patients requiring splenectomy decreased from 24% to 4%.[48] In addition, splenic function after nonoperative treatment of segmental splenectomy appears to be preserved.[16]

Increasingly, recent reports in adult patients have emphasized the fact that in highly selected hemodynamically stable patients without other indications for operative intervention, a nonoperative approach may be successful.[60] In a recent multicenter experience with 832 blunt splenic injuries, 112 were managed intentionally by observation.[9] This series suggested that patients with Class I, II, or III splenic injuries after blunt trauma may be candidates for nonoperative treatment if there is (1) no hemodynamic instability after initial fluid resuscitation; (2) no serious associated intra-abdominal injury, and (3) no extra abdominal condition which precludes assessment of the abdomen, e.g. head injury or need for general anesthesia. Failure rates were significantly lower in younger patients (2% versus 17%, $p<0.05$). Patients with low impact, focal left upper quadrant trauma[29] and low Injury Severity Scores may also fare better.[50] These patients are managed in the Surgical Intensive Care Unit on complete bedrest with close monitoring by repeated physical examinations and serial hematocrits. An empiric 4–6 week period of convalescence with reduced activity for 3 months has been recommended. An alternative view is presented in another recent study which reported that delayed operation diminishes the chance for splenorrhaphy, and a greater splenic salvage rate could be achieved by immediate operation with splenorrhaphy.[43]

Splenic conservation (either nonoperative or splenorrhaphy) may require blood transfusion. Recognition of transfusion associated risks have prompted one author[42] to suggest that when greater than 2 units of blood are transfused, the relative mortality risks of transfusion and post-splenectomy sepsis are equivalent. Using a conditional probability model, a recent estimate of the post-transfusion death rate (due to hepatitis) per unit of blood was reported to be 0.14%. The death rate from overwhelming post-splenectomy sepsis in children was calculated at 0.052% and in adults at 0.026%.[30]

Operative Management

Despite careful selection of patients for conservative treatment, however, other institutions have found that 70% of adult patients ultimately require laparotomy for control of splenic hemorrhage.[4,32] This difference in the adult population may be attributed to a proportionate decrease in smooth muscle and elastic fibers in the splenic capsule and around parenchymal blood vessels with advancing age. With nonoperative management of splenic rupture, there may also be delayed recognition of associated intra-abdominal injuries, which occur more often in adults than in children. Livingston found associated intra-abdominal injuries in 48% of patients with blunt and 92% of patients with penetrating splenic injuries. They warned that nonoperative management may result in a high incidence of missed intra-abdominal injuries.[28]There may also be delayed rupture of the spleen or the development of post-traumatic splenic cysts. If operation is necessary, techniques for splenorrhaphy and segmental resection have enabled surgeons to conserve the spleen in many instances (Fig. 8.10).

Splenic salvage rates in community hospitals (Level II Trauma Centers) of 38% compare favorably with other reported series in Level I institutions where splenorrhaphy is accomplished in approximately 50% of patients.[37] Grade I injuries are usually amenable to hemostatic agents alone; grades II and III injuries to suture or mesh enclosure; grade IV disruptions generally require anatomic splenic resection for hemorrhage control; and grade V injuries are technically irreparable.[49] Both penetrating and blunt injuries may be managed by one of the methods of splenic preservation with a minimum of postoperative morbidity,[14] but experience is an important factor in accomplishing a successful splenorrhaphy.

A midline incision is generally selected for rapid access and ready ability to deal with associated injuries identified at the time of laparotomy (Fig. 8.11). If the patient is hemodynamical-

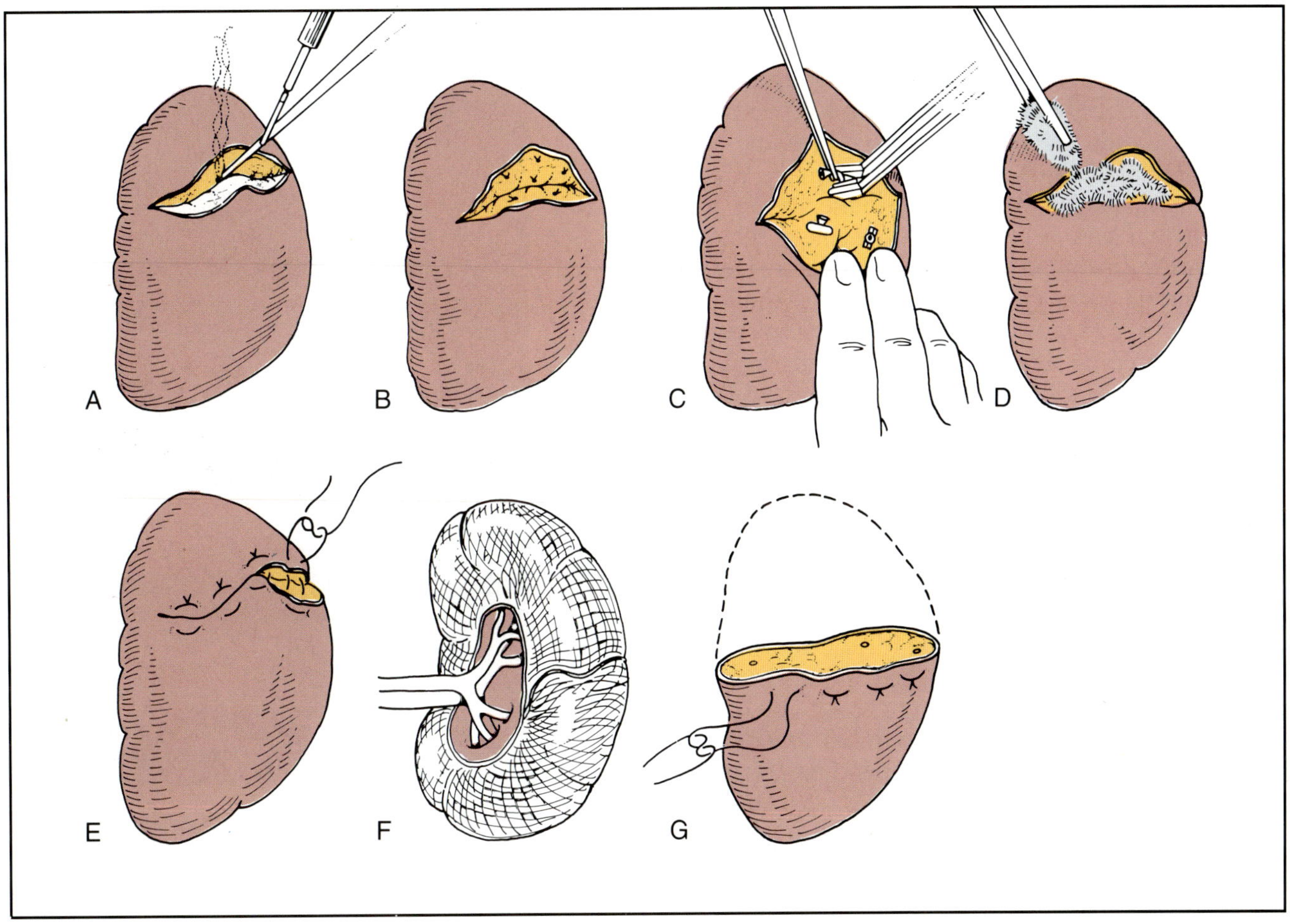

FIGURE 8.10 Techniques for splenorrhaphy. **A** Application of the electrocautery. **B** Suture ligation of the parenchymal vessels. **C** Application of hemoclips to the bleeding vessels. **D** Microfibrillar collagen applied to the splenic laceration. **E** Mattress suture closure of the splenic capsule. **F** Absorbable polyglycolic acid mesh wrap of the injured spleen. **G** Hemisplenectomy.

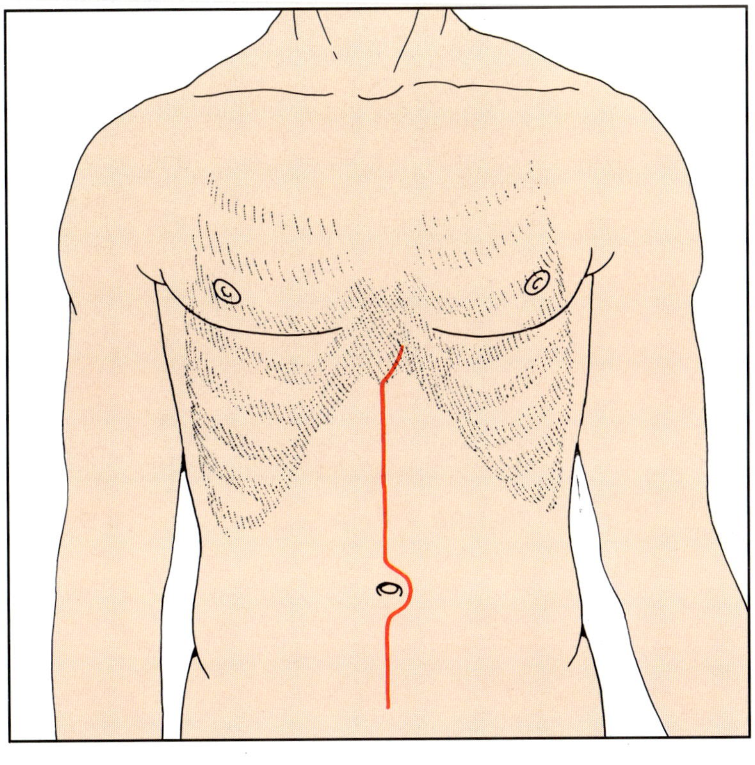

FIGURE 8.11 Midline incision for a splenectomy.

ly unstable, the first priority is to stop the bleeding and control shock. In patients with blunt trauma, for example, bleeding from the liver may need to be controlled before splenectomy is done, if the spleen is not the source of active bleeding. One must be aware that a large retroperitoneal hematoma in the left upper abdomen is more likely to be from the kidney or the aorta than from the spleen. Figure 8.12 *A* shows the spleen removed from a young man following a motorcycle accident. He was rushed to the operating room with hypotension after the initial resuscitation. Figure 8.12 *B* shows that although the spleen was fragmented, life-threatening hemorrhage was coming from the fractured kidney. The extent of his hypotension precluded any attempt at nonoperative management of the renal trauma. Splenectomy was obviously more appropriate than an attempt at splenic salvage, both because of his instability and because an initial, quick splenectomy improved access to the kidney.

After controlling the hemorrhage, the next priority is to stop peritoneal soiling from any wounds of the gastrointestinal tract. Packs, Allis forceps, or running, locked absorbable sutures may be used for temporary control, depending on the number and magnitude of injuries and the stability of the patient. Finally, all injuries must be located and treated appropriately. The operating surgeon must be satisfied that the number and type of wounds correlate with the mechanism of wounding before the abdomen is closed.

Operative Technique

The operative technique depends to some extent on the status of bleeding from the spleen, and a qualified assistant should be present if the patient is unstable. If there is brisk arterial bleeding, the injury usually involves the pedicle, and the first step is to control the bleeding manually. Using both hands, one retracts the gastric cardia medially, slightly caudally, and against the spine and the splenic flexure of the colon downwards; this maneuver allows the operator to see the area of bleeding, assess the status of the splenic parenchyma, and plan the method of controlling the bleeding.

If the spleen is somewhat mobile or has been partially mobilized by blunt trauma, there may be enough room to pass the flat of the left hand behind the spleen. If so, the thumb is brought anteriorly so that the pedicle can be compressed between the thumb and fingers. It may be necessary, however, to use the right hand for additional mobilization of the spleen by blunt dissection posterior to the spleen, after which the left hand is used for pressure to free the right hand for dissection. Should the bleeding be from arterial branches in the hilum, the lesser omental sac in the area can be opened to give best access to the upper aspect of the body of the pancreas, which is often in the thin, avascular omentum along the lesser curvature of the stom-

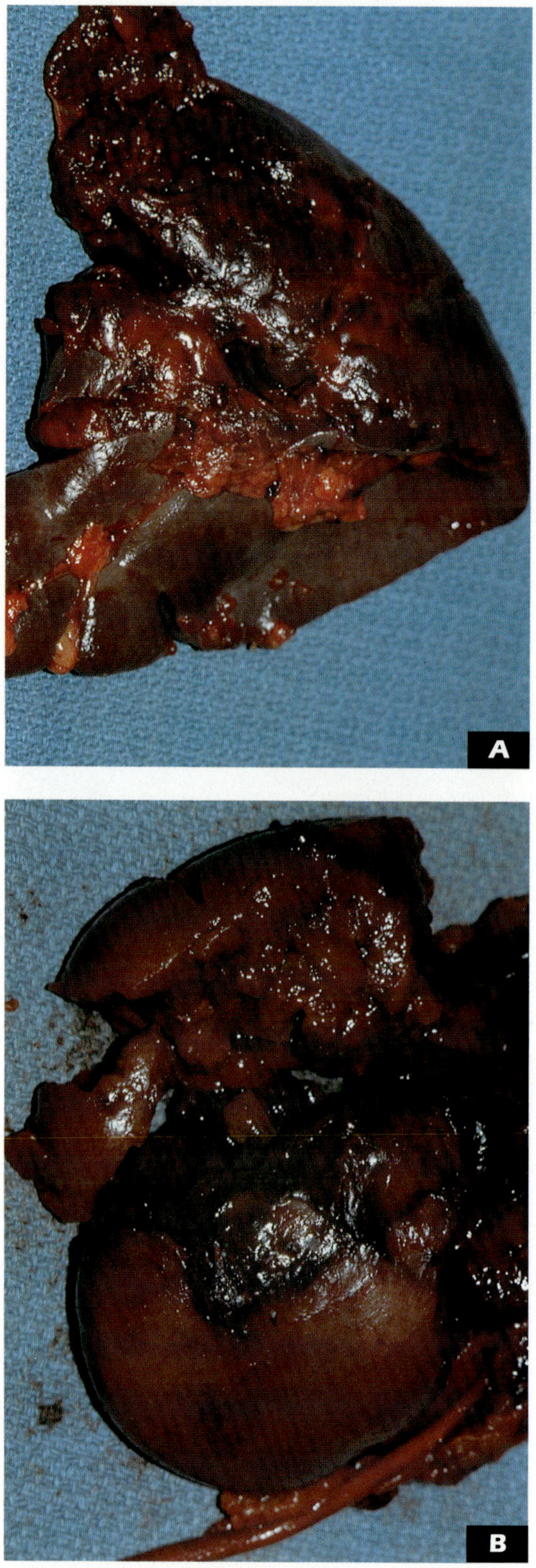

FIGURE 8.12 A Ruptured spleen. **B** Fractured kidney.

ach. This maneuver allows manual compression of the splenic artery in its course along the cephalad portion of the pancreas. The artery can then be traced distally and ligated near the tail of the pancreas, thus controlling exsanguinating hemorrhage and freeing the operator for the proper dissection of the spleen. These maneuvers are used only when it is necessary to control brisk bleeding, which is relatively uncommon in splenectomy for trauma. They are understood more easily by the surgeon with a thorough knowledge of the attachments of the spleen and experience in splenectomies and in visualizing these attachments, because the variability in size and position of the spleen and pancreas make it impossible to give dogmatic rules for every case. Approaching the splenic artery as it courses above the tail of the pancreas, for example, is best done in some patients by entering the lesser sac through the greater omentum at the midpoint of the greater curvature of the stomach, but in other patients through the lesser omentum medial to the lesser curve. This technique should be known to all surgeons managing splenic trauma, although it is rarely used. Manual compression is the quickest and most useful method for control of bleeding, and should not involve the application of clamps except where easy and obvious.

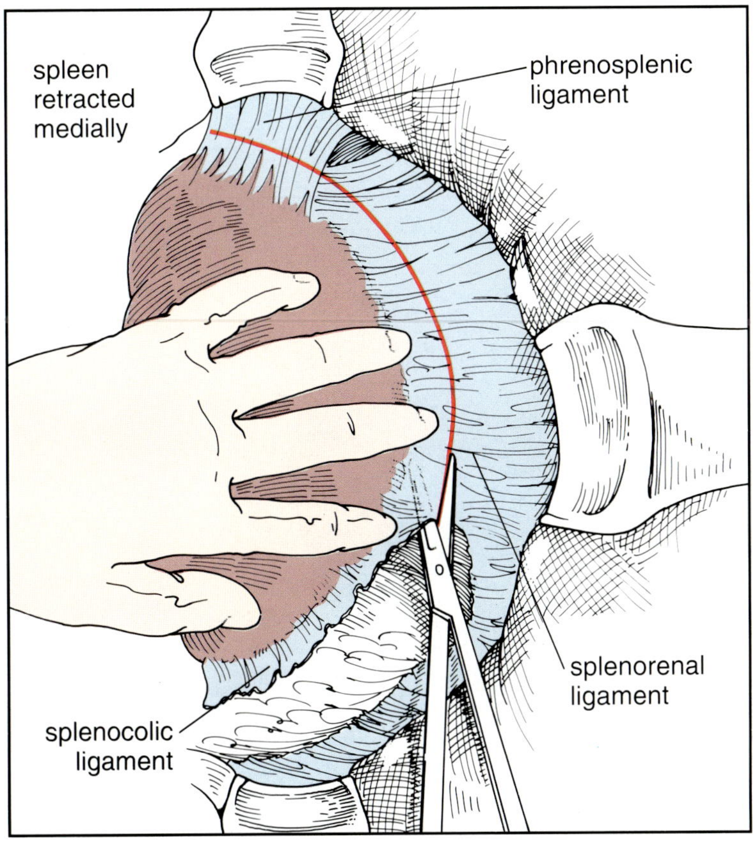

FIGURE 8.13 Initial mobilization of the spleen from its bed.

Once splenic hemorrhage is controlled, one should assess the anatomical relationships of the spleen, pancreas, stomach, omentum, and splenic flexure. At that point, a preliminary decision to preserve or remove the spleen should be made and operative dissection planned. The details of our method are outlined in the following paragraphs.

A self-retaining retractor secured to the table (such as the Bookwalter or upper hand) is applied to provide optimal visualization of the left upper quadrant. With the left hand, the stomach is gently retracted toward the right and clot evacuated from the region of the spleen.

Once the surgeon has ascertained that the spleen has been injured, and that there is active bleeding, mobilization of the spleen from its bed is essential in performance of any of the techniques described here. Nonbleeding injuries may be managed by topical agents or left alone. The spleen is cupped in the left hand and gently retracted toward the patient's right. An incision is made in the peritoneum lateral to the spleen with Metzenbaum scissors and the incision lengthened to parallel the longitudinal axis of the spleen (Fig. 8.13). If this incision is made too close to the spleen, capsular stripping may occur and increase the extent of injury and even preclude the possibility of repair. If there are attachments of the lower pole to the greater omentum, it may be preferable to divide these prior to mobilization of the spleen, or additional trauma may be incurred. It may also be necessary to divide the lowermost vasa brevia before mobilization, especially if the gastrosplenic ligament is short.

Once the peritoneum has been incised, gentle blunt dissection is begun with the fingers of the right hand posterior to the spleen. As the dissection proceeds medially, the left hand is cupped over the superior pole of the spleen and draws it downward and medially, toward the right iliac crest. This maneuver exposes the peritoneal attachments to the lateral aspect of the upper pole of the spleen so that they can be cut. If the line of this incision follows the curve of the upper pole of the spleen, there is less tendency to tear the splenic capsule at the junction of the upper pole with the body of the spleen. After this incision is carried beyond the highest peritoneal attachment of the spleen, the gentle downward and medial traction will free the spleen, the tail of the pancreas, and the lateral aspect of the stomach, allowing them to be brought up into the wound where the entire surface of the spleen can be examined and injuries treated. Gentle, steady traction is the key; undue traction will tear the splenic capsule or veins.

A Frazier tip or Poole tip suction without the guard is very helpful in providing clear exposure of the raw splenic surface. Bleeding from capsular avulsions may be controlled by high voltage electrocautery, arcing the current to the splenic surface, or by applying the cautery to the suction tip or forceps as they are touched to the surface of the spleen. The argon beam coagulator may also be useful in these situations. Microcrystalline collagen is particularly useful for controlling oozing from raw, wet surfaces, and its effectiveness is dependent upon platelet trapping and activation. It may be applied with blunt forceps in powder form or in a sheet. Pressure should then be applied with a dry sponge, which is held in place for 5 minutes. Microfibrillar collagen may be difficult to control, and some authors have recommended a "sandwich" or "cigarette" technique using oxidized cellulose as the outer layer and the microfibrillar collagen as the inner layer.[52] Topical thrombin, provided as a powder, should be reconstituted and then applied as a liquid to the bleeding surface; a spray applicator may also be helpful. Oxidized cellulose is an additional hemostatic agent that may be useful, and fibrin glue surface activation or intraparenchymal injection may result in effective control of surface oozing.[25] Fine vascular suture (5-0 or 6-0) may be used to reapproximate the margins of minor parenchymal disruptions.

In the treatment of more extensive splenic injuries, initial control of the vascular pedicle may be helpful. The most satisfactory control may be achieved by wide exposure through the gastrocolic omentum. A vessel loop should be doubly passed around the splenic artery (Fig. 8.14). No attempt should be made to isolate the vein during splenorrhaphy as it is unnecessary and easily results in injuries. Vascular control can most easily be achieved, however, by manual compression of the vessels in the hilum of the spleen, and if complex splenic repairs are not contemplated, this method will usually suffice. Hematomas should be evacuated from deeper parenchymal lacerations and vessels controlled using hemoclips, cautery, or suture, followed by reapproximation of the capsule with 3-0 absorbable suture in a horizontal vertical mattress or a running locked stitch. Cautery applied to the needle may reduce parenchymal bleeding at the site of passage through the tissue, and packing of lacerations with microfibrillar collagen or omentum may be helpful. Some prefer to use chromic catgut for closure of the capsule because it has some elasticity and less drag in tissue, but application of electrosurgical current to the needle detaches the catgut.

More extensive lacerations or segmental hilar injuries require partial splenectomy, oriented along the transverse planes of the internal vascular architecture of the spleen (Fig. 8.15). The best estimate of the splenic mass necessary to ensure protection against infection is about 30% of the spleen.[20] Once initial control of the main splenic artery has been obtained, individual ligation of segmental arterial branches can be performed. For injuries to the superior pole, the superior polar artery should be ligated and divided. Similarly, for lower pole injuries, the appropriate segmental vessels should be tied. The vessels selected for ligation will depend upon the branching of the splenic artery, the nature of the traumatic injury, and the extent of resection planned.

Ligation of segmental arteries results in almost immediate demarcation of the parenchyma, and incision may then be made through

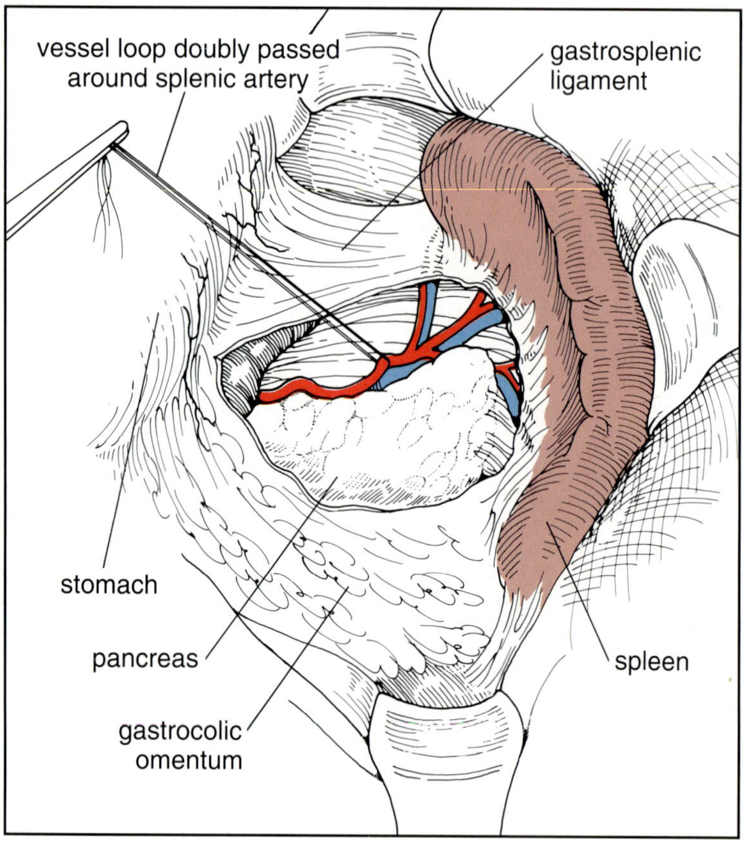

FIGURE 8.14 Control of the splenic artery in the lesser sac.

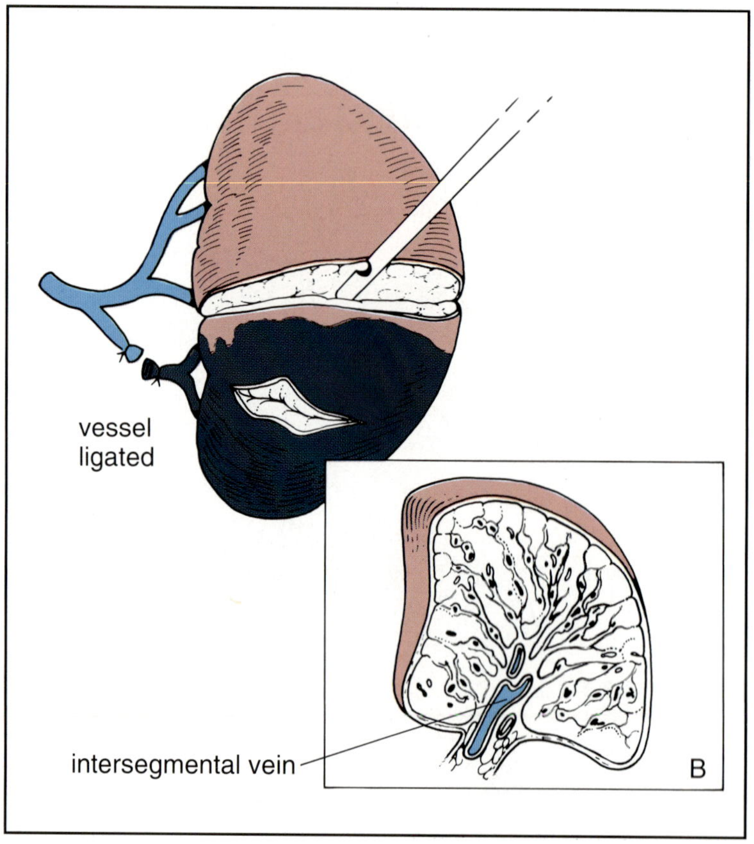

FIGURE 8.15 Technique for segmental splenectomy.

the capsule and into the superficial parenchyma. The plane of dissection should gradually be advanced through the splenic parenchyma using the knife handle, a dissecting peanut sponge, or the suction tip. Vessels should be clipped and divided. The large veins found in the intersegmental planes should be preserved.

After completion of transection of the splenic parenchyma, remaining small arterial "bleeders" should be clipped or oversewn with 4-0 or 5-0 arterial suture in a figure-of-eight fashion. Some bleeding from venous tributaries may persist because of slitlike defects in the wall of the vessel; these defects may be closed with a running vascular suture. Although the parenchyma has very little substance, bites taken securely in the vessel wall will hold. Any remaining oozing from the cut surface of the spleen is due to sinusoidal bleeding, which may be controlled with microfibrillar collagen. Through-and-through parenchymal sutures should be placed only if hemostasis is incomplete.[40] A 2-0 chromic catgut suture on a straight needle may be used or sutures placed using the technique described by Lynn,[6] wherein a number 20 spinal needle is passed through perpendicular to the plane of transection or injury, cauterized, and a 3-0 absorbable suture threaded through it. The sutures are then tied together at each end. It is unnecessary to reapproximate the margins of the splenic capsule. Mattress sutures may be tied over pledgets of Teflon felt, absorbable gelatin sponge, or oxidized cellulose to minimize cutting through the tissue. Buttressing of repairs and resections with omentum has also been described, and free peritoneal grafts may also be used to aid in hemostasis. If a choice exists as to which remnant can be preserved, the upper pole is considered more suitable, since it lies anatomically in the left upper quadrant against the undersurface of the diaphragm.

The recent development of prepackaged absorbable polyglycolic acid mesh may improve splenic salvage by tamponade of bleeding from large surface areas or deeper parenchymal injuries.[26] Although some authors have reported ligation of the main splenic artery just proximal to its terminal bifurcation,[30] this technique is not recommended because it may result in impairment of the normal phagocytic function of the spleen. Splenic infarction manifested by pain and fever has been reported with patients subsequently requiring splenectomy. It is estimated that approximately 6% of patients will have inadequate collateral, and patients who have had extensive mobilization of the spleen are not candidates for this procedure.

Splenorrhaphy is contraindicated in patients with multiple injuries who are unstable, or who show extensive devascularization or fragmentation of the spleen. In these instances, splenectomy is indicated. The initial mobilization of the spleen is similar to that described for splenorrhaphy. The splenic vessels are then sequentially clamped, divided, and secured individually with suture ligatures of 2-0 and 3-0 silk (Fig. 8.16).

Ligating large masses of tissue saves little time, provides insecure hemostasis, and has the potential for injuring adjacent

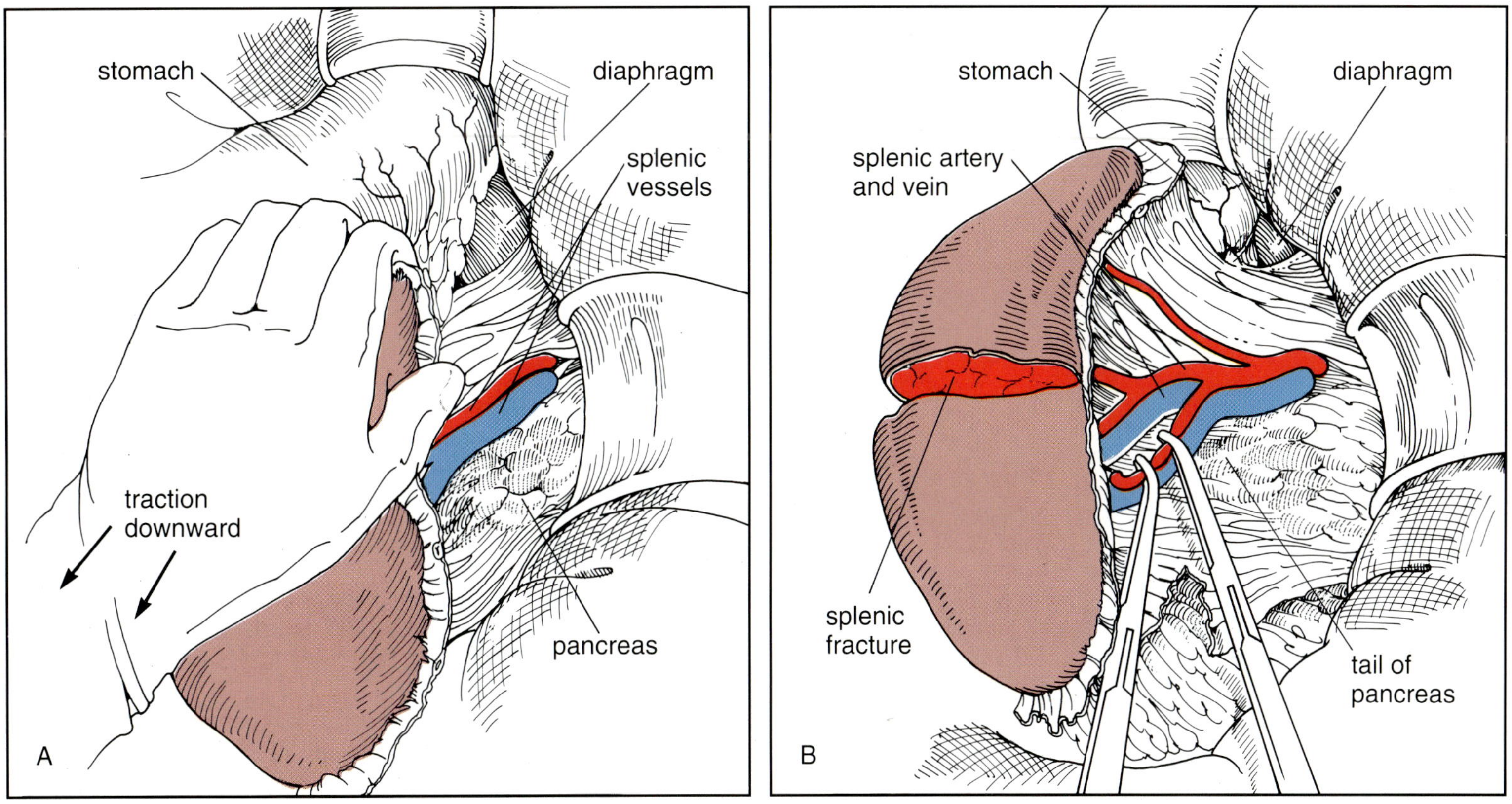

FIGURE 8.16 Technique for emergency splenectomy. **A** Left hand draws down and medially to free spleen, tail of pancreas, and stomach for examination. **B** Clamping and division of splenic vessels in the splenic hilum.

organs. The tail of the pancreas is within 1 cm of the splenic hilum in approximately 15% of patients, and one can determine whether or not the pancreatic capsule is intact at the end of the case by simple inspection, providing mass ligatures on the splenic hilum have not been used. The stomach is another organ that may be injured by improper ligature technique. When one dissects the short gastric vessels, for example, there is a tendency to place the hemostats at the borders of free tissue, leaving the skeletonized vessels between the clamps for ease in cutting. Placing a ligature on the full thickness of the gastric wall can cause necrosis and a postoperative gastric fistula (Fig. 8.17). The greater curvature of the stomach should always be examined before closure to ensure that this error has not been made. At the conclusion of the procedure, the ligatures in the tail of the pancreas should also be re-examined for hemostasis. A folded laparotomy sponge placed in the left upper quadrant and rolled up, out, and over the splenic bed will aid in identifying any source of continued bleeding.

Patients who have been hypotensive and have received large volumes of blood and fluid often have a coagulopathy, and drainage is frequently considered. It should not be used as a replacement for inadequate hemostasis, however. Whereas unnecessarily slow techniques are to be avoided in these patients, secure hemostasis is generally a benefit that outweighs the risk of any extra time required to obtain it. If there is persistent oozing or if there is concern over injury to the tail of the pancreas, closed suction drainage of the left upper quadrant is performed. Drains should be removed as soon as drainage ceases or by the fifth postoperative day to avoid subphrenic infection.[45]

In an attempt to preserve splenic function, some authors have recommended reimplantation of splenic fragments. In the omental pouch technique described by Williams, two or three cross sections of tissue are harvested from the central portion of the spleen. These should be approximately 3 mm thick, with a total weight of about 20 g. The omentum is spread out on the abdominal wall and then folded back on itself and sutured along its edges to form a pocket. The splenic slices are then placed side by side in the pocket and additional sutures close it. The omentum is then replaced in the abdomen.[47]

Implantation of these slices in the omentum preserves the sinusoidal architecture of the spleen and maintains its portal circulation, which may be important for function. These fragments are visible on a later splenic scan, and phagocytic functions of the spleen do appear to return. However, their ability to protect against the development of postsplenectomy sepsis is unproven.

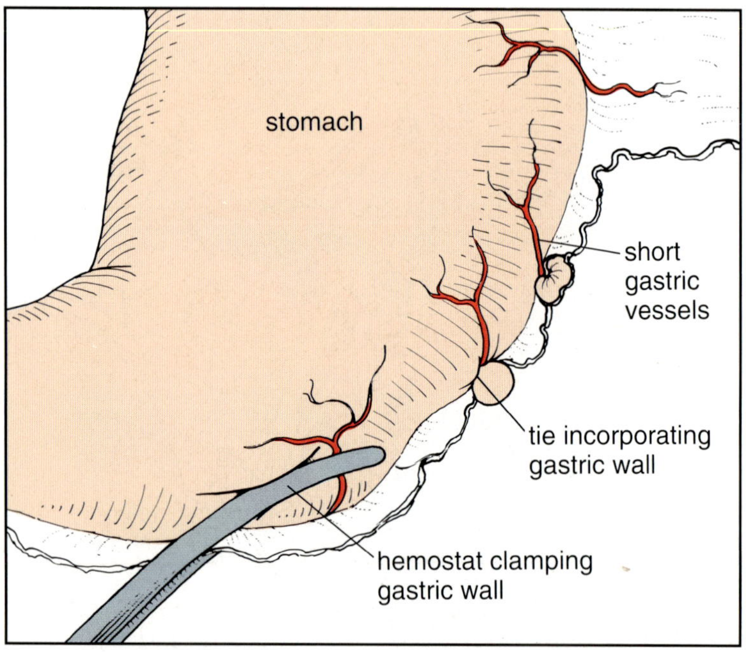

FIGURE 8.17 Ligatures or clamps placed incorrectly cause injury to the gastric wall during splenectomy.

Postoperative Management

Routine postoperative care should be provided. A careful intake and output record is kept, and maintenance fluid requirements administered. Nasogastric suction is continued until bowel function returns and the patient passes flatus. The presence of multiple injuries may prolong the duration of postoperative ileus. In the absence of other injuries, early ambulation is encouraged.

The most common complication following splenectomy is persistent intra-abdominal bleeding. Re-exploration may be required if bleeding persists after clotting studies return to normal. One cannot overemphasize the importance of obtaining hemostasis during the initial operation, especially in multiply injured patients. Morbidity is increased if re-exploration is required.

Devascularization of the greater curvature of the stomach may be catastrophic and may result in subphrenic abscess and gastric fistula. Plication of the greater curvature has been recommended to reduce this complication,[18] but it is best to prevent it by careful technique when dividing the short gastric vessels. Pancreatitis may occur due to operative manipulation or direct trauma and can usually be managed nonoperatively with nasogastric suction and hyperalimentation. Infectious complications may also be increased in these patients.

Patients who have undergone splenectomy or sustained massive splenic injury are at risk of developing postsplenectomy sepsis and should receive immunization with Pneumovax. Currently available vaccines provide protection against 85-90% of pneumococcal isolates. However, impaired IgM and IgG responses identified using enzyme-linked immunosorbent assay (ELISA) testing in splenectomized patients reveal diminished response to antigenic challenge, and the vaccines may not be completely protective.[19] *Hemophilus influenzae* vaccine (type B) and meningococcal vaccines should be added to the prophylactic regimen of splenectomized children 18 months or older. Revaccination may be required.[21] Asplenic patients respond well to antigens administered by the subcutaneous route; those receiving vaccine within 72 hours of splenectomy have a response equal to that of control patients.[7] Because of the high incidence of reactions following revaccination, only an initial vaccination is currently recommended.[10] Ampicillin prophylaxis is recommended for children less than 4 years of age and penicillin for those older than 4 years. However, use of long-term prophylactic antibiotics may lead to the development of resistant organisms. We recommend that all patients be told of the signs and symptoms of post-splenectomy infection and be advised that they should see their physician immediately for any febrile illness, at which time they should be thoroughly evaluated and administered antibiotics.

Following splenectomy for trauma, some patients may develop splenosis, wherein splenic fragments that have become implanted in the peritoneal cavity undergo enlargement. However, these implants are incapable of restoring total splenic function.[27] The amount of splenic tissue and the circulatory pattern to these segments are important factors in the prevention of postsplenectomy infection.

The thrombocytosis following splenectomy is thought to predispose the patient to an increased risk of thrombotic complications, and some authors advocate the use of aspirin or low-dose heparin for prophylaxis.[58] Intraoperative use of pneumatic compression boots might also be considered, but there are no prospective studies to show the efficacy of either technique.

Finally, the patient must understand that the end of the acute phase of the trauma is the beginning of a much longer phase requiring increased, but not neurotic, attention to his health. If a splenectomy was done, the patient must be educated about reasonable attention to the possibility of infections. If splenic salvage was done, periodic evaluations should be made for late complications of these procedures. In either case, if the patient received blood, he should be evaluated for the development of hepatitis and for other complications associated with homologous transfusion.

REFERENCES

1. Alyono D, Morrow CE, Perry JF: Reappraisal of diagnostic peritoneal lavage criteria for operation in penetrating and blunt trauma. Surgery 92:751–757, 1982
2. Austrian R: Prevention of fatal bacterial infection in patients with anatomical or functional asplenia. Ann Intern Med 96:117–119, 1982
3. Awe WC, Eidemiller L: Selective angiography in splenic trauma. Am J Surg 126:171–175, 1973
4. Bitseff EL, Adkins RB: Splenic trauma: A trial at selective management. South Med J 77:1286–1290, 1984
5. Buntain WL, Gould HR, Maull KI: Predictability of splenic salvage by computed tomography. J Trauma 28(1):24–34, 1988
6. Buntain WL, Lynn HB: Splenorrhaphy: Changing concepts for the traumatized spleen. Surgery 86:748–760, 1979
7. Caplan ES, Boltansky H, Snyder MJ et al: Response of traumatized splenectomized patients to immediate vaccination with polyvalent pneumococcal vaccine. J Trauma 23:801–805, 1983
8. Chen L: Microcirculation of the spleen: An open or closed circulation? (abstr) Science 201:157, 1978
9. Cogbill TH, Moore EE, Jurkovich GJ, et al: Nonoperative management of blunt splenic trauma: a multicenter experience. J Trauma 29(10):1312–1317, 1989
10. Committee on Immunization: Council of Medical Societies Guide for Adult Immunization, p 69. Philadelphia, American College of Physicians, 1985
11. Conti S: Splenic artery ligation for trauma: An alternative to splenectomy. Am J Surg 140:444–446, 1980
12. Eichner HR: Splenic function: Normal, too much and too little. Am J Med 66:311–320, 1979
13. Federle MP, Griffiths B, Minagi H, et al: Splenic trauma: evaluation with CT. Radiology 162:69–71, 1987
14. Feliciano DV, Bitondo CG, Mattox KL, et al: A four-year experience with splenectomy versus splenorrhaphy. Ann Surg 201(5):568–575, 1985
15. Fitzgerald JB, Crawford ES, DeBakey ME: Surgical considerations of non-penetrating abdominal injuries: An analysis of 200 cases. Am J Surg 100:22–29, 1960
16. Goldthorn JF, Schwartz AD, Swift AJ, et al: Protective effect of residual splenic tissue after subtotal splenectomy. J Pediatr Surg 13:587–590, 1978
17. Harrison HR, Fulginiti VA: Bacterial immunizations. Am J Dis Child 134:184–193, 1980
18. Harrison BF, Glanges E, Sparkman RS: Gastrin fistula following splenectomy: Its causes and prevention. Ann Surg 185:210–213, 1977
19. Hosea SW, Burch CG, Brown EJ, et al: Impaired immune response in splenectomized patients to polyvalent pneumococcal vaccine. Lancet 1:804–807, 1981
20. Justicz AG, Skandalakis TN, Skandalakis LJ: Management of Splenic Trauma in Adults. In Nyhus LM, Skandalakis JE, Gray SW, eds. Problems in General Surgery—The Spleen. Philadelphia, JB Lippincott, pp.135, 1990
21. Kafidi KT, Rotschafer JC: Bacterial vaccines for splenectomized patients. Drug Intell and Clin Pharm 22:192–197, 1988
22. Kakkasseril J, Stewart D, Dox J et al: Changing treatment of pediatric splenic trauma. Arch Surg 117:758–759, 1982
23. King DR, Lobe TE, Haase GM, et al: Selective management of injured spleen. Surgery 90:677–682, 1981
24. King H, Shumacker HB: Splenic studies: I. Susceptibility to infection after splenectomy performed in infancy. Ann Surg 136:239, 1952
25. Kram HB, DelJunco T, Clark SR, et al: Techniques of splenic preservation using fibrin glue. J Trauma 39(1):97–101, 1990
26. Lange DA, Zaret P, Merlotti GJ, et al: The use of absorbable mesh in splenic trauma. J Trauma 28(3):269–275, 1988
27. Livingston CD, Levine BA, Lecklitner ML et al: Incidence and function of residual splenic tissue following splenectomy for trauma in adults. Arch Surg 118:617–620, 1983
28. Livingston CD, Sirinek KR, Levine BA: Traumatic splenic injury: its management in a patient population with a high incidence of associated injury. Arch Surg 117:670–674, 1982
29. Longo WE, Baker CC, McMillen MA, et al: Nonoperative management of adult blunt splenic trauma: criteria for successful outcome. Ann Surg 210(5):626–629, 1989
30. Luna GK, Dellinger EP: Nonoperative observation therapy for splenic injuries: a safe therapeutic option? Am J Surg 153:462–468, 1987
31. Lutzker LG: Radionuclide imaging of the injured spleen and liver. Semin Nucl Med 13(3):184–198, 1983
32. Mahon PA, Sutton JE: Nonoperative management of adult splenic injury due to blunt trauma: A warning. Am J Surg 149:716–722, 1985
33. Malangoni MA, Levine AW, Droege EA et al: Management of injury to the spleen in adults. Ann Surg 200:702–705, 1984
34. McVay CB: The spleen. In McVay CB (ed): Surgical Anatomy, p 679. Philadelphia, W B Saunders, 1984
35. Meakins JL, Hohn DC, Simmons RL, et al: Host defenses. In Simmons RL, Howard RJ, eds. Surgical Infectious Diseases. Norwalk, CT. Appleton and Lange, pp. 659–680, 1988
36. Mirvis SE, Whitley NO, Gens DR: Blunt splenic trauma in adults: CT-based classification and correlation with prognosis and treatment. Radiology 171(1):33–39, 1989
37. Molin MR, Shackford SR: The management of splenic trauma in a trauma system. Arch Surg 125:840–843, 1990
38. Moore EE, Moore JB, Van DuzerMoore S, Thompson JS: Mandatory laparotomy for gunshot wounds penetrating the abdomen. Am J Surg 140:847–850, 1980
39. Moore EE, Shackford SR, Pachter HL, et al: Organ injury scaling:

40. Morgenstern L, Shapiro SJ: Techniques of splenic conservation. Arch Surg 114:449–454, 1979
41. Morgenstern L, Uyeda RY: Nonoperative management of injuries of the spleen in adults. Surg Gynecol Obstet 157:513–518, 1983
42. Mucha P, Daly RC, Farnell MB: Selective management of blunt splenic trauma. J Trauma 26(11):970–979, 1986
43. Nallathambi MN, Ivatury RR, Wapnir I, et al: Nonoperative management versus early operation for blunt splenic trauma in adults. Surg Gynecol Obstst 166:252–258, 1988
44. Naylor R, Coln D, Shires GT: Morbidity and mortality from injuries to the spleen. J Trauma 14:773, 1974
45. Olsen WR, Beaudoin DE: Wound drainage after splenectomy. Am J Surg 117:615–620, 1969
46. Olsen WR, Polley TZ: A second look at delayed splenic rupture. Arch Surg 112:422–425, 1977
47. Patel J, Williams J, Schmigel B, Hinshaw J: Preservation of splenic function by autotransplantation of traumatized spleen in man. Surgery 90:683–688, 1981
48. Pearl RH, Wesson DE, Spence LJ, et al: Splenic injury: a 5-year update with improved results and changing criteria for conservative management. J Pediatr Surg 24(1);121–125, 1989
49. Pickhardt B, Moore EE, Moore FA, et al: Operative splenic salvage in adults: a decade perspective. J Trauma 29(10):1386 –1391, 1989
50. Rappaport W, McIntyre KE, Carmona R: The management of splenic trauma in the adult patient with blunt multiple injuries. Surg Gynecol Obstet 170:204–208, 1990
51 Rosoff L, Cohen JL, Telfer N, Halpern M: Injuries of the spleen. Surg Clin North 52:667–684, 1972
52 Rush DS, Bivins BA: The avitene sandwich method for handling hemostatic agents. Surg Gynecol Obstet 154:729, 1982
53. Rutkow I: Rupture of the spleen in infectious mononucleosis: A critical review. Arch Surg 113:718–720, 1978
54. Schwartz SI: Spleen. In Schwartz SI (ed): Principles of Surgery, p 1446. New York, McGraw-Hill, 1989
55. Schwartz SI: The spleen. In Schwartz SI, Ellis H (eds): Maingot's Abdominal Operations, p 1671. Norwalk, CT, Appleton-Century-Crofts, 1989
56. Sherman R: Management of trauma to the spleen. Adv Surg 17:37–71, 1984
57. Singer DB: Postsplenectomy sepsis. Perspect Pediatr Pathol 1:285–311, 1973
58. Steele M, Lim RC: Advances in the management of splenic injuries. Am J Surg 130:159–165, 1975
59. Thal ER: Evaluation of peritoneal lavage and local exploration in lower chest and abdominal stab wounds. J Trauma 17:642–648, 1977
60. Villalba MR, Howells GA, Lucas RJ, et al: Nonoperative management of the adult ruptured spleen. Arch Surg 125:836–839, 1990
61. Wesson DE, Filler SG, Ein B et al: Ruptured spleen—When to operate? J Ped Surg 16:324–326, 1981
62. Zarrabi MH, Rosner F: Serious infections in adults following splenectomy for trauma. Intern Med 144:1421–1424, 1984
63. Zucker K, Browns K, Rossman D et al: Nonoperative management of splenic trauma. Arch Surg 119:400–404, 1984

gastrointestinal trauma

John J. Ferrara
P. William Curreri

During the acute stage of management, traumatic injury to the intra-abdominal alimentary canal (including pancreas) is rarely, in and of itself, a threat to either the patient's life or the viability of the damaged organ. Injury to neighboring structures such as spleen, liver, kidney, aorta, vena cava, and portal vein are more likely life-threatening. With a few notable exceptions, surgical correction of alimentary canal injuries can be accomplished with relative ease. In accordance with the principles of managing a patient with multiple organ injuries, correction of damage to the alimentary canal is usually deferred until initial control of life-threatening injuries has been completed. Despite the benign nature of alimentary canal trauma, diligent assessment of injury and sound surgical judgment are required in order to prevent unnecessary postoperative morbidity and mortality.

This chapter will present general perioperative principles utilized by the trauma service at the University of South Alabama Medical Center to manage patients suspected of sustaining an intra-abdominal injury. Specific care guidelines will be introduced for each blunt and penetrating injury of the alimentary canal organs: stomach, pancreas, duodenum, mesenteric small intestine, abdominal colon, and anorectum.

PERIOPERATIVE MANAGEMENT GUIDELINES

To the extent possible, pre-anesthetic hemodynamic stabilization of the patient using crystalloid and blood replacement is desirable, although it should not interfere with the overriding principle of surgical control of hemorrhage. A minimum of two large-bore (14-gauge) intravenous cannulae should be available to accomplish resuscitation. A urinary drainage catheter is inserted to monitor renal output and confirm the absence of hematuria. The risk of aspiration pneumonitis may be diminished by emptying the stomach of its contents by a large-bore gastric tube.

While characteristic signs of visceral perforation may be preoperatively identified (i.e., pneumoperitoneum on the chest roentgenograph), whether the alimentary canal has been violated is usually uncertain. It is well documented that in contaminated abdominal cases, surgical wound and infection rates are decreased when any of a variety of antibiotic regimens are preoperatively administered. Trauma victims should receive a preoperative dose of a moderately broad spectrum antibiotic (usually a cephalosporin); if no hollow visceral injury is identified, further antibiotic therapy is immediately discontinued.

Under most circumstances, at least one member of the surgical team is fully gowned and gloved prior to induction of anesthesia, prepared to intervene should the patient demonstrate signs of hemodynamic instability during administration of the anesthetic agents. Chest, abdomen, and groin are painted with tincture of iodine, and sterile drapes applied to ensure a wide field. A generous midline celiotomy is the preferred approach to the abdominal cavity, because it allows both maximal exposure and a quick, essentially bloodless plane of dissection. In addition, extension to the thorax may easily be accomplished by median sternotomy in order to expose the anterior heart, subdiaphragmatic liver, and retrohepatic vena cava. If gross hemoperitoneum is identified, the clot is rapidly evacuated and large laparotomy sponges are packed into each of the four quadrants. The entire abdomen is then inspected to assess the severity of organ injury.

As mentioned before, the priority of injury management is dictated by severity with respect to life and to subsequent viability of the injured organ. Repair of alimentary canal injury is often delayed, resulting in prolonged exposure of the abdominal cavity to bacterial, enzymatic, and particulate contamination. Unless time is of the essence, the abdomen should be irrigated with several liters of warm saline solution prior to fascial closure. With a few notable exceptions, the placement of "prophylactic" active or passive drainage systems in an attempt to drain the peritoneal cavity is rarely indicated. There has been little experimental evidence to refute John Yates's data, reported in 1905, upon which he concluded that "drainage of the peritoneal cavity is physically and physiologically impossible." Rather, there is a considerable body of clinical[43] and experimental[61] information that would suggest such attempts result in an increased incidence of wound and intra-abdominal infections, anastomotic dehiscence, and abscess formation.

Fascial closure may be safely achieved in a variety of ways. Experimental data suggest that the use of nonabsorbable sutures offers no additional wound closure security over absorbable material, and there is no difference in fascial dehiscence rates between continuous and interrupted suture techniques. These data are difficult to assess when there are so many factors in emergency surgery over which there is little control and that are associated with poor wound healing; examples include shock, bacterial contamination, age of patient, and coexistent illness. Proper, meticulous surgical technique is, however, quite controllable. Regardless of the method or material chosen, the completed closure should not take on the configuration of a parallel set of seams, with evenly spaced fascial purchases. Rather, there should be a staggered look to the closure so that the fascia cannot be weakened by suture penetration in the same plane throughout the length of the wound. Unless attempting to ease the tension of a tight abdominal closure, the addition of retention sutures is not necessary.

Subcutaneous tissues are not approximated over the fascial closure. Although it may be permissible to close the skin following repair of certain types of alimentary canal injuries, most wounds are left open and allowed to heal secondarily or closed 3 or 4 days after surgery (delayed primary closure) with interrupted cutaneous sutures.

GASTRIC TRAUMA

Blunt Gastric Injury

Injury to the stomach secondary to blunt forces is distinctly uncommon, owing in large part to the inherent strength of the gastric wall reinforced by a strong submucosa and three muscular coats. In addition, the stomach is naturally fixed in position solely by the pylorus and esophagus, thereby allowing considerable mobility. Protection of the adult stomach is afforded by the overlying rib cage and well-developed abdominal musculature. These features are less prominent in children, which may account for the increasing number of reports documenting blunt gastric injury in younger age groups.

The mechanism of injury is felt to be one of sudden gastric compression between the anterior parietes and vertebral column due to a sharp epigastric blow. Yajko, Seydel, and Trimble[112] have proposed that a sudden increase in either intraluminal or wall tension will cause rupture at the point of greatest radius, that is, the greater curvature of the stomach, in accordance with the law of Laplace. Although many injuries do occur in this region, injuries have been documented at virtually all topographical areas of the stomach. Other factors must be considered, such at fixation points at sites of weakness when stressed with shearing forces, regional differences in mural thickness, and the position of the stomach overlying the vertebral column at the time of injury.

The injury to the stomach may be of partial or full thickness. Experimental studies using canine stomachs exposed to blunt trauma[89] have shown that tears generally initiate in the seromuscular layer and are followed by mucosal injury. Ultimately, submucosal tears will occur. Clinical correlation is found in reports documenting several different types of gastric injury that resulted from blunt trauma in humans. These may be classified according to extent of mural damage, as follows:

Mucosal/submucosal lacerations
Devascularization injury
Perforations

Each injury has its own characteristic set of clinical manifestations, pertinent diagnostic tests, and management recommendations.

MUCOSAL/SUBMUCOSAL LACERATIONS

The stomach has a rich vascular supply reinforced with multiple anastomotic channels. Even a small laceration in the mucosa or submucosa may result in massive hemorrhage requiring prompt recognition and treatment in order to avert exsanguination. While hematemesis may be the presenting clinical feature, the diagnosis is typically considered when blood is seen in the aspirate of a gastric lavage tube inserted during the course of managing a blunt trauma victim. The likely source of bleeding in such circumstances is proximal to the stomach, the blood having been swallowed. A careful inspection of the face and oral cavity for signs of trauma must be undertaken. Iatrogenic injury may also be at fault, so endotracheal or nasogastric intubation should be checked. Hemorrhage from all but the most severe orofacial injuries usually ceases spontaneously or can be readily controlled; hence, the continued deglutition of blood is limited, if not prevented. Subsequent lavage of the stomach with room-temperature normal saline clears residual blood. A diagnostic gastric lavage is then performed using 250 ml of normal saline. Return of clear fluid rules out significant gastric injury; the presence of blood-tinged aspirate mandates further evaluation (Fig. 9.1).

If the patient remains hemodynamically stable, flexible esophagogastrodudenoscopy is indicated. Unless surgical intervention for concomitant injuries is contemplated, the procedure may be performed at the patient's bedside following the intravenous administration of meperidine and midazolam. A careful, thorough inspection of a maximally insufflated stomach is required. Lacerations may be small or hidden between the rugae; multiple tears are frequent. While most are found along the magenstrasse, Mallory-Weiss–type tears have been documented.

Not all lacerations require emergency surgical intervention.[96] A trial of nonoperative management for gastric mucosal tears is indicated either when nonbleeding lacerations alone are visualized or when no bleeding site is identified and there is no evidence of blood pooling within the stomach. Under these circumstances, a small-bore nasogastric tube is inserted and placed to institute gravity drainage. Diagnostic saline lavages are repeated at 4- to 6-hour intervals for 24 hours; if the aspirates remain free of blood, the nasogastric tube is removed and feedings begun when bowel functions return. Since lacerations may take 6 weeks to heal, some investigators recommend histamine-2 receptor antagonist therapy during this period, which would be discontinued once endoscopic documentation of healing has been achieved.

The indications for surgical intervention for mucosal/submucosal lacerations are:

Massive gastric hemorrhage with hemodynamic instability
Endoscopic visualization of an actively bleeding laceration
Endoscopic evidence of active blood pooling in the stomach despite the inability to visualize a specific bleeding point
Recurrent hemorrhage despite medical management

Two surgical approaches have been proposed. Harrison and Debas[34] place a noncrushing clamp across the midstomach from lesser to greater curvature, thereby dividing it into two compartments. A distal gastrotomy is made and clot evacuated. Using a sterile flexible endoscope, the stomach is inspected and bleeding points oversewn. A second gastrotomy is then made in the proximal compartment and the procedure repeated. While this approach has the advantage of having only two small gastric incisions, we feel that the urgency of the situation usually mandates a generous longitudinal midbody gastrotomy.

In a few instances, hemorrhage is not so massive as to preclude an attempt at intraoperative endoscopic localization of the bleeding site. In this instance, we prefer the standard peroral route immediately following gastric lavage, rather than the intraoperative procedure described above. After gastrotomy, all clot is evacuated and large moist sponges placed into the proximal and distal stomach. Distal sponges are removed initially, because most tears are found in this area. All lacerations are oversewn from within, using a running 2-0 or 3-0 absorbable suture placed at a depth necessary to incorporate both mucosal and submucosal layers. The distal stomach is then irrigated with normal saline to ensure that no sources of hemorrhage have been missed. The identical protocol is then repeated as the more proximal portion of the stomach is inspected. Once hemostasis has been achieved, the gastrotomy is closed with a running 2-0 absorbable suture for the inner layer, followed by an outer layer of interrupted 3-0 silk seromuscular Lembert sutures. External drains are not indicated for this specific injury. A nasogastric tube is positioned in the antrum to monitor the stomach for rebleeding and to decompress it until bowel function returns.

DEVASCULARIZATION INJURY

Ischemic necrosis of a segment of the gastric wall is an exceedingly rare complication of blunt abdominal trauma. It is far more likely that any force great enough to interrupt the vascular supply to a portion of the stomach wall will also cause coincidental gastric perforation. Nonetheless, the serious consequences of gastric devascularization injury are well documented[26] and underscore the necessity for aggressive surgical management once this condition is recognized. The clinical manifestations of gastric devascularization injury are dependent upon whether the diagnosis is made in the immediate postinjury period (when the gastric wall is merely ischemic), or several days following injury (when full-thickness, segmental gastric necrosis has become established).

The presence of bloody gastric aspirate without extragastric sources of bleeding (such as swallowed blood) should alert the clinician to the possibility of acute segmental gastric ischemia. The etiology of gastric bleeding is more likely due to mucosal or submucosal lacerations. The diagnosis of acute segmental gastric ischemia is typically unsuspected until emergency celiotomy is performed for blunt trauma. At that time, careful examination of the stomach wall reveals segmental pallor. This most often occurs along the greater curvature; a hallmark of injury at this site is avulsion of the gastroepiploic vessels. Should the diagnosis remain in question, peroral endoscopic examination is indicated, to search for areas devoid of gastric mucosa, corresponding to the areas of serosal pallor.

Treatment mandates aggressive debridement of nonviable as well as questionably viable segments. The resultant gastric defect is then tailored and closed in two layers. The mucosa and submucosa are approximated using a running 2-0 absorbable suture, and integrity of the stomach is re-established with a series of inter-

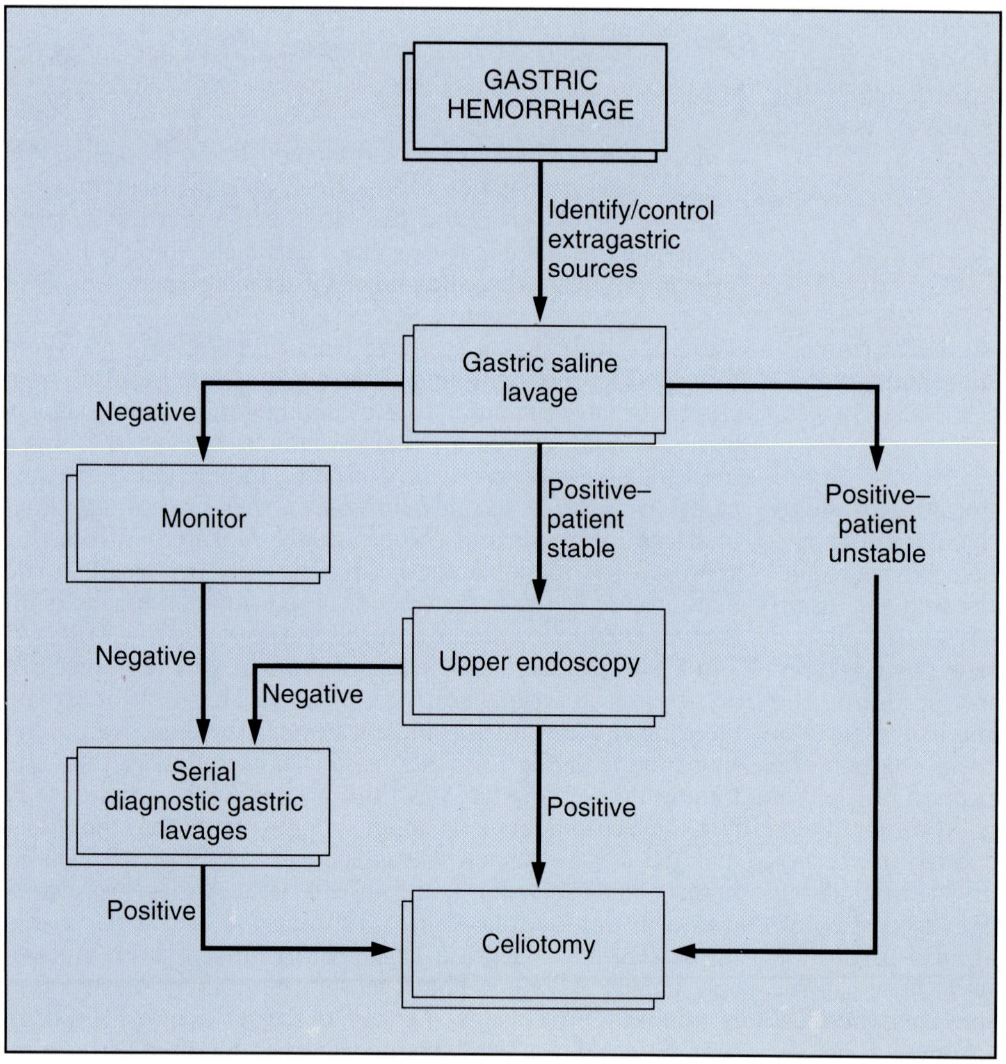

FIGURE 9.1 Management guidelines for a blunt trauma victim with signs or symptoms of gastric hemorrhage.

rupted 3-0 silk Lembert sutures. Because of the large surface area of the stomach, closure may be achieved without significantly narrowing its lumen. Placement of external drainage systems is not indicated. Nasogastric decompression is continued in the postoperative period until bowel function returns.

Failure to recognize or surgically manage acute segmental gastric ischemia will allow progression to full-thickness gastric necrosis. A pattern of intra-abdominal sepsis typically ensues several days postinjury, culminating in exploratory celiotomy. Alternatively, massive gastrointestinal hemorrhage from denuded vessels, situated along the line of demarcation between viable and nonviable gastric wall, may mandate emergency surgery. At operation the gastric segment will demonstrate obvious necrosis with associated perforation, abscess formation, and dense visceral adhesions. Again, aggressive debridement of the involved wall and closure of the defect must be performed exactly as described above. Placement of closed-system drainage devices in residual abscess cavities is recommended; postoperative gastric decompression is mandatory. Despite aggressive surgical management and intense perioperative care, the overall prognosis of these patients is poor.

PERFORATION

Perforation of the stomach is thought to occur in less than 1% of patients who undergo surgical intervention for suspected intra-abdominal injury secondary to blunt trauma.[15,112] Two types of perforation are described: partial transection, or rupture and complete gastric transection.

PARTIAL TRANSECTION

The more common injury is partial transection, which typically occurs in association with a stomach distended by a recently ingested meal.[11] Under these circumstances, a well-placed (often trivial) blow will compress the stomach enough to cause a blowout perforation—not unlike the results of suddenly compressing a blown-up balloon. While perforations of this type have been clinically described in virtually every anatomical area of the stomach, most are found on the anterior surface of the stomach along its greater curvature. In contradistinction to partial transection, complete division of the stomach is exceedingly rare. For this to occur, a tremendous force must be applied to an empty stomach[54,84]; this sudden impaction of the stomach against the vertebral column results in the characteristic vertical orientation of the transection line.

The diagnosis of gastric perforation is rarely made prior to surgical intervention. Rather, it is the deleterious effects of intra-abdominal gastric contents that lead one to suspect a serious intra-abdominal injury and the need for emergency celiotomy. The majority of the patients present with severe diffuse abdominal pain in close temporal association with receiving an epigastric blow. Although most victims describe a severe impact force (as would occur in an automobile or bicycle accident), gastric rupture has been reported to occur following cardiopulmonary resuscitation, a slight fall, and a series of push-up exercises. Abdominal examination reveals diffuse tenderness, guarding, and rigidity. Hypotension and tachycardia without obvious signs of blood loss should alert the clinician to the possibility of intra-abdominal fluid sequestration secondary to chemical peritonitis. The diagnosis of an acute surgical abdomen may remain unclear; helpful adjunctive tests in these instances include an upright chest roentgenograph (for pneumoperitoneum), Gastrografin swallow, and peritoneal lavage.

At celiotomy, the diagnosis of gastric perforation is self-evident. Ruptures are typically solitary, linear defects less than 10 cm in length. Careful debridement of the edges should be performed prior to completing a standard two-layer closure. Use of warm saline irrigation of the abdominal cavity is done to remove spilled gastric secretion and particulate matter. Placement of drainage systems is not recommended for an isolated injury of this type. Gastric decompression is continued in the perioperative period until bowel function returns. Mortality rates for this injury approach 10%, due largely to coexistent organ damage.

COMPLETE TRANSECTION

Complete transection of the stomach is a far more serious injury, carrying a much higher mortality (approximately 50%) than partial transection. In most instances, the vertically oriented transected margins can be debrided and reapproximated using standard technique. The injury may be too extensive or in too close proximity to the pylorus to obtain a primary reanastomosis. Closure of the proximal stomach is quickly achieved using a TA-90 autostapling device; the distal segment is debrided to a point beyond the pylorus, then closed with a TA-55 autostapling device. A gastrojejunostomy is fashioned to restore gastrointestinal continuity. Again, despite heroic efforts mortality remains high, owing in large part to extensive coexistent organ injury.

Penetrating Gastric Injury

Penetrating gastric injury occurs with much greater frequency than blunt gastric trauma. The large surface area of the stomach (particularly when distended by recently ingested foodstuff) in combination with its mobility and ventral position within the abdominal cavity, predisposes it to injury from frontal assault. In the majority of cases a single small gastrotomy will be visualized on the anterior surface of the stomach. It is rarely deemed an immediate threat to the patient's life, particularly when caused by a stab wound or low-velocity firearm. There is usually little tissue destruction, and bleeding from severed gastric mural vessels is both minimal and readily controlled by suture ligation. Repair of this type of gastric injury may be deferred until completion of a thorough abdominal examination for identification and management of more serious injury. Temporary control of leaking gastric contents can be achieved by approximating the wound edges with a Babcock clamp.

Closure of these types of gastric wounds is achieved with ease, using previously mentioned gastric suturing techniques. The single most important principle in managing this injury is diligent inspection of the entire surface of the stomach; in many instances (up to half the cases) at least one additional gastrotomy will be found. The lesser sac must be opened through the gastrocolic omental attachments in order to visualize the posterior wall of the stomach. The greater and lesser curvatures must be carefully examined, because mesenteric fat may conceal an injury. If uncertainty regarding coexistent injury remains, all identified gastrotomies are closed. Normal saline solution is then instilled into the stomach through a nasogastric tube. The integrity of the gastric wall is then tested by firm manual compression of the stomach.

Once a secure closure of the stomach is achieved, the nasogastric tube is positioned in the most dependent portion of the stomach. The abdominal cavity is freed of particulate matter through liberal irrigation prior to completion of the procedure. External drainage devices are not indicated.

When a shotgun has been used to inflict injury, damage to the stomach is severe, and multiple gastrotomies may be encountered. The best method of securely closing those within a few centimeters of each other is by debriding the residual gastric wall between them. This maneuver essentially converts multiple defects into a linear gastrotomy, which is then closed using standard two-layer techniques. One should also keep in mind the large reservoir size of the stomach. Time should not be wasted closing multiple gastrotomies when there are large areas of devitalized gastric tissue and concomitant extragastric injuries. Under these circumstances, segmental gastric resection is the preferred technique.

DUODENAL TRAUMA

Blunt Duodenal Trauma

Several factors are thought to account for the relatively common occurrence of blunt injury to the duodenum. Foremost is that the duodenum is literally draped around the upper lumbar vertebrae, predisposing it to a crushing type of injury from blunt forces. Its mobility is limited by the overlying peritoneum; further fixation is afforded by the pylorus, ligament of Treitz, and overlying mesenteric vessels. Owing in large part to its retroperitoneal position, serious injury to the duodenum may pass undetected for a prolonged period, particularly if the physician relies solely on clinical signs and tests that are suggestive only of intraperitoneal visceral injury. Since delay in definitive therapy is a prime factor in morbidity and mortality associated with blunt duodenal injury,[20] the diagnosis must be assiduously pursued when clinical conditions favoring this possibility exist.

There are basically two types of blunt injury to the duodenum: contained intramural hematoma, and full-thickness laceration. Because of the unique diagnostic and therapeutic features of these injuries, each will be discussed separately.

CONTAINED INTRAMURAL HEMATOMA

In the gastrointestinal tract alone, the duodenum is the most common site of clinically significant intramural hematoma. Though reported to occur in virtually all age groups, children are particularly at risk, most likely because of their lack of well-developed abdominal musculature, their flared costal margins, and proximity of the anterior abdominal wall to the lumbar spine.

The most common mechanism of injury is a powerful blunt force applied to the anterior abdomen, as would occur upon impact with a steering wheel or as a result of a severe bludgeoning assault. While some investigators have suggested that the injury is a consequence of disruption of a closed loop (the pylorus and ligament of Treitz acting as potential sites of partial obstruction), most believe that the varying levels of tensile strength of the duodenal wall predispose weaker segments to injury by shearing forces that disrupt intramural vessels.[80]

There are two distinct clinical scenarios associated with duodenal hematoma. An acute onset of severe epigastric discomfort and abdominal tenderness, in close temporal relationship to a traumatic insult, occurs most frequently in the adult population. In children, the development of symptoms is more insidious and is characterized by the gradual onset of abdominal pain followed by protracted vomiting. Several days may pass before the patient is brought to the attention of a physician. Furthermore, if one is not careful to elicit a history of even remote trauma in these victims, an initial impression of gastroenteritis may delay the correct clinical diagnosis. Physical examination typically reveals mild abdominal tenderness, gastric succussion splash, and an abdominal mass (present in up to 40% of cases).[46] Laboratory analysis is generally nonspecific, although the presence of an elevated amylase should alert one to the possibility of pancreaticoduodenal injury. Plain abdominal roentgenographs are often nonspecific, but the classic indications are the presence of a large gastric bubble, little or no distal intestinal gas, and absence of the right psoas muscle shadow. Peritoneal lavage is indicated only when there is concern for acute significant concomitant intra-abdominal injury in patients who do not otherwise meet standard clinical criteria for emergency celiotomy. The lavage may often be negative in the presence of isolated duodenal hematoma, because of a typical pattern of retroperitoneal confinement.

In the past, the diagnostic procedure of choice in stable patients has been a water-soluble or barium contrast upper gastrointestinal series. The roentgenographic finding of a "coiled spring" appearance of the duodenum, secondary to the stacking of its mucosal folds that have been elevated by clot from the underlying muscularis, is virtually diagnostic of duodenal hematoma. More recently, computed tomography (CT) of the abdomen (Fig. 9.2) has become a popular initial diagnostic test by virtue of its capacity to investigate additional retroperitoneal structures heretofore hidden from conventional nonsurgical diagnostic tests.

The treatment of patients with obstructing duodenal hematomas, particularly those who have suffered through a protracted course of vomiting, is initially directed towards volume and electrolyte replenishment in combination with nasogastric decompression. Following resuscitation, controversy exists as to whether urgent celiotomy is indicated in a patient who, but for the presence of the hematoma, would not require surgical intervention. In a review of the literature on this topic reported in 1971, Jones, Hardin, and associates[46] found that while almost 20% of those who underwent surgical intervention required reoperation, almost 90% of those initially managed nonoperatively ultimately required surgical management of the hematoma. For this reason, early surgical intervention was felt to be the option of choice. In a separate review reported by Janson and Stockinger,[42] the results of nonoperative therapy were not as dismal, with over one-third of patients successfully managed without surgical intervention. The authors noted that at least 2 weeks of nasogastric decompression and fluid administration were required prior to the resolution of obstructive symptoms in those patients. Nonoperative therapy appears particularly attractive in children. Touloukian[101] prospectively managed 12 children possessing obstructing duodenal hematomas with a combination of nasogastric aspiration and parenteral nutrition. Two-thirds of the patients were able to resume oral intake within 1 week, with the remainder requiring a little over 1 month prior to symptomatic resolution of the obstruction. None required surgical intervention and there was virtually no associated morbidity.

Based on these data, it would appear that a 2-week trial of nonoperative management consisting of continuous nasogastric aspiration and nutritional support is warranted in patients with isolated duodenal hematomas. Weekly evaluation of the degree of obstruction, by either upper gastrointestinal series or CT scan should be performed. Failure to achieve clinical improvement within that time frame, particularly in adult patients, should be considered an indication for surgical correction.

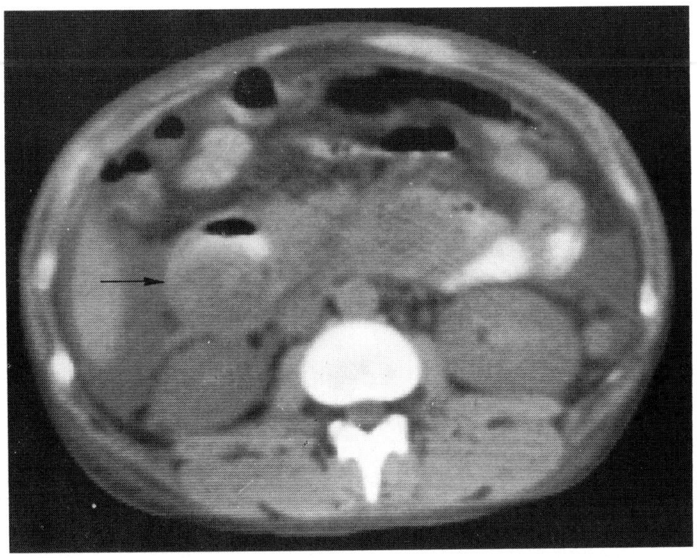

FIGURE 9.2 Duodenal hematoma visualized by oral contrast-assisted abdominal CT scan. Note the air contrast level in the lumen of a duodenum almost completely obstructed by the hematoma (arrow).

At surgery, the duodenum must be carefully mobilized by a wide Kocher maneuver and the entirety of the duodenum inspected for evidence of transmural perforations. If none is found, an incision is made directly over the hematoma along the longitudinal axis of the duodenum, and the clot evacuated. While some surgeons feel that nothing further needs to be added to the procedure, others find security in reapproximation of the incised duodenal wall with a series of simple interrupted 3-0 absorbable sutures, followed by placement of a soft drain several centimeters from the site of the duodenal closure.[34] There are no clear-cut data that either method has advantage over the other; a success rate approaching 90% can be expected.[42,46]

Owing in large part to concerns that obstruction would not universally be relieved by simple evacuation of a duodenal hematoma, it has been proposed that gastrojejunostomy alone or in concert with evacuation of the hematoma be performed. Unfortunately, a high percentage of patients in whom gastrojejunostomy is performed require reoperation, either for malfunction of the anastomosis or for marginal ulceration. For these reasons, gastrojejunostomy is generally reserved for patients who remain obstructed following an initial attempt at simple evacuation of the hematoma. In such patients, truncal vagectomy should be performed in addition to gastrojejunostomy in order to reduce the risk of jejunal ulceration.

While morbidity appears to vary according to the manner of treatment, exceedingly low mortality (under 3%) should be expected using the aforementioned protocols.

FULL-THICKNESS LACERATION

Duodenal lacerations secondary to blunt trauma generally test the diagnostic acumen and therapeutic mettle of even the best clinician. While diagnosis may be as difficult to secure as that of duodenal hematoma, delay in surgical intervention in those with lacerations carries a far higher risk of lethal consequences,[54] including gas gangrene,[114] despite standard salvage efforts.

The etiologic agent of a duodenal laceration is typically a severe frontal force applied to the upper abdomen. This may result in transmural shearing of the duodenum at points of fixation: the pylorus, ligament of Treitz, or overlying superior mesenteric vessels. More often, the duodenum is literally crushed between the vertebral column and the impacting force, the latter being a steering wheel,[20] seat belt,[38,58] or swift kick.[46]

Though retroperitoneal containment may initially cause a delay in the onset of symptoms, the majority of patients will complain of acute abdominal and back pain, which may radiate to the right side of the groin. Unless intra-abdominal contamination has occurred at the time of injury, peritoneal signs will initially be absent despite the presence of diffuse tenderness and decreased bowel sounds. Only after significant diapedesis of spilled duodenal contents into the peritoneal cavity will abdominal rigidity be present. By that time, systemic signs indicative of serious abdominal injury or infection are present as well, leading to emergency celiotomy. In some patients, a sensorium altered by alcohol or a central nervous system injury will cloud the clinician's initial evaluation. In these instances, extreme restlessness or agitation upon abdominal examination is not to be passed off as indicative of primal responses to "head trauma." Rather, more invasive investigation is mandatory.

As in most cases of blunt abdominal injury, laboratory analysis offers little specific diagnostic help. Leukocytosis and hyperamylasemia are often present with duodenal lacerations, but are so nonspecific as to be generally unrewarding. Although noncontrast abdominal films are normal in up to one half of cases,[20] the findings of either free intraperitoneal air or retroperitoneal gas outlining the kidney or right psoas muscle mandate emergency celiotomy. Failing this, diagnostic peritoneal lavage, particularly in those with altered sensorium, is a valuable adjunct to ruling out serious abdominal injury. For reasons previously stated, a negative lavage does not rule out retroperitoneal injury.[20] Should symptoms persist, repeat the lavage at 12 to 24 hours, by which time an elevated amylase concentration in the returned fluid may first become apparent. As previously mentioned, the abdominal CT scan may ultimately prove to be the technique of choice in evaluating patients suspected of having incurred a retroperitoneal injury.[48] Because of the lethal consequences associated with a missed retroperitoneal injury, clinical suspicion of such must not be tempered by a series of negative or inconclusive tests. Under these circumstances, exploratory celiotomy remains a valid diagnostic procedure.

During surgery, duodenal injury should be suspected when blood- or bile-stained fluid is found lateral and inferior to the duodenum. If a significant quantity of air has escaped from the blowout, retroperitoneal crepitus may be felt. In all cases of known or suspected duodenal trauma, the entirety of this structure must be evaluated. Inspection of the superior and descending portions of the duodenum requires a wide Kocher maneuver. Adequate visualization of the transverse and ascending portions can be achieved by reflecting the right and transverse colon upward and to the left of midline; the ligament of Treitz must be taken down as well. The pancreas and distal common bile duct are carefully assessed for concomitant injury, since the choices regarding surgical repair are just as dependent upon the condition of these structures as they are to the severity of duodenal injury.

The vast majority of blunt duodenal lacerations are small, isolated injuries with minimal associated mural devascularization. Primary closure may usually be achieved without tension on the suture line. While closure of small lacerations along the longitudinal axis of the duodenum will not result in luminal compromise, it is generally best to complete closure in the transverse axis. An inner running or interrupted layer of 3-0 absorbable suture is used to approximate the mucosa; tensile strength of the repair is supplied by an outer layer of interrupted 3-0 silk Lembert sutures. Some surgeons abhor the use of external drainage devices placed near the duodenal repair, for fear of promoting anastomotic breakdown or paraduodenal abscess formation.[104] Others favor routine placement of such devices in proximity to the repair, thereby allowing ready escape of duodenal contents in the event of an anastomotic breakdown. While this controversy has yet to be adequately studied, most surgeons favor the latter method.

At the completion of the duodenorrhaphy, the wound is liberally irrigated prior to fascial and skin closure. Nasogastric decompression is maintained until there is clear-cut evidence of restoration of upper gastrointestinal function. Drainage devices are eased out once the patient tolerates a diet. Postoperative complications include a significant incidence of traumatic pancreatitis, which almost uniformly resolves with continued fluid administration and nasogastric intubation. Fistulization from the repair alone or in concert with a paraduodenal abscess is rare. External control of the fistula, in combination with judicious use of antibiotics and total parenteral nutrition, is usually rewarded by spontaneous closure. Despite these complications, the mortality of small duodenal lacerations is minimal, unless there has been a delay in surgical intervention or there are serious concomitant intra-abdominal injuries. Levison, Petersen, and coworkers[55] have confirmed data from other investigators who found a significantly higher mortality rate when definitive repair of blunt duodenal lacerations was delayed beyond 24 hours.

In a distinct minority of patients, the traumatic duodenotomy is large, and secure primary closure cannot be achieved without luminal compromise. These unpleasant circumstances are often made more unfavorable by the presence of significant injury to the pancreas. Successful management of these more serious wounds requires a familiarity with the variety of surgical options that have been devised primarily for the treatment of penetrating duodenal wounds.

Penetrating Duodenal Injury

For several reasons, surgeons are not often faced with perioperative management of penetrating duodenal wounds. The duodenum's small size and limited surface area make it at best a difficult target to hit. By virtue of its position deep within the abdomen, it is protected to some degree in front by overlying viscera and from behind by the vertebral column and paraspinous muscles. The duodenum lies in close proximity to any number of large-caliber blood vessels, including inferior vena cava, portal vein, superior mesenteric vessels, and aorta. Injury to these structures will often result in exsanguination prior to or concomitant with surgical attempts to rectify the situation. When celiotomy confirms the diagnosis of a duodenal wound, the surgeon must keep in mind these general principles:

1. Assess the severity of duodenal injury.
2. Establish the presence and severity of injury to other viscera including pancreas, colon, and common bile duct, which are known to increase morbidity and mortality in the presence of duodenal injury.
3. Remember that there is no uniform way to manage duodenal injuries.
4. Select the option for safe repair that is the least elaborate, accepting the risk of a higher postoperative morbidity as fair exchange for lower perioperative mortality.

During surgery, the presence of blood, bile-stained fluid, or palpable crepitus in the retroperitoneal tissue to the right of and inferior to the duodenum are signs suggestive of penetrating duodenal injury. Unlike blunt trauma, in which the finding of retroperitoneal blood is usually suggestive of hemorrhage from the duodenum itself, in this case it may herald significant concomitant vascular injury (in up to 40% of cases).[90] Mobilization of the duodenum must be performed with the understanding that proximal and distal control of major vessels may be urgently required when the tamponade effect of the retroperitoneum has been released. Once vascular injury has been excluded or effectively treated, the entire duodenum is examined through a combination of a wide Kocher maneuver and extensive reflection of the right and transverse colon. The path of the projectile should be traced until it has clearly passed beyond harm's way; a search for injury to structures in proximity to the duodenum (particularly the pancreas, common bile duct, colon, and kidney) must be completed prior to contemplating repair of the duodenum.

In the majority of patients a small, single or through-and-through wound to the duodenum will be identified. Following debridement, primary closure along the transverse axis with the same two-layer suture techniques used for blunt duodenal lacerations can in most instances be achieved with acceptable morbidity and mortality rates.[2,55,90] Surgeons have historically positioned soft rubber drains near the duodenorrhaphy, in order to control the potentially lethal postoperative complications of paraduodenal abscess or anastomotic breakdown with fistulization. It was not until recent years that primary closure with external drainage was systematically challenged. Stone and Fabian[93] found that external drainage of a duodenal suture line resulted in a 23% incidence of fistulization. Primary closure alone failed in 18%, leading to fulminant sepsis and peritonitis in all, and death in one-third. Because of what was felt to be an excessive morbidity and mortality, the investigators began to employ routine decompression of the duodenum in conjunction with duodenorrhaphy. This was accomplished by constructing a Witzel jejunostomy, then threading a (14-French) catheter in retrograde fashion into the duodenum. A second (feeding) jejunostomy and (Stamm) gastrostomy were routinely added to the procedure. External drainage devices were used only when deemed necessary for concomitant organ injuries, such as to the pancreas and liver. These maneuvers were associated with a decrease in the fistulization rate to under 0.5% and a coincident decrease in mortality. For these reasons, the authors encouraged routine duodenal decompression when primary closure of duodenal wounds is contemplated.

While these results were initially confirmed by others,[22,35] the routine use of duodenal decompression has come under challenge. Ivatury and co-workers[40] analyzed patients with comparably severe duodenal and associated injury, who differed only in respect to method of duodenal repair. Those who underwent duodenorrhaphy alone were found to have a lower postoperative morbidity rate than did the group who, in addition to primary repair, had insertion of a decompressive enterostomy tube. In an expanded patient follow-up study of similar design, Ivatury and colleagues[41] found that in addition to the increased morbidity associated with decompressive enterostomy, mortality was also significantly higher. The authors concluded that routine decompression is not warranted. Others echo this opinion,[2,90] adding that decompressive enterostomy might best be reserved for patients in whom, following closure of the duodenotomy, either residual wall is somewhat contused or in whom the lumen is felt to be minimally compromised. Under these circumstances, duodenal decompressive procedures may be used in favor of more complex attempts at reconstruction.

In hopes of decreasing the risk of duodenorrhaphy dehiscence without resorting to more complex procedures, several suture-line reinforcement techniques were devised. The simplest involves tacking a pedicle of omentum over the duodenorrhaphy in a fashion similar to the modified Graham patch. Alternatively, several investigators proposed the technique of serosal jejunal onlay. Following completion of the duodenorrhaphy, a loop of proximal jejunum is brought up to the injury site in retrocolic fashion. Then, using a series of interrupted 4-0 silk seromuscular sutures, the jejunum is secured to both sides of the duodenal closure. With either technique, a large-bore nasogastric tube is threaded through the pylorus to effect duodenal decompression. More recent data suggest that such reinforcement procedures add little more than time to the overall operation[40,68] and should, generally, be abandoned.

At times, the duodenal injury will be so severe as to preclude secure primary closure alone or in concert with duodenal decompression. Reconstructive options are often limited by coexistent damage to the common bile duct or severe pancreatic injury, but the injury may appear either isolated to the duodenum or associated with a minor pancreatic injury that is treatable by the insertion of external drainage devices. When such conditions exist, several viable surgical reconstruction modalities are available. One is circumferential resection of the damaged duodenal wall with primary end-to-end anastomosis. Injuries to the third and fourth portions of the duodenum are particularly amenable to this procedure. The blood supply to the duodenum is less precarious and the pancreas is not as densely adherent in these areas, allowing completion of a tension-free vascularized anastomosis with standard two-layer suture techniques. Kelly and associates[50] noted that too liberal an attempt to strip the pancreas off the duodenum is discouraged in favor of dissecting away only that amount necessary to secure an enteric anastomosis. Insertion of gastrostomy and duodenostomy tubes as well as external drainage catheters in proximity to the anastomosis are recommended.

A second method, recommended for large isolated defects of the lateral wall of the descending duodenum, employs side-to-(functional)end, Roux-en-Y duodenojejunostomy. Following debridement of the duodenotomy, the distal (closed) end of a previously transected segment of jejunum is brought up in retrocolic fashion to the injury site. Longitudinal antimesenteric jejunotomy is made to approximate the length of the duodenotomy, and standard two-layer duodenojejunostomy is performed. A jejunojejunostomy 40 cm distal to the initial anastomosis restores gastrointestinal continuity. Again, external drainage devices, gastrostomy, and decompressive duodenostomy are recommended.

Successful management of some duodenal wounds, by virtue of extensive mural damage or coexistent injury to the head of the pancreas or the distal common bile duct, requires surgical techniques other than those outlined above. Until recently, the sole viable option appeared to be pancreatoduodenectomy, although its reported mortality rates approached 30%.[71] In 1974 Berne and colleagues[8] reported results of 50 patients who underwent duodenal diverticulization for these types of injuries (Fig. 9.3). Standard components of this procedure include vagectomy, antrectomy, gastrojejunostomy, duodenorrhaphy with proximity drainage, tube duodenostomy, and external drainage of the pancreas as indicated. Drainage of the biliary radicals by a cholecystostomy or choledochostomy was performed if injury to the distal duct system was confirmed or suspected. Using these techniques, their overall mortality rate was 16% (8); four deaths occurred within 24 postoperative hours due to severe associated injuries. While there was a high rate of pancreatic (10%) and duodenal (14%) fistula, all closed spontaneously. In this regard, it is well known that few (20%) lateral duodenal fistulas will heal without surgical intervention;[62] mortality directly related to lateral fistula is reported to be as high as 40%. By performing diverticulization, the investigators noted that in the event of a breakdown of the duodenorrhaphy, the resultant fistula is functionally an end fistula, which is more likely to undergo spontaneous closure. Based on these data, the authors recommended that duodenal diverticulization be performed when there has been either severe duodenal or pancreaticoduodenal injury not amenable to simple closure, although pancreatoduodenectomy would not appear necessary for purposes of debridement.

While success with diverticulization procedures was confirmed elsewhere, there remained concern regarding the complexity and time-consuming nature of this procedure in already critically ill patients. In an effort to simplify matters, Jordan and colleagues[105] developed the technique of pyloric exclusion (Figs. 9.4 and 9.5). Following repair of the duodenal injury, a greater curvature gastrotomy is positioned to accommodate a gastrojejunostomy. The pylorus is identified through the gastrotomy and closed with a running 2-0 absorbable suture, such as polygalactin 910. Side-to-side gastrojejunostomy is then performed to com-

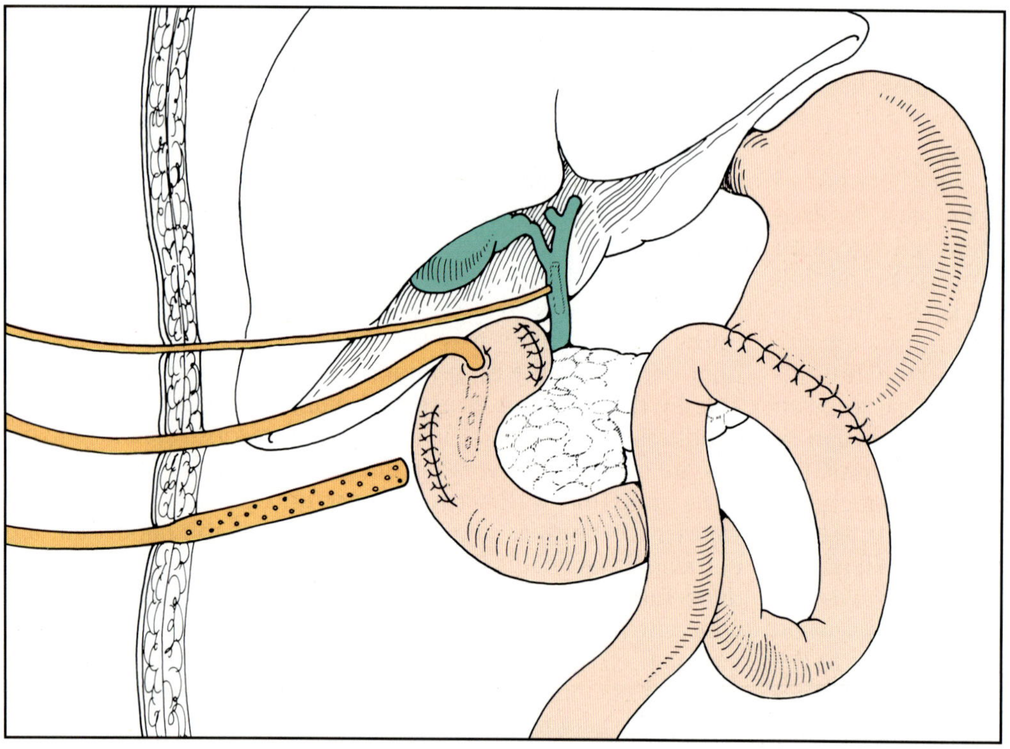

FIGURE 9.3 Diverticulization procedure. Primary closure of the duodenal laceration has been achieved. Multiple closed-drainage system devices are placed in proximity to the injury. Tube duodenostomy has been inserted through an uninjured site of the duodenum. Foley catheter, T-tube, or Malecot catheter are commonly used for decompressive purposes. Choledochostomy was performed, out of concern for distal common bile duct injury. Vagectomy, antrectomy, duodenal stump closure, and gastrojejunostomy have been performed to divert gastric contents from the injury site.[8]

plete the procedure. Considering the lethal nature of these types of injuries, a perioperative mortality rate of 19% (almost half occurring within 36 postoperative hours) was considered at least on a par with other reports. Duodenal fistulization occurred in only 5% of patients; all but one spontaneously healed. Long-term follow-up obtained on many of these patients documented a return of normal gastrointestinal physiologic function within months of the initial procedure. Three patients did develop symptomatic marginal ulcers several months after their injury; two required surgical intervention. Although the authors were somewhat dismayed by this complication, the rate was felt to be too low to recommend adding vagectomy to their procedure. A longer follow-up of these patients will be required since, from a historical perspective, gastrojejunostomy alone performed in patients with peptic ulcer disease has been associated with a 20% rate of marginal ulceration; many occurred several years after the initial procedure. Despite the aforementioned concerns, these and other investigators[49] assert that the benefits associated with pyloric exclusion—that is, avoidance of gastric resection, return of normal gastrointestinal function, low risk of duodenal fistulization—favor its use in patients with severe duodenal or combined pancreaticoduodenal injuries.

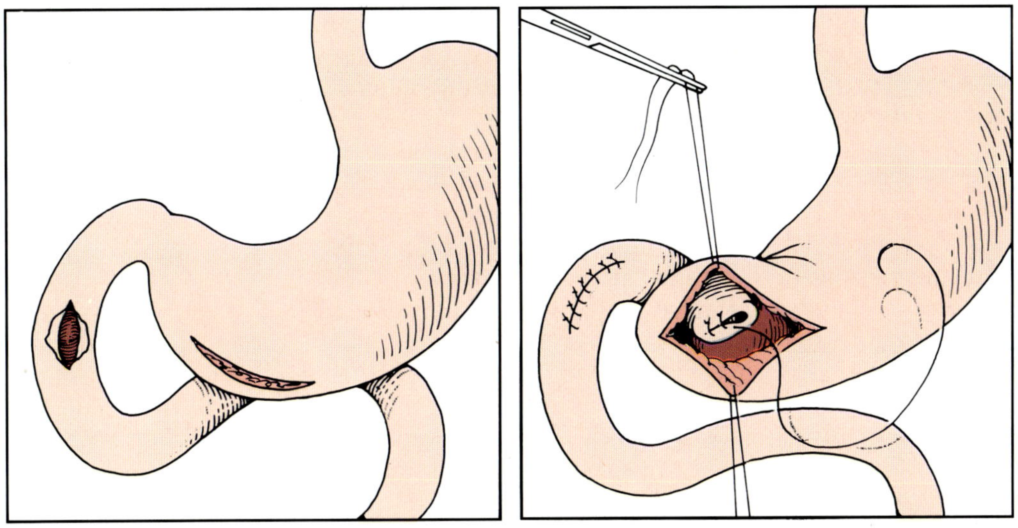

FIGURE 9.4 Pyloric exclusion technique. Following closure of the duodenotomy, a distal greater curvature gastrotomy is made large enough to oversew the pylorus from within. Absorbable suture with a long half-life (polyglycolic acid, polygalactin 910, polydioxanone) is recommended.[105]

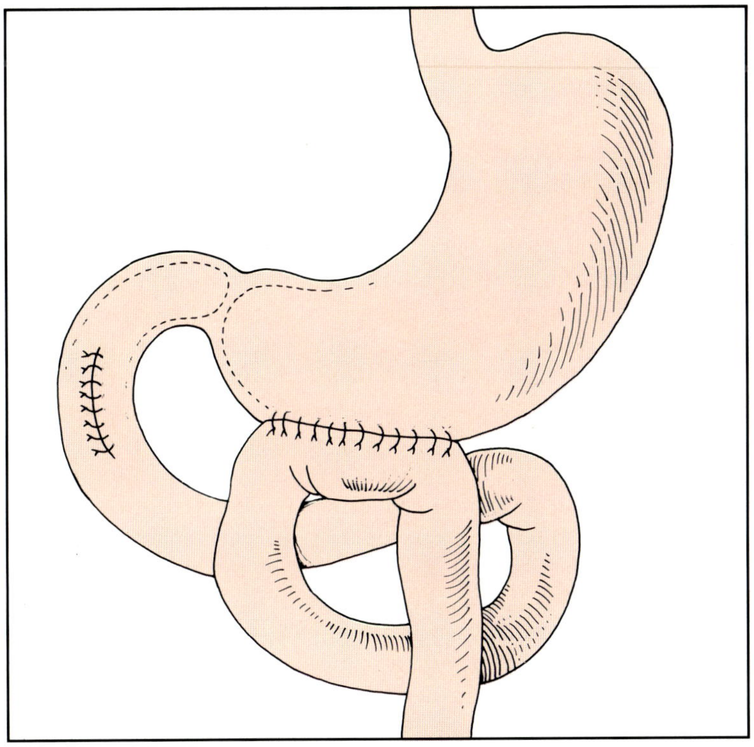

FIGURE 9.5 Pyloric exclusion is completed by a gastrojejunostomy. For injuries of this severity, closed drainage devices are placed near the site of the duodenotomy.[105]

It must always be kept in mind that neither duodenal diverticulization nor pyloric exclusion are to be performed, in lieu of pancreatoduodenectomy (Whipple's operation), for massive devascularization injuries of the duodenum or head of the pancreas.[50] Despite the high associated mortality with the Whipple procedure, it remains the operation of choice to effectively debride massive amounts of devitalized tissue and to control exsanguinating hemorrhage from either injured tissue or associated vascular structures (portal vein, mesenteric vessels).

Institutions with vast experience in managing the entire spectrum of penetrating and blunt duodenal injuries report mortality rates between 10% and 30%. At least half of the deaths occur within 48 postoperative hours, and are usually due to ongoing sepsis or exsanguination. The major contributing factors to this early mortality are the number of associated organ injuries and delay in surgical intervention.[55,90] Survival beyond that point is to a great extent dependent upon the success with which associated organ injuries were managed. If the above surgical precepts are followed, duodenal mortality should account for only a small fraction of the total.

The morbidity associated with duodenal injury does pose a significant problem, particularly when there is a breakdown of the duodenorrhaphy. In the absence of prior insertion of duodenal drainage devices, a clinical pattern of hemodynamic instability, consistent with septic shock that suddenly interrupts a fairly smooth postoperative course, should alert the clinician to the possibility of an anastomotic leak. Radiologic evaluation is usually not necessary to confirm that suspicion and should certainly not delay emergency celiotomy following volume resuscitation. Reclosure of the duodenal wound is generally unrewarding; placement of multiple drains followed by generous peritoneal irrigation is usually the best one can do for these critically ill patients.

If proximity drains were placed, duodenal fistulization is easily recognized as a sudden increase in drainage output several days following the initial repair. Signs of hemodynamic instability are present only when there is an associated paraduodenal abscess. Nonoperative control of both is generally achieved simply by maintaining the position of drainage catheters and judicious use of antibiotics. Surgical intervention may be indicated to establish better drainage of an abscess cavity.

Once control of sepsis or the fistula has been achieved, the site and type of fistula must be defined. Water-soluble contrast fistulography or upper gastrointestinal series will usually be successful in this regard. As mentioned previously, an end duodenal fistula will usually close spontaneously; nasogastric decompression and parenteral nutritional support are to be instituted during the healing period. Lateral duodenal fistulas rarely close, but it is reasonable to institute a short trial of nonoperative therapy to allow the patient time to recover from earlier traumatic insults. Ultimately, surgical intervention will usually be required. Malangoni and co-workers[62] found that procedures designed to convert lateral to end duodenal fistula were associated with a high degree of success. This was generally achieved by modifications of duodenal diverticulization techniques: partial gastrectomy (with or without vagectomy), gastrojejunostomy, duodenal decompression, and wide paraduodenal drainage. The 3 surgical failures (21%) in their study were associated with an attempt at definitive repair of the fistula in the face of uncontrolled local infection; one patient died following such an attempt. From these experiences, a two-stage approach to the treatment of lateral duodenal fistula is recommended:

1. Control the fistula and drain any surrounding septic foci.
2. Surgically convert a lateral to an end-duodenal fistula.

PANCREATIC TRAUMA

Blunt Pancreatic Injury

The pancreas, unlike the duodenum, is a solid organ incapable of dispersing shock waves by luminal decompression. This factor, in combination with its proximity to lumbar vertebrae, increases the organ's susceptibility to crushing injury by blunt forces. With the gradual rise in serious automobile accidents, the improvement in prehospital and hospital management of trauma victims, and the availability of more accurate diagnostic tests (such as abdominal CT scan), blunt injury to the pancreas is being identified more frequently.

There are 3 general patterns of injury to the pancreas, depending upon the vector of frontal force applied to the gland in relationship to the spine.[72] When applied to the right of the spine, injury to the head of the pancreas and to the duodenum can be expected. Midline forces will result in disruption of the body, while those to the left of midline will cause damage to the tail of the pancreas, often resulting in splenic injury as well. The site of injury is prognostically important because damage to the pancreatic head has a mortality rate double that of either body or tail injury.[47,72]

The diagnosis is often made difficult by initially minimal or absent symptoms of abdominal pain particularly when dealing with an isolated pancreatic injury. A sensorium altered by associated head trauma or substance abuse may further cloud the findings. If there is no significant surrounding retroperitoneal tissue injury to activate pancreatic enzymes, days may pass before the buildup of pancreatic secretion results in symptoms suggestive of pancreatitis or pseudocyst formation. Serial abdominal examinations are mandatory because physical findings in the acute postinjury phase may also be misleading, and because mild diffuse tenderness and decreased bowel sounds are so nonspecific as to be initially unimpressive. The majority of patients will ultimately develop significant epigastric pain, often radiating to the back; nausea, vomiting, and tenderness to deep palpation should alert the clinician to the possibility of pancreatic injury.

While serum amylase is often normal in the immediate posttrauma period,[12] it will be elevated in at least 70% of patients with later proven blunt pancreatic injury.[45,72] An elevated level is not to be interpreted as an indication for surgical intervention; corroborative evidence for significant abdominal injury is generally required. Diagnostic peritoneal lavage may be of particular value in this regard since many patients with serious pancreatic injury have associated visceral damage that will result in a positive lavage. The finding of an elevated amylase in the lavage fluid is once again suggestive of significant pancreatic injury, although a normal level does not rule out that possibility.[12]

Diagnosis of blunt pancreatic injury is at times difficult because of the nonspecific nature of clinical findings and laboratory tests. Noncontrast abdominal roentgenographs are of little help in this case. If the patient does not otherwise possess standard criteria for celiotomy, an abdominal CT scan may be employed to assess the status of retroperitoneal structures. Initial data suggest that, using CT scanning, the chance of a false negative result for the serious pancreatic injury is negligible, while a positive scan has excellent surgical correlation.[23]

Operative management of blunt pancreatic injury requires an adequate exposure of the entire pancreas. To that end, four separate techniques are necessary: (1) a Kocher maneuver, (2) complete mobilization of the spleen, (3) exploration of the lesser sac, readily achieved by division of the gastrocolic omentum, and (4) incisions of the retroperitoneal attachments inferior to the pancreas to allow mobilization of the body for purposes of inspection and bimanual palpation of that part of the gland not previously exposed.

Treatment options vary with both the site and severity of pancreatic injury. Lucas[59] developed the following classification for pancreatic injury:

Class I: Contusions or abrasions to any part of the pancreas, but not involving the main ducts
Class II: Severe distal pancreatic lacerations or disruptions with known or suspected ductal injury, but no duodenal injury
Class III: Class II type of injury only to proximal rather than distal pancreas
Class IV: Severe combined pancreaticoduodenal injury

Since class III injuries rarely occur in association with blunt trauma, and class IV blunt pancreatic injuries are managed in a fashion identical to those that occur with penetrating trauma, further discussion of these will be deferred to the section on penetrating trauma.

Class I Injuries The most common type of injury and the easiest to treat is class I. Hemorrhage from superficial pancreatic vessels is usually the major feature, and control is achieved with direct, shallow, simple or mattress 4-0 silk sutures. Absorbable suture material has a shortened life span in the presence of pancreatic enzymes and is to be avoided. No attempts to clamp bleeding vessels should be made prior to ligation because of the inevitable crushing of surrounding pancreatic parenchyma. Wide-based, deeply placed sutures may injure major ductal or vascular structures, further complicating matters. If one is unable to identify a specific bleeding point, surrounding tissue may be selectively debrided to gain adequate exposure. Once hemostasis is achieved, drainage devices are placed along the injury sites and brought out through separate lateral flank incisions. Some investigators prefer soft passive systems (such as Penrose drains) to reduce the risk of erosion of the drain into nearby hollow viscera. Most now favor closed drainage devices because they have been shown to result in markedly less morbidity when compared with open passive systems.[94] Finally, regardless of the drainage system used, it is generally recommended that any disrupted capsule overlying the pancreatic injury not be reapproximated, so that any residual pancreatic secretion has ready access to the drainage catheters. Closure of the capsule might build up fluid beneath, risking formation of a pancreatic pseudocyst. At completion of the procedure, the abdomen is liberally irrigated, and fascia and skin closed in the usual fashion for an isolated injury of this type.

The postoperative course of patients with isolated class I injuries is generally benign, with virtually no mortality and a 2% to 20% occurence of morbidity. During the recovery phase, the output from the pancreatic drains is observed for both quantity and appearance. Serous or serosanguineous discharge is expected, but the presence of a cloudy or milky white effluent should raise suspicion of a developing pancreatic fistula. As a matter of routine, then, amylase levels of the drainage material should be intermittently obtained; results should roughly approximate simultaneously obtained serum levels. In the absence of clinical concern for development of a pancreatic fistula, most investigators agree that a minimum of 7 to 10 postoperative days should pass, and a regular dietary intake established without a change in the type or quantity of drainage effluent prior to removing the drains. If these criteria are met, the drains are to be advanced from the abdomen over a period of several days to allow progressive healing to occur from within the drainage tract site.

Between 2% and 15% of the patients with a class I injury will develop a pancreatic fistula, but fortunately most are of low output (<500 ml/day), minimally affected by oral intake, and able to close spontaneously within 2 weeks. Treatment revolves around ensuring adequate nutrition, controlling the fistula, and preventing skin excoriation by keeping the enzymatic effluent from bathing the skin surrounding the drainage tract. Intravenous nutrition will be required when the fistula is of high output or increases with oral intake, or if it fails to close within 2 weeks. Even under these circumstances, surgical intervention is rarely required; a minimum of 3 months should pass prior to this consideration.

Class II Injuries Major lacerations of the body and tail of the pancreas are best treated by distal pancreatectomy and wide drainage.[9] Attempts to preserve distal pancreatic tissue through the use of elaborate Roux-en-Y pancreaticojejunostomy procedures alone, or in concert with primary repair of a transected pancreatic duct, are both unnecessary and dangerous.[5,94] As long as the line of the proposed pancreatic resection lies to the left of the superior mesenteric vessels, endocrine pancreatic insufficiency rarely occurs[45] and should not be considered a contraindication to pancreatic resection.

During distal pancreatectomy, the spleen and tail of the pancreas should be liberally mobilized ventral and to the right in order to allow adequate visualization, and to ensure that there are no areas of damaged or devitalized tissue in that part of the proximal pancreas to be salvaged. At this point, a decision regarding removal of the spleen in conjunction with distal pancreatectomy must be made. Some investigators, concerned with the consequences of postsplenectomy sepsis, have successfully preserved the otherwise undamaged spleen.[83] Individual ligation of the many arteries and veins coursing between splenic vessels and pancreas is so time-consuming as to make such an attempt very difficult, and visualization of the splenic vessels is often obscured by surrounding retroperitoneal peripancreatic hematoma. Splenectomy is usually required during the course of distal pancreatectomy, with care taken to perform individual suture ligation of the splenic artery and vein using nonabsorbable material. Attempts to preserve the spleen are best reserved for isolated, clean injuries to the pancreas, particularly in children, in whom the risk of postsplenectomy sepsis is well documented.

Once pancreatic mobilization and splenectomy are accomplished, a pair of noncrushing vascular clamps are placed across the pancreas proximal to the injury, and the distal segment is amputated in such a fashion as to allow a 5-mm cuff of normal pancreatic tissue to extrude beyond the remaining proximal clamp. The main pancreatic duct is then identified and suture ligated with 4-0 silk. Using a series of interrupted overlapping 4-0 silk horizontal mattress sutures, the pancreatic cuff is oversewn. The vascular clamp is then released, and the gland is examined for points of hemorrhage that require additional suture control. Once hemostasis is maintained, closed drainage devices are positioned in the pancreatic bed.

As an expedient alternative, several investigators have utilized an autostapling device to secure the residual pancreatic parenchyma with a double staggered row of staples.[4] The speed and excellent hemostatic qualities of this procedure are clear advantages. Once again, closed-system drainage devices are placed in the pancreatic bed prior to fascial approximation.

While postoperative morbidity and mortality are slightly higher when pancreatic resection is required, this is in great part attributable to the common occurrence of co-morbid injuries. Regardless, the primary pancreas-related complication, fistulization, is more common in class II than in class I injuries. While management is identical, with similar satisfactory results, it is important from the standpoint of morbidity to accurately distinguish between the two classes. This may be difficult to achieve. Recognizing that the focal point of differentiation is the integrity of the main pancreatic duct, it has been suggested that intraoperative pancreatography be performed when doubt exists as to the class of injury. Two approaches to the duct are described: lateral duodenotomy with cannulation of the ampulla of Vater and resection of the distal tip of the pancreas with retrograde ductal cannulation. The principal advantage of the former approach is related to the relative simplicity by which it is accomplished. Violation of the gastrointestinal tract may counterbalance any perceived benefit.[25] The latter approach, while more difficult, causes no harm when distal pancreatectomy is required. On the other hand, if the pancreatogram is normal, this method unnecessarily violates the main pancreatic duct, however distal it may be. Using either approach, a 5-French feeding catheter is inserted into the duct and 3 ml to 5 ml of radiopaque contrast material slowly injected. Main ductal disruption of the pancreatic body remains a clear-cut indication for distal pancreatectomy (Fig. 9.6). A normal pancreatogram is consistent with a class I injury treatable by drainage alone.

Penetrating Pancreatic Injury

Patients afflicted with a penetrating injury to the pancreas are likely to die because the majority are victims of gunshot, rather than typically less injurious stab wounds. A missile reaching the pancreas was either fired from close range or was of relatively high velocity. Significant injury often occurs to nearby organs as the missile passes into or out of the gland. Finally, if any of the major vascular structures that lie close to the pancreas are damaged, rapid exsanguination may well preclude any serious efforts toward preoperative resuscitation.

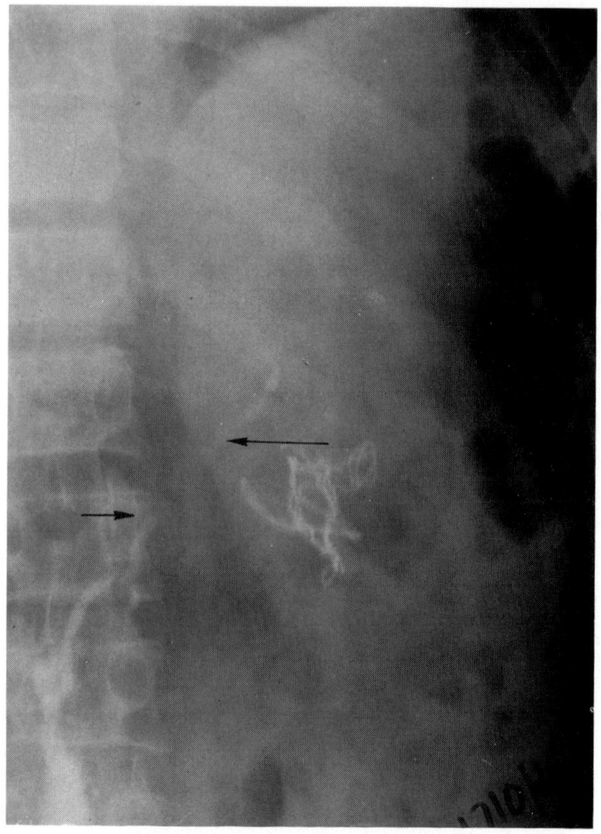

FIGURE 9.6 Intraoperative transduodenal pancreatogram performed on a patient with suspected pancreatic duct transection. Note the interruption (short arrow) to flow of contrast material. Since only the posterior aspect of the duct was violated, contrast material did reach the distal pancreatic duct (long arrow). Distal pancreatectomy was required.

There is generally little doubt regarding the necessity for emergency celiotomy in patients fortunate enough to survive the initial injury. Operative procedure is no different from that mentioned previously: control life-threatening injuries first, define remaining visceral and structural damage, and repair each in order of decreasing threat to the life of the patient. If injury to the pancreas is known or suspected, complete mobilization of the gland by means of the maneuvers described previously is needed. Class I and class II pancreatic injuries secondary to penetrating trauma are managed the same way as blunt injuries to the pancreas. The more serious class III and IV injuries are approached differently.

Class III Injuries Severe damage to the head of the pancreas, even in the absence of duodenal injury, is particularly serious. Hemorrhage from the portal vein, vena cava, aorta, or mesenteric vessels will often result in exsanguination during or shortly after surgical attempts at control of the injuries.[94] Presuming that such injuries either are not present or are adequately controlled, the options available for management of the pancreatic injury are somewhat controversial. Lucas[59] suggests that the procedure chosen is dependent upon first establishing integrity of the main pancreatic duct. Unless a duct injury is clearly identified at surgery, intraoperative pancreatography should be performed. If the major duct has not been violated, duodenal diverticulization in combination with wide pancreatic drainage is warranted.

In the presence of a major duct injury, a more aggressive surgical approach is favored by Lucas. Resection of the damaged pancreas is achieved with care to avoid injury to the distal common bile duct while performing debridement of more proximal pancreatic tissues. As long as a 2-cm cuff of pancreas abutting the duodenum is preserved, their shared blood supply will remain intact. Closure of the transected proximal end of pancreas is achieved by a series of overlapping horizontal 3-0 silk mattress sutures following suture ligation of the pancreatic duct. The residual distal segment of pancreas is then debrided back to viable tissue, preserving its vascular attachments arising from the splenic vessels. A standard retrocolic Roux-en-Y pancreaticojejunostomy is then performed to that distal segment; a series of simple interrupted 3-0 silk sutures are used, with care to ensure that the seromuscular jejunal "bites" are secured to the capsule of the pancreas around the entire anastomosis. Again, wide drainage of the pancreatic bed is indicated.

Initial enthusiasm for these Roux-en-Y procedures [30,59,72] has recently waned. Reports [94] have documented a high incidence of serious postoperative complications related to these procedures, particularly sepsis from anastomotic leaks. Others have found that, regardless of the status of the pancreatic duct, the primary goal of the Roux-en-Y procedure—preservation of pancreatic tissue—can be achieved by wide drainage of the pancreas alone. Postoperative control of the almost inevitable pancreatic fistula will generally be rewarded by spontaneous closure, particularly if the initial surgical procedure includes some form of duodenal diverticulization. For these reasons, it is felt best to limit use of the Roux-en-Y procedures to class III injuries with clean, complete parenchymal transections of the pancreas that occur to the right of the mesenteric vessels, as might occur with blunt, rather than penetrating, traumatic forces.

Class IV Injuries More common than class III injuries, severe combined pancreaticoduodenal injuries are associated with serious perioperative morbidity and mortality, regardless of the methods chosen to manage the injury. From a historical perspective, pancreatoduodenectomy appeared to be the sole option in the management of these injuries. A few studies [57,76,95] lent support to the role of emergency pancreatoduodenectomy despite postoperative mortality rates of up to 40%. Perioperative management and nutritional support of such patients has improved markedly during the past two decades. These advances appear to allow surgeons to perform less radical operations (such as diverticulization) and accept a higher risk of postoperative complications (that is, sepsis, fistulization) that, while serious, no longer carry the high life-threatening potential they had in the past. For these reasons, it is now felt that pancreatoduodenectomy should be reserved for patients with avulsion-type pancreatic injuries in order to achieve adequate debridement of devitalized tissue. In less severe class IV injuries, wide drainage of the pancreas and duodenum together with duodenal diverticulization procedures may be preferred. The wide variety of perioperative complications associated with duodenal diverticulization procedures (usually amenable to medical management) may be acceptable in institutions where pancreatoduodenectomy has been associated with mortality rates greater than 10%.

TRAUMA TO THE SMALL INTESTINE

Blunt Small Intestine Injury

The jejunoileum is freely suspended from the posterior abdominal wall by the fan-shaped mesentery. This affords considerable mobility to the small intestine, allowing it to escape serious injury from most externally applied blunt forces. The extensive series of anastomotic vascular arcades within the mesenteric folds serve to help preserve intestinal viability by carrying blood distally to damaged segmental vessels. Injury to the mesenteric small intestine secondary to blunt trauma is uncommon, occurring in only 5% to 10% of patients who undergo surgery for suspected intra-abdominal injury.[17]

Several theories exist regarding the mechanism of blunt injury. The time-honored theory relates small bowel injury to shearing forces applied to the small intestine at the ligament of Treitz and the cecum. There, the mesentery supporting the proximal jejunum at one end and terminal ileum at the other is foreshortened when compared to mesentery along the remaining small intestine. Damage would be suspected to occur at these points because of the limited mobility; several retrospective clinical studies have demonstrated an increased incidence of injury to small intestine at those fixed points. Additional credence to the shearing theory can be found in the many case reports documenting injury to small intestinal segments held in fixed position by a variety of means such as adhesions,[109] groin hernias,[19] and terminal ileitis.[86] Other investigators found that injury occurs not only at the proximal jejunum and terminal ileum, but more evenly throughout the small intestine.[17] They support the theory that many injuries are due simply to compression of intestinal segments positioned between the instrument of applied force (such as a steering wheel) and the lordotic lumbosacral spine. Williams and Sargent [110] have demonstrated this mechanism of action experimentally in a canine blunt trauma model. Their finding supports clinical data regarding small intestine injury found to occur when automobile seat belts without accompanying shoulder straps are employed.[85] In these cases, the lap belt was applied across the abdomen without support from the bony pelvis. When the victim was forcibly thrust forward, as would occur in a front-end collision, the seat belt would literally crush the small intestine between it and the lumbosacral spine.

The most controversial theory of injury is that of rupture of a distended segment of small intestine. Robbs, Moore, and Pillay[82] felt this was the mechanism of injury in many patients who suffered intestinal perforations after having been struck in the abdomen with a large blunt object. On the other hand, Williams and Sargent [110] presented experimental data that found that blunt abdominal forces transmitted to a given segment of small intestine were harmlessly channeled through the lumen of the remaining small bowel.

The diagnosis of blunt injury to the small intestine is difficult to make on purely clinical grounds, although suspicion should be raised when the victim relates being thrust forward, hitting the abdomen against an immovable object (such as a steering wheel or handlebars of a bicycle or tricycle). Free perforation of the small intestine, upon physical examination, characteristically reveals tachycardia, fever, and a diffusely tender abdomen with decreased or absent bowel sounds. A reliable history or physical examination may not be possible because of impairment of the patient's central nervous system function from closed head injury. Tenderness secondary to intra-abdominal injury may be difficult to differentiate from abdominal wall trauma. It may take several hours before classic signs of peritonitis are evident,[79] given the typically slow leakage of intestinal contents, which are minimally irritating to the peritoneum. Many cases of "delayed" small intestinal perforation have been reported, with involved segments undergoing ischemic necrosis over a period of hours to days.[82,97]

In hopes of improving diagnostic accuracy, several different tests have been proposed. An upright chest roentgenograph will reveal pneumoperitoneum from visceral rupture in 20% to 50% of cases.[66,79,82] While helpful when positive, a negative examination clearly does not rule out significant intestinal injury. Peritoneal lavage appears to offer a much higher diagnostic yield. Again, a negative lavage does not rule out small intestine injury, particularly if there is delayed intestinal rupture or if the lavage was performed so early in the postinjury setting that minimal peritoneal soilage had occurred. Phillips and Brotman[79] found a false-negative peritoneal lavage rate of 25% for this specific injury. The authors concluded that serial clinical examinations are mandatory, complemented as necessary by repeated diagnostic peritoneal lavage.

Marx, Bar-Or, and co-workers[63] improved diagnostic accuracy of small intestine injury by obtaining an alkaline phosphatase level of the lavage fluid. When performed on patients with a negative lavage, by criteria of cell counts and amylase, an alkaline phosphatase level of 3 IU/liter was a sensitive indicator of small intestine injury. As yet, this test has not gained widespread use.

The diagnosis of mesenteric small intestine injury must be pursued with vigor, because the associated morbidity and mortality are to a great extent related to the rapidity with which surgical management is undertaken. Carswell[10] reported a 50% rate of mortality with this injury when there was a 12-hour delay in surgical intervention. Other investigators[82] found a similar mortality rate when there was a 24-hour delay; no deaths occurred when surgical treatment was instituted within 1 day. Survivors of delayed surgical intervention experience a much higher incidence of serious postoperative morbidity (up to 70%) compared with those treated earlier.[87] This data must be tempered with the knowledge that associated injuries also increase patient morbidity and mortality,[17,82] although even in these patients prompt surgical intervention remains critical.

The entire small intestine must be carefully examined from the ligament of Treitz to the ileocecal valve, including all mural surfaces and mesenteric attachments. In general, three types of injury will be identified: perforation, mural damage without perforation, and mesenteric hematoma. In all three the principles of management are debridement of nonviable tissue, followed by restoration of small intestinal continuity. Exteriorization of the small intestine is to be reserved for the patient so critically ill that additional operative time to achieve alimentary continuity is deemed to be life-threatening.

PERFORATION

In most instances of small bowel perforation, inspection will reveal a small (1-cm) clean enterotomy along its antimesenteric surface. Closure following debridement of the borders of the defect is achieved by a seromuscular layer of interrupted 3-0 silk Lembert sutures. If necessary, for hemostatic purposes, the mucosal edges may first be approximated with a continuous inner layer of 4-0 absorbable suture. Since bacterial colonization increases in variety and density from jejunum to ileum, it is thought best to direct attention toward more distal injuries first.

Although larger lacerations are closed in identical fashion, there is an added risk of luminal compromise. This is particularly important when, following debridement, the length of the enterorrhaphy approximates half that of the luminal diameter. Primary closure may still be safely achieved if the closure line is oriented along the transverse rather than longitudinal axis of the intestine. More extensive lacerations necessitate complete resection of involved intestine and enteroenterostomy. Following completion of any of these procedures, the peritoneal cavity should be liberally irrigated and particulate matter removed. Drains are not indicated. While the fascia is closed in the usual fashion, subcutaneous tissue and skin are best left open. Robbs, Moore, and Pillay[82] found that when these layers were closed in primary fashion, a high incidence of septic complications ensued. Since the authors related this morbidity to wound closure, they have recommended that closure by secondary intent be used.

MURAL DAMAGE WITHOUT PERFORATION

Partial-thickness injury to the intestinal wall presents a greater challenge to the surgeon than does perforation. It may be inviting, for instance, to "oversew" limited serosal tears beneath which lies an intact bowel wall. This procedure should be discouraged for at least two reasons: the suture line may act as focus for the development of adhesions, and the intestinal lumen may be entered during placement of the sutures. If mural integrity can be confirmed (distension by firm manual compression of the intestine proximal and distal to the injury site), serosal tears are best left alone.

The management of contusions and intramural hematomas of the small intestine requires first weighing the risks of leaving a potentially nonviable segment of intestine *in situ* against that of exposing the patient to the morbidity associated with resection of potentially viable intestine. In this regard, several methods of assessing intestinal viability beyond simple inspection have been proposed. By placing a sterile Doppler ultrasound probe over the site of injury, one can listen for both arterial and venous pulsations. Marzella, Brotman, and associates[64] demonstrated that the viability of previously traumatized segments of rat small intestine could be accurately predicted at surgery following the intravenous administration of fluorescein (10–15 mg/kg). Segments that were later proven to meet histopathologic criteria for viability were seen at surgery to have fluoresced when exposed to a Wood's lamp; lack of fluorescence was indicative of necrosis. There is often a transition zone of decreased or mottled fluorescence that corresponds to areas of questionable viability, so the fluorescein test has not gained widespread clinical acceptance.

Lacking clear-cut objective means of assessing intestinal viability, clinical judgment remains paramount in the management of this type of injury. Small (<1 cm) nonexpanding mucosal hematomas may be "turned in" with a series of interrupted 3-0 silk Lembert sutures placed, if possible, along the transverse axis of the intestine. Exploration of these lesions is not indicated, since it poses the threat of inadvertent enterotomy. In most other situations, it is prudent to err on the side of transmural debridement or segmental intestinal resection rather than risk leaving *in situ* a segment of questionably viable intestine. This is particularly so when the hematoma is positioned at the mesenteric border, precluding adequate inspection of the adjacent intestinal wall.

MESENTERIC HEMATOMA

Successful treatment of a mesenteric hematoma requires accurate assessment of several characteristics. One must define whether the hematoma is small, stable, and contained as opposed to large, expanding, or uncontained, with rupture of the mesenteric folds. Hematomas possessing the former qualities may be managed without opening the mesentery, while exploration and careful vascular control is indicated in the latter. Hematomas positioned toward the root of the mesentery, although more likely to expand owing to involvement of larger vessels, may remain stable in size; operative exploration could lead to further vascular damage. Anastomotic vascular collaterals within the undamaged mesenteric folds distal to the hematoma may be adequate to maintain intestinal viability. This will more likely occur when the hematoma is located in the ileal mesentery, since the number of vascular (particularly venous) arcades increases as one progresses down the mesentery from the ligament of Trietz. In contradistinction, hematomas closer to the intestinal wall often stabilize due to limited small vessel damage. Nonetheless, collaterals distal to the hematoma will be fewer, such that intestinal viability becomes a more serious concern.

Within this framework, the initial goal in managing a mesenteric hematoma is to be certain that there is no ongoing hemorrhage. Should it become necessary to explore a hematoma, the uninvolved mesentery proximal to it toward the base should be examined, and a site of vascular control identified, if possible. Manual compression is then applied to that point while the mesentery is incised over the length of the hematoma, bisecting it. Following careful evacuation of clot, bleeding points are individually controlled with 3-0 or 4-0 silk suture ligatures. Indiscriminate placement of mass suture ligatures is to be avoided, since damage to previously unharmed vessels may occur, further risking intestinal ischemia. Once control of hemorrhage has been accomplished, viability of intestine distal to the area of vascular damage must be determined. Resection of clearly nonviable as well as questionably viable intestine should be performed.

Patients with isolated, blunt mesenteric small intestinal injury generally experience a rapid recovery with minimal postoperative morbidity, and a mortality rate below 5%.[77] Morbidity and mortality increase dramatically when there are associated injuries or when the vascular supply is transected at the very base of the mesentery.[17] Because abdominal infections are usually cited as the major contributing factors to postoperative morbidity, patients must be observed carefully for signs and symptoms of wound or intra-abdominal sepsis.

Penetrating Small Intestine Injury

In contradistinction to injury from blunt forces, penetrating injury to the small intestine carries a much more favorable prognosis, whether the damage is isolated or associated with other visceral injury.[32] This is largely because patients who survive the initial penetrating insult are generally operated upon earlier and suffer less of a traumatic insult than those requiring surgery secondary to injury by blunt forces.

The conduct of celiotomy is similar to that detailed for blunt small intestinal injury. The bowel and mesentery are carefully examined for evidence of perforation and intramural or mesenteric hematoma. Mesenteric hematomas are managed in a fashion identical to those occurring secondary to blunt abdominal trauma. The other two types of injury require additional comments.

PERFORATION

Because of its superficial position in the midabdomen, the small intestine is frequently perforated by objects that penetrate the abdominal wall. Any number of enterotomies may be found; it is no longer felt necessary to identify an "even" number (that is, for every entrance there is an exit intestinal wound), as tangential injury to the intestinal wall is known to occur. It is far more important to carry out an assiduous inspection of the entire small intestine, particularly along its mesenteric border, and to identify all injuries. When the clinician is unable to rule out full-thickness penetration of an injured segment, manual compression of the intestinal wall proximal and distal to the injury site should be attempted. Leakage of intestinal contents through the area in question confirms the diagnosis of perforation. Partial-thickness injuries require no suture. Once the number and extent of enterotomies have been defined, the more distal ones should be managed first. Intestinal clamps or Babcock clamps may be utilized to limit intra-abdominal soilage from remaining enterotomies until definitive repair can be undertaken.

The majority of enterotomies, particularly those caused by low-velocity missiles or stab wounds, are so small that they can be closed with a few 3-0 or 4-0 silk Lembert sutures. The wall between two small enterotomies in close proximity can often be resected and closed along the transverse axis of the intestine. Larger wounds or those caused by high-velocity missiles may require a more vigorous effort to achieve mucosal hemostasis following debridement of the wound edges. A two-layer closure oriented along the transverse diameter of the intestine can be used if the wound measures less than half the diameter of the involved intestine.

Segmental intestinal resection should be reserved for large lacerations that, if closed, would compromise the luminal diameter; wounds requiring extensive mural debridement; and multiple enterotomies in a short segment of intestine. While a standard one or two-layer, end-to-end anastomosis will certainly suffice, many prefer a functional end-to-end anastomosis using autostapling devices (Fig. 9.7). The ease and rapidity with which this latter anastomosis can be performed makes it a useful technique in the management of patients with any injury to the small intestine requiring resection.

INTRAMURAL HEMATOMA

The management of intramural hematomas secondary to penetrating trauma presents a difficult challenge. In a study of experimentally induced missile injuries in pigs, Johansson, Norrby, and Lennquist [44] demonstrated that the risk of delayed perforation of intramural hematomas was high if the following clinical criteria were present at initial inspection: serosal tear, palpable defect of the involved intestinal wall, and a hematoma diameter of 1 cm. There were many segments of intestine meeting these criteria that, following resection, were found to be histologically viable. In addition to these criteria, if the intestine did not fluoresce within 5 minutes of the intravenous administration of fluorescein, the diagnostic accuracy improved considerably. Even adding this criterion does not achieve the sensitivity and specificity required for uniform application to human injury. Clinical judgment remains paramount. Again, one should err on the side of resecting what would prove to be a viable segment of intestine, rather than risk leaving *in situ* a potentially necrotic area.

The postoperative management of small intestine injuries is similar for blunt and penetrating trauma. A high index of suspicion for intra-abdominal sepsis must be maintained, particularly when there are associated intra-abdominal injuries, prolonged exposure of the abdomen to leaking intestinal contents, multiple enterorrhaphies or resections, and intestinal or mesenteric hematomas left *in situ*. Despite the high morbidity associated with reoperation of such critically ill patients, surgical intervention may be urgently required as both a diagnostic and therapeutic maneuver.

ABDOMINAL COLON TRAUMA

Blunt Colonic Injury

Significant injury to the abdominal colon secondary to blunt trauma is unusual. Of patients who undergo celiotomy for injuries sustained by blunt forces, less than 5% will have damage to the colon. The injury is rarely isolated; the vast majority of patients will be found to have suffered serious injuries to other intra-abdominal structures, which underscores the tremendous force generally required to injure the abdominal colon. The mortality and morbidity rates of those fortunate enough to survive the initial traumatic insult are surprisingly low, if proper diagnostic and therapeutic intervention is undertaken. Most importantly, the morbidity and mortality rates are not often attributable to the colon injury itself, unless a significant delay in recognition or treatment of that injury occurred.

Three separate mechanisms have been proposed to account for blunt injury to the abdominal colon.[91] A crush injury appears to be the most common mechanism, occurring when the colon hits the vertebral column or pelvis, following a severe blunt assault directed to the anterior abdomen. As evidence for this, the majority of injuries occur in the transverse and sigmoid colon; many patients with injuries in these areas also present with vertebral and pelvic fractures. Those with transverse colon damage have a high incidence of concomitant injury to that portion of the pancreas overlying the lumbar vertebrae.[37]

Shear injuries are less common, occurring at sites where the fixed retroperitoneal portions of the colon assume an intraperitoneal position and are suspended from a mesentery. In this regard, avulsion injuries at the hepatic and splenic flexures, cecum, and sigmoid colon are well documented. Additional fixation points of the colon, such as adhesions and hernias, have also been associated clinically with shearing injuries secondary to blunt abdominal trauma.

Sudden compression of a fluid-filled segment of colon that is at least partially occluded at either end may account for injury to that segment. It is suspected that this bursting-type of injury rarely, if ever, occurs. Rather, the pressure will more likely be dissipated through even a partially occluded lumen, since it offers far less resistance than the colonic wall itself.

The diagnosis of colon injury secondary to blunt trauma is rarely secured prior to examination of the organ by a celiotomy. Analysis of retrospective studies of patients who suffered such an injury suggests that clinical suspicion should be aroused in the presence of the following circumstances: deceleration injury, particularly when the victim is thrown against a steering wheel or is wearing only a lap restraint; coexistent injuries such as pelvic or lumbar vertebral fractures; or retroperitoneal paracolic air visualized upon abdominal roentgenographs.

Physical examination is helpful only insofar as it is a valid assessment of the necessity for surgical intervention, although the presence of blood in the rectal vault should raise suspicion for serious injury to the alimentary tract. Serologic tests are of little diagnostic benefit. While peritoneal lavage is often positive, the results do not assist in the specific preoperative diagnosis of colon injury. Finally, both delayed presentation of acute colonic injury[37] and delayed perforation of the colon[91] are well-documented phenomena. Prolonged clinical follow-up of patients who suffer severe blunt abdominal trauma is mandatory. Clinical deterioration in the patient's status, increased abdominal tenderness, an evolving pattern of sepsis, and development of paralytic ileus or mechanical obstruction are common findings in patients with either a missed colonic injury or delayed perforation. Under these circumstances, prompt celiotomy is felt to be the single most important step in minimizing patient morbidity and mortality.

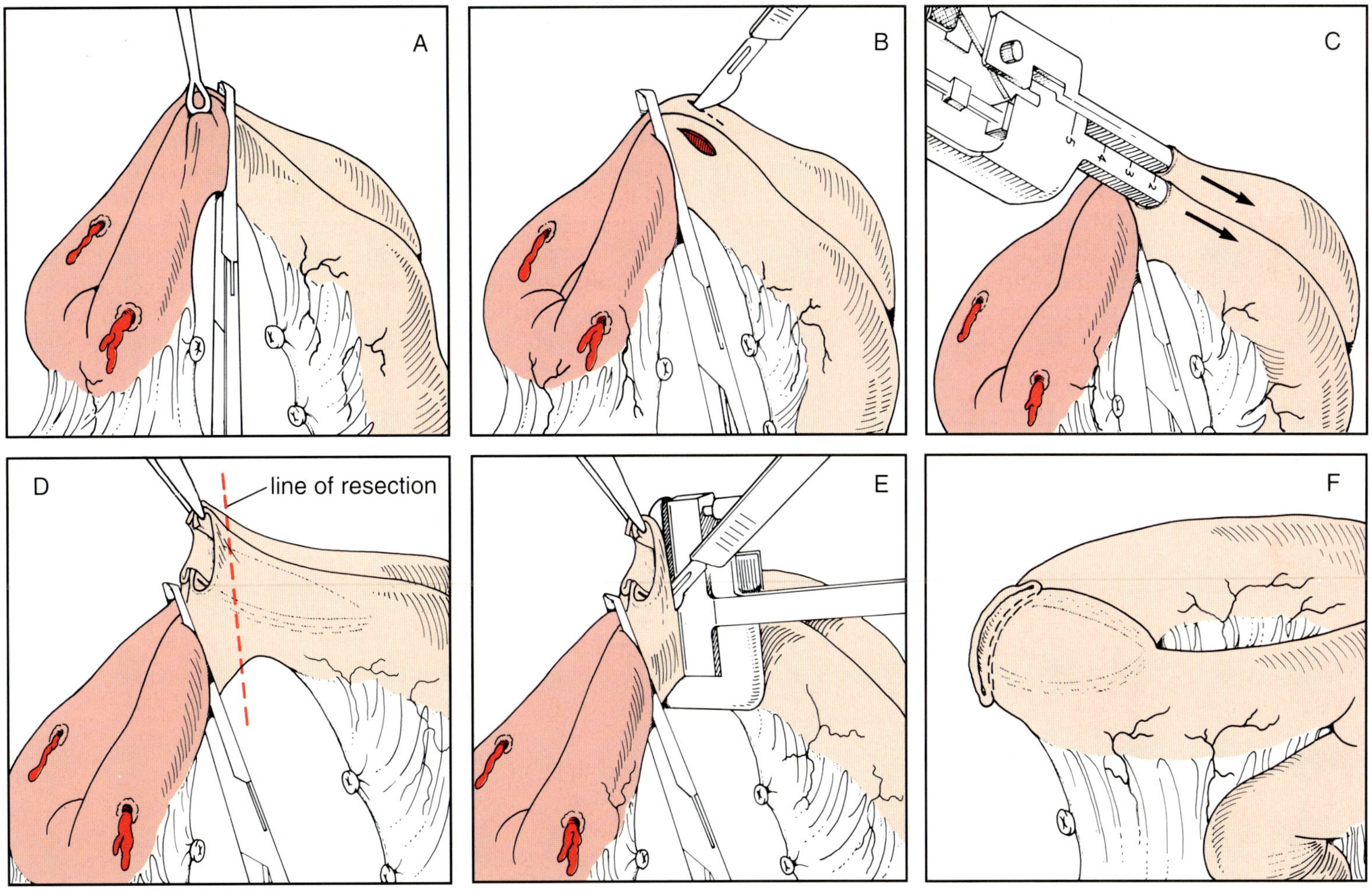

FIGURE 9.7 Small bowel resection with functional end-to-end anastomosis. **A** Antimesenteric borders of the intestine to be resected are approximated with a Babcock clamp. A Kocher clamp is placed across the intestinal loop just beyond the proposed line of resection. **B** Using a knife or cautery instrument, a stab wound is made into the lumen of both proximal and distal intestinal limbs. **C** One fork of the open GIA (gastrointestinal anastomosis) instrument is placed entirely within each lumen. Following assurance that mesentery will not become entrapped within the instrument, it is closed and engaged. Two double staggered rows of staples join the bowel walls; the knife of the GIA instrument is then used to cut between the staple lines, creating the anastomosis. The instrument is then disengaged and removed, and the anastomosis inspected for hemostasis. **D** The intestine is grasped with forceps so that the neostoma is held in the open position. **E** The TA-55 autostapling instrument is placed around proximal and distal segments and the staples engaged. The unwanted specimen is amputated using the TA-55 edge as a cutting guide. **F** Completed anastomosis. As an alternative, the injured intestine may be first resected and each end oversewn. A GIA stapled anastomosis is completed in a fashion identical to that outlined above. The pair of small intestine stab wounds are then closed in standard fashion.

In a fashion similar to that of a small intestine injury, surgical management of blunt colon injury is dependent upon both the extent of colon damage and the presence of coexistent injuries. Several points that distinguish colon from small intestine injury deserve emphasis. The arterial supply to the colon compared to the small intestine has only a few anastomotic arcades (Fig. 9.8); the colon possesses watershed areas (the points of Griffith and Sudeck) where the blood supply to the colon is at best adequate, so segmental devascularization of the colon can be achieved with a small vascular injury. Because the luminal bacterial content of the colon increases in logarithmic fashion as one moves distally from the ileocecal valve, the likelihood of serious bacterial contamination is higher in colonic than in small intestine injury. Experimental data demonstrates a significant decrease in the healing of primarily repaired colon injuries in the presence of additional blunt intra-abdominal trauma.[39] These points, together with the fact that most patients with blunt trauma to the colon have a high incidence of coexistent injuries, limit the options available for management; in fact, fewer options exist than for either blunt small intestine or penetrating colonic injury. Primary repair of blunt colonic injury can rarely be achieved with an adequate margin of safety, with two possible exceptions: minimal injury to the colon with no co-morbid conditions, and injury to the right colon with minimal associated injuries, permitting right hemicolectomy with iliotransverse colostomy.

Isolated linear serosal tears of the colon with an intact mucosal barrier are the most common type of injury and the easiest to repair.[17] Primary seromuscular reapproximation by means of several interrupted 3-0 Lembert silk sutures achieve nearly uniform success.

Injuries of a more serious nature mandate an aggressive surgical approach. Intramural hematomas, particularly those involving the transverse colon, may have a rather benign appearance. It may seem preferable to leave these untouched, particularly if transmural perforation cannot be demonstrated. Some will reabsorb without incident, but an unknown quantity will rupture secondary to infection of the hematoma or to compromise of mural blood supply because of compression by the hematoma. A certain percent of hematomas that heal will do so by scarification, resulting in clinically significant colonic stricture. Unless the hematoma is small and stable in size, a "let it be" attitude cannot be condoned.

Solitary hematomas of moderate size, particularly when located in the transverse or sigmoid colon, may be managed by exteriorization of the involved segment through a separate abdominal incision. This is a particularly attractive alternative, since it avoids violation of the gastrointestinal tract. The treatment of multiple or large colonic hematomas requires aggressive debridement of even questionably devitalized colon wall. Following this, a proximal colostomy and distal mucous fistula are fashioned through separate abdominal incisions. While the fascia is

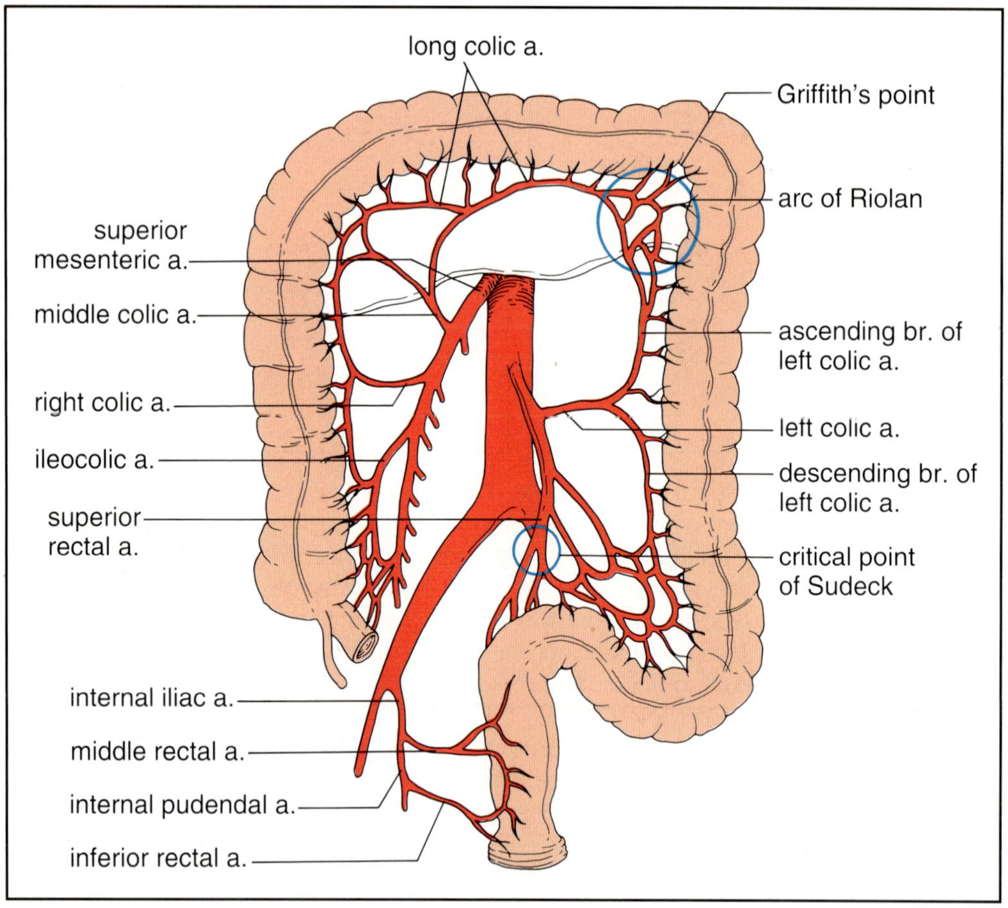

FIGURE 9.8 Schematic representation of arterial supply to the colorectum.

approximated in the usual fashion, subcutaneous tissues and skin are best left open in these and other more serious injuries.

A hematoma that arises from the blood supply to the colon is a particularly treacherous injury because of the poorly developed collateral vascular system. Following control of hemorrhage (as described for managing those of the mesenteric small intestine), viability of the colon must be carefully assessed. While both Doppler ultrasound and intravenous fluorescein injection have been proposed to assist in this decision-making process, clinical judgment remains paramount. One must clearly take an aggressive approach toward excising even questionable areas of viability rather than risk leaving an ischemic segment of colon *in situ*. Again, proximal colostomy and distal mucous fistula are required.

Management of an acute perforation or transection of the colon is extremely uncommon, since the force necessary to cause this injury is usually lethal. In patients fortunate enough to survive until celiotomy, the colon wall surrounding an acute perforation will generally appear devascularized. Generous resective debridement is needed, followed by proximal colostomy and distal mucous fistula.

Colonic perforation has been reported to occur several days to weeks following the initial traumatic insult. It is usually due to the progression of the initially ischemic segment of colon to gangrenous infarction. Morbidity and mortality rates are extremely high with this injury, and are usually secondary to septic complications. Survival is uniformly dependent upon prompt recognition of an intra-abdominal focus of sepsis, followed by immediate surgical intervention. A treatment of radical debridement of necrotic debris, complete fecal diversion, and drainage of abscess cavities will afford the best chance for survival.

The postoperative management of a patient with significant blunt colon trauma can be extremely difficult, especially when injury to other major organ systems, such as the cardiorespiratory or central nervous system, has occurred. In addition to intense perioperative hemodynamic and nutritional support, a constant surveillance of the patient for signs and symptoms of sepsis must be maintained. This is particularly important in light of the well-documented incidence of postoperative colonic rupture occurring several days to weeks following the initial insult.[91] Should a pattern of sepsis develop when all extra-abdominal sources have been satisfactorily excluded by radiologic and microbiologic analysis, urgent celiotomy should be considered as a diagnostic and therapeutic maneuver.

Penetrating Colonic Injury

Approximately 20% of patients who suffer penetrating abdominal trauma will have a colon injury. In the vast majority, the injury is confined to a limited segment of the colon, though widely separated injuries can occur.[108] When the colon is injured, concomitant organ injury is present at least 70% of the time—more so if the injuries are secondary to a gunshot or shotgun (80%), less if they are results of stab wounds (50%). The intraoperative assessment of the severity of these coexistent injuries is extremely important in determining which of several available surgical options affords the lowest mortality with acceptable morbidity. With proper judgment along established surgical guidelines, mortality rates—at one time more than 50%—can be extremely low; recent accumulated studies report rates well under 10%.[1,99,108] Analysis of the deaths in these studies suggests that the vast majority were due to complications arising from associated injuries rather than either the colon injury itself or the type of repair used.[78] Despite the improvement in mortality, patient morbidity remains high (30%); individual rates vary widely and are clearly dependent upon the surgical technique used. From this perspective, the principles of managing a colon injury should be (1) to select the surgical technique that ensures a low mortality risk, and (2) given a choice of techniques with equivalent mortality rates, to select the one that affords the lowest morbidity.

In order to better understand how various techniques for managing penetrating colon injury were developed, a brief historical review[1] is helpful. Prior to recent decades, most knowledge of these injuries was gained through military experience. During the early stages of World War II, mortality rates secondary to colon injury were more than 50%. It was not until the management principles espoused by Ogilvie,[74] Hamilton,[33] and a host of other surgeons were employed that mortality from this injury decreased appreciably. These physicians individually developed the concept that exteriorization of the colon injury is of primary importance. If not possible, the injured segment should be either resected and a colostomy performed, or defunctionalized by proximal diverting colostomy. After several months, gastrointestinal continuity would be restored. With further improvement in perioperative management of trauma victims, application of these operative principles to victims of more recent military conflicts reduced the mortality rate to 10%, despite more virulent weaponry.

The remarkable improvement in military injury survival led to establishing these principles as the standard of care in civilian practice. As early as 1951, Woodhall and Ochsner[111] reported their experience with selective primary closure of penetrating colon wounds in civilians. By reserving primary closure for patients demonstrating hemodynamic stability, small wounds to the colon with minimal intraperitoneal contamination, and virtually no associated injuries, they were able to achieve mortality rates similar to those for exteriorization of the colon wound. Due to the low morbidity associated with primary closure versus exteriorization (that is, secondary operative procedure required), the authors concluded this to be a viable alternative in the management of civilian colon injury. Despite this data, majority opinion clearly favored exteriorization until later reports reaffirmed the selective role of primary closure of colon wounds in both civilian[78] and military[73] practice. There was some initial evidence that primary repair might best be reserved for right-sided colon injury[56] because of its favorable characteristics of liquid content with both fewer and less diverse microorganisms, better blood supply, and larger luminal diameter. It has since been demonstrated that despite such differences, penetrating trauma to the right and left hemicolon can be managed in similar fashion.[99]

Many surgeons were still hesitant to accept primary closure techniques (for fear of the mortality associated with breakdown of the repair), so a compromise procedure evolved.[75] Following primary repair of the colon injury, that segment would be exteriorized through a separate abdominal incision for purposes of observation. If the colon repair failed, the patient would be no worse off than if the wound had simply been exteriorized, but if the repair remained intact for several days, the segment of colon could be returned to the abdomen. This is still safer than restoring gastrointestinal continuity following open exteriorization procedures. Exteriorized repair of colon injuries became an acceptable alternative in select cases of penetrating colon injury because of these advantages.[7]

It would appear from available data that a uniform approach to the management of penetrating abdominal colon injury is unnecessary. Given proper patient selection, the mortality rates for primary repair, closed exteriorization, and open exteriorization/resection will be similar. In terms of individual patient morbidity, the risk: benefit ratio of each procedure must be properly assessed to determine the best way to manage a given colon injury. The following discussion summarizes the conditions and technical considerations under which each of the three general approaches to the management of a colon injury might best be applied.

Primary Repair Over the past several years, circumstances under which primary repair of a colon injury might better be deferred have been fairly well established:[108]

- Prolonged or persistent hypotension
- Greater than 6-hour delay between injury and surgical intervention
- Gross fecal spillage
- Extensive damage to abdominal or retroperitoneal muscle
- Significant hemoperitoneum
- Multiple coexistent visceral injuries or serious injury to the liver, spleen, pancreas, or kidney

Though age and associated medical illnesses such as cirrhosis, diabetes mellitus, and atherosclerotic vascular disease are not absolute contraindications, they must be considered in the overall decision-making process. The vast majority of patients who suffer penetrating colon injury in civilian life, fortunately, are otherwise young and healthy.

Intraoperative evaluation of the colon injury itself is as well extremely important. The Flint classification[24] and Denver colon injury severity score [88] have been devised in an attempt to grade the severity of injury. Based on results of patients with penetrating colon injury graded by either classification, initial contemplation of primary repair should be reconsidered if any of the following conditions are found at celiotomy:

- Devitalization of more than one-fourth of the colon wall;
- Impairment of the blood supply to the injured segment;
- More destructive colon injury than a simple through-and-through perforation.

Given appropriate regard to the aforementioned, it is estimated that at minimum one-half of patients will be candidates for primary repair of a penetrating colon injury.[3,70,92,99,108] The technique begins with thorough and meticulous debridement of the wound edges. Most surgeons then employ a standard two layer closure (an inner layer of simple running or interrupted 4-0 absorbable suture to invert the mucosa, followed by an outer seromuscular row of interrupted 3-0 silk Lembert sutures to turn in the inner layer). More recently, however, the use of a single layer anastomosis employing a 2-0 or 3-0 polypropylene (or polydiaxonone) suture has gained popularity. The establishment of proximal "protective" diverting colostomy defeats most of the advantages of primary repair. Prior to fascial closure, the abdomen is liberally irrigated with saline and all particulate matter removed. "Sentinel" drains placed at or near the site of a primarily closed colon wound are not indicated. Wide debridement of any tract created by a missile after it exits the colon is uniformly indicated.[23] Although several authors have reported that skin and subcutaneous tissues can be primarily closed,[3] others [36,107] have found this maneuver to result in excessively high wound infection rates, and recommend closure by delayed primary methods (if not by secondary intent).

When the aforementioned principles are strictly observed, the mortality rate associated with this injury has been reported to average 5%.[3,70,88,92,99] The majority of deaths were due to causes unrelated to the colon injury itself. Stone and Fabian [92] indicated that the infectious morbidity associated with primarily closed colon wounds was actually lower than a matched group who had a colostomy fashioned as well. Patients who undergo primary repair are spared a second major surgical procedure, that of colostomy closure. For these reasons, it is concluded that primary repair is both a safe and effective means of managing many penetrating colon injuries.

Exteriorized Repair Despite the reports that appeared in the surgical literature in the 1970s demonstrating the efficacy of selective primary closure of penetrating colon wounds, some surgeons felt that the risk:benefit ratio was too high to support its utilization. Others who performed selective primary repair found, on the one hand, that under certain conditions the repair was insecure; on the other hand, formation of a colostomy was felt to be overly aggressive. For these reasons, a compromise procedure called exteriorized repair, based on earlier descriptions by Mason [33] and Colcock,[13] was brought to the forefront. This procedure involves meticulous debridement of the colon wound followed by careful two-layer anastomosis. The injured segment of colon is then mobilized and brought out through an incision separate from that of the celiotomy wound. There can be no tension exerted on the repair once the exteriorized segment is supported by a rod on the abdominal wall. Fascial closure is achieved in the usual fashion; skin and subcutaneous tissues are left open. The exteriorized segment is kept moist within a colostomy bag by covering it with petroleum jelly–impregnated fine mesh gauze.

Use of this technique enables 50% to 75% of patients to undergo early "internalization" of the involved colon segment.[3,7,16,70,72,100] While this second procedure may require a general anesthetic, the segment of colon can usually be freed up from surrounding structures and returned to the abdomen using local anesthetic agents supported by intravenous administration of meperidine or diazepam. This procedure is done from 5 to 14 days following the initial colon repair, after the complete return of bowel function. Additional support for this interval is found in a review of 32 exteriorized repairs performed for penetrating colon injuries. Of the 16 that failed, 11 occurred within 7 postoperative days; the remaining 5 breakdowns happened by the ninth day.[100] Based on this data, the authors recommended a 10-day period of observation prior to internalizing a colon repair. Critics of exteriorized repair note both the high associated failure rate and the increased number of other complications (such as wound infection) when compared with either primary repair or colostomy. There is also a general impression that repair breakdown is a predictable result of the inhibitory effects on wound healing secondary to a serositis that typically develops when the colon is exposed to the outside air for even a short period. In animal studies that examined exteriorized colon anastomoses, healing was virtually uniform.[51] While perhaps not as successful in the clinical setting of emergency surgery in humans, it is clear that at least some patients who underwent emergency exteriorized repair were spared a colostomy. Furthermore, those who experienced breakdown of the repair were likely no worse off than if they had received a formal colostomy in the first place. It would therefore appear that, under limited circumstances, exteriorized repair belongs in the armamentarium of treatment options for penetrating abdominal colon injury.

Open Exteriorization/Resection There is little doubt that the standard treatment of colon injuries as originally espoused by Ogilvie and others remains the treatment of choice in severely injured patients with penetrating colon wounds. While some authors[14] maintain that these principles should be applied to virtually all penetrating colon injuries, acceptance by surgeons of selected primary closure or exteriorized repair has resulted in a decrease in the use of open exteriorization/resection procedures to 25% to 50% of all civilian wounds. The fundamental principles behind this technique have remained essentially unchanged over the years. For small, isolated colon wounds, the involved segment is first mobilized and then exteriorized through a separate abdominal incision in order to function as a colostomy. Large wounds, multiple wounds, or wounds resulting in a major area of devascularized colon require segmental colon resection with proximal diverting colostomy and distal mucous fistula, fashioned again through separate abdominal incisions. Following liberal saline lavage of the abdominal cavity, fascia is approximated in the usual fashion; skin and subcutaneous tissues are left open.

These techniques are associated with a mortality rate comparable to that of methods previously described for managing penetrating colon injury. Both immediate and delayed morbidity do appear to be higher. Some authors have reported an increased number of early postoperative complications related directly to the use of colostomy procedures, but Stone and Fabian[92] found that when patients with favorable injuries are randomly given either primary closure or colostomy, no difference in early postoperative morbidity (other than a shortened hospital stay in primarily closed patients) was identified. It would be reasonable to assume that the higher number of complications with colostomy (reported in other studies) reflects the known bias favoring the use of colostomy procedures in more seriously injured patients.

The major morbidity associated with colostomy is that requiring reconstitution of the gastrointestinal tract in a second major operative procedure. The timing of this operation is important to minimize the associated surgical morbidity. Thal and Yeary [99] have found that colostomy closure at 1 to 2 postoperative months is associated with a lower morbidity (4%) compared to that which occurs when the operation is performed between 2 and 12 months (10%–15%). It would certainly appear that, in otherwise healthy patients who experience an uncomplicated initial postoperative course, delay of colostomy closure beyond 3 months in order to allow further resolution of residual inflammatory processes is unwarranted.[60]

Mention must be made of specific conditions under which more extensive colon injuries can be managed by means other than resection with proximal diversion. These circumstances are especially favorable when the site of colon injury is in the right hemicolon and the patient otherwise exhibits conditions that, with the exception of the severity of the colon injury, would favor an attempt at primary repair. Given these conditions, right hemicolectomy with primary ileotransverse colostomy has been performed by many surgeons, with morbidity and mortality rates equivalent to those of primary repair of less extensive injuries. The major advantage of this procedure is that it avoids the fluid and electrolyte complications known to occur with an ileostomy. However, as clearly pointed out by Walt,[108] no compromise of established surgical principles for managing a colon injury should be made in an attempt to spare the patient from the morbidity of a temporary ileostomy. With this caveat, right hemicolectomy with primary anastomosis may ultimately become the preferred method of managing penetrating right colon injuries.

Selection of the technique that best fits a given injury requires an accurate assessment of the patient's clinical status and a familiarity with the conditions under which each procedure can safely be applied. In this light, there has been a clearcut preference toward the performance of primary repair of colon injuries. In 1984, Adkins, Zirkle, and Waterhouse reported that, despite the increased rate of primarily repaired colon wounds, the percentage of colostomies remained fairly constant, while exteriorized repairs decreased. This finding was felt to underscore the continued respect on the part of surgeons for the principles under which primary repair is not indicated. Since morbidity rates were not appreciably altered, the authors implied that the trend toward primary repair was most likely due to a learning curve—as surgeons acquiesced to the guidelines established for performing that procedure, rather than compromise them by choosing exteriorized repair.

More recently, Fabian and colleagues[27,28] analyzed their experience in managing colon injuries from both retrospectively and prospectively collected data. These investigators once again found that the perioperative morbidity and mortality rates associated with primary closure of colon injuries were no different than those associated with open exteriorization/resection. In all patients, the complication rates were clearly increased in the face of prolonged hypotension, significant fecal contamination, multiple transfusions, etc.—factors mentioned earlier in this chapter that would cause one seriously to reconsider a decision to primarily close a colon wound. However, the complications that occurred in patients with primarily closed colon injuries were a consequence of the severity of the injuries themselves rather than technical problems with the colonic suture line (e.g., anastomotic leak). Given these data, it was concluded that virtually all colon injuries, regardless of severity or anatomic site, were amenable to primary closure with or without resection. While many surgeons feel this posture is a bit too liberal, the general consensus appears to be leaning towards a more aggressive approach to primarily close colon injuries—at least to the exclusion of closed exteriorization procedures.

The postoperative course of patients with penetrating abdominal colon injury is dependent upon the extent of associated injuries. Morbidity, particularly of an infectious nature, is related directly to the existence of co-morbid conditions, such as the number and extent of intra-abdominal and retroperitoneal injuries. Close clinical observation for signs of wound or intra-abdominal sepsis must be maintained. Despite leaving skin and subcutaneous tissue open and postoperative continuation of broad-spectrum antibiotic therapy, wound infection rates associated with colon injuries are known to approach 20%.[107] More importantly, the presence of infection in an open wound is associated with an intra-abdominal abscess in almost three-fourths of the cases reported in that study, so simply establishing drainage of an apparently superficial wound abscess is not sufficient. All efforts must be geared toward the identification of a more deeply seated infection requiring reoperation if it is found to be inaccessible to percutaneous drainage.

ANORECTAL TRAUMA

Blunt Anorectal Injury

Injury by blunt forces to that part of the large intestine below the peritoneal reflection is unusual, because of the protection offered by the bony pelvis. While anorectal injury can be secondary to abdominal trauma,[69] it more commonly occurs in conjunction with a blunt force applied directly to the pelvis of such magnitude as to result in extensive fractures of the bony ring as well as perineal lacerations. The extensive network of arteries and veins that course along the pelvic side walls cause massive retroperitoneal hemorrhage to frequently accompany this injury. Patients fortunate enough to survive the initial traumatic insult will often be afflicted with coexistent injuries to the central nervous system, lungs, abdominal viscera, bladder, and long bones,[81] challenging the physician's resuscitative efforts and diagnostic acumen. In this setting, failure to identify or adequately treat an anorectal or perineal injury will severely compromise any initial success in managing the patient past the acute phase of injury. For bacterial contamination of a devascularized, blood-laden retroperitoneum/perineum will almost uniformly result in sepsis (necrotizing fasciitis) that will proceed uncontrolled despite heroic efforts.

The diagnosis of anorectal injury alone or with a perineal laceration should be entertained whenever there is clinical or roentgenographic evidence for significant pelvic trauma. The cause of the injury is typically a crushing or compressive force applied to the pelvis, as would occur when the victim has been struck or run over by a motor vehicle. In these instances, examination of the skin overlying the lower abdomen and pelvis for ecchymosis may further raise suspicion of pelvic fracture. The stability of the pelvic ring can be assessed by gently applying pressure to both iliac crests. All clothing must be removed and the perineum closely examined for evidence of laceration.

Rectal examination is extremely important. A mobile prostate is presumptive evidence for urethral injury. Presence of heme-positive stool mandates further evaluation by proctosigmoidoscopy; despite an examination compromised by the presence of residual stool in the rectal vault, the site of anorectal injury can often be identified. Due to the morbid consequences associated with missing an anorectal injury, a negative examination should not override clinical concern that an injury requiring early and aggressive surgical management has in fact occurred. Such patients must be rapidly assessed for the following:

- Injury to other organs, particularly intra-abdominal viscera, that mandates urgent surgical intervention
- Presence and extent of pelvic ring fracture
- Perineal injury that has converted a closed pelvic fracture to an open one
- Violation of the closed retroperitoneal space by a deep perineal laceration
- Presence or suspicion of anorectal injury

Whether or not the anorectum has been violated, it is clear that in the absence of significant intra-abdominal sources of hemorrhage, early mortality in patients with massive pelvic injury is related directly to fracture-associated hemorrhage. The task of maintaining an adequate blood volume and normal coagulation profile is made more difficult when the patient has suffered a concomitant deep perineal laceration, violating the retroperitoneal space. As a result, there is a loss of the tamponade effect of that closed space, which would otherwise limit blood loss from a pelvic fracture. If emergency surgery is not otherwise indicated, a graded series of maneuvers to achieve control of pelvic hemorrhage is recommended:

1. Application of pneumatic antishock garment to both stabilize the pelvic fracture and supply external tamponade
2. Angiographic embolization of clot into bleeding pelvic arteries
3. External fixation of the pelvic fractures with orthopaedic appliances
4. Surgical ligation of hypogastric vessels
5. Exploration of the pelvic hematoma itself with direct suture ligation
6. Abdominoperineal resection with subsequent gauze packing of the pelvis

The availability at most institutions of vast quantities of blood and blood products has allowed nonsurgical methods to be used successfully to control hemorrhage in most instances. Despite institution of the full gamut of heroic measures to control hemorrhage in patients with pelviperineal injuries, the early mortality rate from hemorrhage is reported to be 10% to 33%.[52,67,81]

Even with patient survival beyond the stage of massive hemorrhage, efforts to rule out anorectal injury beyond reasonable doubt must persist, lest the patient become a victim of septic complications from a missed or incorrectly managed injury. Early definitive surgical management, consisting of total fecal diversion, should be encouraged in any patient with one of the following conditions:

- Endoscopically visualized anorectal injury, regardless of associated injuries

A possible anorectal injury, clinically suspected but not identified
Open pelvic fracture, whether or not anorectal injury has been identified

While the first two indications are self-explanatory, the final one deserves further attention. Several investigators have noted that, while 31% to 67% of patients with open pelvic fracture have an anorectal injury lending itself to definitive surgical therapy, failure to totally divert the fecal stream (even in the absence of the anorectal injury) resulted in a high rate of septic morbidity and mortality. Since the authors relate these complications to continued fecal soilage of the pelviperineal injury, immediate and complete fecal diversion in all cases of open pelvic fracture is recommended.[52,67,81]

The favored surgical approach to achieve total fecal diversion is lower midline celiotomy with the patient in a slight lithotomy position. Once an assessment of intra-abdominal viscera has been made, the sigmoid colon is mobilized with care to avoid intra-abdominal violation of the retroperitoneal space. The colon is then divided between the intestinal clamps and each end brought out through separate abdominal incisions. Once fascial closure is completed, skin and subcutaneous tissue are packed open and then isolated from the neostomas with wound dressings. The intestinal clamp on the distal segment of the sigmoid colon is removed and intubated with a large-bore (28-French) catheter. After an assistant dilates the anus from below, several liters of saline solution are instilled through the catheter, irrigating the distal colon until clear; manual transanal disimpaction may be required. While some surgeons prefer to reapply the intestinal clamp to the mucous fistula and delay formal maturation of both stomas for several days in order to minimize contamination,[67] others find no disadvantage to immediate stomal maturation.

In cases where an anorectal injury is found to be readily accessible to a transanal approach, wound approximation using a single layer of running 3-0 absorbable suture may be attempted. Injuries in the area of the anorectal junction are particularly amenable to repair. Attempts to identify whether the sphincter mechanism has been violated should be made. If such an injury is found, muscular reapproximation is performed using interrupted horizontal mattress techniques with a 3-0 absorbable suture. The mucosa is reapproximated over this repair using a continuous 3-0 absorbable suture; the anal mucocutaneous junction is left open for drainage purposes. It is important to recall that primary closure of any anorectal wound from blunt trauma does not obviate the need for a totally diverting colostomy. Debridement of nonviable tissue from any existing perineal wounds is mandatory. All patients with blunt anorectal injuries should have insertion of at least two presacral retrorectal drains. There is no role for draining perineal wounds through a transperitoneal approach.

Sepsis is the primary source of delayed morbidity and mortality in patients with these types of injury. It usually occurs within the pelvic retroperitoneal hematoma, particularly when there has been an associated perineal laceration, rectal injury, or urinary disruption. Retrospective analysis [52,67,81] of patients who suffered these injuries indicates that in most instances, failure to control sepsis could be traced to at least one of the following errors in judgment: delay in performance of colostomy, failure to perform a totally diverting colostomy, failure to complete a rectal washout, or failure to utilize liberal presacral drainage. Strict adherence to the aforementioned surgical guidelines is associated with the lowest incidence of septic morbidity and mortality.

Even with proper fecal diversion, the postoperative management of these patients must be oriented toward early identification and aggressive treatment of septic foci. While pulmonary and intra-abdominal infections are common co-morbid conditions, the most likely source of sepsis remains the pelviperineal injury. Residual infection may require several sessions of intraoperative debridement in order to control sepsis, even with the insertion of multiple active and passive presacral drainage devices, effective use of antibiotics, and bedside efforts to mechanically debride these wounds. Hemipelvectomy has been required in more serious cases as a lifesaving maneuver. Septic bouts in most patients are well controlled with far less drastic surgical procedures, and gradual recovery can be expected in the majority. Colostomy closure in these patients should not be contemplated until all fractures are healed, wounds have closed, and residual hematoma has been resorbed. Completion of this process may take several additional months following clinical recovery.

Penetrating Anorectal Injury

Virtually everything, from bicycle seats[30] to enema tips[18] and unusual attempts at sexual gratification,[18] has been implicated as the causative agent of penetrating anorectal injury. Gunshot or shotgun wounds remain the most common cause. The presence of buckshot wounds in the thighs, perineum, buttocks, or lower abdomen should alert the clinician to this injury possibility. The path of one or several gunshot missiles may be estimated if entrance and exit wounds can be lined up; a projectile that is estimated to have crossed the midline in the perineal/pelvic area mandates further evaluation of the anorectum. Bullets do not uniformly travel in straight lines; they may tumble as they strike various tissues and cause considerable damage at a distance from the proposed missile tract. It is best to proceed with further evaluation of the anorectum if there is any evidence of missile proximity. In this regard, digital rectal examination is required; the presence of blood in the stool is presumptive evidence of alimentary canal injury, usually to the distal colon. Proctosigmoidoscopy should be performed in all patients suspected of having suffered anorectal injury, regardless of the findings on rectal examination. In the majority, the site of injury will be identified; in a few, the presence of blood in the upper rectal vault will be the only evidence of injury requiring surgical intervention.[103]

If time permits and there remains uncertainty regarding the possibility of anorectal injury, anterior-posterior and lateral lower abdominal roentgenographs may be helpful, particularly when no exit wound is identified or the patient has incurred a shotgun injury. The presence of missiles lodged below the peritoneal reflection, particularly if they appear to have crossed the midline, is cause for concern. Laboratory analysis is of little benefit. Hematuria may be indicative of bladder or urethral injury; and since both structures are in close proximity to the anorectum, concomitant injury to the latter should be suspected. Peritoneal lavage is rarely indicated in these patients, as most with penetrating injury otherwise meet conventional criteria for urgent celiotomy.

The principles of surgical management for penetrating trauma to the anorectum are similar to those detailed for treatment of blunt injury. Midline celiotomy with the patient in mild lithotomy position is used to gain maximal exposure. An injury to the lower rectum that is accessible by a transanal approach should be repaired using techniques identical to those outlined above. Those beyond a transanal approach should be identified transabdominally by incising the peritoneum just lateral to either side of the rectum, and mobilizing that segment. Upon identifying the site of injury, the wound edges are debrided and standard two-layer closure of the colotomy performed. Any missile tract found at celiotomy to approach the rectum should be carefully traced until satisfied that its course presents no potential for visceral injury. Failure to visualize an injury should not override clinical concern that one has in fact occurred. On the contrary, suspicion of anorectal injury based on proximity alone is a clear-cut indication for definitive therapy.[102]

Treatment of anorectal trauma requires a diverting (sigmoid colon, if possible) colostomy. Initial enthusiasm [6,31] for selective primary repair alone of these injuries has dimmed, due to the high postoperative complication rate. It would appear that total diversion of the fecal stream rather than closure of the enterotomy is the most important principle in management. In a series of rectal injuries reported by Tuggle and Huber,[103] whether or not primary closure was used in colotomy made no difference in postoperative morbidity provided that diversion of the fecal stream was performed. Distal colon washout remains an important feature in the care of these patients, despite some evidence that it was of no benefit in so-called "minimal" injuries.[103] To the contrary, several investigators [51,106] have found a significantly higher rate of septic complications when colon washout did not accompany diversion in patients with penetrating anorectal trauma. Insertion of active and passive presacral drains, to be left in place for several postoperative days, is clearly warranted.

As an expedient alternative to the standard diverting colostomy techniques described previously, stapled loop colostomy has been utilized to deal with some anorectal injuries. Ideal candidates for this procedure are those with a small clean proximal rectal injury that is readily approximated by standard closure techniques; and those suspected of anorectal injury on the grounds of proximity, but without identified colonic mural damage. The technique (Figs. 9.9 and 9.10) basically involves mobilization of a loop of sigmoid colon through a separate (lateral) abdominal incision. After the segment is stabilized on the abdominal wall by a rod passed through the colonic mesentery, a stapling device (TA-55 or TA-90) is applied across the colon, functionally diverting fecal flow from the distal colon. After fascial closure, the midline wound is isolated with dressings from the colostomy and a 3-0 absorbable purse-string suture is placed in that part of the colon distal to the staple line. A colotomy is then made within the purse-string and an irrigating catheter inserted for distal colonic washout. The purse-string is drawn up and secured after the catheter is withdrawn. A series of interrupted 3-0 silk Lembert sutures are then used to turn in the purse-string suture. The rapidity with which this procedure can be performed makes it an ideal alternative to conventional tech-

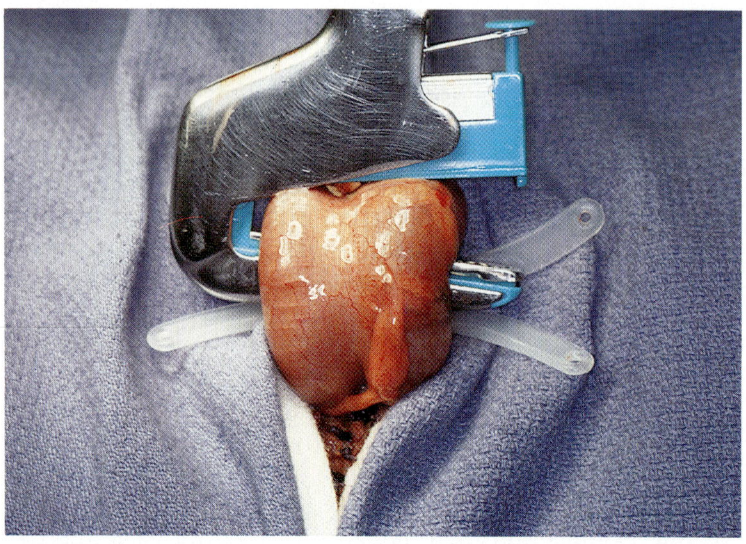

FIGURE 9.9 Stapled diverting colostomy. The sigmoid colon has been exteriorized, supported on the abdominal wall by a plastic rod. A TA-90 autostapling device is placed across the colon. Engagement of the device will result in functional division of the colon.

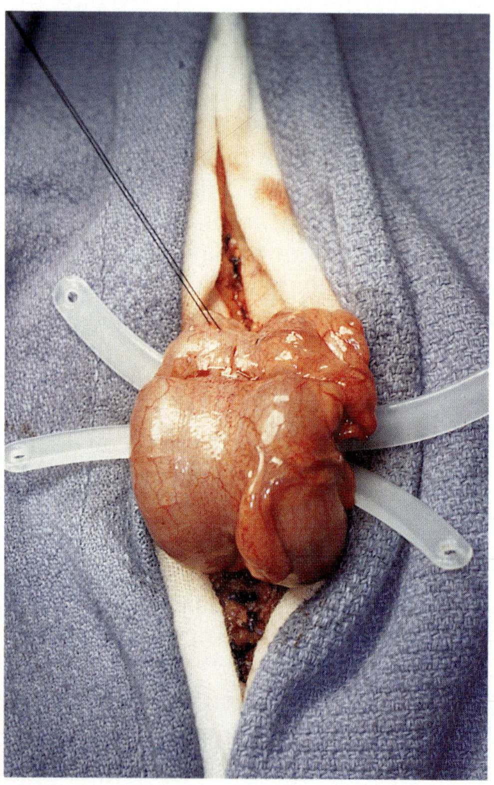

FIGURE 9.10 A doubled staggered row of stainless steel staples is shown. A purse-string suture placed in the distal colonic segment allows controlled colotomy and irrigation of the distal colorectum. Following catheter removal the suture is secured and turned in with interrupted 3-0 silk Lembert sutures, recreating total fecal diversion.

niques. The major theoretical concern is that, should the purse-string colotomy repair break down, total diversion would be difficult to maintain. This concern has yet to achieve clinical significance, and stapled colostomy remains an attractive option, given selective circumstances, that has considerable support in the literature.[67]

As in blunt trauma, the most common complication associated with penetrating anorectal trauma is that of pelviperineal sepsis. A low threshold for surgical exploration of the presacral space, despite the presence of drainage systems, must be maintained in order to minimize infection-related morbidity. If proper surgical technique is combined with aggressive perioperative care, morbidity in patients with penetrating anorectal injuries should be no more than 10%.[53,102,103,106]

REFERENCES

1. Abcarian H, Lowe R: Colon and rectal trauma. Surg Clin North Am 58(3):519–537, 1978.
2. Adkins RB, Keyser JE III: Recent experience with duodenal trauma. Am Surg 51:121–131, 1985.
3. Adkins RB, Zirkle KP, Waterhouse G: Penetrating colon trauma. J Trauma 24(6):491–499, 1984.
4. Andersen DK, Bolman RM, Moylan JA: Management of penetrating pancreatic injuries: Subtotal pancreatectomy using the auto suture stapler. J Trauma 20(4):347–349, 1980.
5. Balasegaram M: Surgical management of pancreatic trauma. Am J Surg 131:536–540, 1976.
6. Bartzial JF, Boyd DR, Folk FA et al: A initial review of management of 392 colon and rectal injuries. Dis Colon Rectum 17:313–318, 1974.
7. Barwick WJ, Schoffstall RO: Routine exteriorization in the treatment of civilian colon injuries: A reappraisal. Am Surg 44:716–722, 1978.
8. Berne CJ, Donovon AJ, White EJ, Yellin AE: Duodenal "diverticulization" for duodenal and pancreatic injury. Am J Surg 127:503–507, 1974.
9. Berni GA, Bandyk DF, Oreskovich MR, Carrico CJ: Role of intraoperative pancreatography in patients with injury to the pancreas. Am J Surg 148:602–605, 1982.
10. Carswell JW: Small gut injuries in blunt abdominal trauma: 18 cases from Uganda. Injury 5:233–236, 1974.
11. Case MES, Nanduri: R: Lacerations of the stomach by blunt trauma in a child: A case of child abuse. J Forensic Sci 28(2):496–501, 1983.
12. Cogbill TH, Moore EE, Kashuk JL: Changing trends in the management of pancreatic trauma. Arch Surg 117:722–728, 1982.
13. Colcock BP: Injuries of the colon and rectum. Surg Clin North Am 76:665, 1946.
14. Cook I, Levine BA, Rusing T et al: Traditional treatment of colon injuries. Arch Surg 119:591–594, 1984.
15. Courcy PA, Soderstrom C, Brotman S: Gastric rupture from blunt trauma: A plea for minimal diagnostics and early surgery. Am Surg 50:424–427, 1984.
16. Dang CV, Peter ET, Parks SN, Ellyson JH: Trauma of the colon: Early dropback of exteriorized repair. Arch Surg 117:652–656, 1982.
17. Dauterive AH, Flancbaum L, Cox EF: Blunt intestinal trauma: A modern-day review. Ann Surg 201(2):198–203, 1985.
18. Davis JH: Self-inflicted injuries of the anus, rectum and perineum. Am J Proctol 20(3):209–213, 1969.
19. Evans JP: Traumatic rupture of the ileum. Br J Surg 60(2):119–121, 1973.
20. Fabian TC, Mangiante EC, Millis M: Duodenal rupture due to blunt trauma: A problem in diagnosis. South Med J 77(9):1078–1082, 1984.
21. Federle MP, Crass RA, Jeffrey RB, Trunkey DD: Computed tomography in blunt abdominal trauma. Arch Surg 117:645–650, 1982.
22. Flint LM, McCoy M, Richardson JD, Polk HC: Duodenal injury: Analysis of common misconceptions in diagnosis and treatment. Ann Surg 191:697–702, 1980.
23. Flint LM, Voyles CR, Richardson JD, Fry DE: Missile tract infections after transcolonic gunshot wounds. Arch Surg 113:727–728, 1978.
24. Flint L, Vitale GC, Richardson JD: The injured colon: Relationship of management of complications. Ann Surg 193:619–623, 1981.
25. Freeark RJ, Moss GS, Sheldon G, Walt AJ: AAST Panel: Controversies in management of duodenal injuries. J Trauma 24(6):481–485, 1984.
26. Garfinkle SE, Matolo NM: Gastric necrosis from blunt abdominal trauma. J Trauma 16(5):406–407, 1976.
27. George SM, Fabian TC, Mangiante, EC: Colon trauma: further support for primary repair. Am J Surg 156:16-20, 1988.
28. George SM, Fabian TC, Voelle GR, Kudsk KA, Mangiante EC, Britt LG: Primary repair of colon wounds: a prospective trial in nonselected patients.Ann Surg 209(6):728-734, 1989.
29. Gourdie AL: Penetrating rectal wound from a bicycle saddle. Br J Accident Surg 16(6): 409–410, 1985.
30. Graham JM, Mattox KL, Vaughan D, Jordan GL: Combined pancreatoduodenal injuries. J Trauma 19(5):340–346, 1978.
31. Haas PA, Fox TA: Civilian injuries of the rectum and anus. Dis Colon Rectum 22(1):17–23, 1986.
32. Hall A, Angles A: Traumatic injuries to the small intestine. Am Surg 35(2):130–134, 1969.
33. Hamilton JE: War wounds of the colon and rectum. NY State J Med 44:2706–2712, 1944.
34. Harrison RC, Debas HT: Injuries of the stomach and duodenum. Surg Clin North Am 52(3):635–648, 1972.
35. Hasson JE, Stern D, Moss GS: Penetrating duodenal trauma. J Trauma 24(6):471–474, 1984.
36. Haygood FD, Polk HC: Gunshot wounds of the colon: A review of 100 consecutive patients, with emphasis on complications and their causes. Am J Surg 131:213–218, 1976.
37. Howell HS, Bartizal JF, Freeark RJ: Blunt trauma involving the colon and rectum. J Trauma 16(8):624–632, 1976.
38. Hudson I, Kavanagh TG: Duodenal transection and vertebral injury occurring in combination in a patient wearing a seat belt. Br J Accident Surg 15(1):6–9, 1983.
39. Irvin TT, Hunt TK: The effect of trauma on colonic healing. Br J Surg 61:430–436, 1974.
40. Ivatury RR, Gaudino J, Ascer E et al: Treatment of penetrating duodenal injuries: Primary repair vs. repair with decompressive enterostomy/serosal patch. J Trauma 25(4): 337–341, 1985.
41. Ivatury RR, Nallathambi M, Gaudino J et al: Penetrating duodenal injuries. Ann Surg 20:153–158, 1985.
42. Janson KL, Stockinger F: Duodenal hematoma; Critical analysis of recent treatment techniques. Am J Surg 129:304–308, 1975.
43. Jepsen OB, Larsen SO, Thompson VF: Postoperative wound sepsis in general surgery: II. An assessment of factors influencing the frequency of wound sepsis. Acta Chir Scand (Suppl) 396:80, 1969.
44. Johansson L, Norrby K, Lennquist S: Fluorescein angiography in the elevation of intestinal intramural hemorrhage after trauma. Acta Chir Scand 150:57–61, 1984.
45. Jones RC: Management of pancreatic trauma. Ann Surg 187(5):555–564, 1978.
46. Jones WR, Hardin WJ, Davis JT, Hardy JD: Intramural hematoma of the duodenum: A review of the literature and case report. Ann Surg 173(4):534–544, 1971.
47. Karl HW, Changler JG: Mortality and morbidity of pancreatic injury. Am J Surg 134:549–554, 1977.
48. Karnaze GC, Sheedy PF II, Stephens DH, McLeod RA: Computed tomography in duodenal rupture due to blunt abdominal trauma. J Comput Assist Tomogr 5(2):267–269, 1981.
49. Kashuk JL, Moore EE, Cogbill TH: Management of the intermediate severity duodenal injury. Surgery 92(4):758–764, 1982.
50. Kelly G, Norton L, Moore G, Eiseman B: The continuing challenge of duodenal injuries. J Trauma 18(3):160–164, 1978.
51. Kirkpatrick JR, Rajpal SG: Management of a high risk intestinal anas-

tomosis. Am J Surg 125:312–315, 1933.
52. Kusminsky RE, Shbeeb I, Makos G, Boland JP: Blunt pelviperineal injuries: An expanded role for the diverting colostomy. Dis Colon Rectum 25(8):787–790, 1982.
53. Lavenson GS, Cohen A: Management of rectal injuries. Am J Surg 122:226–230, 1971.
54. Leddy JE, Frew EMS: Complete transection of the body of the stomach resulting from blunt trauma. Can J Surg 20:264–266, 1977.
55. Levison MA, Petersen SR, Sheldon GF, Trunkey DD: Duodenal trauma: Experience of a trauma center. J Trauma 24(6):475–480, 1984.
56. LoCicero J, Tajima T, Drapanas T: A half century of experience with management of colon injuries: Changing concepts. J Trauma 17:554–556, 1977.
57. Lowe RJ, Saletta JD, Moss GS: Pancreatoduodenectomy for penetrating pancreatic trauma. J Trauma 17(9):732–741, 1977.
58. Lubbers EJC: Injury of the duodenum caused by a fixed three-point seatbelt. J Trauma 17(12):960, 1977.
59. Lucas CE: Diagnosis and treatment of pancreatic and duodenal injury. Surg Clin North Am 57(1):49–65, 1977.
60. Machiedo GW, Casey KF, Blackwood JM: Colostomy closure following trauma. Surg Gynecol Obstet 151:58–60, 1980.
61. Magee C, Rodeheaver GT, Golden GT et al: Potentiation of wound infection by surgical drains. Am J Surg 131:547–549, 1976.
62. Malangoni MA, Madura JA, Jesseph JE: Management of lateral duodenal fistulas: A study of fourteen cases. Surgery 90(4):645–651, 1981.
63. Marx JA, Bar-Or D, Moore EE, Tercier JA: Utility of lavage alkaline phosphates in detection of isolated small intestinal injury. Ann Emerg Med 14(1):10–14, 1985.
64. Marzella L, Brotman S, Mayer J, Cowley RA: Evaluation of injured intestine with the aid of fluorescein. Am Surg 50:599–602, 1984.
65. Mason JM: Surgery of the colon: The forward battle area. Surgery 18:534, 1945.
66. Maull KI, Reath DB: Impact of early recognition on outcome in nonpenetrating wounds of the small bowel. South Med J 77(9): 1075–1077, 1984.
67. Maull KI, Sachatello CR, Ernst CB: The deep perineal lacerations. An injury frequently associated with open pelvic fractures: A need for aggressive surgical management. J Trauma 17(9):685–696, 1977.
68. McInnis WD, Aust JB, Cruz AB, Root HD: Traumatic injuries of duodenum: A comparison of 1° closure and the jejunal patch. J Trauma 15(10):847–853, 1975.
69. Morton JH: Perineal and rectal damage following nonpenetrating abdominal trauma. J Trauma 12(4):347–352, 1972.
70. Nallathambi MN, Ivatury RR et al: Aggressive definitive management of penetrating colon injuries: 136 cases with 3.7 per cent mortality. J Trauma 24(6):500–505, 1984.
71. Nance FC, DeLoach DH: Pancreaticoduodenectomy following abdominal trauma. J Trauma 11(7):577–585, 1971.
72. Northrup WF, Simmons RL: Pancreatic trauma: A review. Surgery 71(1)27–43, 1972.
73. Nwafo DC: Selective primary suture of the battle-injured colon: An experience of the Nigerian Civil War. Br J Surg 67:195–197, 1980.
74. Ogilvie WH: Abdominal wounds in the western desert. Surg Gynecol Obstet 78:225–238, 1944.
75. Okies JE, Bricker DL, Jordan GL et al: Exteriorized primary repair of colon injuries. Am J Surg 124:807–810, 1972.
76. Oreskovich MR, Carrico CJ: Pancreaticoduodenectomy for trauma: A viable option? Am J Surg 147:618–623, 1984.
77. Orloff MJ, Charters AC: Injuries of the small bowel and mesentery and retroperitoneal hematoma. Surg Clin North Am 52(3):729–734, 1972.
78. Parks TG: Surgical management of injuries of the large intestine. Br J Surg 68:725–728, 1981.
79. Phillips TF, Brotman S: Perforating injuries of the small bowel from blunt abdominal trauma. Ann Emerg Med 12(2):75–78, 1983.
80. Prathikanti V, Bhuta I: Intramural hematoma of the duodenum. South Med J 69(4):490–492, 1976.
81. Raffa J, Christensen NM: Compound fractures of the pelvis. Am J Surg 132:282–286, 1976.
82. Robbs JV, Moore SW, Pillay SP: Blunt abdominal trauma with jejunal injury: A review. J Trauma 20(4):308–311, 1980.
83. Robey E, Mullen JT, Schwab CW: Blunt transection of the pancreas treated by distal pancreatectomy, splenic salvage and hyperalimentation. Ann Surg 196(6):695–699, 1982.
84. Rooney JA, Pesek IG: Transection of the stomach due to blunt abdominal trauma. J Trauma 8(4):487–492, 1968.
85. Rouse T, Collin J, Darr A: Isolated injury to the intestine from blunt abdominal injury. Br J Accident Surg 16(2):131–133, 1984.
86. Rowlands BJ: Intestinal injury due to nonpenetrating abdominal trauma. Injury 8(4):284–289, 1977.
87. Schenk WG, Lonchyna V, Moylan JA: Perforation of the jejunum from blunt abdominal trauma. J Trauma 23(1):54–56, 1983.
88. Shannon FL, Moore EE: Primary repair of the colon: When is it a safe alternative? Surgery 98(4):851–859, 1985.
89. Silbergleit A, Berkas E: Neonatal gastric rupture. Min Med 49:65–67, 1966.
90. Snyder WH, Weigelt JA, Watkins WL, Bietz DS: The surgical management of duodenal trauma: Precepts based on a review of 247 cases. Arch Surg 115:422–429, 1980.
91. Stahl KD, Geiss AC, Bordan DL et al: Blunt trauma and delayed colon injury. Curr Surg 42(1):4–9, 1985.
92. Stone HH, Fabian TC: Management of perforating colon trauma: Randomization between primary closure and exteriorization. Ann Surg 190:430, 1979.
93. Stone HH, Fabian TC: Management of duodenal wounds. J Trauma 19(5):334–339, 1979.
94. Stone HH, Fabian TC, Satiani B, Turkleson ML: Experiences in the management of pancreatic trauma. J Trauma 21(4):257–262, 1981.
95. Sturm JT, Quattlebaum FW, Mowlem A, Perry JE: Patterns of injury requiring pancreatoduodenectomy. Surg Gynecol Obstet 137:629–632, 1973.
96. Tan DTD, Kim HS, Richmond D: Gastric mucosal lacerations from blunt trauma to the abdomen. Am J Gastroenterol 63(3):246–248, 1975.
97. Taylor GJ: Delayed presentation of small intestine damage due to closed abdominal trauma. Br J Surg 69:55–57, 1982.
98. Thal R, Yeary EC: Morbidity of colostomy closure following colon trauma. J Trauma 20:287–291, 1980.
99. Thompson JS, Moore EE, Moore JB: Comparison of penetrating injuries of the right and left colon. Ann Surg 193:414–418, 1980.
100. Thompson S, Moore EE: Factors affecting the outcome of exteriorized colon repairs. J Trauma 22(5):403–406, 1982.
101. Touloukian RJ: Protocol for the nonoperative treatment of obstructing intramural duodenal hematoma during childhood. Am J Surg 145:330–334, 1983.
102. Trunkey D, Hays RJ, Shires GT: Management of rectal trauma. J Trauma 13(5):411–415, 1973.
103. Tuggle D, Huber PJ: Mangement of rectal trauma. Am J Surg 148:806–808, 1984.
104. Vargish T, Urdaneta LF, Cram AE, Jochimsen PR: Duodenal trauma in the rural setting. Am Surg 49(4):211–213, 1983.
105. Vaughan GD, Frazier OH, Graham DY et al: The use of pyloric exclusion in the management of severe duodenal injuries. Am J Surg 134:785–790, 1977.
106. Vitale GC, Richardson JD, Flint LM: Successful management of injuries to the extraperitoneal rectum. Am Surg 49(3):159–162, 1983.
107. Voyles CR, Flint LM: Wound management after trauma to the colon. South Med J 70(9):1067–1069, 1977.
108. Walt AJ: Management of injuries of the colon and rectum. Adv Surg 16:277–297, 1983.
109. Weiss M, Dreiling DA: Small bowel perforation in blunt trauma. Am J Gastroenterol 50(4):279–288, 1968.
110. Williams RD, Sargent FT: The mechanism of intestinal injury in trauma. J Trauma 3:288–294, 1963.
111. Woodhall JP, Ochsner A: The management of perforating injuries of the colon and rectum in civilian practice. Surgery 29(2):305–320, 1951.
112. Yajko RD, Seydel F, Trimble C: Rupture of the stomach from blunt abdominal trauma. J Trauma 15(3):177–192, 1975.
113. Yates JL: An experimental study of the local effects of peritoneal drainage. Surg Gynecol Obstet 1:473–492, 1905.
114. Yeo CK, McNamara J: Retroperitoneal rupture of duodenum with complicating gas gangrene. Arch Surg 106:856–857, 1973.

pediatric trauma management

Howard C. Filston

What kills kids? How long it has taken for the facts related to this question to penetrate our awareness! Infections used to kill kids, but immunizations and antibiotics have reduced these deaths remarkably. Complications of prematurity and congenital anomalies still account for infant deaths, but these numbers have been reduced as well. Cancer still takes its toll at all ages (approximately 3000 deaths a year in children from the age of 1 to 14).[35] As medicine has won the battle with many of the above killers, it has long neglected what is now and has been for several decades the number-one killer of children and young adults–trauma. Trauma deaths among the young are actually increasing.[32]

The care of the child trauma patient has lagged behind improvements in the management of adult trauma patients, but is now gaining ground, led by pediatric and trauma surgeons throughout the country. The statistics show 12,000 trauma deaths a year in children 1 to 14 years of age.[32] Some suggest 25,000 deaths in children each year[29]; of these, 4,700 are motor vehicle related.[32] Twelve to fifteen million injuries (some estimates are nearly 25 million[30]) occur in this age group each year. An estimated 100,000 of these injuries will result in lifetime debilities. Holmes and Reyes[19] surveyed a 2-year period at the Cook County Hospital (4/1/79 to 3/31/81), during which 719 pediatric patients with trauma were admitted to the institution. Forty-six percent had lacerations, fractures, or wringer injuries. Isolated head injuries were present in 35%, and 10% had multiple injuries including head injuries. Only 2.2% had gunshot wounds and 1.1% stab wounds. Blunt trauma related to automobile accidents, falls, and assaults made up 94.3% of all injuries.

The excellent salvage rates for battlefield injuries in recent wars put to shame the failures being experienced in trauma care in civilian patients. Civilian care has gradually improved, with organization and identification of regional trauma centers and improved on-site emergency care and transportation. Trauma specialists have realized that mobile ambulance services and emergency medical technicians, trained and directed by cardiologists to handle myocardial problems, must be retrained and reorganized to manage the trauma patient effectively. The pediatric trauma specialist must also become involved at this level to modify protocols to provide appropriate care for the pediatric trauma patient.

The maxim that the child is not "a little adult" applies as fully to the pediatric trauma victim as to the neonate with a surgically correctable congenital anomaly. Ramenofsky, citing National Highway Safety Council data, reports that 25,000 children die annually due to accidental injury.[29] The majority of the deaths were not in the hospital. This may account for some of the disparity in numbers from other reports extrapolated from hospital deaths. Most of the deaths were in children under 6 months of age, and an estimated 50% of the deaths were preventable with proper care; in 79% of deaths, the injury was not identified. Seidel and associates,[33] in 1984, reported a survey of Los Angeles County in which they found that 10% of paramedic calls were for pediatric trauma: the majority were less than 13 years of age, 25% less than 3 years of age and 10% less than 1 year of age. Death rates from trauma were noted to be higher for children than for adults, particularly in relation to head trauma. Overall, 12% of children versus 7% of adults died in the emergency room or the hospital. Holmes and Reyes[19] noted that all of the deaths in their series at Cook County Hospital were in patients who were transferred to Cook County Hospital from other hospitals, rather than being brought directly to Cook County Hospital by the emergency service. Haller and associates[16] have taken a preliminary look at the results of a regionalized pediatric trauma program in Maryland, in which approximately 25 children each month are admitted to the Regional Trauma Center. They have noted improved outcomes in children with pelvic trauma and head trauma, and of equal importance, have raised important questions and identified areas for scientific studies in the management of pediatric trauma in general.

That pediatric trauma care is finally reaching a level of sophistication worthy of recognition is attested to by the overwhelmingly successful First National Conference on Pediatric Trauma sponsored by the well-organized Kiwanis Regional Trauma Program at the Tufts New England Medical Center in 1985.[18] Subsequent Trauma conferences have been met with equal enthusiam, and there is now a separate "Trauma Session" during the Annual Meeting of the American Pediatric Surgical Association. It is hoped that increased attention at this level will result in reduced numbers of pediatric trauma victims as preventive measures are instituted. For those children who are seriously injured, better methods of care and rehabilitation at special centers throughout the country will produce improved survival and less debility. Standards of care for the pediatric trauma victim have been set forth, and it is hoped they will be increasingly achieved throughout the United States.[30]

Together with regional trauma centers, it is essential to identify independent regional pediatric trauma centers. These may be the same institutions, but in areas of dense population, there may be several major adult trauma facilities, but only one center capable of care for seriously injured pediatric patients. EMTs and other transporters must be aware of these centers and required to selectively convey child trauma patients to the appropriate center. Ramenofsky and Morse[31] estimate that only 3% to 4% of the 25 million children injured annually will require admission to any hospital; only a small fraction of these are critically injured and require admission to a major children's trauma center. However, it is in the latter group that the deaths occur; it is toward this group of patients that the sophisticated children's trauma center must address itself.

This chapter will address special problems of childhood trauma. Rather than repeat the discussions of each injury in each organ system, it will contrast pediatric trauma management with management of similar injuries in adults, emphasizing the differences attributable to the child's anatomy, physiology, the factors of growth, and the resiliency of a still-developing organism.

A final word of introduction to pediatric trauma must address the monetary and philosophical costs of childhood trauma to our society. The permanently impaired child trauma survivor represents a lifetime of expense to society, and an equal number of productive years lost. It behooves all of us to achieve maximum prevention and ideal resuscitation and rehabilitation for these young patients.

ETIOLOGY AND PREVENTION

Trauma is an unfortunate fact of our highly technical modern life. The most common source of injury in children is the motor vehicle. The child may be victimized as an occupant, a pedestrian, or while bicycling or playing with other mobile toys. Extensive studies have concluded that the majority of children killed as passengers in motor vehicles would survive if properly restrained. Ninety percent of infants under 1 year of age and greater than 50% of older children in motor vehicle accidents as passengers would live if properly restrained. In fact, Rivara[32] estimates that 90% of children less than 4 years of age who die as occupants in motor vehicles could be saved with proper restraint systems. Much of this information is based on the fact that children frequently die in accidents in which adults survive, often with minimal injury. The unrestrained child becomes a missile in the rapidly decelerating vehicle. Baker[1] notes that the youngest children have the highest death rates. The peak is at two to three months of age, with a rate of 9/100,000 infants under 6 months of age. By 1 year of age the rate falls to 4.5/100,000 and it remains at 3/100,000 between 6 and 12 years of age.

Other common sources of trauma to children are falls, especially from heights, bicycling injuries and those related to such motorized vehicles as motor scooters and "all-terrain vehicles" (ATVs), drownings, poisonings, burns, and asphyxiation. Fortunately, stabbings and gunshot wounds are among the less common causes of childhood trauma. However, among teenagers, homicide and especially suicide take an appreciable toll, the latter often involving ingestions and gunshots.

Recent campaigns in most states have achieved some protection for children in motor vehicles by mandatory seatbelt statutes. However, in general, education of parents as to the importance of preventive measures will go much further than statutory efforts to eliminate those risks. Nevertheless, Barlow and associates,[2] surveying 10 years of experience with falls from heights in children at Harlem Hospital, noted that there was a 96% decrease in the incidence of children falling from heights after legislative institution of mandatory safety bars on windows in rental apartments. Rivara[32] has listed the following injury sources and solutions:

Motor vehicles: Infant seat restraints, seatbelts, airbags
Motorcycles and pedal cycles: Helmets
Poisoning: Expansion and enforcement of Poison Prevention Packaging Act
Drownings: Barriers around pools
Fire and flames: Self-extinguishing cigarettes, smoke detectors
Firearms (non-intentional, homicide, suicide): Elimination of handguns
Choking or suffocation: Heimlich maneuver and Consumer Product Safety Commission regulations
Falls: Window bars

Finally, a recent article by Tanz and Christoffel[36] points out that more children are injured as pedestrians than as motor vehicle passengers. As the death rate for motor vehicle passengers falls owing to increased use of restraints, the importance of pedestrian injuries by motor vehicles will become apparent.

PREHOSPITAL RESUSCITATION

Life-threatening effects from trauma relate to head and spinal injuries, shock from blood loss, hypoxia from airway obstruction or loss of central respiratory drive. At the scene of the accident, care should consist of control of hemorrhage, protection of the spinal cord, securing an airway, and initiation and maintenance of ventilation. Ideally, if blood loss has occurred, vascular access should be accomplished and volume replacement should be initiated.

The smaller and younger the child the more difficult it is to secure the airway and achieve vascular access. Thus, the debate rages as to whether to "scoop and run" or resuscitate and stabilize. Military experience proves that rapid transport to a sophisticated treatment facility will save more lives than prolonged care in the field. More time may be spent gaining vascular access than is needed to airlift the patient to the facility, so rapid transport should be the goal. The spine must be stabilized, the airway secured, ventilation dependable, and bleeding controlled. Most children have resilient-enough vascular systems to tolerate well a short period of hypovolemia. Thus, education of emergency medical technicians (EMTs) is better directed toward skill at intubation and ventilation than toward techniques of vascular access.

Initial control of the airway requires clearing the mouth and hypopharynx of food or vomitus and breathing by mask when ventilation is inadequate. The infant and young child are best ventilated in the "sniffing" position: the head is in a neutral position with the face forward. Neck extension pushes the larynx behind the base of the tongue and results in obstruction. The mandible must be lifted up into the mask to bring the tongue forward, clearing the pathway to the larynx. The fact that the neck need not be extended is advantageous in protecting the spinal cord against a possible cervical spine fracture. This injury is, fortunately, rare in children, but the mishandling of it is so devastating (resulting in almost certain quadriplegia) that all patients in whom the possibility of such an injury exists should be managed as though it is present until it is ruled out.

The infant or young child is intubated in the same "sniffing" position using a straightbladed laryngoscope (Fig. 10.1). The tip of the scope is advanced into the mouth until it touches the uvula, and then the handle is pushed toward the child's feet parallel to his body, causing the epiglottis to be exposed. A slight additional push and lift will then expose the cords. Suctioning capability is essential during attempts at intubation. A straight uncuffed tube should fit loosely through the cords so that air leaks back around it. Unlike in the adult airway, the cricoid ring is the narrowest diameter of the child's and infant's airway; a tube fitting snugly at the cord level will be too tight at the cricoid level and cause pressure necrosis of the mucosa and subsequent subglottic stenosis.

The tube is best advanced until breath sounds decrease in the left chest, indicating entry of the tube into the right main-stem bronchus. The tube is then retracted until clear sounds are heard again on the left; the tube is then secured dependably. Occasionally, preferential entry is into the left main bronchus, requiring reversal of the procedure.

Care should be taken to ventilate infants properly. Slow deep ventilation is inappropriate. The infant should be ventilated about 40 breaths/min with about half the volume used for adults. Comfortable but not excessive expansion of the chest is the best guide. Tidal volume is 7 cc/kg/breath, but usually 10 cc to 15 cc/kg/breath are needed to allow for loss in the tubing and around the endotracheal tube. Good ventilation is important not only to sustain normal oxygenation of blood, but also to control cerebral perfusion. Decreasing $PaCO_2$ will decrease cerebral blood flow, a factor that may help to lessen intracerebral pressure and brain swelling in cases of serious head injury.

EMTs must be trained to handle infant and child trauma victims appropriately, and this will come about only if pediatric trauma specialists involve themselves in the training, certification, and continuing education of the community EMTs. Knowledge of normal vital signs in infants is essential. Newborns and infants have heart rates of 120 to 160 beats/min. Rates of less than 100 beats/min usually represent bradycardia, implying hypoxia or hypovolemia. Infants' hearts are unable to compensate for increased demands by increasing stroke volume; therefore, bradycardia invariably reduces cardiac output.

Normal systolic blood pressure in a full-term newborn is 80 mm Hg; premature neonates have correspondingly reduced levels of 50 to 60 mm Hg, depending on their weights. A rough rule of thumb for infant systolic blood pressure is 80 mm Hg plus twice the age in years. This is a minimum level, however, as many infants have systolic pressures of up to 100 mm Hg. It is essential to train EMTs and others involved in infant transport not to overload infant trauma victims with fluids while trying to push their pressures up to 100 to 120 mm Hg. Futhermore, trauma scoring systems must be modified for pediatric victims to account for the differences in the normal ranges of vital signs.

EMERGENCY ROOM CARE

Whether the trauma center is an independent children's hospital or a general hospital, appropriate equipment and experienced personnel must be available at all times to receive the critically injured child.[30] A specially equipped area for children is essential, with scales, an overhead warmer, appropriate-size monitoring equipment, and a variety of vascular access devices and airway equipment for children. Immediately after arrival, the ABCs of trauma care must be achieved: Airway, Breathing, and Circulation. As these are being attended to, the cervical spine must be protected with traction, sandbags, or a collar until a spinal fracture is ruled out. Although a rare injury in childhood, spinal fracture must be thought of whenever the mechanism of injury could have produced cervical spine injury, or when the mechanism of injury is uncertain.

Ventilation

Mechanical ventilation, if needed, should be attempted first by mask and bag, assuming that the patient has not already been intubated at the accident scene; but if this is not successful, intubation should be expeditiously accomplished by someone

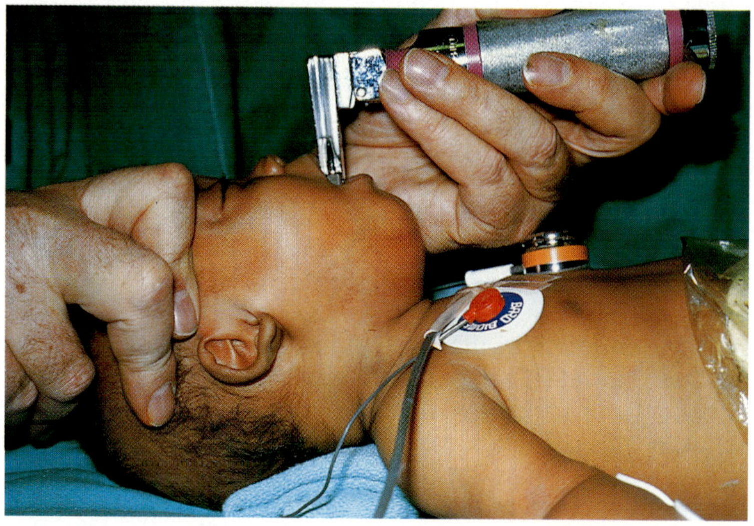

FIGURE 10.1 The "sniffing position" for intubating an infant. The baby's face is forward. The laryngoscope blade is advanced until it touches the uvula, and then the handle is pushed toward the baby's feet and lifted slightly to expose the epiglottis.

who is skilled at infant and child intubation. This may be an anesthesiologist, emergency pediatrician, pediatric surgeon, respiratory therapist, or trauma nurse. All of these individuals should be trained and experienced in this technique.

If translaryngeal intubation proves impossible or unsatisfactory, a needle cricothyroidotomy using a 12-, 14-, or 16-gauge needle or plastic vascular access cannula may buy time until satisfactory endotracheal intubation or a formal incisional tracheostomy can be achieved. Emergency incisional tracheostomy is a hazardous and uncertain procedure and should be avoided if possible. Incisional cricothyroidotomy is also risky in the infant and young child and often results in permanent injury to the airway.

Once a stable airway is achieved, adequate ventilation should be attained by manual bagging or mechanical ventilation. The position of the endotracheal tube should be carefully checked to assure good ventilation bilaterally. Most inexperienced personnel ventilate infants too slowly and too deeply. Rates of 40 to 60 breaths/min are needed for babies and 30 to 40 breaths/min for infants and children. The chest should rise and fall easily, not excessively. If lung compliance is normal, peak pressures of 15 to 20 cm H_2O should be sufficient.

If good ventilation is not achieved after intubation and proper tube positioning, the clinican should suspect esophageal intubation, tension pneumothorax, or a major tracheobronchial disruption. Proper position of the tube through the cords can be viewed with a laryngoscope, and pneumothorax can be confirmed by chest radiograph. However, severe tension pneumothorax can produce such severe respiratory compromise that "blind" tube thoracostomy may be essential without waiting for x-ray film confirmation. This procedure can be achieved quickly with a vascular needle-stylet plastic cannula and may provide adequate relief of the tension to then allow radiographic confirmation of the pneumothorax followed by careful, less urgent, tube placement.

If proper intubation of the airway and tube thoracostomies to relieve tension pneumothorax still do not result in adequate ventilation, a major tracheobronchial disruption probably exists and requires urgent thoracotomy and restoration of continuity of the airway.

Volume Restoration

Once respiratory integrity is assured, volume restoration and circulation must be attended to. The most rapid and dependable site for vascular access in a hypovolemic patient is the saphenous vein at the ankle, which is cannulated by incisional cutdown. A venous tourniquet is placed at mid-calf level or lower, and a 1-cm incision is placed 1 cm superior and 1 cm anterior to the medial malleolus. A curved mosquito hemostat is used to dissect deeply into the tissues at one corner of the incision. It is then firmly scraped across the depth of the wound and brought out the opposite corner and opened. Adventitious tissue will fall away or separate as the clamp is opened, leaving the more elastic vein lying in the curve of the instrument. This maneuver should be repeated until the vein is identified. A ligature is placed under the vein to use temporarily for traction; it is not tied. A percutaneous cannula is inserted under direct vision, but without incision into the vein. A larger bore cannula can be placed into a blood-distended vein than into one emptied by incision prior to cannulation. The ligature is removed, the incision closed with one suture, and the cannula secured with tape.

Individuals skilled at percutaneous vascular access in infants may be able to achieve access without cutdown if the child is not severely hypovolemic; undue time lost attempting this must be avoided, however. Similarly, percutaneous subclavian access may be gained quickly if personnel with vast experience at this technique are available. It is not generally as expeditious and dependable as ankle cutdown in emergencies, however. Intraosseous access (into the marrow cavity of the tibia) may prove to be the most expeditious and easily mastered technique for those who do not work with children enough to become sufficiently skilled at vascular access.[34]

Restoration of circulation should be achieved by bolus administration of crystalloid solutions and blood. It has been repeatedly demonstrated that normal children with normal vascular volumes will tolerate a rapid 25% expansion of vascular volume. Newborns and infants have a blood volume equal to 8% of body weight or 80 ml/kg, so that a bolus administration of 20 ml/kg (25% of 80 ml/kg) of lactated Ringer's solution or normal saline should initiate circulatory resuscitation while awaiting blood matching. This volume push is repeated once; if the blood pressure remains unstable, 20 ml/kg of blood is then administered. Continued instability after this volume replacement, which represents 75% of the child's blood volume, indicates ongoing significant hemorrhage. These volume recommendations are appropriate throughout childhood; they presume that all external sources of blood loss were initially controlled.

It is important to realize that the young infant, unlike the adult or teenager, can occasionally lose enough blood into the expandable cranium from intracranial hemorrhage or into a thigh from a femoral fracture to result in severe hypovolemia. Recognition of such injuries should lead to proper vascular access and circulatory volume restoration before embarking on further investigation of these injuries. Children have died of hypovolemic shock in the radiographic suite when sent there unresuscitated from such injuries.

Another maxim in pediatric trauma care is that intrinsic cardiac dysfunction is rare. Therefore, poor cardiac output or unstable blood pressure is almost invariably due to hypoxia or hypovolemia. Direct myocardial injury occasionally occurs, as does tamponade from buildup of pericardial blood, but hypoxia and hypovolemia should be suspected first.

Cardiac arrest, if it occurs in the infant, requires attention to the restoration of ventilation, oxygenation, and circulatory volume. A hypoxic heart will not resume normal function, nor can the heart perfuse the tissues when vascular volume is severely depleted. The infant heart requires a rapid massage rate to achieve output, but great care must be taken in allowing time for diastolic filling. Complications of a cardiac arrest such as persistent asystole and arrhythmias are handled the same as for adults, but a list of drug doses on a weight scale such as outlined in Fig. 10.2 is essential information for any pediatric trauma center.

VOLUME RESTORATION

Infant blood volume

$$8\% \times \text{Body weight} = 80 \text{ ml/kg}$$

Tolerable fluid "push"

$$1/4 \text{ blood volume} = 20 \text{ ml/kg}$$

Bolus fluid restoration

$$20 \text{ ml/kg} \times 2\ (D_5\%/LR^*) = 40 \text{ ml/kg}$$

$$20 \text{ ml/kg whole blood} = 20 \text{ ml/kg}$$

$$\text{Total} = 60 \text{ ml/kg}^\dagger$$

* Normal saline or lactated Ringer's solution
† 75% of blood volume

Initial Assessment

With the ABCs attended to, a rapid but thorough system-by-system assessment should now be accomplished. The child should be maintained in a warm environment, preferably under an overhead heater. Since all therapies in children are related to weight, either an accurate estimation or direct determination of weight is essential.

Serious trauma to children is most frequently blunt trauma, and head injury is a frequent (60%–80%) and serious component of life-threatening injuries. Early evaluation of the level of consciousness and computation of the Glasgow coma scale are essential (Fig. 10.3). Of equal importance in the care of the brain-injured child are early intubation with adequate hyperventilation to lower $PaCO_2$ and reduce cerebral blood flow and a careful assessment for other major injuries that might result in severe or prolonged hypoxia or hypovolemia, both of which may contribute to worsening of the brain injury. In fact, it has been observed that for children sustaining brain injuries that are not immediately fatal, a large percentage of the deaths and permanent debilities are due to the secondary effects of increased intracranial pressure, hypoxia, and hypovolemia, rather than to the initial damage. Thus, proper care of injuries to other systems is also protective of the intracranial injury.

Injuries discovered at this initial assessment should be attended to appropriately. Fractures should be splinted and extremity circulation assessed. Open wounds should be cleaned, hemorrhage controlled, and preparations made for debridement and closure if appropriate. External wounds to the chest and abdomen should be noted and attention directed to intrathoracic and intra-abdominal injuries.

Remember that multiple system or organ injury is the rule in the critically injured patient, so appropriate suspicion and adequate assessment are essential. The chest is best assessed by a plain radiograph and the abdomen by careful physical examination followed by computed tomography (CT) scan when injuries are suspected. Spine, pelvis, and extremity bone films will confirm or discover fractures, but the discovery of fractures, especially rib and pelvic fractures, should also suggest adjacent soft tissue injuries. When head injury is present or suspected, skull films and CT scan are mandatory, the latter being more urgent and more diagnostic of brain injury.

Double-contrast CT scanning is the method of choice for evaluating blunt trauma.[21] Since the mere demonstration of blood in the peritoneal cavity is no longer an indication for operative intervention in the child trauma patient, peritoneal

FIGURE 10.2
DRUGS FOR CARDIAC RESUSCITATION

DRUG	DOSAGE
Sodium bicarbonate (1mEq/ml)	1 mEq/kg
Epinephrine (1:10,000)	0.1 ml/kg
Atropine	0.01–0.03 mg/kg
Calcium chloride (100mg/ml)	0.1–0.25 ml/kg
Calcium gluconate (100 mg/ml)	0.3 ml/kg
Lidocaine 2%	0.5–1.0 mg/kg/dose, slow IV push
Dopamine	2–10 µg/kg/min
Isuprel	0.1 µg/kg/min
Defibrillation	2 watt-sec/kg*

*Double and repeat prn.

FIGURE 10.3
GLASGOW COMA SCALE

FUNCTION	RESPONSE	RATING
Best motor response	Obeys	M6
	Localizes	5
	Withdraws	4
	Abnormal flexion	3
	Extensor response	2
	Nil	1
Verbal response	Oriented	V5
	Confused conversation	4
	Inappropriate words	3
	Incomprehensible sounds	2
	Nil	1
Eye opening	Spontaneous	E4
	To speech	3
	To pain	2
	Nil	1

*Double and repeat prn.

lavage or the peritoneal tap should be used only when there are specific indications. It is most useful where rapid assessment for intraperitoneal bleeding is essential and an abdominal CT scan is not readily available, or when the patient is too unstable to allow time for a CT scan. Indications for peritoneal lavage include the following:

Severe brain or spinal cord injury requiring emergency surgery, where responses to abdominal examination are undependable;

Unexplained hypovolemic shock after adequate volume replacement or when there has been no external blood loss;

Suspected or possible intra-abdominal injury when the patient must undergo emergency surgery for other system injuries and will be unavailable for careful reevaluation for intra-abdominal injury for a crucial period of time, and

Physical examination suggesting peritonitis in a patient with a negative CT scan and no evidence of intraperitoneal bleeding. In this case, finding bacteria, leukocytes, or fecal contents would be very useful in diagnosis and treatment.

Relative indications for peritoneal lavage include:

Uncooperative conscious patient,
Inexperienced examiner, and
Nonavailability of abdominal CT scanning.

The latter two indications probably would be better resolved by transfer to a more sophisticated trauma center than by peritoneal lavage.

HOSPITAL CARE

The patient who remains unstable after initial volume resuscitation or in whom an injury requiring operative correction is identified should be transported to the operating room for surgical correction. Others with life-threatening or multiple injuries should be admitted to an acute care unit that is experienced in the care of pediatric trauma victims. Multiply injured patients should be admitted to the general pediatric surgical or trauma service initially, as should patients with unstable respiratory or circulatory systems. Patients with clearly defined injuries involving single subspecialty services may be admitted directly to the care of those services. If there is suspicion of or potential for significant injury in other systems, initial admission to the general service is wise; transfer to the subspecialty can be accomplished safely after 24 to 48 hours of stability.

Ventilatory Support

If the child is intubated, ventilation is accomplished with pressures set as low as possible to avoid unnecessary barotrauma. Attention must be given to the special considerations for infants outlined in the section on resuscitation: the tube should fit loosely and there should be an air leak around the tube. Cuffed tubes are rarely needed for preteenage children. Usually, volumes of 10 cc to 15 cc/kg/breath are adequate to ventilate children with normal compliance (tidal volume is 7 cc/kg/breath); this should result in peak pressures of 15 cm to 18 cm H_2O. Lung expansion is maintained with 3 cm to 5 cm of positive end-expiratory pressure (PEEP) to avoid atelectasis. Considerably higher levels of PEEP may be needed when lung compliance is reduced by injury, such as contusion with hemorrhage or by interstitial edema resulting from capillary damage or intravascular oncotic deficits.

Ventilatory rates for infants should be 40/min, reducing to 30/min for 1-year-olds and 20/min for 2-year-olds. Muscle relaxants may be added if the child "fights the ventilator" and is inadequately ventilated. Sedation should be added if not contraindicated by a head injury.

Secretions must be cleared from intubated patients by careful suctioning. The patient should be "preoxygenated," if possible, before each suctioning episode. The suction catheter should be passed gently, but fully, in infants; too-forceful passage of the suction catheter may perforate the pulmonary parenchyma and lead to tension pneumothorax. The patient should be bag-ventilated after suctioning to overcome any atelectasis produced by the suctioning.

Oxygenation and ventilation should be monitored by frequent arterial blood gas sampling. Hypoxia should be quickly corrected by increasing inspired O_2, and then increasing mean airway pressure by adding additional end-expiratory pressure. Atelectasis is the usual cause of hypoxia in the adequately ventilated patient; increased inspired oxygen actually enhances atelectasis because oxygen diffuses across the alveolar-capillary membranes (versus inert nitrogen when inspired oxygen is lower). PEEP distends the alveoli, adding surface area for gas diffusion.

Patients should be actively and rapidly weaned from the ventilator and tube to limit barotrauma. As long as loosely fitting tubes are used, tracheostomy need not be performed for prolonged intubation alone. Obviously, when intubation will be required indefinitely, tracheostomy may be elected to allow oral feeding, speech, and resumption of normal activities.

Fluid and Electrolyte Management

Once stability is achieved with normal blood pressure and pulse, rapid administration of volumes of balanced electrolyte solutions should continue until a stable urine output of 1 ml to 2 ml/kg/hr (40–50 ml/kg/day maximum) is established. Additional fluid requirements will then be the same for postoperative and non-operated trauma patients with consideration of the following categories of fluid needs.

MAINTENANCE

Free water is a requirement for everyone each day. Insensible losses from the lungs and skin surface, together with an obligatory urine volume requirement to allow excretion of the daily metabolic wastes, demand administration of approximately 1000 ml/m^2 every 24 hours. Two commonly used formulas for calculating this requirement in children are as follows:

100 ml/kg up to 10 kg; + 50 ml/kg from 11 to 20 kg; + 20 ml/kg over 20 kg = M
(100 ml − 3 × age in years) × wt. in kg = M

Adults require 1500 ml to 2000 ml (1730 ml for the average adult of 1.73 m^2). We arbitrarily hold the upper limit of maintenance in children to 1500 ml when the child is hypovolemic and requiring additional fluids for volume replacement to avoid the inefficiency of diluted solutions that leak from the capillaries along the osmotic concentration gradient.

Dextrose should be added to provide at least minimal calories in the form of a 5% to 10% concentration in the free water. This allows the Krebs cycle to function and avoids lysis of red blood cells, which would occur if free water were actually administered intravenously. For full nutrition, the child actually requires calories equal to the free water calculated by the previously noted formulas, that is, 100 cal/kg for infants, and so on.

Electrolytes, particularly Na^+, K^+, and Cl^-, are needed to restore those lost in urine and stool. Infants require 3 mEq/kg/day of $Na^+ + Cl^-$ and 2 to 3 mEq/kg/day of K^+. A solution containing 3 mEq NaCl/100 ml is 1/5th normal saline (1/5 × 15.4 mEq NaCl/dl). The requirement for Na^+, Cl^-, and K^+ reduces with size as does that for water and calories, so that calculating the requirement in 1/5th normal saline (NS) will achieve reduction to the 45 to 60 mEq/day NaCl requirement for adults. It is important to recognize that 1/5th or 1/4th NS is just a convenient combination of the day's free water and electrolyte requirements. Thus, for the patient who starts out hyponatremic and hypochloremic, additional electrolytes are required to correct them to normal levels. These should also be added to the free water and the nearest appropriate electrolyte solution chosen.

Example: A 10.kg infant with serum electrolytes Na^+ = 130 mEq/liter, Cl^- = 90 mEq/liter. To correct chloride (a total body water ion, or TBW) requires 15 mEq NaCl/liter of TBW (to correct from 90 mEq to 105 mEq). Liters TBW = 60% × weight = 60% × 10 kg = 6 liters. Correction = 15 mEq/liter × 6 liters = 90 mEq.

This child requires 90 mEq NaCl to correct his deficiency + 3 mEq NaCl/kg for maintenance = 90 mEq + 30 mEq = 120 mEq. His free water requirement is 1000 ml (100 ml/kg). Thus, he requires 1 liter of solution containing 120 mEq/liter NaCl. This is D_5%/4/5th NS.

Other maintenance requirements to remember are multivitamins, calcium, phosphorus, magnesium, and vitamin K, which can be rapidly depleted when enteral feedings are withheld.

MEASURED LOSSES

Measured losses are usually gastrointestinal, most frequently gastric. Gastric losses are replaced volume-for-volume with D_5%/1/2 NS + 30 mEq KCl/liter. This solution provides 77 mEq Na^+, 107 mEq Cl^-, and 30 mEq K^+/liter, a reasonable approximation of gastric juice. Losses distal to the pylorus are similar in content to extracellular fluid and are replaced with D_5%/lactated Ringer's solution. Long-term enteral losses should be analyzed for exact content and replacement solutions chosen accordingly.

THIRD SPACE REPLACEMENT VOLUMES

There are important losses from the circulatory volume that can occur during and after surgery and as a result of trauma, whether treated operatively or nonoperatively. They can occur most seriously as a result of capillary membrane damage that may result from vasoconstrictive shunting during hypovolemic shock, from hypoxia, and from endotoxic damage during sepsis. Other extravascular shifts occur as a result of fluid sequestration in the bowel lumen from ileus or obstruction, and fluid sequestration in the form of inflammation, ascites, or edema. Any or all of these sources may be active in the trauma patient at some stage.

The amount of fluid required must be seen initially as a guess. As such, errors are expected, and therefore monitoring is essential. The correct amount of *third space replacement fluid* is the amount of balanced salt solution that, when added to the volumes of maintenance fluid and measured losses, results in a urine output of 1 ml to 2 ml/kg/hr for 24 hours. Thus, establishment and maintenance of the optimal urine output is the primary monitoring guide for fluid administration. The urine output, once established, is an excellent guide to the rate of fluid administration required. A lack of urine output may have multiple causes, including reduced cardiac output, inappropriate antidiuretic hormone, renal insufficiency, and sepsis, in addition to hypovolemia. In that case, a monitor of vascular volume status in the form of central vascular access becomes essential.

For patients having abdominal surgery, we have found a "quadrant scheme" helpful in refining the guess for third space requirements.[11] This scheme suggests that for each quadrant of the abdomen involved in an inflammatory or obstructive disease process or significantly explored by the surgeon, one fourth of the maintenance volume will be required as third space fluid in the form of balanced salt solution with or without colloid. Thus, peritonitis would require an additional full maintenance volume; a cholecystectomy would require one-fourth extra maintenance volume. This guideline does not eliminate the need for careful adjustments based on hourly urine volumes. An estimate of third space requirements in abdominal trauma could be based on a similar scheme taking into account the extent of the abdomen involved in the traumatic process. The scheme is, of course, useful after surgery for abdominal trauma.

As urine output exceeds the optimal maximum of 2 ml/kg/hr, the fluid administration rate is reduced until the hourly rate is equal to that required to administer maintenance plus measured losses, at which point the balanced salt solution for third space replacement is discontinued.

Support After Significant Hypovolemic or Hypoxic Injury

If the child has sustained a significant hypovolemic or hypoxic injury, multisystem dysfunction should be anticipated. Despite their healthy hearts, children will show myocardial insufficiency after generalized stress and often need inotropic support. Dopamine usually suffices and should initially be instituted at levels that will sustain or augment renal and mesenteric perfusion. This generally is less than 8 μg to 10 μg/kg/min but often 4 μg to 5 μg/kg/min will suffice.

Ventilatory support should be instituted at the least suggestion of insufficiency, and PEEP used liberally to counter atelectasis. Central venous monitoring can be achieved by percutaneous subclavian access even in the smallest infants, providing good monitoring of volume restoration.[12]

Particularly in young infants, hypoxic and hypovolemic insults can result in severe over-reaction of the splanchnic flow, with vasoconstriction and shunting producing ischemic bowel injury. Rapid restoration of circulatory volume and maintenance of good oxygenation are essential to minimize damage to the bowel.

Once stability is achieved, rapid weaning may be possible, but adequate levels of PEEP and dopamine should be maintained to avoid backsliding with atelectasis and increasing inspired oxygen requirements to maintain PaO_2 at adequate levels. Inspired oxygen should be reduced well down toward room air before reducing the level of PEEP required to achieve stable oxygenation. Also, too-early withdrawal of dopamine support may again produce splanchnic flow reductions. When blood pressure is stable and urine output adequate, dopamine can be reduced to levels of 4 μg to 5 μg/kg/hr; 24 to 48 hours of additional time at these levels may allow myocardial recovery and improved output.

Nutritional Support

Plans for nutritional support should be formulated early in the overall planning of therapy, but initiation of nutritional support can await complete circulatory stabilization. With major head, blunt abdominal, or burn trauma, a period of ileus is common and must first be resolved, best judged by resumption of gastric emptying. Particularly in young infants who commonly have gastroesophageal reflux as a physiologic deficiency, inadequate gastric decompression will lead to reflux and aspiration. Once the gut is functioning, enteral feeds can be resumed by oral, nasogastric, or duodenal tube access. Enteral feeding is always preferable, but when the gut is injured or has sustained significant ischemia, parenteral support may be required. The central access monitoring line, if present, can be converted for TPN use. A balanced nutritional solution is best, one that contains 2.5 g/kg protein, glucose concentrations of 25% to 30%, and lipid emulsion supplying about one third of the total calories. Infants require 100 kcal to 120 kcal/kg for growth and weight gain. The baseline calories for other age children can be calculated from the maintenance fluid formulas discussed previously. With severe multisystem trauma, especially when complicated by sepsis, a hypermetabolic state may develop and require considerably increased calorie administration.

Limiting the TPN administration to about 18 of each 24 hours may help to reduce the severity of liver damage from long-term TPN, as may the provision of at least a small portion of the intake enterally when possible. The etiology of TPN-related liver injury is unclear; direct toxicity from protein or fat,[37] overwork from continuous high-level caloric infusions, and cholestasis from taurine deficiency,[9] or a lack of gut hormone stimulators of cell secretion and biliary contraction have all been implicated.[20]

Vitamins, minerals, and trace elements are added daily as needed, and careful monitoring of electrolytes, clotting functions, bilirubin, and liver enzymes at least weekly should be routine. Weight stability and gain are the most direct indicators of adequate nutritional support, assuming that there is no reason for inappropriate fluid retention.

The risk of sepsis mandates a careful program of catheter usage and care; signs of sepsis should lead to a careful evaluation of all sources of infection including peripheral and central blood cultures, the latter drawn through the central line. Should the signs of infection fail to resolve in 24 to 36 hours after instituting appropriate antibiotic therapy for a line-related septic episode, the line should be removed. Whenever the gut is available for nutritional support, it is the preferred route. Early resumption of enteral feeds is facilitated by tube-feeding regimens, even in the unconscious patient and those on prolonged ventilatory support.

Control of Infection

Infection is a constant threat to the seriously injured child. Consequently, the support of a knowledgeable pediatric infectious disease specialist is essential to the trauma team. Infection problems include specific abscesses related to collections of blood and other fluids or necrotic debris from injured organs, pulmonary complications from aspiration or poorly cleared secretions, central line-related bacterial sepsis, enterocolitis from antibiotic-induced gut flora changes, and of course burn wound sepsis. Other sources of infection complicating trauma care are the routine illnesses to which all children are subjected. These may be of increased severity in the debilitated trauma patient. We have seen life-threatening viral tracheobronchitis develop in debilitated infants requiring antiviral agents for resolution.

Unique to the infant-toddler age group is the ease with which meningitis may develop, either complicating other bacterial infection or as an isolated entity. Cerebrospinal fluid analysis and culture should be a routine test in infants with fever of unknown origin.

Great care is required in the use of antibiotics to avoid the emergence of resistant organisms. For prophylaxis, short courses (24–48 hours) of coverage, best begun before contamination of tissues, are ideal. Such prophylaxis is especially important for newborns who are immune-deficient hosts with little or no prior antigenic exposure.

Control of Analgesia

Children are generally very straightforward about pain—they either hurt or they don't—there is rarely much psychologic overlay. Many will not complain of pain, but also will not be as mobile as is desirable without adequate analgesia. There are fears that the child will become addicted to analgesics.

Even the tiniest infants have some obvious discomfort after major surgery; all children should be liberally provided with analgesia immediately after trauma or surgery, and then tapered off rapidly after 24 to 48 hours. Since most children fear and hate shots more than any other aspect of medical care, it is nice to provide them with intravenous analgesia, especially in the intensive-care setting where they can be adequately monitored for any respiratory depression.

Parental Visiting

Children need the support of their families, and highly restrictive visiting regulations are not supportive of the needs of either the child or the parents. There must obviously be time for hospital "work rounds" and procedures, and there are situations in which most parents do not do well, such as during life-threatening catastrophies in their child's course or that of others in the ACU. At other times, however, visiting should be encouraged. Some restrictions at night are helpful to allow sleep time for the child—and the parents, who need to be relieved of the feeling that they must remain at constant vigil by the bedside. Provision of sleep rooms near the unit for parents of critically injured children is certainly ideal support in the early hours and days after the injury when the outcome is uncertain.

SPECIFIC ORGAN INJURIES DUE TO BLUNT TRAUMA

Only those injuries in which there are specific pediatric factors will be addressed.

Head Injuries

Bruce and associates[4] note that there are 5 million cases of head trauma in children in the United States each year, but that fewer than one in ten suffers a significant brain injury. Unique childhood injuries include subarachnoid hemorrhage from birth trauma (which usually presents secondarily as hydrocephalus), and hemorrhage in the less-than-1-year-old infant caused by violent shaking by the parent or caretaker; this latter results in tearing of the parasagittal bridging veins with subdural hemorrhage.[4] Most other cases of head trauma in children are due to blunt trauma.

Obvious skull fractures indicate a strong probability of intracranial injury, but often blunt trauma from an acceleration-deceleration injury produces brain injury without external signs. Every blunt trauma patient should be assessed initially for level of consciousness and scored with the Glasgow coma scale if unconscious (see Fig. 10.3). Changes from baseline are important signs of severe or worsening brain trauma.

Injury to the brain occurs from direct contusion, contracoup contusion against the opposite bony vault, hemorrhage with pressure and ischemia to compressed tissue, and brain swelling secondary to injury or ischemia. The direct injuries may be so severe as to be lethal, but progressive injury often results from ongoing hemorrhage with compression and herniation, ischemia secondary to inadequate ventilation and hypoxia, poor perfusion from hypovolemic shock from blood loss due to other system injuries, and edema secondary to brain injury, hypoventilation with increased cerebral perfusion, or inappropriate fluid management. The secondary injuries to the brain are preventable by careful attention to the general management of the trauma victim and some specific therapies directed against the effects on the brain of injuries in other systems. Severe brain trauma may break down the auto-regulation of blood flow to the brain, resulting in increased flow with increased systemic flow or pressure.[4]

Early intubation and hyperventilation of the brain-injured patient will maintain good oxygenation and lower $PaCO_2$; the result is lower volume flow to the brain, thus offsetting brain swelling. At the same time careful attention to volume restoration will avoid shock and resultant hypoxia and acidosis.

Unique to the brain-injured infant is the expandable cranium. It allows greater intracranial blood volumes to be lost so that the infant may actually be in shock from intracranial losses (an unlikely occurrence in older individuals). Also unique is the child's ability to recover function after severe brain injury, frequently to a remarkable degree. Thus, short of electroencephalographic evidence of brain death, recovery from seemingly overwhelming brain injury is the rule in the young child. Unfortunately, this recovery rarely is complete and many children are left with cognitive and affective disabilities and some with motor dysfunction as well.

Mahoney and associates[25] evaluated the long-term outcome of children with severe head trauma in prolonged coma at the Regional Trauma Center at Johns Hopkins University. They noted that 200,000 children with head trauma are hospitalized each year, with 4,000 deaths and 15,000 prolonged hospitalizations. Half of those patients who remain in coma for over 24 hours will have major neurologic sequelae. However, they noted that the outcome after head trauma is far better in children than in adults. In their study of 91 patients with significant head trauma, 46 were in coma for over 24 hours. Those children dying in the emergency room or dying in less than 24 hours were not included. Of the 46 patients in coma more than 24 hours, 12 died (a mortality rate of 38%). The coma in the survivors lasted an average of 15.5 days.

The outcome was encouraging. Twenty-nine percent were considered entirely normal. Fifty-three percent returned to school without significant motor deficits, but with mild behavioral or cognitive problems. Some of these had had prior problems of this sort. Nine percent showed motor dysfunction without an intellectual deficit (one because of a spinal cord injury). Only 9% had major motor and intellectual deficits. Nine of 14 children who were in coma for more than 2 weeks had minimal residual deficits. Importantly, infants showed a poorer outcome than children in the age group of 5 to 20 years of age. The study also noted continued improvement from months to years following head trauma in children, whereas adults rarely improved after 6 months.

EVALUATION

After neurologic physical examination, assessment of the level of consciousness, and calculation of the Glasgow coma score, an enhanced brain CT scan is the standard method of evaluation. This will demonstrate hemorrhage, edema, ischemia, and many fractures. Bruce and colleagues[3,4] note the presence of a mass lesion (hematoma) in 20% to 30% of unconscious children sustaining blunt trauma to the head. The CT scan has obviated exploratory burr holes. Skull films and facial bone films can be obtained later to search for additional specific fractures.

MANAGEMENT

Children with head injuries who are obtunded or comatose should have gastrointestinal decompression by nasogastric tube to prevent vomiting with aspiration and respiratory tract injury. Newborn infants should have orogastric tubes to avoid occlusion of the nares, since they are obligate nasal breathers.

Management of cerebral edema is crucial in avoiding secondary brain injury from swelling and resultant ischemia. Placement of a ventricular "bolt" or intraventricular catheter for monitoring intracerebral pressure is a useful aid in this management. Cerebral perfusion pressure equals arterial blood pressure minus intracerebral pressure; this value must be above 40 torr to avoid brain ischemia.[23] Improved perfusion pressure is best achieved by normalizing arterial pressure and reducing intracerebral pressure. Edema causing increased intracerebral pressure can be lessened by elevation of the head, reduction of $PaCO_2$ to 25 torr or less, diuresis with furosemide or mannitol, and barbiturate "coma" to reduce brain metabolism; the value of barbiturates and steroids is unproven.

Obvious blood accumulations in the epidural, subdural, or interparenchymal spaces discovered by a CT scan should be evacuated and hemorrhage controlled. Thus, CT scanning allows definitive diagnosis and specifically directed operative therapy.

RESULTS

Proper management can result in greater survival and less permanent severe debility by avoiding secondary damage after the initial injury. With the capacity for recovery of the head-injured child, proper management can often salvage a person who can be a useful and independent member of society rather than one who exists only in a vegetative or highly dependent state. Since blunt trauma is the most common method of injury of children, and severe head trauma is the most serious injury in 60% to 80% of critically injured children, proper management of all aspects of the trauma patient that affect the brain injury is essential to improved outcome.

Injuries to the Thorax

Blunt trauma to the chest may produce bony injury. Multiple rib fractures may result in flail chest. These injuries, common in adults, are infrequent in children because their ribs are flexible and bend with the blow. Penetrating injury to the lung by a fractured rib with hemopneumothorax is less likely to occur in the child. However, direct contusion of lung tissue is common in children, because the flexible bony cage affords less protection to the underlying soft tissues. Similarly, direct contusion of the myocardium may occur.

Realization that lung contusion is a common and somewhat unique injury in childhood trauma should lead to careful assessment of respiratory function and early baseline chest radiographs. More importantly, continual reassessment is essential because lung contusion may cause little initial respiratory embarrassment, but result in a progressive loss of functional capacity as hemorrhage and edema accumulating in the contused tissues alter compliance and contribute to physiologic "dead space" or unventilated, perfused lung tissue.

EVALUATION

Thorough assessment of respiratory function by physical examination and arterial blood gases, followed by appropriate corrections for hypoxia and inadequate ventilation, are part of the initial ABCs of trauma care. Failure to normalize and stabilize with proper resuscitation suggests pneumothorax. Failure to correct after tube thoracostomies suggests a major airway disruption. Chest radiographs provide baseline and follow-up assessment of the soft tissue structures of the chest, and interval blood gas determinations will demonstrate progressive respiratory deficiency.

MANAGEMENT

Tube thoracostomy will usually stabilize hemopneumothorax so that operative intervention is rarely required. Trauma sufficient to disrupt the aorta is rare in childhood and usually results in instant death. However, the mechanism of injury, such as a teenage driver who hits the steering wheel, may suggest such an injury and in such an instance it must be looked for and ruled out. Traumatic aneurysms are rarely seen as late sequelae of trauma in childhood. Emergency bronchoscopy and thoracotomy must be provided when a major airway disruption is suspected.

Most instances of injury and respiratory deficiency from blunt chest trauma can be managed with mechanical ventilatory support, adequate inspired oxygen, increased distension pressure using appropriate levels of PEEP, and good airway clearing through careful, gentle sunctioning. Secondary barotrauma from mechanical ventilation cannot always be avoided, but it can be lessened by careful management of mechanical ventilation using loosely fitting tubes, minimum peak pressures and inspired oxygen levels, and careful monitoring for improvements that will allow reductions in the mechanical support.

Abdominal Injuries

Blunt trauma to the abdomen is the second most common major nonskeletal injury in childhood trauma; it should be suspected in all motor vehicle accidents and significant falls. Occasionally, isolated trauma to the abdomen occurs, such as in falls on bicycle handlebars or when a shovel or lawnmower handle slips through the child's hands and strikes the epigastrium. External signs of trauma are more often absent than present.

Intra-abdominal organs are injured by direct contusion and by deceleration with tearing of the organ from its attachments. Solid organ injury is far more common than is injury to the bowel or bladder. Kidneys are injured more frequently in infants and children than in adults because of less muscle and bony skeletal protection.

EVALUATION

A nasogastric tube should be placed early in the course of treatment for all suspected abdominal injuries. Careful, gentle physical examination of the abdomen is the first line of assessment.

Liver dullness should be noted; its absence suggests hollow viscus rupture with pneumoperitoneum. Alterations of bowel sounds provide little useful information in assessing the abdomen for injury. Palpation to elicit tenderness, guarding, and spasm is most useful. Frequent reassessment is essential.

Suspicion of intra-abdominal injury based on positive findings on physical examination, unexplained significant blood loss or hypovolemia, or simply a strong probability of injury due to the source of trauma should indicate an abdominal CT scan. A plain abdominal radiograph is generally first obtained, but rarely identifies significant injury. An upright or cross-table lateral film would be useful in demonstrating pneumoperitoneum from a hollow viscus rupture. The CT scan is excellent for demonstrating disruption of liver, spleen, or kidney and the presence of fluid col-

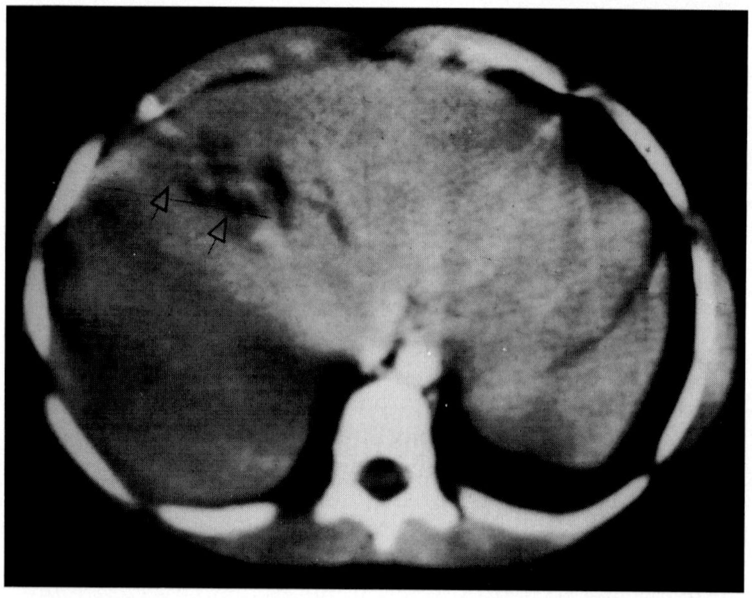

FIGURE 10.4 CT scan shows laceration deep in the liver parenchyma (arrows). (Courtesy of Dr. Donald R. Kirks, Durham, North Carolina.)

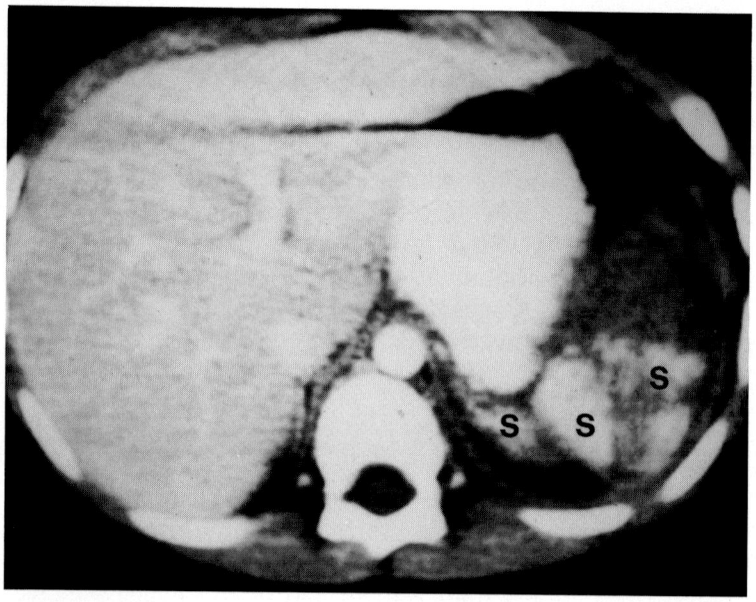

FIGURE 10.5 CT scan shows fractured spleen with multiple splenic fragments (S). (Courtesy of Dr. Donald R. Kirks, Durham, North Carolina.)

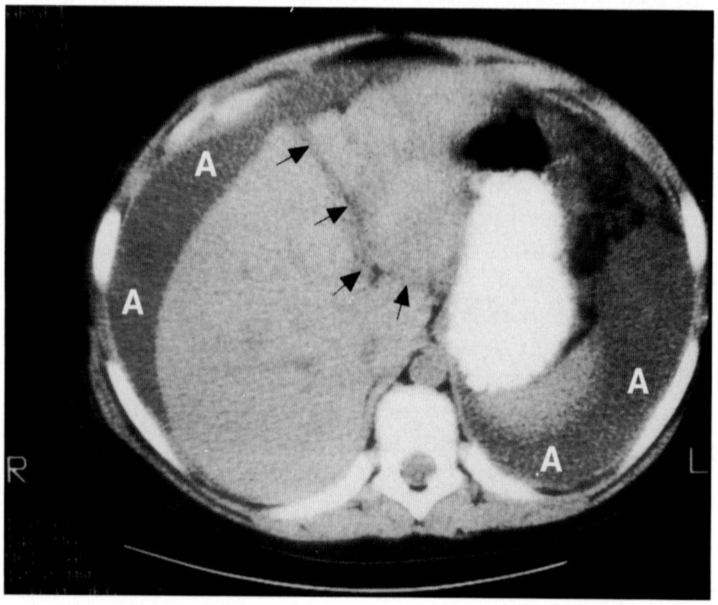

FIGURE 10.6 Liver laceration and bile ascites by CT scan. Bile ascites (A) are seen surrounding the liver and spleen. There is a linear laceration (arrows) through the liver and gallbladder fossa.[24]

lections, presumably hemorrhage (Figs. 10.4–10.6). Alternative methods of evaluation are ultrasonography and radionuclide liver spleen scan (Fig. 10.7). The former is highly dependent on the skill and experience of the operator, and the latter gives little information about organs other than the liver and spleen. The role of peritoneal tap and lavage was discussed earlier; there are specific indications for its limited use in childhood trauma.

Ultrasound may be very useful in evaluating the pancreas, particularly in providing a baseline for subsequent recognition of an evolving pseudocyst (Fig. 10.8). It may also demonstrate fluid in the pelvis and is occasionally more accurate than the CT scan in demonstrating injury to pelvic organs. Contrast gastrointestinal radiography is rarely used to assess initial injury from blunt trauma to the abdomen.

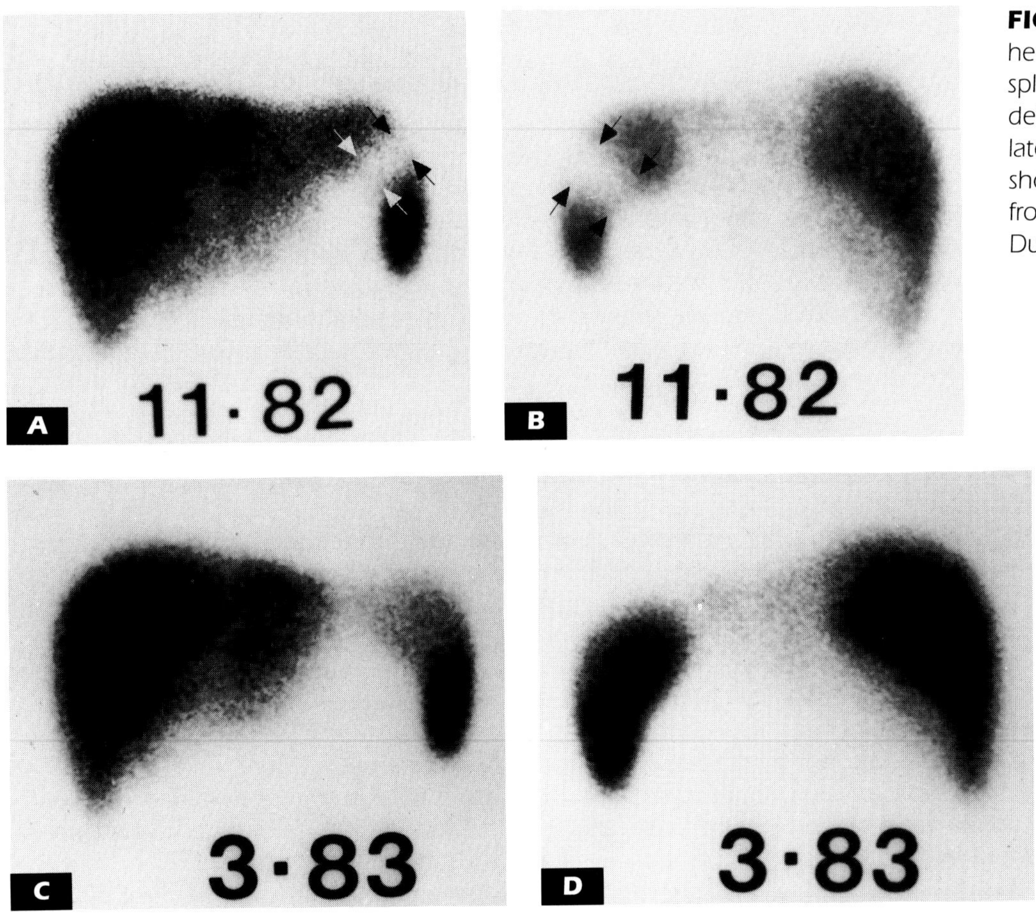

FIGURE 10.7 Splenic laceration and hematoma. In **A** anterior and **B** posterior liver-spleen nuclear scintigraphy, there is a broad defect (arrows) in the spleen. Four months later, the **C** anterior and **D** posterior views show healing of the disrupted spleen. (A, B from [24]; C, D courtesy of Dr. Donald R. Kirks, Durham, North Carolina.)

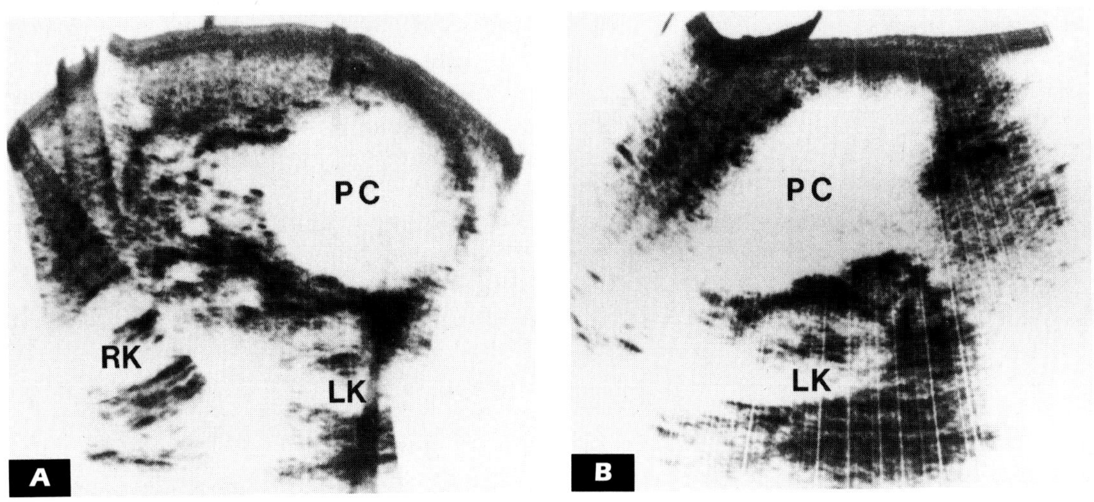

FIGURE 10.8 Pancreatic pseudocyst. **A** Transverse ultrasonography. There is a large anechoic cystic mass (PC) in the left upper quadrant. RK, right kidney; LK, left kidney. **B** Longitudinal ultrasonography. The pancreatic pseudocyst (PC) is ventral to the left kidney (LK).[24]

MANAGEMENT

Pediatric surgeons have led the way in demonstrating that many injuries to solid organs in the abdomen are best treated nonoperatively or with reparative rather than excisional surgery. It must be clearly understood that a decision against laparotomy can be considered only in an unquestionably stable patient. Excessive emphasis on nonoperative management is to be condemned, but appropriate conservative management by surgeons in the easily stabilized patient may be very beneficial.

Certain factors weigh in favor of nonoperative management for the child. First, a child's healthy vascular system is such that hemorrhage is unlikely to produce the cardiovascular or cerebrovascular catastrophes that are common in older adults with degenerative diseases. Thus, the child managed nonoperatively in a sophisticated center capable of intensive electronic monitoring and continuous evaluation by experienced, trauma-oriented pediatric intensive care nursing personnel can tolerate a secondary hemorrhage without life-threatening vascular calamities if properly resuscitated. This risk is therefore acceptable. When the child is severely brain injured, however, the cerebrovascular effects of secondary hemorrhage may add further insult to the injured brain if hypoperfusion or ischemia result from the secondary hemorrhage in the abdomen. Thus, reasoned, balanced judgment is essential to choose the safest course.

Nevertheless, it has been clearly shown that highly selective nonoperative management of major splenic and hepatic disruptions is possible and that outcomes are highly favorable. Advantages of nonoperative management include avoiding the ever-present temptation to manage hemorrhage with excisional surgery, as in splenectomy; avoidance of the deleterious effects of anesthesia and of incisional pain on respiratory function; and elimination of the long-term risks of adhesion-caused bowel obstruction from the incision and exploratory procedures. Disadvantages include delayed recurrent hemorrhage, infection of undrained fluid collections, and missed perforation of a hollow viscus, such as the intestine or gallbladder. Fortunately, such hollow viscus injuries in childhood blunt trauma are rare, and gallbladder injury can usually be demonstrated by CT scan or ultrasonography.

Increasing numbers of injuries to the intestines, especially the transverse colon and mesentery, are being seen in restrained children who sustained injury to the intestine from the seatbelt. This may result in acute perforation, delayed stenosis, or adhesive bowel obstruction. Ischemia is the common etiology.[6,17]

Careful reassessment of the abdomen is essential if nonoperative therapy is selected. However, fever, tenderness and leukocytosis commonly accompany solid viscus injury and intraperitoneal hemorrhage; peritoneal lavage is indicated if hollow viscus disruption is suspected.

Conservative operative treatment is an alternative to nonoperative management and should be selected for the unstable patient or one with multiple intra-abdominal injuries. Splenic injuries can be controlled by partial resection, suture control of hemorrhage or cauterization, and the use of hemostatic materials. Only a totally shattered or devascularized spleen should be removed. The risk of postsplenectomy sepsis mandates splenic preservation whenever possible.

When splenectomy is elected, consideration should be given to immunizing the patient against pneumococcal and meningococcal infections with appropriate vaccines and daily, life-long penicillin therapy, as has been suggested for patients after splenectomy for hematologic or oncologic indications. Remember that the vaccines do not cover all strains of the organisms and that organisms not covered by the vaccines can cause postsplenectomy sepsis.

Clearly only a small minority of patients are dependent on the spleen for significant immunologic protection, but since this minority cannot yet be identified, and since splenic salvage procedures have proven to be so satisfactory in children, the indications for total splenectomy should be few.

NONOPERATIVE MANAGEMENT

When nonoperative management is elected for demonstrated solid organ disruptions, the patient should be initially cared for in a pediatric intensive care setting in a center capable of full operative, anesthetic, and blood-product support for any complications that may ensue. Nasogastric decompression is essential for the frequently accompanying ileus, and intravenous glucose/electrolyte support is given. If central vascular access has been achieved, early nutritional support may be useful. A short course of antibiotics may provide prophylaxis, but the efficacy of this has not been proven. Prolonged broad-spectrum coverage is contraindicated as it may produce a resistant flora more difficult to control. Specifically identified infection should, of course, be treated vigorously.

As noted, the patient with a lacerated liver or spleen and extravasated blood or bile in the peritoneal cavity will often have tenderness, guarding to palpation, fever, and leukocytosis. These may last for a week or more. The patient is generally very stable, appears well, and improves daily. Signs of generalized sepsis or toxemia, lethargy, or altered consciousness should suggest infection of the extravasated fluids and lead to surgical drainage, although this is rarely necessary.

Bedrest should be continued for several days and then judicious ambulation begun. Once totally stable with no evidence of bleeding for 48 hours, the patient may be transferred to an intermediate-care bed. (The hematocrit is the best monitor of recurrent bleeding.) Feedings may resume when the ileus resolves. After 10 days, the patient may be discharged home with limited activity for another 2 weeks, followed by return to school with physical education restrictions up to 12 weeks. This schedule should provide adequate insurance against inadvertent reinjury.

The lesion should be followed at increasing intervals by CT scan or ultrasound to provide evidence of resolution and a baseline in the event of a subsequent injury. Karp and associates[22] found on CT scans that most injuries were healed by 3 to 4 months.

The liver injury most amenable to nonoperative management is the subcapsular hematoma.[5] Small lacerations with minimal fluid collections may also respond nicely to this approach. Large lacerations with extensive extravasation of blood and bile may be managed by conservative surgery, debridement of devitalized tissue as necessary, hemostasis by electrocoagulation or suture, evacuation of extravasated blood and bile, and effective drainage. Penrose drains in the laceration and sump drain catheters in the collecting area usually suffice.

Increasingly, authors are reporting significant numbers of patients with major hepatic injuries managed without surgery. Giacomantonio and associates[13] from Toronto's Hospital for Sick Children reported 32 cases of blunt hepatic trauma treated between 1974 and 1982; 23 were due to motor vehicle accidents (Fig. 10.9). Eighteen were treated surgically, seven urgently for massive bleeding. There were seven deaths in this group, five from uncontrollable bleeding and two from head injuries. Fourteen of their patients were treated nonoperatively. All were diagnosed by liver/spleen scan. Five required blood transfusion of an average of 33 ml/kg. There were no late complications. Follow-up liver/spleen scans were performed in 11 patients, all showing resolution.

Karp and associates[22] also reported a series of 17 patients managed nonoperatively. The patient's clinical course, not the presence of blood in the abdomen, determined the necessity for operative intervention. They noted that in reports emphasizing conservative surgery for hepatic blunt trauma, 20% to 67% of patients had stopped bleeding by the time of laparotomy. They had no infection, hemobilia, or delayed hemorrhage. Two patients continued to bleed and one of them required operation. Twelve patients required transfusion; three had associated renal and splenic injuries. These authors outlined the healing stages as noted by CT scan:

- Resorption of blood and injured tissue by 10 to 14 days;
- Coalescence of stellate injuries to one large lesser density area by 1 month;
- Increasing density and decreased size from 1 to 3 months; and
- Reduction in size and restored parenchymal homogeneity by 3 to 4 months (2–6 months depending on the extent of the injury).

These same authors[21] reported their results with computed tomography and the evaluation of blunt trauma in children. Of 46 children evaluated, all were stable. Seventy-four percent showed positive results on the CT scan with 12 showing genitourinary trauma, 11 of which were managed nonoperatively. Two severe injuries were not found on intravenous pyelogram. There were 13 splenic lacerations, nine of which were treated nonoperatively. The authors cited the advantages of CT scanning as visualization of all organs, demonstration of the relationships to surrounding structures, demonstration of intraperitoneal fluid (presumably blood), and the ability to follow the course of healing long term. Their criteria for contrast-enhanced CT scanning of the abdomen included stable vital signs, a suspected intra-abdominal injury, a slowly declining hematocrit or the need for only mild fluid resuscitation, a neurologically injured patient, the presence of multiple injuries requiring general anesthesia, the presence of multiple bleeding sources, or the presence of hematuria.

Grisoni and associates[14] from Case Western Reserve University reported 20 patients with liver injury, 16 of whom were treated nonoperatively. None had peritoneal lavage. There were no delayed complications. Of the 20 patients, eight were operated on for a transfusion requirement of over 50 ml/kg, and one for an associated intra-abdominal injury.

Surgeons from the Toronto Hospital for Sick Children have been in the forefront of nonoperative treatment of splenic injuries.[10] In 1981, Wesson and associates[38] reported 63 patients with splenic injuries treated from 1974 to 1979. Forty-four of these were treated nonoperatively. Sixteen of the nonoperative patients required transfusions averaging 31.2 ml/kg. There were no late ruptures and no deaths. Of the 19 patients treated operatively, 19 required transfusions averaging 80.4 ml/kg preoperatively and an average of 175 ml/kg throughout their course. Fifteen of these patients had splenectomy, two partial splenectomy, and one splenorrhaphy; one patient's spleen was not bleeding at the time of operation. All patients were operated on by 16 hours postinjury and there was no major bleeding after 24 hours. These patients were diagnosed by liver/spleen scan and not by CT scan. A 1989 follow-up report from the same institution gave even more convincing results. Of 75 patients admitted with splenic injuries between 1981 and 1986, 10 underwent surgery (only one total splenectomy); three died, none from splenic trauma. Only 23 percent of nonoperated patients required blood transfusions. Total hospital stay was reduced to seven days on the average for patients with isolated splenic injury. Of 45 children with isolated splenic injuries, only one required laparotomy; none required splenectomy; and only six required transfusions. The hemoglobin threshold for transfusion was 80 g/1.[27]

FIGURE 10.9
LIVER TRAUMA MANAGEMENT AND OUTCOME[13]

DRUG	NUMBER OF PATIENTS	SURVIVAL	MORTALITY
Nonoperative	14	14	0
Drainage alone	3	3	0
Suture and drainage	6	5	1
Debridement	2	2	0
Lobectomy	4	1	3
Uncontrolled bleeding	3	0	3
Total	32	25 (78%)	7 (22%)

Recent studies have been directed at the best operative treatment for the injured spleen.[8] Preservation of as much of the spleen with an intact blood supply as possible gives the best postoperative immune function. In laboratory experiments, splenic artery ligation is superior to autotransplantation of splenic slices and creation of intraperitoneal splenosis, because these latter modalities do not provide adequate clearing of organisms by the splenic implants.

An interesting study from the Children's Hospital of Cincinnati by Oldham and his associates[27] indicates that the hepatic enzymes serum glutamic -oxaloacetic and -pyruvic transaminase (SGOT and SGPT) may be indicators of significant hepatic injury. The authors studied 100 children with blunt abdominal trauma by CT imaging, 95 of whom were hemodynamically stable. Forty-four showed an immediate rise of hepatic enzymes above 30 immunizing units (IU). Nineteen of these had significant hepatic injury. All children with injuries showed SGOT levels above 200 IU and SGPT above 100 IU. Of the 31 children who had SGOT and SGPT levels above 100 IU, 19 were injured, for a specificity of 62%. Thus, the authors felt that a significant rise in SGOT/SGPT in children sustaining blunt abdominal trauma was an indication of probable liver injury and thereby an indication for CT scanning.

Pancreatic Injuries

Most pancreatic injuries can be treated nonoperatively initially, but careful follow-up is essential to recognize a developing pseudocyst. Major lacerations may require drainage, and uncontrollable hemorrhage may require resection and internal intestinal anastomosis, or even a pancreatoduodenectomy for severe crush injury. Aggressive surgery for pancreatic injuries is rarely indicated, however. A baseline ultrasonogram should be obtained, and weekly follow-ups provided for 4 to 6 weeks, looking for an evolving pseudocyst.[7] If one develops, internal drainage into the stomach or a Roux-en-Y jejunal loop is the preferred treatment. Traumatic pancreatitis should be managed with rest, gastric decompression, and nutritional support with TPN until symptoms abate and serum and urinary amylase levels normalize. Clinical judgment is important, however, because amylase levels may remain misleadingly high for long periods.

Duodenal Hematoma

A related injury that is almost unique to childhood is the duodenal hematoma. This frequently occurs when a narrow object such as a bicycle handlebar or shovel strikes the epigastrium. Typically, the child is asymptomatic for 24 hours, then develops epigastric pain and vomiting. Contrast upper GI radiography will demonstrate partial obstruction of the duodenum in the third to fourth part by a submucosal hematoma impinging on the lumen (Fig. 10.10). A classic radiographic appearance confirms the diagnosis.

Treatment is bowel rest with decompression and nutritional support until the hematoma resolves enough in 7 to 10 days to allow resumption of feedings. Surgery is rarely indicated.

Renal Injuries

Injury to the kidney from blunt trauma is more common in childhood because there is less bony and muscular protection for the kidney and less perinephric fat. The kidneys can be evaluated by CT scan, if one is already indicated to evaluate liver or splenic injury, or an intravenous pyelogram can be obtained. The latter will rule out a severely disrupted renal pedicle and a major crush with extravasation of urine, but may not rule out minor lacerations or disruptions.

Treatment of renal injuries has undergone wide swings of philosophy in the past decade. Individualization is probably best, because it allows exploration and revascularization of a major pedicle injury but avoids disruption of a stable hematoma contained by the perinephric tissue with consequent nephrectomy for hemostasis.

Careful follow-up of renal injuries is essential. Extravasated blood and urine may become infected and require drainage; devitalized areas of renal tissue may require delayed partial nephrectomy.

Another feature of renal trauma unique to childhood is the possibility of an underlying renal tumor or congenital anomaly.

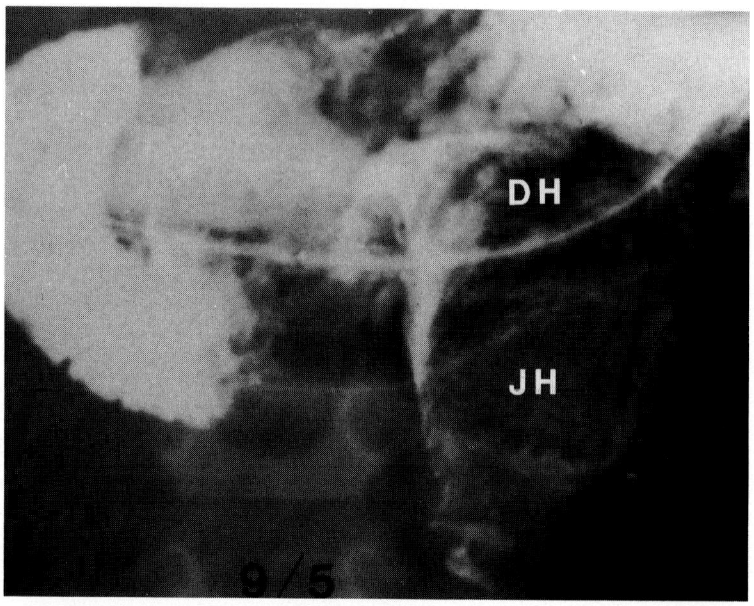

FIGURE 10.10 Duodenal hematoma, upper GI series. There is a large hematoma of the distal duodenum (DH) and jejunum (JH). The "coiled-spring" appearance is most marked in the proximal jejunum (JH).[24]

Incidence of this combination has been estimated to be 2% to 15% of traumatized kidneys.[26] This possibility should be considered especially when the traumatic event seems insufficient to produce the degree of renal injury.

Pelvic Fractures

The rather elastic growth centers and ligaments of the child's pelvis account for the fact that pelvic fracture is less common in childhood, but the admonition to look for soft tissue injuries is still appropriate. A careful rectal examination is mandatory, and the urethra should be investigated by meatal insertion of contrast material prior to attempts at bladder catheterization; the reason is that catheterization without examination first may complete the disruption of a partially divided urethra.

Extremity and Long Bone Fractures

One feature of extremity fractures unique to children, especially to infants, is the possibility of sufficient hemorrhage occurring into the soft tissues around a fracture, such as of a femur, to result in shock. Infants with no other injury than a fractured femur have been sent to the radiology suite for routine extremity films without vascular access having been obtained. One such infant sustained a cardiac arrest from which he was unable to be resuscitated before irreversible brain death occurred. At post mortem examination, only a fractured femur with massive hemorrhage was confirmed. Infants with major extremity fractures should be carefully evaluated for circulatory stability, and secure vascular access should be provided prior to further evaluation of the fracture. Monitoring for impending circulatory collapse should be continued while radiographic evaluations are being done, and adequate replacement volumes should be given in a timely fashion.

The other unique feature of extremity fractures in children is the presence of the growth center in the bones. The growth plate may be directly involved in the fracture or growth may be affected by vascular changes related to the fracture. The influence of fractures on the child's subsequent growth and function mandates that they be cared for by an orthopedic specialist experienced in the special problems of fracture care in children.

OTHER INJURIES

Burns

A general principle of burn injury management in children is that children survive with greater percentages of body surface involvement and greater depths of burn injury than do adults. Children with 90% of their surface area burned have survived. Of course, the price for this in terms of debility, disfigurement, psychic trauma, and endurance of painful reconstructive procedures is tremendous. Nevertheless, the high survival rate for massive burn injuries in childhood underscores the need for aggressive skillful management.

EVALUATION

An accurate assessment of burn injury in infants and young children, is based on the knowledge that body parts do not represent the same percent of total surface area in infants as in adults. The head and trunk of children make up a relatively larger percentage of body surface area and the extremities, especially the lower extremities, a relatively smaller percentage. Charts and diagrams are available to aid in calculating surface area involvement for fluid volume restoration (Fig. 10.11).

In calculating fluid volume requirements, the child's daily maintenance must also be considered, and this is figured by one of the formulas given earlier in this chapter under "Fluid and Electrolyte Management." This volume is frequently ignored in the adult, in whom it is about 25 ml/kg per day; infants have a maintenance requirement of 90–100 ml/kg/day. This volume must not be ignored.

Whether to use high volumes of isotonic salt solutions or a balanced fluid program of colloid and isotonic salt solutions has been debated for years. It has been my observation that infants tolerate a balanced program better and develop less edema with added colloid, but the important factor is early adequate fluid resuscitation to insure tissue perfusion and avoid hypovolemia with its attendant shunting, tissue hypoxia, and capillary membrane damage. The latter results in massive fluid shifts to the interstitium throughout the body, even in nonburned, uninvolved areas, thus compounding the fluid requirements.

Unlike older children and adults, infants with second- and third-degree burns involving less than 20% of the body surface may require hospitalization or, at the very least, close observation. Their increased maintenance requirement (see above) makes them more subject to dehydration if their intake is reduced by the burn wound trauma. They will frequently develop an ileus and vomit, therefore failing to consume enough fluid orally to protect them from hypovolemia, even though the expected loss from the burn wound would seem to be manageable without hospitalization and intravenous fluid administration. As a result, many of those infants will return in 24 to 48 hours in near shock, having been released from the emergency room by an inexperienced physician.

A common cause of burns in infants is a container of hot liquid, such as coffee or tea, which has been pulled from a table or stove by its electric cord onto the toddler or infant below. These are usually "splotchy," medium-to-deep, second-degree burns and are efficiently managed by a covering of fine meshed gauze soaked with povidone-iodine solution, which is dried in place to form a scab-like covering similar to the donor site of a skin graft; silver sulfadiazine cream (*Silvadene*, Marion Laboratories) may also be used.

BURN ESTIMATE AND DIAGRAM
AGE vs. AREA

Area	Birth–1 yr.	1–4 yr.	5–9 yr.	10–14 yr.	15 yr.	Adult	2°	3°	Total
Head	19	17	13	11	9	7			
Neck	2	2	2	2	2	2			
Ant. Trunk	13	13	13	13	13	13			
Post. Trunk	13	13	13	13	13	13			
R.Buttock	2 1/2	2 1/2	2 1/2	2 1/2	2 1/2	2 1/2			
L.Buttock	2 1/2	2 1/2	2 1/2	2 1/2	2 1/2	2 1/2			
Genitalia	1	1	1	1	1	1			
R.U. Arm	4	4	4	4	4	4			
L.U. Arm	4	4	4	4	4	4			
R.L. Arm	3	3	3	3	3	3			
L.L. Arm	3	3	3	3	3	3			
R. Hand	2 1/2	2 1/2	2 1/2	2 1/2	2 1/2	2 1/2			
L. Hand	2 1/2	2 1/2	2 1/2	2 1/2	2 1/2	2 1/2			
R. Thigh	5 1/2	6 1/2	8	8 1/2	9	9 1/2			
L. Thigh	5 1/2	6 1/2	8	8 1/2	9	9 1/2			
R. Leg	5	5	5 1/2	6	6 1/2	7			
L. Leg	5	5	5 1/2	6	6 1/2	7			
R. Foot	3 1/2	3 1/2	3 1/2	3 1/2	3 1/2	3 1/2			
L. Foot	3 1/2	3 1/2	3 1/2	3 1/2	3 1/2	3 1/2			
						TOTAL			

AGE ____________________
SEX ____________________
WEIGHT ____________________

NAME ____________________
VUH# ____________________

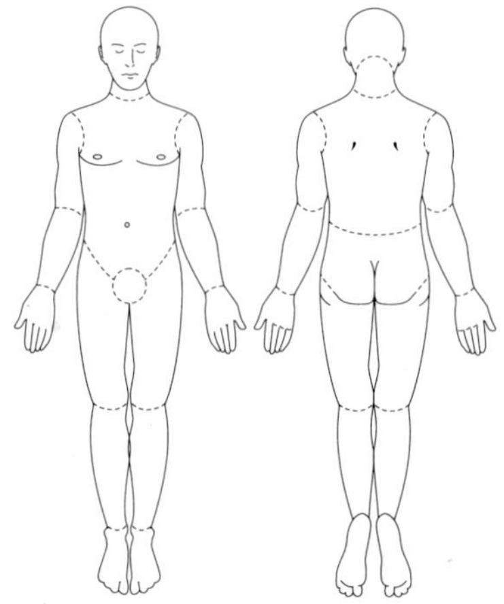

FIGURE 10.11 Estimations of total surface area (in percentages) at various ages of childhood are used in calculation of percentage of surface area burned. (Reproduced with permission from O'Neill, J.A., Jr.: Burns, in Ravitch, M.M., et al. [eds.]: Pediatric Surgery, 3rd edition, Vol. 1. Copyright © 1979 by Year Book Medical Publishers, Inc., Chicago.)

ELECTRICAL BURNS

Another burn most frequently seen in infants is the electrical burn, usually as the result of the toddler biting an exposed electrical cord. This burn must always be considered to be worse than it initially appears. Often deep tissues about the mouth and face are destroyed. The child should be hospitalized until the burn demarcates and the extent of the injury is determined.

Wringer Injuries

Wringer injuries used to be a common reason for hospitalization on pediatric surgical services. As the wringer washing machine fades into antiquity, this injury has become less common. However, when seen, the degree of injury must be appreciated. Often the injury is compounded by the mother pulling the child from the wringer with the rollers engaged and still rolling, which creates a severe crush injury extending from the palm to above the elbow in many cases. Initially the injury may not appear significant and the inexperienced physician may discharge the child. Resultant swelling may create a compartment syndrome with ischemic necrosis of the distal forearm and hand. Children with wringer arm injuries should be admitted, with the wound loosely dressed, elevated, and observed carefully over the next 24 hours. If there is no evidence of compartment syndrome, the child may then be discharged, to be followed up carefully over the next several days.

Bicycle Spoke Injuries

A bicycle spoke injury is similar to the wringer injury in the degree of crush and resultant swelling. However, it is frequently associated with a distally based skin-flap laceration. Again, this is an injury that may be mismanaged by the inexperienced physician. The distally based skin-flap laceration has a poor blood supply and may undergo necrosis. In addition, the crushed tissues may swell extensively, again with ischemic necrosis of distal tissues. The severity of the injury should be explained to the parents initially and careful follow-up provided. The distally based skin flap should be debrided and closed and should be followed up carefully in case necrosis ensues. The fact that the child may often be incapacitated for as long as 6 weeks by the crush injury should indicate the need for careful follow-up.

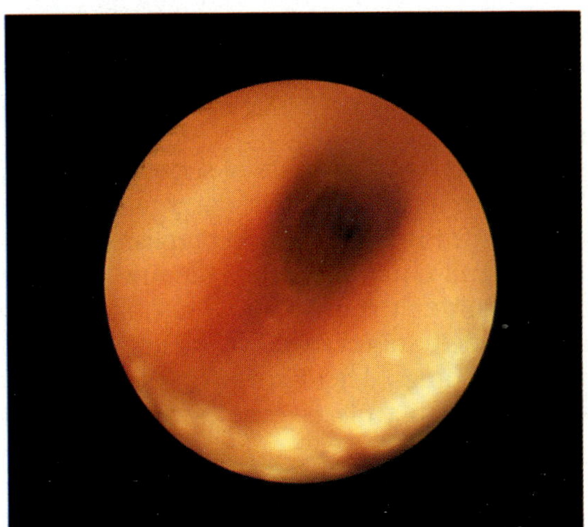

FIGURE 10.12 Subglottic airway injury from lye aspiration during lye ingestion. The marked subglottic narrowing required frequent dilatations following tracheostomy.

Ingestions

The curiosity of the infant, toddler, and young child leads him or her to sample the environment in a variety of ways, most often orally. Thus, the child tends to taste and ingest liquids and powders that are found about the house. Add to this tendency the carelessness, ignorance, and occasional frank stupidity of the child's caretakers, and ingestion of poisonous and injurious agents is unfortunately common. Poisonings are best managed by saving the container and any remaining material and immediately consulting the regional poison control center for advice.

The most common injurious agents ingested by children are cleaning products, most frequently those containing strong alkali. These can be highly destructive of the hypopharynx, esophagus, and laryngotracheobronchial tree. Emphasis in regard to alkali ingestion is usually placed on the destruction of the esophagus, to the neglect of the potential injury to the larynx and trachea. The child with a history of alkali ingestion should be very carefully observed for development of airway edema. The epiglottis and larynx should be viewed to be certain they are not burned. (Fig. 10.12).

If the child is to be transferred to a distant center for care of a suspected esophageal injury, attention must be given to the possibility of an evolving airway injury. A serious airway injury that compromises either air exchange or the protective glottic mechanism against aspiration requires early intubation. If full-thickness damage to the epiglottis, larynx, or cords has occurred, tracheostomy may be required.

Management of suspected esophageal burns is still subject to some differences of approach, but several points of agreement can be offered. Mouth burns may be present or absent in association with severe esophageal injury; initial esophageal contrast studies may not define the extent of injury; and esophagoscopy is mandatory to define the seriousness of the damage.

Still in debate is the use of antibiotics and steroids. Well-controlled studies have never been achieved, but the most widely followed regimen is the use of early and prolonged antibiotics and steroid therapy based on clinical and laboratory observations by Haller and his associates at John Hopkins University.[15] Our regimen has been to begin amoxicillian or ampicillin and prednisone (2 mg/kg/day) or equivalent intravenous steroids if necessary. The patient is examined with an esophagoscope at the next regular operating room time (avoid emergency esophagoscopy in a patient with a stomach full of alkali and food). If serious injury is not present, the antibiotics and steroids are discontinued, but when significant esophageal damage is found, antibiotics are maintained for 10 days and steroids for 3 weeks. Dilatations, if needed, are begun after this period, facilitated by a gastrostomy; a string covered with Silastic tubing is then passed through the esophagus and out the gastrostomy to facilitate retrograde dilatations, which are safer.

The use of steroids does not seem to avoid strictures and the need for dilatations, but it does seem to have reduced the need for esophageal replacement. However, this latter observation may be the result of fewer ingestions and reduced strength of commonly used household products containing alkali.

BIRTH TRAUMA, CHILD ABUSE, AND HOMICIDE/SUICIDE

Birth Trauma

Birth trauma is, of course, always mentioned in conjunction with trauma in childhood, but significant trauma to the infant during the birth process is remarkably rare. Most commonly there is battering of the cranium against the cervix and pelvis which often results in cephalohematomas but rarely in brain injury or skull fracture. Abnormal presentations such as breech, footling, and arm may result in stretching of nerve roots, producing damage to the brachial plexus and occasionally to the adjacent phrenic nerve. Direct injury to internal organs, such as the liver or spleen, is even less common, but should be considered in any newborn infant with a falling hematocrit, unexplained shock, or abdominal distention without gaseous bowel distention.

CHILD ABUSE

Child abuse is widespread in our society and has attracted significant media attention recently. Physical abuse of children results in death and serious injury to untold numbers of infants and children each year. Characteristically, a history of abuse cannot be obtained from the child because of fear and guilt. It should be suspected whenever children present with injuries in late evening or night and with unlikely stories for the etiology of the injury. Marks from beatings or cigarette burns are warning signs, but the most significant sign of abuse is radiographic evidence of numerous fractures in various stages of healing.

Care must be taken to rule out osteogenesis imperfecta and other collagen deficiency states associated with multiple spontaneous fractures. Also remember that children do sustain strange injuries because of their curiosity and adventurousness.

In most states, the physician is legally protected and in fact legally required to report suspected abuse. Many major medical centers have SCAN (Suspected Child Abuse and Neglect) teams made up of physicians, psychiatrists, social workers, and often legal counsel to facilitate investigation of suspected abuse. Suspected abuse is an indication for protective hospitalization until the issue is resolved.

Shaking small infants can tear bridging meningeal vessels and result in serious cerebral hemorrhage and brain damage. Other common injuries due to abuse include beatings, cigarette burns, head injuries, fractures, scald burns, and blunt abdominal trauma. Appropriate early use of newer diagnostic imaging modalities may help to offset the high mortality rate from serious blunt abdominal trauma.[24]

Suicide and Homicide

Suicide attempts are often drug-related and frequently overdosing is the mechanism of suicide chosen by children and teenagers. Gunshots, usually to the head, are second in frequency. Care of the victim is not unique in this age group, but preventive methods need to be addressed in our society.

EMOTIONAL SUPPORT OF THE CHILD TRAUMA VICTIM

One of the unique aspects of trauma to the child is the meaning of the injury to the child. Most children have received repeated warnings from their parents throughout childhood in an attempt to heighten their awareness of the dangers in the environment and encourage their self-protective actions. They have been told repeatedly that if they do (or do not do) such and such a thing, they will be injured. Thus, when a child is injured, he frequently feels very guilty, associating the injury with some failure on his part. This often leads to fear and anger and a seemingly hostile attitude toward family and caretakers. Understanding this guilt association is important, for the child needs much reassurance that the trauma was not his fault and that he is not being punished for his own wrongdoing. Parents will often be baffled by a child's behavior following trauma; they may recognize a significant personality change and fear that their child has serious brain injury. Both the child and parents need reassurance and help to work through the child's guilt and anxiety.

As we strive to improve the care of seriously injured pediatric trauma victims, we must also direct our attention to preventive measures. Some measures are best accomplished through education of parents and children; others require legislative efforts, such as those requiring the use of child restraints in motor vehicles and attempting to discourage driving under the influence of alcohol and other drugs. The carnage on our highways must be recognized for what it truly is—the number one killer of our children.

REFERENCES

1. Baker SP: Motor vehicle occupant deaths in young children. Pediatrics 64:860–865, 1979.
2. Barlow B, Niemirska M, Gandhi RP et al: Ten years of experience with falls from a height in children. J Pediatr Surg 18:509–511, 1983.
3. Bruce DA: Manipulation of intracranial pressure. In Harris BH (ed): First National Conference on Pediatric Trauma, p 135. Boston, Kiwanis Pediatric Trauma Institute, 1985.
4. Bruce DA, Schut L, Sutton LN: Pediatric head injury. In Wilkins RH, Rengachary SS (eds): Neurosurgery, p 1600. New York, McGraw-Hill, 1985.
5. Cheatham JE, Smith EI, Tunnel WP et al: Non-operative management of subcapsular hematomas of the liver. Am J Surg 140:852–856, 1980.
6. Cobb LM, Vinocur CD, Wagner CW, et al: Intestinal perforation due to blunt trauma in children in an era of increased non-operative treatment. J Trauma 26:461–463, 1986.
7. Cooney DR, Grosfeld JL: Operative management of pancreatic pseudocysts in infants and children: A review of 75 cases. Ann Surg 182:590–596, 1975.
8. Cooney DR, Michalek WA, Michalek DM, Fisher JE: Comparative methods of splenic preservation. J Pediatr Surg 16:327–337, 1981.
9. Cooper A, Betts JM, Pereira GR et al: Taurine deficiency in the severe hepatic dysfunction complicating total parenteral nutrition. J Pediatr Surg 9:462–466, 1984.
10. Douglas GJ, Simpson JS: The conservative management of splenic trauma. J Pediatr Surg 6:565–570, 1971.
11. Filston HC, Edwards CH, Chitwood WR Jr et al: Estimation of postoperative fluid requirements in infants and children. Ann Surg 196:76–81, 1982.
12. Filston HC, Grant JP: A safer system for percutaneous subclavian venous catheterization in newborn infants. J Pediatr Surg 14:564–570, 1979.
13. Giacomantonio M, Filler RM, Rich RH: Blunt hepatic trauma in children: Experience with operative and nonoperative management. J Pediatr Surg 19:519–522, 1984.
14. Grisoni ER, Gauderer MW, Ferron J et al: Nonoperative management of liver injuries following blunt abdominal trauma in children. J Pediatr Surg 19:515–518, 1984.
15. Haller JA Jr, Andrews HG, White JJ et al: Pathophysiology and management of acute corrosive burns of the esophagus: Results of treatment on 285 children. J Pediatr Surg 6:578–584, 1971.
16. Haller JA Jr, Shorter N, Miller D et al: Organization and function of a regional pediatric trauma center: Does a system of management improve outcome? J Trauma 23:691–696, 1983.
17. Hardacre JM II, West KW, Rescorla FR, et al: Delayed onset of intestinal obstruction in children after unrecognized seat belt injury. J Pediatr Surg 25:967–969, 1990.
18. Harris BH (ed): Progress in Pediatric Trauma: Proceedings of the First National Conference on Pediatric Trauma. Boston, Kiwanis Pediatric Trauma Institute, 1985.
19. Holmes MJ, Reyes HM: A critical review of urban pediatric trauma. J Trauma 24:253–255, 1984.
20. Hughes CA, Talbot IC, Ducker DA et al: Total parenteral nutrition in infancy. Effect on the liver and suggested pathogenesis. Gut 24:241–248, 1983.
21. Karp MP, Cooney DR, Berger PE et al: The role of computed tomography in the evaluation of blunt abdominal trauma in children. J Pediatr Surg 16:316–323, 1981.
22. Karp MP, Cooney DR, Pros GA et al: The nonoperative management of pediatric hepatic trauma. J Pediatr Surg 18:512–518, 1983.
23. Kasdon DL: Physiology of the nervous system. In Harris BH (ed): First National Conference on Pediatric Trauma, p 8. Boston, Kiwanis Pediatric Trauma Institute, 1985.
24. Kirks DR: Radiological evaluation of visceral injuries in the battered child syndrome. Pediatr Ann 12:888–893, 1983.
25. Mahoney WJ, D'Souza BJ, Haller JA et al: Long-term outcome of children with severe head trauma and prolonged coma. Pediatrics 71:756–762, 1983.
26. Miller RC, Sterioff S Jr, Drucker WR et al: The incidental discovery of occult abdominal tumors in children following blunt abdominal trauma. J Trauma 1:99–106, 1966.
27. Oldham KT, Guice KS, Kaufman RA et al: Blunt hepatic injury and elevated hepatic enzymes: A clinical correlation in children. J Pediatr Surg 19:457–461, 1984.
28. Pearl RH, Wesson DE, Spence LJ, et al: Splenic injury: A five-year update with improved results and changing criteria for conservative management. J Pediatr Surg 24:121-125, 1989.
29. Ramenofsky ML: Trauma scores and outcome studies. In Harris BH (ed): Progress in Pediatric Trauma: Proceedings of the First National Conference on Pediatric Trauma, p 50. Boston, Kiwanis Pediatric Trauma Institute, 1985.
30. Ramenofsky ML, Morse TS: Standards of care for the critically injured pediatric patient. J Trauma 22:921–933, 1982.
31. Ramenofsky ML, Morse TS: Reply to Letters to Editor. J Trauma 9:849, 1983.
32. Rivara FP: Traumatic deaths of children in the United States: Currently available prevention strategies. Pediatrics 75:456–462, 1985.
33. Seidel JS, Hornbein M, Yosheyama KE et al: Emergency medical sources and the pediatric patient: Are the needs being met? Pediatrics 73:769–772, 1984.
34. Seigler RS, Tecklenburg FW, Shealy R: Pre-hospital intraosseous infusion by emergency medical services personnel: a prospective study. Pediatrics 84:173–177, 1985.
35. Sutow WW, Vietti TJ, Fernbach DJ (eds): Clinical Pediatric Oncology, 2nd ed, p 4. St. Louis, CV Mosby, 1977.
36. Tanz RR, Christoffel KK: Pedestrian injury: The next motor vehicle injury challenge. Am J Dis Child 139:1187–1190, 1985.
37. Vileisis RL, Imwood RJ, Hunt CE: Prospective controlled study of parenteral nutrition-associated cholestatic jaundice: Effect of protein intake. J Pediatr 96:893–897, 1980.
38. Wessen DE, Filler RM, Ein SH et al: Ruptured spleen—when to operate? J Pediatr Surg 16:324–326, 1981.

11

genitourinary trauma

David F. Paulson

Traumatic injury to the genitourinary tract accounts for less than 3% of all trauma admissions in the civilian population.[26] For the purposes of this discussion, genitourinary tract trauma will be subdivided into upper urinary tract trauma (trauma involving the kidney or its vascular supply), trauma to the drainage system from the kidney (the renal pelvis and ureters), trauma to the bladder, and trauma to the external genitalia.

Traumatic injury to the renal parenchyma and its vasculature, the ureters, and bladder may be classified as internal trauma, because the extent of injury may not be readily apparent to the examining physician. Many patients who receive traumatic injury to the kidney, ureters, or bladder also have severe associated intrathoracic, intra-abdominal, or pelvic trauma, which may direct attention from these genitourinary organ sites.

RENAL TRAUMA

Renal trauma may be subdivided into renal vascular and renal parenchymal trauma, and those further subdivided into penetrating and nonpenetrating injury. However, awareness of the possibility of trauma to the kidney as a unit should promote an early attempt to confine the extent of injury. The dominant clinical sign of injury to the renal unit is hematuria. Blood in the urine, either gross or microscopic, almost always occurs with renal injury. However, failure to define blood in the traumatized patient does not exclude the possibility of trauma to the renal unit. Vascular injury that disrupts renal perfusion may produce loss of all renal function in the absence of hematuria. Similarly, complete and total rupture of the renal unit itself secondary to severe blunt trauma may result in renal failure. Last, severe associated injuries that produce marked contraction of the intravascular volume may precipitate acute renal ischemia in the absence of direct renal trauma, but with the end result of anuria.

An examination of the traumatized patient for the presence of injuries known to be associated with renal trauma should prompt an assessment of renal function. Injuries to the lower chest, flank, or upper abdomen are frequently associated with renal parenchymal damage. Penetrating abdominal injuries involve the kidney in approximately 8% of all cases.[22] Radiographic evidence of lower rib fractures or avulsion of the transverse lumbar processes frequently confirms associated renal damage.

Diagnosis

Various imaging modalities exist to determine the nature of the upper tract injury. A plain film of the abdomen permits the physician to examine the bony structures surrounding the renal units. Lateral distortion of the spine (scoliosis with concavity directed toward the site of injury) is frequently noted. Failure to define the radiographic margins of the kidney itself or the psoas shadow are indicators of either blood or urine in the retroperitoneum. Displacement of bowel from the suspected area of trauma frequently indicates an expanding retroperitoneal mass.

The degree of injury to the vasculature or parenchyma and other diagnostic information may be assessed by use of the intravenous pyelogram in the patient who is hemodynamically stable. However, this study in a patient who is hemodynamically unstable may, because of the absence of adequate renal perfusion, fail to identify the renal unit and the degree of damage. Nonvisualization of the kidney should prompt suspicion of renal vascular injury, major renal parenchymal disruption, or obstruction of the urinary tract itself. This simple screening study does provide at the least a basis from which to proceed.

Renal Vascular Injuries

The lack of renal function in the patient who is hemodynamically stable should raise the issue of damage to the renal pedicle.

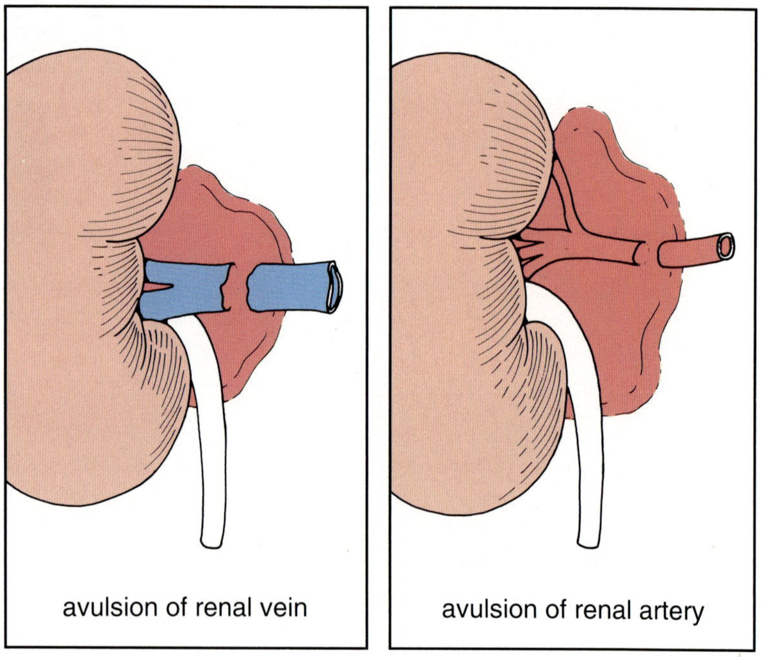

FIGURE 11.1 Schematic drawing demonstrating avulsion of either the renal vein or artery. Often complete disruption of the vasculature results in vascular spasm with minimal bleeding during the immediate post-trauma period. Failure to visualize the kidney during contrast study should raise the possibility of vascular injury.

Although technetium-99 pertechnetate may be employed to demonstrate the integrity of the renal vascular supply, it seems more appropriate to proceed directly to renal arteriography to determine the extent of the renal artery or venous lesion. Also, when hemorrhage and cardiovascular instability is an accompanying phenomenon, temporary balloon occlusion of the bleeding vessels may very well enhance the margin of safety prior to active surgical control.

PENETRATING

Injuries to the renal artery and vein most often accompany penetrating abdominal wounds.[9] Penetrating and lacerating injury to the renal artery and vein (Fig. 11.1) are usually associated not only with injury to other surrounding vascular structures, but also frequently with significant hypovolemic shock of such severity that patient salvage supersedes the ordering of preoperative imaging studies. However, when the patient can be stabilized, these studies should be acquired.

In any event, whether the lesion is defined preoperatively or whether immediate exploration is required for patient salvage, the patient is best opened through a midline incision (Fig. 11.2). The vasculature is exposed through an extended incision in the posterior peritoneum, a hematoma evacuated, and the renal vessels controlled with noncrushing vascular clamps. Anatomic distortion and bleeding may be such that blunt control of the aorta and vena cava above and below the renal vasculature is necessary, not only in order to stem the hemorrhage, but also to give definitive control of the great vessels above and below the renal vasculature in order to permit careful and exact assessment of the degree of vascular injury.

Repair with salvage of the renal unit or nephrectomy is dependent upon the degree of damage produced. Massive destruction of the renal vasculature or recognition of a preexploration prolonged ischemia time often may mandate immediate nephrectomy, rather than a heroic attempt at repair with subsequent delayed nephrectomy. Replantation of the vasculature or use of an associated autologous vein or artery may be necessary for repair. It rarely is advisable to seek autotransplantation except in those instances in which it is necessary for the preservation of a single remaining renal unit. *In situ* perfusion with an appropriate cooling solution or cooling the kidney in slush may provide an enhanced period for repair when the conditions so dictate.

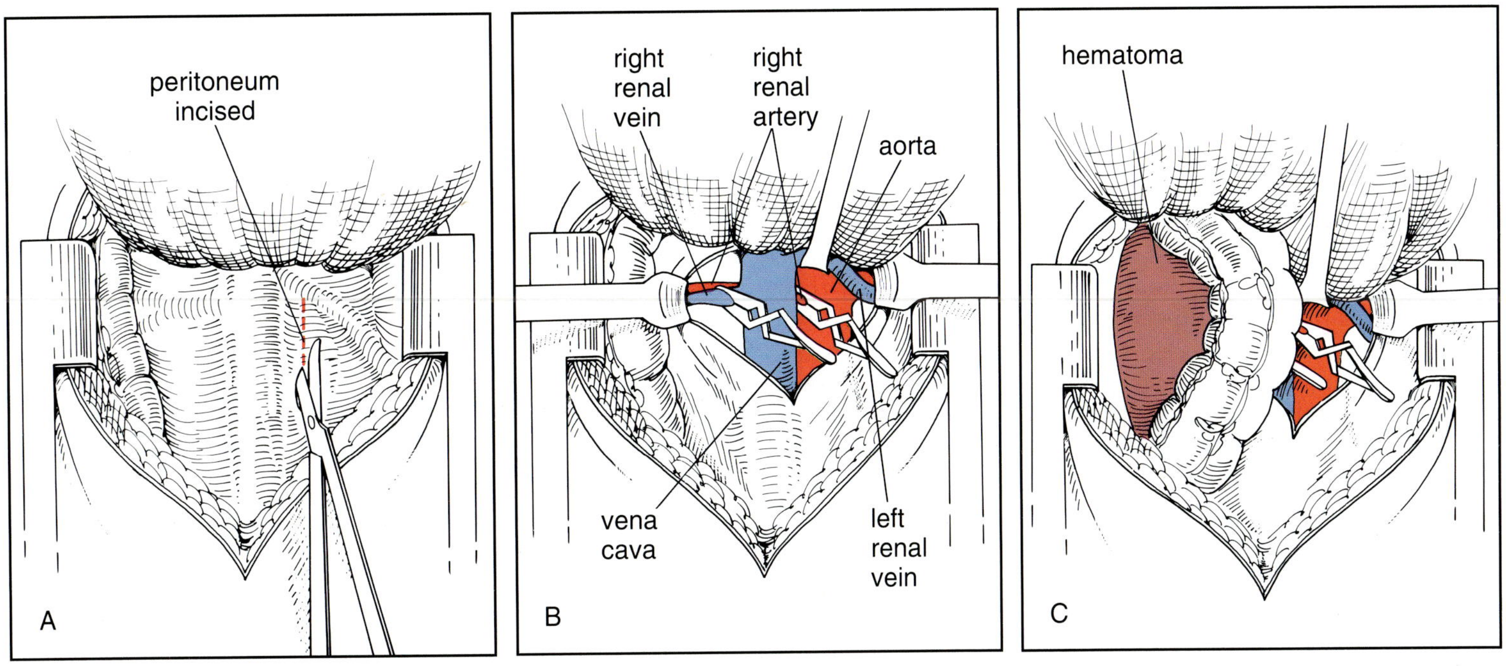

FIGURE 11.2 Surgical approach to the injured kidney: **A** incision in the parietal peritoneum over the aorta; **B** exposure of the renal arteries and application of vascular clamps; **C** incision in the colic gutter to expose the hematoma within Gerota's fascia. (Adapted from Carlton CE: Renal trauma. In Glenn JF [ed]: Urologic Surgery, 3rd ed, p 267. Philadelphia, JB Lippincott, 1983.)

NONPENETRATING

The renal artery may be injured by a non-penetrating trauma usually produced through contrecoup (Fig. 11.3). This injury is produced through excessive stretching of the renal artery with disruption of the renal intima, subsequently followed by thrombosis of the renal artery.[4,9,13,20] The patient who presents with severe nonpenetrating abdominal or back trauma, any auto–pedestrian injury, or severe deceleration injury, should be suspected of having a renal artery injury and undergo evaluation by high-dose urography. As indicated above, failure of renal visualization should prompt immediate renal angiography. Repair of the injury is accomplished by excision of the damaged segment, limited arteriotomy with intimal repair, or replacement of the injured segment with an autologous vein or arterial graft.

Renal Parenchymal Injuries

PENETRATING

Penetrating injuries can be managed on a conservative basis so long as these injuries do not involve other intra-abdominal structures and so long as there is no contamination of the traumatized area by bowel contents. The penetrating injuries therefore usually segregate themselves into either blast or stab injuries. When the patient is hemodynamically stable, and when the traumatologist is certain that direct injury of the renal vasculature has not occurred, conservative observation has the greater chance of providing salvage of the maximal amount of functioning renal tissue than does hasty and heroic surgical intervention.

NONPENETRATING

The management of nonpenetrating blunt renal injury is perhaps the most controversial area in genitourinary trauma. Although it had been the practice to explore most of these bluntly traumatized renal units surgically, the current trend is to reserve surgical exploration for those patients who have hemodynamic instability secondary to continued parenchymal bleeding or massive urinary extravasation with loss of urine into the abdominal cavity. Current thinking would also permit the observation and delayed surgical exploration of the patient with massive retroperitoneal urinary extravasation, as long as the patient remained uninfected and urine could be demonstrated to pass down the ureter itself. The principle that primary healing of any injured tissue is enhanced by early debridement, hemostasis, and primary repair before the onset of necrosis and urinary extravasation may not hold in closed renal injuries.

Closed renal injuries may be grouped into four types, as illustrated in Figure 11.4. Their characteristics are as follows:

Contusion. A contusion or a bruising of the renal parenchyma. This is usually visualized on the intravenous pyelogram as an area of decreased function.

Minor cortical laceration. A laceration of the renal parenchyma with or without disruption of the renal capsule. The laceration extends no deeper than the corticomedullary junction. There is no evidence of urinary extravasation or the development of a large perirenal hematoma. There may be a subcapsular hematoma.

Major cortical laceration. A laceration in which there is transcapsular disruption that extends deep within the corticomedullary junction. Major cortical lacerations are usually associated with urinary extravasation and the development of a large perirenal hematoma.

Multiple lacerations. More severe injuries may be multiple lacerations in both the upper or lower poles of the kidney or total maceration of the renal unit itself.

Little controversy exists as to the management of either major or minor blunt renal injury. Between 70% to 90% of all nonpenetrating blunt renal injuries may be characterized as minor, with mild or transient hematuria, normal radiographic studies or ones that show some delay in concentration or excretion, and systemic vital signs that are stable or readily stabilized (Fig. 11.5). These injuries are best treated by observation rather than by operative intervention.

Major blunt renal injuries are characterized by severe and unremitting hematuria or by no hematuria secondary to total absence of renal function due to complete disruption of the renal parenchymal unit. Radiographic studies consistently fail to show nonfunction; moreover, the patients are unstable from a cardiovascular standpoint and cannot be managed by massive transfusions. As previously mentioned, these patients often are best evaluated by renal angiography (Fig. 11.6). Again, balloon

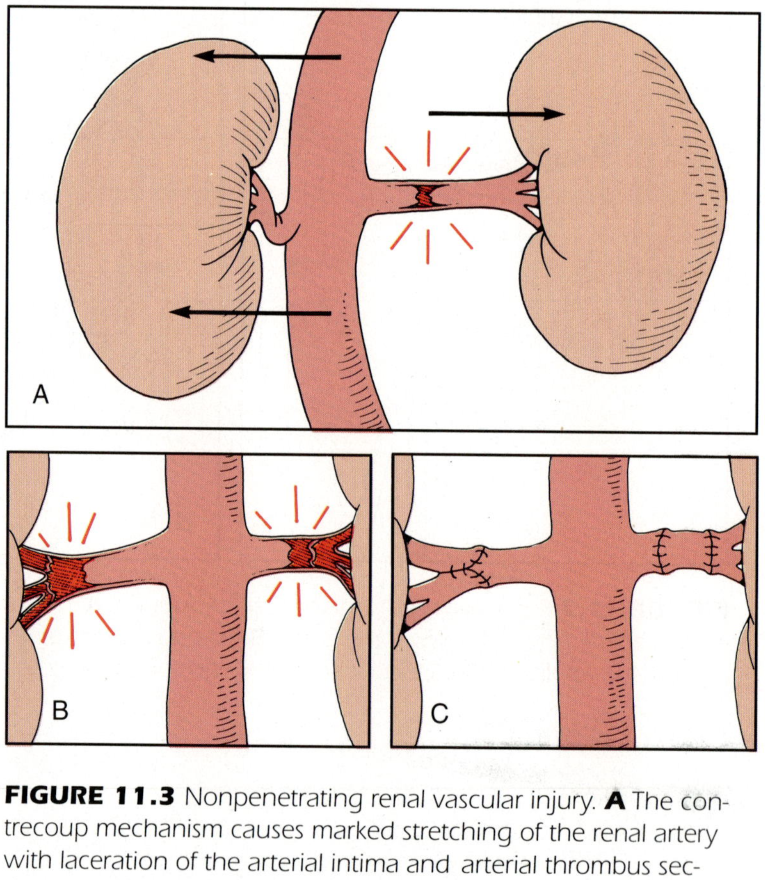

FIGURE 11.3 Nonpenetrating renal vascular injury. **A** The contrecoup mechanism causes marked stretching of the renal artery with laceration of the arterial intima and arterial thrombus secondary to laceration of the intima. **B** and **C** show common locations of intimal laceration and techniques of repair. (Adapted from Carlton CE: Renal trauma. In Glenn JF [ed]: Urologic Surgery, 3rd ed, p 265. Philadelphia, JB Lippincott 1983.)

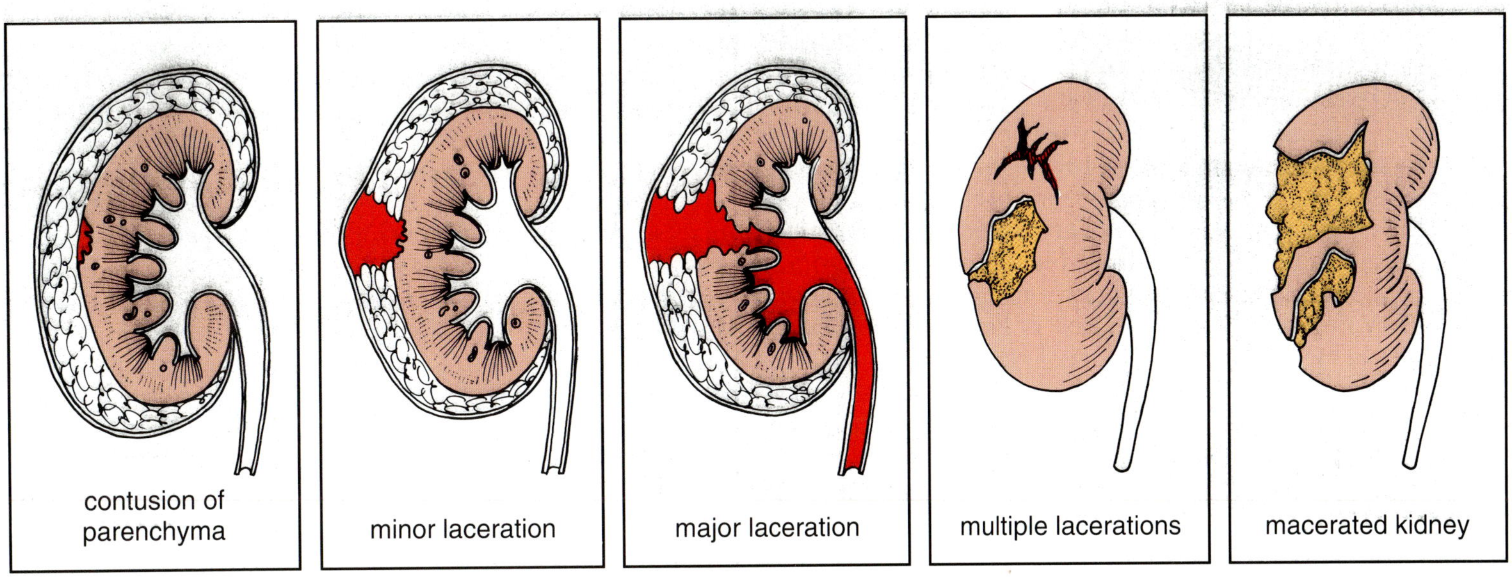

FIGURE 11.4 Classification of renal injury by extent of injury.

FIGURE 11.5
BLUNT RENAL INJURIES

	MINOR	INTERMEDIATE	MAJOR
Hematuria	Mild, remitting		Severe, unremitting; or none
Urography	Normal, delayed/diminished function		Nonfunction
Vital signs	Normal, stable		Unstable, unacceptable

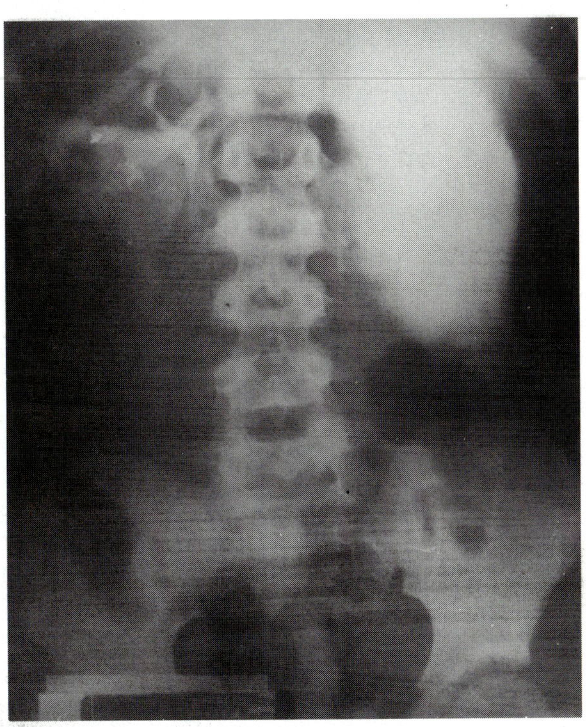

FIGURE 11.6 Intravenous pyelogram after nonpenetrating trauma to the left flank. Note that the contrast is entirely contained within Gerota's fascia. There is massive extravasation on this side, indicating that despite the injury, there is functioning renal parenchyma.

occlusion of the renal artery may stabilize the patient prior to operative intervention. Either prompt operative exploration to determine the extent of injury and the possibility of repair or nephrectomy is appropriate. The peritoneal cavity is entered through a long midline incision, the bowel eviscerated, and the posterior peritoneum overlying the great vessels incised through the midline. The origin of the renal artery and vein are rapidly identified and these vessels controlled with either noncrushing clips or with surgical tape. An additional margin of safety can be obtained by prolonging the tolerated ischemia time through cooling the kidney either by direct renal perfusion with lactated Ringer's solution, or by surrounding the kidney with slush. Once vascular control has been established, the kidney can be exposed by careful removal of the surrounding hematoma and evaluated for the degree of renal injury and the decision for either repair or nephrectomy (Fig. 11.7).

When an attempt is made to salvage the kidney, these principles of surgical management apply: debridement of all devitalized renal parenchyma, meticulous hemostasis, watertight closure of the collecting system, and primary approximation of the debrided margins, with obliteration of dead space using viable tissue such as omentum or perirenal fat. Any renal tissue suspected of devitalization is debrided by sharp excision. The veins and arteries may be identified and oversewn using figure-of-eight sutures of absorbable catgut. When all visible vasculature has been controlled, the occluding clamp may be removed and additional bleeding points similarly closed. When the cut margins of the renal parenchyma cannot be closed by primary approximation of the renal capsule, occasionally the dead space may be obliterated by using mattress sutures over Gelfoam pledgets to prevent tearing of the renal parenchyma. When this cannot be accomplished, it is preferable to mobilize a segment of the omentum, tacking vascularized omentum within the defect and then wrapping the defect with vascularized omentum. This not only prevents fixation of the kidney in the traumatized renal bed, but also provides internal drainage.

Major lacerations of the upper or lower pole often are best treated by guillotine amputation of the injured segment. The renal capsule surrounding the injured segment is mobilized and retracted over the viable kidney. The traumatized segment of the renal unit is amputated, the vessels controlled, and the retracted capsule brought over the amputated segment of the renal unit. Again, the cut margin should be protected either with vascularized perirenal fat or with a vascularized omental graft.

The current controversy in management concerns those patients who have blunt renal injury of an intermediate nature. These patients and patients with minor injury of a debatable degree previously underwent exploration on the basis of the degree of urinary extravasation. Urinary extravasation may be categorized as shown in Figure 11.8. Grade I extravasation is intraparenchymal and confined to the renal capsule; grade II urinary extravasation penetrates the renal capsule but is confined within Gerota's fascia, while grade III extravasation is extensive retroperitoneal extravasation outside Gerota's fascia. Grade I or grade II urinary extravasation may not need prompt exploration in the patient who is hemodynamically stable, whose ureter can be visualized, and who shows evidence of unobstructed ureteral drainage. Under these circumstances, many recommend observation for grade III urinary extravasation as well, with surgical exploration reserved for those patients who either become infected or continue to show a progressive increase in the amount of retroperitoneal extravasation, and in whom extravasation produces metabolic disruption. Any indication that the urinary extravasation is infected or that there is obstructed ureteral drainage should prompt an initial attempt to relieve the ureteral obstruction with appropriate percutaneous or open operative drainage of the infected urinoma.

It is no longer felt that parenchymal fracture alone in the presence of hemodynamic stability is an indication for exploration. The current thinking would indicate that parenchymal fracture or laceration develops according to those shearing forces that are transmitted between tissues of different density within the renal parenchyma. Because the kidney is composed of four tissue compartments (renal capsule, collecting system, vascular system, and parenchyma), and because the latter offers the bulk of the system and the least resistance to traumatic injury, blunt or tangential forces tend to produce fracture lines parallel to the vascular planes. The result is a tendency for continued vascularization and function of the fractured fragments despite their wide separation. With time, gradual reabsorption of the bridging hematoma and a progressive loss of the separation between the fractured renal units occur, with ultimate restoration of a more normal renal architecture.[12,14,19,22]

Current thinking would prompt observation of patients with closed renal injury who are hemodynamically stable and who fail to demonstrate vascular injury by appropriate study. Demonstration of a vascular injury may prompt immediate exposure in hopes of either establishing hemodynamic control or renal salvage. Conservative management of the traumatized renal unit, even when this trauma is of mild or intermediate nature, frequently results in salvage of the maximal amount of functioning renal tissue.

URETERAL TRAUMA

Ureteral injuries are most commonly iatrogenic, produced during the course of operative procedures. Ureteral injuries secondary to nonoperative trauma are extremely rare. Fewer than 100 ureteral injuries were reported during World War I, World War II, and the Korean conflict combined.[8,18] The small size of the ureter and its position in the flank and posterior abdomen reduce the probability of injury from penetrating injuries of the flank or abdomen. Fewer than 10% of all ureteral injuries occur secondary to blunt trauma.[25] In children, muscular development at the attachments of the ureter to the renal pelvis and of the renal pelvis to the parenchyma is less, making them more susceptible to ureteral avulsion in severe blunt trauma. Blunt or penetrating ureteral injury is rarely accompanied by gross or

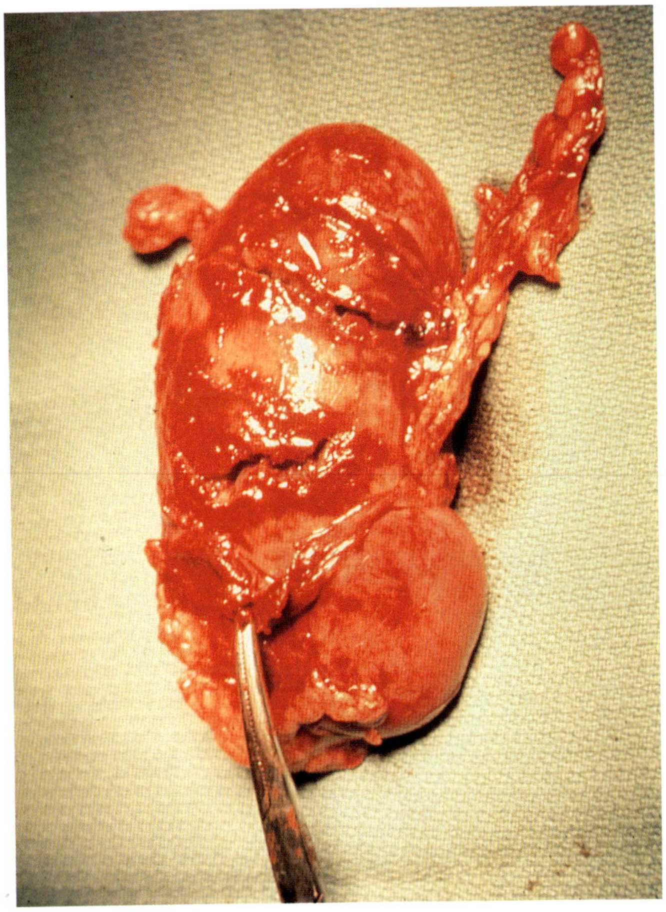

FIGURE 11.7 A severely lacerated kidney that required nephrectomy. Note that there are multiple lacerations in the renal parenchyma. This kidney was removed because of uncontrollable bleeding. Extravasation alone in the presence of hemodynamic stability does not demand removal.

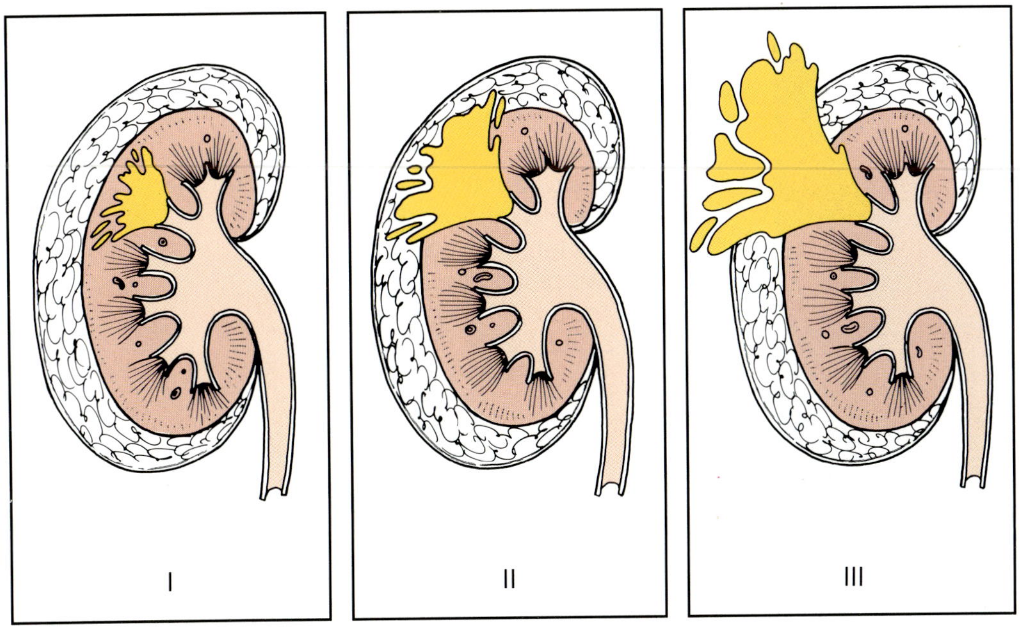

FIGURE 11.8 Grading of urinary extravasation: I, intraparenchymal II, extracapsular; III, retroperitoneal. (Adapted from Peterson NE: Intermediate-degree blunt renal trauma. J Trauma 17[6], © 1977, The Williams & Wilkins Co, Baltimore.)

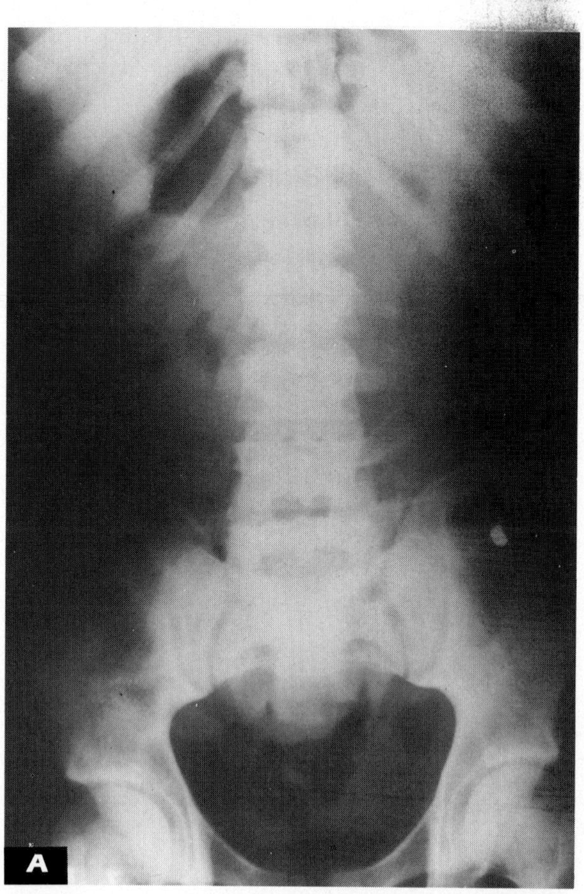

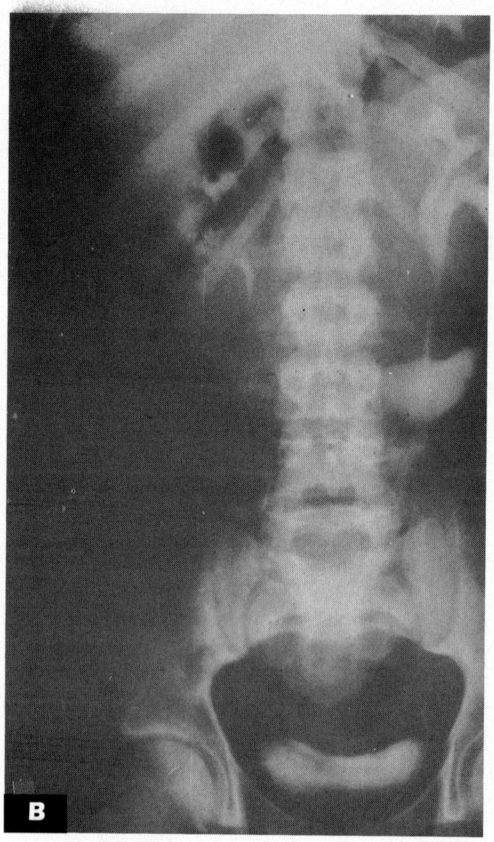

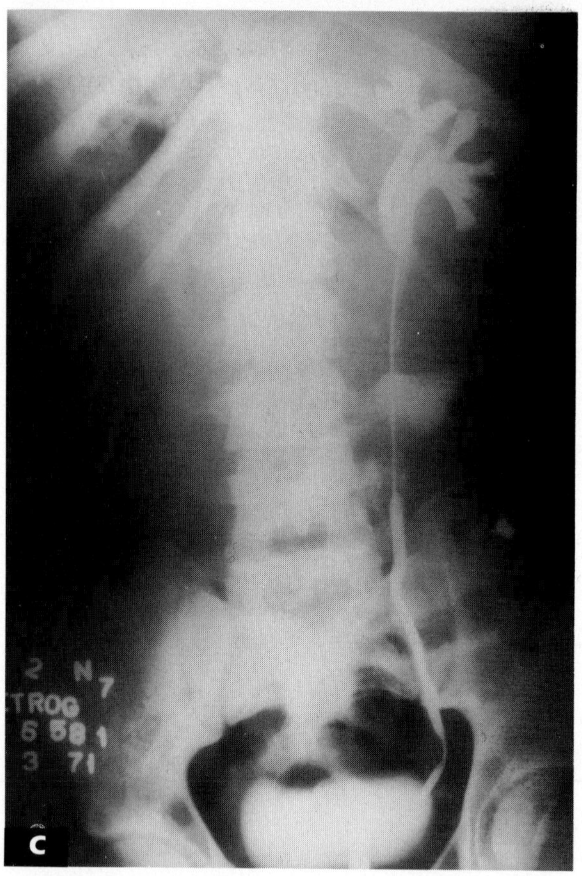

FIGURE 11.9 A A plain film on a patient who was shot in the lower abdomen. Urinalysis did not show hematuria. A subsequent intravenous pyelogram **B** demonstrated extravasation of contrast in the region of the midureter on the left, and a retrograde pyelogram **C** confirmed extravasation of urine and the level of injury. Note that a catheter has been passed up into the renal pelvis past the area of injury, indicating that the ureter was only partially transected by the missile.

microscopic hematuria; therefore, the examining physician must rely on clinical suspicion in diagnosing this injury (Fig. 11.9). Children or adults who present with penetrating wounds of the back or abdomen and those who have severe bony trauma to the spine or vertebral bodies or ped-icles should undergo intravenous pyelography to determine the integrity of the ureters bilaterally. Only approximately one third of ureteral injuries are recognized at the time of presentation, resulting in delayed treatment by nephrectomy in the remaining two thirds. Nephrectomy occurs three times more frequently when recognition of ureteral injury is delayed.[8] In the patient who does not have immediate recognition of either the operatively or accidently injured ureter, the presentation is usually one of progressive flank pain, fever, and either an expanding flank or abdominal mass or a urinary fistula (if a penetrating wound has occurred).

When either penetrating or nonpenetrating injury to the ureter has been identified, surgical exploration of the extent of damage is appropriate. Most of the principles that will be discussed for management of intraoperative damage to the ureter may be applied to the repair of the accidentally traumatized ureter. Ureters that are sharply transected by knife wound may be primarily joined. The traumatized margins should be sharply cut back to clean and healthy tissue. The severed ends of the ureter should be spatulated and a direct anastomosis accomplished over a stenting catheter, using a multiple interrupted 4-0 or 5-0 absorbable suture. Every attempt should be made to make this closure watertight. The closure suture should not be running, but interrupted. Drainage of the repaired site by either Penrose drains or a suction drainage is appropriate. The traumatized site may be wrapped in omentum to support the repair and provide internal drainage.

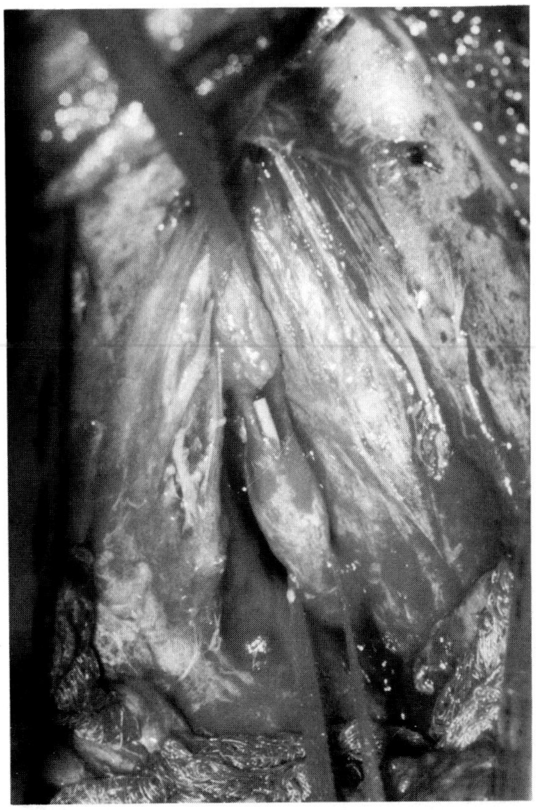

FIGURE 11.10 This photograph is of the gunshot injury of Figure 11.9 taken 10 days after the injury occurred. Note that a portion of the ureteral wall has been blown away by the blast injury. The area of injury would not heal spontaneously and resection with reanastomosis was necessary.

Blast or gunshot injuries to the ureter are more difficult to repair (Fig. 11.10). The blast injury frequently produces microvascular damage at points distant from the disrupted ureteral margins, and the extent of this damage often cannot be assessed at the time of immediate exploration. Thus, when one is confronted with this sort of injury, a more aggressive excision of ureteral margins both proximal and distal to the site of damage is advised. Even then, it must be recognized that all of the damaged ureter may not be removed. When a segment is removed, such as to place the anastomosis on tension, additional length may be obtained by mobilizing the kidney in its retroperitoneal bed and dropping it into the retroperitoneum. Frequently, as much as 5 cm to 6 cm of additional ureteral length can be obtained in this way.

The traumatized patient may benefit from surgical techniques that have been devised to manage the patient who is injured in the course of another planned procedure. These techniques are detailed below.

Lower Ureteral Injuries

Extraperitoneal exposure of the lower ureter is preferred in managing extensive injury to the lower third of the ureter.

URETERAL REIMPLANTATION

Traumatic injuries of the paravesical ureter less than 3 cm to 5 cm from the ureterovesical junction may best be repaired by mobilization of the lower ureter and immediate ureteroneocystostomy. The distal portion of traumatized ureter may be left in place, preferably with the bladder side ligated with absorbable suture. The proximal portion of the ureter is mobilized and brought into the bladder close to the midline but above the interureteric ridge. While it is preferable to create a submucosal tunnel by fixing the ureter to the detrusor musculature with multiple interrupted 4-0 chromic catgut sutures, a nontunneled anastomosis may be necessary. A pediatric feeding tube may be placed across the anastomosis and up the ureter, being brought out through a small vesical stab wound and left for 5 to 7 days to provide adequate drainage. When the ureteral injury is so extensive that the proximal ureter cannot be brought to the bladder without tension, the bladder should be mobilized and secured with the psoas muscle on the side of the defect, above

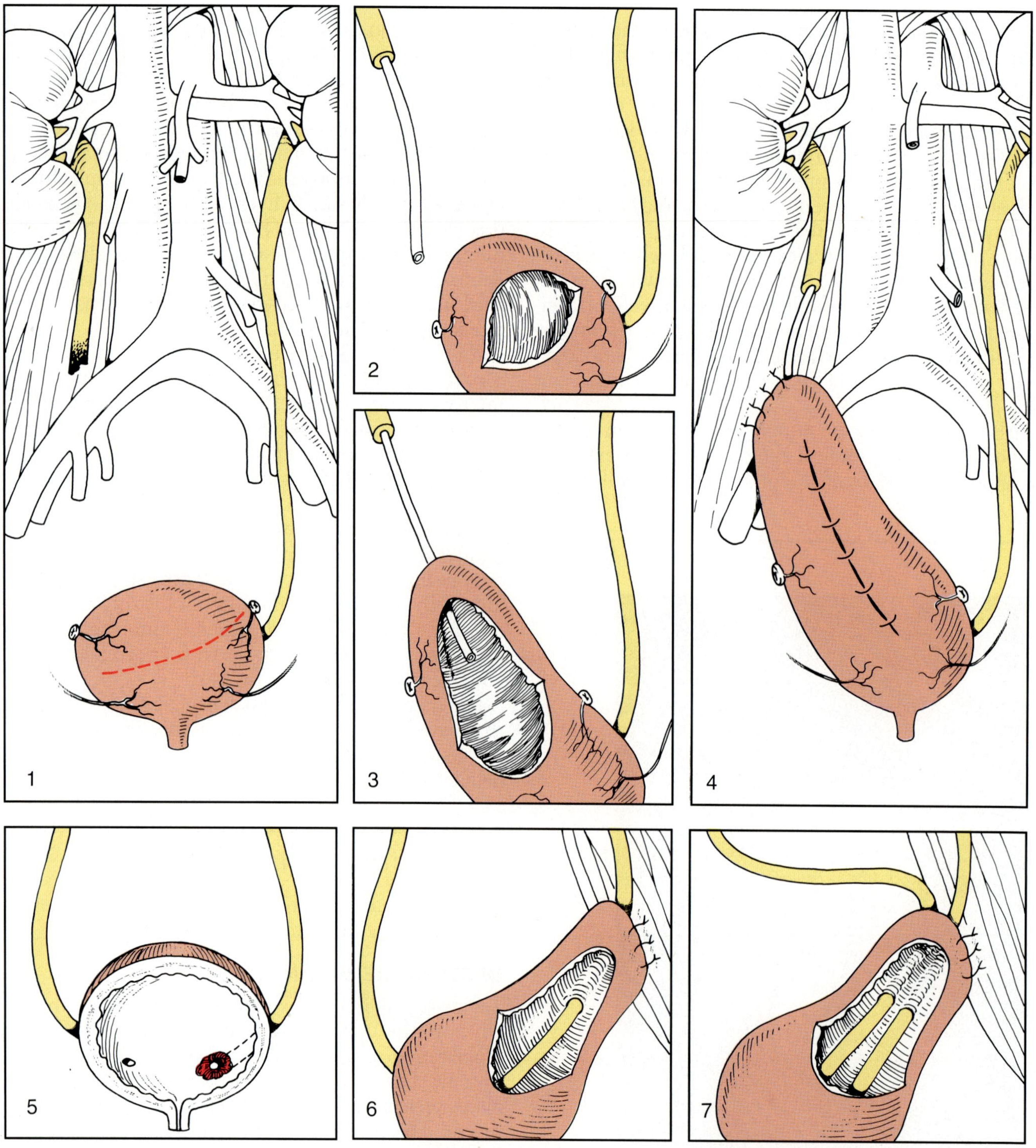

FIGURE 11.11 Surgical technique for psoas hitch and distal ureteroneocystostomy. The bladder is mobilized, opened transversely, and sutured above the iliac vasculature. When the distal ureter at the level of entry into the bladder is injured, the bladder may be mobilized (as in the bottom row of diagrams), the ureter reimplanted with a psoas hitch, and the primary defect of the posterior wall of the bladder closed. Alternatively, both ureters may be reimplanted into the "hitched" bladder.

the external iliac vasculature using multiple interrupted 1-0 chromic catgut sutures (Fig. 11.11). This "psoas hitch" can be used to bridge defects of the lower third of the ureter. The distal ureter is brought into the bladder, a submucosal tunnel created, and the ureter secured to the detrusor musculature with several interrupted 4-0 chromic catgut sutures.

Occasionally, the entire ureter may be damaged, either from extensive blast injury or from extensive surgically induced injury. In these instances, it may be necessary to replace the ureter, either partially or totally, with an ileal segment. The ileal segment may be either anastomosed between the remaining renal pelvis and the bladder, or sutured to the lower caliceal system and then to the bladder. In these instances, hitching the bladder to the psoas musculature above the iliac vasculature may be helpful.

TRANSURETEROURETEROSTOMY

More extensive damage to the lower ureter may require a transureteroureterostomy.[1,5,10,21,23,27] A modification of this maneuver may be accomplished when an upper ureteral unit is lost secondary to trauma but the lower ureteral segment is preserved, or when the contralateral lower ureter is traumatized but the upper renal unit is preserved. Crossover from the preserved lower ureter to the contralateral upper renal unit may be accomplished directly, bridging the traumatized defect and providing adequate drainage.

A transureteroureterostomy requires a midline transperitoneal incision. The donor ureter is mobilized lateral to the colon after incision of the lateral peritoneal reflection (Fig. 11.12). The healthy portion of the ureter is mobilized and divided distally, in order to permit transfer of the ureter beneath the mesentery sufficiently that tension on the anastomosis does not occur. It is preferable that the crossing be made above the inferior mesenteric artery to prevent sharp angulation or kinking of the ureter at this level. The distal end of the involved ureter is spatulated for a distance of 1.5 cm to 2.0 cm and sutured to the recipient ureter using a longitudinal ureterotomy of similar size.

Upper Ureteral Injuries

Massive injuries to the upper ureter require more drastic maneuvers. When the upper third or a major portion of the midureter has been lost traumatically, it may be best to ligate the residual ureteral stump and to drain the kidney through a percutaneous nephrostomy tube. This will permit the traumatized patient to recover from his associated injury and permit delayed repair utiliz-

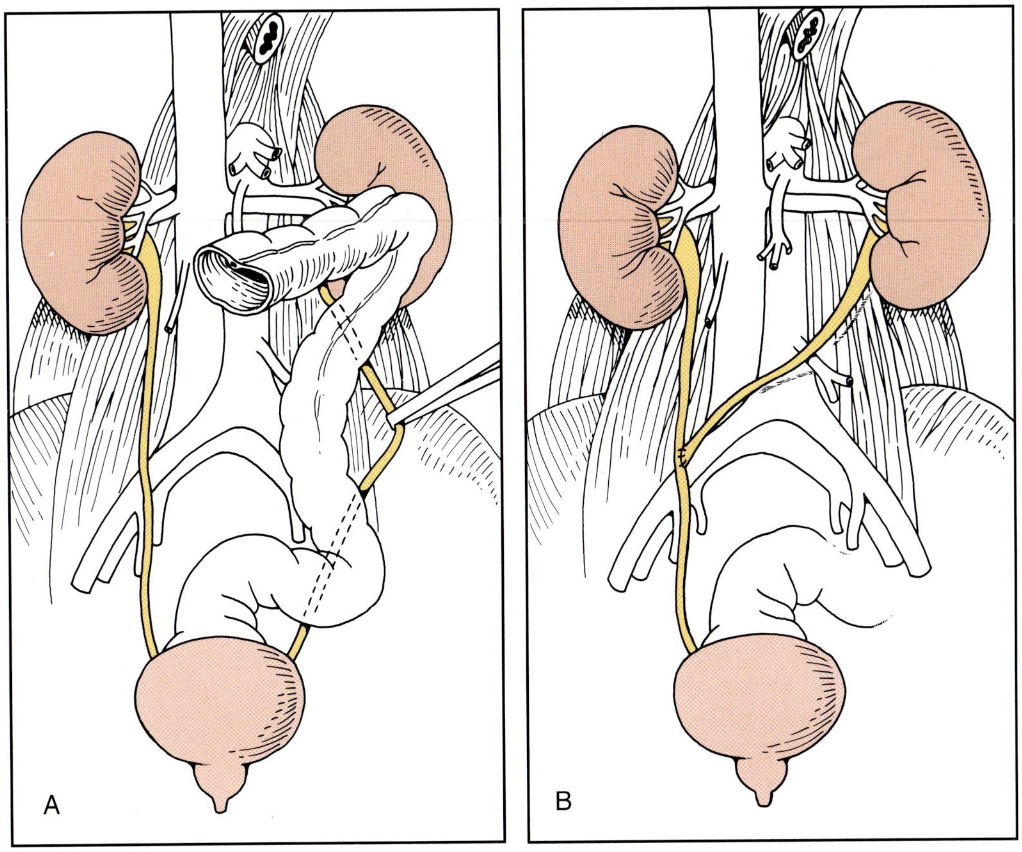

FIGURE 11.12 A Transureteroureterostomy funnel is developed by gentle, blunt retroperitoneal dissection after exposure of upper ureter lateral to colon. **B** Ureter is brought across retroperitoneal space above level of inferior mesenteric artery to avoid tension to anastomosis. (Adapted from Zinman L, Libertino JA: Surgery of the midureter. In Libertino JA, Zinman L [eds]: Reconstructive Urologic Surgery: Pediatric and Adult, pp 97–117. © 1977, The Williams & Wilkins Co., Baltimore.)

ing a long bowel segment to connect the renal pelvis to the bladder or to accomplish delayed autotransplantation (Fig. 11.13).

BLADDER TRAUMA

Traumatic injury to the bladder may be either penetrating or nonpenetrating (Fig. 11.14). Blunt abdominal trauma is the more prevalent, occurring in 80% to 85% of such cases.[3,26] Approximately 70% of all blunt trauma to the bladder is associated with pelvic fractures.[18] Bladder injuries may be classified as follows:

Contusion or ecchymosis of the intact bladder wall with microscopic or gross hematuria

Extraperitoneal rupture with laceration of the bladder below the pelvic peritoneum. Contrast cystography will demonstrate extravasation of the contrast agent around the bladder and outside of the peritoneal cavity (Fig. 11.15).

Intraperitoneal rupture with rupture of the bladder into the peritoneal cavity. Contrast examination will demonstrate extravasation into the peritoneal cavity (Fig. 11.16).

Combined extraperitoneal and intraperitoneal rupture in which both extravesical and intravesical contrast can be identified. Retroperitoneal and intraperitoneal contrast can be identified.

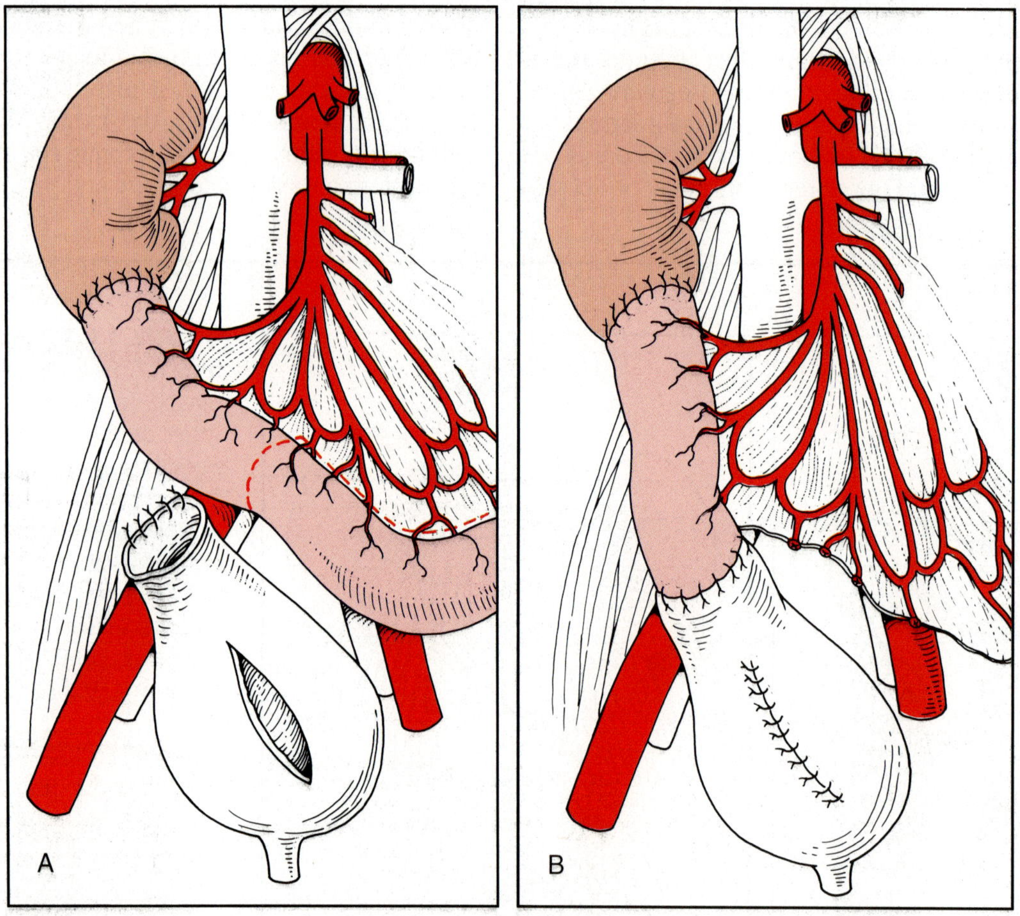

FIGURE 11.13 The importance of the vesical psoas hitch for ileal ureteral substitution. Note how much additional redundant ileum can be sacrificed, leaving a shorter ileal segment. **A** The bladder is hitched above the iliac vasculature and an isolated segment of ileum is anastomosed to the lower collecting system. **B** The proximal end of the ureter may be attached directly to the "hitched" bladder. Alternatively, the ileal segment can be tapered prior to implantation into the bladder.

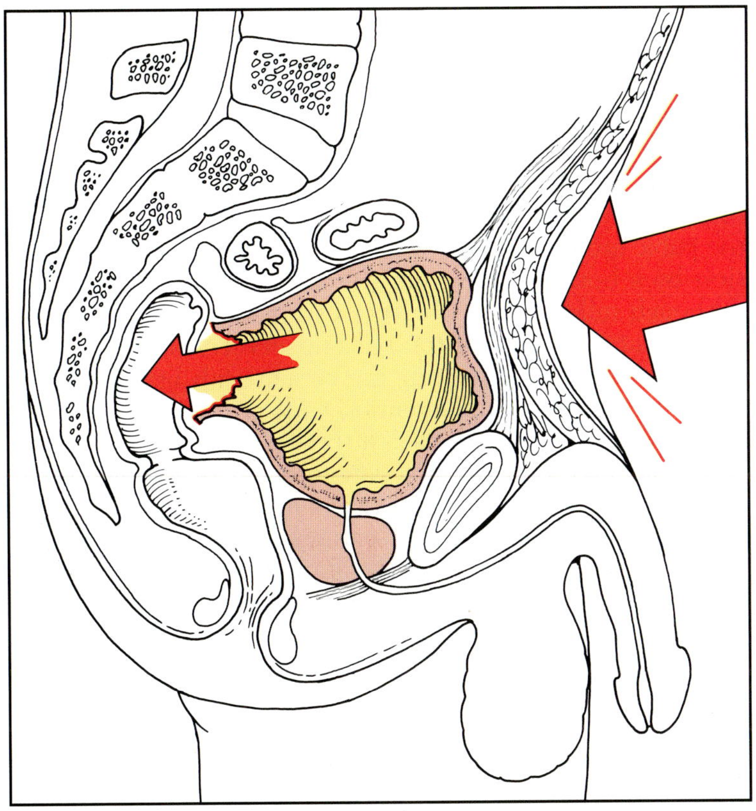

FIGURE 11.14 Blunt trauma to the lower abdomen when the bladder is full may result in disruption of the bladder beneath the peritoneal reflection, shown here, producing extraperitoneal or intraperitoneal extravasation.

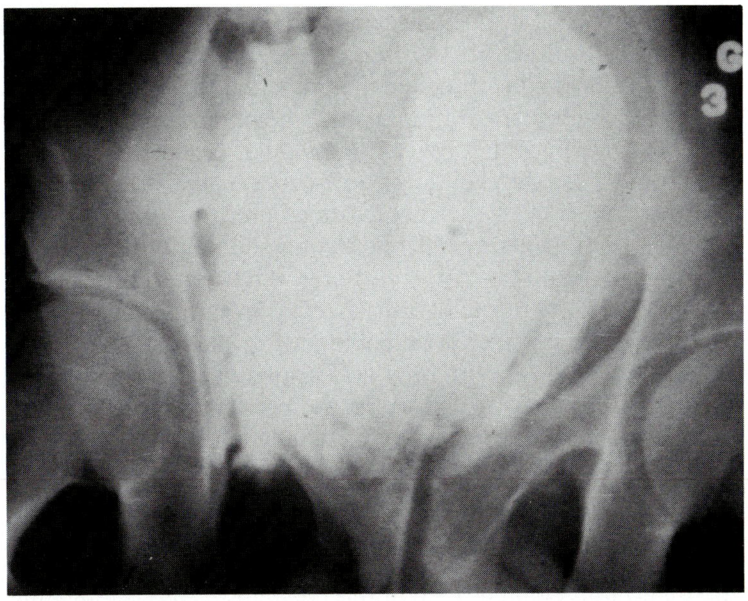

FIGURE 11.15 Cystogram demonstrating extraperitoneal extravasation of contrast material. Note the feathery appearance of contrast material in the pelvis. The bladder is also distorted, having been pushed into the contralateral side of the pelvis and elongated.

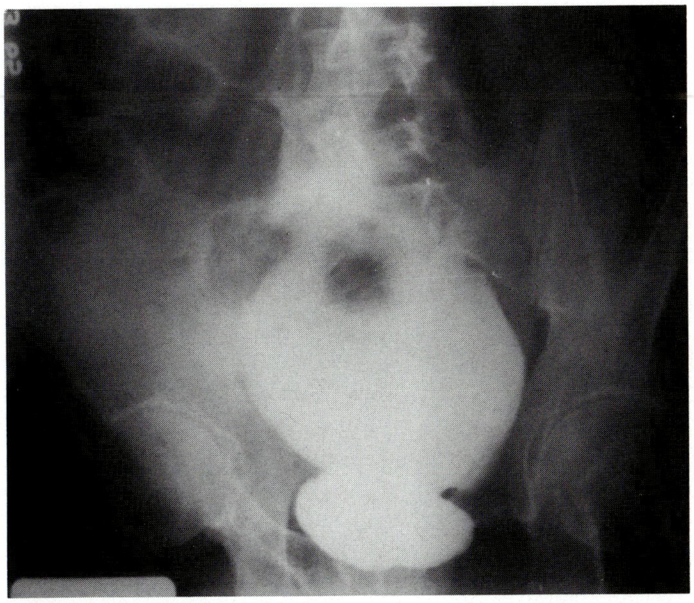

FIGURE 11.16 This is the classic "hourglass" appearance of intraperitoneal rupture.

The findings of cystography are summarized in Fig. 11.17. A word of caution about the presence of vesical injuries: nearly 70% are associated with pelvic fractures, and these fractures may also produce associated injury to the membranous urethra. The urethra is fixed at the level of the muscular perineal diaphragm. Accordingly any deceleration injury may very well produce traumatic transection of the membranous urethra. Therefore, the patient who presents with pelvic trauma should not immediately have placement of a Foley catheter. The more conservative approach is to perform an initial rectal examination to determine that the prostate is palpable and in place. If so, a Foley catheter may be gently passed and urine obtained. However, if the prostate cannot be defined in the pelvis on rectal examination, there is a good possibility of traumatic disruption between the apex of the prostate and the urethra. As a means of confirmation, a retrograde urethrogram must be obtained. If such disruption is confirmed the statements that follow are not applicable.

There are certain classic symptoms of bladder injury: hematuria, lower abdominal pain, urinary frequency, and the inability to void. However, these symptoms may be masked by the associated symptoms that accompany intra-abdominal pelvic trauma. The diagnosis of vesical rupture or perforation is made by contrast cystography. The cystogram is performed by placing 250 mg to 300 mg of the contrast agent into the bladder through a urethral catheter; films are taken, the bladder is drained, and a postoperative film obtained. When rupture is identified, repair is appropriate.

Bladder contusions, indicated by hematuria and no demonstrated extravasation of contrast material, are best treated by rest and catheter drainage. This will allow healing of the bladder wall until bleeding stops. The more seriously traumatized bladder may rupture either intraperitoneally or extraperito-neally; approximately 75% of all ruptures are extraperitoneal.[17] A distended bladder is more susceptible to injury because as it enlarges, its walls become thinner and less able to withstand injury. The empty bladder, which enjoys some protection from the pubic arch, is usually perforated in an extraperitoneal position by a bony spicule from the associated pelvic fracture. Although mild degrees of either extraperitoneal or intraperitoneal rupture may be treated conservatively by catheter drainage alone while treating the patient with broad-spectrum antibiotics, operative intervention with primary closure of the defect is usually recommended. If those patients who are treated conservatively show signs and symptoms of pelvic inflammation or infection, or prolonged evidence of intra-abdominal irritation secondary to prolonged urinary extravasation, then the decision for operative exploration and operative closure is warranted. All penetrating wounds of the bladder should be explored and primarily closed.

Operative closure of a bladder defect should be made through a lower midline incision (Fig. 11.18). This will provide easy access for complete abdominal exploration to identify any associated injuries. A small incision in the peritoneum should be made to determine if there is intraperitoneal blood. If so, a complete abdominal exploration must be conducted. If no intra-abdominal injury is detected, the dissection then may be carried extraperitoneally. If the defect in the bladder is not evident upon paravesical exploration, a vertical midline incision should

FIGURE 11.17
CYSTOGRAPHIC FINDINGS IN BLADDER INJURIES

CONTUSION	EXTRAPERITONEAL RUPTURE	INTRAPERITONEAL RUPTURE
Teardrop-shaped bladder	Pattern of extavasated dye ranges from small lines or streaks to large stellate or sunburst	Hourglass pattern when the extravasated contrast medium layer is in the dependent portion of the peritoneal cavity
Elevation of bladder	Base of the bladder obscured by dye	Gas-containing small bowel loops surrounded by opaque contrast material
Obliteration of the soft tissue planes in the pelvis by hematoma		Colon outlined by the contrast medium in an irregular fashion, resulting in a scalloped appearance
Deviation of the bladder laterally		Opaque linear bands along the peritoneal reflections of the paracolic recesses
Absence of extravasation of contrast materials		Contrast medium outline of portions of the diaphragm, liver, and spleen

be made above the bladder neck to provide access to the lumen. No attempt should be made to dissect laterally, because this may disrupt the tamponading effect of any paravesical hematoma. The area of bladder disruption can be identified from within. The margins of the disruption should be freshened and the defect closed in two layers with running absorbable sutures. The first layer should be a muscular layer only, and the second layer should approximate both mucosa and muscularis. The bladder may be drained with a suprapubic tube; however, this is frequently not necessary and the bladder may be drained appropriately with a urethral catheter. While the bladder is open, both ureteral orifices should be observed for bloody efflux and, if any suspicion of ureteral injury exists, a small ureteral catheter should be passed up either ureter. If the laceration is posterior or posterolateral, direct drainage of this area may not be possible without disrupting the paravesical hematoma. However, if a drain can gently be placed in this area and left in place for 48 to 72 hours, or until drainage ceases, it is preferable. The cystotomy wound should be closed in two layers with running absorbable suture and drained appropriately. If extensive pelvic hematoma formation has occurred as a result of pelvic fracture formation, and if hemostasis is secure because of formed clot in the paravesical area, exploration in this area is best avoided, since bleeding may be initiated and be difficult to control. (Fig. 11.19) If extensive and rapid bleeding occurs during the time of this exploration, the bleeding vessels can occasionally be identified and oversewn; fortunately, this is rare. When it does occur, and the urethra is intact and a Foley catheter has been passed per urethra into the bladder, a large-volume Foley balloon filled to approximately 50 ml with mild tension on the Foley catheter will force the bladder and prostate into the pelvis and assist in hemostasis. Penetrating injuries of the bladder may require wide debridement because of devitalized tissue. In these instances, care should be taken to determine that ureteral injury and posterior penetration of bowel structures have not occurred. When in doubt, sigmoidoscopy should be conducted on the operating table, and if perforation of the colon has occurred, a proximal diverting colostomy should be established.

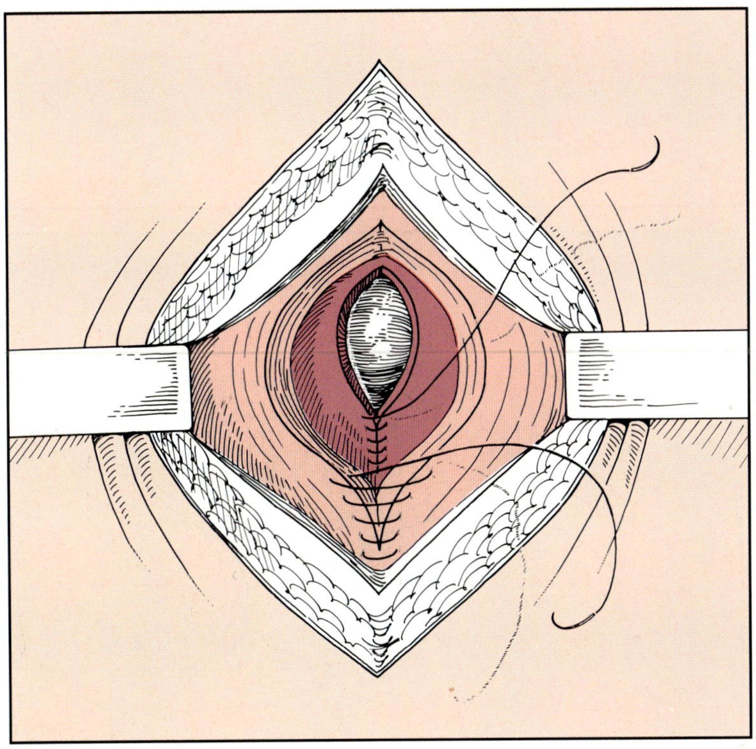

FIGURE 11.18 Diagrammatic rendering of the two-layer bladder closure. Note that the mucosal suture alone should result in a watertight closure. Buttressing of this first layer is accomplished by continuous or interrupted sutures incorporating the entire thickness of the bladder adventitia and muscularis down to, but not including, the mucosal layer. The defect in the bladder should be identified, the edges freshened, and a two-layer closure accomplished. These may be overlying suture lines, at right angles if possible. The suture material should be absorbable. The bladder should be drained per urethra or by a suprapubic tube for 5 to 7 days to permit adequate healing.

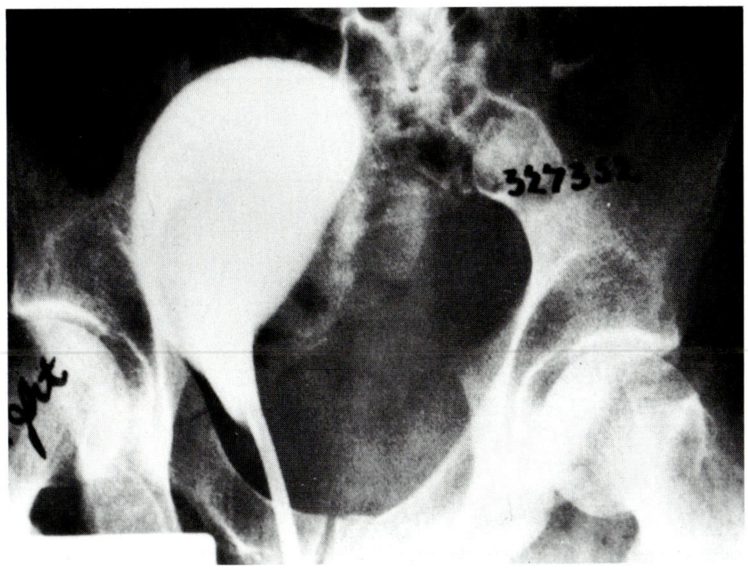

FIGURE 11.19 This cystogram demonstrates superior and lateral displacement of the bladder secondary to a large pelvic hematoma. Note the transurethral Foley catheter. The urethra has been markedly lengthened secondary to bladder displacement. The catheter should be left in place and, as the hematoma resolves, the bladder will assume a normal position.

POSTERIOR URETHRAL TRAUMA

In pelvic trauma or rapid deceleration injuries involving the pelvis, injury to the posterior urethra most frequently occurs in the membranous portion (Fig. 11.20). The urethra is ruptured from its prostatic attachments at the urogenital diaphragm (Fig. 11.21). Rectal examination will reveal that the prostate has been displaced superiorly and inferiorly. When urinary extravasation occurs, it is almost always extraperitoneal. However, bladder rupture and disruption of the urethra can simultaneously occur.[7,15,16] In the emergency situation, when the prostate cannot be palpated in its normal position, or when it is obscured by periprostatic hematoma, it is best to perform a ret-

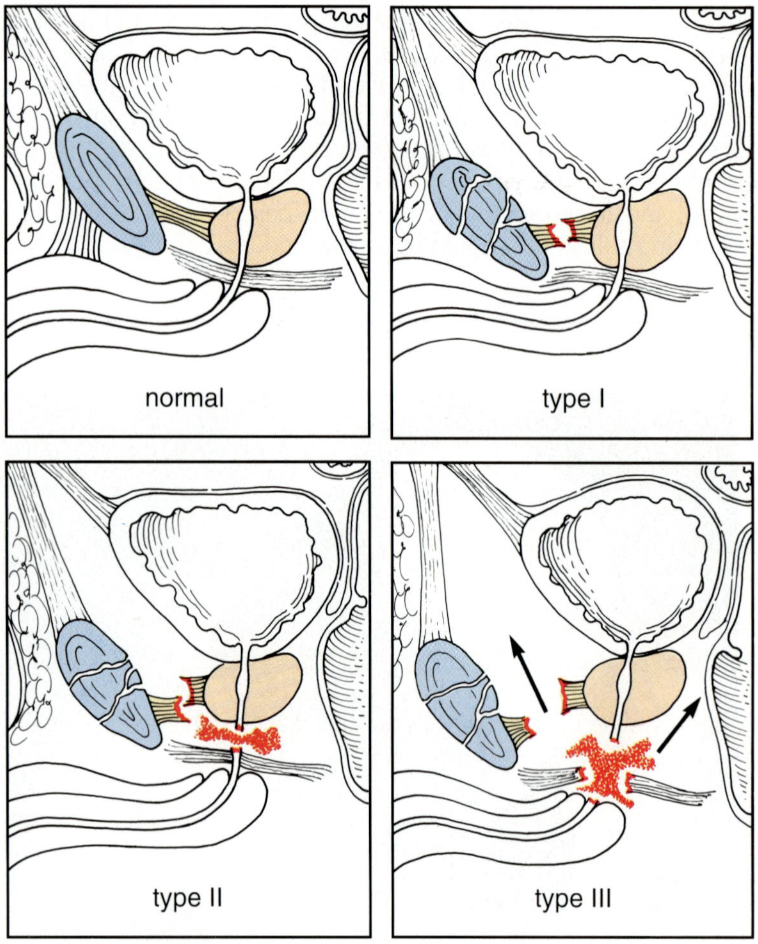

FIGURE 11.20 Classification of prostatomembranous urethral injury from pelvic fracture. Type III is most common.

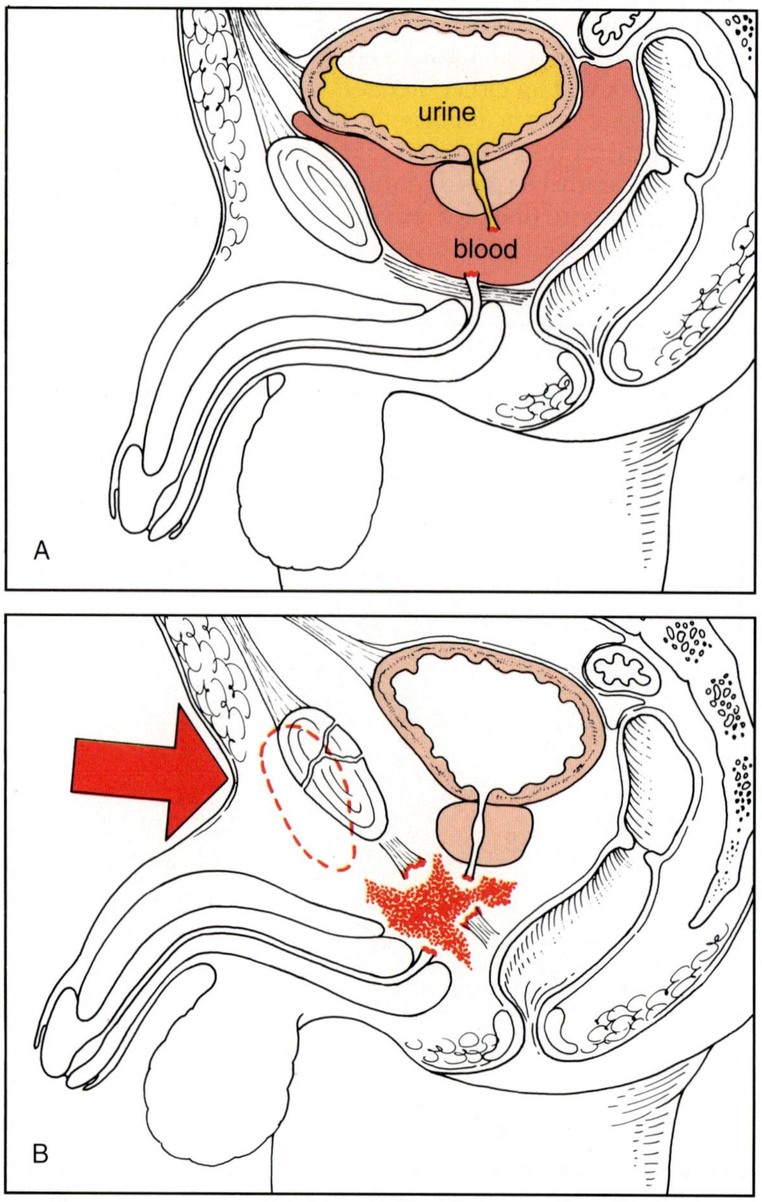

FIGURE 11.21 A The prostate is fixed on the membranous urethra in the pelvis. A deceleration injury may produce a shearing of the prostatic urethra from the membranous urethra. Associated bleeding within the pelvis will then effect displacement of both bladder and prostate. **B** Alternatively, a crush injury involving any portion of the bony pelvis may disrupt the perineal diaphragm and the membranous urethra.

rograde urethrogram before attempting to pass a catheter retrograde into the bladder (Figs. 11.22 and 11.23). If total or partial disruption of the urethra is identified by extravasation of the contrast material on the retrograde urethrogram, it is best to make a small suprapubic incision and to insert a suprapubic catheter. This should be left in place until the patient has recovered from all associated injuries and the disrupted urethra has repaired itself. Acute management of the urethral disruption frequently results in scarring that prevents successful secondary repair. In addition, an emergency attempt at repair may result in disruption of the corporal nerves and subsequent erectile impotence.

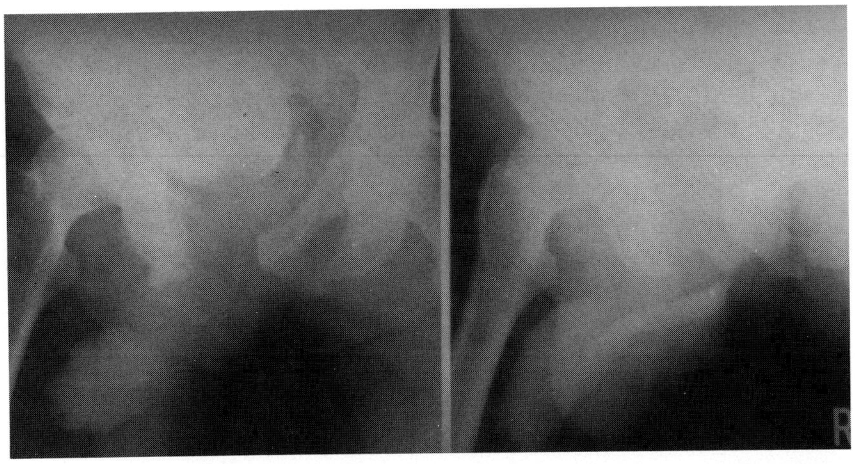

FIGURE 11.22 The left panel demonstrates pelvic fracture with displacement of the bladder. Note the contrast material–filled bladder is no longer in its normal position in the pelvis. The right panel is a retrograde urethrogram demonstrating disruption of the urethra at the point at which the perineal diaphragm was torn.

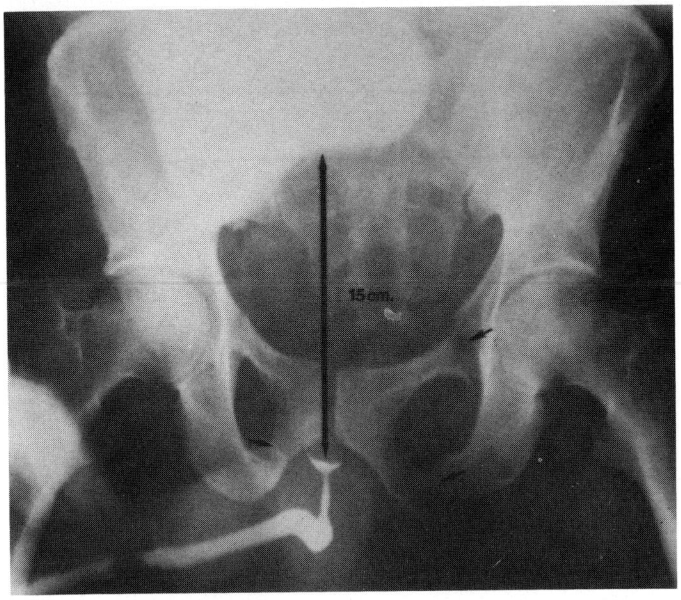

FIGURE 11.23 A combined cystogram and retrograde urethrogram shortly after butterfly fracture of the pubic rami with total disruption of the prostatomembranous urethra. An approximately 15-cm separation due to large pelvic hematoma is evident. (Webster GD: The urethra. In Paulson DF [ed]: Genitourinary Surgery, p 459. New York, Churchill Livingstone, 1984, by permission.)

ANTERIOR URETHRAL TRAUMA

Straddle Injuries

The anterior urethral injury may be traumatized iatrogenically or by straddle injury (Fig. 11.24). The mechanism for the straddle injury is trauma to the perineum that occurs as the patient falls astride any firm object.[2,24] The urethral tear may be either partial or complete. The patient usually presents with a perineal hematoma or perineal bruising. There may be associated evidence of urinary extravasation into the perineum, scrotum, or pelvis. The area of extravasation is a function of the level of damage (Figs. 11.25 and 11.26). The diagnosis must be suspected before it may be confirmed by retrograde urethrography. Patients who have inflammatory stricture in this area may have traumatic disruption or penetration of the urethra, as a result of forced urethral dilation and attempts to pass a sound or catheter into the bladder. In most cases there is no permanent damage, except for profuse bleeding when the catheter or sound is withdrawn. However, in most instances the bleeding stops spontaneously. If a catheter cannot be passed with guidance or under direct vision into the bladder itself, the patient is best treated conservatively by open placement of a suprapubic catheter.

Finally, the traumatologist must deal with external genital injuries, most of which are war-time wounds. However, in peace time there may be many external genital injuries inflicted by gunshot.

Penile Injuries

Penile injuries are of six types: strangulation, cutaneous, circumcision-induced, penile skin avulsion, penile fracture, and penile amputation.

Penile strangulation usually occurs secondary to voluntary (occasionally involuntary) placement of some constricting apparatus around the penis. When it occurs in the infant, it may be due to a piece of string or hair that has wound itself around the base of the penis truly accidentally. When identified, the hair or the string should just be removed and the patient treated conservatively until the edema subsides. However, in adolescents and young adult males, a number of devices are placed around the base of the penis to maintain erection for an extended period.[11] These constricting devices often cannot be removed by voluntary means, and significant edema and swelling of the penis distal to the constricting device occurs. Upon arrival of the patient, every attempt should be made to remove the constricting device. This often requires either sawing off or clipping the constricting metal device; usually the device cannot be removed by pulling it over the distal end of the penile shaft. Occasionally, the edema will be so severe that vascular perfusion of the penis will be compromised. The progressive gangrenous death of the penis will be evident by violaceous changes initially in the skin, followed by infarction, usually only of the superficial tissues. It is rare that the corpus spongiosum and the contained urethra become necrotic; however, this may occur and a urethral fistula at the level of the constricting device may be a delayed result.

Therapy should be directed only to removal of the constricting agent with debridement, following only upon specific identification of the demarcated dead-skin area. Debridement is often best accomplished by alternating wet and dry soaks, with the removal of the dry soak accomplishing the debridement.

Cutaneous injuries usually include simple lacerations, zipper injuries, circumcision injuries, or similar superficial injuries. These are best treated in a conservative manner.

Skin avulsion or the "power take-off" injury usually occurs when the material of the pants or trouser is caught in the power take-off of industrial or farm machinery. Once the material becomes engaged in the machinery, the loose scrotal and penile skin are entrapped with the fabric and, as the fabric is carried away with the machinery, the skin of the penis and scrotum, separately or together, are avulsed, leaving the testes and penile shaft bare of their skin covering (Fig. 11.27). The skin of the glans penis is tightly adherent at the level of the coronal sulcus and consequently the glans remains covered with the skin as the shaft is "degloved."

These injuries are best treated initially by saline soaking until the area is clean and granulating. The testicles may be maintained in saline soaks until the injured area is clean; since the vascular supply usually remains intact for a matter of days. The testes may then be placed in subcutaneous pouches on the inner thigh and maintained there until scrotal reconstruction occurs. From a technical aspect, it is best that the testicles be placed at

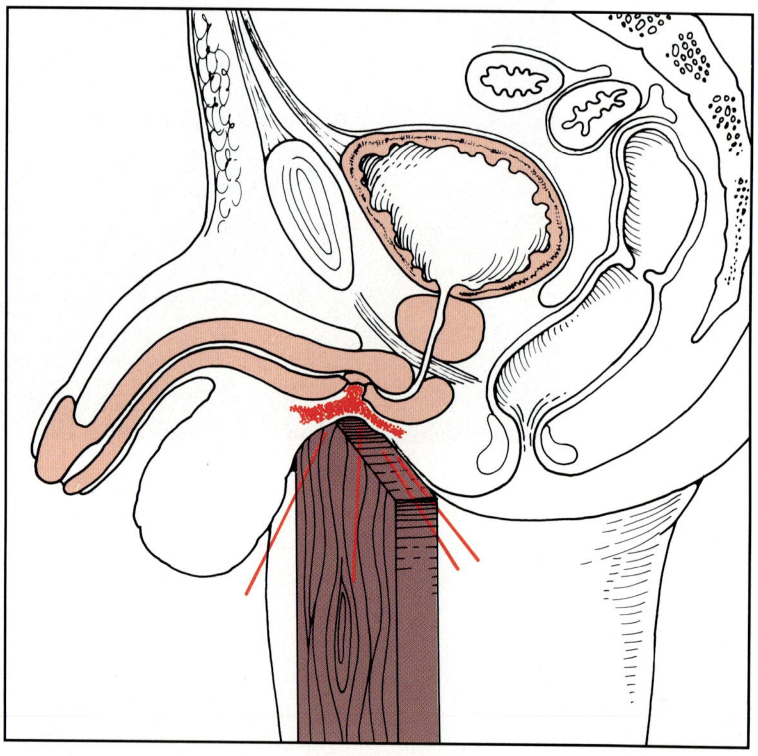

FIGURE 11.24 "Fall-astride" injury trapping the urethra beneath the symphysis pubis. (Adapted from Webster GD: The urethra. In Paulson DF [ed]: Genitourinary Surgery, p. 453. New York, Churchill Livingstone, 1984, by permission.)

different levels in the thigh in order to prevent their rubbing together with motion and walking.

Penile fracture is a very infrequent injury, usually caused by blunt trauma to the erect penis. Approximately one third of the injuries occur during coitus.[5] The patient usually complains of a cracking sound, followed by pain, marked rapid detumescence of the penis, distortion, and angulation of the penis to the side opposite the injury. There is rapid extravasation of blood into the subcutaneous tissues and marked discoloration of the penile shaft itself because of a rupture of the tunica albuginea. The ure-

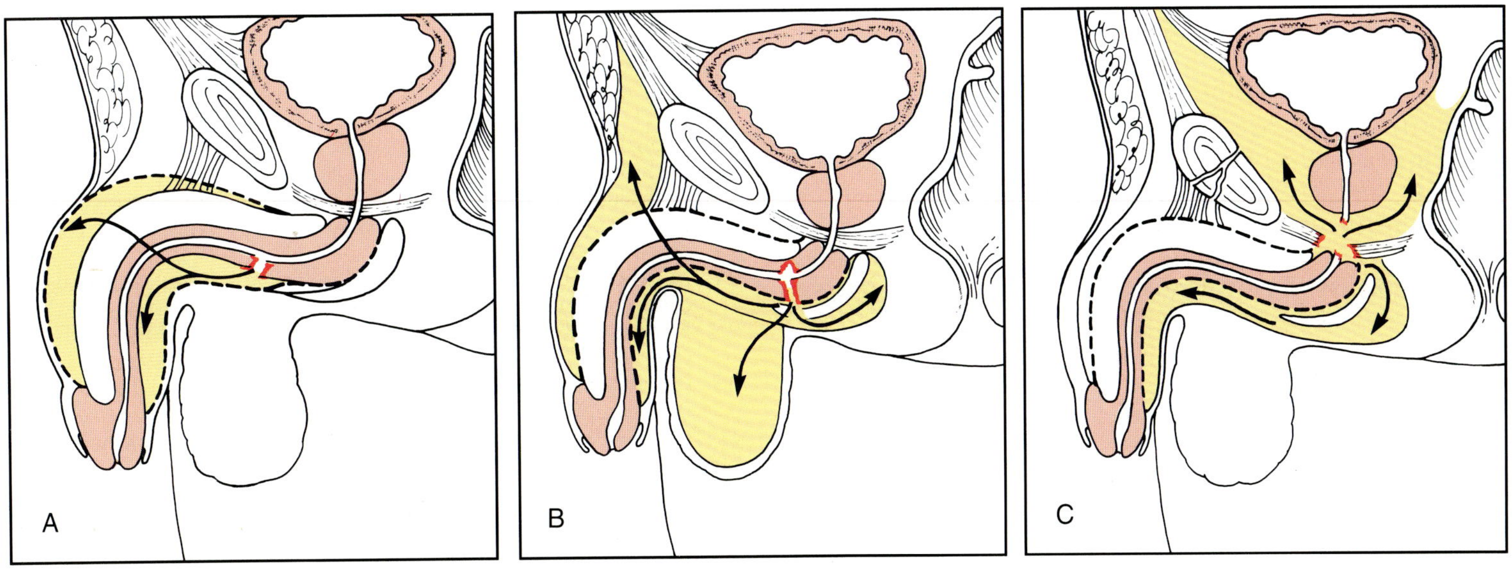

FIGURE 11.25 The type of urethral injury and the attachments of the fascial layers of the perineum and genitalia will determine the pattern of urinary extravasation and hematoma following urethral trauma. **A** Anterior urethral injury with intact Buck's fascia (dotted line) results in extravasation limited to the space around the erectile bodies and corpus spongiosum. **B** More severe anterior urethral injury with tearing of Buck's fascia. Extravasation is now limited by the attachments of Colles', dartos, and Scarpa's fascia. **C** Prostatomembranous urethral injury most commonly disrupts the entire urogenital diaphragm. Extravasation occurs into the pelvis and into the subdiaphragmatic spaces enclosed by Colles', dartos, and Scarpa's fascia. (Adapted fromWebster GD: The urethra. In Poulson DF [ed]: Genitourinary Surgery, p 453. New York, Churchill Livingstone, 1984, by permission.)

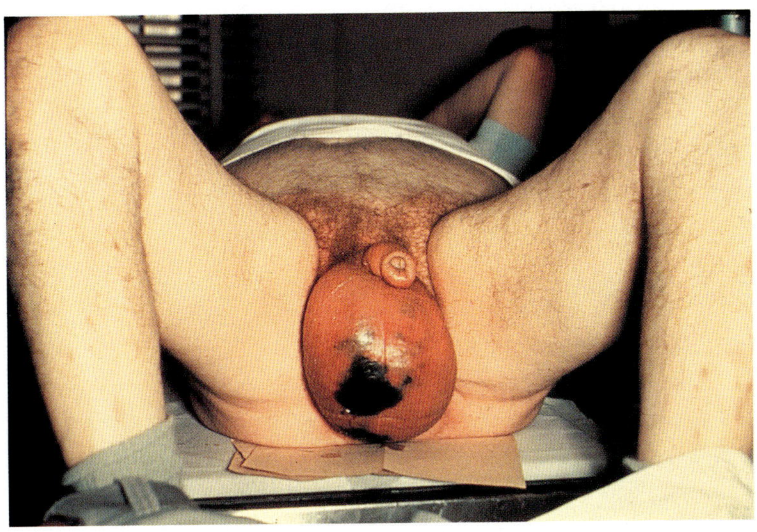

FIGURE 11.26 This man incurred a "fall-astride" injury to the urethra, initially unrecognized, and the partial disruption allowed extravasation of urine within the confines of Colles' and dartos fascia of the perineum and scrotum. (Courtesy of E. E. Anderson, M.D.)

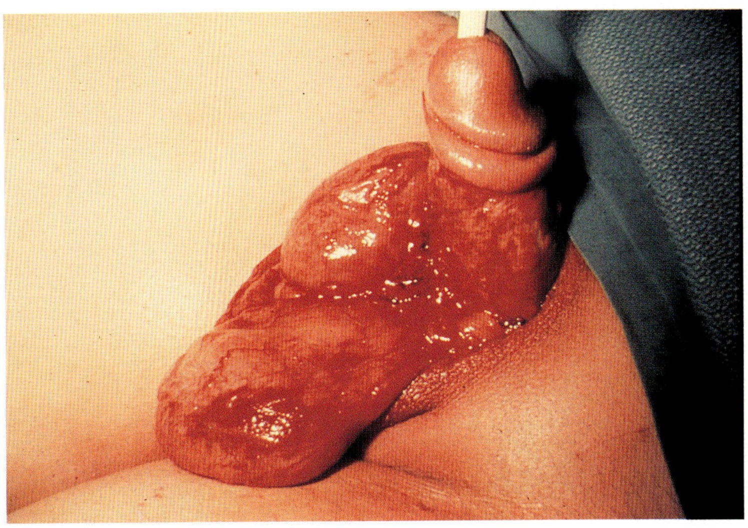

FIGURE 11.27 This is an avulsion injury of the scrotal and penile skin. This is also known as the "power take-off" injury in which the loose skin of the scrotum becomes entrapped and is pulled off from its attachment at the perineum.

thra is infrequently involved, being simultaneously fractured in only about 20% of patients.

Penile fractures may be managed conservatively by packing the penis in ice and administering analgesics. Alternatively, acute surgical intervention, with minimal debridement of the area but immediate resuturing of the corpora cavernosa may result in a shortened hospital stay. The surgeon, however, should be aware that aggressive debridement of the injured area may not only inhibit subsequent erectile function, but also result in deviation of the penis to the side of repair with subsequent erections.

Penile amputation usually occurs in patients with significant psychiatric disturbance. When the penile remnant and the patient appear within a reasonable period, appropriate management is to directly resuture the penis and to perform microvascular reconstruction of the dorsal artery and vein and of the cavernosal structures in the urethra. The incidence of these injuries is too few to provide statistics with respect to success of repair.

REFERENCES

1. Barnasconi F, Colombino S: Contribution `a l'e´tude du traitement des blessures de l'uretere aucours des interventions chirurgicales. Ann Mal Org Genito-Urin 22:1361, 1905.
2. Blumberg N: Anterior urethral injuries. J Urol 102:210, 1969.
3. Brosman SA, Fay R: Diagnosis and management of bladder trauma. J Trauma 13(8):929–939, 1973.
4. Cornell SH, Reasa DA, Culp DA: Occlusion of the renal artery secondary to acute or remote trauma. JAMA 219:1754, 1972.
5. DeWeerd JH: Management of injuries to the bladder, urethra and genitalia. Surg Clin North Am 39:973, 1959.
6. Ehrlich RM, Skinner DG: Complications of transureteroureterostomy. J Urol 113:467, 1975.
7. Gibson GR: Impotence following fractured pelvis and ruptured urethra. Br J Urol 42:86, 1970.
8. Grant RP, Gifford RW, Pedvan WR et al: Renal trauma and hypertension. Am J Cardiol 27:173, 1971.
9. Guerriero WG, Carlton CE, Scott R et al: Renal pedicle injuries. J Trauma 11:53, 1971.
10. Hodges CV et al: Clinical experiences with transureteroureterostomy. J Urol 90:552, 1963.
11. Hoffman HA, Colby FH: Incarceration of the penis. J Urol 54:391, 1945.
12. Krahn HP, Axenrod R: The management of severe renal lacerations. J Urol 109:11, 1973.
13. Leandoer JL, Tremann JA, Oishi RH et al: Bilateral renal artery thrombosis following blunt trauma: Report of two cases. J Trauma 12:166, 1972.
14. Lucey DT, Smith MJV, Koontz WW: A plea for the conservative treatment of renal injuries. J Trauma 11:390, 1971.
15. Mitchell JP: Injuries to the urethra. Br J Urol 40:649, 1968.
16. Morehouse DD, Belitsky P, Mackinnon KJ: Rupture of the posterior urethra. J Urol 107:255, 1972.
17. Morehouse DD, MacKinnon KJ: Urological injuries associated with pelvic fractures. J Trauma 9:479, 1969.
18. Peters PC: Trauma to the genitourinary system. In Shires GT (ed): Care of the Trauma Patient. New York, McGraw-Hill, 1966.
19. Peterson NE: Intermediate-degree blunt renal trauma. J Trauma 17(6). Baltimore, Williams & Wilkins, 1977.
20. Ross R, Ackerman E, Pierce JM: Traumatic subintimal hemorrhage of the renal artery. J Urol 104:11, 1970.
21. Sandoz IL, Paull DP, McFarlane CA: Complications with transureteroureterostomy. J Urol 117:39, 1977.
22. Scott R, Carlton CE, Goldman M: Penetrating injuries of the kidney. J Urol 101:247, 1969.
23. Sharpe NW: Trans-uretero-ureteral anastomosis. Ann Surg 44:687, 1906
24. Sterioff S, Izant RJ, Persky L: Perineal injuries in children. J Trauma 9:56, 1969.
25. Walker JA: Injuries to the ureter due to external violence. J Urol 102:410, 1969.
26. Waterhouse K, Gross M: Trauma to the genitourinary tract: A five-year experience with 251 cases. J Urol 101:241, 1969.
27. Zinman RM, Libertino JA, Roth RA: Management of operative ureteral injury. Urology 22(3), 1978.

peripheral vascular injuries

Richard L. McCann
Raymond G. Makhoul

1 2 6 3 7 11 4 8 12 16 5 9 13 17 10 14 18 15 19 20

Between 1% and 5% of trauma cases involve injury to a major vascular structure.[49] The lives and limbs put in jeopardy by these vascular injuries often belong to young people; their salvage may mean many years of satisfactory function. It is estimated that in excess of 1% of persons currently 10 to 34 years old will die of injuries before the year 2000.[9] Traumatic injury continues to be the leading cause of death for persons 1 to 44 years old. Thus even without armed military conflict, there is a role for efficient and effective surgical management of traumatic vascular injuries.

Most advances in the treatment of major vascular injuries have evolved from military experience, in which large numbers of patients were treated in relatively short periods. Many of the lessons learned have been incorporated into modern civilian practice, including the use of trained technical personnel in the field to triage and resuscitate victims at the scene, the use of efficient ground and helicopter transportation, and the centralization of resources into trauma treatment centers. The high frequency of traumatic injuries and the fact that efficient and skillful treatment can save many lives and limbs make treatment of the injured an important area for every surgeon.

HISTORY

The first consideration in the treatment of vascular injury is the control of hemorrhage. Ancient physicians and surgeons used a number of methods to achieve this, including cautery, hot and cold applications of oil and other substances, and ligature. The last, however, did not become firmly established until the 16th century when Paré demonstrated that amputation for battlefield injury could be accomplished above the level of gangrenous demarcation if the artery were first held in a clamp, and then ligated with a linen ligature (Fig. 12.1).

The first repair of an arterial injury is credited to Hollowell, an English surgeon, who treated a laceration of the brachial artery that resulted from deliberate bleeding. The vessel walls were approximated by driving a pin through both edges and holding these together with a figure-of-eight wrap of thread (Fig. 12.2). A second successful arterial repair[55] was reported 127 years later, by Postemski in 1886. A number of attempts at lateral vascular repairs were reported both in humans and in experimental animals in the remainder of the 19th century.[12] These methods included the use of tubes of ivory, glass, and even magnesium as well as several different suture techniques, among them passage of the suture through only part of the vessel wall.

Success in vascular repair and anastomosis was, however, inconsistent until the pioneering work of Carrel after the turn of the century. [12] Carrel's advances are perhaps no less important today than they were 90 years ago. In the laboratory he was able to suture both large and small vessels, arteries and veins, with remarkable patency rates. Carrel discarded the surgical instruments that were available in his day because they were far too gross and harmful to tissues. Instead he advocated extreme gentle surgical technique and cautioned particularly against crushing and stretching vascular structures. The needles of the day were exceedingly large and, finding them unsuitable for use on small vascular structures, Carrel is said to have purchased his needles from the fine embroidery shops, for which the city of Lyon was known more than for its medical school. He developed very fine noncrushing surgical techniques of joining blood vessels in experimental animals, using frequent irrigation with physiologic saline and very fine suturing with thin needles and threads. With ease and routine success he was able to transplant thyroid glands, kidneys, and other organs. His achievements are all the more dramatic when it is remembered that they were performed prior to the availability of heparin or any other clinical anticoagulant.

Despite these tremendous strides in the laboratory, there were few practical applications during the first two major military conflicts of the 20th century. Bernhard Bernheim, inspired by Carrel's work, and with the encouragement of William S. Halstead, pioneered the clinical use of vascular surgery at Johns Hopkins University in the early part of the century. Bernheim actually went to Europe during the First World War with the intention of establishing vascular repair in the treatment of battle casualties. However, he found that the rate of infection was so high, in part because of the length of time required for evacuation, that a surgeon "would have been a foolhardy man (to) have essayed suture of arterial or venous trunks in the presence of such infections."[4] The great frequency with which these military wounds met with severe infection is well documented in the careful and comprehensive analysis of 2471 vascular injuries occurring during World War II by DeBakey and Simeone.[18] This remarkable study revealed that gas gangrene caused nearly as many amputations as vascular injuries. Although suture of vascular injury was attempted in just 81 cases, it improved the limb salvage rate over ligation only from 51% to 64%. It might also be noted that insertion of the then-popular Vitallium tubes lined with autogenous vein grafts (Fig. 12.3) without suturing actually resulted in a lower rate of limb salvage than debridement and ligation.

It was clear that the difficulties imposed by battle conditions interfered wiith effective treatment of vascular injuries. Many of the objections to vascular repair were overcome in the next major military conflict, the Korean War. During this conflict, medical facilities were well organized and centralized and were placed relatively close to the front, and helicopter evacuation was used for the first time. These factors reduced the average time from injury to operation to less than 10 hours.[30,31] These factors combined to reduce the amputation rate for vascular injuries from 50% to 12.5%.[31] The techniques initially developed during the Korean conflict were refined and expanded during the Vietnam War. It is fortunate that the surgical experience with vascular injuries during that war has been so well documented by Rich and Spencer[49] and others.[46] In 1000 major arterial injuries extracted from the Vietnam Vascular Registry, ligation was employed in only 15 cases (1.5%). Of 1000 major vascular injuries, there was only a 1.7% mortality rate and limb salvage was greater than 85%. These results were achieved in spite of the high-velocity missiles and other highly destructive weapons characteristic of modern warfare.

The principles learned during these military conflicts which are immediately applicable to civilian practice include the early treatment of vascular injuries before distal thrombosis or irre-

FIGURE 12.1
HISTORY OF TREATMENT OF VASCULAR INJURIES

CONTRIBUTOR	CONTRIBUTION	DATE	REFERENCE
Ambrose Paré	Ligature	1552	48
Lambert-Hollowell	Closure of arterial wound	1759	48
Alexis Carrel	Technique of vascular suture	1902	12
Bertram Bernheim	Vascular injuries, WWI	1920	4
DeBakey and Simeone	Vascular injuries, WWII	1946	18
C. W. Hughes	Vascular injuries, Korea	1958	30
Rich, Baugh, and Hughes	Vascular injuries, Vietnam	1970	45

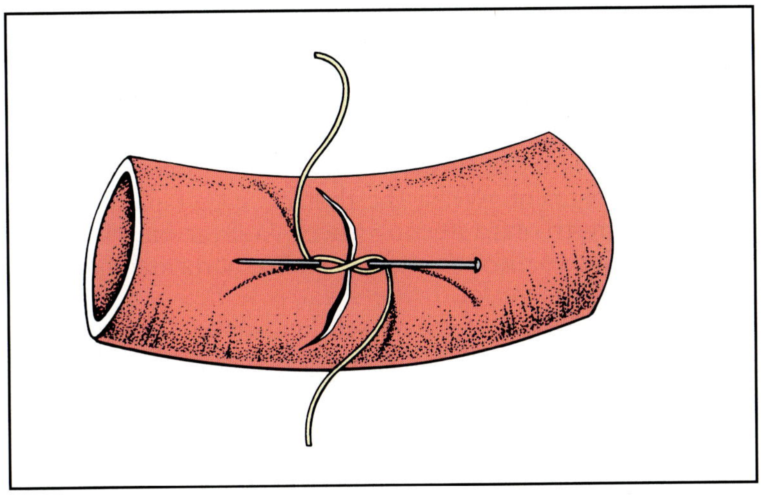

FIGURE 12.2 Hollowell's repair of an injured brachial artery in 1759. This method was adapted from a technique used to treat cleft lip.

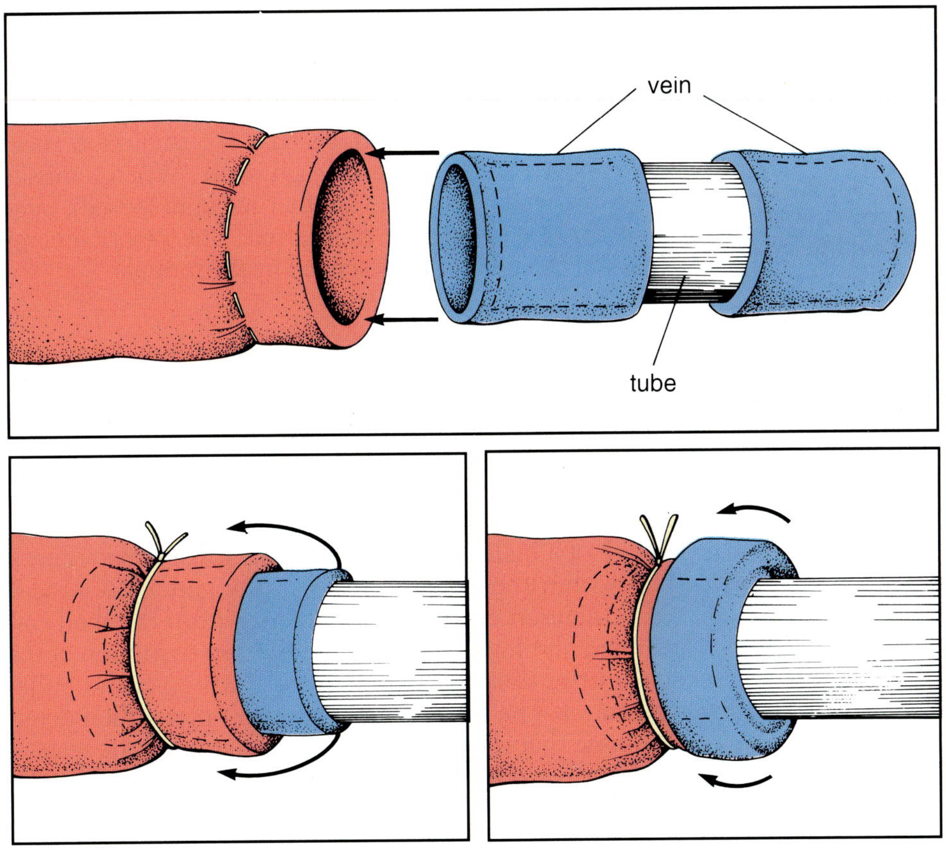

FIGURE 12.3 Depiction of the use of a rigid/tube lined with a vein graft for vascular repair. The vein is everted over each end of the tube. The ends of the tube are then inserted into the artery and secured with a circumferential ligature.

versible neurologic or muscular injury occurs. The use of autogenous tissue grafts to bridge extensive arterial defects is another valuable lesson widely practiced today. Also of importance is the concept of wide debridement of all devitalized tissue and adequate coverage of vascular anastomoses and grafts by muscle or fascial tissues, even if it requires flap rotation or extra-anatomic routes for blood flow.

EPIDEMIOLOGY

The largest number of vascular injuries in the United States is treated today in our major urban trauma centers. A report from the early 1980s describes management of 456 cardiovascular injuries in a single year.[20] All but 12.8% of these injuries were due to acts of violence and the majority of these (68%) were due to gunshot wounds or shotgun blasts, the remainder being due to stab wounds. In this urban series, blunt injuries caused only 2.9% of the total vascular injuries. Lacerations from sharp objects and medical therapeutic mishaps were responsible for the remaining 9.9% of injuries.

While the largest number of vascular injuries is seen at major urban institutions, the unrelenting increase in automobile and other types of accidents (*e.g.*, those resulting from industrial and farm equipment, skiing, and falls) will continue to provide a source of vascular injuries for medical centers in smaller cities and even rural areas. Since the first recorded death from an automobile accident in 1898,[66] more than 1.6 million people have died on the nation's highways. Blunt trauma is responsible for from 2% to 50% of vascular injuries, depending upon the geographic location and the patient population studied.[5,10,20,44,64]

The treatment of injuries requires more than 3.6 million hospital admissions annually in this country. One of every ten admissions to a short-stay hospital is for treatment of injury. For all age groups combined, the number of admissions for treatment of injuries is exceeded only by admissions for treatment of digestive and circulatory system diseases. Injuries are responsible for more years of life lost than all other causes of death combined.[2] Motor vehicle crashes alone are responsible for more than 500,000 hospital admissions averaging 8 days in length during a single calendar year. While 52,000 of these patients will die, the well-being of the remainder will be dependent upon prompt and skillful medical care, which must therefore be available within a reasonable distance. For these reasons it is imperative that skilled surgical care be available not only in the major urban trauma centers but geographically distributed throughout the country.

It is estimated that the cost to society of all injuries during a recent year was in the range of 75 to 100 billion dollars. These startling costs relate only to economic values. One must also consider the pain, grief, and social and psychological effects of disfigurement and long-term disability that may result from severe injuries.[16]

BALLISTICS AND MECHANISMS OF INJURY

Blunt trauma causes vascular injury by placing excessive tensile or shear strain on vascular tissues. *Tensile strain*, or excessive longitudinal force, may result in frank vessel rupture, or more frequently, in rupture of the intima leaving only the more elastic layers of the vessel wall intact (Fig. 12.4). If the intimal fracture is severe, it will expose a large surface which is rich in collagen and other thrombogenic substances to the flowing blood, often resulting in local thrombosis. Alternatively a weakened section of vessel wall may create a false aneurysm which may subsequently enlarge or experience delayed rupture.

Shear strain results from lateral forces acting on the vessel wall (Fig. 12.4). It frequently occurs in deceleration-type injuries, in which a portion of the vessel is fixed while an adjacent segment is less tightly attached to the bony skeleton. A good example is the thoracic aorta, in which the segment at the level of the arch vessels is more firmly fixed to the spine than is the descending segment. When the thoracic cage rapidly decelerates—as with striking a steering wheel—a shear stress is applied at the junction of the arch and descending aorta and may result in tearing of the vessel. If the shear is sufficient to tear the entire circumference of the vessel, immediate exsanguination may occur. In 10% to 20% of cases, however, the adventitia remains intact, at least for a time, thus allowing the possibility of a surgical correction.

Penetrating injuries cause damage to vascular structures by two mechanisms (Fig. 12.5). Stab wounds and low-velocity missile wounds may result in direct damage to vascular structures. In these cases, the penetrating instrument or missile must pass directly through the vascular tissue to cause injury. A high-velocity missile, on the other hand, may cause injury to vessels and tissue not directly in its path, because of a cavitation effect caused by passage of the missile through tissue. When a missile passes from one medium (air) to another medium (tissue), large amounts of kinetic energy are transferred. The kinetic energy (KE) possessed by an object is described by the formula

$$KE = \frac{\text{Mass} \times \text{Velocity}^2}{g}$$

Thus, the amount of kinetic energy, and therefore potential destructive power, possessed by a missile increases proportionately with its velocity. Very small missiles traveling at high speeds are more destructive than larger missiles traveling more slowly. The velocity of a bullet is a function of the force imparted to it while it is within the firing chamber of the gun. This force is achieved by ignition of the powder charge within the shell casing. The rapid burning of this powder results in expansion of the gases within the shell casing, which in turn push the bullet along the barrel. The length of the weapon's barrel then determines the time that these expanding gases act upon the mass of the bullet and thus the acceleration of the missile to its final (muzzle) velocity. This acceleration can be described mathematically as the force applied divided by the mass. Thus with a given force, the smaller the mass the faster is the maximum velocity that can be achieved. It follows, then, that a smaller missile can be imparted a much greater velocity and thus more destructive power than can a larger missile, given the same amount of exploding charge.

Once the missile leaves the barrel of the gun, a number of other factors that also affect its destructive power act upon it. Once the velocity and momentum have been imparted to the missile by the expanding gases of the charge, they are removed (deceleration) by the medium through which the missile passes. The decelerating or drag forces are analogous to friction and are a function of the density of the medium and the profile of the missile; air removes very little of the kinetic energy while soft

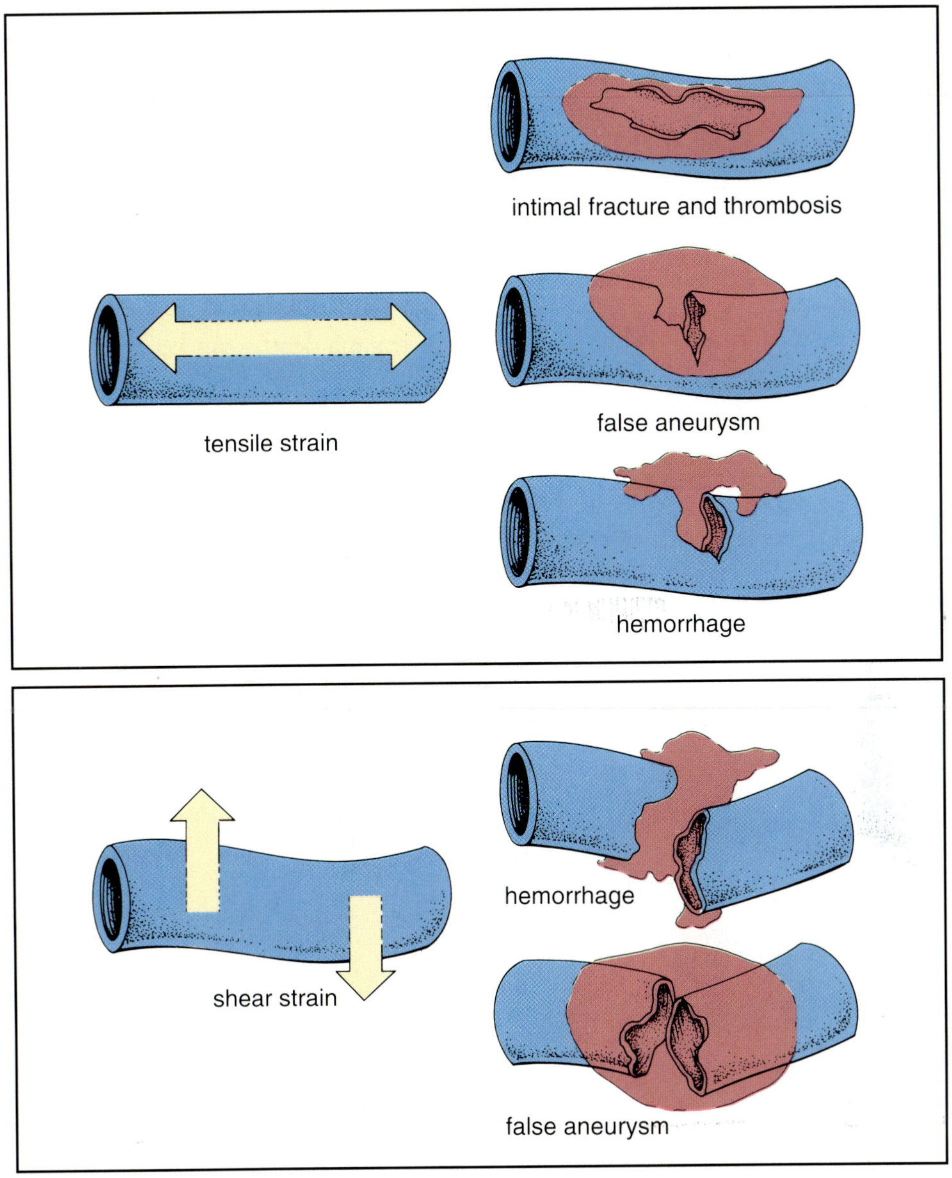

FIGURE 12.4 Mechanisms of vascular injury due to blunt trauma. Trauma places excessive tensile or shear strain on vascular tissues.

tissues remove more, and bone may be so dense that all the kinetic energy is given up and the missile stops. The geometry of the missile also contributes to the amount of drag present as the missile passes through any medium. Bullet shape and launching point just reduce these drag forces. *Yaw* refers to the deviation of the missile from its longitudinal axis during its flight. The tendency toward yaw and even its extreme, tumbling, is dependent upon the density of the medium. Thus a missile entering tissue may rapidly increase the surface area and the transfer of kinetic energy by exaggerated yaw or tumbling. This tendency explains the remarkable destructive power of the so-called hollow-point bullets with soft tips, which immediately deform upon striking tissue. As the missile passes through tissue it continuously transfers kinetic energy and causes the particles that it encounters to accelerate at an angle identical to that of incidence. It is this transfer of energy that creates the cavitational effect and that, in fact, is responsible for the majority of the destructiveness of high-velocity missiles.

The clinical significance of these concepts is that simple stab wounds and small-caliber, low-velocity bullets will cause only local injuries. A bullet of higher velocity or greater mass passing through the tissues will result not only in a permanent cavity or tract, but also in a much larger temporary cavity in which there is extreme tissue destruction due to the "secondary" missiles created by the transfer of energy to the matter encountered. Thus, severe vascular injury as well as injury to other tissues may occur even when a missile passes near these structures and not directly through them.

BALLISTIC FACTORS DETERMINING TISSUE DAMAGE

- Velocity
- Mass
- Profile

PRINCIPLES OF MANAGEMENT

The outcome of the management of vascular injuries depends upon prompt evaluation, accurate diagnosis, and skillful technical management. Failure in any one of these areas will result in increased limb loss and possibly in increased mortality. Trunkey[61] has suggested that trauma deaths can be divided into

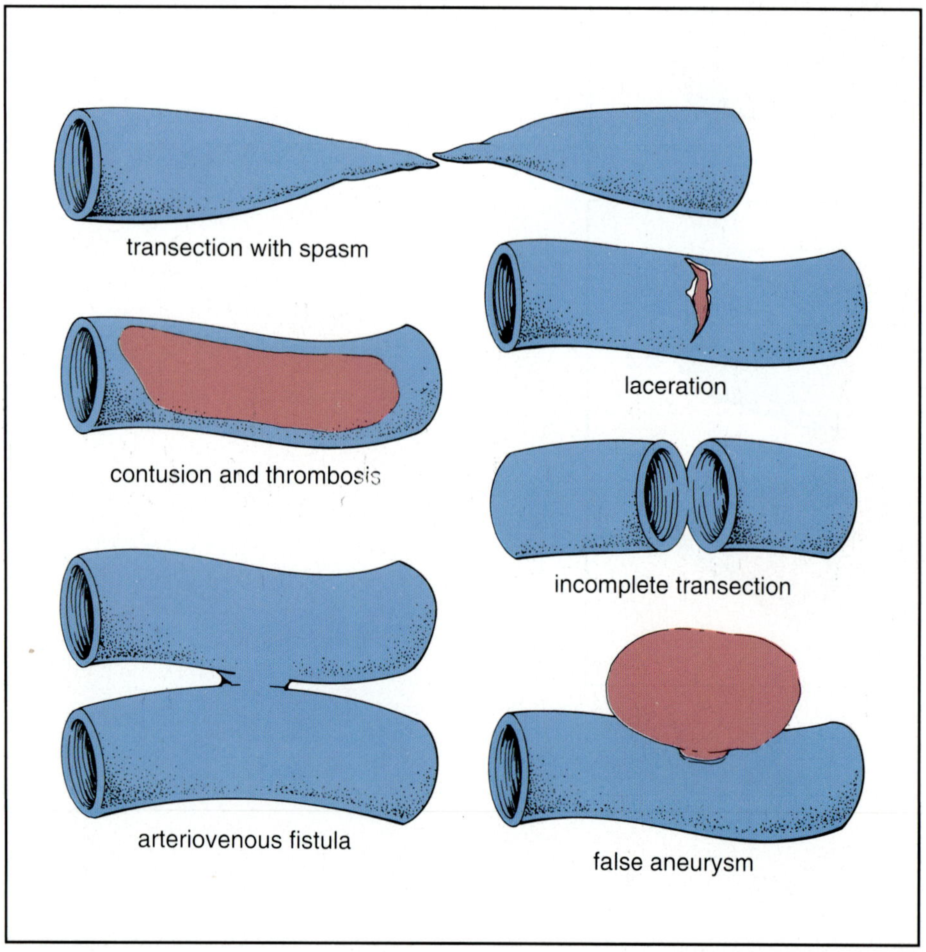

FIGURE 12.5 Mechanisms of vascular injury due to penetrating trauma.

immediate, early, and late categories, depending upon the amount of time elapsed from the injury. Immediate deaths are due to massive central nervous system injury or to injury of a major cardiovascular structure with exsanguinating hemorrhage. Even if prompt resuscitation and surgical treatment are available, only a small percentage of this group may be saved. Thirty percent of trauma deaths fall into the early category. The cause of death in these patients is also injury to the nervous system or hemorrhage. Prompt surgical intervention can influence the loss from hemorrhage. Even in cases of severe hemorrhage with bleeding of up to 100 ml/min, if treatment is begun within 30 minutes of injury, survival is likely. Such rapid treatment is now available in many communities by trained emergency medical technicians who may inititate intravenous therapy in the field. Rapid transportation to medical facilities specially equipped and staffed for the treatment of the injured is now also available in many communities. More than 30 years after its efficacy was demonstrated by the military in the Korean War, air transportation by helicopter is becoming increasingly available in the civilian sector. This has proved to be highly efficacious and has markedly reduced the length of the prehospital phase in semi-urban and rural areas.

Finally, the late deaths from vascular injuries are usually due to infection and multiple organ failure. These are the sequelae of profound and prolonged shock. Reduction of these unfavorable outcomes will be achieved by more speedy and aggressive treatment of the injured.

PRINCIPLES OF TREATMENT OF VASCULAR INJURIES

- Early treatment before distal thrombosis
- Wide debridement of devitalized tissue
- Bridge arterial defects with grafts
- Cover grafts with viable musculofacial tissue

EMERGENCY ROOM MANAGEMENT AND INITIAL EVALUATION

Triage

Treatment priorities must be established for trauma patients arriving in the emergency department. First priority is given to arresting obvious hemorrhage, establishing and maintaining an airway and adequate respiration, and stabilizing the cervical spine if necessary. Once immediate vital functions are ensured, a more detailed secondary evaluation is carried out followed by or concurrent with initiation of definitive management. The secondary evaluation is conveniently divided into penetrating trauma and blunt trauma injury evaluation. As noted above, penetrating injuries are the most common form of vascular injury in most medical centers. An important principle in treating these injuries is to recognize that penetrating wounds, particularly high-velocity ones, in the vicinity of a major vascular structure must be treated as if that structure is damaged until proven otherwise. The consequences of late diagnosis and delayed treatment of extremity vascular injuries have been described.[51] In one study of 30 patients with delayed diagnosis of vascular injury, major amputation was required in a third of the patients; other complications included coagulopathy, secondary hemorrhage, sepsis, and compartment syndromes. Thus the severe consequences of delayed treatment are almost completely avoidable by maintaining a high index of suspicion.

The purpose of the emergency room evaluation is to gather as much information as possible about the injuries that have occurred without delaying their definitive management. In patients who arrive in severe shock from hemorrhage, an operation may be performed or at least begun in the emergency department to stop continuing hemorrhage from the heart or other major vascular structure. This may be accomplished by cardiorrhaphy or, in cases of injury to major abdominal vascular structures with intractable shock, by clamping the descending aorta and then taking the patient to the operating room for more definitive repair of the injury site.

For patients with major hemorrhage but less severe distress, resuscitation should be initiated in the emergency center while preparations are being made for surgery. Vascular access is of paramount importance in these patients and may be difficult to achieve if shock is present. Large-bore catheters in central veins are required for rapid volume administration to replace blood loss and ongoing hemmorrhage. When there is blunt or penetrating abdominal injury, only the upper extremities and neck should be used for vascular access, because major caval injury in the abdomen would result in loss of fluids administered through the lower extremities through the injury itself and thus not be effective. The easiest and most definitive access site for patients in shock is the subclavian vein beneath the clavicle. The internal jugular vein may be collapsed and difficult to catheterize in the patient in shock even in the Trendelenburg position. In experienced hands, catheterization of the subclavian vein in these patients is reliable and relatively safe.[56] At the time of venous catheterization, blood should be drawn for typing. Fluid resuscitation is initiated with a balanced salt solution, usually Ringer's lactate, and blood when it becomes available. Uncross-matched O-negative blood should be reserved for the patient whose blood pressure does not respond to rapid infusion of 2 liters of Ringer's lactate.

EMERGENCY ROOM EVALUATION

Primary

- Assure airway
- Arrest hemorrhage
- Stabilize spine

Secondary

- Initiate resuscitation
- Complete examination
- Begin diagnotic studies

Vascular Survey

Once resuscitation is under way, the vascular survey can be completed. This includes an evaluation of signs of blunt injury, as well as examination of entrance and exit sites of bullets or other missiles. The entire body must be examined to ensure that no injuries are missed. Most weapons today have more than one bullet, and victims are often shot more than once. One must make every effort to try to determine the nature of the weapon used, the number of injuries sustained, and the potential paths of the missiles involved. This is particularly important in the case of high-velocity missiles, which do not have to directly traverse vascular structures in order to injure them. The vascular examination is completed by searching for evidence of ischemia in the form of absent pulses or diminished distal Doppler occlusion pressures. Other evidence of significant vascular injury includes pulsatile hematomas and bruits or thrills suggesting the presence of an acute arteriovenous fistula.

The value of arteriography in vascular injury remains a controversial subject. A number of factors must be considered in deciding whether to obtain a preoperative anteriogram. One of the most important is the amount of time that has elapsed since injury occurred. As a general rule, extremity tissues will tolerate four to six hours of ischemia before irreversible damage occurs. This general rule is tempered by considerations of the amount of collateral circulation available and the degree of other tissue damage that may have occurred. While collateral circulation to the upper extremity is excellent and ischemia will not be severe or time-limiting if the injury involves only the axial vessels and spares the major collateral pathways, the same is not true of the lower extremity. For example, in injury to the popliteal artery resulting in thrombosis, collateral circulation is insufficient to maintain viability, and irreversible tissue injury will occur in four to six hours if revascularization is not achieved during that period. Thus if a patient arrives several hours following injury to the popliteal artery and ischemia of the lower leg is obvious, then a formal preoperative arteriogram is superfluous and possibly dangerous because it delays the indicated treatment.

More complex is the patient who presents with palpable distal pulses and penetrating or blunt trauma in the region of a major artery. It has repeatedly been demonstrated that palpable pulses may be documented in the presence of a significant vascular injury in up to 30% of patients.[5,19,45,50] Diagnosis hinges on a high index of suspicion.

We continue to feel that arteriography is indicated if time and the general condition of the patient allow, and if there has been penetrating trauma in the vicinity of an artery or blunt trauma over it. The opposite tack of exploring all these wounds seems to result in an excessively high negative exploration rate.[57,67] Modern biplane cut film arteriography is remarkably reliable in excluding the presence of significant vascular injury. The arteriographic manifestations of these vascular injuries may be subtle (Fig. 12.6). Digital subtraction angiography has been proposed as a screening test for patients with possible vascular injury. Although continued improvements in image quality are likely, the current images are not sufficiently detailed to compare with cut film angiograms. In addition the small field size does not allow for complete examination of the arterial tree (Fig. 12.7). Therefore, we feel strongly that if angiography is indicated, the most sensitive technique, the cut film method, should be used.

Seventy-three patients were evaluated at Duke University Medical Center over a period of four years. Applying the above criteria, the rate of positive angiograms in these patients was 33%. Twenty-two percent of patients who had diminished distal pulses or decreased Doppler pressures were found to have intact vasculature (Fig. 12.8). In this study there were no false-negative arteriograms.[63] Because of this experience we continue to rely heavily upon arteriography both to demonstrate accurately and precisely the nature of vascular injuries and to exclude patients from needless surgical exploration if the arteriogram fails to demonstrate a significant vascular injury.

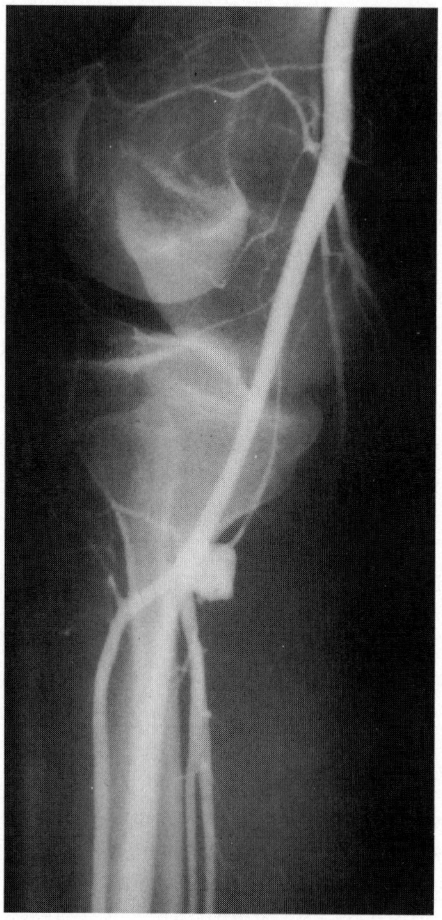

FIGURE 12.6
Preoperative arteriogram of a patient shot in the leg. Distal pulses were easily palpable. The arteriogram shows an acute false aneurysm of the popliteal artery and illustrates that significant vascular injury often exists in the presence of normal distal pulses.

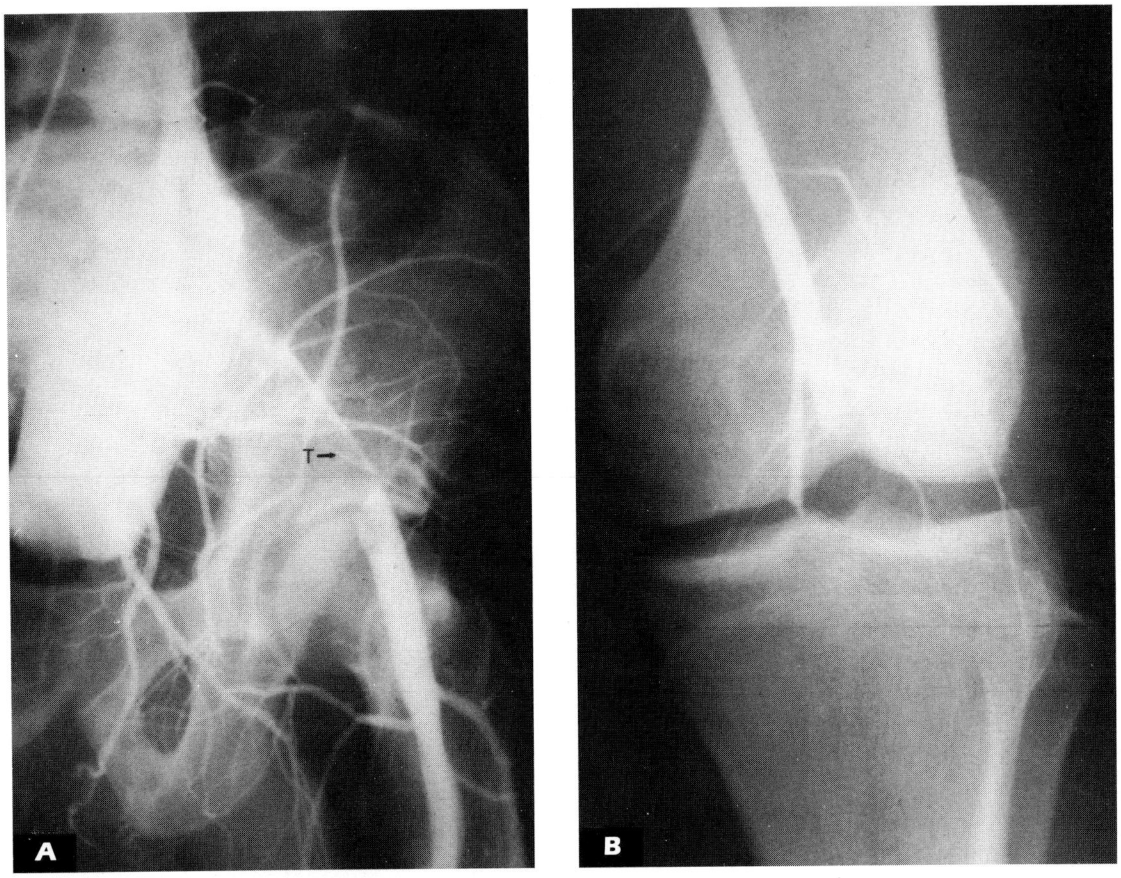

FIGURE 12.7 This patient had blunt trauma and absent left leg pulses. **A** The external iliac thrombus (T) due to intimal fracture. **B** A sharp cutoff in the popliteal artery is due to distal embolization of a portion of the thrombus. This important lesion would have been missed without complete angiography.

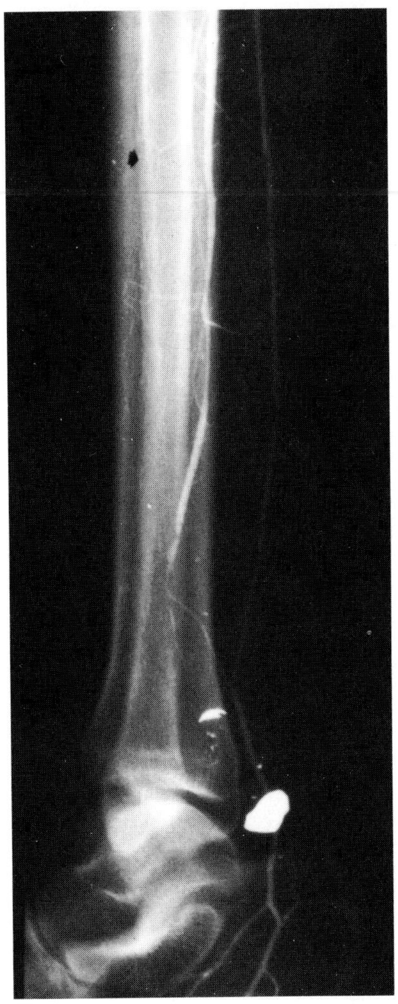

FIGURE 12.8 This angiogram is from a patient with a gunshot wound in an ischemic-appearing leg. There is direct injury to the peroneal artery and spasm of the anterior tibial artery (arrow). The posterior tibial artery is intact. Fasciotomy of the anterior compartment is all that was required for complete recovery. This illustrates the role of angiography in avoiding major vascular exploration.

OPERATIVE TECHNIQUES

The goals of the operative management of vascular injuries are to effect efficient and rapid revascularization with a vascular repair that is both durable and infection resistant.

Time factors are critical in terms of the operative plan and efficiency. In managing vascular injuries in the operating room, proximal and distal control of the injured vascular structures should be efficiently and rapidly obtained through adequate incisions. The area of vessel injury should then be explored through the same or another generous incision. There is no substitute for exposure, and small, cosmetic-type incisions are inadequate. All devitalized tissue must be meticulously debrided. If there is a concomitant long bone fracture, the vascular repair is usually done first to provide revascularization of the ischemic distal tissues, and then the fracture is stabilized by the orthopedic members of the trauma team. In certain circumstances, particularly when a considerable amount of orthopedic manipulation that would jeopardize a tenuous vascular repair is anticipated, it may be advisable to provide temporary revascularization with an indwelling shunt until the bone is stabilized[13] (Fig. 12.9). At that time the shunt can be removed and the vessel repaired. Since a graft is almost always necessary, it may be possible to harvest that simultaneously from the opposite extremity while the fracture is being reduced.

Probably the most common reason for failure of vascular anastomoses in the trauma setting is tension on the suture line. Since most of the vessels encountered are otherwise normal, a high patency rate should be expected. It is important that vascular repairs be performed in areas where the vessels are completely normal. The principle of debridement of devitalized tissue is just as important as selection of the arterial tree. Failure to adhere to this principle by using a section of less-damaged but nevertheless abnormal artery risks thrombosis of the reconstruction. Often several centimeters beyond the area of externally obvious injury must be resected in order to obtain thin, glistening, nonthrombogenic adherent intima. This is particularly true for the small vessels of the extremities.

Systemic heparinization is usually contraindicated by the associated soft tissue injuries. Often distal thrombosis due to stasis can be prevented, however, by local injections of dilute heparin solutions.

Vascular repair may be effected by lateral suture, by short resections with mobilization of the proximal and distal ends with primary anastomosis, or by the use of interposition grafts of autogenous or synthetic material. Lateral suture may be appropriate for low-velocity missile or edged-instrument injury to the larger blood vessels, but it is seldom appropriate for the smaller vessels of the extremity. The smaller vessels are more likely to be narrowed by such a technique. In Gorman's study of popliteal artery injuries, all vessels that had been closed with lateral suture required reexploration.[27] Small noncircumferential wounds with minimal longitudinal arterial damage may be closed with a patch or with local resection and reanastomosis. The latter technique, however, often results in significant tension on the suture line. The advantage of using only a single suture line in this procedure (two are needed for a graft) is completely lost if there is any tension whatsoever on the suture line. We and others have found this only rarely applicable to vascular injuries, however, and we are more likely to employ an interposition graft.

Considerable controversy surrounds the proper graft material to use in cases of vascular injury. We strongly prefer the use of autogenous tissue for replacement of small-to medium-size vessels. The most appropriate graft in these circumstances is the contralateral saphenous vein. If for some reason this vein is not available, the ipsilateral vein may be used or, less favorably, the cephalic vein. Larger-caliber vessels may be replaced with the internal jugular vein or with the distal left renal vein. The use of autogenous arterial grafts such as the hypogastric or the external iliac, which are then replaced by a synthetic conduit, has been described, but indications for use of these techniques should be exceedingly rare.

The one disadvantage of the saphenous vein is its behavior in severe infection. The vein may completely disintegrate if it becomes infected, resulting in massive hemorrhage. Lau and coworkers[36] have expressed preference for synthetic grafts because infection of these tubes often presents with a sentinel hemorrhage that allows time for treatment. Moreover, with proper attention to wound care, and coverage of vein grafts with muscle tissue, including rotation flaps when necessary, the incidence of direct infection of vascular repairs should be infrequent enough not be a major deterrent to selecting the saphenous vein.

METHODS OF VASCULAR REPAIR
- Lateral suture
- End-to-end anastomosis
- Interposition graft

MANAGEMENT OF SPECIFIC VASCULAR INJURIES

Neck Injuries

Vascular injuries of the neck involve trauma to the carotid and, to a lesser extent, the vertebral arteries. Although the majority of the injuries result from penetrating trauma, injuries due to blunt trauma have increased in frequency. The possibility of irreversible neurological damage and the close association of these vessels to other vital structures in the neck make their diagnosis and management vital.

PENETRATING TRAUMA

When wounds to the neck that penetrate the platysma are routinely explored, injury to the carotid or vertebral arteries will be found 6% to 17% of the time.[33,39,52,53] Injury to the common carotid artery is more frequent than is injury to the internal carotid. In one of the largest reported studies of carotid injuries by Brown and associates,[7] injury to the common carotid artery accounted for 72% of the total injuries. Of 143 carotid artery injuries, 84 involved the left side and 59 the right side. This predilection for the left side might be related to the greater number of right-handed assailants. Thirty percent of the patients had associated injuries of the internal jugular vein, while there was a much smaller incidence of injuries to the pharynx, esophagus, trachea, larynx, and thyroid gland.

Gunshot wounds are by far the most common cause of injury to the carotid artery, being responsible for 68% to 75% of the injuries.[22,34,59] Most of the rest are due to stab wounds. (Blunt injury to the vessels of the neck are relatively rare and will be dealt with separately.) The type of injury sustained by the vessel is dependent upon the mode of injury. Civilian gunshot wounds are from low-velocity bullets, which usually cause complete transection of the artery or tangential injury with tissue loss. Stab wounds may result in lacerations or perforations. The formation of arteriovenous fistulas between the carotid and the adjacent internal jugular vein has also been described.

Bright red bleeding, an expanding hematoma, and a palpable thrill or bruit are all suggestive of major vascular injury in the neck. However, many vascular injuries may be missed because the bleeding may be tamponaded or temporarily sealed by a thrombus. Therefore, any penetrating wound to the neck must be considered serious. The management of asymptomatic neck wounds is controversial. Some advocate exploration of all wounds which traverse the platysma, while others feel observation is sufficient. Arteriography is a valuable diagnostic tool in penetrating neck wounds (Fig. 12.10). Again, there is controversy regarding its use. Some feel that all stable patients should undergo arteriography, even if signs of vessel injury are present. In a study by McCormick and associates,[41] arteriography was performed in 91 wounds of the neck and extremities, regardless of physical findings. The physical findings were often found to be unreliable, yielding a false negative result in 20% and a false positive result in 42%. Furthermore, arteriography may provide valuable decision making information regarding operative repair, such as delineating internal carotid artery injuries at the base of the skull. The major drawback to routine arteriography is the delay to operation, which may result in bleeding or neurologic deterioration. When arteriography is performed, all four vessels should be visualized. In addition to arteriography, plain radiographs of the neck may reveal soft tissue injuries, tracheal deviation by hematoma, or foreign bodies.

The major goals in the treatment of vascular injury in the neck are the avoidance of exsanguinating hemorrhage and of permanent neurologic deficit. Initially, the patient's airway should be assessed. An expanding hematoma may cause tracheal compression and respiratory compromise. Massive active bleeding should be controlled by direct pressure. Large-bore catheters are inserted for the administration of intravenous fluids. Penetrating wounds of the neck that are not actively bleeding should not be probed in the emergency room, because this may dislodge a thrombus and initiate bleeding. Similarly, nasogastric tubes are to be placed with caution, because coughing or gagging may also result in bleeding. A thorough neurologic examination is extremely important. Neurologic deficits due to cerebral ischemia or infarction are differentiated from those which may be due to associated head trauma or spinal cord injuries.

The best incision for operative exploration of vascular wounds in the neck is a diagonal one, along the medial border of the sternocleidomastoid muscle. If possible, control of the vessel proximal and distal to the suspected site of injury should be obtained before the hematoma is entered. In some cases, control of bleeding with direct digital pressure or a Fogarty balloon catheter placed intraluminally may be necessary.

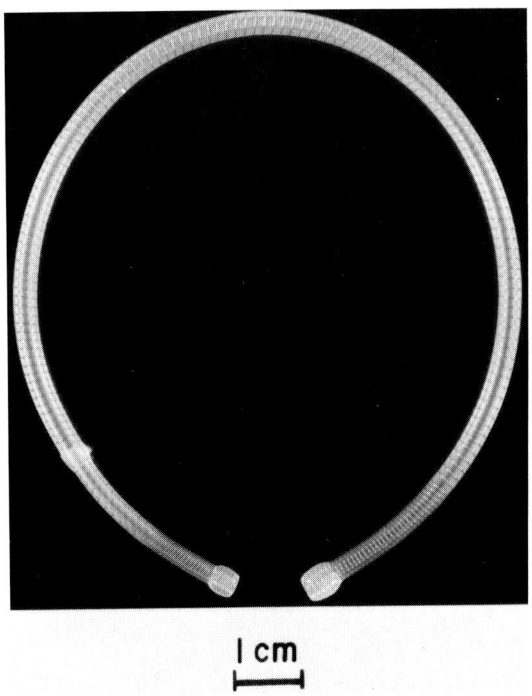

FIGURE 12.9
One type of shunt that may be used for temporary revascularization in complex injuries. The flow surface is heparin-bonded so that systemic heparinization is not required.

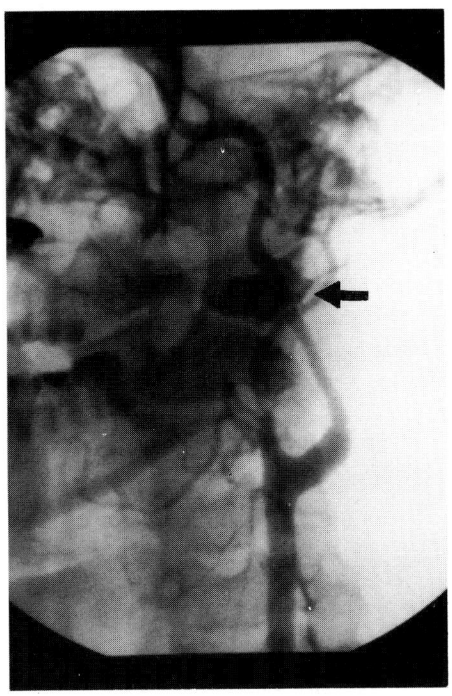

FIGURE 12.10
Injury to the high internal carotid with acute false aneurysm. Distal carotid control was not possible, so this lesion was treated by gradual ligation with a Crutchfield clamp with continuous (awake) clinical evaluation and EEG monitoring.

The various methods of repair of carotid injuries include lateral arteriorrhaphy with or without a vein patch, end-to-end anastomosis, interposition vein graft, prosthetic graft interposition, and ligation with or without bypass (Fig. 12.11). Lateral arteriorrhaphy may be performed in many instances where there is a simple laceration due to a stab wound. With many low-velocity gunshot wounds there are defects in the arterial wall which must be debrided until normal-appearing vessel is reached. An end-to-end anastomosis or an interposition graft is then used to repair the defect. The use of prosthetic grafts should be avoided and an autogenous saphenous vein used whenever possible. Penetrating injuries of the internal carotid artery at the base of the skull may be difficult to expose and adequate distal control of the vessel for repair may prove impossible. Gewertz and others[26] described five such patients who underwent extracranial-intracranial bypass. This involves the construction of an end-to-side anastomosis between a branch of the external carotid artery and a cortical branch of the middle cerebral artery. When technical considerations necessitate ligation of the internal carotid artery, this type of bypass may prevent ischemic neuronal dysfunction.

Concomitant injury to a vein, usually the internal jugular, may safely be ligated. For small lacerations of this vessel, however, suture repair may be possible. Associated injuries to neck structures such as the trachea and esophagus, should be identified. Repair of an esophageal injury should include drainage, which is best accomplished on the side opposite the arterial repair.

The majority of patients presenting with carotid arterial trauma will not have a neurologic deficit, and the management of these cases should consist of repair whenever technically possible. The proper management of patients with a neurologic deficit, however, is controversial. During and after the Korean War vascular repair was the accepted form of management for almost all patients. Bradley,[6] however, reported on five patients with preoperative hemiplegia or quadriplegia who underwent vascular repair. All five died in the postoperative period with clinical evidence of brain stem herniation. Autopsies performed on two of these patients showed extensive hemorrhagic infarction of the revascularized lobe. Based on these findings, along with the results of surgical revascularization in patients with acute strokes, Wylie[66] cautioned against revascularization in patients with neurologic deficits because of concern that the reconstitution of flow would result in hemorrhagic infarction. A military report based on the Vietnam experience by Cohen and others[15] also emphasized the significant morbidity and mortality in these patients.

In contrast to these findings, Liekweg and Greenfield,[38] in a review of 233 cases of carotid trauma, stated that patients with all grades of neurologic deficit short of coma should have primary vascular repair. They found the morbidity and mortality rates

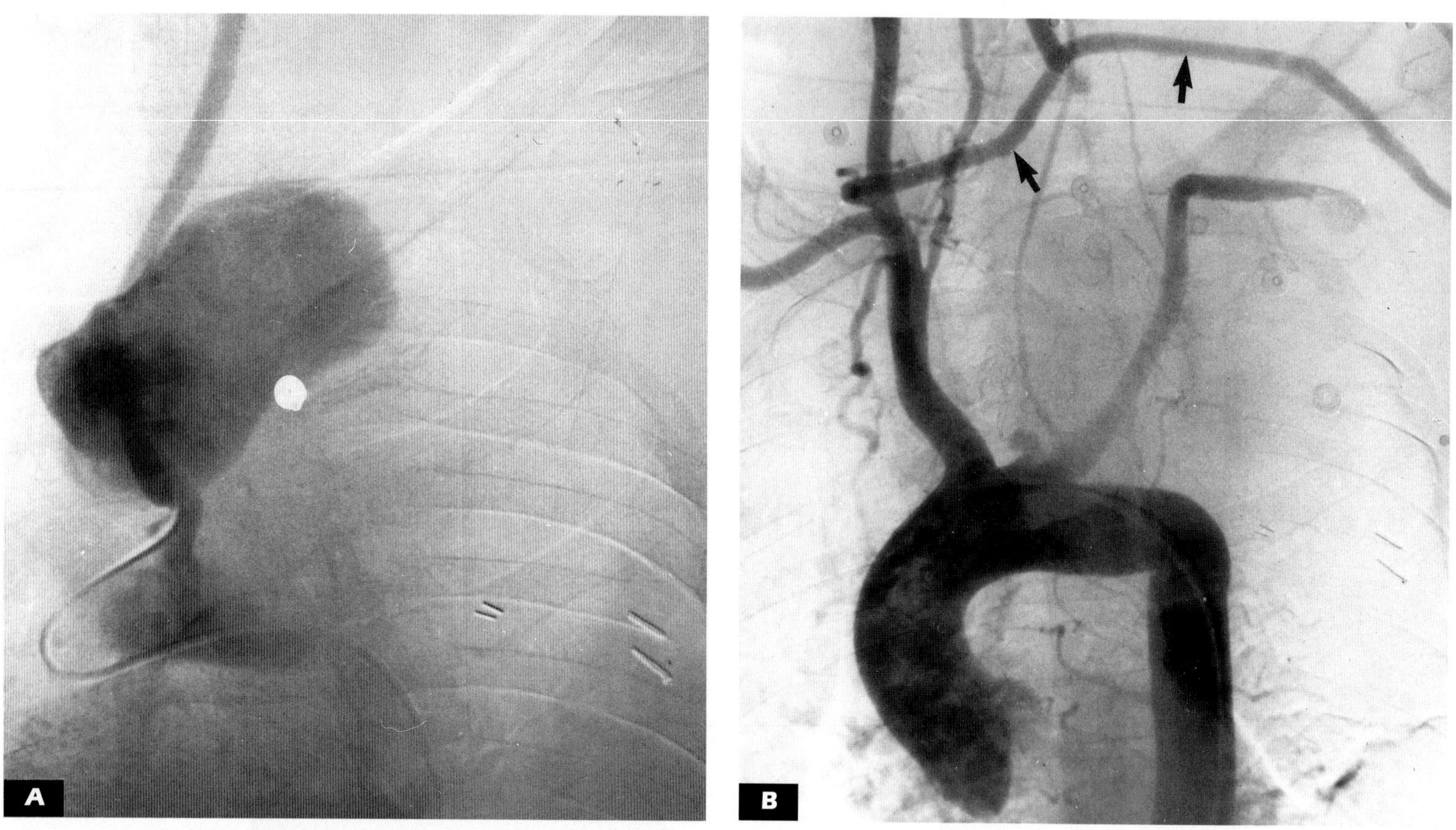

FIGURE 12.11 A Late false aneurysm of the left common cartoid artery discovered as a mediastinal mass seven years after a stab wound. **B** This injury was treated with ligation and bypass from the right cartoid using an autogenous saphenous vein graft.

were significantly less following repair than with ligation (15% vs. 50%). In patients with coma, the type of management had no effect on the eventual result. Similarly, Unger and associates[62] reviewed the English-language literature and found that of 186 patients presenting with severe neurologic deficits after carotid trauma, 34% improved following repair, whereas only 14% improved with ligation. Ledgerwood and colleagues[37] reported that of five patients who presented with deficits and subsequently died following repair, none exhibited hemorrhagic infarction at postmortem examination. In summary, the current evidence suggests that penetrating injuries to the carotid artery should be repaired in all instances. Ligation should be used only when repair is technically impossible or when the patient's overall condition does not allow for repair.

BLUNT TRAUMA

Blunt trauma to the carotid artery accounts for only about 5% of carotid injuries, but carries a mortality rate of 30% to 40%. In contrast to penetrating injuries, blunt trauma to the carotid most often involves the carotid bifurcation or the internal carotid artery. Four sources of trauma to the carotid artery have been described:

Direct blow to the neck, which most frequently injures the carotid bifurcation
Blow to the head resulting in abrupt extension and rotation of the neck, which stretches the internal carotid artery across the transverse processes of the first three cervical vertebrae
Intraoral trauma by foreign objects that injure the internal carotid artery posterior to the tonsillar fossa
Basilar skull fractures that traumatize the petrosal segment of the internal carotid artery[17]

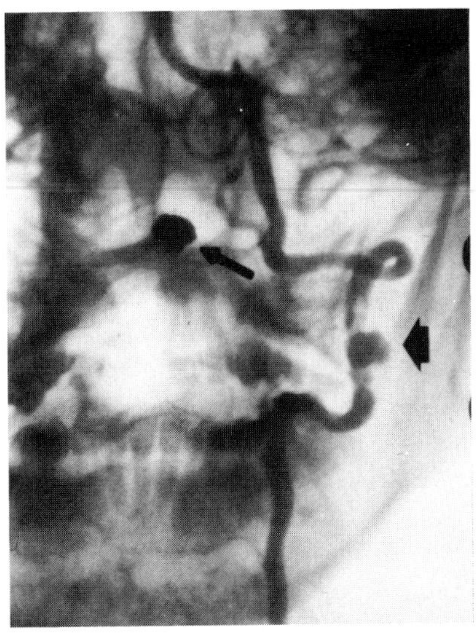

FIGURE 12.12 Injury to the cervical vertebral artery identified by use of complete angiography. Short arrow indicates extravasation from the vertebral artery. Long arrow indicates the bullet.

In a review by Krajewski and Hertzer,[35] the most common source of trauma was vehicular accident (55%), followed by falls (17%), objects striking the head or neck (15%) and brawls (10%).

The pathophysiology involved in blunt carotid trauma involves disruption of the intima with the subsequent development of thrombosis and eventual occlusion. Distal embolization or subintimal dissection may also occur from this injured area. The clinical diagnosis of this condition may be difficult. Often there are associated closed head injuries that may obscure the picture. Jernigan and Gardner[32] have described a set of clinical features which may aid in the diagnosis. These include a significant hematoma in one of the upper anterior triangles of the neck; Horner's syndrome, due to trauma of the superior sympathetic chain and the first ganglion; transient ischemic attacks; an interval between the time of injury and the development of severe neurologic symptoms (usually occurring in the first 24 hours); and finally, monoparesis or hemiparesis in an alert patient. Since this type of injury may be difficult to diagnose initially, arteriography is invaluable.

Injury to the vertebral arteries is rare, but it is recognized with increasing frequency because of the routine use of four-vessel angiography in neck trauma (Fig. 12.12). Meier and associates[42] reported that in a 16-year period from 1957 to 1973 only seven vertebral artery injuries were found. However, during a 3-year period from 1976 to 1979 after the institution of routine four-vessel angiography, 13 patients were diagnosed with this type of injury. In this study, all injuries were the result of penetrating trauma, the majority of which were located in the C6 area. Treatment consisted of proximal and distal ligation in eight patients, proximal ligation in three patients, Gelfoam embolization in one patient, and observation in one patient. These authors could attribute no morbidity or mortality to ligation of the vertebral artery. However, others have reported that unilateral vertebral artery ligation has been followed by fatal midbrain or cerebellar necrosis. It has been estimated that 3.1% of patients with a left vertebral ligation and 1.8% of patients with a right vertebral ligation will develop an acute midbrain necrosis.[60] This led Monson and his colleagues[43] to recommend that if a hypoplastic or anomalous contralateral vertebral artery is seen on arteriography, an attempt should be made to repair the injured vertebral artery rather than ligate it.

Venous Injuries

The diagnosis and management of vascular trauma has long emphasized arterial injuries. Proper treatment of venous injuries, however, is also important. Injuries to major veins, such as the inferior vena cava, carry a significant mortality rate, while the improper management of peripheral venous injuries may lead to amputation or significant long-term morbidity.

As with arterial injuries, the etiology of venous injuries may be penetrating or blunt trauma. In a review of 115 civilian venous injuries, Agarwal and co-workers found gunshot wounds responsible for 52%, stab wounds for 36%, blunt trauma for 7%, and shotgun wounds for 5% of venous injuries.[1] Iatrogenic causes occurring during surgical procedures or vascular instrumentation have also been reported. Rich and associates found that venous injuries occurred concomitantly with acute arterial injuries 38% of the time.[46] The most frequently injured veins are the superficial femoral vein, the inferior vena cava, and the internal jugular vein. The iliac veins, popliteal veins, portal venous system, and subclavian vein are less commonly involved.

The clinical diagnosis of venous injury is often more difficult than the diagnosis of arterial trauma. Massive venous hemorrhage may consist of a steady flow of dark blood, which may be accompanied by shock, depending on the size of the involved vessel. The presence of large hematomas is also often associated with venous bleeding. Acute venous insufficiency within the first 24 hours after injury is characterized by massive edema and a cool, bluish extremity. The most important diagnostic tool in the evaluation of venous injury is venography. This was shown by Gerlock and associates in a study of 30 consecutive cases of acutely injured extremities.[25] Five of these patients had positive venograms and the findings were confirmed at surgical exploration. The venous abnormalities that can be diagnosed with this modality include traumatic occlusions, thrombosis, and lacerations with hemorrhage. Postoperatively, venography is important in the evaluation of extremity edema and suspected deep venous thrombosis, and in examining the venous repair. Doppler ultrasound, impedance plethysmography, phlebogram, and radionuclide studies may also be useful.

Management of venous injuries depends on the location, severity of injury, and association with other trauma. Surgical principles include the use of pressure or packing to control hemorrhage initially and the use of a longitudinal incision along the course of the vein to provide adequate exposure for proximal and distal control. In cases of associated arterial injury, the artery is usually repaired first to minimize hemorrhage and anoxia to the distal extremity. Occasionally, the vein must be dealt with initially in order to clear the field for adequate arterial repair.

Treatment of the venous injury may consist of ligation, repair with lateral suture with or without a vein patch, reconstruction with an end-to-end anastomosis, or the insertion of a vascular graft. In the past the most common and, in fact, preferred treatment was ligation. Venous repair was often avoided because it was thought that there would be a high incidence of thrombophlebitis and possibly pulmonary embolism associated with it. Results from civilian studies as well as the Vietnam Vascular Registry have not borne this out, however. Rich and associates had no instances of clinical pulmonary embolism in 124 patients who underwent repair of venous injuries.[48] Gaspar and Treiman had no cases of thrombophlebitis in patients undergoing repair, but they documented three such cases in patients who had venous ligation.[24]

There are a number of clinical and experimental studies which document the deleterious effects of venous ligation and the importance of repair. Sullivan and colleagues reported in a study of 26 patients with popliteal vein injury, venous insufficiency (judged by massive edema and tense fascial compartments) did not occur in any of the 21 patients who had primary vein repair, but did occur in four of five patients who did not.[58] In another series, Rich and associates evaluated 110 patients with only popliteal vein injuries; they found a 51% incidence in edema of the involved extremity following ligation, compared to only 13% after repair.[47] Experimental studies in dogs[3] and baboons[68] have demonstrated that when the femoral vein is ligated, there is a significant (50% to 75%) reduction in femoral arterial flow accompanied by an increase in venous pressure and in femoral vascular resistance. Femoral arterial flow does not return to normal until 72 hours after the occlusion. The reduction in flow to the limb during this period might add an ischemic insult to an already traumatized extremity, or threaten the patency of the arterial repair. Thus, clinical and experimental evidence suggest that venous repair should be attempted if at all possible.

Before repairing the vein, the vessel should be explored for thrombi. If found, they should be gently extracted. Meticulous surgical technique is mandatory. Fine suture on a small needle should be used and the suture line should be left under less tension than with arterial repairs to avoid constriction. When a vein graft is necessary for repair, autogenous vein is the best replacement in all sites. Construction of panel grafts from autogenous vein is often required to create grafts that are of the same diameter as the native vein. The use of synthetic grafts has not been very encouraging. Adjunctive measures to enhance patency, such as the creation of arteriovenous fistulas and the use of anticoagulant and antiplatelet drugs, may be useful in selected circumstances.

Visceral Blood Vessel Injuries

CELIAC TRUNK AND BRANCHES

Injuries to the celiac trunk are infrequent due to its well-protected position and short length. The preferred method of dealing with injuries to the celiac trunk is repair, but sufficient collateral channels exist between the visceral arteries to allow for acute ligation. Hepatic arterial injuries may be treated by ligation, since the portal vein provides 80% of the total hepatic blood flow. If possible, ligation should be performed proximal to the gastroduodenal artery to allow this large vessel to serve as a collateral to supply arterial blood not only to the liver, but also to the bile duct. Busuttil and associates,[11] in a report of 21 patients with injuries to the porta hepatis, recommended that if the injury involves only the common hepatic artery or its primary branches, and if repair is not very straightforward, then ligation should be performed. In a patient suffering injury to both the hepatic artery and the portal vein, and if one vessel is to be repaired, the artery should be ligated and an attempt made at portal vein repair. Finally, injuries to the left gastric artery and splenic artery may be treated with ligation.

SUPERIOR AND INFERIOR MESENTERIC ARTERIES

Almost all of the injuries to the superior mesenteric artery are due to penetrating trauma. Rarely, blunt trauma may injure the artery at the point where it passes from beneath the pancreas.

In their report of eight patients with penetrating injuries to the superior mesenteric arterial circulation, Fullen and associates[23] developed a classification based on anatomical grounds and on the extent of ischemia. Zone I is from the superior mesenteric artery trunk of the aorta to the first branch, usually the inferior pancreaticoduodenal artery. Injuries here usually result in ischemia of the jejunum, ileum, and ascending colon and variable involvement of the transverse colon. Associated pancreatic trauma is common with zone I injuries. Zone II is the superior mesenteric artery trunk distal to the inferior pancreaticoduodenal artery and proximal to the middle colic artery. Injuries in zone II produce ischemia similar to that in zone I. Zone III is the superior mesenteric artery trunk distal to the middle colic artery. Injury at this level produces a widely variable extent of ischemia. Zone IV injury involves the segmental jejunal, ileal, or colic branches, and often results in minimal or no ischemia.

Exposure of zone I injuries is best accomplished by medial rotation of the spleen, pancreas, and kidney and the descending colon, following incision of the peritoneum lateral to the left paracolic gutter. Zone II of the superior mesenteric artery is exposed by opening the gastrocolic omentum or by a direct approach through the transverse mesocolon. Both zone I and zone II injuries require restoration of flow in order to avoid small bowel ischemia. This may be accomplished with lateral arteriorrhaphy, end-to-end anastomosis, or an interposition vein graft. Injuries in zone IV usually involve ligation and bowel resection. Almost all injuries to the inferior mesenteric artery can be treated with ligation.

PORTAL VENOUS SYSTEM

Injuries to the portal venous system include trauma to the portal, superior mesenteric, inferior mesenteric, and splenic veins. While the incidence of these injuries is relatively low, they carry a high mortality rate—50% to 70% in injuries to the portal vein. The reasons for this are the often difficult exposure, problems in controlling hemorrhage, and the high association with other vascular, enteric, and pancreatic trauma. In a review of 94 patients with 98 portal venous injuries, Graham and associates[28] found the highest mortality associated with portal vein injuries (51%), followed by superior mesenteric vein injuries (31%). None of the patients with inferior mesenteric vein or splenic vein injuries died. The etiology of these injuries is most commonly gunshot wounds, followed by stab wounds and blunt trauma.

Control of bleeding in portal and mesenteric vein injuries must be obtained before repair can be performed. This may be accomplished using the Pringle maneuver (clamping the hepatoduodenal ligament). The liver should not be deprived of blood flow for greater than 15 minutes in the normothermic patient or 45 minutes in the hypothermic patient. Methods of dealing with portal vein injuries include lateral venorrhaphy, end-to-end anastomosis, graft interposition (autologous vein or synthetic material), superior mesenteric vein to splenic vein anastomosis, ligation of the portal vein with portosystemic shunt, and ligation of the portal vein alone.[21]

Since 80% to 90% of the oxygen and nutrients to the liver are supplied by the portal vein, restoration of portal venous flow is the preferred method of management. Although ligation can be tolerated in most individuals, problems with intestinal infarction and chronic portal hypertension have been reported. When ligation is performed, a second-look procedure 24 hours later should be done to exclude retrograde thrombosis of the superior mesenteric vein and small bowel infarction. In addition, large amounts of fluid may be needed to replace fluid sequestered in the splanchnic bed after ligation. The use of portosystemic shunts has been associated with a high rate of encephalopathy.[65] Injuries to the superior mesenteric vein should be repaired, since ligation will result in massive edema of the small intestine. Ligation with splenectomy is usually required for splenic vein injuries, while injuries to the inferior mesenteric vein are almost always treated by ligation.

RENOVASCULAR INJURIES

The incidence of renovascular injuries is relatively low, and injury to these vessels is often associated with other severe abdominal injuries. The cause in most cases is penetrating trauma but blunt injury of the vascular pedicle may also occur. Brown and colleagues,[8] in a review of 154 patients with renovascular trauma, reported blunt trauma responsible for 16% of the injuries. The mechanism of injury to the renal artery in blunt abdominal trauma is felt to be from a sudden deceleration of the abdomen, which sets the kidney in motion and stretches the vascular pedicle. This causes an intimal tear with subsequent thrombosis.

The diagnosis of renal vascular injury by the presence or absence of hematuria is not reliable. Up to 20% of patients with renal injury will not have hematuria. The intravenous pyelogram is a useful test. In a review by Clark and colleagues,[14] only 3% of patients with renal artery trauma had normal pyelograms. In addition the functional state of the contralateral kidney can be ascertained. Selective renal arteriography may be valuable, especially in patients with blunt trauma. Intraoperatively, injury to the kidneys or renal vasculature should be suspected if a retroperitoneal hematoma is seen.

Management of renovascular injuries is either by reconstruction or nephrectomy. The mode of management chosen is dependent upon the extent of associated injuries, hemodynamic stability of the patient, and damage to renal vessels and parenchyma, as well as the functional status of the other kidney and the duration of renal ischemia. Of 154 patients with renovascular injuries reviewed by Brown and colleagues,[8] only 24% had attempted revascularization; the majority underwent nephrectomy or ligation. Only 16 of 27 renal artery injuries were successfully repaired and resulted in kidney salvage.

Surgical management depends on the type of injury. In blunt trauma with renal artery thrombosis, isolation of the vessel and thrombectomy may be the treatment of choice. At the time of thrombectomy, any intimal tears should be identified. Other alternatives for revascularization include bypass from the abdominal aorta to the distal renal artery, and autotransplantation.

Renal vein injuries should be repaired when possible. The left renal vein can be safely ligated near the inferior vena cava as there is adequate collateral drainage through lumbar, adrenal, gonadal, and capsular vessels. On the right side, however, collaterals are usually not present and ligation cannot be tolerated.

Extremity Injuries

The two most important factors in the management of wounds of the extremities are the time from initial injury to the performance of definitive repair and the extent of associated nervous, bone, joint, and soft tissue injuries.

The recognition of vascular injury in the extremity may be difficult (Fig. 12.13).[54] Tangential wounds may not result in diminution of distal pulses or the appearance of ischemia even though significant vascular injury has occurred. Conversely, if associated significant extravascular trauma is present with swelling, hypovolemia, fracture, and perhaps associated head injury, the determination of adequacy of the distal circulation in an injured extremity may be quite difficult. The Doppler velocity detector may be helpful in this regard when pulses are difficult to palpate. A difference in pressure between the injured and uninjured extremity of more than 10 mm Hg is considered significant. A high index of suspicion for vascular injury should be maintained in cases of penetrating trauma to the extremities, particularly if the projected path of the bullet is in proximity to a major vascular channel (Fig. 12.14).

Considerations regarding angiography have already been discussed. It should always be kept in mind that if arteriography is deemed necessary but one is reaching the limits of tolerable ischemia time, a "one-shot" percutaneous arteriogram can be performed by the surgeon, either in the emergency room or preferably on the operating table with portable equipment. Although not as elegant as a formal arteriogram, an emergency angiogram may provide sufficient information to plan to vascular repair (Fig. 12.15).

Equally important is the decision not to attempt revascularization of an injured extremity. If concomitant bone, joint, skin, muscle, and nervous injuries are so severe that a functional limb cannot be achieved, then there is no point in the technical exercise of repairing the injured vasculature. Unfortunately, it is often difficult to determine the ultimate outcome beforehand. Robbs and Baker have reported revascularization of extremities with anesthesia, paralysis, extreme hypothermia, skin mottling, and increased muscle turgor, and have achieved a viable functional limb in nearly two thirds of cases.[51] Although revascularization was associated with myoglobinuria, disseminated intravascular coagulation, and secondary hemorrhage with extensor compartment infarction, none of these patients died. These results argue for an aggressive attitude toward treatment of vascular injuries, particularly in the young, who are more likely to withstand such serious complications (Fig. 12.16).

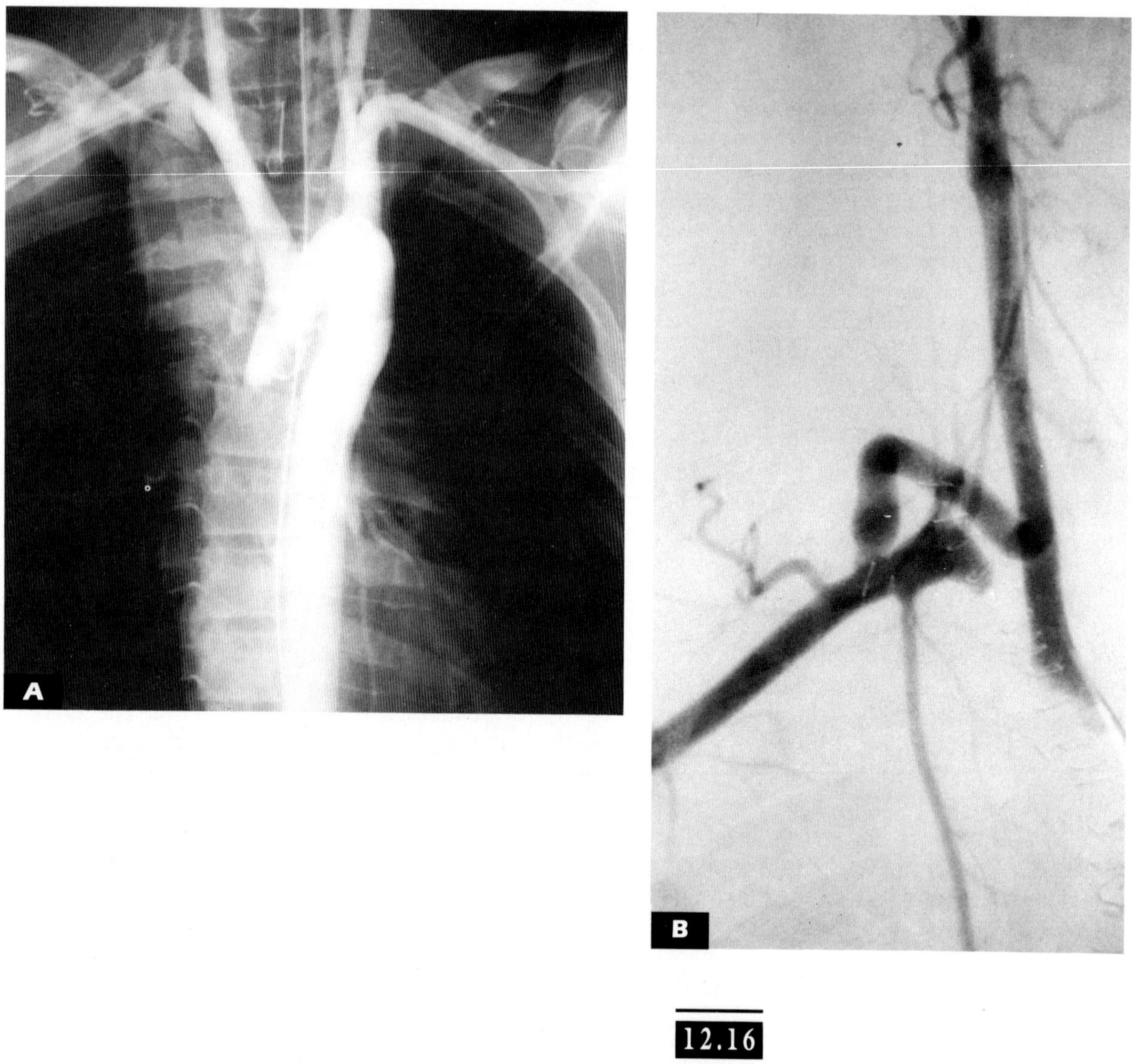

FIGURE 12.13 A This patient presented with normal upper extremity pulses but a widened mediastinum on chest x-ray after blunt chest trauma. **B** An arch angiogram demonstrates the injury to the right subclavian artery treated with saphenous vein bypass from the adjacent carotid artery.

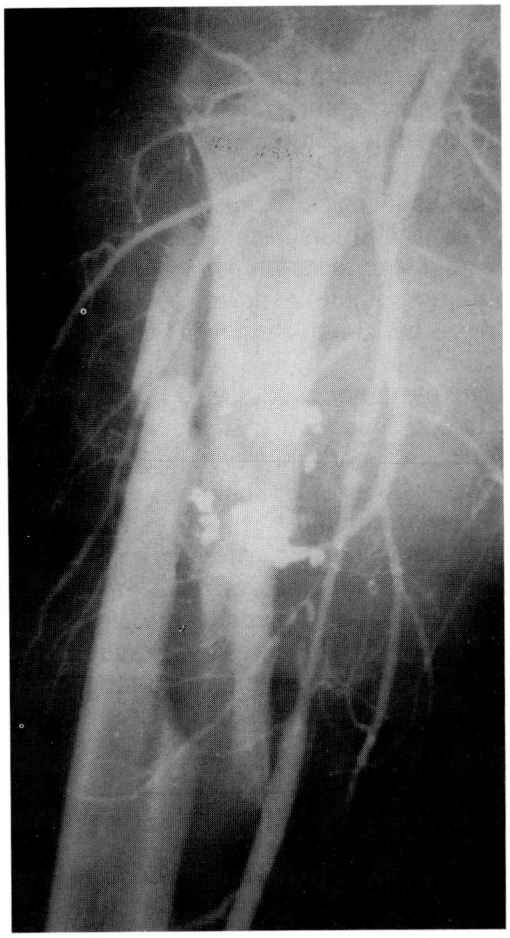

FIGURE 12.14 Large-caliber gunshot wound to the thigh. The shock wave of the missile has caused intimal disruption and dissection of the femoral artery. The angiogram demonstrates not only the presence of the vascular injury but also the extensive segment of femoral artery that must be replaced.

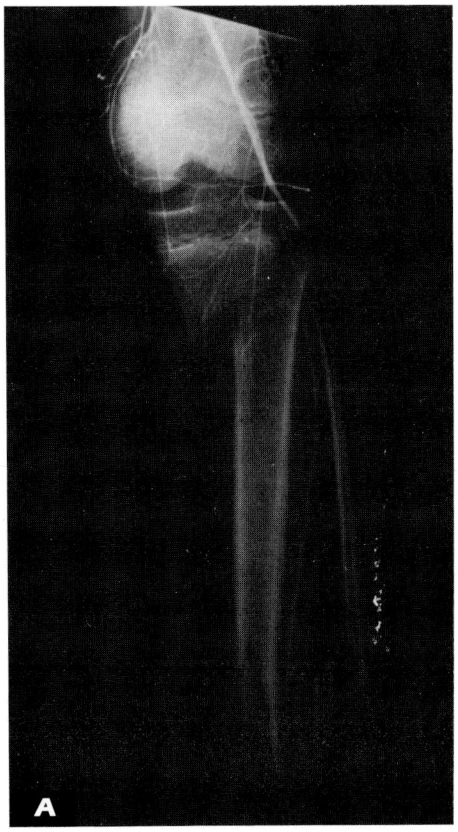

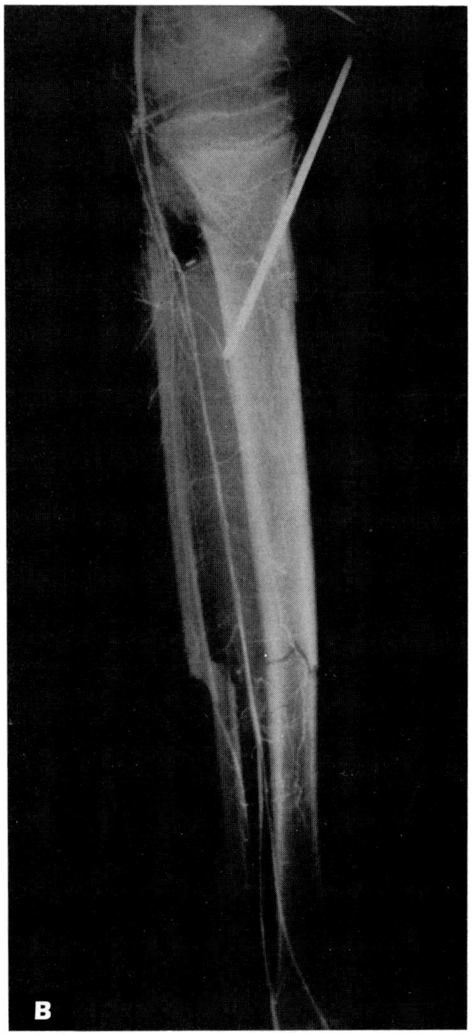

FIGURE 12.15 A Operative arteriogram of a child with blunt leg trauma and distal ischemia. Sharp cutoff at the fracture site identifies the trapped popliteal artery. **B** After the vessel is released and the fracture is reduced, a repeat arteriogram shows satisfactory flow into the leg.

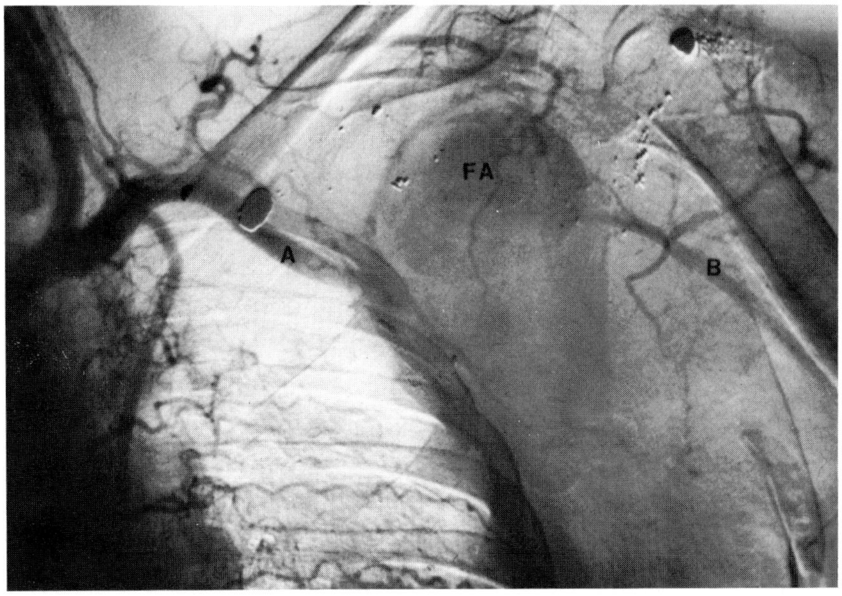

FIGURE 12.16 Late sequelae of vascular injury. This patient presented with a pulsating mass in the shoulder six months after having been shot multiple times in the chest. Cords of brachial plexus are in the wall of the false aneurysm (FA) between the axillary (A) and brachial (B) arteries, significantly complicating its operative management.

In most cases general anesthesia is preferred for the operative management of extremity injuries. Although regional anesthesia or even local anesthesia may be appropriate in selected cases, most procedures are of sufficient duration that general anesthesia is preferred. The extremities are widely prepared for complete and total access to the entire limb. In lower extremity injuries the opposite limb is also prepared for surgery, so that if a saphenous vein graft is required, it can be harvested from the uninvolved extremity. This reduces the likelihood of the development of venous insufficiency in the involved extremity. Similarly, in upper extremity injuries at least one leg is prepared as well for the same reason. Proximal and distal control are achieved before disturbing the perivascular hematoma and exploring the injury. Common femoral or proximal superficial femoral injuries in the groin may require a separate inguinal incision through which the external iliac artery is approached extraperitoneally to ensure proximal control. Popliteal injuries can be approached medially or posteriorly. The medial approach is more versatile and can be used in combination with orthopedic repair of the joint in cases of posterior dislocation. Injuries to a single tibial vessel do not require repair, but can be safely ligated. If two or more vessels are injured in the calf, however, an attempt should be made to repair at least one of them.

Systemic heparinization is often inadvisable if there is associated extensive soft tissue trauma. Local heparin administration, however, can be applied. After assuring patency of the distal arterial tree by passage of a Fogarty catheter, the vessels should be irrigated with a heparinized saline solution.

Distal pulses will be available in the completely prepared extremity. If these are not easily palpable, one should suspect an additional site of injury or distal thromboembolism. Even if pulses are palpable, an operative arteriogram is advisable upon completion. This takes only a few minutes to do and is used not only to check the vascular repair but also to ensure patency of the distal arterial tree.

Occasionally with relatively minor injuries, either lateral arteriorrhaphy or local resection, mobilization, and primary anastomosis can be performed. More frequently, however, an interposition graft will be required. Autogenous tissue should be used whenever feasible and should be excised from the opposite extremity.

Revascularization of a severely ischemic extremity can result in tremendous local swelling. This swelling can result in compression of nervous structures resulting in permanent damage and can also aggravate ischemic injury. This excessive pressure can be released by an appropriate fasciotomy. We prefer a long lateral incision down to the fibula, with incision of the fascia separating

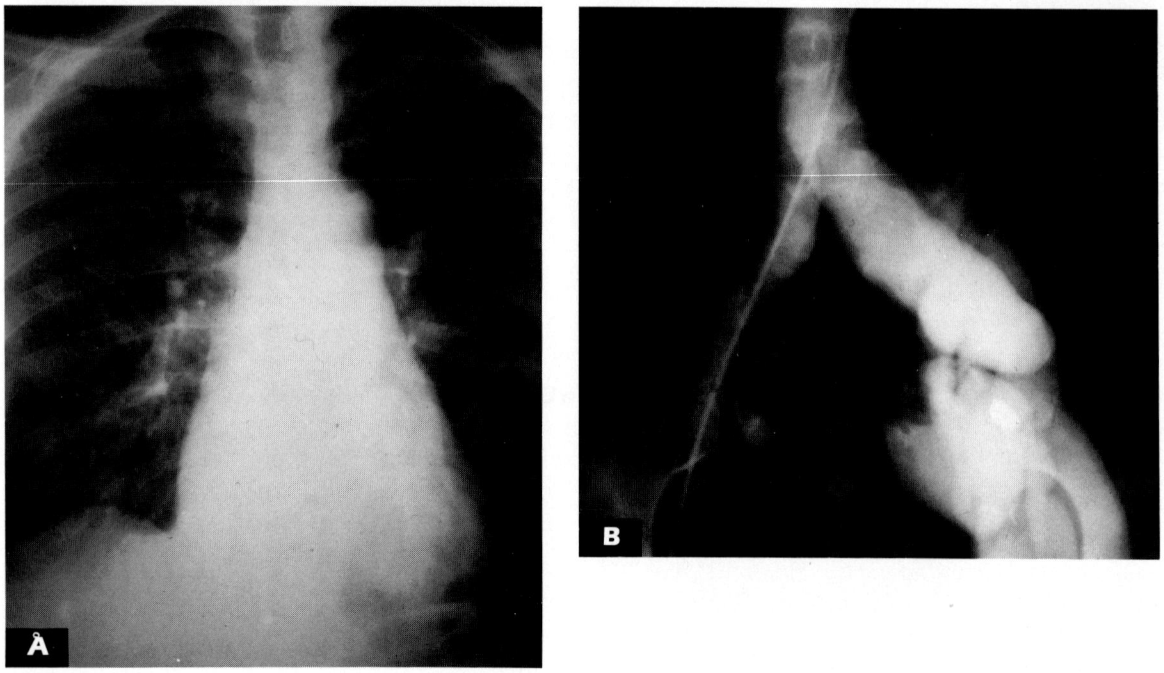

FIGURE 12.17 This patient's complaint was shortness of breath due to heart failure. He had been shot 15 years earlier which accounted for the iliac arteriovenous fistula. **A** Enlarged cardiac silhouette. **B** Iliac arteriovenous fistula.

the anterior peroneal, deep posterior, and superficial posterior compartments. Actual resection of the fibula is not required.

Arteriovenous Fistulas

An injury that produces concomitant penetration of adjacent arteries and veins may result in the formation of an endothelialized connection between these two vascular structures. When this occurs the rapid flow of blood to the low-pressure venous circuit tends to keep the lesion open. The deleterious hemodynamic effects of the fistula require some time to become manifest (Fig. 12.17).[40] The hypovolemia, fluid retention, and ultimate heart failure are usually seen in fistulas that were not immediately recognized and were presented for treatment months or even years after the original injury (Fig. 12.18).

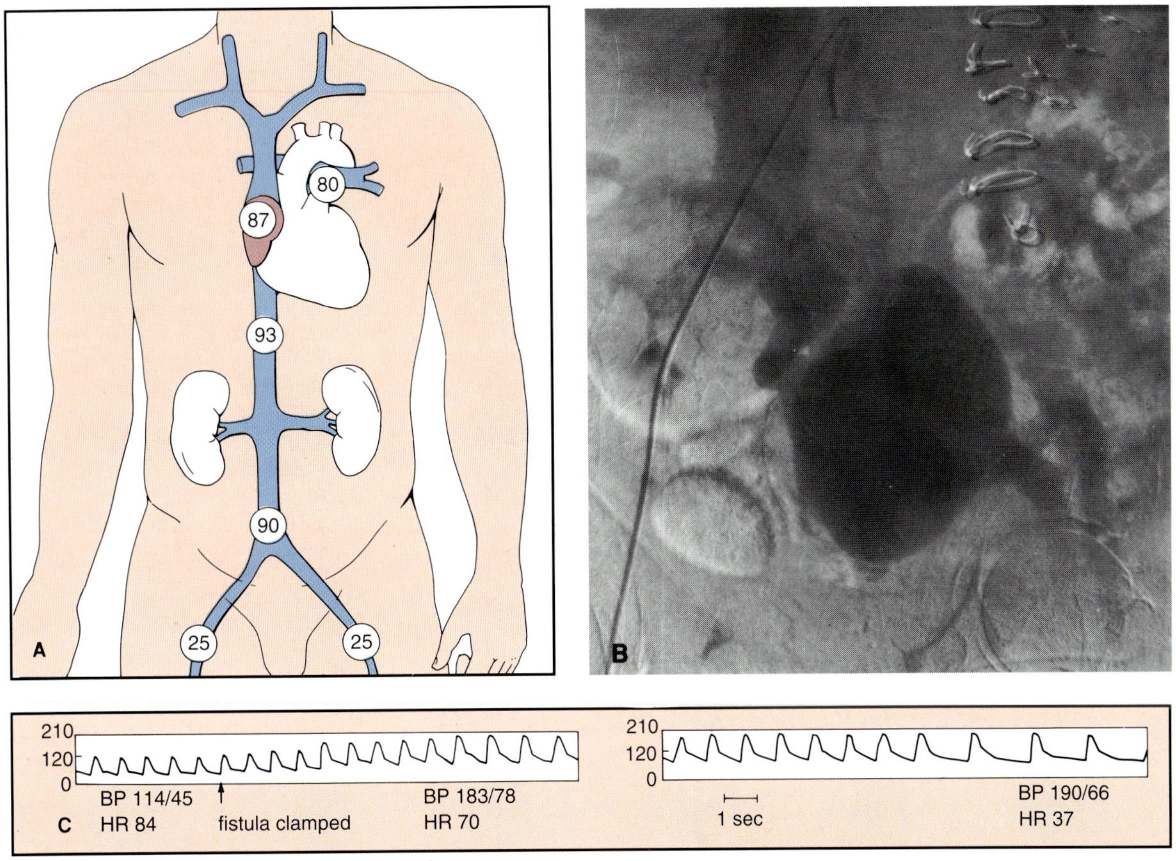

FIGURE 12.18 A Diagnosis of arteriovenous (AV) fistula by measurement of venous oxygen saturation. A Swan-Ganz catheter was passed from the groin and measurements of venous oxygen saturation made at various points. The step-up at the IVC level was due to a left iliac AV fistula. **B** Limited angiographic demonstration of the AV fistula is shown. **C** Blood pressure recording made during closure demonstrates the hemodynamic consequences of the large AV fistula. The marked flow through the fistula is compensated for by acquired hypervolemia. This extra volume immediately expands the vasculature when the fistula is suddenly closed, causing hypertension and reflex bradycardia (Branham's sign). (McCann RL, Makhoul RG, Damiano R: Diagnosis of arteriovenous fistula by venous oxygen saturation: A case report. J Vasc Surg 3:921–923, 1986.)

Arteriovenous fistulas should be closed when recognized. This is easier to accomplish in the acute setting before the development of significant collateral flow. Proximal and distal control must be achieved of all four poles of the fistula before opening it. Additional small collateral flow can be controlled by insertion of balloon catheters, if necessary, to produce a dry field. Repair is usually accomplished by lateral arteriorrhaphy and, when indicated, venorrhaphy. Interposition of extraneous muscular fascial tissue is not necessary if a satisfactory repair has been achieved. In chronic fistulas, the proximal arterial tree may be tremendously enlarged. This enlarged segment may not regress following closure of the fistula (Fig. 12.19) and indeed this vessel should be observed subsequently for the development of significant aneurysmal change.[29]

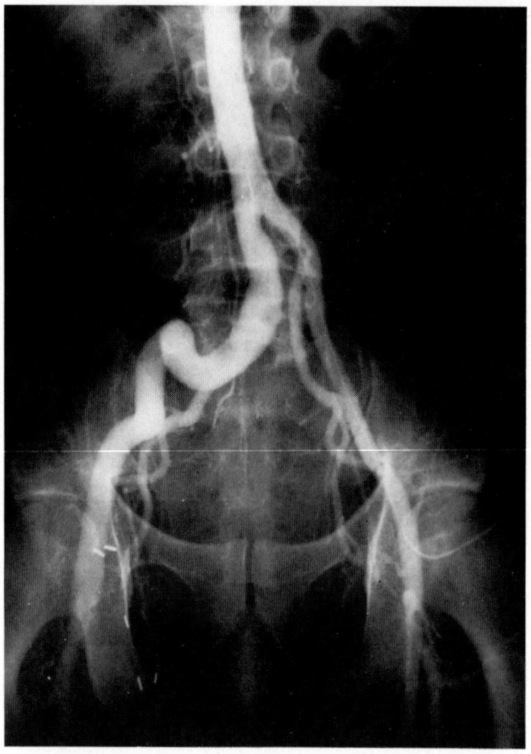

FIGURE 12.19 Ten years following closure of a femoral arteriovenous fistula, the proximal iliac artery remains dilated and tortuous.

REFERENCES

1. Agarwal S, Shah P, Clauss RH et al: Experience with 115 civilian venous injuries. J Trauma 22:827–832, 1982.
2. Baker SP, O'Neill B, Karpf RS: The Injury Fact Book. Lexington, MA, Lexington Books, 1984.
3. Barcia PJ, Nelson TG, Whelan TJ: Importance of venous occlusion in arterial repair failure: An experimental study. Ann Surg 175:225–227, 1972.
4. Bernheim BM: Blood vessel surgery in the war. Surg Gynecol Obstet 30:564–567, 1920.
5. Bole PV, Purdy RT, Munda RT et al: Civilian arterial injuries. Ann Surg 183:13–23, 1976.
6. Bradley EL: Management of penetrating carotid injuries: An alternative approach. J Trauma 13:248–255, 1973.
7. Brown MF, Graham JM, Feliciano DV et al: Carotid artery injuries. Am J Surg 144:748–753, 1982.
8. Brown MF, Graham JM, Mattox KL et al: Renovascular trauma. Am J Surg 140:802–805, 1980.
9. Budnick LD, Chaiken BP: The probability of dying of injuries by the year 2000. JAMA 254:3350–3352, 1985.
10. Burnett HF, Parnell CL, Williams GD, Campbell GS: Peripheral arterial injuries: A reassessment. Ann Surg 133:701–707, 1976.
11. Busuttil RW, Kitahama A, Cerise E et al: Management of blunt and penetrating injuries to the porta hepatis. Ann Surg 191:641–648, 1980.
12. Carrel A: The surgery of blood vessels etc. Johns Hopkins Hospital Bull 18:18–28, 1907.
13. Chitwood WR, Rankin JS, Bollinger RR, Moylan JA: Brachial artery reconstruction using the heparin-bonded Sundt shunt. Surgery 89:355–358, 1981.
14. Clark DE, Georgitis JW, Ray FS: Renal arterial injuries caused by blunt trauma. Surgery 90:87–92, 1981.
15. Cohen A, Brief D, Malhewson C: Carotid artery injuries: An analysis of eighty-five cases. Am J Surg 120:210–214, 1970.
16. Committee on Trauma Research, Commission on Life Sciences, National Research Council and the Institute of Medicine: Injury in America, A Continuing Public Health Problem. Washington, National Academy Press, 1985.
17. Crissey MM, Bernstein EF: Delayed presentation of carotid intimal tear following blunt craniocervical trauma. Surgery 75:543–549, 1974.
18. DeBakey ME, Simeone FA: Battle injuries of the arteries in World War II, an analysis of 2471 cases. Ann Surg 123:534–579, 1946.
19. Drapanas T, Hewitt RL, Weichert RF, Smith AD: Civilian vascular injuries: A critical appraisal of three decades of management. Ann Surg 172:351–360, 1970.
20. Feliciano DV, Bitondo CG, Mattox KL et al: Civilian trauma in the 80's, a 1 year experience with 456 vascular and cardiac injuries. Ann Surg 199:717–724, 1984.
21. Fish JC: Reconstruction of the portal vein: Case reports and literature review. Am Surg 32:472–478, 1966.

22. Fry RE, Fry WJ: Extracrainal carotid artery injuries. Surgery 88:581–587, 1980.
23. Fullen WD, Hunt J, Altemeier WA: The clinical spectrum of penetrating injury to the superior mesenteric arterial circulation. J Trauma 12:656–664, 1972.
24. Gaspar MR, Treiman RL: The management of injuries to major veins. Am J Surg 100:171–175, 1960.
25. Gerlock AJ, Thal ER, Snyder WH: Venography in penetrating injuries of the extremities. Am J Roentgenol Radiumther Nucl Med 126:1023–1027, 1976.
26. Gewertz BL, Samson DS, Ditmore QM, Bone GE: Management of penetrating injuries of the internal carotid artery at the base of the skull utilizing extracranial-intracranial bypass. J Trauma 20:365–369, 1980.
27. Gorman JF: Combat wounds of popliteal artery. Ann Surg 168:974–980, 1968.
28. Graham JM, Mattox KL, Beall AC: Portal venous system injuries. J Trauma 18:419–422, 1978.
29. Graham JM, McCollum CH, Crawford ES, DeBakey ME: Extensive arterial aneurysm formation proximal to ligated arteriovenous fistula. Ann Surg 191:200–203, 1980.
30. Hughes CW: Arterial repair during Korean War. Ann Surg 147:555–561, 1958.
31. Jahnke EJ, Seely SF: Acute vascular injuries in the Korean War: An analysis of 77 consecutive cases. Ann Surg 138:158–177, 1953.
32. Jernigan WR, Gardner WC: Carotid artery injuries due to closed cervical trauma. J Trauma 11:429–435, 1971.
33. Jones RF, Terrell JC, Salyer KE: Penetrating wounds of the neck: An analysis of 274 cases. J Trauma 7:228–236, 1967.
34. Karlin RM, Marks C: Extracranial carotid artery injury: Current surgical management. Am J Surg 146:225–227, 1983.
35. Krajewski LP, Hertzer NR: Blunt carotid artery trauma: Report of two cases and review of the literature. Ann Surg 191:341–346, 1981.
36. Lau JM, Mattox KL, Beall AC et al: Use of substitute conduits in traumatic vascular surgery. J Trauma 17:541–546, 1977.
37. Ledgerwood AM, Mullens RJ, Lucas CE: Primary repair vs ligation for carotid artery injuries. Arch Surg 115:488–493, 1980.
38. Liekweg WG, Greenfield LJ: Management of penetrating carotid arterial injury. Ann Surg 188:587–592, 1978.
39. Markey JC, Hines JL, Nance FC: Penetrating neck wounds: A review of 218 cases. Am Surg 41:77–83, 1974.
40. McCann RL, Makhoul RG, Damiano R: Diagnosis of arteriovenous fistula by venous oxygen saturation: A case report. J Vasc Surg 3:921–923, 1986.
41. McCormick TM, Burch BH: Routine angiographic evaluation of neck and extremity injuries. J Trauma 19:384–387, 1979.
42. Meier DE, Brink BE, Fry WJ: Vertebral artery trauma: Acute recognition and treatment. Arch Surg 116:236–239, 1981.
43. Monson DO, Saletta JD, Freeark RJ: Carotid vertebral trauma. J Trauma 9:987–997, 1969.
44. O'Neill JA Jr: Traumatic vascular lesions in infants and children. In Dean RH, O'Neill JA (eds): Vascular Disorders of Childhood. Philadelphia, Lea & Febiger, 1983.
45. Perry MD, Thal ER, Shires GT: Management of arterial injuries. Ann Surg 173:403–408, 1971.
46. Rich NM, Baugh JH, Hughes CW: Acute arterial injuries in Viet Nam: 1000 cases. J Trauma 10:359–369, 1970.
47. Rich NM, Hobson RW, Collins GW, Anderson CA: The effect of acute popliteal venous interruption. Ann Surg 183:365–368, 1976.
48. Rich NM, Hughes CW, Baugh JH: Management of venous injuries. Ann Surg 171:724–730, 1970.
49. Rich NM, Spencer FC (eds): Vascular Trauma. Philadelphia, WB Saunders, 1978.
50. Robbs JV, Baker LW: Arterial trauma involving the lower limb. J Trauma 18:324–328, 1978.
51. Robbs JV, Baker LW: Cardiovascular trauma. Curr Prob Surg 21:1–87, 1984.
52. Roon AJ, Christensen N: Evaluation and treatment of penetrating cervical injuries. J Trauma 19:391–397, 1979.
53. Saletta JD, Lowe RJ, Lim LT et al: Penetrating trauma of the neck. J Trauma 16:579–587, 1976.
54. Schwartz LB, McCann RL: Traumatic false aneurysm of the common carotid artery presenting as a mediastinal mass: A case report. J. Vasc Surg. 10:281-286, 1989.
55. Shumaker HB: Arterial suture techniques and grafts; past, present and future. Surgery 66:419–433, 1969.
56. Simpson ET, Aitchison JM: Study of subclavian venipuncture in 172 shocked patients. J Trauma 22:781–784, 1982.
57. Snyder WH, Thal ER, Bridges RA et al: The validity of normal arteriography in penetrating trauma. Arch Surg 113:424–428, 1978.
58. Sullivan WG, Thorton FH, Baker LH et al: Early influence of popliteal vein repair in the treatment of popliteal vessel injuries. Am J Surg 122:528–531, 1971.
59. Thal ER, Snyder WH, Hays RT, Perry MO: Management of carotid artery injuries. Surgery 76:955–962, 1974.
60. Thomas GI, Anderson KN, Hain RF, Merendino KA: The significance of anomalous vertebral-basilar artery communications in operations of the heart and great vessels. Surgery 46:747–757, 1956.
61. Trunkey D: Trauma. Scientific American 249:28–35, 1983.
62. Unger SW, Tucker WS, Mrdeza MA et al: Carotid arterial trauma. Surgery 87:477–487, 1980.
63. Van Trigt P. Unpublished data.
64. Villavicencio JL, Gonzales-Cerna JL: Acute vascular problems of children. Curr Prob Surg 22(8):1–85, 1985.
65. Voorhees AB, Chaitman E, Schneider S et al: Portal-systemic encephalopathy in the non-cirrhotic patient. Arch Surg 107:659–664, 1973.
66. Waller, JA: Injury Control, p 107. Lexington, MA, Lexington Books, 1984.
67. Warden MJ, Machiedo GW, Swan KG et al: Management of penetrating vascular injuries to the extremities. In: Hobson RW II (ed): Venous Trauma Pathophysiology, Diagnosis and Surgical Management. Mount Kisco, NY, Futura, 1983.
68. Wright CR, Hobson RW: Hemodynamic effects of femoral venous occlusion in the subhuman primate. Surgery 75:453–460, 1974.
69. Wylie EJ, Hein MF, Adams JE: Intracranial hemorrhage following surgical revascularization for treatment of acute strokes. J Neurosurg 21:212–215, 1964

13

wound care

Basil A. Pruitt, Jr.
Cleon W. Goodwin

Wound healing begins at the time of tissue injury. In the initial care of the wounded patient, emphasis must be placed on prevention of further injury, prompt correction of shock, prevention of organ failure, and restoration of a physiologic wound environment. Wound care that meets all of these requirements permits uncomplicated wound healing, while failure of any aspect of treatment may exaggerate tissue damage, delay healing, and predispose the patient to local and systemic sepsis, organ dysfunction, and even a fatal outcome.

The goals of surgical wound care include preservation of tissue, prevention of infection, maintenance of function, and timely closure. To prevent further loss of tissue, the injury process should be interrupted as rapidly as possible by removing the patient from contact with the injuring agent or vice versa. Hemorrhage must be controlled and hypovolemia and hypoxemia corrected immediately to prevent extension of tissue damage and the occurrence of organ failure. When the patient has been stabilized, the wound should be cleansed, irrigated, and debrided to reduce the microbial density, remove foreign bodies, and excise all nonviable tissue to minimize the risk of infection. Thereafter, desiccation and secondary contamination of extensive open wounds and burns should be prevented by closure or, alternatively, application of appropriate dressings, topical antimicrobials, or a biologic dressing. Perioperative antibiotics, begun upon admission, are employed to reduce risk of wound and intracavitary infections in patients with penetrating wounds.

Maintenance of function is achieved by conservation of all viable tissue, prevention of infection, immobilization in a position of function, if necessary, and the institution of physical therapy at the earliest possible time. Wounds from which all nonviable tissue and foreign bodies can be removed within 10 hours of injury can be closed primarily.[5] Delayed primary closure, secondary closure by suture or grafting, and even closure by scarification are used for other wounds depending upon the adequacy of debridement, the microbial status of the wound, and the extent of the tissue defect.

CAUSES OF IMPAIRED WOUND HEALING

Ischemia

An adequate blood supply that delivers sufficient oxygen and nutrients to a sufficiently immobilized wound free of bacteria permits unimpeded wound healing, characterized by an orderly sequence of cellular changes, tissue maturation, and increase in tensile strength. Ischemia can result from microvascular thrombosis secondary either to physical injury of the vasculature by the initial trauma or to hypovolemic shock resulting from initial blood loss or plasma volume deficits later in the post-injury period. Both inadequate blood flow and impaired oxygenation of the blood due to pulmonary dysfunction can cause wound hypoxia that, if severe enough, will result in necrosis. In addition to causing hypovolemia, wound edema can increase tissue pressure to levels above those of venous pressure, thus augmenting edema formation and further impairing tissue blood flow. Moreover, by increasing intercapillary distance, edema may further reduce tissue oxygen tension.

Maintenance of adequate intravascular volume is the single most effective measure for preventing wound ischemia and infection.[26] Aulick and associates have shown that the vascular bed of a large granulating wound is essentially parasitic to the circulatory system of the intact organism.[8] Perfusion of a healing wound appears to vary primarily with changes in systemic pressure and cardiac output. The new blood vessels in the wound are denervated, without neurogenic vasoconstriction tone, and unresponsive to variations in oxygen or substrate delivery. The vascular smooth muscle in the granulation tissue neovasculature responds to alpha but not beta agonists, whether from endogenous or exogenous sources, and therefore will vasoconstrict in response to such stimuli as hemorrhage, spinal anesthesia, hypothermia, or intravenous injection of epinephrine or norepinephrine. Obviously, such vasoconstriction in the wound reduces its blood flow, and these stimuli can be expected to be detrimental to wound healing and resistance to infection. An adequate intravascular volume and increased cardiac output are necessary to meet the high blood flow requirement of the wound and provide sufficient substrate for its predominant glycolytic metabolic pathways.[9]

To provide the optimum environment for wound healing, hypovolemia should be corrected by appropriate transfusion and fluid therapy. In patients with extensive wounds, volume replacement restores blood pressure, pulse rate, urine output, and sensorium before cutaneous perfusion. Conversely, the onset of hypovolemia triggers compensatory mechanisms that divert blood flow away from the wound and cutaneous vascular bed to maintain flow to vital tissues, such as the heart and brain. Volume replacement should restore not only the usual vital signs, but also peripheral circulation, as evidenced by normal skin temperature and vigorous capillary refill.

A number of local and systemic factors predispose wounds to ischemia and infection. Wound edema leads to increased tissue pressure and subsequent reduction in microvascular blood flow. Edema should be minimized by positioning and, if possible, active motion of the involved part.[102] Escharotomy may be necessary to maintain adequate blood flow in a limb with encircling full-thickness burns, and fasciotomy may be required in patients with deep burns or mechanical injury, in whom edema has increased subfascial tissue pressures to levels that compromise the microcirculation (Fig. 13.1). Blood flow is reduced in traumatized but still viable tissue, whether caused by the initial injury or by rough handling of tissue by the surgeon; such tissue heals slowly and is more susceptible to infection.[17] Tissue in which the microcirculation is compromised should be debrided to reduce the likelihood of wound infection. Inappropriately placed ligatures encompassing large amounts of tissue, and sutures under undue tension can also produce ischemic tissue necrosis and adversely affect wound healing.[41] The location of the wound influences the rate of healing. Wounds in areas of high tissue vascularity, such as the face and neck, heal quickly, while those in locations with less vascularity, such as thick layers of adipose tissue or the distal regions of the extremities, heal more slowly and are more prone to infection. Muscle, with a very high capillary density, seldom becomes infected and heals quickly. Drying of exposed wound surfaces damages the underlying small blood vessels and leads to the formation of a nonviable neoeschar (Fig. 13.2).

Systemic factors may potentiate wound ischemia, impair subsequent healing, and increase susceptibility to infection. Diabetes mellitus causes regional ischemia by producing both large and small-vessel occlusive disease and by promoting capillary basement membrane thickening. Higher local perfusion pressures are needed in diabetic patients to heal lower extremity wounds.[10] In diabetic animal models, collagen synthesis is significantly decreased; however, since insulin administration improves this deficit, ischemia may play only a partial role.[30] In similar studies of incisional wounds, tensile strength was reduced in diabetic rats.[33]

Atherosclerotic peripheral vascular diseases may produce ischemia in tissues distal to the site of a vascular obstruction. While perfusion may be sufficient for intact tissues, a superimposed injury may impose a demand for blood flow that exceeds the supply capacity of the obstructed vessels. Such tissues, often in the distal portions of the lower extremities, almost always become necrotic and infected. Wound repair is often impossible until adequate blood flow is restored by a peripheral vascular reconstruction. Irradiated tissues are also prone to ischemic damage following injury. This susceptibility appears to be due to the obliterative arteritis caused by radiation.[111]

Hypoxia

Blood flow determines the rate of oxygen delivery to tissue, and the effects of hypoxia on wound healing to a large extent must be interpreted in terms of perfusion and wound microvascular integrity. The healing wound can be viewed as an organ in which anaerobic metabolism predominates. The wound consumes large quantities of glucose and produces lactate and pyruvate, without a proportionate increase in oxygen utilization.[118] The oxygen consumed by the wound appears to be used by the inflammatory cells responsible for initiating the healing process and controlling infection.

Tissue perfusion seems to be more important for wound healing than the oxygen-carrying capacity of the blood. Anemia (within certain bounds) does not appear to affect wound healing. As long as circulating blood volume is sufficient to ensure adequate tissue perfusion, increasing the hematocrit does not directly improve wound healing.[40] Conversely, patients with stable cyanotic congential heart disease, even those with marked systemic hypoxemia, exhibit only a moderate slowing of an ultimately intact healing process. However, at the level of the wound tissue, hypoxia produces markedly deleterious effects on collagen synthesis, fibroblast replication, angiogenesis, and epithelialization. Although the initial hypoxia caused by the injury *per se* has been cited as the stimulus that initiates tissue repair,[43] sufficient oxygen is thereafter necessary to support the cellular activity essential for wound healing.[76]

Collagen synthesis is critically dependent on the availability of molecular oxygen for the hydroxylation of proline and lysine, which is necessary for cross-linking newly made collagen trimers.

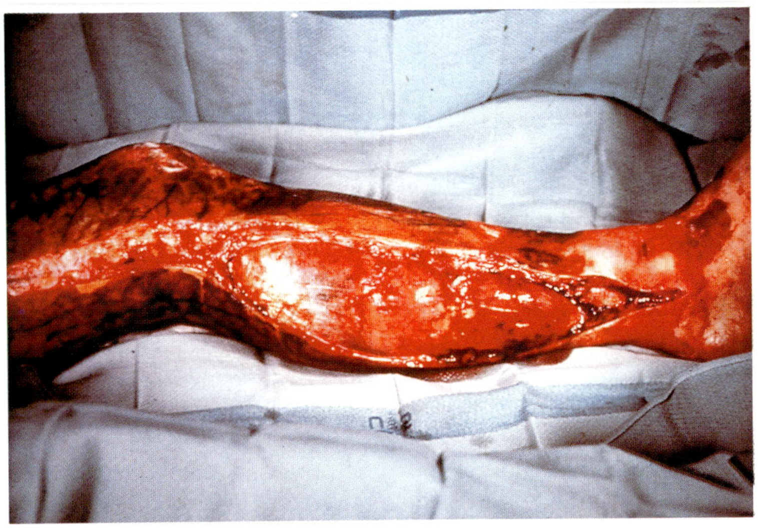

FIGURE 13.1 Subfascial edema in this deeply burned leg made the initially placed escharotomy incision, extending proximally and distally from the exposed muscle, ineffective in restoring nutrient blood flow to unburned tissues. Fasciotomy was required to reduce the elevated tissue pressure. Note the dark foci of thermal discoloration on the surface of the proximal portion of exposed muscle that bulges above the cut edges of the fascia.

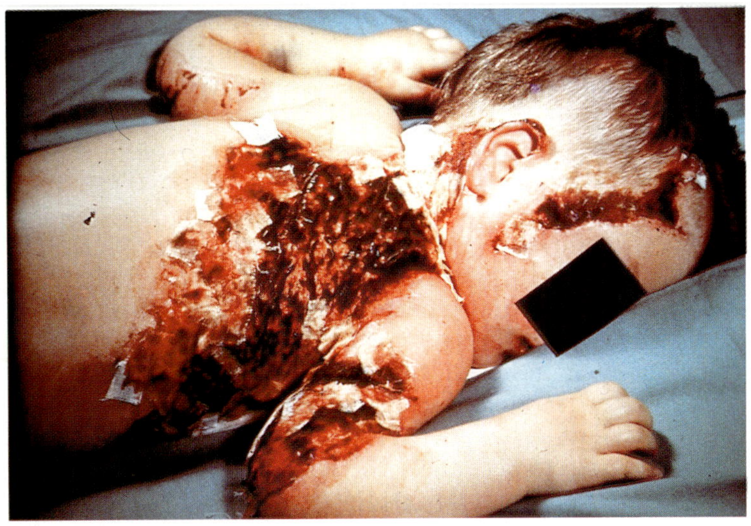

FIGURE 13.2 Following separation of the eschar from the burn wounds of this child, desiccation of the exposed immature granulation tissue led to formation of the dark neoeschar in which infection rapidly developed.

Hypoxia results in less stable collagen with reduced tensile strength.[107,116] Fibroblast proliferation is proportional to oxygen availability; the optimal PO_2 for replication of fibroblasts is approximately 30 to 40 torr.[75] Likewise, new vessel formation in the healing wound is sensitive to tissue oxygen levels and appears to proceed down a steep oxygen gradient.[52] Oxygen also appears to regulate the rate of epithelialization.[66] Wounds in poorly perfused hypoxic tissues are prone to infection.

Hunt and associates were able to decrease tissue infection by increasing oxygen concentrations in inspired gases, and subsequently in the blood supplied to the wound.[44] This effect appeared to be related to elevated tissue PO_2 levels and not to major changes in wound perfusion and has led those investigators to promote oxygen as an antibiotic.[53] In general, maximal wound healing can be accomplished by maintaining an adequate intravascular volume and a hematocrit level that does not increase cardiac work. Oxygen and mechanical ventilation should be administered as necessary to maintain the arterial PO_2 in the range of 80 to 90 torr.

Motion

Excessive motion can also impair wound healing and result in wound dehiscence or graft loss. The injured parts should, if anatomically possible, be elevated to prevent or limit edema formation and be placed at rest to reduce tension on the wound edges and prevent application of shear stress to a skin flap or a skin graft. The patient should be immobilized with the wounded part in the position of function to minimize subsequent functional deficits. The degree of immobilization required may range from simple restriction of activity for a wound of limited extent that does not involve a functional area, to rigid total immobilization for an extensive wound or one that involves deep tissues, such as muscles, tendons, or bone. Immobilization in the latter case requires application of a splint or cast that fixes the joints above and below the wound or grafted area.

Infection

Infection as a result of inadequate debridement of contaminated tissue is another common cause of impaired wound healing. The risk of wound infection is related to the level of contamination and the type of organisms present in the wound (see Microbial Factors in Wound Infection). Traumatic wounds are invariably contaminated, and both the density of the microbial population and the type of organisms present determine the incidence and characteristics of infection.[89] The initial contaminating organisms are predominantly the gram-positive resident skin flora and those organisms from the environment, gram-positive, gram-negative, and fungal, that have been carried into the tissue by the wounding agent or other foreign bodies, such as clothing or soil. The number of organisms, initially low, increases with time in untreated wounds. Prompt cleansing and debridement are essential to reduce the number of microorganisms in the wound and to remove all nonviable tissue and foreign bodies that predispose to persistence and proliferation of microorganisms (Fig. 13.3).

The wound flora also ,changes in character to become predominantly gram-negative within 5 to 10 days.[99] Generic and strain-specific properties of microorganisms are important in terms of both local and systemic effects. Streptococci elicit an intense local inflammatory reaction that expands by contiguous spread and by way of lymphatics, with little tendency to deep tissue invasion. Staphylococci have a greater propensity to involve deep tissues, but the intensity of the evoked inflammatory reaction often leads to formation of a thick inflammatory membrane that retards extension of the abscess and also limits the effectiveness of systemic antibiotic therapy. Staphylococcal toxins may also exert systemic effects of variable severity, such as the toxic shock syndrome attributed to toxic shock syndrome toxin-1 (TSST-1) production. Enzymes and metabolites produced in varying amounts by various gram-negative organisms exert cytotoxic effects that promote local invasion and systemic effects that may impair the function of remote organs, for example, endotoxin, exotoxins, extracellular polysaccharides, vascular permeability factors, collagenase, elastase, lipase, nucleases, and hemolysins.[88]

Anaerobic organisms are common in heavily contaminated wounds, particularly those in which the gastrointestinal tract has been violated. Clostridial organisms proliferate rapidly in nonviable tissue, and their toxins produce marked systemic effects. Other anaerobes appear to increase synergistically the invasive potential of aerobic organisms and typically produce infections that burrow along or across tissue planes. Nonbacterial organisms may also impair wound healing and cause genera-specific wound infections. *Candida* species frequently colonize burns and other wounds but seldom invade. Infections caused by *Aspergillus* species and *Fusarium* species are usually confined to the subcutaneous tissues, but they may invade even deeper tissues in the compromised host (Fig. 13.4). The *Phycomycetes* are aggressive invaders and readily traverse tissue planes to infect tissues beneath the investing fascia, necessitating radical debridement or even amputation to control the septic process.[90]

The risk of gas gangrene and all other wound infections is reduced by prompt debridement of all necrotic and heavily contaminated tissue. Additional protection is provided by the application of a topical antimicrobial agent to a burn wound and, in patients with significant penetrating wounds, prophylactic administration of systemic antibiotics started on admission, supplemented intraoperatively, and discontinued after one postoperative dose. Immunization, active or passive depending upon the patient's immunization status, eliminates the risk of tetanus.

In wounds that cannot be closed primarily, the success of subsequent closure is influenced by microbial density. The presence of 10^5 or more organisms per gram of tissue is associated with a high rate of subsequent wound infection or graft failure. The identification of bacteria on a specifically prepared smear of a homogenized biopsy specimen has been equated with a microbial density of greater than 10^5 organisms per gram of tissue and used as an indication that further preparation is required before a wound is closed.[101] In wounds requiring secondary closure, the type of organism present is of lesser importance in terms of success of closure, but streptococci in small numbers can cause postclosure cellulitis and even the rapid lysis of skin grafts.

MICROBIAL FACTORS IN WOUND INFECTION

- Density of microorganisms > 10^5 per gram of tissue
- Proliferation of organisms on foreign bodies
- Lack of microbial competition
- Time-related changes in microbial flora
- Microbial toxins and enzymes
- Endotoxin
- Exotoxins
- Vascular permeability factor
- Extracellular polysaccharides
- Collagenase, elastase, proteases, lipase, nucleases, hemolysins
- Microbial motility
- Antibiotic resistance
- Intrinsic
- Antibiotic-induced

Nutritional Deficits

Nutritional deficits may also impair wound healing, as is made manifest by the higher wound infection rates in patients who are significantly overweight or malnourished before injury.[1] Following injury, sufficient calories, nitrogen, essential fatty acids, minerals, and vitamins (particularly vitamin C) must be provided by the enteral or parenteral route to satisfy the elevated nutritional needs of the hypermetabolic injured patient and to provide the substrates required for tissue repair and wound healing.[98]

WOUND MANAGEMENT

Wound Cleansing and Debridement

Although lightly regarded by some, wound debridement tests the skills of even the most accomplished surgeon. As described earlier, rapid population of the newly created wound bed by fibroblasts is a critical step in normal healing. Any factor that delays this normal response predisposes the wound to infection and compromises wound integrity. Necrotic tissue impairs host resistance in the wound by inhibiting leukocyte bacterial phagocytosis and killing. Severely contused but viable tissue is more prone to infection than is uninjured or minimally injured tissue.[17] Foreign bodies in contaminated wounds lower the number of bacteria necessary to cause tissue infection. Such foreign bodies include not only the usual debris accompanying blunt and penetrating trauma, but also suture material and surgical drains.[24] Hematomas that are often associated with severe wounds also potentiate infection and retard effective wound healing. All of these detrimental factors, when present, should be removed by careful wound debridement.

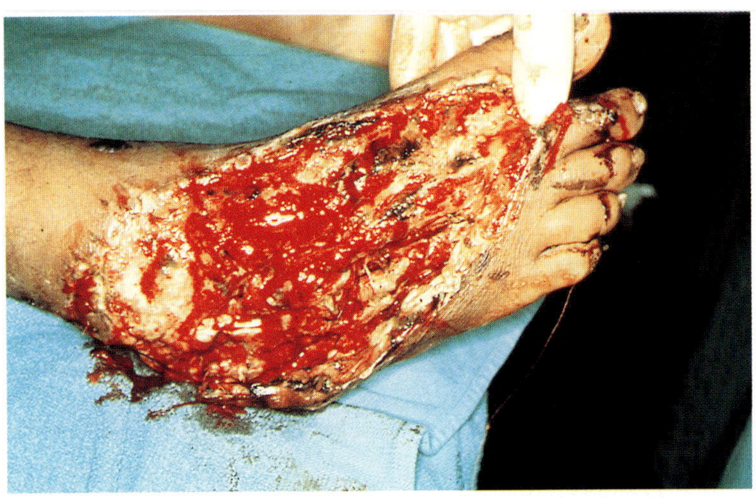

FIGURE 13.3 Inadequate debridement and primary closure of a large flap of ischemic, partially avulsed skin was followed by infection, which necessitated excision of the necrotic skin. Note the dark blood clot occupying the base of the wound just distal to the ankle and the darker colored focal areas of necrosis of the tissue overlying the heads of the first and second metatarsals.

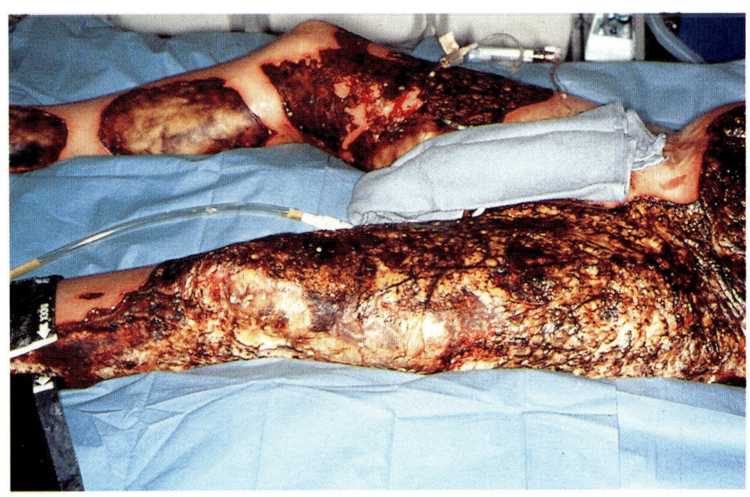

FIGURE 13.4 Generalized, invasive fungal burn-wound infection has caused the discoloration and necrosis evident in both the unexcised burn wounds on the medial aspect of the right leg and the previously excised burn wounds of the right thigh, left leg, and left thigh.

The goals of wound debridement are reduction of bacterial load and the removal of debris that can serve as a nidus for infection. By using sterile technique and appropriate anesthesia, all foreign and necrotic tissue is meticulously removed from the wound. Loose debris and free fluid can be removed by irrigation and gentle suction, but adherent eschar and dead tissue often require sharp excision down to the level of viable uninfected tissue. Severely contused tissue should also be removed if such structures are expendable; however, nonexpendable structures such as major nerves, tendons, and facial features should be preserved while any perfusion remains. Fortunately, areas such as the face that are richly vascularized are often ensured of survival. In long-standing wounds, fibrotic granulation tissue must be excised if collapse of the wound to eliminate dead space is required. Following debridement, bleeding from small vessels is controlled by direct pressure; larger vessels should be electrocoagulated and major vascular structures ligated with a minimal amount of nonreactive suture material.

Effective debridement requires considerable judgment and experience on the part of the surgeon. A tissue depth with circulation adequate to resist infection and to support wound healing is indicated by brisk bleeding and the typical appearance normally expected for that tissue in its uninjured state. Such signs are subject to misinterpretation by inexperienced operators. Especially in muscle, small patent blood vessels may traverse grossly necrotic tissue, and cut surfaces may bleed briskly. However, the cyanotic appearance and lack of contraction on electrical stimulation verify that the muscle is not viable. In addition to removing necrotic tissue and foreign material, wound debridement effectively reduces the degree of bacterial contamination of the wound. Often, debrided wounds can then be closed without subsequent infection.

However, clinical assessment of wound integrity is often erroneous, and decisions of which wounds to debride and how extensive a debridement to carry out, if wrong, will be attended by the development of wound infection. Wound biopsy with both quantitative bacterial cultures and histologic examination allows differentiation of colonization from invasive infection.[85] Histologic confirmation of invasive infection in the wound bed that is not readily controlled by antibiotic therapy alone is an indication for surgical excision of the involved tissue. Closure without subsequent infection can be guided by quantifying bacterial contamination in the wound. Wounds with bacterial densities greater than 10^5 organisms per gram of tissue should usually not be closed, since the incidence of wound infection in such situations is 50% to 100%.[101] Lesser magnitudes of bacterial contamination generally are associated with successful wound closure, unless the patient has impaired host resistance. Group A β-hemolytic streptococci are a major exception to the above guideline on quantitative bacterial counts. These organisms are much more virulent than other bacteria because they produce cytolytic enzymes. Relatively low numbers of these organisms can produce a wound infection characterized by rapidly spreading cellulitis and lymphangitis.

Topical Application of Antimicrobial Agents

The role of topical antimicrobial agents in controlling wound infection is well established in burn wounds and will be discussed later. However, the place of such agents in the management of other types of wounds is uncertain. In theory, topical application of antimicrobial agents produces high drug concentrations in the immediate vicinity of the wound and should lower bacterial density chemotherapeutically by direct physical contact. Unfortunately, with the exception of mafenide (Sulfamylon), most topical antimicrobial agents penetrate poorly into tissue and probably do little to reduce bacterial counts below the wound surface. Those agents that do penetrate, such as neomycin, have severe systemic toxicity and cannot be used. Efficacy studies of topical antimicrobial agents usually evaluate combined topically and systemically administered agents; most trials have been unable to demonstrate any added advantage of topical therapy in preventing infection in closed wounds.[12] Systemically administered antibiotics remain the most effective method of controlling propagation of infection into surrounding tissues.

Topical antimicrobial agents do appear to play an effective role in the control of bacterial proliferation in contaminated wounds undergoing active serial debridement, in fresh clean wounds that cannot be immediately closed (such as large soft tissue defects for which there is no tissue available for immediate closure), and in contaminated surface wounds closed with meshed split-thickness skin grafts. In each of these situations topical antimicrobial agents are employed to limit microbial proliferation and reduce the bacterial density of contaminated wounds. Topical antimicrobial agents do not permit closure of heavily contaminated wounds which should be left open until all necrotic tissue had been removed and the microbial burden reduced.

McManus and colleagues have recently reviewed the most commonly used topical antimicrobial agents, which include gentian violet, hypochlorite solution, penicillin, polymyxin B, mafenide, gentamicin, povidone-iodine, silver sulfadiazine, and chlorhexidine compounds.[60] As mentioned above, mafenide, either as cream or as a solution, is uniquely effective because of its wide antibacterial spectrum, high tissue penetration, and low incidence of antimicrobial resistance. The aminoglycosides are much less useful because of their high rate of microbial antibiotic resistance and low therapeutic ratio. Solutions of povidone-iodine, silver nitrate, and hypochlorite are cytotoxic and mildly impair epithelialization when used in their usual clinically effective concentrations. However, this drawback is primarily important for partial-thickness, skin surface wounds. In order to deliver adequate concentrations of antimicrobials to the wound bed, these agents must be suspended in an aqueous solution or a water-miscible base. The use of oil-based suspension media prevents effective delivery of the active agent to the wound.

Wound Closure

The degree of bacterial contamination and extent of tissue viability determine the timing of safe wound closure. The premature closure of dirty, ischemic wounds is invariably followed by wound breakdown and sepsis. While most clean, relatively atraumatic wounds may be closed soon after their occurrence, those characterized by large quantities of necrotic debris and purulent drainage may require many weeks to heal completely.

PRIMARY CLOSURE

Primary closure (also called *per primam* closure and healing by primary intention) involves reapproximation of full-thickness wound edges soon after the wound has been created. Granulation tissue formation between the wound's coapted edges is minimal and wound contraction usually does not occur. Epithelium spreads across the small exposed surface within 24 to 48 hours and serves to seal the wound from bacterial contamination, although it provides no strength to the closed wound. Primarily closed wounds are either sterile or contain very low densities of bacteria. The interval that can elapse between wounding and final closure before increasing bacterial contamination makes infection likely depends on the clinical circumstances, but varies between 6 and 12 hours. Most incisions used in elective surgical procedures and many accidental lacerations are closed primarily.

DELAYED PRIMARY CLOSURE

Delayed primary closure was introduced in World War I as the best method for treating wounds that were heavily contaminated or severely traumatized.[13,108] At the time of initial debridement soon after injury, foreign material and contused or nonviable tissues are removed, and hemostasis is obtained. As originally described, the wound is then left open and is packed with gauze dressings. Unless infection develops, this wound dressing is left in place until the closure procedure.[18,35] Three to seven days later, the original dressing is removed and the wound, if clean, is closed. Delayed primary closure does not delay the development of wound strength.[42] An example of a wound treated by this method is the skin incision for surgery of perforated diverticulitis with fecal spillage. When the wound is closed on the third or fourth postoperative day, it has the same tensile strength on the seventh postoperative day as a primarily closed incision.

Current usage of delayed primary closure employs a modification of the above-described technique. The wound dressings are changed several times, even daily, instead of leaving the packing in until anticipated closure. In this manner, any residual necrotic tissue can be debrided, thus removing potential foci of infection. Further control of bacterial proliferation can be obtained by using dressings saturated with topical antibacterial solutions. Robson and Heggers advocate the use of quantitative wound biopsy to assess readiness of wounds for closure.[101] However, most surgeons rely on the physical appearance of the wound to determine the timing of the closure procedure. Using this technique of serial dressing changes, with or without topical antimicrobial solutions, complete healing without infection is much more likely than with the original wartime method of passive observation of the packed wound for several days.

SECONDARY CLOSURE

Secondary closure (also called healing by third intention) involves reapproximation of the surfaces of a granulating wound. Such conditions occur when a primarily closed wound breaks down and is resutured later, after granulation tissue has formed on its surface or when a deep wound has not been sutured primarily. In this latter case, the wound has been left open beyond the time interval for primary closure (more than 4 or 5 days). Because granulation tissue is present, scarring and contraction are much more extensive in the healed wound.

A number of methods for secondary closure are available. The most frequently used is suture approximation. Apposition of the wound surfaces can be difficult because of the presence of relatively nonpliable fibrotic granulation tissue. Even when the wound appears sealed at skin level, large dead spaces frequently remain and these dead spaces may become infected. However, the use of layered suture closure to obliterate dead space potentiates wound infection at a higher rate than otherwise occurs in the dead spaces that the buried sutures attempt to address.[20] Granulating wounds with exposed flat surfaces, such as an open skin incision, can be temporarily closed with biologic dressings, such as cadaver allograft or porcine xenograft.[32] These biologic dressings have the added advantage of reducing bacterial density in the granulating wound bed and of preparing the wound bed for secondary suture or autografting. For large soft tissue defects, split-thickness skin autografts can provide effective permanent closure. Meshing the skin graft allows drainage of fluid collections beneath the graft and penetration of topical antibacterial solutions. It should be realized that, in addition to its tendency to produce noncollapsing dead spaces, granulation tissue causes extensive scarring and weaker wound healing. All of those drawbacks can be avoided by excising the granulating wound margins, when possible, down to normal tissue. Such wounds can then heal with less scarring and subsequent contracture.

CLOSURE BY SECONDARY INTENTION

Closure by secondary intention is healing by biologic processes without surgical intervention. A wound defect is first covered by granulation tissue and then closed by contraction and secondary ingrowth of epithelium. Contraction plays a major role by bringing dermal structures together and reducing the surface area of the wound. The growth of epithelium over granulation tissue slows the contraction process, and large areas of scar covered only by epithelium tend to be unstable. While healing by secondary intention usually is undesirable, large areas of tissue loss not amenable to surgical closure will ultimately close if the defect is allowed to fill with granulation tissue and to contract. Such wounds usually arise from severe trauma with massive tissue loss, or from primarily closed wounds which have become infected and dehisced.

WOUND DRAINAGE

Wound drains may be required when less than ideal obliteration of wound dead space is obtained by primary closure. Drainage is employed for four general reasons: (1) to obliterate dead space (or potential dead space), which is prone to fluid collection and infection; (2) to drain cytotoxic fluids leaking from injured organs, such as liver or pancreas; (3) to drain areas of established infection; and (4) to drain sites of injury or prior surgery which are prone to continued bleeding. Wound drains are foreign bodies and can promote wound infection.[59] Passive drains, such as Penrose drains, are particularly prone to infectious complications and should not be used alone. Closed suction drains minimize bacterial contamination of the wound along the drain tract and are most effective in collapsing dead space in the wound. Wound drains should be brought out through the skin at a site distant from the skin incision.

Specific Tissues

TENDON INJURY

The objective of tendon repair is the restoration of tissue continuity with high tensile strength, but without excessive scar formation that will impair gliding motion within the tendon sheath. Very rarely is a tendon injured in an isolated fashion, but rather in a more complex injury involving skin, subcutaneous fat, bone, blood vessels, and nerves. This compound wound, including the damaged or repaired tendon, heals together as a unit—"one wound, one scar," as described by Peacock.[81] Thus, the tendon can be entrapped in the scar generated by the injury.

A mature tendon and its surrounding sheath contain few cells active in producing fibrous proteins for scar formation. Most are inactive spindle cells resembling inactive fibroblasts. Following injury, blood-borne inflammatory cells migrate into the area of damage. There, the cells initiate the synthesis and deposition of collagen. Thus, an intact blood supply to the tendon is critical for the formation of the dense fibrous reaction involved in tendon healing.[79]

During the first weeks after tendon injury, collagenolysis predominates over collagen synthesis. Cut ends of the tendon become rounded and decrease in size. If the cut ends remain separated by a long gap, scar tissue forms within the tendon sheath. Although closely resembling a tendon, this tissue is not a regenerated tendon. Rather, this pseudo-tendon is anatomically distinct from the true tendon and the surrounding sheath, adds little strength to the muscle-tendon-joint complex, and restricts gliding motion.[80]

Scar formation at the site of tendon damage or repair affects gliding motion in a complex fashion. A small gap between cut ends can be bridged, but direct coaptation produces the least amount of scar. For a tendon to glide through its sheath, secondary remodeling of the newly formed fibrous scar must occur to decrease the restrictive qualities of the scar. Adhesions almost invariably form at the site of repair, but reduction in lateral cross-linking during remodeling promotes elongation of adhesive bands and mobility of the tendon. These elongating adhesions resemble peritenon, which is immediately adjacent to these adhesions. In fact, preservation of peritenon is important; if lacking, adhesions formed at the site of repair remain unstretchable and restrict gliding motion.

Principles of surgical tendon repair are complex and have been reviewed by Peacock.[82] In general, primary repair soon following injury should be carried out whenever possible. However, secondary tendon repair is common for many injuries in which other treatment requirements take precedence over tendon repair, and the wound is initially closed at the level of the integument. Later, repair is readily accomplished without disadvantage to the integrity of the repair. Considerable experience is required in making the judgment between primary and secondary repair.

The repair itself is straightforward. Following exposure of the damaged region, the fibrous tendon sheath around the area of anastomosis should be removed, since the tendon repair swells as the scar matures. A minimal amount of nonabsorbable, monofilament suture is required. The suture is placed transversely through the tendon and its sheath, away from the anastomotic site. The suture ends then are crisscrossed across the junction of the cut ends and placed through the opposite tendon in a similar fashion. Inclusion of the tendon sheath in the suture path adds early strength to the repair and immobilizes the tendon in its sheath. A fine continuous (6-0 or 7-0) monofilament suture is placed circumferentially for meticulous apposition of the severed edges of the tendon sheath.

NERVE INJURY

Following nerve damage, repair is directed toward restoring nerve continuity so that regeneration of the interrupted segments can occur. If a nerve cell is destroyed, it is permanently lost; after birth, no new nerve cells are formed. If a nerve fiber (which is a cytoplasmic extension of the nerve cell) is damaged, regeneration is frequently possible. Nerve repair takes advantage of this possibility.

The anatomical structure of nerve trunks has important implications for the surgical techniques of nerve repair. Individual axons with their Schwann's cell envelopes are surrounded by an endoneurium, a connective tissue sleeve composed of fibroblasts, collagen, and capillaries. Bundles of these fibers are in turn surrounded by a similarly constituted perineurium, which also forms fibrous septa in the nerve trunk itself. Surrounding the entire nerve is the epineurium, which contains the major vascular supply of the nerve. Removal of the epineurium for more than a few centimeters renders the nerve avascular.

When a nerve is severed, the nerve cell body proximal to the injury usually survives, while the distal portion of the axon undergoes Wallerian degeneration. Unmyelinated fibers degenerate faster than myelinated fibers. The axoplasm in the distal segment condenses and is absorbed, leaving an empty channel. Schwann's cells proliferate in the area of injury, become mobile, and form dense cords along the tracts of the degenerated axons. Within two days of nerve transection, sprouting of nerve fibers occurs at the proximal end of the divided nerve. These regenerating nerve fibers then extend along the new fibrous tracts formed by the Schwann's cells until complete restoration of the nerve trunk has been accomplished.

Surgical repair seeks to optimize realignment of the ends of the severed nerve. Timing of nerve repair depends on the nature of the entire wound and the clinical condition of the patient. Primary repair is most appropriate when a clean soft tissue laceration has produced a relatively atraumatic transection of the nerve and the patient is sufficiently stable to tolerate the time required for the surgical procedure. Further, the function served by the nerve will influence the decision for primary repair. Major motor nerves should be repaired primarily, if possible. Degeneration of motor end plates occurs soon after nerve division and the denervation changes in the muscle may become irreversible after several months. By contrast, repair of a sensory nerve may well restore sensation years after the initial injury.

If the nerve is involved in a blast or crush injury, the associated soft tissue and bone destruction precludes primary repair. Secondary repair allows the surgeon time to assess the proximal extent of neuronal damage following the injury. This is particularly helpful if the nerve has been stretched, compressed, or contused. Delay for several weeks allows identification of the proximal extent of injury, so that the nerve repair is not carried out at a more distal, nonviable site. When secondary repair is planned, it is advisable at the time of initial wound exploration, when possible, to reapproximate the severed nerve ends with a single suture so that nerve length is preserved. Interestingly, when the secondary repair is carried out later, the nerve ends are commonly found to be in perfect cross-sectional alignment. Nerve repair ideally coapts the divided ends as accurately as possible so that axonal flow can continue down distal neurilemmal tracts. As little suture material as possible should be used in order to minimize the amount of scar tissue induced by these foreign bodies. Tension on the nerve or anastomosis restricts axonal regeneration and nerve repair.[114] An adequate length is best obtained by positioning of the extremity when feasible, rather than by longitudinal dissection, which may strip the nerve of its blood supply. If the nerve is being secondarily repaired, the neuromas at the severed ends of the nerve should be cleanly resected. Following orientation of the nerve ends to each other, epineural edges are coapted by very fine (7-0 or 8-0) monofilament sutures. The suture should not pass deeply into the epineurium but should be placed instead in the more superficial loose connective tissue. As few epineural sutures as possible to ensure *en face* reapproximation should be used to minimize scarring. Young and co-workers have demonstrated no clinical advantage in funicular repair as compared to simple epineural repair.[121] Following completion of the nerve repair, the involved area should be immobilized for three weeks so that stretching of the involved segment is avoided. Following nerve anastomosis, at least five to six weeks elapse before any evidence of regeneration can be detected.

BONE INJURY

Although healing of bone resembles that of skin, tendon, and other soft tissues, its complex structure is dictated by several features related to its weight-bearing function. In long bones, the ends are composed of spongy, or cancellous bone, which is composed of columns of trabeculated bony substance. The columns follow lines of stress and redistribute weight along the load-bearing surfaces of the bone. The shaft of long bones is composed of compact bone, which is traversed by haversian canals. These canals interconnect with each other and the main marrow cavity. The bone is surrounded by the periosteum, composed of a fibrous outer layer and an inner, or cambrium, layer. The cambrium can form new bone cells and is important in fracture healing. A similar membrane, the endosteum, lines the marrow cavity. Bone is composed of matrix and deposited calcium salts. The matrix consists primarily of type I collagen, which is very similar to tendon and skin collagen; smaller amounts (less than 5%) of mucopolysaccharides and glycoproteins provide ground substance to the matrix. The calcium salt crystals in mature bone are composed almost entirely of hydroxyapatite, a crystalline form of calcium and phosphate.

Two types of cells are involved in bone formation and remodeling. Osteoblasts form matrix and thus are important for new bone formation. They are similar to fibroblasts and synthesize collagen. Osteoblasts are located predominantly on the surface of bone, in the cambium of the periosteum, and in the endosteum. Osteoblasts are also present in large numbers at fracture sites, where these multinucleated cells are involved in bone resorption and remodeling. Osteocytes can behave both as bone-forming cells and bone-resorbing cells. Most osteocytes reside as quiescent cells in the haversian canals.

Bone heals either by endochondral ossification or intramembranous ossification. In endochondral ossification, repair is preceded by the formation of cartilage, which is subsequently replaced by bone. This is the same process by which bone growth occurs at epiphyseal plates following birth. In intramembranous ossification, bone is laid down directly by bone-forming cells without cartilage formation. The actual mechanism operating at any fracture site depends on local vascularity, compression, mobility of fragments, and systemic factors (particularly oxygen availability).

When a bone is fractured, hemorrhage occurs at the site of injury and a blood clot forms. Like injured tissue elsewhere, the hematoma and wound debris initiate the local proliferation of inflammatory cells and activation of osteoblastic activity. Within several days, the osteoblasts begin to synthesize a fibrous collagen matrix, or callus, which is similar to granulation tissue in soft tissue wounds. Callus has a rich capillary network, and maintenance of its vascular integrity is essential for fracture healing.[115] In long bones the majority of the vascular supply to the fracture site derives from the medullary cavity, the remainder from the periosteum. The density of the blood supply to the fracture site callus determines the kind of healing that will take place. In areas of rich blood supply, such as at the endosteal and periosteal surfaces adjacent to the fracture, osteoblasts form bone directly. In areas of restricted perfusion, osteogenic cells first differentiate into chondroblasts and form cartilage. Later, as neovascularization proceeds, the cartilage calcifies and is converted into bone. Oxygen tension governs in large part which process dominates: low oxygen concentrations favor endochrondral ossification, while higher tensions promote direct intramembranous ossification.[11] In long-bone fractures, both types of healing occur, depending on the distance of the callus from its blood supply.

By 3 to 4 days after fracture, highly vascularized endosteal and periosteal bone begins to appear at the site of callus. Parietal bone, such as in the skull, forms little callus at a fracture site and heals almost entirely by intramembranous ossification. Soon after the onset of fracture repair, remodeling by the fracture callus begins. This process is mediated by osteoblasts, which contain a collagenase active against bone matrix collagen. The trabeculated bone is resorbed and replaced by new cancellous compact bone. Remodeling also reshapes the bone at the fracture site in an attempt to return to the original alignment of that structure.

Fracture treatment includes initial stabilization, generally achieved in the case of long bones by the application of traction. Following restoration of organ function and treatment of other life-threatening conditions, the primary aim of fracture care, is immobilization of the fracture fragments to prevent further local tissue injury, prevent extension of the fracture hematoma, restore length, reduce the risk of fat embolus, and reduce pain. Depending upon the age of the patient, the location and character of the fracture, and the location of associated injuries, external or internal fixation is used to immobilize the fracture (Fig. 13.5). Following fixation by means other than balanced skeletal traction, patient activity is progressively increased, the ultimate goals being ambulation and self-sufficiency. Such treatment minimizes fracture-associated systemic complications and muscle atrophy secondary to disuse.

MUSCLE AND FASCIA INJURIES

Most muscle injuries occur following free rupture or division by a sharp object (including the surgeon's scalpel). Although formation of new muscle cells does not occur, existing cells have the ability to regenerate. If the gap between severed ends is small and sufficiently clean, old myofibrils reestablish connections across the wound. Therefore, injured muscle should be repaired as soon as possible. Delay allows the formation of fibrous scar between the wound edges, preventing the regeneration by the muscle cells. Further, as this scar matures, it stretches or thins out, leaving a defect in the area of the old injury. Any repair should begin with removal of necrotic or scarred wound margins. To obtain strong reapproximations, the suture should be placed in fibrous septa in or around the muscle, rather than in the muscle itself.

Fascia heals in a fashion closely akin to that of skin and tendon. Fibrous protein is synthesized in the junction between apposed fascial edges, and the scar of remodeled collagen is dense and usually of high tensile strength. Fascia has no ability to regenerate itself, and once a defect appears it is permanent. Either transplant of fascia from another location or suture approximation of the wound edges is necessary to close the defect. Clinically, the most common fascial defects are the various types of hernias. The most catastrophic failure of fascial healing is abdominal wound dehiscence. Wound dehiscence in other locations, although a major complication with morbidity, usually does not have the high incidence of sepsis and fatality that occurs with abdominal wound disruption.

Wound Dehiscence

Abdominal wound dehiscence is the separation of the fascial layers of the abdominal wound with either imminent or actual expulsion of the intra-abdominal contents. Many factors detrimental to effective wound healing are present in patients with this complication: bacterial contamination of the wound, inability to obliterate dead space, compromised tissue perfusion, malnutrition, and impaired host defense mechanisms. Although these systemic factors have received much of the blame for wound failure, dehiscence in the vast majority of instances occurs because of technical errors.[2] Tensile strength of wound closures is reduced in patients with hypoproteinemia and anemia, but many other complications are present in these patients, including sepsis and low flow states.[31] On the other hand, patients with cancer, burns, diabetes mellitus, and long-term steroid treatment (unless dosage is massive) experience little difficulty with wound closure and healing.[78,109] Contrary to initial impressions, midline vertical and other incisions heal as well as other wounds; however, many studies continue to report the relative weakness and increased dehiscence rate of paramedial incisions.[32,47,113]

The technical aspects of wound closure are of paramount importance. Studies in animal models have documented that an

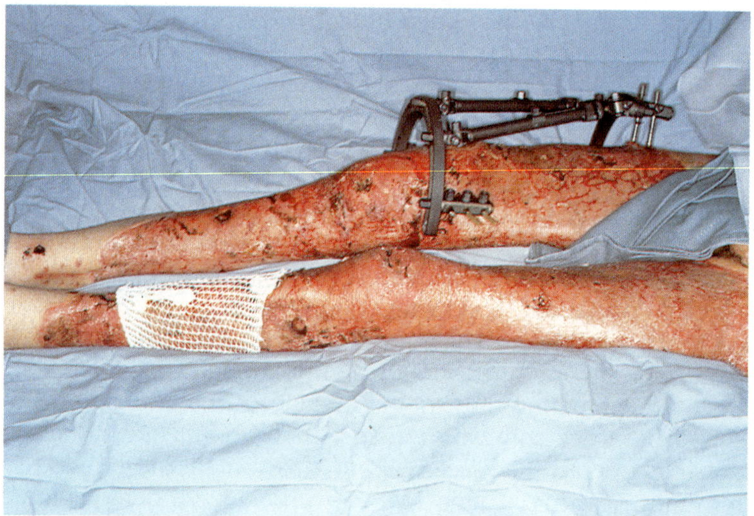

FIGURE 13.5 The external fixation device shown here immobilized the distal femoral fracture that underlay full-thickness burns of the thigh. The use of such devices avoids the risk of infection associated with devices implanted during open reduction and internal fixation, permits movement of the patient as necessary for general care, and allows free access to the burn wound for application of topical antimicrobial agents, excision of the burn wound, and skin graft application.

abdominal incision elongates in the immediate postoperative period, thus expanding the distance between sutures.[23] Further, sutures placed near the wound edge or tied sufficiently tight to strangulate the encircled tissue commonly pull through the tissue. Mass sutures, placed 1.5 cm to 3 cm back from the wound margin and approximately 1.5 cm to 2 cm apart so as to include all fascial layers and adjacent muscle, form the strongest closure.[21,47] The use of mass sutures in numerous clinical populations has drastically reduced the incidence of dehiscence, regardless of the incision used and the associated clinical conditions. Closure of the peritoneum is unimportant and does not affect the dehiscence rate.

The ultimate test of an abdominal closure occurs in severely burned patients undergoing laparotomy. In a series of 103 massively burned patients requiring 149 intra-abdominal procedures, dehiscence occurred in 33 patients.[32] Almost all were due to technical factors, including broken sutures if polypropylene was used, employment of paramedian incisions, and inadequate tissue bites during suture placement. The presence of burn wound on the abdominal wall did not affect the incidence of dehiscence. These critically ill patients were capable of adequate wound healing. When disrupted wounds were reclosed with retention sutures, none subsequently dehisced, confirming the impression that technical failure was responsible for wound separation. None of the incisions that were closed with mass sutures failed. Use of this technique, placing the suture through all muscle and fascial layers of the abdominal wall, should be routinely employed for closure of all abdominal incisions in burn patients, especially those who are critically ill.

BURN WOUND CARE

The burn patient differs from other wounded patients in terms of the extent of cutaneous injury, the length of time during which the skin defect persists, and the magnitude and duration of injury-related impairment of the immune and other organ systems. Exposure of tissue to temperatures above 45°C causes coagulation necrosis, with the severity of injury related to both the temperature and duration of exposure.[69]

Local Effects of Burn Injury

In areas of full-thickness injury, coagulation involves all skin appendages (hair follicles and sweat glands) and is associated with immediate microvascular thrombosis and permanent occlusion of the local blood supply (Fig. 13.6). In partial-thickness burns the zone of coagulation involves only a fraction of the dermis and a variable number of viable skin appendages persist from which spontaneous reepithelialization may occur. The zone of coagulation is surrounded by a concentric zone of stasis in which the cellular injury and compromised blood supply are potentially reversible if hypovolemia is promptly corrected, desiccation of the wound surface avoided, and infection prevented. A zone of hyperemia characterized by vasodilatation and increased blood flow surrounds the zone of stasis (Fig. 13.7).[41] In tissues subjected to temperatures over 43°C, permeability edema occurs as a

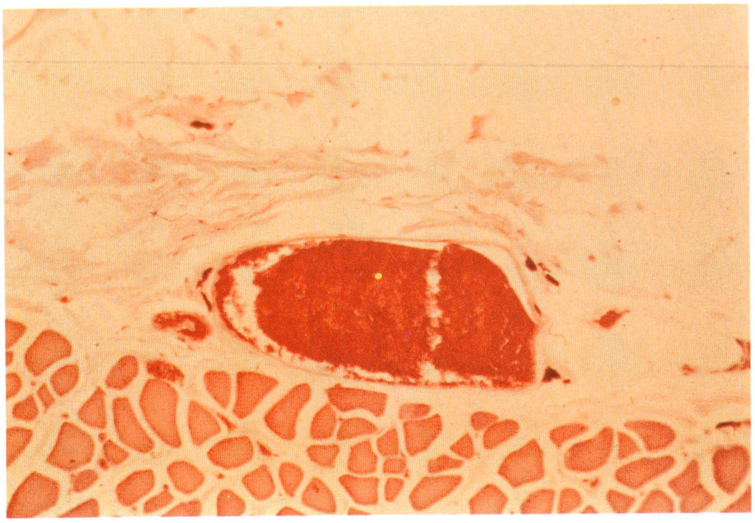

FIGURE 13.6 Histologic examination of this full-thickness or third-degree burn reveals coagulation necrosis of muscle, with edema and microvascular thrombosis evident in the overlying areolar tissue.

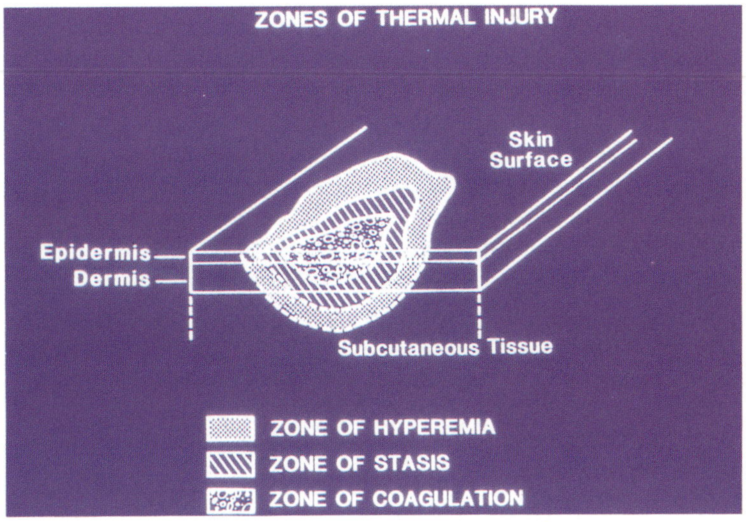

FIGURE 13.7 Concentric hemispheroidal zones of progressively less severe tissue injury extend outward from the area of cell death characterized by coagulation necrosis.

result of vascular endothelial injury.[74] The edema that forms in the injured tissue may further compromise local blood flow and tissue oxygenation. Physiologically active materials, such as histamine, serotonin, prostaglandins, and leukotrienes, as well as products of coagulation and complement activation liberated from the damaged tissue, exert effects both locally and systemically that can exaggerate edema formation and further compromise an already impaired circulation.

Systemic Effects of Burn Injury

A broad spectrum of systemic effects is elicited by burn injury, the magnitude and duration of which are in direct proportion to the extent of the burn. The loss of fluid from the vascular compartment in the immediate postburn period results in hypovolemia with a resultant decrease in cardiac output and a compensatory rise in peripheral resistance that preferentially restricts peripheral blood flow to protect visceral blood flow.[7,95] Pulmonary vascular changes elicited by the burn *per se* and inflammatory changes of the airway elicited by inhalation injury (a common accompaniment of burn injury) can impair oxygenation of the blood and reduce the amount of oxygen delivered to the wound.[6,91] Burn size-related impairment of the host defense system also predisposes the burn patient to infection in the burn wound as well as other sites.[86]

Initial Care of the Burn Injury

Prevention of further injury is the goal of initial burn wound care. The role of cold applications in the treatment of burn injury is limited. The application of ice packs or cold soaks will unquestionably relieve the pain and discomfort associated with partial-thickness burns, and this therapy can be employed for the symptomatic treatment of partial-thickness burns involving 20% or less of the total body surface. In patients with more severe injury in whom tissue temperatures are still elevated (usually those encountered within 10 minutes of injury), cold applications may also reduce tissue damage. Tissue that has already been coagulated will not be influenced by such treatment, but extension of necrosis in areas of lesser tissue injury may be reduced. Cold applications should be continued only long enough to effect pain relief and reduce local tissue temperature, lest cardiac arrhythmias be induced and the peripheral vasoconstriction elicited by hypovolemia be accentuated by systemic hypothermia.

In order to prevent extension of the zone of stasis, the blood and plasma volume losses secondary to edema formation should be corrected and minimized by the intravenous administration of fluids, as guided by any of several commonly used resuscitation formulas. Adequate oxygen delivery to the injured tissue should be ensured by ventilatory support, the need for which is determined by physiological monitoring of pulmonary function. Elevation and periodically scheduled active motion are used to reduce edema formation in the burned parts.

ESCHAROTOMY AND FASCIOTOMY

In patients with encircling full-thickness burns of the limbs or trunk, circulation and ventilation are compromised when edema increases tissue pressure to a level that impairs nutrient blood flow to the tissue underlying or distal to the circumferential limb burn, or that restricts the ventilatory excursion of the chest wall. Edema and coolness of unburned skin in a circumferentially burned limb are not indications of circulatory embarrassment, but cyanosis and impaired capillary refilling in unburned skin, and neurologic change in the limb—in particular, progressively severe paresthesias and unrelenting deep tissue pain—are. All such clinical indications are less reliable in assessing the circulatory status of a burned limb than ultrasonic flowmeter examination, which can verify lack of pulsatile flow in distal arteries, that is, the posterior tibial or palmar arch vessels, or progressive diminution of the flow signal on serial examination.[72] The ultrasonic flowmeter can also be used to determine adequacy of blood flow in the digital arteries of burned fingers and toes.

Escharotomy, carried out as a ward procedure, relieves the circulatory impairment caused by encircling burns. The escharotomy incision, placed in the mid-lateral or mid-medial line of the involved limb or digit, should extend from the distal to the proximal margin of the burn and be carried across the involved joints (Fig. 13.8). The escharotomy incision need not extend into the deep subcutaneous tissue and need only transect the underlying superficial fascia to permit separation of the cut edges of the eschar. Brief application of a pressure dressing or electrocoagulation readily controls the bleeding from a properly performed escharotomy. Neither general nor local anesthesia is required for an escharotomy because the incision transects only insensate third-degree burn. If the burn

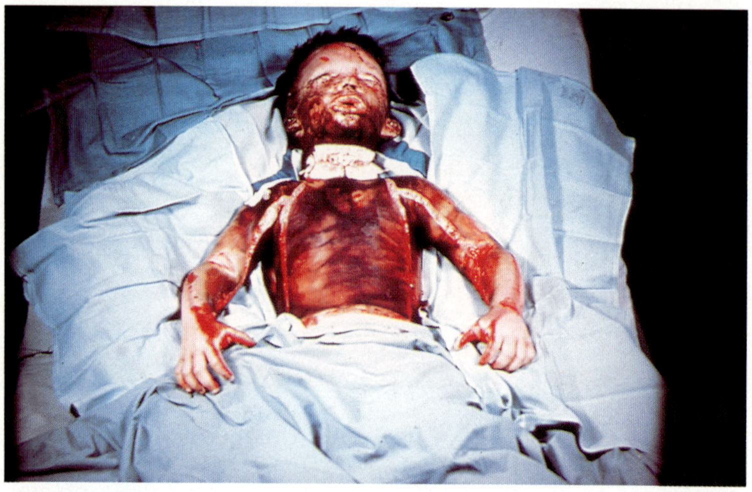

FIGURE 13.8 Escharotomy incisions were placed in the mid-medial lines of both upper limbs and the anterior axillary lines to relieve the vascular and respiratory compromise caused by the encircling full-thickness burns of the arms and trunk of this patient.

or an associated injury has produced edema beneath the investing fascia, an escharotomy will be inadequate to restore blood flow to unburned tissue in that limb; instead, a fasciotomy performed in the operating room with appropriate anesthesia will be necessary.

Escharotomy is also indicated for the relief of ventilatory restriction caused by an encircling full-thickness burn of the trunk.[83] Chest wall escharotomy incisions should be placed in the anterior axillary line bilaterally, with those incisions connected by a costal margin incision if the eschar involves a significant amount of the anterior abdominal wall. The tissues exposed by escharotomy incisions are readily colonized by microorganisms from the adjacent eschar and should be protected by liberal application of the topical chemotherapeutic agent used for treatment of the burn wound.

ASSESSMENT AND INITIAL CARE OF THE BURN WOUND

The extent of the burn determines the magnitude of organ dysfunction and the patient's resuscitation needs, but the depth of the burn influences the type of wound care required, the need for skin grafting, and the ultimate functional result. Third-degree or full-thickness burns, characterized by destruction of all skin appendages and an increased risk of infection as compared with partial-thickness burns, require skin grafting for closure even when infection does not occur. Partial-thickness or second-degree burns, if protected from infection, heal spontaneously by proliferation and spread of epithelial cells from surviving skin appendages and do not require skin grafting for closure.

Clinical characteristics helpful in differentiating full-thickness from partial-thickness burns are listed in Figure 13.9. Unequivocal full-thickness burns are easily differentiated from superficial partial-thickness burns that heal within 3 weeks, but it is often difficult to differentiate them from deep second-degree burns that involve the thicker skin of the back, face, and scalp and require more than 3 weeks for spontaneous healing. Deep partial-thickness burns are commonly treated as if they were full-thickness burns in patients whose burns are of limited extent, but in patients with burns involving more than 50% of the total body surface deep partial-thickness burns are more often allowed to heal spontaneously so that the donor sites that are available can be used for coverage of the full-thickness burns that are present.

The differentiation of burn depth is relatively imprecise in children and the elderly, in whom the skin is thinner. In those patients, burns that are initially bright to dark red and initially exude large volumes of serous fluid may be erroneously classified as partial-thickness, and only later, when the surface becomes dry and dark red or brown in color, are they recognized as full-thickness injuries. In the immediate post-burn period, these same wounds have diminished pinprick sensitivity and are leathery to the touch.

Following resuscitation, the burn wounds should be cleansed using any available surgical detergent, loose nonviable skin debrided, and the body hair shaved from the wound and from a 3-cm to 4-cm peripheral margin of unburned skin. The rupture of bullae greater than 2 cm in diameter is so common that they

FIGURE 13.9
CLINICAL CHARACTERISTICS OF PARTIAL- AND FULL-THICKNESS BURN WOUNDS

	PARTIAL-THICKNESS BURNS	FULL-THICKNESS BURNS
Cause	Hot Liquids Flashes of flame Brief exposure to dilute chemicals	Flame High-voltage electricity Exposure to concentrated chemicals Contact with hot metal
Color	Pink Mottled red	Pearly white or charred Translucent and parchment-like
Surface	Blisters Moist and weeping	Dry with shreds of nonviable epidermis Thrombosed vessels visible
Texture	Pliable	Inelastic and leathery
Sensation	Hypersensitive	Hypalgesic
Healing	10–35+ days	Grafting required

should be excised to prevent the proliferation of colonizing bacteria in the protein-rich exudate trapped between the collapsed nonviable epidermis and the wound surface; smaller bullae may be left intact. Burn wound complications are related to both the depth and extent of the burn. Topical antimicrobial therapy is unnecessary for most patients with partial-thickness burns of less than 10% of the total body surface, since the risk of infection is low. Following initial cleansing and debridement, such limited burns can be treated by exposure if the burns are so located that they do not involve joints and are not subject to abrasion by clothing.

Limited burns that involve a joint or would be irritated by contact with clothing or bedclothes can be covered by an occlusive dressing, consisting of an innermost layer of fine-mesh gauze thinly impregnated with petrolatum, over which absorbant gauze sponges are held in place by a semielastic roller gauze or an elastic wide-mesh tubular dressing. For the first 3 to 5 days postburn, the outer layers of the dressing should be removed daily with the inner layer of fine-mesh gauze left undisturbed. If there is no evidence of infection, fresh outer layers are reapplied and the dressing is reconstituted. Excessive wound exudation or displacement of the inner layer of fine-mesh gauze necessitates complete dressing renewal. If evidence of infection, such as erythema or suppuration, is noted, the wound should be cultured and thereafter treated by the exposure technique with a topical antimicrobial agent. The occurrence of a wound infection in those patients who are being treated as outpatients (adults with burns of less than 15% and children with burns of less than 10% of the body surface) may necessitate admission to the hospital. In those patients in whom healing proceeds uneventfully, the inner layer of fine-mesh gauze spontaneously separates as partial-thickness burns reepithelialize.

Patients with full-thickness burns of less than 2% of the total body surface can be treated on an outpatient basis until eschar separation and wound maturation occur. At that time, depending upon the location of the burn, it may be necessary to admit the patient to the hospital for wound closure. Prophylactic systemic penicillin (or an alternative antibiotic in patients allergic to penicillin) is not administered to burn patients treated in the hospital, but is commonly employed for 3 to 5 days postburn in patients treated as outpatients, particularly burned children in whom b-hemolytic streptococci are frequently recovered from the oropharynx.

If a burn patient has soft tissue lacerations or avulsions due to associated mechanical trauma, the high risk of wound infection caused by the organisms colonizing the burn contraindicates primary closure of such defects. Lacerations in unburned skin should be dressed following cleansing and debridement and later closed in delayed primary or secondary fashion. Lacerations in the burn wound proper should be treated with a topical agent applied to the burn and closed secondarily. Avulsions in unburned areas can be covered with a temporary biologic dressing to prevent desiccation of deep tissues, such as vessels and nerves, and later closed by autografting or by transfer of local or remote tissue. If the tissue exposed by the avulsion has been burned, it is treated in the same manner as other burn wounds. If a patient with burns requires an abdominal operation, the risk of wound infection and dehiscence is so high that retention sutures should always be used and the skin edges and subcutaneous tissue left unsutured and covered if necessary with a biologic dressing[32] (Fig. 13.10).

Pathogenesis of Burn Wound Infection

The risk of burn wound infection increases as the extent of burn injury increases, and patients with more extensive burns are best cared for in the hospital.[122] The occurrence of invasive infection is promoted by an imbalance between host defenses and microbial invasiveness. Local wound factors that permit the proliferation of colonizing microorganisms and invasion of viable tissue include abrogation of the mechanical barrier function of the skin; the presence of the protein-rich coagulum or eschar on the wound surface, which serves as a pabulum for microbial proliferation; and the avascularity of the eschar, which limits the delivery of either the humoral or cellular components of the immune system and delivery of parenterally administered antibiotics.[77] The importance of the local blood supply is indicated by the conversion of partial-thickness burn wounds and even split-thickness skin-graft donor sites to full-thickness injury and the subsequent occurrence of invasive wound infection in patients in whom hypotension occurs following resuscitation. Other local factors that predispose the burn wound to invasive infection include maceration of tissue, the presence of foreign bodies, temperature-related reduction of local blood flow due to surface cooling, and tissue acidosis. The latter favors the development of fungal infection.

Immunosuppression proportional to burn size and affecting the entire immune system also predisposes the burn patient to the development of wound and other infections.[87] In the immediate postburn period, circulating levels of the immunoglobulins and fibronectin are depressed in association with elevation of circulating levels of components indicating activation of the alternative complement pathway. All cells of the host defense system are altered in patients with extensive burns as indicated by indiscrete margination of neutrophils,[123] impairment of neutrophil oxygenation activity,[4] chemotaxis,[117] phagocytosis and bactericidal capacity,[3] alteration of lymphocyte populations with significant decrease in helper T cells,[16] depressed interleukin-II production by T-lymphocytes,[119] impaired macrophage activity,[54] and impairment of the reticuloendothelial system.[56]

The small number of predominantly gram-positive cocci that initially colonize a burn wound are gradually supplanted by gram-negative organisms that proliferate within and penetrate through the eschar if topical antimicrobial therapy is not utilized.[99] Those organisms then proliferate in the subeschar space to effect eschar separation by lysis of the denatured collagen. If the microbial density exceeds the capacity of host defenses, invasion of the viable tissue underlying the burn wound occurs; 10^5 organisms per gram of tissue appears to be the critical level associated with increased likelihood of invasion, but in a compromised host, infection may occur at lesser microbial densities.[70] Other microbial factors that predispose to burn wound infection include the previously noted production of enzymes and toxins, motility,[62] and both intrinsic and induced antibiotic resistance.

Topical Burn Wound Therapy

Topical chemotherapy controls the proliferation of microorganisms on and in the nonviable eschar of the burn wound. Extensive clinical use has verified the effectiveness of three topical antimicrobial agents in controlling the bacterial density in burn wounds and reducing the occurrence of invasive burn wound infections.[28,71,97]

Sulfamylon burn cream, an 11% suspension of mafenide acetate, is active against a broad spectrum of bacteria including virtually all strains of *Pseudomonas*. A thin, approximately 1/8-inch coating of this cream is applied to the entirety of the burn wound being treated by the exposure technique (Fig. 13.11). The water solubility and tissue diffusibility of mafenide acetate, which permit it to penetrate and establish an effective bacteriostatic level throughout the burn eschar and at the nonviable/viable tissue interface, are the principal advantages of Sulfamylon burn cream, particularly for treatment of a referral population in whom delayed or ineffective topical therapy has permitted a sizable intraeschar bacterial population to develop. The principal disadvantages of Sulfamylon burn cream are the pain upon application to partial-thickness burns, and mafenide acetate inhibition of carbonic anhydrase, predisposing the patient to a usually mild acidosis.

Dilute silver nitrate solution (0.5%) also has a broad spectrum of antimicrobial activity. This agent is applied to the wound in the form of many-layered, occlusive soak dressings, and although it is painless when applied to the wound, there is discomfort when the dressings are changed two to three times each day. The absence of hypersensitivity reactions and the reduction of heat loss by the occlusive dressings are considered to be the principal advantages of silver nitrate soak therapy. The rapid inactivation of this agent by precipitation upon contact with chloride ion or protein prevents its penetration into the eschar and confines its antimicrobial action to the surface of the burn wound. Additionally, this treatment regimen is associated with the development of electrolyte deficits as a result of leeching of sodium, potassium, and calcium through the burn wound into the hypotonic dressing. Such deficits are prevented or corrected by administration of appropriate supplements.

Silvadene burn cream, a 1% suspension of silver sulfadiazine, also has a broad antibacterial spectrum. Silvadene burn cream is applied in the same manner as Sulfamylon burn cream. Burn wounds to which Silvadene has been applied are commonly treated by the exposure technique, although the use of overlying occlusive dressings has been described. Lack of electrolyte disturbances and of pain upon its application to the burn wound are the principal advantages of Silvadene burn cream. Its principal disadvantages are the resistance of certain gram-negative organisms, an apparently batch-related neutropenia, and a sulfonamide resistance plasmid that confers resistance to multiple antibiotics.

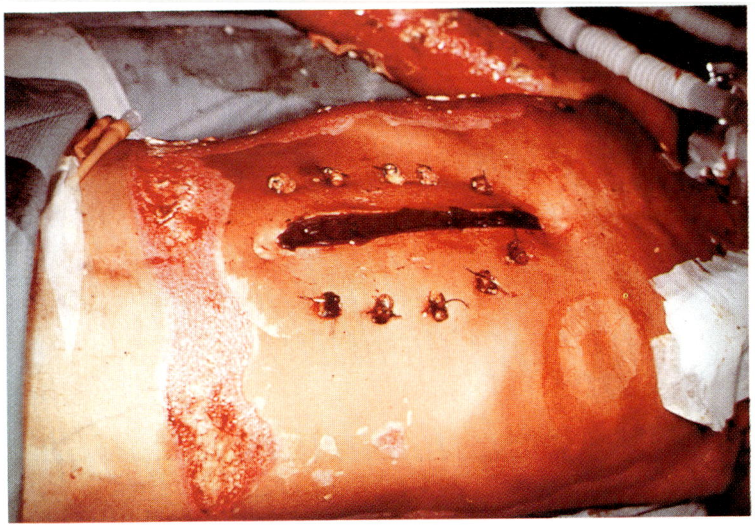

FIGURE 13.10 The risk of infection and dehiscence of abdominal incisions in burn patients mandates use of allograft skin to cover the subcutaneous tissues that are left unsutured and the placement of retention sutures.

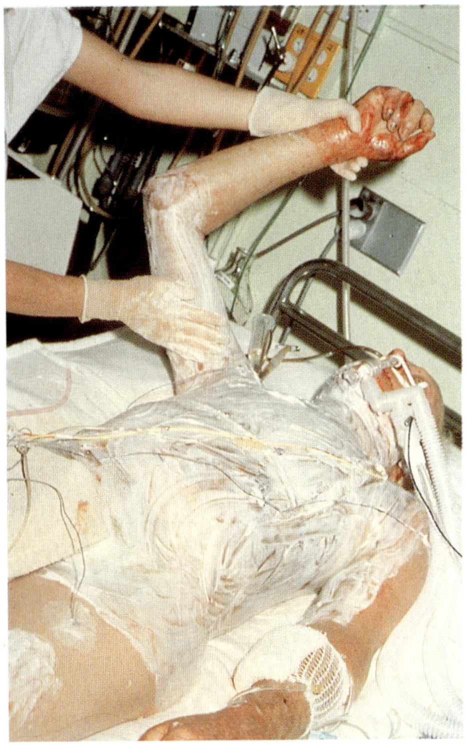

FIGURE 13.11 Topical chemotherapy, using Sulfamylon-brand burn cream, limits microbial proliferation in the burn wound. As shown here, the gloved hand is used to apply a thin coating of the cream, following which the wound is left exposed.

The advantages and disadvantages of each of the available topical agents (Fig. 13.12) must be kept in mind in order to individualize wound care and meet each patient's specific needs. Since the activity of 0.5% silver nitrate soaks is limited to the wound surface and the solubility of the sulfadiazine in Silvadene is poor, they are less effective than Sulfamylon burn cream in controlling intraeschar proliferation of microorganisms. Silvadene burn cream and 0.5% silver nitrate soaks are thus most effective when they can be begun immediately after burn injury to control the surface flora on the burn wound and prevent heavy colonization of the eschar. At the present time our regimen of topical therapy for patients without evidence of burn wound infection consists of an application of Sulfamylon burn cream following the daily wound cleansing and the application of Silvadene burn cream 12 hours later. This alternate application of agents reduces the occurrence of agent-specific complications, and the evening application of Silvadene burn cream causes little wound discomfort and minimizes sleep disturbance.

Sulfamylon burn cream is used exclusively on those patients in whom delay in topical therapy has permitted development of a high density of intraeschar bacteria and on patients with burn wound infection. The thinness of auricular skin and the limited blood supply of the auricular cartilage make the burned ear susceptible to invasive infection and mandate the exclusive use of Sulfamylon burn cream; the mafenide acetate readily diffuses into those tissues and reduces the incidence of auricular chondritis. Several other topical agents have been used in the treatment of burn wounds, but the effectiveness of such agents remains unverified.

Regardless of the topical antimicrobial agent utilized, the entirety of the burn wound of each patient should be examined each day and evaluated for the presence of infection. Dilute (0.5%) silver nitrate soak therapy obviates cleansing of the wound, but the unburned skin of such patients should be cleansed daily. Ambulatory patients treated with topical antimicrobial creams can go to the shower and cleanse their own wounds under appropriate supervision, and the wounds of nonambulatory patients can be cleansed with the patient in bed or while suspended on a slanted plinth over a Hubbard tank, using a gentle spray to remove the topical agent. Following cleansing

FIGURE 13.12
ADVANTAGES AND DISADVANTAGES OF COMMONLY USED TOPICAL ANTIMICROBIAL AGENTS

	SULFAMYLON BURN CREAM	SILVADENE BURN CREAM	0.5% SILVER NITRATE SOAKS
Advantages	Mafenide acetate difffuses into and penetrates eschar Wound exposed—readily inspected Easily applied Excellent activity against gram-negative organisms, particularly Pseudomonas sp. Joint motion maintained	Painless Wound exposed—readily inspected Easily applied Active against yeasts Joint motion maintained	Painless upon application No hypersensitivity Excellent activity against gram-negative organisms Occlusive dressings reduce heat loss
Disadvantages	Pain upon application to the partial-thickness burns Accentuation of postburn hyperventilation Early bicarbonate diuresis Hypersensitivity in 6–7% of patients Delayed eschar separation	Poor penetration of eschar Hypersensitivity—infrequent Bone marrow suppression Resistance of certain gram-negative organisms Sulfonamide resistance plasmid confers resistance to multiple antibiotics Delayed eschar separation	No penetration of eschar Induces deficits of sodium, potassium, and calcium Methemoglobinemia—infrequent Dressings impede joint motion Discolors environment

and removal of residual topical agent, the wound is inspected and any indicated cultures or biopsies are obtained. At this time any loose eschar can be removed and debridement carried out to the point of bleeding or pain. The entirety of the burn wound is then covered with a topical antimicrobial cream and 12 hours later the second of the twice daily applications is made. In the immediate postburn period the topical agent may be rapidly displaced from the wound surface by serous exudate and more frequent application of the agent may be necessary. In active young children, the topical agent may be removed by contact with the bedclothing and more frequent application of the topical agent may also be required.

Effective topical chemotherapy has significantly decreased the incidence of invasive burn wound infection. Concomitantly, the mortality of patients with burns involving up to 70% of the total body surface has significantly decreased.[93] Although the mortality rate of patients with more extensive burns remains unchanged, invasive wound infections have been significantly reduced in those patients. The topical antimicrobial agents limit intraeschar microbial proliferation but do not sterilize the burn wound.[70] Consequently, invasive burn wound infection still occurs in certain patients, usually those with burns involving more than 30% of the total body surface.

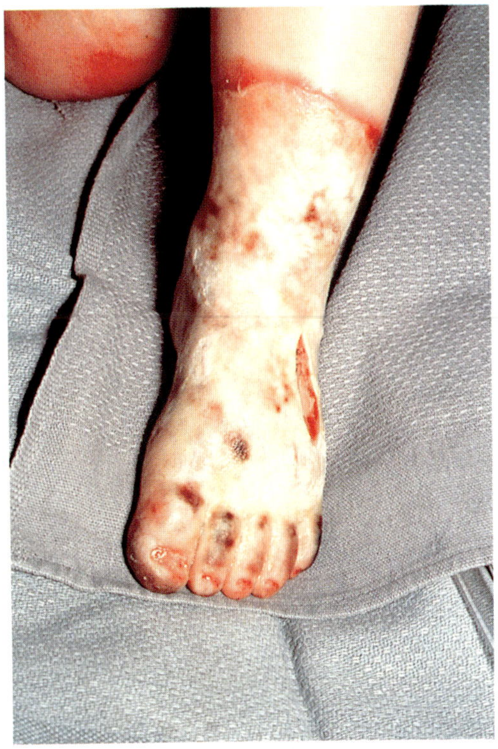

FIGURE 13.13 The focal areas of discoloration in the full-thickness wounds on the dorsum of the foot and anterior surface of the leg are characteristic of Pseudomonas burn wound infection. Note the elliptical biopsy wound on the lateral aspect of the dorsum of the foot.

Diagnosis and Treatment of Burn Wound Infections

DIAGNOSIS

The imperfect protection provided by topical agents necessitates daily examination of the entire burn wound to identify signs of infection at the earliest possible time.[86] Focal dark-red, brown, or black discoloration of the eschar is the most common wound change indicative of infection but such color change is nonspecific, since intraeschar hemorrhage due to minor trauma may produce wound changes of similar appearance (Fig. 13.13). The most reliable sign of burn wound infection is the rapid conversion of an area of partial-thickness injury to full-thickness necrosis, a change that may occur with striking rapidity and be of surprising magnitude in fungal infections, particularly those caused by *Phycomycetes*.[90] Invasive burn wound fungal infection may cause unexpectedly rapid separation of the eschar, but such separation may also occur where the burn is of sufficient depth to cause liquefaction of the subcutaneous fat.

The unreliability and imprecision of local signs and symptoms requires that other methods be used to diagnose burn wound infection. Although surface culture techniques may be useful in epidemiologic monitoring and in characterizing the microbial flora of burn wounds, the frequency of falsely negative and falsely positive results makes even quantitative culture techniques unreliable in diagnosing burn wound infection. The discordance of quantitative culture results in paired samples documents the severe limitations of quantitative cultures of even burn wound biopsy specimens.[120] Although there appears to be a generally good correlation between low wound biopsy microbial density and negative biopsy histology, there is a very poor correlation between microbial densities higher than 10^5 organisms per gram of tissue and histologic evidence of wound invasion.[61]

The most reliable means of differentiating microbial colonization of nonviable tissue from microbial invasion of viable tissue–and thus diagnosing burn wound infection–is the histologic examination of a burn wound biopsy.[92] Wound biopsies have also been used for the diagnosis of infection in other than burn wounds. Earlier diagnosis and improved survival have been attributed to the use of wound biopsy for histologic diagnosis in patients with necrotizing fasciitis.[106]

A burn wound biopsy is obtained by using a scalpel to excise from that area of the wound showing the most prominent changes indicative of infection a 500-mg lenticular tissue sample that includes underlying unburned subcutaneous tissue (Fig. 13.14). A portion of the specimen is sent unfixed to the microbiology laboratory to identify and determine the antibiotic sensitivities of the organisms present. The remainder of the biopsy sample is processed using either rapid section technique or a newly described frozen section technique, by which slides can be prepared for histologic examination within 30 minutes.[50,51] The identification of microorganisms (bacteria, fungi, or viruses) in viable tissue confirms the diagnosis of invasive burn wound infection (Fig. 13.15). The other signs listed below are less specific but should heighten the index of suspicion and prompt a meticulous examination of the histologic sections. Erroneous histologic interpretation or harvest of the biopsy specimen from a nonrepresentative area of the wound can both result in falsely negative histologic readings. Conversely, a falsely positive biopsy diagnosis may result from erroneous histologic interpretation or by examination of only the bacteria-laden eschar in a biopsy specimen that does not include unburned tissue.

The burn patient's general condition must always be considered in interpreting the results of histologic examination of a biopsy specimen. A repeat biopsy should be obtained when the biopsy report is negative in a patient with systemic sepsis. If the repeat biopsy is also negative, a search should then be made for infection in a site other than the burn wound.

The microbial status of the burn wound can be graded according to the density and depth of penetration of microorganisms, as shown in Figure 13.16. A histologic classification of Stage II confirms the presence of invasive burn wound infection. A histologic grading of Stage IIc correlates closely with systemic spread of infection and a fatal outcome. Even in the absence of invasive infection, the histologic grade assigned to a biopsy should be compared with the grade assigned to prior or subsequent biopsies. A progressive increase in the numerical grading of serial biopsy specimens is indicative of inadequate control of the microbial population of the burn wound, in which case wound care should be changed; that is, applications of a topical agent with limited diffusibility should be discontinued and Sulfamylon topical therapy instituted.

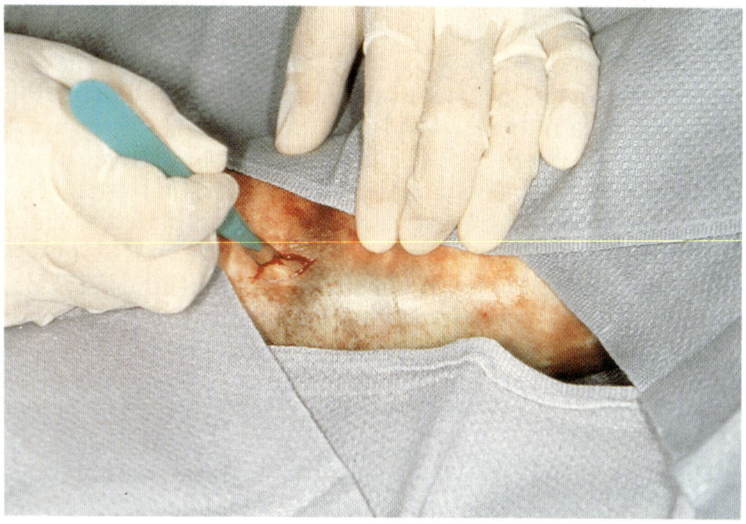

FIGURE 13.14 A burn wound biopsy is performed by using the scalpel to excise a 500-mg lenticular sample of discolored eschar and underlying unburned subcutaneous tissue.

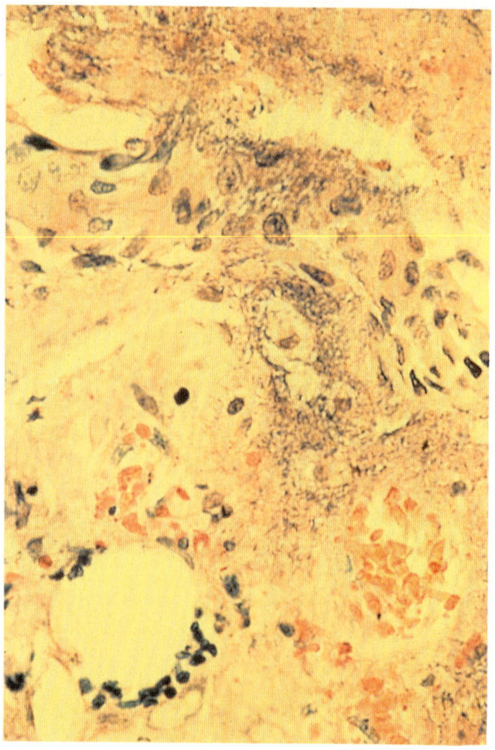

FIGURE 13.15 The presence of microorganisms in viable tissue confirms the diagnosis of invasive burn wound infection. Note the coagulation necrosis of the eschar in upper one third of this section and the presence of dark-staining bacilli in the unburned underlying tissue, the viability of which is indicated by the presence of inflammatory cells.

CLINICAL SIGNS OF INVASIVE BURN WOUND INFECTION

- Focal areas of dark-red, brown, or black eschar discoloration
- Conversion of partial-thickness injury to full-thic kness necrosis
- Rapid separation of eschar*
- Hemorrhagic discoloration of subeschar tissue
- Green pigment visible in subcutaneous fat†
- Edema or violaceous discoloration of unburned skin at wound margin
- Erythematous necrotic lesions (ecthyma gangrenosa) in unburned skin†
- Rapid centrifugal expansion of subcutaneous edema with central necrosis*
- Vesicular lesions in healing or healed partial-thickness burns‡
- Crusted serrated margins of partial-thickness burns of face

* Characteristic of fungal infection
† Characteristic of *Pseudomaonas* infection
‡ Characteristic of herpes simplex infection

HISTOLOGIC SIGNS OF BURN WOUND INFECTION

- Microorganisms present in unburned tissue
- Heightened inflammatory reaction in unburned tissue
- Hemorrhage present in viable subeschar tissue
- Small vessel thrombosis and ischemic necrosis in unburned tissue
- Dense microbial growth along hair follicles and sweat glands
- Intense microbial proliferation in subeschar space
- Intracellular viral inclusions

TREATMENT

Biopsy confirmation of invasive burn wound infection necessitates changes in both systemic and local therapy. General supportive measures should be employed to maintain or restore cardiac, pulmonary, and metabolic function. Systemic antibiotic therapy should be initiated based on organism prevalence and antibiotic sensitivity as determined by the institution's microbial surveillance program. The antibiotic regimen is subsequently adjusted on the basis of sensitivity testing of the organisms recovered from the biopsy material. If another topical agent is being used, it should be stopped and Sulfamylon burn cream applied to the burns twice a day.

Organism-specific characteristics of the septic process determine the local care necessary to treat a burn wound infection. Staphylococcal burn wound infections typically present as multiple, superficial small abscesses initially confined to the dermis that, if untreated, may expand. Simple unroofing of staphylococcal microabscesses often controls the septic process, but tangential excision of extensive areas of the eschar may be necessary to drain multiple small abscesses. More extensive excision at or below the level of the investing fascia may be needed to remove larger penetrating abscesses and the inflammatory tissue that surrounds such lesions.

Gram-negative bacteria, particularly *Pseudomonas* organisms, are much more commonly the cause of invasive burn wound infections. Such infections spread rapidly into viable tissue and may disseminate both regionally and systemically by way of both the lymphatic and vascular systems.[112] As soon as the patient's general condition will permit, the infected tissue should be excised. To minimize intraoperative hematogenous dissemination of the infecting bacteria and the metabolic products of such bacteria, an antibiotic-containing solution should be infused into the area of infection and the immediately surrounding subcutaneous tissues 6 to 12 hours before and immediately prior to excision.[63] One-half of the daily dose of a broad spectrum penicillin, such as piperacillin suspended in 1000 ml. of normal saline, should be infused into the infected areas of the wound using a #20 spinal needle to minimize the number of injection

FIGURE 13.16
HISTOLOGIC GRADING OF MICROBIAL STATUS OF BURN WOUNDS

STAGE I	STAGE II
Burn Wound Colonization	Burn Wound Invasion
Ia. Superficial: Organisms present on wound surface	IIa. Microinvasion: Small foci of microorganisms in the most superficial viable tissue
Ib. Penetrating: Variable penetration of eschar by microorganisms	IIb. Generalized invasion: Multifocal or generalized spread of microoganisms into viable tissue
Ic. Proliferating: Dense population of microorganisms at the nonviable-viable tissue interface	IIc. Microvascular involvement: Microorganisms present in small blood vessels and lymphatics

sites. Thereafter a scalpel or an electrocautery device is used to remove the infected tissue. All tissue superficial to the investing fascia is removed and, if the infection has penetrated deeper tissues, they too are excised. In patients whose general condition will not permit surgical debridement of the infected tissue, such subeschar antibiotic injections are repeated twice a day. In a small number of patients with focal and even multifocal *Pseudomonas* burn wound infection of limited extent, the subeschar infusion of antibiotics has arrested the septic process, as indicated by cessation of lesion expansion and desiccation of the necrotic tissue.

If one is uncertain regarding the adequacy of excision of an infected burn wound, the wound should be covered with dressings saturated with an antimicrobial solution. (We use a 5% solution of mafenide acetate, but it is not generally available.) The dressings are changed daily and, if persistent infection is noted at the time of dressing change, further excision should be carried out. Alternatively, if one is confident that all infected tissue has been removed at the time of the original excision, the surgical wound can be covered with a biologic dressing and thereafter examined daily for evidence of residual infection. If no residual or new foci of infection are apparent at the time of a dressing change, the wound can then be closed by autografting.

The survival of patients with generalized burn wound infection, particularly those with systemic dissemination, is virtually nil. McManus and colleagues have demonstrated the importance of the early diagnosis of invasive burn wound infection in a group of 19 extensively burned patients with histologically verified *Pseudomonas* burn wound infection who were treated by subeschar antibiotic infusion and, when possible, surgical excision of the infected tissue.[64] Nine patients died of uncontrolled infection. In ten patients, five of whom died later due to other causes without evidence of persistent wound infection, the septic process was controlled. The diagnosis of infection in the five patients who survived was made before the septic process had gained access to the general circulation. All blood cultures obtained prior to excision of the infected tissue were negative.

ANAEROBIC INFECTIONS

Anaerobic burn wound infections are exceedingly rare, as would be anticipated in wounds where the damage is confined to the surface. Although clostridial myositis has been reported in patients treated with occlusive 0.5% silver nitrate soaks, the circumferential distribution and depth of the burn may have caused ischemic necrosis of deep tissues as a result of vascular compromise.[68]

FUNGAL INFECTIONS

Nonbacterial organisms may also invade the burn wound. *Candida* species frequently colonize the wound but infrequently invade deeper tissues.[14] Recent experience shows that even though the topical application of antifungal agents, such as clotrimazole, may clear the burn wound of *Candida* organisms, the patient's outcome is unaltered. Burn wound infections caused by *Aspergillus* and *Fusarium* species, characteristically localized and superficial to the investing fascia, should be treated by local excision.[86] As previously noted, phycomycotic burn wound infections spread rapidly and frequently traverse fascial planes, necessitating radical excision and even amputation to control the septic process (Fig. 13.17). Systemic amphotericin-B in combination with 5-fluorocytosine is indicated in patients with evidence of progressive local extension or systemic spread of a fungal infection.[90]

VIRAL INFECTIONS

The most frequently encountered viral infections of the burn wound are those caused by herpes simplex virus.[27] The most reliable means of diagnosing cutaneous viral infections in the burn patient is the microscopic examination of lesion scrapings or lesion biopsies. Herpes simplex infections of the cutaneous type do not require specific treatment. Systemic herpetic infections, which may involve liver, spleen, bone marrow, and adrenals should be treated with parenterally administered adenine arabinoside, but the effectiveness of that agent remains unconfirmed.

Burn Wound Excision

Surgical excision with immediate grafting of the excised wound has long been used for the treatment of full-thickness burns of limited extent (1% or less of the total body surface). The standard treatment of more extensive burns prior to the 1970's consisted of topical antimicrobial chemotherapy with daily debridement of the margins and other areas of the eschar that were easily removed without significant bleeding or pain. When the burn eschar spontaneously sloughed or was removed by such daily debridement, the exposed mature granulation tissue was

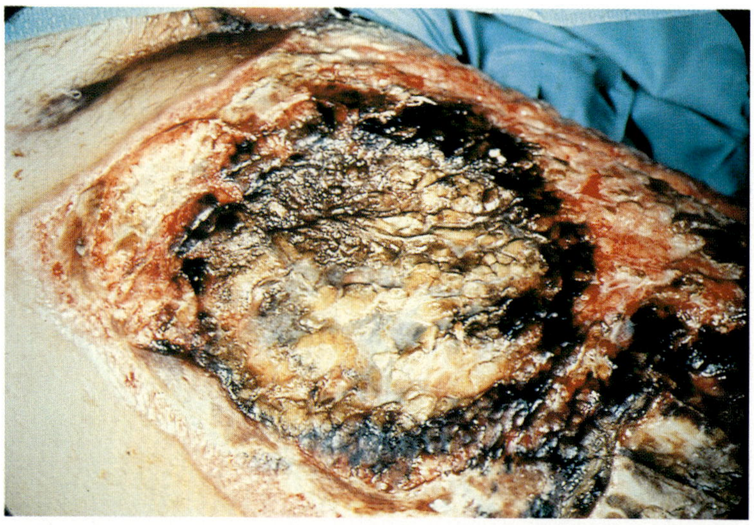

FIGURE 13.17 Invasive phycomycosis of the burn of this thigh has caused rapidly expanding necrosis of unburned subcutaneous tissue. Note edema of tissue at the darkly discolored margins of the two rounded lesions and involvement of fascia evident at right lower corner of photograph.

covered with split-thickness cutaneous autografts. Immature granulation tissue was protected and prepared for grafting by serial applications of a biologic dressing.

In 1956, Macmillan et al reported that scalpel excision of full-thickness burns at the level of the investing fascia could safely be carried out in patients with extensive burns, but they found no improvement in survival.[57] Since the procedure was associated with extensive blood loss and necessitated the use of large amounts of allograft skin when the area of the excision exceeded that of available donor grafts, it was performed infrequently. In 1970, Janzekovic described the technique of tangential excision by which successive thin layers of nonviable tissue are removed from the wound, until a bed of viable tissue with uniformly dense capillary bleeding is developed, then closed by the immediate application of split-thickness auto graft skin.[46] A guarded skin knife or dermatome can be used to perform tangential excision (Fig. 13.18). This technique was originally used for the treatment of partial-thickness burns but has now been extended to the treatment of deeper burns.

Full-thickness burns, in which there is significant thermal injury of subcutaneous fat, are usually best managed by scalpel or electrocautery excision at the level of the investing fascia (Fig. 13.19). If the thermal injury involves the investing fascia or deeper tissues, they too should be excised. As noted above, tangential excision is the treatment of choice for partial-thickness burns and may be used for full-thickness burns in which a variable fraction of the subcutaneous tissue superficial to the investing fascia has been injured. Staged or sequential excision is a variant of tangential excision designed to reduce the associated blood loss. When using this technique, successive layers of nonviable tissue are excised only to that level where bleeding is first encountered.[67] The procedure is then terminated and the wound is covered either with dressings moistened with a topical chemotherapeutic agent or, if little nonviable tissue is present, with allograft skin. A gauze dressing is changed daily, biologic dressings changed as dictated by submembrane exudation or suppuration. The patient is returned to the operating room in 3 to 7 days, and further excision of nonviable tissue is carried out if necessary, the wound autografted if no nonviable tissue remains.

Limitations of excision include the susceptibility of the excised wound to colonization and infection by the microorganisms present on adjacent unexcised burns, sacrifice of viable skin elements in areas of deep partial-thickness burn when full-thickness burns are excised by scalpel technique, and the loss of autograft skin applied to burned subcutaneous fat erroneously assessed as viable. Blood loss, the most significant limitation of the excision procedures, is least with electrocautery excision at fascial level and greatest with tangential excision. Snelling and associates have reported blood loss exceeding 9% of the blood volume for each 1% of the body surface area excised by the tangential technique.[104] Blood loss associated with excision of a burn wound at the fascial level on a limb can be reduced by use of a tourniquet and the blood loss associated with the other techniques of excision can be minimized by the use of topical thrombin or local subeschar injection of ornithine vasopressin.[19] To minimize the physiologic impact of blood loss, no more than 20% of the body surface should be excised at a single sitting. To limit general physiologic stress, total operating time should be limited to 2 hours if possible. The usefulness of excision is also limited in patients with massive burns in whom the paucity of available donor sites makes it impossible to effect immediate, definitive closure of the wound following excision.

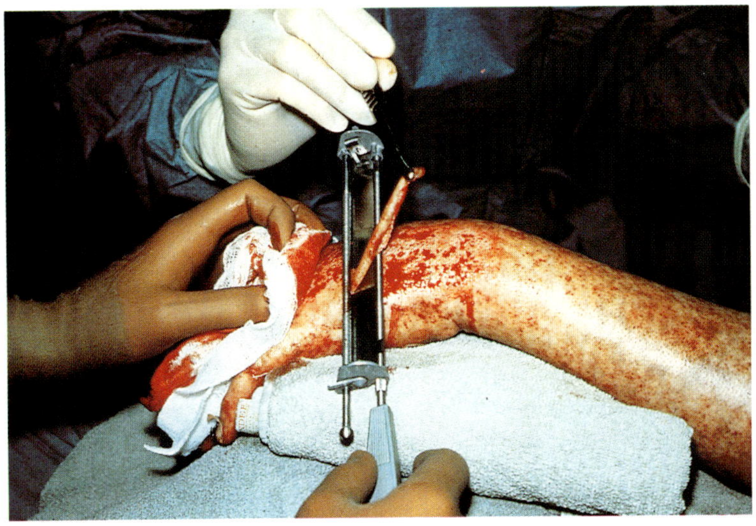

FIGURE 13.18 A guarded skin knife can be used to tangentially excise nonviable tissue from a deep second-degree burn of the dorsum of the hand. The excised tissue is being elevated by the assistant. Note the punctate capillary bleeding from the excised wound bed to the right of the knife.

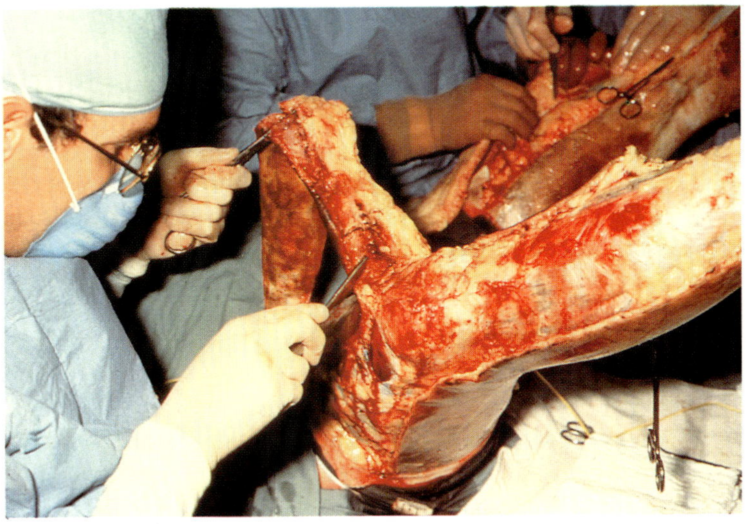

FIGURE 13.19 Scalpel excision at the level of the investing fascia is used to remove full-thickness burns in which there is significant thermal damage of the underlying subcutaneous tissue. Two teams of surgeons are used, as shown here, to reduce operating time when burns on both legs must be excised.

Another hazard associated with burn wound excision is that of mechanically induced bacteremia. Positive blood cultures can be recovered from 20.6% of patients during wound care procedures with the recovery rate related to both total extent of the burn and the intensity of wound manipulation.[103] This risk of hematogenous dissemination of bacteria by manipulation of the wound speaks for performance of excision before the wound is heavily colonized. Even so, the often densely mixed polymicrobial flora of the burn wound justifies the perioperative systemic administration of antibiotics active against both gram-positive and gram-negative organisms at the time of burn wound excision or an extensive debridement.

During the resuscitation period, the hemodynamic effects of anesthesia and the excision procedure should not be imposed on an extensively burned patient in whom physiologic compensation is at the maximum. Burn wound excision should also be delayed in patients with profound pulmonary insufficiency due to inhalation injury or other pulmonary complication until improvement in pulmonary function will permit the patient to tolerate transport to the operating room and the imposition of the pulmonary effects of anesthesia on already injured lungs. In elderly burn patients, in whom post-excision pulmonary and hemodynamic complications are most likely to occur, burn wound excision should only be employed when physiologic status has been optimized and when a careful weighing of the advantages and limitations of excision favors operation.

A review of 381 patients with burns covering over 30% of the body surface treated at the U.S. Army Burn Center during a recent 5½ year period revealed that burn wound excision had been carried out in 93% of the surviving patients. However, excision had been precluded by pulmonary insufficiency, hemodynamic insufficiency, or sepsis-related intravascular coagulation in 51% of the 146 patients who died. In addition to those complications that had precluded excision, a temporary delay in excision was necessary in certain patients to control burn wound cellulitis or to correct electrolyte and acid-base disorders.

The use of historic controls and the non-random selection of patients have flawed many studies of burn wound excision outcome and a beneficial effect of the procedure on the burn patient mortality rate remains unconfirmed. A randomized control study of excision in patients with burns on up to 20% of the total body surface demonstrated that burn wound excision reduced the occurrence of complications, shortened hospital stays, lowered the cost of care, and permitted earlier and more likely return to work.[25] In 2 studies of patients with burns involving more than 20% of the body surface, randomized as to excisional or non-excisional therapy, burn wound excision shortened hospital stay but did not effect mortality.[34,105] A 3 year follow-up to one of those studies revealed that burn wound excision did not alter scar formation or the need for reconstruction.[48] Recent laboratory and clinical studies on excision have demonstrated a salutary effect on indices of immune function and a reduction in the occurrence of sepsis and pneumonia.[49,110]

Studies of the effect of excision on post-injury hypermetabolism have indicated that excision of the entirety of the burn wound and immediate closure by grafting were necessary to reduce the elevated metabolic rate characteristic of burn patients.[55] Even in the absence of documented mortality reduction, burn wound excision can be justified on the basis of reducing the duration and cost of hospital care, decreasing the risk of burn wound and other infections, and reducing the duration of burn-associated physiologic stress.[38,39,65]

Enzymatic Debridement

As an alternative to mechanical debridement many enzymatic debriding agents have been used to hasten eschar removal. To date no agent has uniformly lysed all the nonviable tissue or produced in a brief period of time a reliably graftable wound bed. Local and systemic toxicity as well as wound bleeding and an increased risk of infection are additional limitations to the use of the enzymatic debriding agents.

Burn Wound Closure

Following slough or surgical removal of the nonviable tissue, definitive closure of a full-thickness burn wound is achieved by split-thickness autografting. The absence of nonviable or infected tissue and the presence of bright red, nonedematous, finely granular granulation tissue are clinical indications that a burn wound is ready for autograft closure. A density of less than 10^5 organisms per gram of tissue in a biopsy of the wound bed provides laboratory confirmation of the clinical assessment. As noted previously, uniform adherence of a biologic dressing to the burn wound confirms the readiness of the wound for autograft closure and ensures an excellent autograft take.

Thin split-thickness skin grafts should be used to ensure optimum take in patients with extensive burns while, in patients with limited burns, thicker split-thickness grafts will optimize cosmetic results. Meshed autografts, which increase the wound surface that can be covered by up to ninefold, can be used to partially overcome the shortage of available donor sites in patients with extensive burns[22] (Fig. 13.20). Mesh grafts expanded to up to a 3:1 ratio are frequently used, but mesh grafts expanded to a 6:1 or 9:1 ratio are seldom used because the time required for epithelialization of the interstices is so long. Mesh grafts should be covered to prevent desiccation of the wound bed, exposed until the interstices close by epithelial spread. The risk of rapid lysis of any freshly applied split-thickness cutaneous autograft skin justifies perioperative systemic administration of penicillin or, in a penicillin-allergic patient, another antibiotic active against β-hemolytic streptococci at the time of skin grafting.

Biologic Dressing and Skin Substitutes

If a burn or other wound cannot be closed by application of cutaneous autografts or transfer of autogenous tissue from adjacent or remote sites, a biologic dressing will provide temporary coverage of any open wound prior to definitive coverage. Biologic dressings can also be used to accelerate and improve the quality of healing of superficial partial-thickness burns, accelerate the healing of deep partial-thickness burns, effect debridement of residual nonviable tissue following excision or eschar slough, provide immediate coverage following burn wound excision, protect granulation tissue between "crops" of autograft in patients with extensive burns, and serve as test material to determine the readiness of a burn wound for autografting (Fig. 13.20). The beneficial effects of biologic dressings include reduction of evaporative water and heat loss from the burn wound, prevention of wound desiccation, limitation of bacterial growth and proliferation on the wound surface, reduction of exudative protein and red cell loss, reduction of wound pain and facilitation of motion of involved joints, and promotion of angiogenesis in granulation tissue. Viable cutaneous allograft is the most frequently used and effective biologic dressing.[94] Other biologic dressings, such as lyophilized allograft, cutaneous xenograft, and amnion, do not form a true biologic union with the wound bed and are consequently less effective than viable allograft skin.[84] The limitations of biologic dressings, principally the difficulty in matching supply with demand, complex storage requirements, finite shelf life, possibility of disease transmission, and cost have led to the development of skin substitutes designed to mimic the morphology and function of skin.

The desirable properties of a skin substitute include tissue compatibility; absence of toxicity, antigenicity, and microorganisms; sufficient drapability to conform to minute irregularities of the wound surface; sufficient tensile strength to resist linear and sheer stress; permeability to water vapor; low cost; minimal storage requirements; and indefinite shelf life. A skin substitute should promote the reduction of the bacterial population on the wound surface in order to limit submembrane bacterial proliferation and should permit the establishment of biologic union between the wound bed and the membrane. A bilaminate structure appears to be necessary for a skin substitute to function optimally.[94] The inner layer, or dermal analogue, should be of sufficient porosity to permit biologic union by the ingrowth of fibrovascular tissue, and the outer layer, or epidermal analogue, should have pores sufficiently small to serve as a microbial barrier yet permit passage of water vapor. None of the presently available skin substitutes possess all of the desirable properties.

Available skin substitutes consist of either collagen-based bilaminate membranes or culture-derived epidermal sheets. A clinical evaluation has shown that as a wound dressing, Biobrane, a collagen-based composite is indistinguishable from porcine cutaneous xenografts[100] (Fig. 13.21). Integra® consists of a collagen-based dermal analogue enriched with chrondroitin-6-sulfate and

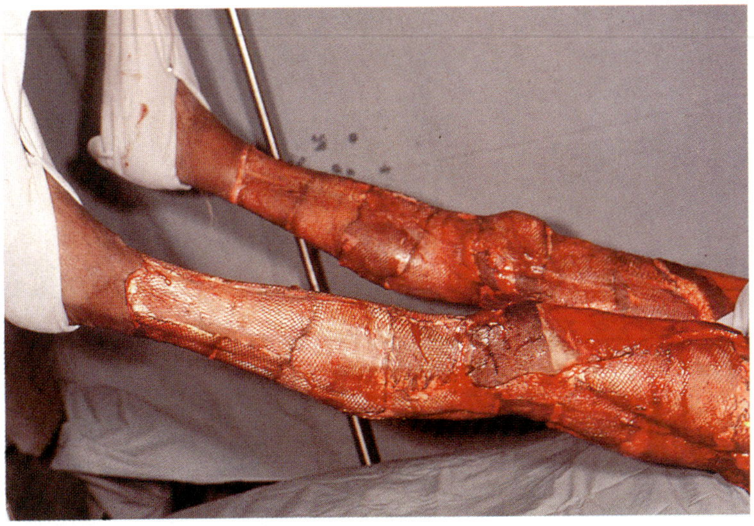

Figure 13.20 Limited availability of donor sites necessitated use of meshed autograft skin expanded at a 3:1 ratio to cover the burn wounds of both legs of this patient.

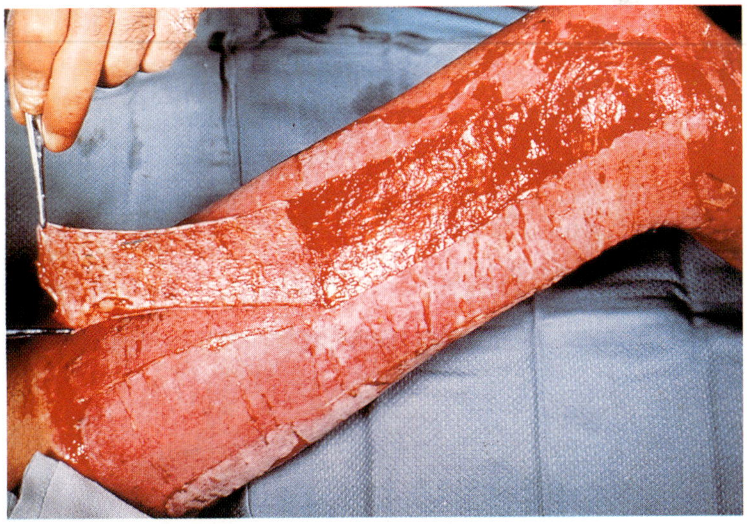

FIGURE 13.21 Removal of well-vascularized, uniformly adherent cutaneous allografts applied to test the readiness of this burn wound reveals bright-red, richly vascular granulation tissue, which ensures that subsequently applied autografts will take.

a thin Silastic epidermal analogue. When the dermal analogue of that material has been well vascularized as the result of granulation tissue ingrowth, the Silastic membrane is removed and the wound closed by application of a thin split-thickness autograft to the vascularized dermal analogue[15] (Fig. 13.22). Heimbach, et al, on the basis of a multi-institutional study of this material, have reported that when the material was applied to the wound bed immediately after excision, the "take" of the dermal analogue was slightly less than that of autograft skin but equivalent to that of allograft and xenograft skin and synthetic dressings.[37] In that study, coverage of the vascularized dermal analogue was achieved by application of split-thickness skin grafts that averaged 0.006 inches in thickness. One year after discharge, there appeared to be less hypertrophic scarring of the

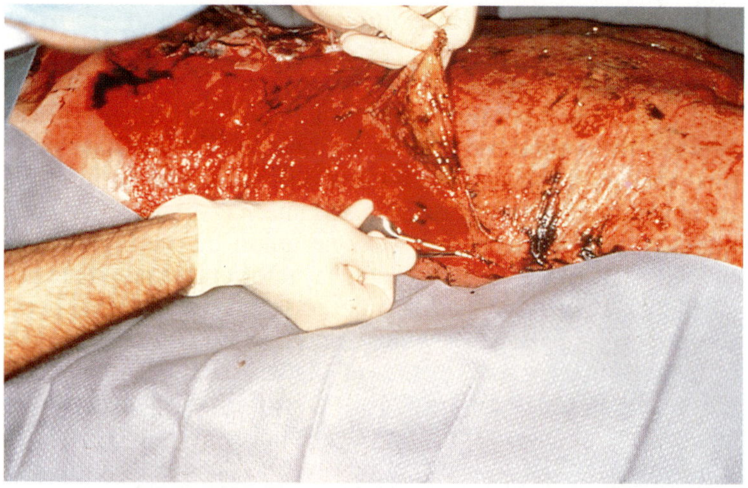

FIGURE 13.22 A collagen-based bilaminate skin substitute, Biobrane, has been used to cover the wounds on the back of this patient following burn wound excision. The wound of the upper back (to the right of the surgeon's hand), readily visible through the well-adherent membrane, is obviously free of suppuration. Note the healthy appearance of the wound bed from which the intact membrane is being removed.

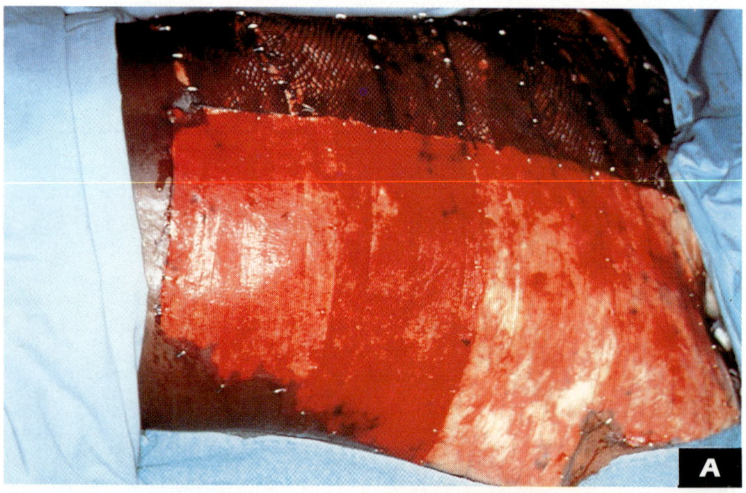

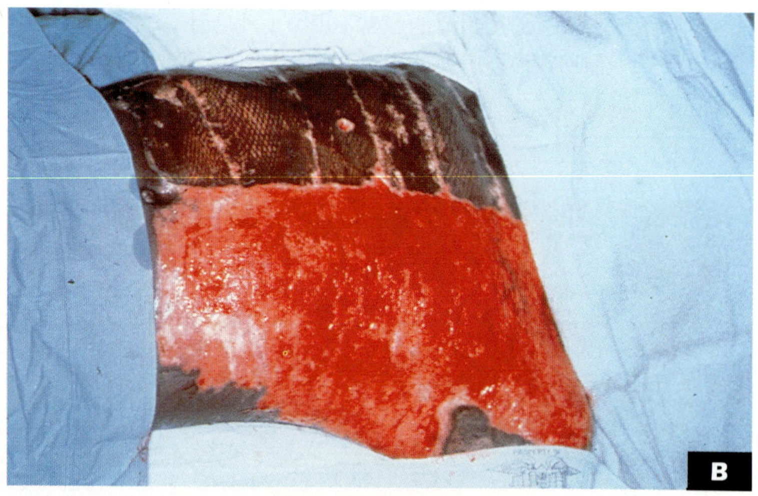

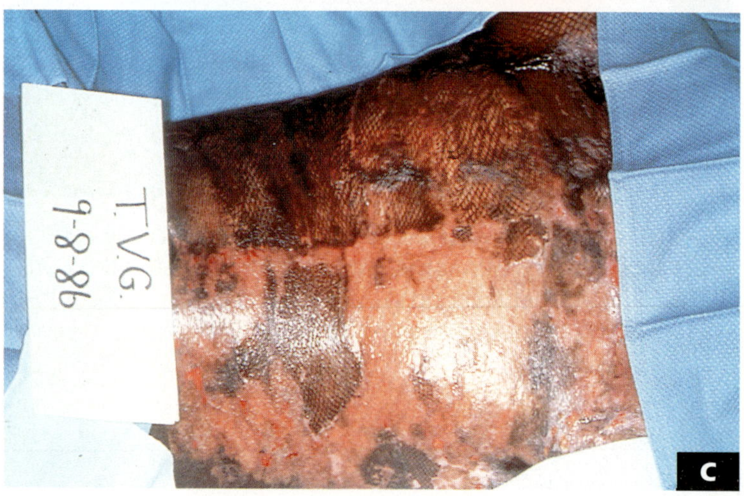

FIGURE 13.23 A Following tangential excision, the wound on the right chest of this patient was covered with meshed split-thickness autografts and the wound on the left chest with the bilaminate skin substitute, Integra. **B** The silastic epidermal analogue can be removed when the dermal analogue is well vascularized, as shown here 14 days after the membrane was applied. The wound is then closed by application of thin split-thickness autografts to the surface of the "neo-dermis". **C** A secure take of the thin cutaneous autografts provides satisfactory functional and cosmetic closure of the wounds.

wounds treated with the artificial dermis as compared to wounds treated with other materials, even though all of the treatments studied became more equivalent over time.

Epidermal sheets, produced by the culture of disaggregated epidermal cells (either autogenous or allogenic), have also been used for burn wound closure following excision[29] (Fig. 13.23). In a recent study of seven patients, with a mean burn size of 69.6% of the total body surface, Munster, et al, found that the average take of cultured epidermal grafts was 75% as compared to an average 92% take of meshed split-thickness autografts.[73] It was noted that areas grafted with cultured epidermis appeared to blister more readily than those covered with autograft skin, but only during the initial two to three months following application. There were no subsequent differences in tolerance to heat, cold, or pressure garments. Madden and associates have reported that allogeneic epidermal sheets do not survive on a wound bed produced by excision of the full thickness of the dermis, but they do adhere to and promote the healing of wounds in which the dermis remains following excision (Fig. 13.24).[58] The long-term persistence of such allogeneic grafts is unconfirmed

Hansbrough et al have recently developed a bilaminate membrane consisting of a collagen-glycosaminoglycan dermal analogue and a sheet of cultured keratinocytes as the epidemal analogue.[36] This material, the dermal analogue of which is seeded with cultured autologous fibroblasts, is treated with basic fibroblast growth factor immediately prior to application of the composite graft to the recipient wound. The resulting stimulation of angiogenesis and epithelial growth enhances "take" of the tissue composite and is said to accelerate wound closure. Histologic examination of the grafts, two-thirds of which survived, demonstrated that a basement membrane-like structure developed within nine days following application. The long-term adequacy and fate of this composite graft are unknown. The usefulness of epidermal sheets and composite tissue grafts is limited by the time required for their growth in culture (three to four weeks) and by their susceptibility to microbial lysis, low resistance to trauma, and late contraction and scar formation. The usefulness of culture-derived tissue will be significantly increased if the culture time can be shortened and the antigenicity eliminated so that allogeneic tissue will indeed persist indefinitely.

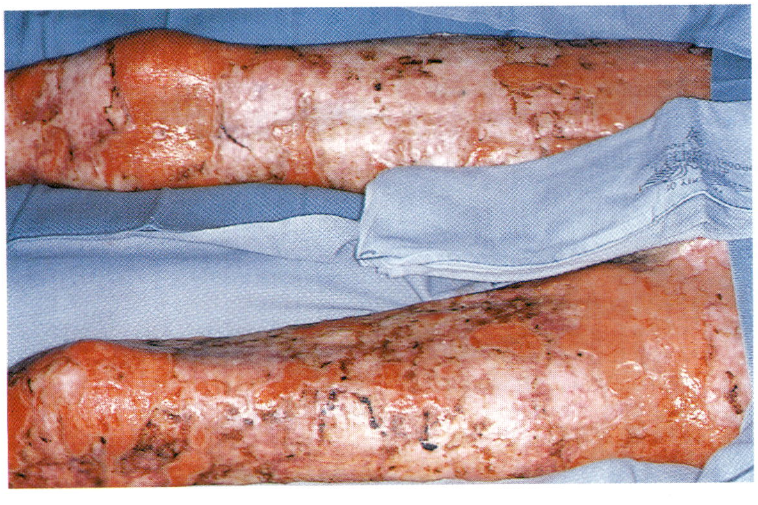

FIGURE 13.24 Following excision of the full-thickness burns of the right leg of this patient, multiple sheets of cultured keratinocytes were applied. At the time of removal of the gauze pledgets, to which the keratinocytes were attached for application, take of the gray-white sheets of keratinocytes to the medial and anterior thigh is apparent.

REFERENCES

1. Ad hoc Committee of the Committee on Trauma, Division of Medical Sciences, National Research Council Report: Postoperative wound infections; the influences of ultraviolet irradiation of the operating room and the influence of various other factors. Ann Surg 160(Aug 1964 Suppl):53–58, 1964.
2. Alexander HC, Prudder JF: The cause of abdominal wound disruption. Surg Gynecol Obstet 122:1223, 1866.
3. Alexander JW, Wixsom D: Neutrophil dysfunction and sepsis in burn injury. Surg Gynecol Obstet 130:431–438, 1970.
4. Allen RC, Pruitt BA Jr: Humoral-phagocyte axis of immune defense in burn patients. Arch Surg 117:133–140, 1982.
5. Altemeier WA, Burke JF, Pruitt BA Jr, Sandusky WR (eds): Manual on Control of Infection in Surgical Patients, p 127. Philadelphia, JB Lippincott, 1976.
6. Asch MJ, Feldman RJ, Walker HL et al: Systemic and pulmonary hemodynamic changes accompanying thermal injury. Ann Surg 178:218–221, 1973.
7. Asch MJ, Meserol PM, Mason AD Jr et al: Regional blood flow in the burned unanaesthetized dog. Surg Forum 22:55–56, 1971.
8. Aulick LH, Baze WB, McLeod CG et al: Control of blood flow in a large surface wound. Ann Surg 191:249, 1980.
9. Aulick LH, Wilmore DW, Mason AD Jr et al: Influence of the burn wound on peripheral circulation in thermally injured patients. Am J Physiol 233:H520, 1977.
10. Barnes RW, Thomhill B, Nix L et al: Prediction of amputation wound healing: Roles of Doppler ultrasound and digital plethysmography. Arch Surg 116:80, 1981.
11. Bassett CAL, Hermann I: Influence of oxygen concentration and mechanical factors on differentiation of connective tissue in vitro. Nature 190:400, 1961.
12. Bergamini TB, Lamont Pm, Cheadle WG et al: Combined topical and systemic antibiotic prophylaxis in experimental wound infection. Am J Surg 147:753, 1984.
13. Bleier E: Delayed suture of simple fresh wounds. Am J Surg 33:178, 1919.
14. Bruck HM, Nash G, Stein JM et al: Studies on the occurrence and significance of yeast and fungi in the burn wound. Ann Surg 176:108–110, 1972.
15. Burke JF, Yannas IV, Quinby WC et al: Successful use of a physiologically acceptable artificial skin the treatment of extensive burn injury. Ann Surg 194:413–428, 1981.
16. Burleson DG, Vaughan GK, Mason AD Jr et al: Use of light scatter in flow cytometry measurements of rat lymphocyte subpopulations after burn injury with infection. Arch Surg (in press).
17. Cardany CR, Rodeheaver GT, Thacker JG et al: The crush injury: A high risk wound. JACEP 5:965, 1976.
18. Churchill ED: The surgical management of the wounded in the

Mediterranean theater at the time of the fall of Rome. Ann Surg 120:268, 1944.
19. Clarke AM, Solomon JR: The use of a new vasoconstricter in the management of burns. Med J Aust 2:361–362, 1972.
20. de Holl D, Rodeheaver GT, Edgerton MT et al: Potentiation of infection by suture closure of dead space. Am J Surg 127:716, 1974.
21. Dennis C, Aka E: The figure-of-8 through-[iw-2]and-through monofilament abdominal wound closure with wound splints: Elimination of evisceration in poor-risk wounds over 25 years. Surgery 73:171, 1973.
22. DiVincenti FC, Curreri PW, Pruitt BA Jr: Use of mesh skin autografts in the burn patient. Plast Reconstr Surg 44:464–467, 1969.
23. Dudley HAF: Layered and mass closure of the abdominal wall: A theoretical and experimental analysis. Br J Surg 57:664, 1970.
24. Edlich RF, Rodeheaver GT, Thacker JC et al: Management of soft tissue injury. Clin Plast Surg 4:191, 1977.
25. Engrav LH, Heimbach DM, Reus JL et al: Early excision and grafting vs. nonoperative treatment of burns of indeterminant depth: A randomized prospective study. J Trauma 23:1001–1004, 1983.
26. Feng LJ, Price D, Mathes SJ: Relationship of blood flow and leukocyte mobilization in infection. Plast Surg Forum 6:128, 1980.
27. Foley FD, Greenawald KA, Nash G et al: Herpesvirus infection in burned patients. N Engl J Med 282:652–656, 1970.
28. Fox CL Jr, Rappole BW, Stanford W: Control of Pseudomonas infection in burns by silver sulfadiazine. Surg Gynecol Obstet 128:1021–1026, 1969.
29. Gallico GG III, O'Conner NE, Compton CC: Permanent coverage of large burn wounds with autologous cultured epithelium. N Engl J Med 311:448–451, 1984.
30. Goodson WH, Hunt TK: Studies of wound healing in experimental diabetes mellitus. J Surg Res 22:221, 1977.
31. Goodson WH, Hunt TK: Wound healing and the diabetic patient. Surg Gynecol Obstet 149:600, 1979.
32. Goodwin CW Jr, McManus WF, Mason AD Jr et al: Management of abdominal wounds in thermally injured patients. J Trauma 22:92–97, 1982.
33. Gottrup F, Andreassen TT: Healing of incisional wounds in stomach and duodenum: The influence of experimental diabetes. J Surg Res 31:61, 1981.
34. Gray DT, Pine RW, Harnar TJ et al: Early surgical excision vs. conventional therapy in patients with 20 to 40 percent burns: A comparative study. Am J Surg 144:76–80, 1982.
35. Grosfeld JL, Solit RW: Prevention of wound infection in perforated appendicitis: Experience with delayed primary wound closure. Ann Surg 168:891, 1968.
36. Hansbrough JF, Boyce St, Cooper ML, et al: Burn wound closure with cultured autologous keratinocytes and fiberblasts attached to a collagen-glycosaminoglycan substrate. JAMA 262:2125–2130, 1989.
37. Heimbach D, Luterman A, Burke J, et al: Artificial dermis for major burns: A multi-center randomized clinical trial. Ann Surg 209:313–320, 1988.
38. Herndon DN, Barrow RE, Rutan RL, et al: A comparison of conservative vs. early excision therapies in severely burned patients. Ann Surg 209:547–553, 1989.
39. Herndon DN and Parks DH: Comparison of serial debridement and autografting and early massive excision with cadaver skin overlay in the treatment of large burns in children. J Trauma 26:149–152, 1986.
40. Heughan C, Crislis G, Hunt TK: The effect of anemia on wound healing. Ann Surg 179:163, 1974.
41. Howe CW: Experimental studies on determinants of wound infections. Surg Gynecol Obstet 123:507, 1966.
42. Hugo NE, Epstein L, Cone A et al: The effect of primary wounding on the tensile strength of secondary wounds. Surg Gynecol Obstet 131:516, 1970.
43. Hunt TK, Halliday B: Inflammation in wounds: From "laudable pus" to primary repair and beyond. In Hunt TK (ed): Wound Healing and Wound Infection: Theory and Surgical Practice, pp 286–287. New York, Appleton-Century-Crofts, 1980.
44. Hunt TK, Linsey M, Grislis G et al: The effect of differing ambient oxygen tension on wound infection. Arch Surg 181:35, 1975.
45. Jackson DM: Second thoughts on the burn wound. J Trauma 9:839–862, 1969.
46. Janzekovic Z: The burn wound from the surgical point of view. J Trauma 15:42–62, 1975.
47. Jenkins TPN: The burst abdominal wound: A mechanical approach. J Surg 63:873, 1976.
48. Kalaja E: Acute excision or exposure treatment? Secondary reconstructions and functional results. Scand J Plast Reconstr Surg 18:95–99, 1984.
49. Kara M, Peters WJ, Douglas LG, et al: An early surgical approach to burns in the elderly. J Trauma 30:430-432, 1990.
50. Kim SH, Hubbard GB, McManus WF et al: Frozen section technique to evaluate early burn wound biopsy: A comparison with the rapid section technique. J Trauma 25:1134–1137, 1985.
51. Kim SH, Hubbard GB, Worley BL et al: A rapid section technique for burn wound biopsy. J Burn Care Rehab 6:433–435, 1985.
52. Knighton D, Silver IA, Hunt TK: Regulation of wound healing angiogenesis—effect of inspired concentration and oxygen gradient. Surgery 90:262, 1981.
53. Knighton DR, Halliday B, Hunt TK: Oxygen as an antibiotic: The effect of inspired oxygen on infection. Arch Surg 119:199, 1984.
54. Kupper TS, Greene DR, Durum SK et al: Defective antigen presentation to a clones T helper cell by macrophages from burned mice can be restored with interleukin I. Surgery 98:199–206, 1985.
55. Lalone C and Demling RH: The effect of complete burn wound excision and closure on postburn oxygen consumption. Surgery 102:862–868, 1987.
56. Lemperle G: Depression and stimulation of host defense mechanisms after severe burns. Plast Reconstr Surg 45:435–440, 1970.
57. MacMillan BG, Moncrief JA, Pillsbury RD, et al: Early excision of extensive areas of full-thickness burns. In US Army Surgical Research Unit: Biennial Report 1955–56, Fort Sam Houston, TX, 1956, pp 29–33.
58. Madden MR, Finkelstein JL, Staiano-Coico L et al: Grafting of cultured allogeneic epidermis on second and third-degree burn wounds in 23 patients. J Trauma (in press).
59. Magee C, Rodeheaver GT, Golden GT et al: Potentiation of wound infection by surgical drains. Am J Surg 131:547, 1976.
60. McManus AT, Denton CL, Mason AD Jr: Topical chlorhexidine diphosphanilate (WP-973) in burn wound sepsis. Arch Surg 119:206, 1984.
61. McManus AT, Kim SH, Mason AD Jr et al: A comparison of quantitative microbiology and histopathology in divided burn wound biopsies. Arch Surg (in press).
62. McManus AT, Moody EE, Mason AD Jr: Bacterial motility: A component in experimental Pseudomonas aeruginosa burn wound sepsis. Burns 6:235–239, 1980.
63. McManus WF, Goodwin CW, Mason AD Jr et al: Burn wound infection. J Trauma 21:753–756, 1981.
64. McManus WF, Goodwin CW Jr, Pruitt BA Jr: Subeschar treatment of burn wound infection. Arch Surg 118:291–294, 1983.
65. Mc Manus WF, Mason AD Jr, Pruitt BA Jr: Excision of the burn wound in patient with large burns. Arch Surg 124:718–720, 1989.
66. Medawar PB: The behavior of mammalian skin epithelium under strictly anaerobic conditions. J Micros Sci 88:27, 1974.
67. Monafo WW, Aulenbacher CE, Pappalardo C: Early tangential excision of the eschars of major burns. Arch Surg 104:503–508, 1972.
68. Monafo WW, Brentano L, Gravens DL et al: Gas gangrene and mixed-clostridial infections of muscle complicating deep thermal burns. Arch Surg 92:212–221, 1966.
69. Moncrief JA: The body's response to heat. In Artz CP, Moncrief JA, Pruitt BA Jr (eds): Burns: A Team Approach, pp 23–35. Philadelphia, WB Saunders, 1979.
70. Moncrief JA, Lindberg RB, Switzer WE et al: Use of topical antibacterial therapy in the treatment of the burn wound. Arch Surg 92:558–565, 1966.
71. Moyer CA, Brentano L, Gravens DL et al: Treatment of large human burns with 0.5 percent silver nitrate solution. Arch Surg 90:812–867, 1965.

72. Moylan JA, Inge WW Jr, Pruitt BA Jr: Circulatory changes following circumferential extremity burns evaluated by the ultrasonic flowmeter: An analysis of 60 thermally injured limbs. J Trauma 11:763–770, 1971.
73. Munster AM, Weiner SH and Spence RJ: Cultured epidermis for the coverage of massive burn wounds. Ann Surg 211:676-680, 1990.
74. Mustafa KY, Selig WM, Burhop KE et al: Hyperthermia-induced pulmonary edema. J Appl Physiol 60:1980–1985, 1986.
75. Niinikoski J: Oxygen and wound healing. Clin Plast Surg 4:361, 1977.
76. Niinikoski J: The effect of blood and oxygen supply on the biochemistry of repair. In Hunt TK (ed): Wound Healing and Wound Infection: Theory and Surgical Practice, pp 56–70. New York, Appleton-Century-Crofts, 1980.
77. Order SE, Moncrief JA: Vascular destruction and revascularization in severe thermal injuries. Surg Forum 15:37–39, 1964.
78. Oxlund H, Fogdestam I, Vidik A: The influence of cortisol on wound healing of the skin and distant connective tissue response. Surg Gynecol Obstet 148:876, 1979.
79. Peacock EE Jr: A study of circulation in normal tendons and healing grafts. Ann Surg 149:414, 1959.
80. Peacock EE Jr: Fundamental aspects of wound healing relating to the restoration of gliding function after tendon repair. Surg Gynecol Obstet 11:241, 1964.
81. Peacock EE Jr: Biological principles in the healing of long tendons. Surg Clin North Am 45:461, 1965.
82. Peacock EE Jr: Wound Repair pp 263–331. Philadelphia, WB Saunders, 1984.
83. Petroff PA, Pruitt BA Jr: Pulmonary disease in the burn patient. In Artz CP, Moncrief JA, Pruitt BA Jr (eds): Burns: A Team Approach, pp 96–97. Philadelphia, WB Saunders 1979.
84. Pruitt BA Jr: The burn patient: II. Later care and complications of thermal injury. Curr Probl Surg 16(5):22–23, 1979.
85. Pruitt BA Jr: Biopsy diagnosis of surgical infections. N Engl J Med 310:1737, 1984.
86. Pruitt BA Jr: The diagnosis and treatment of infection in the burn patient. Burns 11:79–91, 1984.
87. Pruitt BA Jr: Host-opportunist interactions in surgical infection. Arch Surg 121:13–22, 1986.
88. Pruitt BA Jr: Infections of burn and other wounds caused by Pseudomonas aeruginosa. In Sabath LD (ed): Pseudomonas aeruginosa: The organism, diseases it causes, and their treatment, pp 55–70. Berne, Hans Huber, 1980.
89. Pruitt BA Jr: Burns in soft tissues. In Polk HC (ed): Infection and the Surgical Patient, pp 113–131. London, Churchill Livingstone, 1982.
90. Pruitt BA Jr: Phycomycotic infections. In Alexander JW (ed): Problems in General Surgery, pp 664–678. Philadelphia, JB Lippincott, 1984.
91. Pruitt BA Jr, Erickson DR, Morris A: Progressive pulmonary insufficiency and other pulmonary complications of thermal injury. J Trauma 15:369–379, 1975.
92. Pruitt BA Jr, Goodwin CW and Pruitt SK: Burns: Including cold, chemical, and electric injuries. In Sabison DC Jr (ed.): Textbook of Surgery, 14th Edition, W.B. Saunders Company, Orlando, FL, in press..
93. Pruitt BA Jr, Foley FD: The use of biopsies in burn patient care. Surgery 73:887–897, 1973.
94. Pruitt BA Jr, Levine NS: Characteristics and uses of biologic dressings and skin substitutes. Arch Surg 119:312–322, 1984.
95. Pruitt BA Jr, Mason AD Jr, Moncrief JA: Hemodynamic changes in the early postburn patient: The influence of fluid administration and of a vasodilator (Hydralazine). J Trauma 11:36–46, 1971.
96. Pruitt BA Jr, Silverstein P: Methods of resurfacing denuded skin areas. Transplant Proc II:1537–1545, 1971.
97. Pruitt BA Jr, O'Neill JA Jr, Moncrief JA et al: Successful control of burn wound sepsis. JAMA 203:1054–1056, 1968.
98. Pruitt BA Jr and Goodwin CW Jr: Nutritional management of the seriously ill burn patient. In Winters RW, Green HL (eds): Nutritional Support of the Seriously Ill Patient, ch 6, pp 63–84. New York, Academic Press, 1983.
99. Pruitt BA Jr, Lindberg RB: Pseudomonas aeruginosa infections in burn patients. In Doggett RG (ed): Pseudomonas aeruginosa, pp 339–366. New York, Academic Press, 1979.
100. Roberts LW, McManus WF, Shirani KZ et al: Biobrane and porcine xenograft—a comparative study. Presented at the 17th annual meeting of the American Burn Association, Orlando, Florida, March 29, 1985.
101. Robson MC, Heggers JP: Delayed wound closures based on bacterial counts. J Surg Oncol 2:379–383, 1970.
102. Salisbury RE, Loveless S, Silverstein P et al: Postburn edema of the upper extremity: Evaluation of present treatment. J Trauma 13:857–862, 1973.
103. Sasaki TM, Welch GW, Herndon DN et al: Burn wound manipulation-induced bacteremia. J Trauma 19:46–48, 1979.
104. Snelling CFT: The effect of topical epinephrine hydrochloride in saline on blood loss following tangential excision of burn wounds. Plast Reconstr Surg 72:830–834, 1983.
105. Sorensen B, Fisker MP, Steensen JP et al: Acute excision or exposure? Final results of a three year randomized controlled clinical trial. Scand J Plast Reconstr Surg 18:87–93, 1984.
106. Stamenkovic I, Lew PD: Early recognition of potentially fatal necrotizing fasciitis. N Engl J Med 310:1689–1693, 1984.
107. Stevens FO, Hunt TK: Effect of changes in inspired oxygen and carbon dioxide tensions on wound tensile strength: An experimental study. Ann Surg 173:515, 1971.
108. Stokes A, Tytler WH: Primary and delayed primary suture of gunshot wounds. Br J Surg 6:111, 1918.
109. Stone HH, Hoefling SJ, Strom PR et al: Abdominal incisions: Transverse vs. vertical placement and continuous vs. interrupted closure. South Med J 76:1106, 1983.
110. Tchervenkov JR, Epstein MD, Silberstein EB, et al: Early burn wound excision and skin grafting postburn trauma restores in vivo neutrophil delivery to inflammatory lesions. Arch Surg 13:1477-1481, 1988.
111. Telok HA, Mason ML, Wheelock MD: Histopathologic study of radiation injuries of the skin. Surg Gynecol Obstet 90:335, 1950.
112. Teplitz C: Pathogenesis of Pseudomonas vasculitis and septic lesions. Arch Pathol 80:297–307, 1965.
113. Tera H, Aberg C: Tissue strength of structures involved in musculo-aponeurotic layer sutures in laparotomy incisions. Acta Chir Scand 142:349, 1976.
114. Terzis J, Gaibisoff B, Williams HP: The nerve gap: Suture under tension vs. graft. Plast Reconstr Surg 56:166, 1975.
115. Trueta J: An experimental study of the vascular contribution to the callus of fracture. Surg Gynecol Obstet 120:731, 1965.
116. Uitto J, Prockop DJ: Synthesis and secretion of underhydroxylated procollagen at various temperatures by cells subject to temporary anoxia. Biochem Biophys Res Commun 60:414, 1974.
117. Warden GD, Mason AD Jr, Pruitt BA Jr: Evaluation of leukocyte chemotaxis in vitro in thermally injured patient. J Clin Invest 54:1001–1004, 1974.
118. Wilmore DW, Aulick LH, Pruitt BA Jr: Metabolism during the hypermetabolic phase of thermal injury. Adv Surg 12:193, 1978.
119. Wood JJ, O'Mahoney JB, Roderick ML et al: Abnormalities of antibody production after thermal injury: An association with reduced interleukin II production. Arch Surg 121:108–115, 1986.
120. Woolfrey BF, Fox JM, Quall CO: An evaluation of burn wound quantitative microbiology: I. Quantitative eschar cultures. Am J Clin Pathol 75:532–537, 1981.
121. Young L, Wray C, Weeks P: A randomized prospective comparison of fascicular and epineural digital nerve repair. Plast Reconstr Surg 68:89, 1981.
122. Yurt RW, McManus AT, Mason AD Jr et al: Increased susceptibility to infection related to extent of burn injury. Arch Surg 119:183–188, 1984.
123. Yurt RW, Pruitt BA Jr: Decreased wound neutrophils and indiscrete margination in the pathogenesis of wound infections. Surgery 98:191–197, 1985.

maxillofacial trauma

Gregory S. Georgiade
Mark E. Manstein

The face, which plays such a fundamental role in sensory perception, communication, and oral intake, often suffers from its relatively unprotected position. It is frequently exposed to wounding forces that disrupt its delicate architecture. The role of the trauma surgeon in this area is not only to halt bleeding and prevent infection but to recreate and restore normal anatomy and function as much as possible. This chapter will cover the basic management and fundamental reconstructive options of the various aspects of maxillofacial trauma.

ACUTE CARE

Although facial wounds require much skill in reconstruction, they are, fortunately, almost never fatal. Repair of the injuries can often be delayed while attention is shifted to the more crucial issues of airway, bleeding, and cardiovascular status. Until these other life-threatening matters are addressed, the facial wounds can be quickly irrigated and lightly dressed. No magical "golden" period for facial wound closure exists; while wounds should be closed as soon as possible, most can still be repaired primarily 24 hours after insult. (Animal or human bites or traumatic tattoos should be debrided or excised much sooner, however.)

Airway

Obstruction of the airway is the primary potentially life-threatening complication of facial injuries. Except for gunshot wounds to the oropharynx or hypopharynx, obstruction is usually the result of obturation of the airway by emesis, dentures, or foreign bodies rather than by glossal edema or retrusion of the tongue. Hence, the airway can usually be cleared manually. Except in the case of gunshot wounds to the mouth, tracheostomy is seldom indicated. Futhermore, an endotracheal tube should be considered prior to any tracheostomy; high-volume, low-pressure tracheal cuff tubes may be left in place for several weeks without complication. If a tracheostomy must be performed, it should be carried out in the operating room under optimal conditions. A transverse skin incision should always be made except under the most trying of conditions, for it will normally heal well without the need for a scar revision. Of more importance is how the stoma is fashioned; it must be devised so that the cannula could easily be replaced were it to fall out during a vigorous cough. Protection of the airway cannot be overemphasized.

Bleeding

Although the vascularity of the head and neck is quite abundant, most bleeding wounds on the face allow direct visualization of the responsible vessels. They can easily be occluded by direct digital pressure, and then either cauterized or ligated with fine ties. However, deep stab wounds—or gunshot wounds, with their resultant blast effect—create different scenarios. In those cases one must consider the possibility of injury to deeper, larger blood vessels. Arteriography and ligation by radiologic methods are frequently employed in such instances.

DIAGNOSIS

Physical Examination

To accurately assess the injured patient, one must become familiar with the intricate anatomy of the facial skeleton and soft tissues. Significant injuries may not be obvious and may go unrecognized unless specifically sought. An example is the small puncture wound in the cheek that at first glance appears only to have disrupted the dermis. On closer scrutiny, it is often found that the parotid duct and a branch of the facial nerve are severed.

To carry out a thorough examination of the facial structures, one must proceed in a systematic fashion. Usually one starts with the scalp and continues caudally. Fortunately, the face is symmetrical in a sagittal plane, and this allows immediate comparison. The stature or droop of an eyebrow or lip can easily be assessed vis `a vis the contralateral side. Both sensory function and motor function must be evaluated. In addition, the thinness of the facial skin facilitates a thorough examination of the bones. All bony structures must be palpated to uncover fracture "stepoffs," crepitation, tenderness, or mobility. The oral cavity allows several fingers of one hand to be placed behind the lower facial bones so that a thorough bimanual evaluation may be conducted.

The oral examination must be thorough. Mandibular excursion, dental arch symmetry, and dental occlusion must be evaluated. Broken teeth, mucosal tears, or hematomas in the soft tissues over the mandible or maxilla should raise the index of suspicion for a fracture.

Many maxillofacial injuries are in close proximity to the eyes. The presence of visual disturbances and the state of extra-ocular muscle function must be documented. The fundi must be visualized. Enophthalmos and medial canthal deformity must be noted. In the current overly litigious environment, probably all patients with fractures about the orbit should have a formal ophthalmologic evaluation.

Old records may be quite helpful in patient care. Previous dental records or plaster molds may prove invaluable, especially in cases of malocclusion. The physician's awareness of a patient's class III occlusion prior to a midface fracture is crucial to therapy. Old photographs of the patient may likewise prove useful, although reconstruction and cosmesis are limited by the tissues available.

Radiologic Examination

X-rays play a significant role in delineating facial skeletal status in trauma. Soft tissue edema may mask bony abnormalities that may be revealed only radiologically. In addition, the films provide firm documentation and a permanent record of their existence. Sometimes routine facial films may only hint at suspected fractures, and follow-up computed tomography (CT) scans or tomograms may be needed to clarify the issue. (Indeed, new computer-generated three-dimensional imaging is aiding in the planning of surgical reconstruction in which significant bone loss has occurred.)

Despite their limitations, roentgen studies still form the basis of the radiologic evaluation. Although a full "facial series" should be obtained if possible, often in trauma this is not feasible. Unstable patients with tenuous airways should never be sent to the radiology suite for facial x-rays; they can always be obtained later. If there is sufficient time and patient stability for one good film, then it should be the Waters (occipitomental) view. This projection highlights the orbital rims and floor, the maxillary sinuses, and the nasal septum. A large proportion of the maxillofacial skeleton can be scrutinized with a single well-taken Waters view.

If a mandibular fracture is suspected, on the other hand, a Waters view will not be helpful. A good-quality orthopan (panoramic view) will display the entire mandible from condyle to condyle. Unfortunately this film, taken through a special imaging device, is not universally available. If an orthopan cannot be obtained, then a posterior–anterior or, as a second choice, an anterior–posterior view, oblique views of the mandible, and a modified Towne's view will be sufficient.

It must be emphasized that cervical spine injuries coexist in approximately 10% of patients with maxillofacial injuries.[18] High-quality cervical spine films must be obtained prior to any other facial views in all patients with questionable neck trauma. These must clearly show all vertebrae from C1 to C7. If such films cannot be obtained, the patient must be treated for spinal injury in a supportive collar until these x-rays are available.

STRATEGY

On initial arrival of a patient to the emergency room, the maxillofacial injuries should be quickly surveyed, and one should hold off radiologic examination or definitive therapy until all more emergent problems are addressed. Once an adequate airway has been provided, vascular status stabilized, and crucial diagnostic procedures such as peritoneal lavage or arteriography performed, then attention can be turned toward the facial injuries.

Many factors determine when the patient receives treatment. If the patient needs to go to the operating suite for pelvic stabilization under general anesthesia, then that is an opportune time for concomitant repair of a lacerated parotid duct, severed facial nerve, or soft tissue injury. Most maxillofacial injuries do not require an immediate trip to the operating room. In fact, most soft tissue injuries of the face—other than those involving the facial nerve or a duct—can easily be treated in the accident ward under local anesthesia. Furthermore, closed facial bone injuries do not necessitate immediate reduction, and such treatment is commonly delayed several days to allow soft tissue edema to recede. The surgeon may wait up to 2 weeks postinjury with nonopen fractures and still readily reduce a fracture if, for example, hematologic or neurologic problems preclude earlier intervention. (In children, the bones heal much quicker, so fracture reduction should be undertaken within 10 days if possible.) The treatment of open fractures can likewise be delayed by simply closing the skin initially under local anesthesia and returning when the patient is more fit for general anesthesia.

As with all fractures in the body, a fundamental requirement for early sound healing is good soft tissue coverage. A well-vascularized milieu maximizes wound repair. The initial objective must be soft tissue coverage even if the underlying bone is ignored for the moment. This will also serve to minimize skin desiccation and wound contraction. Rarely will a facial wound be so contaminated that immediate closure is deferred. The tremendous vascularity and elasticity of the facial skin allow most wounds to be debrided vigorously or even excised and still be closed primarily.

Because of the abundant vascularity, epinephrine-induced vasoconstriction is commonly employed to assist in the procedure. This is usually mixed with the local anesthetic in a dose of 1:200,000 to 1:300,000 epinephrine. If adequate time for vasoconstriction to occur (7–10 minutes) is provided and the minimal dose of the drug is used, cardiac side-effects can be minimized.

Soft Tissue Injury

GENERAL CARE OF WOUNDS

Once the patient is anesthetized, the wound should be cleaned thoroughly. While antiseptic solutions such as povidone-iodine (Betadine) and chlorhexidine gluconate (Hibiclens) are not toxic to intact keratinized epithelium, they may be injurious to the wound. Saline solution and hydrogen peroxide solution should be the mainstay of irrigation, with the effort aimed at loosening and washing away dirt and foreign tissue. The irrigation may be delivered by a bulb syringe or with the pulsating jet-lavage of a Water-Pik. (However, some critics of the latter device claim that it embeds the dirt into the soft tissue.)

Cleaning the wound also serves to identify more clearly the extent of the injury. Soft tissue trauma has in the past been categorized in the following fashion: contusion, abrasion, puncture wound, laceration, avulsion, and traumatic tattoo.

Contusions and abrasions should be thoroughly cleaned and lightly dressed. Many advocate covering abrasions with an antibiotic cream such as Neosporin to prevent desiccation and speed epithelialization. It has been shown experimentally that epithelialization occurs sooner when a wound is protected by a moist occlusive dressing.

Puncture wounds must be copiously irrigated and probed to determine depth of penetration. If the wound is superficial, it can be completely excised and closed. Deeper wounds must be investigated thoroughly, because a small entrance wound may mask significant injury. (This will be covered in more detail later.)

Simple lacerations should be cleaned and reapproximated if the edges are "sharp," such as caused by metal or glass. If the edges are beveled or irregular, sharp débridement up to an excision of the wound will remove all contaminated tissue and allow a more aesthetic scar. While this is quite functional in small wounds, large wounds allow less tissue débridement. The closure of these large lacerations often results in significant scar formation, which necessitates later scar revision. Stellate lacerations, especially, must be revised, since they compromise the blood supply at the center of the wound and lie counter to Langer's lines.

Basic principles of plastic surgery should be followed in all wound closure. Wound edges should be reapposed, but not strangulated. The minimal amount of suture necessary to align the skin edges should be used. Buried absorbable sutures to minimize tension on the skin edges should be employed. While buried suture may form a nidus for bacterial growth, dead space, with its resultant collection of serum or blood, is a greater deterrent to satisfactory healing. It should be remembered that the finest suture with the smallest "purchase" of tissue needed to close the wound adequately provides the least foreign body reaction and the best scar.

A difficult wound with which to obtain a good cosmetic result is an avulsion injury. This is created by a sharp object striking the skin in an oblique plane and either completely shearing off the soft tissue or leaving a flap held on by a small pedicle. If such a flap is to survive, the pedicle must contain enough nutrient vessels to nourish the flap until it can gain new blood supply through the wound. In many such injuries to the face it may not appear that the pedicle is broad enough to provide for the survival of the entire flap; yet in most cases the flap will survive because of the extensive vascularity of the skin. If the flap is small enough to be excised and closed easily, then it should be done to avoid a "trapdoor" deformity created by circular scar contracture. If the flap is too large to be completely excised, its most distal edge may have to be sharply debrided, for this is the region where the blood supply is most tenuous. Prior to closure, the wound beneath the flap must be cleaned and gently debrided so that no foreign body is left there to foment a focus of inflammation.

Often a sharp avulsive injury completely "fillets" off soft tissue, and it is too large an area to be closed primarily. In such cases a skin graft or a local flap is needed for reconstruction. While it is a primary tenet of plastic surgery to use the simplest, most expedient, and most easily revascularized tissue available, this is not always followed on the face. Because of aesthetic considerations, local pedicle-rotation flaps are commonly employed rather than grafts because of excellent color match, texture, and reliability.

Skin grafts to the face still have an important role and are even sometimes placed as a temporary biologic dressing. Grafts should be full thickness (Wolfe[23] and Krause[24] grafts) unless skin is in short supply (as in a major burn). Full-thickness grafts provide better texture and color match and less contraction than split-thickness grafts. Donor areas for tissue include the supraclavicular region, the preauricular and postauricular regions, and the upper eyelids. None of these areas is ideal, although the preauricular region has the best color match, but it is limited in amount of tissue available. Usually the supraclavicular region is chosen.

Local rotation flaps are easy to design if the defect is small. Larger defects may require distant rotation flaps or free vascularized tissue transfer. Pedicled temporoparietal fascial flaps covered by full-thickness skin grafts have proved quite reliable in recontouring thin, full-thickness avulsions.

Traumatic tattooing occurs when multiple small foreign body fragments become embedded in the soft tissue. These particles must be meticulously removed under magnification by scrubbing with a brush or a dermabrader. Bullet fragments, on the other hand, do not cause tattoos. They are traveling at high speeds, and so, are basically sterile. They react minimally with the soft tissue, penetrate deeply, and are usually quite inaccessible to retrieval. Unless they have injured a major structure and necessitate major surgical explorations, the bullets should be left alone.

SPECIFIC INJURIES

Eyelid Trauma

Eyelid injuries pose a formidable reconstructive challenge because of their complex anatomy and function. Wound closure alone is insufficient therapy if the patient is needlessly left with epiphora or dacryocystitis. A solid review of the orbital anatomy is necessary for any surgeon dealing with injuries in that region. It must be remembered that beneath the skin of the eyelid lies the orbicularis oculi muscle with its attachments to the medial and lateral canthi. Beneath the muscle is the fine septum orbitale, which separates the connective tissue spaces of the lids from those of the orbit. The tarsal plates consist of dense connective tissue and serve as the main structural support of the lids. In the upper lid the septum and the levator palpebrae superioris fuse and attach to the skin at the superior palpebral fold. Reconstruction must take these structures into account.

If the skin of the eyelid is only superficially lacerated, it can be reapproximated with fine, interrupted, nonabsorbable suture. If the tarsal plate is divided, it should be reconstructed in layers with pullout nonabsorbable sutures. Orbicularis muscle should be reapproximated only if there is a large avulsion, with the underlying septum avulsed as well. Otherwise, the muscle can be debrided and loosely reapposed. As long as there is muscle to prevent the orbital fat from herniating, there is no need to repair the septum. In deep penetrating lacerations, there is potential for injury to the levator, rectus, or oblique muscles. These must be sought out and repaired with fine absorbable suture if identified[7] (Fig. 14.1).

Small conjunctival lacerations need not be sutured. If they measure greater than 0.5 cm, they should be reapproximated with 6-0 or 7-0 plain catgut.

Many injuries to the eyelids involve the full-thickness loss of soft tissue. If there is a full-thickness deficit of less than 25% of the lid, the wound can be closed directly. As before, this should be done in layers. Primary closure depends on the laxity of the tissue; older patients have much more lid laxity. If tension on the repair is found to be excessive, a lateral cantholysis with release of the lateral canthal raphe can be performed. This will allow the lid to move in a more medial manner and diminish tension on the suture line. If the defect is too large for direct closure, a flap is needed. The most common flap for upper lid defects is the lower lid in an Abbé-type[1] lid switch. One-quarter of the lower lid may be rotated to the upper one. Lower lid defects, on the other hand, never borrow from the upper lid. They are instead reconstructed by rotation cheek flaps; nasal septal mucosal composite flaps can be used to recreate the tarsal–conjunctival border.[19]

Medial eyelid injuries require special consideration because of the potential involvement of the lacrimal drainage apparatus. At the puncta, the lacrimal canaliculi begin in a vertical position, moving away from the lid margin. After about 2 mm they bend sharply medially, to converge into the lacrimal sac. The sac lies in a fossa on the anteromedial wall of the bony orbit, with its upper end covered by the medial palpebral ligament. The sac then empties into the nasolacrimal duct inferiorly; the duct terminates by passing through the nasal mucosa, to open into the inferior nasal meatus.

If the lacrimal canaliculus or sac is injured, it should be repaired with 7-0 or 8-0 nylon sutures over a stent. The stent is usually passed via the duct out through the nose. It may also be passed through both puncta into the sac. The stent can be a

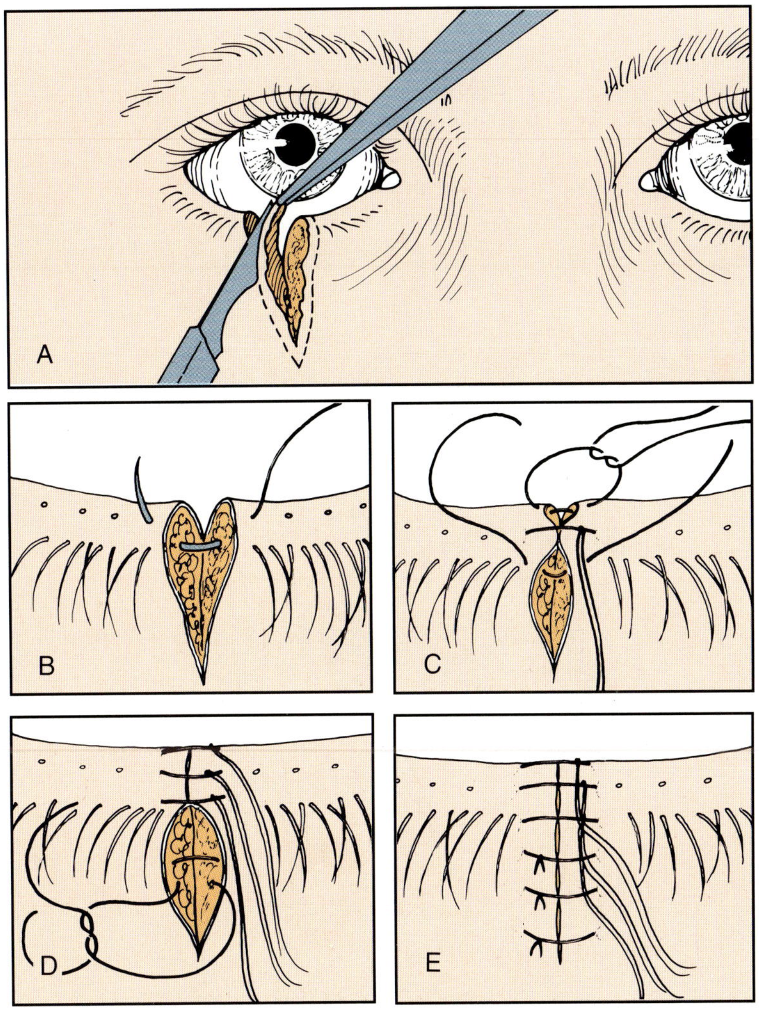

FIGURE 14.1 Repair of lid lacerations. **A** The wound is excised to remove all foreign bodies and damaged tissue and allow a straight surgical scar. **B** The first suture is through the line of the tarsal gland ducts and aligns the margins. **C,D** Additional sutures are made through superior and anterior edges. **E** All sutures are in place.

thin soft polyethylene or Silastic* catheter or a heavy nylon suture if a catheter is unavailable. Whichever is employed, it should be left in place for several weeks. If the injury to the lacrimal system is more extensive, a dacryocystorhinotomy may be necessary[9] (Fig. 14.2).

Ear Injury

The ear, in its exposed position, is frequently abraded, contused, or lacerated. Abrasions are gently cleaned and covered with a light, occlusive dressing to prevent perichondritis. A contusion may result in a hematoma of the auricle, which should be aspirated or evacuated as soon as possible. It may require repeated aspirations or even insertion of a drainage catheter. If the hematoma is left intact, it may go on to organization and eventual "cauliflower" ear deformity.[21]

Ear lacerations can usually be repaired by simple skin approximation. If the cartilage is lacerated, the edges can be gently trimmed but should not be sutured. If the ear is nearly avulsed, with a pedicle of tissue remaining, it should be sewn back into place and supported with a bulky dressing. The ear will usually survive this sort of assault because of its excellent blood supply. If it is totally avulsed, it can be replanted only by microvascular technique. This is possible only if there are vessels of sufficient size (0.4 mm) that have not been damaged too extensively. Because the auricle is primarily skin and cartilage, it will survive an ischemic insult far better than most other organs. A totally avulsed ear should be placed in a plastic bag and kept in ice until revascularization is effected.

If the auricle is unsalvageable, a new external ear can be created using a rib-cartilage scaffold covered by a temporoparietal fascial flap and skin graft.[6] This is usually carried out as a secondary procedure when the injured tissues have healed.

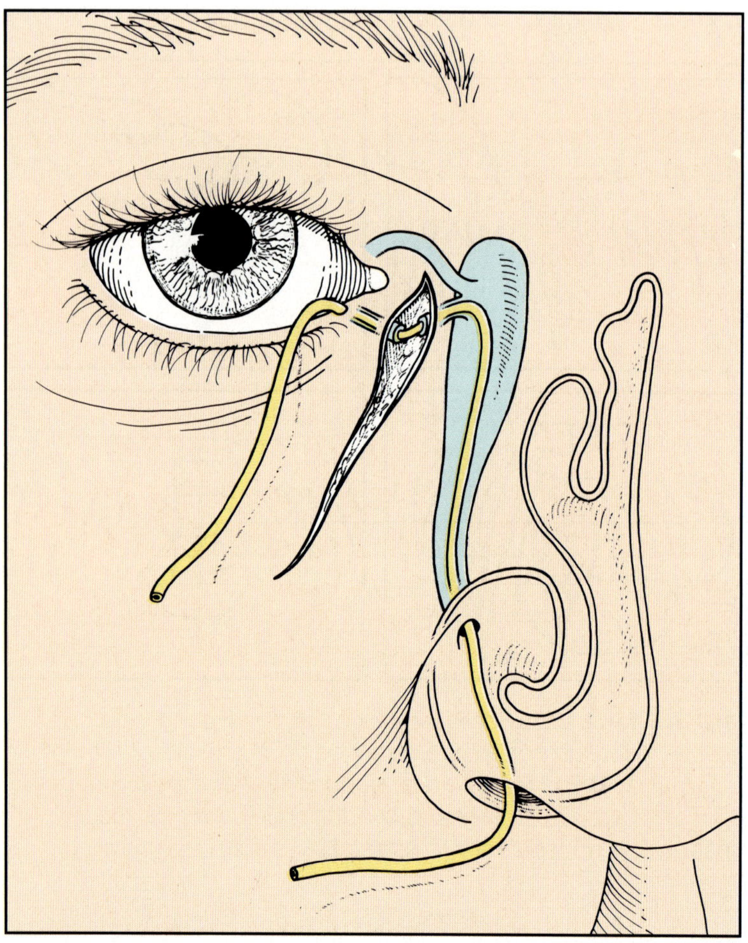

FIGURE 14.2 A silicone catheter or "stent" has been passed through the lower punctum across the lacerated canaliculus, through the lacrimal sac, and down the nasolacrimal duct to emerge out the nostril. The stent aids in suture placement and in prevention of stenosis of the canaliculus.

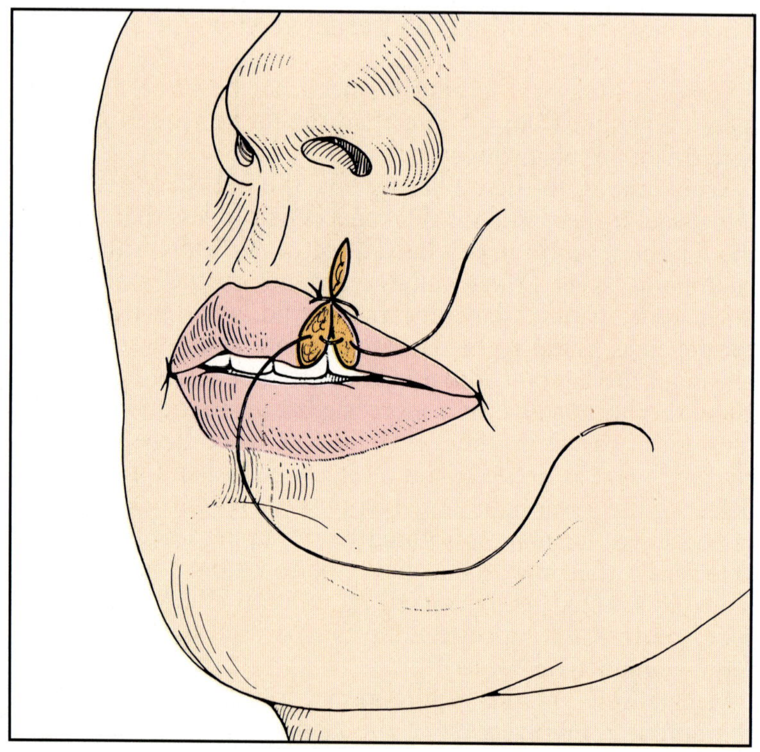

FIGURE 14.3 Repair of lip lacerations. The first suture is placed at the vermilion-cutaneous border to avoid irregularity at the border. The next sutures should be buried absorbable sutures to relieve tension of the skin closure and avoid a dead space.

*Silastic, brand of Dow Corning, Midland, Michigan.

Nasal Injury

Nasal lacerations are usually straightforward. Superficial lacerations should be closed with fine, nonabsorbable suture. Full-thickness defects should be repaired in layers. The inner nasal skin or mucosa should be realigned with 4-0 chromic suture. The cartilage should be reapproximated in proper position and the skin repaired with nonabsorbable suture (preferably subcuticular if feasible).

If a segment or the entire nose has been avulsed, there are a number of means of reconstruction. If the nose is only partially avulsed, it should be sewn back into place. Its blood supply is excellent. If a segment of the nose, such as an alar rim, is completely lost it can be recreated by a composite graft from the helical rim or with a nasolabial flap. Complete loss of the nose necessitates new tissue, and this is usually provided by a forehead flap with cartilage or bone as a framework.[22]

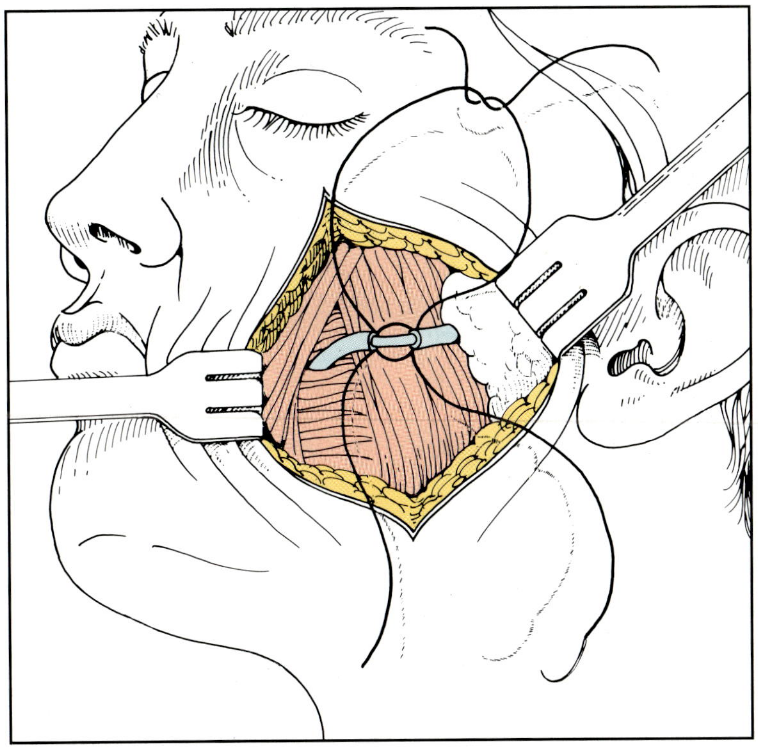

FIGURE 14.4 Repair of a lacerated parotid duct. A Silastic catheter should be passed proximally by way of Stensen's duct orifice in the mouth, and the laceration repaired over the catheter.

Lip Injury

Because of abundant tissue, most lacerations of the lip can be aggressively debrided or excised to obtain the minimal scar. Full-thickness lacerations are quite common because of the close proximity of the lip to the incisor teeth; these wounds should be closed in layers by first lining up the vermilion border with a nonabsorbable skin suture, and then closing the oral mucosa with absorbable suture. The orbicularis oris muscle is then likewise reapproximated with absorbable suture. Fine, nonabsorbable sutures are then used to loosely align the skin edges (Fig. 14.3).

Occasionally a patient arrives in the emergency room with loss of a segment of the lip from a human bite. These mouths can be reconstructed by Abbé,[1] Estlander,[10] or Karapandzic[13] flaps dependent on the location and size of the defect. If the deficit is less than a third of the length of the lip, then the wound can be closed primarily. Otherwise, it will require some sort of lip rotation. In such a case, aggressive débridement is mandatory prior to any closure. It is recommended that the definitive reconstruction be delayed until possible infection from the bite has been ruled out.[16]

Facial Nerve and Parotid Duct Injury

A deep laceration in the mid-cheek will often lacerate both Stensen's duct and a branch of the facial nerve. The duct lies approximately along a plane from the tragus of the ear to the midportion of the upper lip. It empties into the oral cavity via an orifice located in the mucosa opposite the upper second molar.

If a parotid duct laceration is suspected, a small Silastic catheter can be passed through the oral opening and advanced retrograde. If it appears in the wound, there is an obvious disruption; but if it passes easily to the parotid, no injury should be found. If there is ductal laceration, the catheter should be left in place as a stent bridging the severed duct, and the duct repaired with fine, absorbable sutures approximating the severed ends. The catheter should be sewn to the buccal mucosa to preclude its dislodgement (Fig. 14.4). After approximately 2 to 3 weeks, the stent may be removed.[25]

If a laceration on the immediate preauricular region demonstrates clear fluid exiting, most likely the parotid gland itself has been damaged. In this region no repair to the gland should be performed; fistulous drainage will normally cease spontaneously within 3 weeks. What must be determined is whether the facial nerve has likewise been lacerated. (In this particular region the nerve lies quite deep and is most often unharmed.)

The intimacy of the facial nerve and the parotid gland is the reason why concomitant injuries are so common. It is in the midst of the gland that the nerve divides into multiple branches. Although five branches are commonly mentioned, in reality there are many divisions. The five main divisions refer more to regions of distribution than to actual branches.

The temporal branch, which is typically multiple, crosses the zygoma approximately halfway from the tragus to the lateral canthus. It supplies the muscles of the forehead, including the major portion of the orbicularis oculi. The zygomatic branches also supply the orbicularis, as well as nasal and upper lip musculature. The buccal branch supplies the muscles of both lips; this branch normally follows the course of the parotid duct, and usually if the latter is lacerated, so too is the former (Fig. 14.5).

The marginal mandibular branch is classically found within a centimeter of the angle of the mandible. It parallels the body of the mandible until it rises to supply the depressors to the lower lip. Injury to the nerve results in an inability to bring the lower lip downward and laterally or evert the vermilion border. Because the mandibular branch has only a 15% crossover with other branches, function may not be regained spontaneously if it is divided and not repaired.

The cervical branch of the facial nerve supplies the platysma, which is also a depressor of the lower lip but of much less importance. Because loss of the cervical branch is relatively insignificant cosmetically or functionally, it is never repaired.

Lacerations to any of the facial nerve branches medial to the plane of the pupil of the eye are likewise commonly not explored. Not only are the axons small and difficult to identify in this region, but there is frequently cross-innervation from other nearby twigs.

More proximal injuries demand meticulous exploration to identify nerve ends and coapt them. If exploration is carried out within 72 hours of injury, a nerve stimulator will be quite helpful in identifying the distal ends.[4]

Because of the magnitude of the loss to the patient in most cases of facial palsy, nerve coaptation should be performed in the most precise manner possible. At present this is with use of an operating microscope and epineural sutures. Even with the most fastidious repair, it may still be up to 18 months before function is restored.

Bites

Human bites to the face are frequently seen and are often more serious than animal bites. The mixed anaerobic pathogens of the human oral flora are quite virulent. Fortunately most human bites are small. One may be able to totally excise the wound. If not, it should be debrided and left open to limit the likelihood of infection.

Animal bites may be larger, especially dog bites to children's faces. These wounds can be treated more aggressively; that is, debrided and closed. Most bites will require later scar revision.

Skeletal Fractures

FRACTURES IN THE ORBITAL FLOOR

Orbital fractures typically result from local forceful trauma and are characterized by ecchymosis, edema, and discomfort. The eyelids will often be quite swollen, as may be the conjunctiva. Palpation of the orbital rim may demonstrate a "stepoff." These fracture lines usually occur at the thinnest or weakest anatomical sites: the infraorbital foramen, suture lines, and so forth.

Numbness in the region of the upper lip or in the area of the nasolabial fold should suggest contusion or compression (neurapraxia) of the infraorbital nerve from an orbital floor or inferior rim fracture. Similar findings may also result from direct trauma to the nerve as it exits the foramen onto the cheek.

Blowout fractures of the orbital floor result from a blunt force, usually a ball or fist striking the globe directly (Fig. 14.6). This markedly raises intra-orbital pressure, which is released through an out-fracturing of one of the thinnest adjacent bones, the orbital floor. The inferior rim, which is much stronger, remains intact; immediately posterior, the orbital contents are being forced out into the maxillary sinus. If the orbital soft tissue, fat, or muscle become entrapped, several findings may be present. The total volume of orbital contents may be decreased, causing enophthalmos, or the entrapment

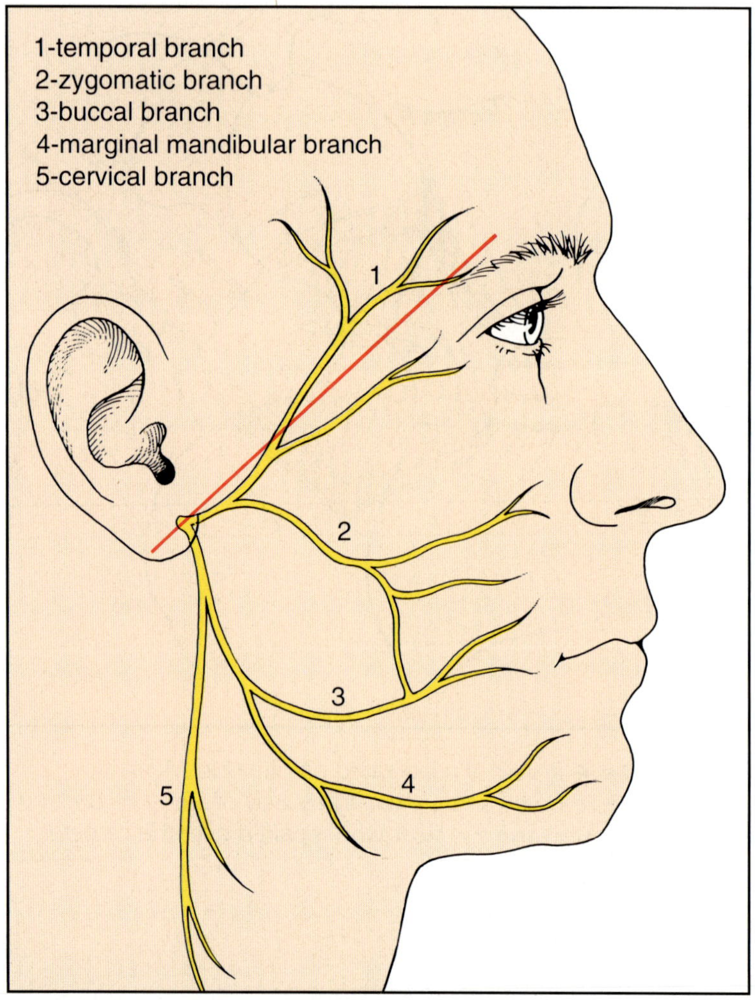

FIGURE 14.5 Branches of the facial nerve. The frontal branch is highlighted and lies in a plane drawn from the lateral eyebrow to the tragus of the ear.

of the extraocular muscle (inferior rectus muscle) may limit globe rotation (particularly upward gaze), causing diplopia. Mere spasm of the muscle alone may cause diplopia. Radiologically, on Waters view, there is characteristic clouding of the maxillary sinus from mucosal disruption of the antral roof, causing bleeding. Often there is also a teardrop-shaped soft tissue shadow hanging from the orbital floor, which signifies the soft tissue trapped through the fracture line. If Waters views are ambiguous, tomograms or CT scans may be needed, and the latter provide the most information.[24]

Indications for surgical exploration include diplopia, extraocular muscle entrapment, enophthalmos, flattening of the malar prominence, or anesthesia in the distribution of the infra-orbital nerve. The usual surgical approach is via a subciliary incision with interosseous wire fixation of the reduced fracture (Fig. 14.7). If bone is missing or too fragmented to be wired together, a thin bone graft or prosthetic wafer of Teflon or Silastic can be used to reconstruct the floor. Rarely, the floor may be so badly shattered that a temporary pack is needed in the maxillary sinus to serve as a splint. This packing is placed via the oral cavity by a Caldwell-Luc antrostomy.

ZYGOMATIC FRACTURES

Often concomitant with an orbital floor fracture is displacement of the zygoma. The zygoma is commonly fractured at the orbital floor and rim, the lateral orbital rim near the frontozygomatic suture line, and in the zygomatic arch. When all three areas are involved, this is referred to as a *tripod* or *trimalar fracture*. There is actually a fourth component, as evidenced by the bone's inferior depression; it has lost its deep lower support.

A zygomatic fracture should be suspected in the presence of periorbital ecchymosis or edema, subconjunctival hemorrhage, arch depression, orbital rim stepoff, intra-oral hematoma in the upper buccal sulcus, and all blowout fracture findings. Appropriate x-rays include a Waters view and a Caldwell view, as well as a submentovertex in order to visualize the arch.

Arch fractures can usually be treated in a closed fashion with a percutaneous bone hook or via a Gillies sub-temporal fascia approach to pop out the depressed bone. Most other zygomatic fractures require an open reduction and interosseous wiring as needed. Two-point fixation is usually sufficient—at the orbital floor and lateral rim. These landmarks are exposed by a subciliary incision and an incision in the lateral eyebrow so that both scars

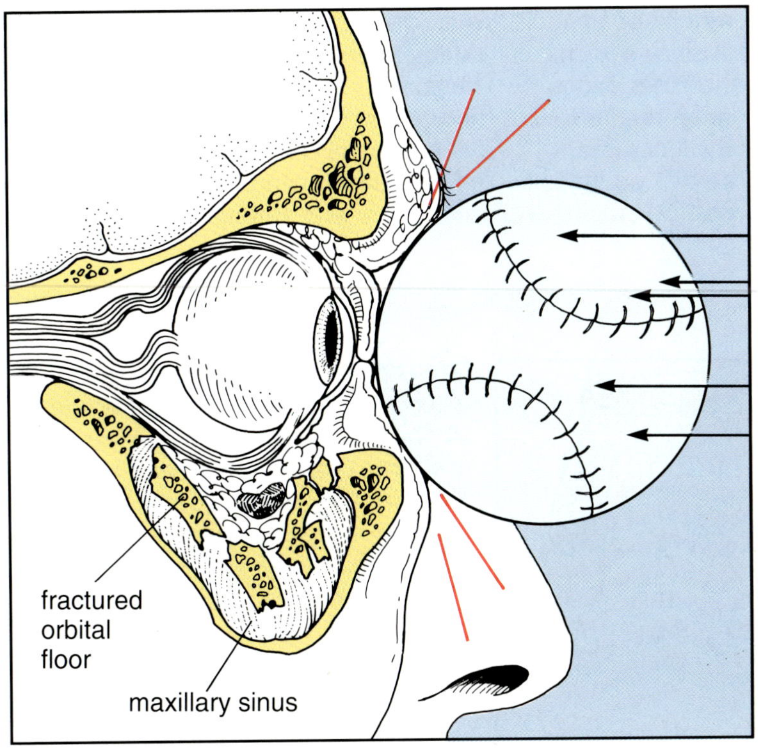

FIGURE 14.6 Blowout fracture of the orbit. External pressure forces the globe downward, fracturing the orbital floor and commonly entrapping periorbital fat and extra-ocular musculature in the maxillary antrum.

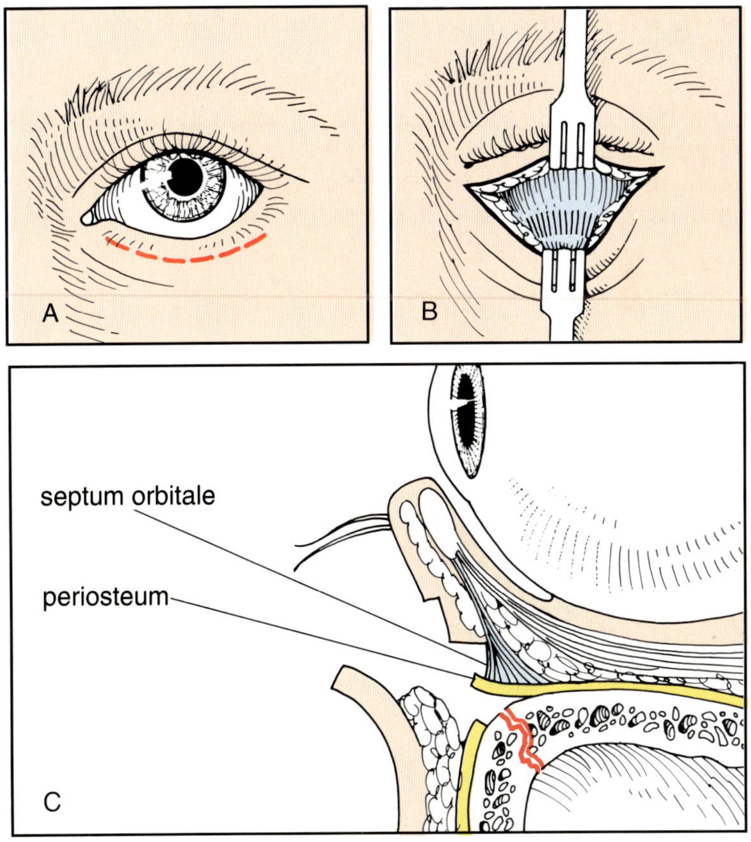

FIGURE 14.7 Exposure of orbital floor. **A,B** An incision is made just inferior to the lower eyelid lashes through a naturally occurring crease. The incision is then carried down to the septum orbitale, which is followed inferiorly to the orbital rim. **C** The periosteum of the orbital floor is elevated, exposing the fracture.

are hidden (Fig. 14.8). If it is apparent that the zygoma is being "flattened" by the pull of the masseter, a third point of wire fixation is needed at the maxillary junction, which is exposed via an upper buccal sulcus incision. Rarely will the zygomatic arch require a fourth point of fixation. In badly comminuted fractures of the zygoma, calvarial bone grafts or split rib grafts may be necessary to provide the needed support and cosmetic projection.

NASAL FRACTURES

The nasal bones, nasal cartilages, and septum may all be injured in nasal fractures. Typically, the diagnosis can be determined on the basis of physical examination alone. The patient will have lateral displacement of the nose with significant tenderness and edema of the dorsum. Bony instability and crepitus will be elicited. There may be airway obstruction on the deviated side, but this may also be due to a septal hematoma. (Septal hematomas must be identified and drained to prevent eventual cartilage destruction and saddle-nose deformity.)

Most nasal fractures that are treated within 2 weeks of injury can be reduced in a closed fashion with digital and instrumental manipulation. Under local and topical anesthesia with diazepam (Valium) sedation, an Asche forceps can be used to reduce nasal bones and septum back into a symmetric position. Intranasal packs and a rigid dorsal splint can then be used to maintain the reduction until union occurs (Fig. 14.9). Fractures older than 2 weeks will most likely need to be treated with osteotomies in a modified rhinoplastic manner.

Nasal fractures in children are diagnosed and treated in the same fashion as those in adults. X-rays, which in an adult are of limited value, are of even less importance in children. Deformity, tenderness, crepitation and periorbital ecchymosis are key criteria in making the diagnosis. It should be pointed out that septal hematomas are even more common in children, and direct nasal speculum examination must be performed to rule this out.[20]

NASO-ETHMOID FRACTURES

In frontal impact nasal fractures in which the nose appears foreshortened, with a dorsal depression, a naso-ethmoid fracture should be suspected. This is especially true if there is profuse nasal bleeding or cerebrospinal fluid rhinorrhea. Telecanthus will probably be present, but this depends on the degree of comminution of the fragments and the integrity of the periosteum. A normal intercanthal measurement does not rule out naso-ethmoid orbital fractures.

Radiologic examination is key to the diagnosis. Facial films will show fractures in the orbital rim, nose, and frontal region, as well as medial orbital wall fractures. There will usually be air-fluid levels in the ethmoid and maxillary sinuses. These films usually fail to provide information about the full extent of the injuries.

CT scans, on the other hand, are essential for delineating the injury and planning therapy. They provide clarity and detail of bone fragmentation. The presence of fractures through the nose and medial and inferior orbital rims is diagnostic of naso-ethmoid fractures. Isolated medial orbital wall (ethmoid) fractures are not naso-ethmoid fractures and do not require reduction.

Treatment should take place as soon as possible, while the fragments are still very mobile. Exposure can be through existing lacerations or by incisions across the root of the nose. Subciliary incisions with medial extension should also be made to provide direct rim exposure. The goals of reduction are to stabilize the orbital rim, as well as the adjacent frontal, zygomatic, and maxillary bones (Fig. 14.10). A transnasal canthopexy must reposition the two orbital rims and the medial canthal ligaments. This is done by looping a stainless-steel wire through the nasal bones

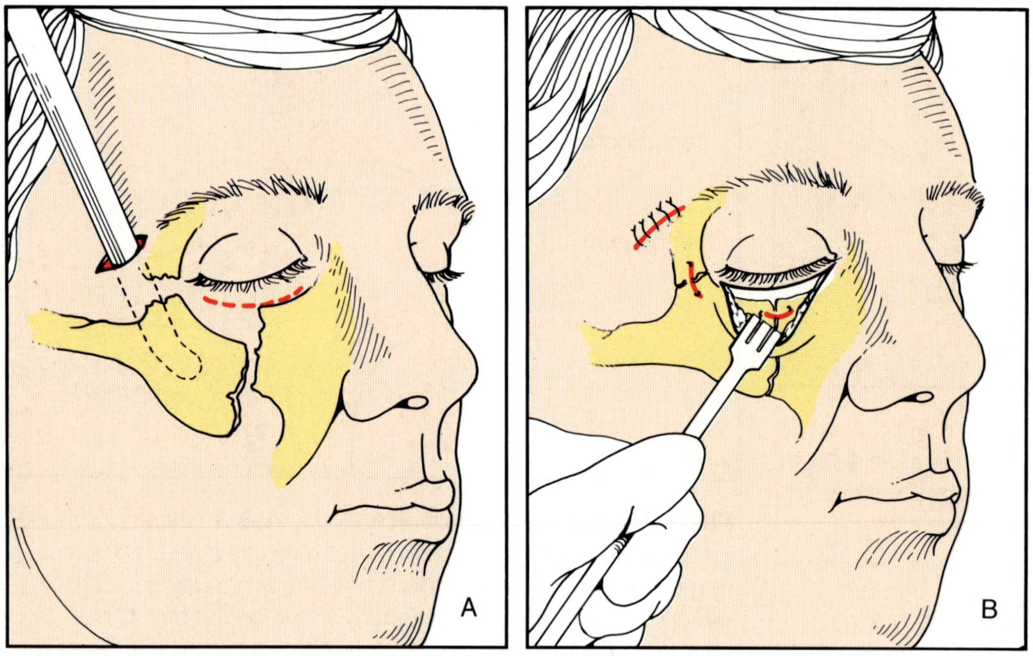

FIGURE 14.8 Open reduction and internal fixation of zygomatic fracture. **A** The zygoma (malar bone) is elevated back into proper position via a lateral brow incision. **B** The zygoma is held in place by interosseous wiring both at the lateral orbital rim and inferior orbital rim. (The exposure of the orbital rim is by a subciliary incision.)

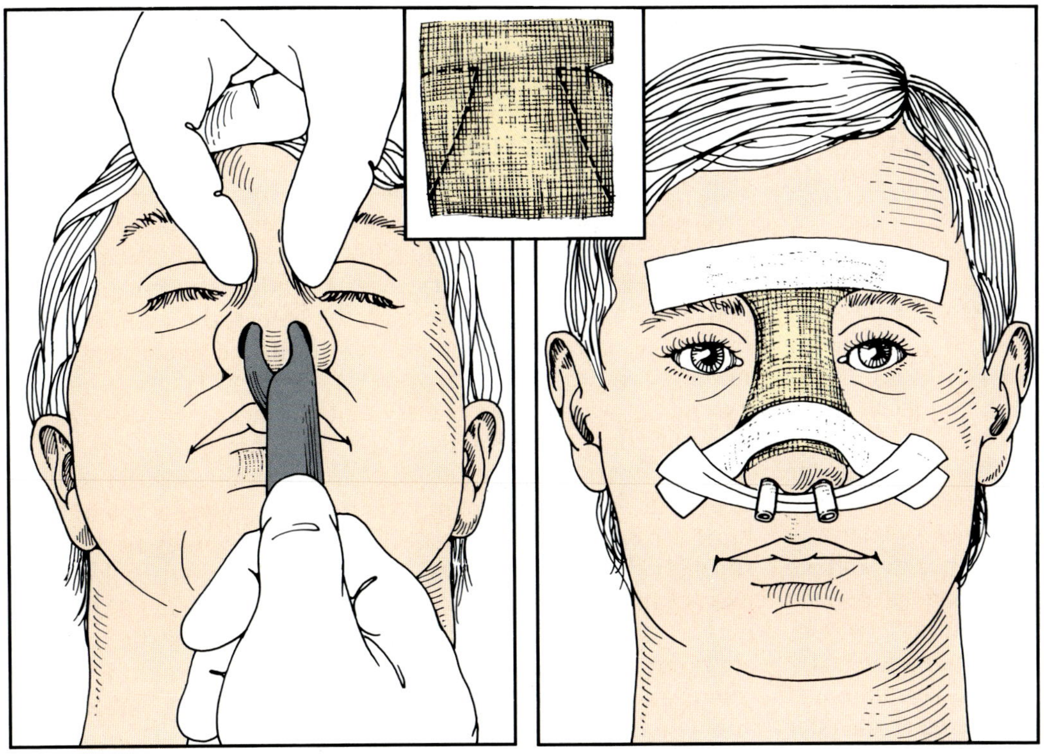

FIGURE 14.9 Closed reduction of nasal fracture. Asche forceps are used to straighten a septal fracture or elevate a depressed nasal bone fracture. Once adequate reduction has been achieved, the nose is splinted with internal petroleum jelly packs and an external plaster splint.

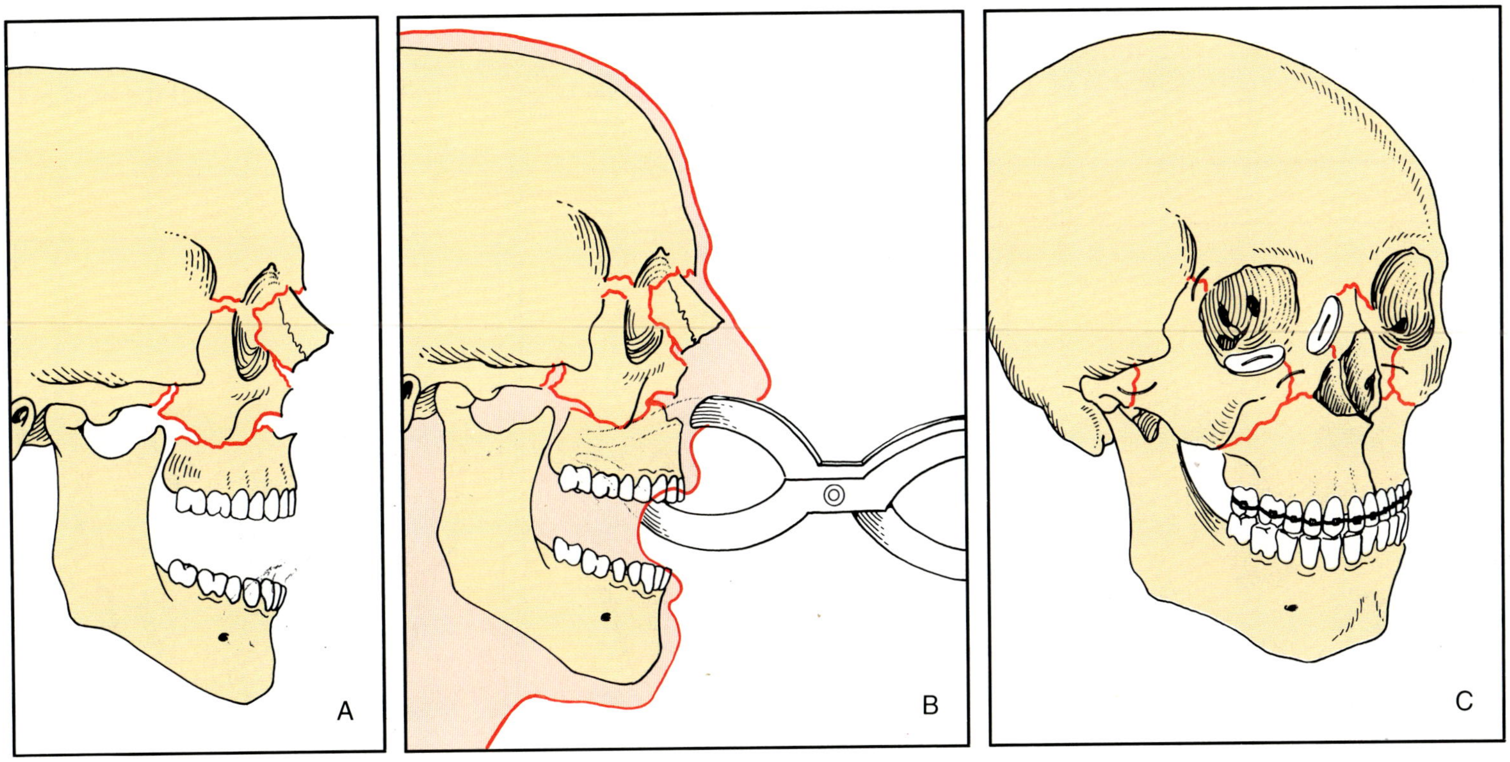

FIGURE 14.10 Complex midface fractures including naso-ethmoid fracture. **A** The bones are impacted inward, flattening the profile. **B** The impacted maxillary fragment is reduced with Rowe-type disimpactors. **C** Fractures have been reduced and stabilized. Note the canthal buttons to aid in reinsertion of the medial canthal tendons into the medial orbital walls. Note also the bone graft or Teflon plate to the orbital floor and the use of a Kirschner wire to help stabilize the zygoma. Miniature compression plates may also be used.

with both ligaments attached. In tightening this wire, one must remember that it is virtually impossible to overshorten the intercanthal distance.[17]

Bone fragments are then reapproximated with interosseous wire. If bone is missing or too fragmented, bone grafts can be used. Because of the proximity of the lacrimal system, it should be visualized and repaired if injured.

FRONTAL BONE FRACTURES

The frontal bone may be fractured in the anterior or posterior walls of the frontal sinus, or both. Often this is an open fracture with a large forehead laceration. CT scans are obtained on all of these patients because of the head trauma, but surgical exploration is mandatory if the fractures are open.

If the forehead laceration is extensive, the injury can be explored through it. Usually a bicoronal incision is necessary, and this provides immediate access to cranial bones for grafting.

Fractures with displacement of only the anterior sinus wall are handled in the following fashion. The depressed bone is elevated and wired in place, and patency of the nasofrontal duct must be ensured. This may necessitate passing a drain down into the nose.

If the posterior wall is fractured, the sinus should be eliminated by cranialization. The mucosa is stripped and ligated at the duct level or invaginated with the duct mucosa into the nose to seal off the nasal cavity. The posterior wall bone fragments are gently removed and can be used to reconstruct the anterior wall if need be. If the bones are too fragmented to be useful and the anterior wall requires a large graft, this should be harvested from the iliac crest. This graft will handle the daily trauma of the forehead better than thinner membranous bone grafts.

MAXILLARY FRACTURES

It is customary to describe fractures in the middle third of the face with respect to Le Fort's classification. Le Fort,[15] in studying skeletal fractures at the turn of the century, found three major patterns of disruption. A Le Fort I fracture extends across the lower maxilla through the base of the pyriform aperture. It separates the alveolar ridge from the remainder of the maxilla. A Le Fort II fracture is a pyramidal fracture that extends upward across the root of the nose. It separates the nasomaxillary segment from the zygomata and orbits. A Le Fort III fracture, or craniofacial dysjunction, separates all of the facial skeleton including the maxillae, zygomata, and nasal bones from the cranial base. The fracture lines here travel through the upper portion of the zygomatic–frontal border, naso-ethmoid region, and orbital floors (Fig. 14.11). Although Le Fort classified these as three separate entities, the fractures are often in combination. Frequently, in severe motor vehicle trauma, a patient will have a Le Fort III on one side of the face and a Le Fort II on the other.

Because in all transverse fractures the maxillary dentition is dissociated from the upper facial or cranial skeleton, the key maneuver in diagnosis is to determine midface mobility. The upper alveolar ridge is grasped with one hand and the head held

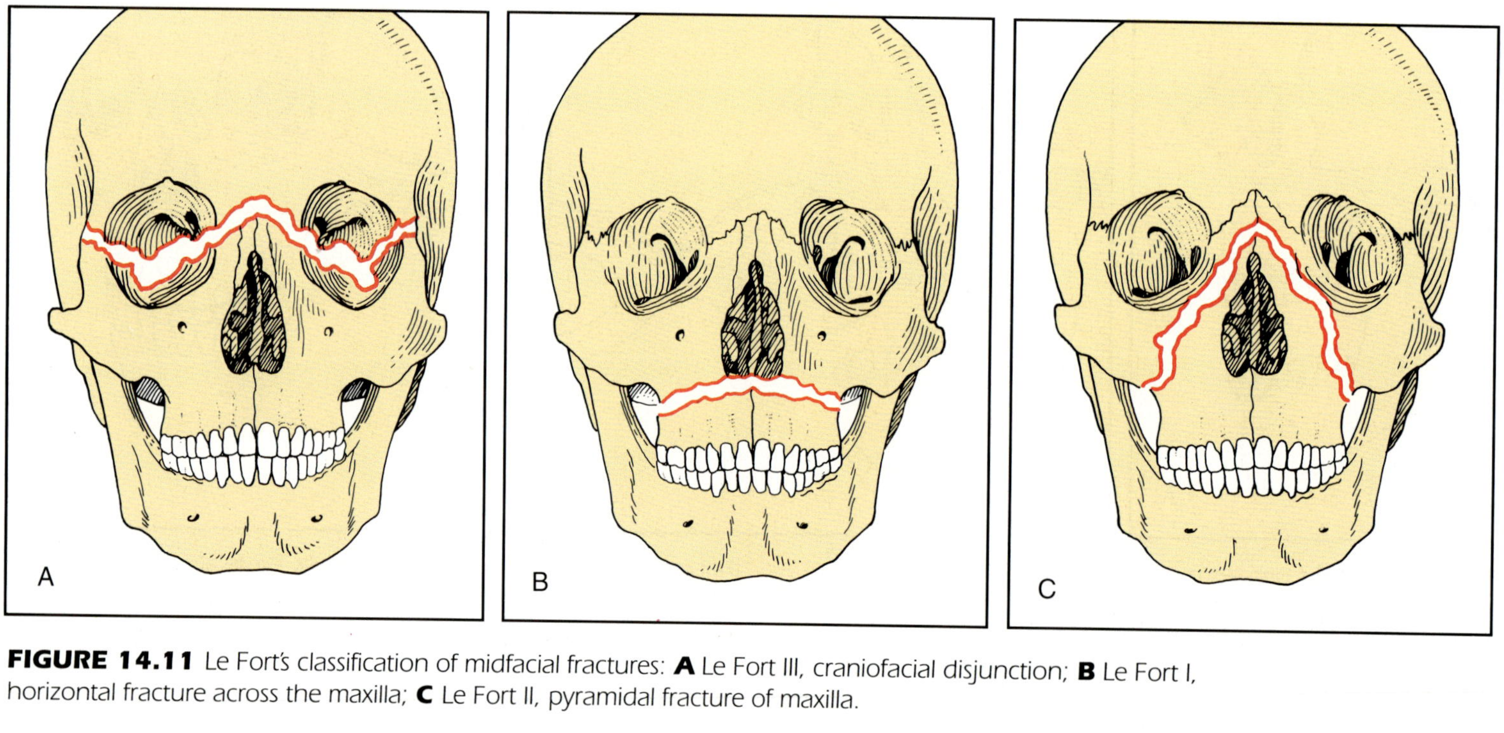

FIGURE 14.11 Le Fort's classification of midfacial fractures: **A** Le Fort III, craniofacial disjunction; **B** Le Fort I, horizontal fracture across the maxilla; **C** Le Fort II, pyramidal fracture of maxilla.

firmly with the other, and skeletal instability is appraised. Often, x-rays will be necessary to determine the exact nature of the fracture because clinically one can only state that skeletal mobility is present and that the patient has malocclusion.[12]

In severe midface trauma, the patient most commonly presents with massive facial edema, "raccoon-eye" ecchymosis, and nasal bleeding. Cerebrospinal fluid rhinorrhea is present in up to 50% of Le Fort II and III fractures. The patient may demonstrate a retruded midface with an anterior open bite due to inferior displacement of the facial skeleton. This is described as a "long face" because the traumatic blow has forced the midface posteriorly and inferiorly.

Again, the Waters view is the single most useful roentgen examination. CT scans, though, are invaluable for clarifying Le Fort II and III fractures, especially at the naso-ethmoid region and orbital floors.

The goals of therapy are to restore proper occlusion and to regain proper projection of the lower midface. If the mandible is unscathed, it serves as the support and guide to proper reduction. In addition, suspension wires from unfractured upper skeletal bones help maintain projection and reduction (Fig. 14.12).

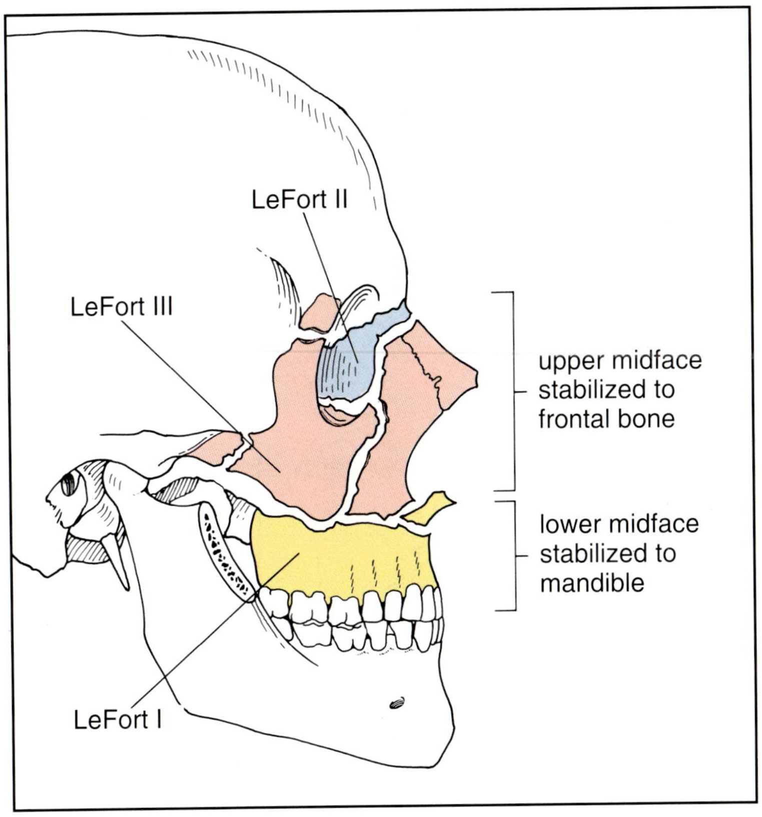

FIGURE 14.12 Stabilization of midface fractures. The mandible, unless also fractured, is held to the cranial base and can be used to stabilize lower midface fractures. Upper midface fractures are stabilized to the frontal bone. If all are fractured, a Georgiade Halo may be used for stability.

Le Fort I fractures can be treated by intermaxillary fixation (IMF), often with suspension wires from the zygomatic arches. Compression bone plates are being used more frequently now to shorten or eliminate the unpleasantness of intermaxillary fixation.

Le Fort II and III fractures require subciliary incisions and bicoronal or eyebrow incisions to get access to fracture lines. Interosseous wires or mini-compression plates may be used, along with IMF to restore occlusion. Cranial suspension wires from the frontal bone may be passed down to the maxillary arch or better yet to the mandibular arch bar, to stabilize the entire complex. Headframes such as the Georgiade Halo**[11] may be necessary with severe midface retrusion despite open reduction. These serve to provide external traction, which brings out the inwardly crushed segments. These headframes make circumferential point contact with the outer table of the skull, balancing the forces, and are useful in patients who have lost frontal cranial support or mandibular supports.

FRACTURES OF THE MANDIBLE

Fractures of the mandible are determined not only by the force and direction of the external blow but also by the position of the teeth. The long cuspid teeth and unerupted third molars create areas of relative weakness; hence, a high percentage of fractures occur at these sites. It should be remembered that since the teeth are a potential source of infection, any fracture occurring through an alveolar socket or the crypt of an impacted tooth should be treated as an open fracture, requiring antibiotics.

Unlike other facial fractures, mandibular fractures may be distracted by the vigorous pull of the muscles of mastication. Depending on the location of the fracture, these muscles may provide strong forces to separate the bone ends. An intact periosteum will serve to prevent major displacement; once the periosteum is disrupted, the bone ends may be free to follow the contracting muscles. In order to properly treat mandibular fractures, one must understand the anatomy and function of the muscles as well.

Fractures of the posterior body or angle of the mandible will tend to be distracted superiorly by the masseter, temporalis, and medial pterygoid musculature, and medially by both the medial and lateral pterygoids. The lateral pterygoid, through its insertion on the condylar neck, will tend to displace the condyle medially if it is fractured.

The anterior mandibular fragment of any body fracture will be depressed inferiorly by the geniohyoid, genioglossus, mylohyoid, and digastric muscles. In the case of a unilateral parasymphyseal fracture, the geniohyoid and mylohyoid muscles will tend to displace the fragments toward the tongue.

The direction of fracture lines may serve to aid or resist distraction. Because of the shape of the mandible as a **U**, fractures may be regarded as favorable or unfavorable in two planes, hori-

**Padgett Instruments, Kansas City, KS.

zontal and vertical (Fig. 14.13). If an anterior oblique body fracture permits unopposed distraction of the posterior segment, it is an unfavorable fracture. If the fracture line is perpendicular to the previously described one, such that with the pull of the masseter and temporalis, the end of the posterior fragment is imbedded into the anterior fragment, it is quite favorable.[8]

The most consistent clinical finding of mandibular fractures is dental malocclusion (Fig. 14.14). There is also pain on biting, deviation of the jaw on opening, and trismus. If the fracture injures the inferior alveolar or mental nerve, there will be anesthesia in the soft tissue supplied by that nerve. The jaw will demonstrate a deformity, often with a stepoff, broken teeth, or a malaligned alveolar ridge. Mucosal lacerations or hematomas may lie over the fracture site.

Radiologically, the most desirable film is the panorex, which demonstrates the entire mandible. If this is unavailable, multiple views including an anterior-posterior of the mandible, lateral oblique shots, and a modified Towne's view should be obtained.

The overriding goal of treatment is to restore a normal occlusive relationship between the jaws and the teeth, with good bony union of the fragments. As with other fractures, the simplest and most effective route is the one to be followed. The most uncomplicated method is IMF, and more than 65% of mandibular fractures can be handled in a closed fashion.[3] There are various techniques for open reduction and internal fixation, the most common being interosseous wiring and use of compression plates. Interosseous wiring still requires IMF, whereas primary osteosynthesis with mini-compression plates may shorten or eliminate the need for IMF. Because the location of the fracture determines therapy, each major region of the mandible will be covered separately.

CONDYLAR FRACTURES

Surgical intervention is rarely used in condylar fractures, in which the aim is to encourage active motion as early as possible and preserve the use of the temporomandibular joint. Hence, in unilateral fractures a soft diet is tried if the patient can bring his teeth into occlusion. If there is too much pain or displacement of the mandible, then IMF is used for a week until muscle spasm has been overcome.

In bilateral cases the resultant shortening of the ramus may necessitate IMF for 3 to 4 weeks. It is recommended that corticosteroids be injected into the glenoid fossa at weekly intervals during fixation to minimize scarring in the joint.

Open reduction is necessary only if the condylar segment is so rotated that it is interfering with jaw movement or if it has pushed up into the cranial fossa, causing neurologic impairment.[5]

BODY FRACTURES

If there is adequate dentition on each side of the fracture, arch bars and IMF are sufficient for stabilization and immobilization.

FRACTURES OF THE ANGLE AND SYMPHYSIS

Angular and parasymphyseal fractures are usually not adequately managed with IMF alone. If the fracture line at the angle is posterior to the last tooth, the lateral fragment is usually distracted

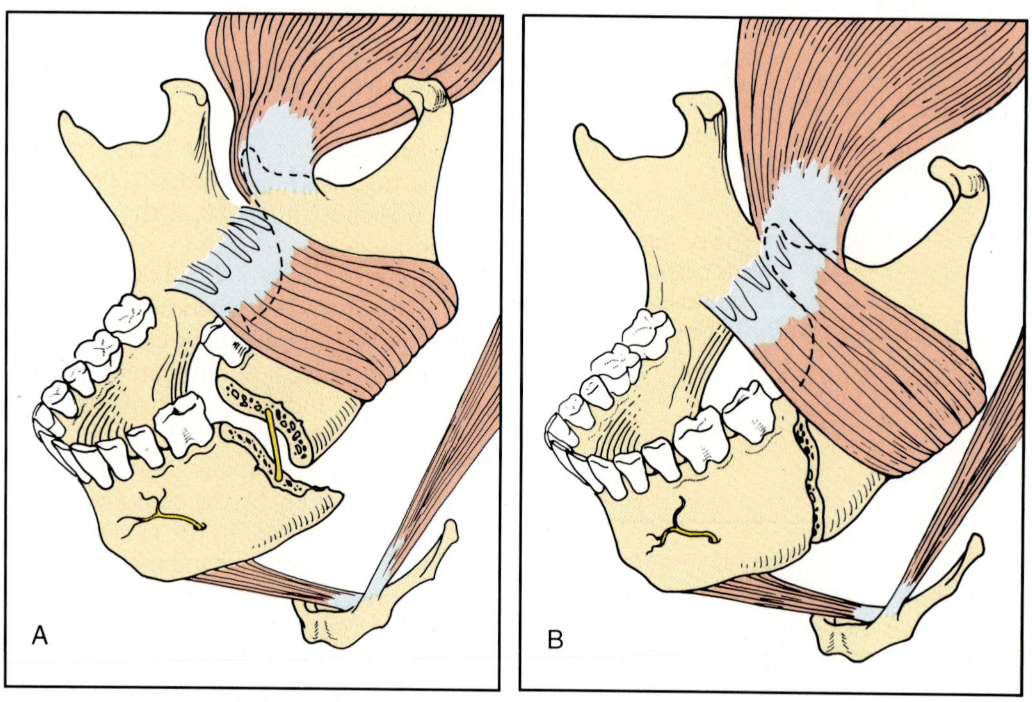

FIGURE 14.13 Influence of the muscles of mastication on mandibular fractures: **A** horizontally and vertically unfavorable fracture; **B** horizontally and vertically favorable fracture. Note in **B** how the masseter and temporalis will pull fragments together.

medially and superiorly. Open wiring or plating is necessary. Likewise, parasymphyseal fractures are displaced inferiorly by the suprahyoid muscles and are rotated medially. For this reason they are best handled by an open reduction and internal fixation. An intraoral approach to the parasymphyseal fractures can avoid a visible scar. Fixation of this type of fracture is aided by the use of a more rigid arch bar (Jalenko).

EDENTULOUS MANDIBULAR FRACTURES

With the loss of teeth comes a resorption of the alevolar bone. The cortex becomes very thin and the marrow wider. The blood supply is then essentially from the periosteal vessels. For this reason, bone healing is frequently fraught with difficulties, and there is a 70% incidence of nonunion.

Because there are no teeth, there is no concern with dental occlusion. Small irregularities in the bony profile can be ignored by the surgeon and taken into account on the base of the dentures. Undisplaced fractures do not require any therapy other than a soft, pureed diet. Minimally displaced fractures can be handled by circummandibular wiring with the patient's lower dentures or an acrylic used as a splint. If there is significant displacement, a Gunning-type splint can be fashioned, with a space left in the incisor region for eating.[3]

MANDIBULAR FRACTURES IN CHILDREN

Fractures of the mandible in children are rare but demand special attention. Children possess bell-shaped teeth that make wiring difficult, and their jaws are full of unerupted teeth. Therefore, children with few permanent teeth are placed in a Gunning-type splint, which is held in place with circumferential wires. If a large number of teeth are available, arch bars may be placed or a plastic splint constructed, with circumferential wires to stabilize the splint, teeth, and mandible. Open reduction is seldom undertaken, though, for fear of injuring developing tooth buds.[2]

Gunshot Wounds to the Face

Gunshot wounds to the face, especially those to the mouth, require special attention because of the frequent discrepancy between apparent damage and actual injury. What may be overlooked in all the soft tissue damage is the overriding need for a good airway. If the patient has survived the blast and the trip to the emergency room, his central nervous system has probably been unharmed. What will now most likely cause his death is the loss of an adequate airway.

As in all injuries, the blood and foreign bodies should immediately be cleared from the oral cavity. If there is significant damage in the oral cavity and/or nasal cavity, consideration of immediate intubation or even tracheostomy must be given. Even if the patient is moving sufficient air on arrival, there is the great potential for soft tissue hematoma and emesis, which can cause respiratory obstruction.

Once a good airway is guaranteed, the patient may be taken to the radiology room for CT scans, cervical spine films, and so

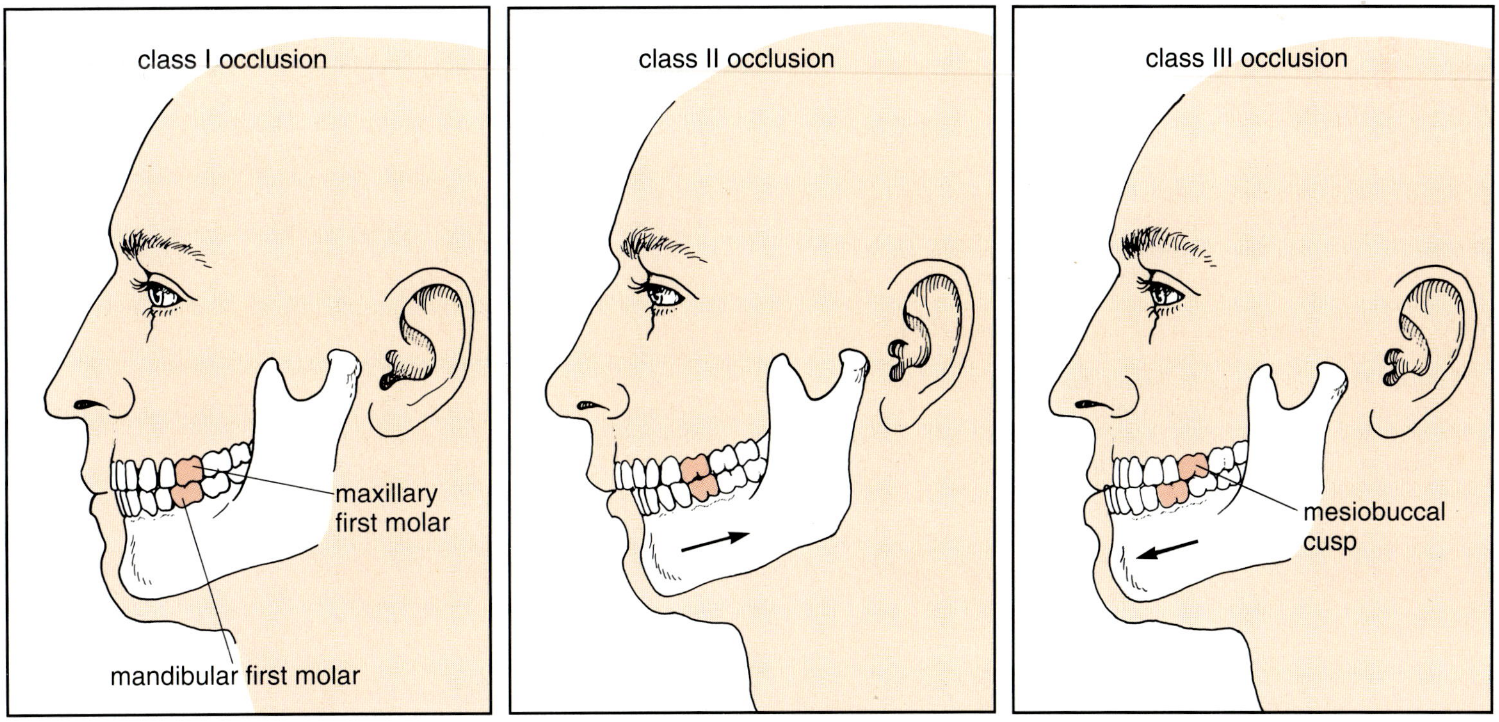

FIGURE 14.14 Angle's classification of malocclusion. The classification is based on the relationship of the mesiobuccal cusp of the maxillary first molar with the mesiobuccal groove of the mandibular first molar. Class I (neutral occlusion) is normal. In class II (distal occlusion) the mandible is retrognathic and the lower face appears recessed. In class III (mesial occlusion) the mandible is prognathic.

forth. A chest x-ray should also be part of the routine to rule out aspiration of a foreign body, or traumatic pneumothorax. Under no circumstances should these studies be done earlier.

If there are no neurologic problems, the patient may then be taken to the operating room for débridement and closure. All obvious nonviable tissue, including small bony fragments, must be removed, as should shotgun wadding or accessible pellets. Although the initial soft tissue injury may appear to be devastating, in reality very little tissue is usually lost. The soft tissue should be reconstructed in layers, and frequently the entire soft tissue envelope is found to be intact. If there are soft tissue segments missing, adequate repair will require flap transfer by either regional flaps or free microvascular flaps.

Bone is a different matter, for if it is hit by a high-speed bullet, there will be significant bone loss. The point of entrance of the bullet will quite often cause less damage than the point of exit, where some of the internal tissues, such as bone, themselves act as missiles. For this reason, once the soft tissue has been reapproximated, a means of bony stabilizing, usually external fixation, should be placed. This maintains the mandibular alignment. Once the soft tissues have healed and there is minimal risk of infection, bone grafts can be placed to reconstruct the bone loss. The external fixators serve to stabilize the mandible through this period of bone grafting. If both significant bone and soft tissue are missing, the mandible and soft tissue can be reconstructed in one stage in a number of ways. Vascularized calvarial bone grafts based on the superficial temporal vessels have recently been described in mandibular reconstruction. Microvascular osteocutaneous groin or scapular flaps are other methods of one-stage composite reconstruction.

REFERENCES

1. Abbé R: A new plastic operation for the relief of deformity due to double harelip. Med Rec 53:477, 1898.
2. Angelillo JC: Fractures of the mandible in children. In Serafin D, Georgiade NG (eds): Pediatric Plastic Surgery, pp 531–551. St Louis, CV Mosby, 1984.
3. Angelillo JC: Management of fractures of the mandible. In Georgiade NG, Georgiade GS, Riefkohl R, Barwick WJ (eds): Essentials of Plastic, Maxillofacial, and Reconstructive Surgery, pp 365–379. Baltimore, Williams & Wilkins, 1986.
4. Barwick WJ, Klein HW: Soft tissue injuries of the face. In Serafin D, Georgiade NG (eds): Pediatric Plastic Surgery, pp 650–654. St Louis, CV Mosby, 1984.
5. Bradley P: Injuries of the condylar and coronoid process. In Rowe NL, Williams JL (eds): Maxillofacial Injuries, pp 337–362. Edinburgh, Churchill Livinstone, 1985.
6. Brent B, Byrd HS: Secondary ear reconstruction with cartilage grafts covered by axial, random, and free flaps of temporoparietal fascia. Plast Reconstr Surg 72:141, 1983.
7. Cole JG: Primary treatment of eyelid lacerations. In Tessier P et al (eds): Symposium on Plastic Surgery in the Orbital Region, pp 39–42. St Louis, CV Mosby, 1976.
8. Converse JM: Surgical Treatment of Facial Injuries, 3rd ed, pp 142–156. Baltimore, Williams & Wilkins, 1974.
9. Converse JM, Smith B: Defects of the lacrimal system. In Converse JM (ed): Reconstructive Plastic Surgery, 2nd ed, pp 980–989. Philadelphia, WB Saunders, 1977.
10. Estlander JA: Classic reprint. Eine methode aus der Einen Lippe Substanz verluste der Anderen zu Erstetzen (A method of reconstructing loss of substance in one lip from the other lip). Translated from the German by Dr. Borje Sundell. Arch Klin Chir 14:622, 1872; Plast Reconstr Surg 42:360, 1968.
11. Georgiade N, Riefkohl R, Georgiade G: Twenty-five year evaluation of external halo fixation for severe maxillofacial injuries. Plast Reconstr Surg 68:444, 1981.
12. Heckler FR, Jabaley ME: Maxillofacial injuries. In Chang WHJ (ed): Fundamentals of Plastic and Reconstructive Surgery, pp 172–173. Baltimore, Williams & Wilkins, 1980.
13. Karapandzic M: Reconstruction of lip defects by local arterial flaps. Br J Plast Surg 27:93, 1974.
14. Krause F: Ueber die transplantation grosser ungestielter hautlappen. Arch Klin Chir 46:177, 1893.
15. Le Fort R: Étude expérimentale sur les fractures de la machoire supérieure. Rev Chir 23:208, 360, 479, 1901.
16. Lesavoy MA: Reconstruction of the Head and Neck, pp 97–116. Baltimore, Williams & Wilkins, 1981.
17. Manson PN, Crawley WA, Yaremchuk MJ et al: Midface fractures: Advantages of immediate extended open reduction and bone grafting. Plast Reconstr Surg 76:1, 1985.
18. Manson PN, French JH, Hoopes JE: Management of midfacial fractures. In Georgiade NG, Georgiade GS, Riefkohl R, Barwick W (eds): Essentials of Plastic, Maxillofacial, and Reconstructive Surgery, pp 349–364. Baltimore, Williams & Wilkins, 1986.
19. Mustardé JC: Repair and Reconstruction in the Orbital Region, pp 92–151. Edinburg, Churchill Livinstone, 1980.
20. Schultz RC: Pediatric facial fractures. In Kernahan DA et al (eds): Symposium on Pediatric Plastic Surgery, pp 255–259. St Louis, CV Mosby 1982.
21. Schultz RC: Basic principles in management of facial injuries. In Georgiade NG, Georgiade GS, Riefkohl R, Barwick W (eds): Essentials of Plastic, Maxillofacial, and Reconstructive Surgery, pp 337–348. Baltimore, Williams & Wilkins, 1986.
22. Stark RB: Total Facial Reconstruction, pp 41–43. New York, Thieme-Stratton, 1984.
23. Wolfe J: A new method of performing plastic operations. Br Med J 2:360, 1875.
24. Zizmor J, Lombardi G: Atlas of Orbital Radiography, pp 21–33. Birmingham, AL, Aesculapius, 1973.
25. Zook EG: The Primary Care of Facial Injuries, pp 4, 146. Littleton, MA, PSG Publishing, 1980.

15

neck injuries

Worthington G. Schenk III

The evaluation of neck injuries is a high priority in the care of the trauma patient, especially the victim of multiple blunt vehicular trauma. Airway maintenance, protection of the axial spine, and prevention/treatment of hypovolemic shock all require some evaluation of the neck in the initial seconds of medical attention. Establishing control of the upper airway is assigned the highest priority in multiple trauma because it is the one therapeutic intervention that has the greatest likelihood of favorably altering an otherwise unfavorable outcome.[1] Although airway management techniques are discussed in Chapter 3, their importance cannot be overemphasized. Airway compromise through direct blunt or penetrating trauma to the upper airway will be covered in this chapter. Protection of the axial spine and spinal cord share top priority in multiple trauma and will be covered primarily in the section on blunt neck injuries. The control and definitive management of hemorrhagic complications is primarily an issue with penetrating neck injuries.

This chapter is organized into discussions of blunt and penetrating neck trauma. Blunt neck trauma most frequently is the result of automotive vehicular accidents, and the approach to its management revolves primarily around protection of airway patency and axial spine integrity. Penetrating neck injuries are usually the result of interpersonal conflict. Gunshot wounds and stab wounds to the neck also require diligent protection of the airway and cervical spine, but the options for diagnosis and surgical management remain controversial.

BLUNT NECK TRAUMA

Every victim of vehicular trauma seeking medical attention is assumed to have a significant neck injury until proven otherwise. The Socratic adage *primum non nocera* is nowhere more applicable than in the management of a patient who potentially has an occult unstable injury to the cervical spine. Through the excellent organized efforts of prehospital care providers over the past 2 decades, stabilization and protection of the axial spine in transport from the scene of the accident has become routine. Fig. 15.1 illustrates the necessary components of this protection. Because a potentially hazardous unstable spinal injury can exist in the complete absence of signs and symptoms, and because the sequelae of iatrogenic spine destabilization can result in quadriplegia or other major permanent disability, there is every reason to apply these protective prophylactic measures to every victim of vehicular, decelerative, or other energy-transfer blunt trauma who is transported to the hospital. The onus is then on the physician who discontinues these protective measures to establish proof that an occult injury to the neck has been ade-

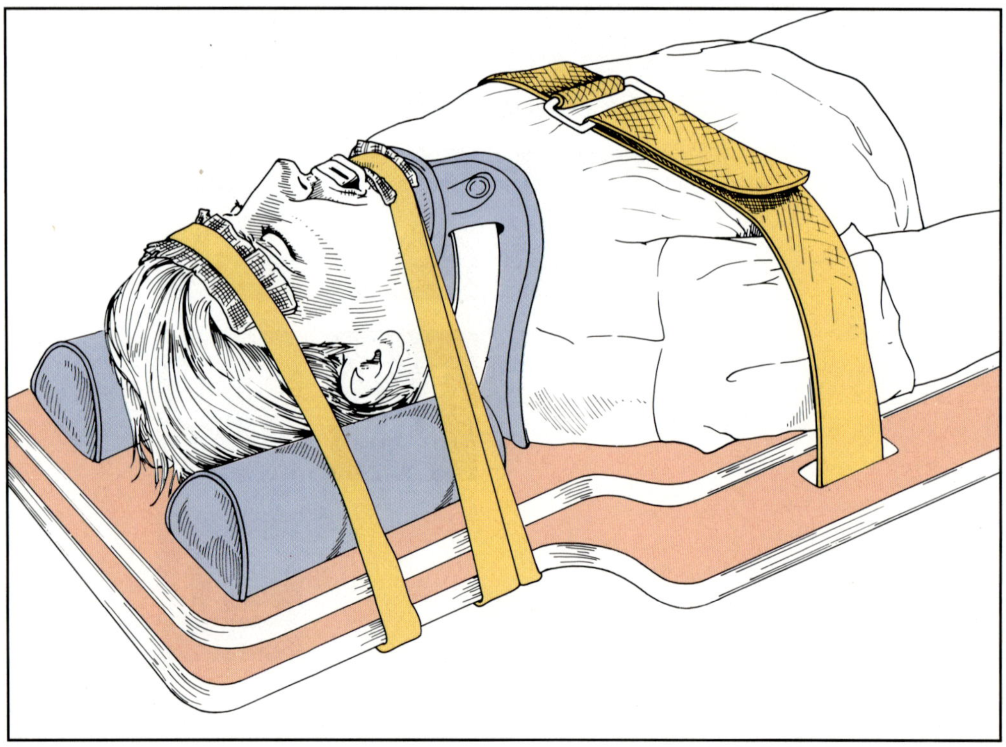

FIGURE 15.1 The essential components of protection of the cervical spine for prehospital transport. Note the short and long spine boards, semirigid collar, sandbags, and straps on the torso, chin, and forehead.

quately, if not completely, disproven. The medicolegal liability of this decision must not be underrated by any physician involved in the immediate evaluation of trauma.

Initial Evaluation

Maintenance of upper airway patency and protection of the cervical spine share top priority in the immediate management of the blunt trauma victim, but they may be mutually antagonistic: manipulation of the airway can be hazardous to an unstable spinal injury, and the axial spine protection measures may interfere with airway management. The protocol for initial airway assessment and management recommended by the American College of Surgeons Committee on Trauma is reproduced in Fig. 15.2.

Portable radiographs of the chest and cervical spine are appropriately completed during this same initial stabilization period. A single screening lateral cervical spine film may alert the physician to the presence of an occult spine injury that needs further protection and evaluation. This finding should lead to enhanced caution when the patient is positioned, transported, or intubated, but the single screening film is not sufficient to exclude a potentially unstable spine injury, since as many as 18% of injuries to the cervical spine will have an unremarkable initial lateral cervical spine film.[4,13] The definitive exclusion of a threat to the upper spinal cord must await the more methodical phase of trauma evaluation, after resuscitation and stabilization

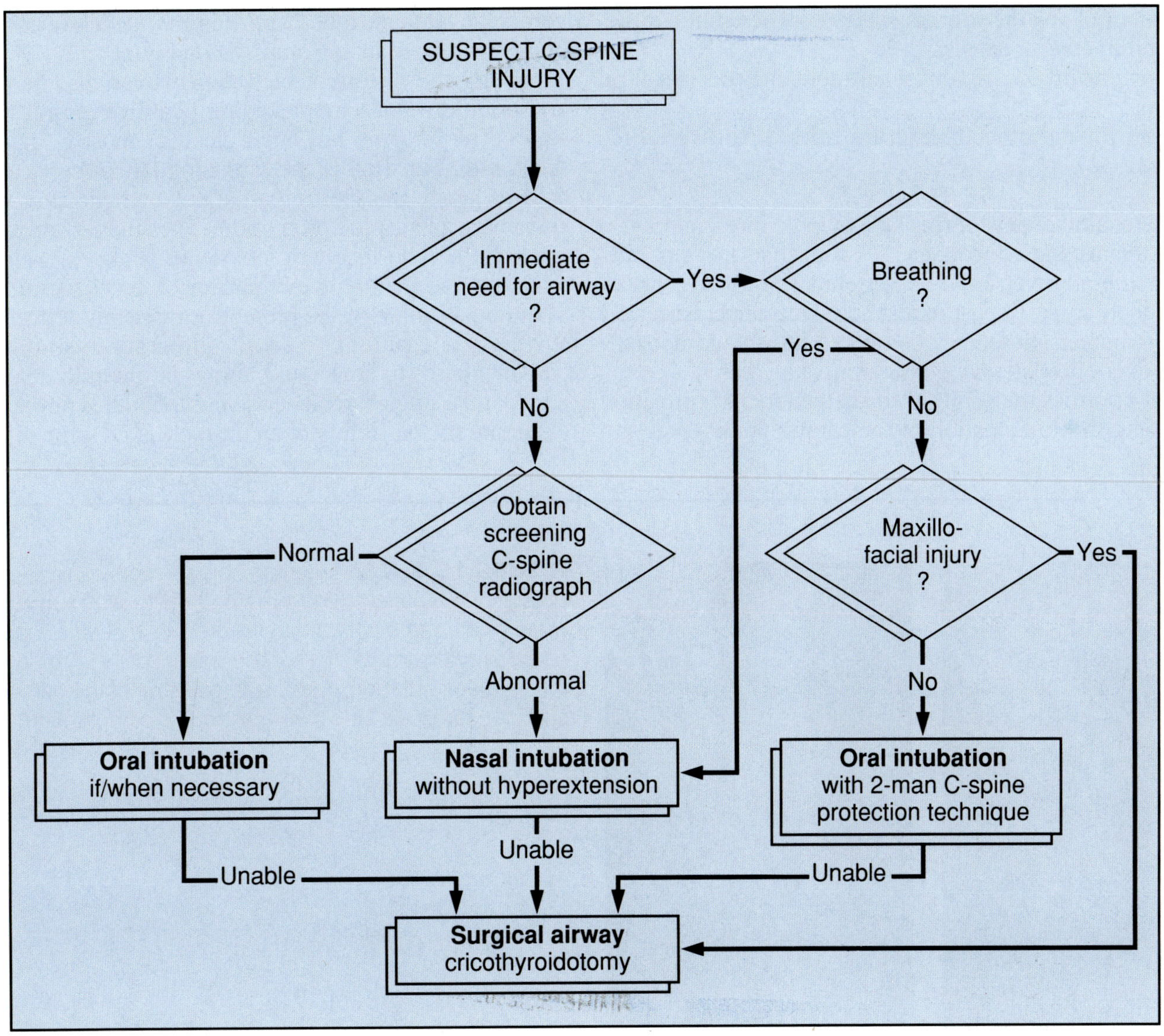

FIGURE 15.2 Protocol for initial airway assessment and management. (Figure based on recommendations of the American College of Surgeons Committee on Trauma: Advanced Trauma Life Support. Chicago, American College of Surgeons, 1984.)

are well under way. The unremarkable screening lateral spine film in Fig. 15.3 is of a patient who had sustained vehicular trauma. However, the myelogram of the same patient demonstrates transection of the spinal cord at the C6 level; this preventable catastrophic complication occurred after relaxation of the axial spine protective measures.

A systematic evaluation of the screening lateral cervical spine film should include:

1. Examination of technical adequacy and visualization of all seven cervical vertebrae and the C7–T1 interspace
2. Examination of soft tissues, visible airway, and abnormal subcutaneous air
3. Measurement of the retropharyngeal airspace to identify abnormal prevertebral soft-tissue swelling
4. Careful inspection of the lines defined by the anterior margin of the vertebral bodies, posterior margin of the vertebral bodies, arches, laminae, and spinous processes
5. Measurement of any offset or angulation of these lines, if present, in millimeters or degrees
6. Special attention to any encroachment on the vertebral spinal canal
7. Inspection for radiolucent fracture lines of the vertebrae themselves.

A good systematic review of this radiographic interpretation is given by Williams and co-workers.[18] A film that does not adequately visualize all seven cervical vertebrae cannot be considered an adequate study. Repeat radiographs with upper extremity traction or swimmers views may be needed but should not take precedence over other lifesaving resuscitative measures.

The initial priorities then shift to the detection and correction of hemorrhagic shock. Palpation of the carotid pulse serves as a rapid evaluation of cerebral perfusion. Intravenous volume replacement may then be required, preferably by peripheral venous access; however, the neck is available for external jugular line placement and, though less immediately desirable, internal jugular catheter placement. Intravenous catheters in the neck should be avoided if possible in the presence of clinically suspected neck injuries.

HISTORY

A direct injury to the neck may occasionally be inferred from the history. High-risk accidents include diving into shallow water, falls with resultant severe angulation of the head and neck, and some sports injuries. It is also generally true that any blow to the head sufficient to warrant evaluation for a possible skull or brain injury is sufficient to produce an occult cervical spine injury. Too often, however, cervical injuries from blunt trauma are occult, asymptomatic, and unsuspected; they must be presumed in all cases involving high-energy transfer, such as vehicular trauma, falls from heights, decelerations, and any blunt trauma producing multisystem injury.

Trusting the history of such patients can also be treacherous; any notation made by preceding healthcare professionals that states "the C-spine has been cleared" must be regarded with skepticism. Fig. 15.4 is the screening lateral cervical spine film used to justify transporting a patient by helicopter without the customary axial spine protection. The study is obviously grossly inadequate. The receiving physician is always well advised to make an independent evaluation of cervical spine stability, assuming an injury to be present until clearly proven otherwise. While it is efficient to send radiographic studies with the patient, these studies should always be carefully reassessed firsthand, and a single lateral cervical spine film is never adequate to eliminate the possibility of an unstable axial spine injury.

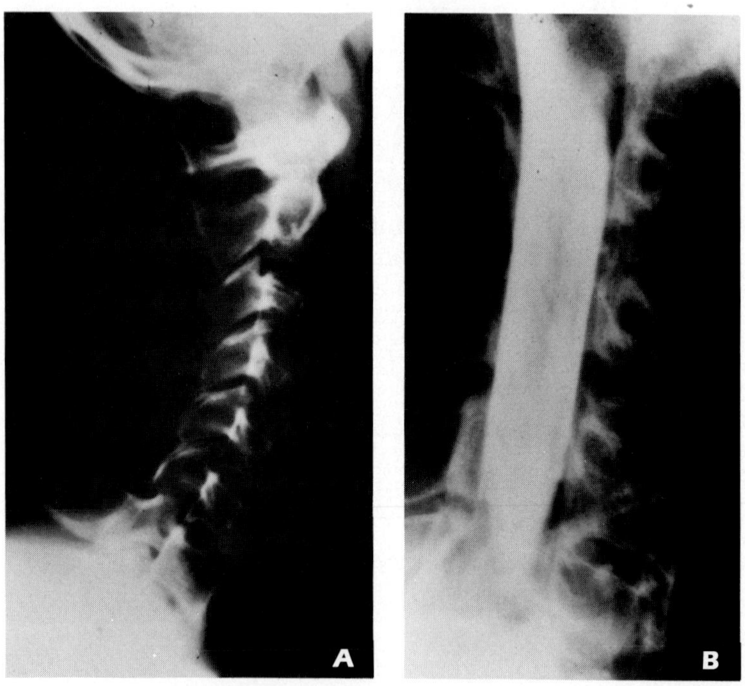

FIGURE 15.3 A An unremarkable screening lateral spine film obtained in a patient who sustained vehicular trauma. **B** A myelogram of the same patient after protective measures had been relaxed reveals transection of the spinal cord at the C6 level. As this sequence demonstrates, a single view of the cervical spine cannot entirely exclude this catastrophic complication.

High-risk mechanisms of injury include vehicular trauma with a flexion-extension "whiplash" mechanism, nonuse of restraint devices, being thrown from the vehicle or into the windshield, and accompanying fatalities in the same accident. There should be careful questioning regarding the apparent neurologic function of the victim since the time of the accident. Complete paralysis since the moment of injury generally suggests an irreversible neurologic injury. Any reliable history that a paralyzed extremity showed any motor or sensory function at any time since the injury is highly significant; paralysis in these instances has some chance of reversibility with prompt and appropriate therapy. Facial trauma is a major risk factor in vehicular trauma, with approximately 20% of significant facial fractures harboring a significant occult cervical spine injury.[9]

PHYSICAL EXAMINATION

The neck of the blunt trauma victim should be carefully inspected for external evidence of trauma such as discoloration, hematoma, edema, and tenderness. Subcutaneous air may be visible or only palpable, and its presence may signify a major airway injury (see Treatment section). Any externally evident edema or hematoma of the neck must be observed closely as a potential source of airway compromise. Carotid pulses should be assessed. Abnormalities in the contour of the thyroid cartilage should be noted by inspection and palpation. The midline position of the trachea in the suprasternal notch should be confirmed.

It is recommended that physical examination of the cervical spine be deferred until the screening cervical spine radiograph has been reviewed. If this study is normal, the protective measures to the axial spine can be removed to allow an examination of the posterior neck. The individual spinous processes should be palpated with notation of any soft tissue swelling, crepitus, stepoff, or tenderness. An adequate neurologic examination including assessment of the motor, sensory, and reflex function of each extremity is appropriate at this point. The discovery of any findings suggesting a cervical spine injury mandates the immediate resumption of all protective measures.

ADDITIONAL DIAGNOSTIC PROCEDURES

Additional diagnostic measures available after the initial stabilization include special radiologic views, tomography, CT scanning, radionuclide imaging studies, and arteriography. These studies should be utilized cost-effectively and for specific indications.

Definitive Management

Definitive evaluation of the axial spine must now be considered. Once the more pressing conditions have been stabilized, the question of an occult spine injury can be laid to rest. Although the initial screening lateral cervical spine film will detect 80% to 90% of clinically important injuries, protective measures cannot be relaxed until a definitive study is completed. This usually involves augmentation of the cross-table lateral film with AP and open-mouth odontoid views. The risk of an unrecognized injury is now well below 1%, and the odds can be further refined by adding oblique films,[5,17] although the necessity and cost-effectiveness of the five-view series over the three-view series may be questioned.[14] The completely asymptomatic alert patient with a normal three-view series probably has no easily measurable benefit from the addition of oblique views, although the cost, time, and radiation exposure are low. Alert patients with uncertain minor degrees of misalignment may benefit from carefully done flexion-extension views.

Special views, tomography, and CT scanning may be necessary to rule out abnormalities in areas that are poorly visualized or in which the routine films are inconclusive. A suggested algorithm

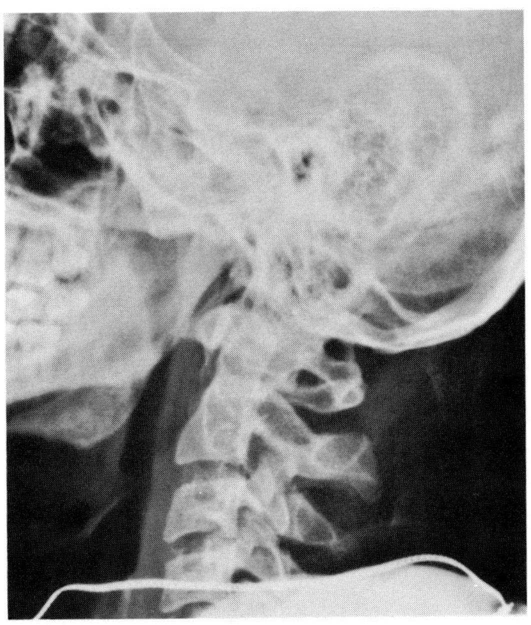

FIGURE 15.4 This radiograph accompanied the patient in transport whose protective measures had been relaxed because "the C-spine had been cleared." The film is obviously grossly inadequate. Even an adequate film that visualized all seven cervical vertebrae and the C7–T1 interspace could not completely have excluded a significant unstable injury. All patients should have the axial spine protected during transport.

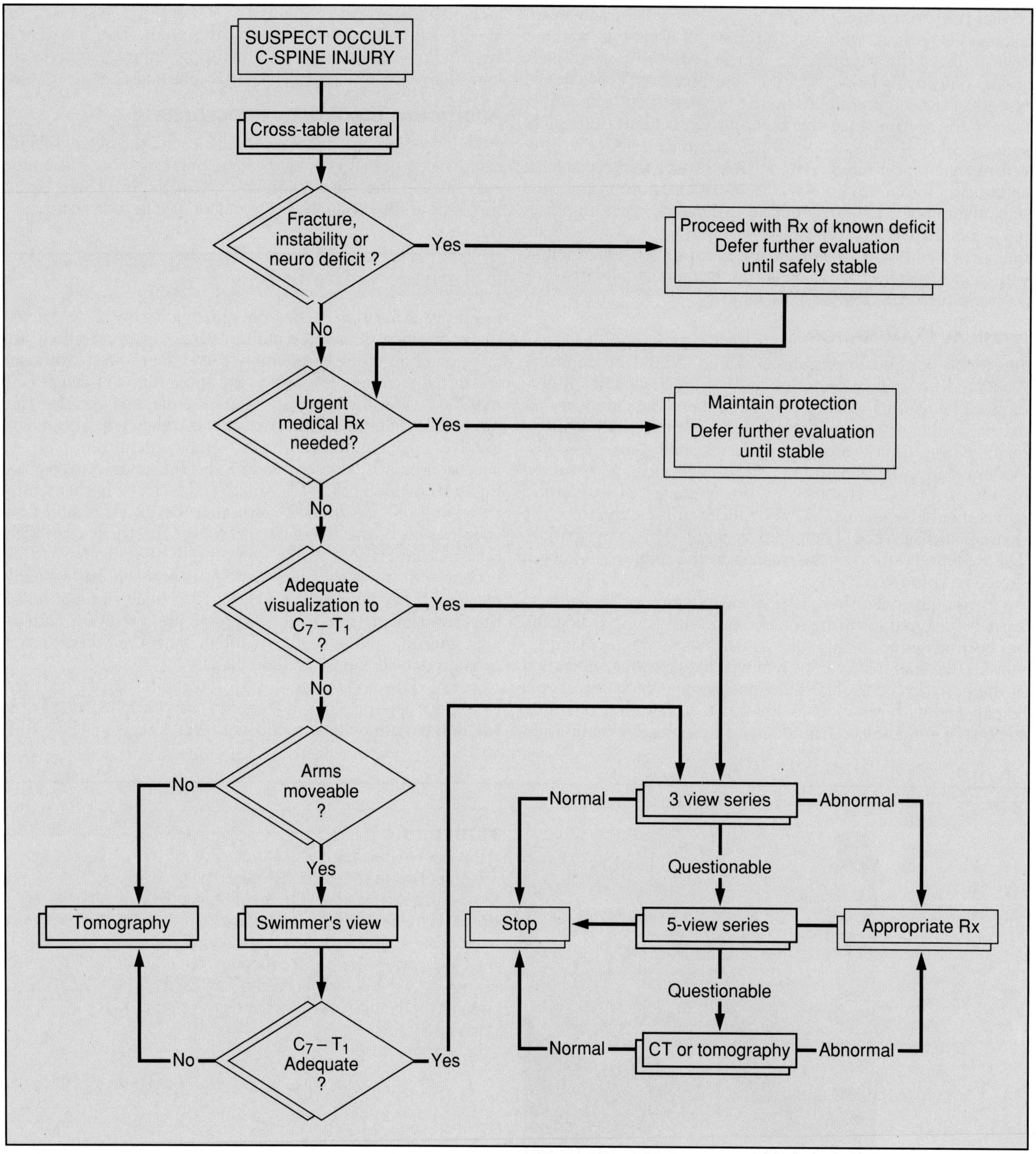

FIGURE 15.5 Suggested protocol for the efficient and cost-effective use of special radiographic studies to rule out an occult cervical spine injury.

for the use of additional studies is given in Fig. 15.5. An example of an abnormality demonstrated by tomography is given in Fig. 15.6 and shows a possible fracture of the odontoid in the unconscious patient, which was suspected on the basis of a minor irregularity seen on the cross-table lateral film. High-resolution CT scanning is capable of providing excellent anatomical detail in some cervical spine fractures. An example of CT demonstration of a burst fracture of C1 is given in Fig. 15.7. The utility of this mode may be somewhat limited in the acute period. Radionuclide bone scanning can image an occult nondisplaced fracture but only after the healing process is well established, typically after 10 to 14 days. Maintenance of cervical spine protection must continue during this interval if the presence of an injury remains uncertain.

Arteriography is occasionally indicated in blunt neck trauma because of false aneurysm formation, bleeding, intimal tear, or thrombosis in the carotid system. A direct blow or stretch injury from forced hyperextension of the head may be the responsible

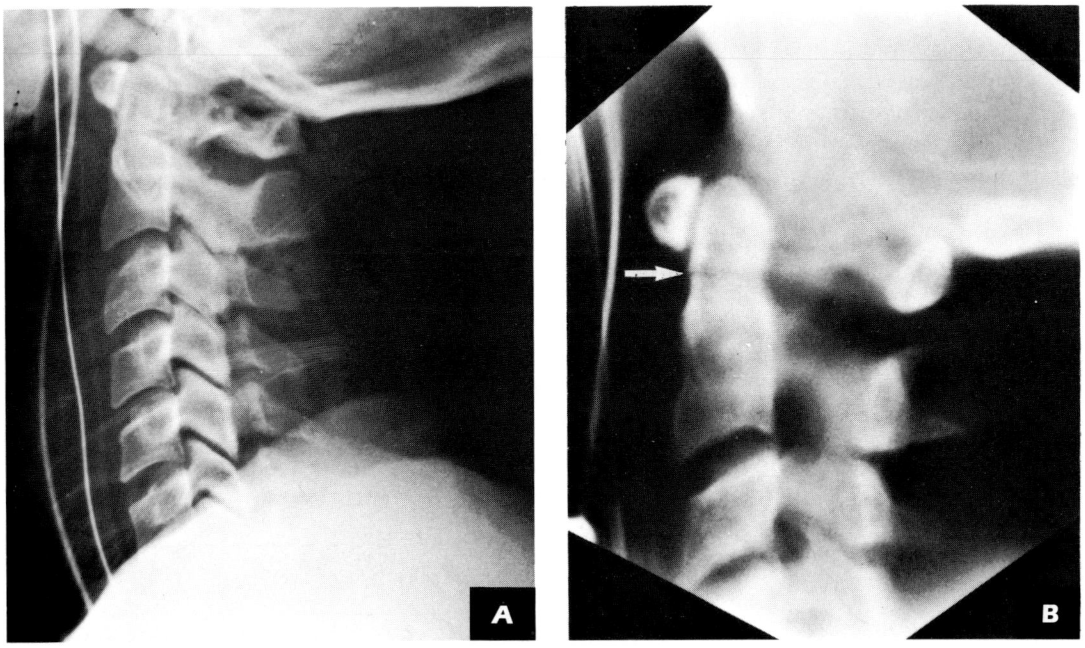

FIGURE 15.6 Use of tomography to rule out an occult cervical spine fracture. **A** An injury was suspected based on a minor irregularity of the odontoid in this screening cross-table lateral radiograph. **B** The tomogram demonstrates the nondisplaced odontoid fracture.

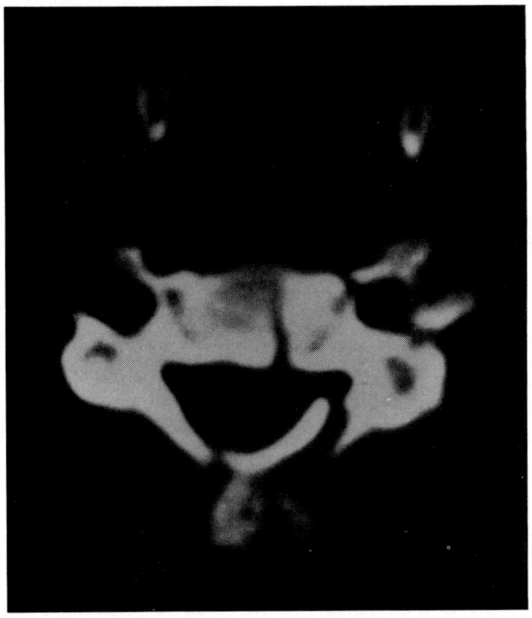

FIGURE 15.7 The precise anatomy of a cervical spine fracture of the body and arch of C5 is well demonstrated by CT.

pathophysiology. Indications include an expansile or pulsatile mass, or a neurologic deficit attributable to an extracranial vascular lesion.

Other endoscopic and contrast studies are more applicable to penetrating neck trauma. These will be discussed below. Endoscopic evaluation may be required in the evaluation of laryngeal trauma, as outlined in the next section.

Treatment

Definitive therapy for blunt neck trauma generally involves care of injuries to the axial spine or upper airway. Trauma to the vasculature or other components of the visceral compartment are much more frequently seen with penetrating trauma.

The immediate treatment of an axial spine injury involves maintenance of the protective measures already described. Patients without a neurologic deficit must be protected from developing one, while those with an established deficit must be protected from further irreversible injury to the central nervous system. The immediate application of longitudinal traction, rather than simple axial stabilization, is controversial. While the placement of a traction device, such as Crutchfield tongs, can be easily mastered, the direction and amount of traction to be applied is most safely accomplished with orthopaedic or neurosurgical consultation. If the patient must be transported to obtain that consultation, it is safer to maintain static stabilization, rather than try to initiate and maintain dynamic traction in transport. The application of a traction device to the head can mechanically destabilize the patient's condition if the traction to that device is not properly applied and maintained.

The rationale, mechanics, and technique of cervical traction depend on numerous factors, including the anatomy of demonstrable fractures, the presence of known or presumed accompanying ligamentous injuries, and the mechanism of injury. Traction may be specifically contraindicated with some mechanisms of injury, such as the distraction-lateral bending mechanism of a hangman's fracture. A tabulation of the frequent mechanisms of injury of the various cervical injuries is given in Fig. 15.8. The pathophysiologic mechanism of injury is complex in many vehicular accidents, as illustrated in Fig. 15.9.

The definitive management of these injuries can be complicated and, though within the purview of the orthopedic or neurologic surgical specialist, it is beyond the realm of this review. Definitive management ranges from the use of a semirigid ("Philadelphia") cervical collar, dynamic skeletal traction, and external stabilization ("four-poster" and others), to operative reduction, fixation, and fusion. Fluctuating neurologic deficit may require more urgent intervention by the nonspecialist. The patient who, by reliable history, has been rendered paraplegic or quadriplegic from the moment of injury is generally considered to have a permanent neurologic deficit and needs only to be protected from further deterioration. The patient who has reliably been observed to have some sensory or motor function that later deteriorates, or who has an incomplete deficit or one that fluctuates, has some hope of restoration of spinal cord function, although the prognosis remains guarded even with the best of treatment. Urgent neurosurgical or orthopedic consultation may provide some hope of neurologic recovery. The patient with a fluctuating neurologic deficit may have a varying degree of cord impingement from an unstable axial spine and may benefit from prompt reduction of fracture dislocations that impinge on the spinal canal. Beyond mechanical reduction, the use of operative decompression and steroids or other medical measures remains controversial. Urgent operative decompression and stabilization is generally considered to be contraindicated in a patient with a fixed stable neurologic deficit. Such patients do, however, frequently benefit from delayed fixation or fusion to permit mobilization and rehabilitation without fear of further spine or cord injury.

Blunt trauma to the upper airway can be a treacherous management challenge. Laryngeal fractures can occur in vehicular trauma, when the front of the driver's neck strikes the upper surface of the steering wheel. Such injuries can also occur with isolated direct blows to the front of the neck. Deceleration injuries with blows to the thoracic inlet can produce blunt transection of the trachea at the level of the cricoid. These injuries can present as critical airway emergencies, or they can present as occult injuries in which mismanagement of the airway may result in catastrophic destabilization.

Patients with some blunt injury to their upper airway usually have signs and symptoms leading one to suspect the presence of the injury: the patient may have hoarseness or stridor, or may have a normal voice that only the patient recognizes as different. Subcutaneous emphysema in the neck may result from dissection of air along mediastinal tissues into the visceral com-

FIGURE 15.8
MECHANISMS OF INJURY IN CERVICAL SPINE TRAUMA[2]

MECHANISM	TYPE OF INJURY
Hyperflexion	Anterior compresson fracture Bilateral locked facets Posterior ligament rupture with subluxation Odontoid fracture Spinous process fracture
Hyperextension	Hangman's (pedicles of C2) fracture Posterior arch fractures Lamina Pedicles Spinous process Anterior body chip fracture
Vertical compression	Burst fracture Jefferson fracture
Flexion-rotation	Unilateral locked facet

partment of the neck from a tracheobronchial injury, or it may occur with a laryngeal fracture with rupture of the mucosa. An expansile quality of crepitant swelling of the neck with breathing is pathognomonic of a laryngeal fracture. Finally, crepitus on palpation of the laryngeal cartilage or loss of the normal anatomic prominence may suggest a fracture of the cartilage. Radiographic confirmation of a laryngeal fracture is illustrated in Fig. 15.10. Recognition of any of these findings demands immediate ENT consultation. If the patient has worsening stridor or other evidence of developing upper airway obstruction, an immediate cricothyroidotomy should be performed without an attempt at direct laryngoscopy and intubation. Blind nasotracheal intubation should never be attempted if an upper airway injury is suspected. The additional caveat is to observe for evidence of airway trauma during intubation of patients not previously suspected of harboring such an injury: if a laryngeal fracture, submucosal hemorrhage or air, or linear tears of the laryngeal mucosa are seen, intubation through the larynx should not be attempted. Endotracheal intubation, or even manipulation by direct laryngoscopy, can aggravate an existing injury and complicate definitive repair. The worst scenario is the patient with blunt transection of the subglottic trachea. Passage of an endotracheal tube can rupture the remaining mucosa and soft tissues, allowing the trachea to retract into the thoracic inlet and rendering all subsequent efforts at establishing an airway impossible. The recommended algorithm for

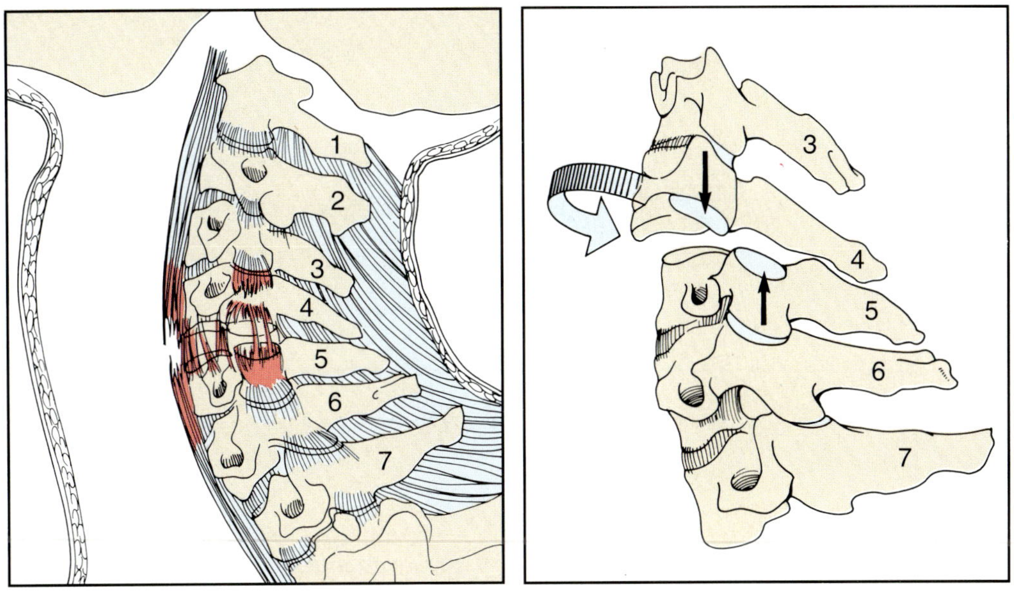

FIGURE 15.9 Many neck injuries probably result from complex mechanisms. The "whiplash" injury illustrated here results in disruption of several longitudinal and collateral ligaments with extension **A**, permitting a unilateral locked facet with subsequent flexion and rotation **B**.

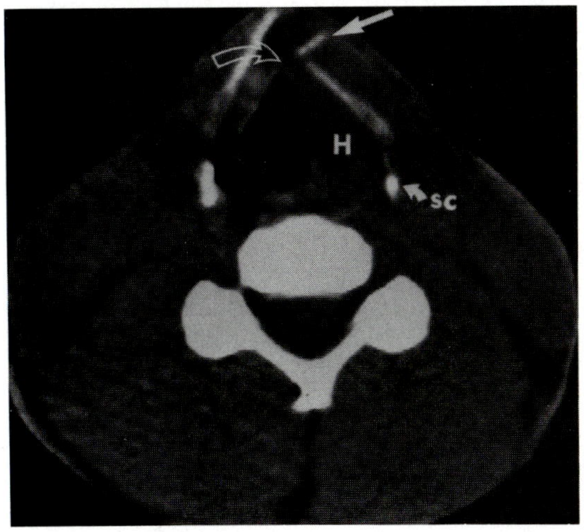

FIGURE 15.10 CT confirmation of a laryngeal fracture. A comminuted fracture of the thyroid cartilage is indicated by the solid arrow. The hematoma (H) involves the left paralaryngeal space and pre-epiglottic space (open arrow). (sc, superior cornua) (Federle MP, Brant-Zawadzki M et al: Computed Tomography in the Evaluation of Trauma. 1986, The Williams & Wilkins Co, Baltimore.)

management of suspected blunt trauma to the upper airway is given in Fig. 15.11. The underlying principle is to obtain immediate specialist consultation as soon as an airway injury is suspected, and to go directly to emergency surgical cricothyroidotomy if inadequate gas exchange demands an immediate airway.

PENETRATING INJURIES

Interpersonal violence accounts for the rise in frequency of penetrating neck wounds, especially in urban centers. Most cities report an increasing proportion of gunshot wounds to stab wounds, probably due to the easy availability of handguns in the United States. Moreover, the dense concentration of vital structures in the visceral compartment of the neck makes it prone to frequent damage requiring surgical correction. The recommendations for evaluation and treatment of these injuries remains an area of active controversy.

Initial Evaluation

PATIENT HISTORY

Civilian penetrating neck trauma usually results from either a gunshot wound or stab wound. Identification of the specific

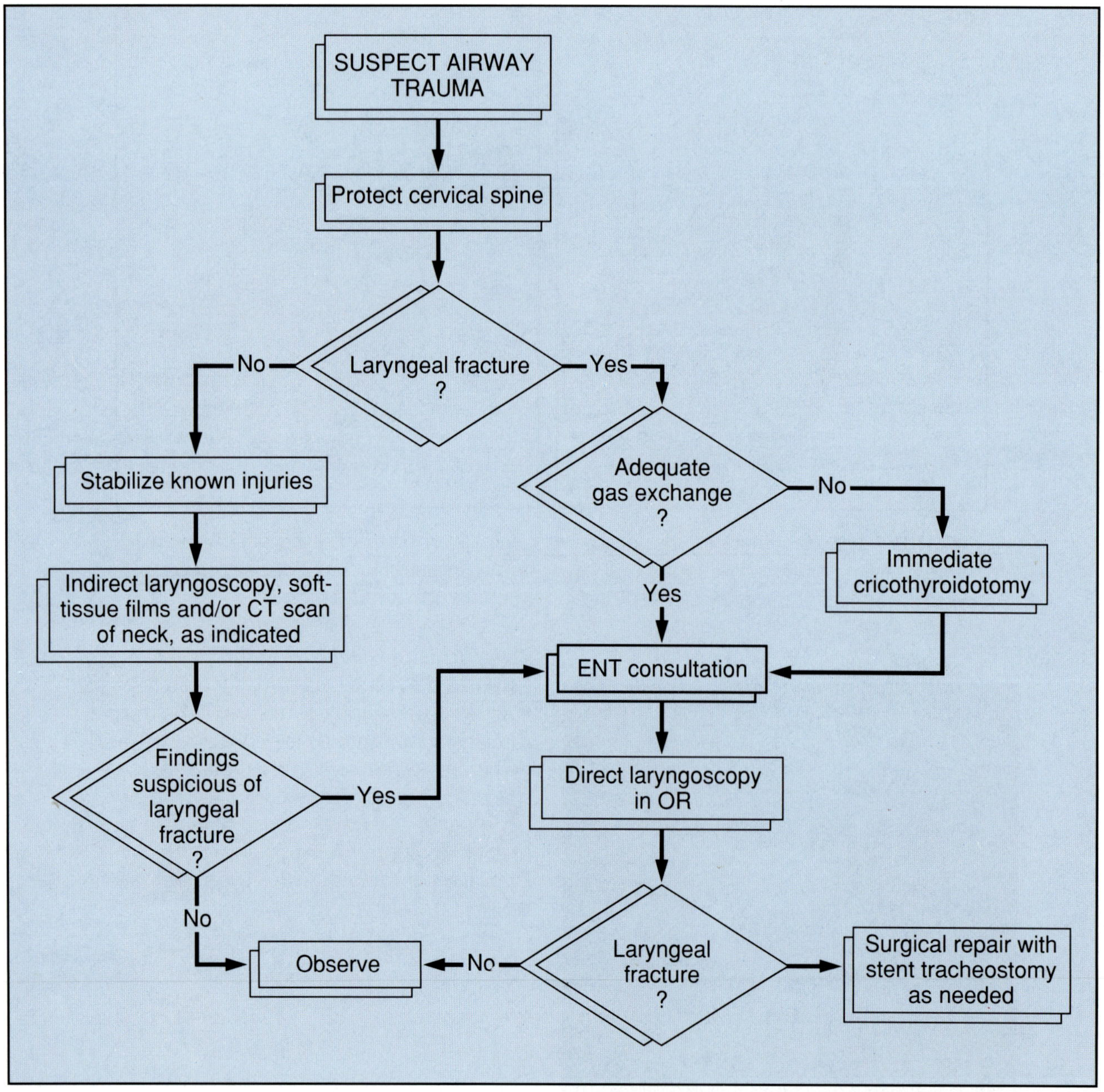

FIGURE 15.11 Protocol for the management of suspected blunt upper airway trauma.

weapon may suggest the anticipated level of energy transfer and tissue destruction. Less commonly, other projectiles or weapons may be involved. Neck penetration occasionally occurs from jagged or exposed metal parts in complex vehicular accidents. Any permanent or transient neurologic deficit attributed to the injury, an alteration in level of consciousness attributable to impairment of cerebral perfusion, and a subjective change in breathing, hoarseness, or quality of the voice are important. Unfortunately, a large fraction of vascular, airway, and esophageal injuries remains treacherously asymptomatic.

PHYSICAL EXAMINATION

The general condition of the patient must be rapidly assessed, as with any form of trauma. Since the majority of penetrating neck wounds occur as isolated injuries, the focus can quickly be shifted to the neck. The patient with a rapidly expanding hematoma in the neck is a candidate for prophylactic endotracheal intubation under the safest of controlled conditions, before airway compromise becomes critical. Subcutaneous emphysema in the neck suggests a perforation of the aerodigestive tract, but urgent intubation is usually not necessary if the patient is breathing comfortably.

DEFINITIVE MANAGEMENT

Two distinctly different schools of thought have emerged over the past two decades regarding definitive management of penetrating neck injuries. Several studies during the 1970s [3,12] advocated a policy of mandatory surgical exploration. The rationale for this policy was that up to 14% of significant visceral neck injuries occurred in the absence of diagnostic signs and symptoms. Missed injuries, particularly those of the pharynx, hypopharynx, and cervical esophagus, were highly morbid, with greater than 50% mortality[15]; therefore, prompt surgical exploration was expeditious, safe, and associated with low operative morbidity.

With mandatory exploration yielding a 40% to 60% negative exploration rate, many trials were undertaken during the 1970s and 1980s to establish criteria for safe, selective exploration to improve cost-effectiveness and reduce the negative exploration rate.[6,11] Selective exploration has proven to be safe and effective, provided that a prospective comprehensive diagnostic protocol is followed compulsively.[10]

Both mandatory exploration and diagnostic evaluation with selective exploration have repeatedly been shown to be effective, and no clear advantage has emerged of one over the other,[10] so that either approach can be justified (Fig. 15.12). Noyes and colleagues have shown that while length of hospital stay may be reduced by an average of one day, the total hospitalization cost is slightly higher in asymptomatic patients undergoing diagnostic workup rather than exploration.[10] Since the medical advantages seem balanced, the choice of policy at a specific center may hinge on other economic, logistical, and convenience factors. It would perhaps be rational to pursue mandatory exploration for gunshot wounds and selective exploration for stab wounds, although this specific recommendation has not been studied. A policy of mandatory exploration may be recommended at centers treating only a small number of penetrating neck injuries, since the need to promptly and reliably exclude an asymptomatic morbid injury could justify the higher negative exploration rate.

It must be emphasized that simple observation without a thorough diagnostic evaluation cannot be recommended; the innocuous-appearing asymptomatic neck penetration must undergo either surgical or nonsurgical evaluation to exclude a hazardous visceral injury. A missed pharyngeal, hypopharyngeal, or esophageal perforation, if allowed to progress to posterior mediastinitis or empyema, will result in death from infectious complications in more than 50% of patients.[15]

MANDATORY EXPLORATION

The protocol of mandatory neck exploration is straightforward, expeditious, and requires no additional specialized diagnostic equipment, technicians, or specialists. The patient is examined as described earlier and evidence of impending airway compromise is treated appropriately. Patients without hoarseness, change in voice, or subcutaneous emphysema may be intubated upon induction of anesthesia, if gas exchange is not compromised. The asymptomatic patient may undergo a superficial wound exploration in the emergency room to confirm penetration of the platysma. If the muscle has not been penetrated, the wound may be treated like any simple skin wound on an ambulatory basis. If mandatory exploration is to follow, most authors recommend foregoing all further preoperative diagnostic studies because they are unnecessary and add no additional useful clinical information.

The use of preoperative arteriography to supplement mandatory exploration has been examined by several authors with similar conclusions: that there are specific topographic zones of injury that mandate preoperative arteriography (Fig. 15.13).[3,7] These zones describe areas of injury where arteriography may avoid intraoperative dilemmas in proximal and distal control in vascular injuries. Gunshot wounds or stab wounds at the thoracic inlet or base of the neck may require vascular control below the level of the clavicles. Conversely, penetrating wounds at the base of the skull can produce an internal carotid artery injury in which extracranial distal control is impossible. The more common zone II injuries can generally be explored without preoperative arteriography, although multiple penetrating injuries in a stable patient may benefit from arteriography to define anatomatical sites of injury. Although preoperative arteriography may precisely localize injuries for the surgeon or identify additional unexpected injuries, it is not widely recommended for zone II injuries because the time required to obtain the study may allow the development of a neurologic deficit, with concomitant major increase in morbidity and mortality. Whether surgical exploration is even worthwhile in the presence of an established neurologic deficit is debatable; Unger and colleagues have reported that although the outlook is grave for patients with a hemispheric neurologic deficit resulting from an extracranial vascular injury, surgical restoration of perfusion can improve neurologic function in survivors.[16] The details of the surgical procedure are outlined below.

SELECTIVE EXPLORATION

The diagnostic evaluation–selective exploration protocol also begins with physicial examination, assessment of the airway, and local wound exploration, if necessary, to exclude superficial preplatysmal injuries. Prompt surgical exploration is then recommended if absolute indications are present, such as airway involvement, subcutaneous emphysema, hoarseness or voice change, an expanding hematoma or arterial bleeding, bleeding in the oropharynx or nasogastric tube drainage, or a neurologic deficit including evidence of a brachial plexus injury or sympathetic chain injury (Horner's syndrome). A suspicious abnormality on routine diagnostic studies, such as pathologic soft-tissue air on neck or chest films, also mandates immediate exploration. In the absence of such findings in the asymptomatic patient, a complete diagnostic evaluation can be undertaken.

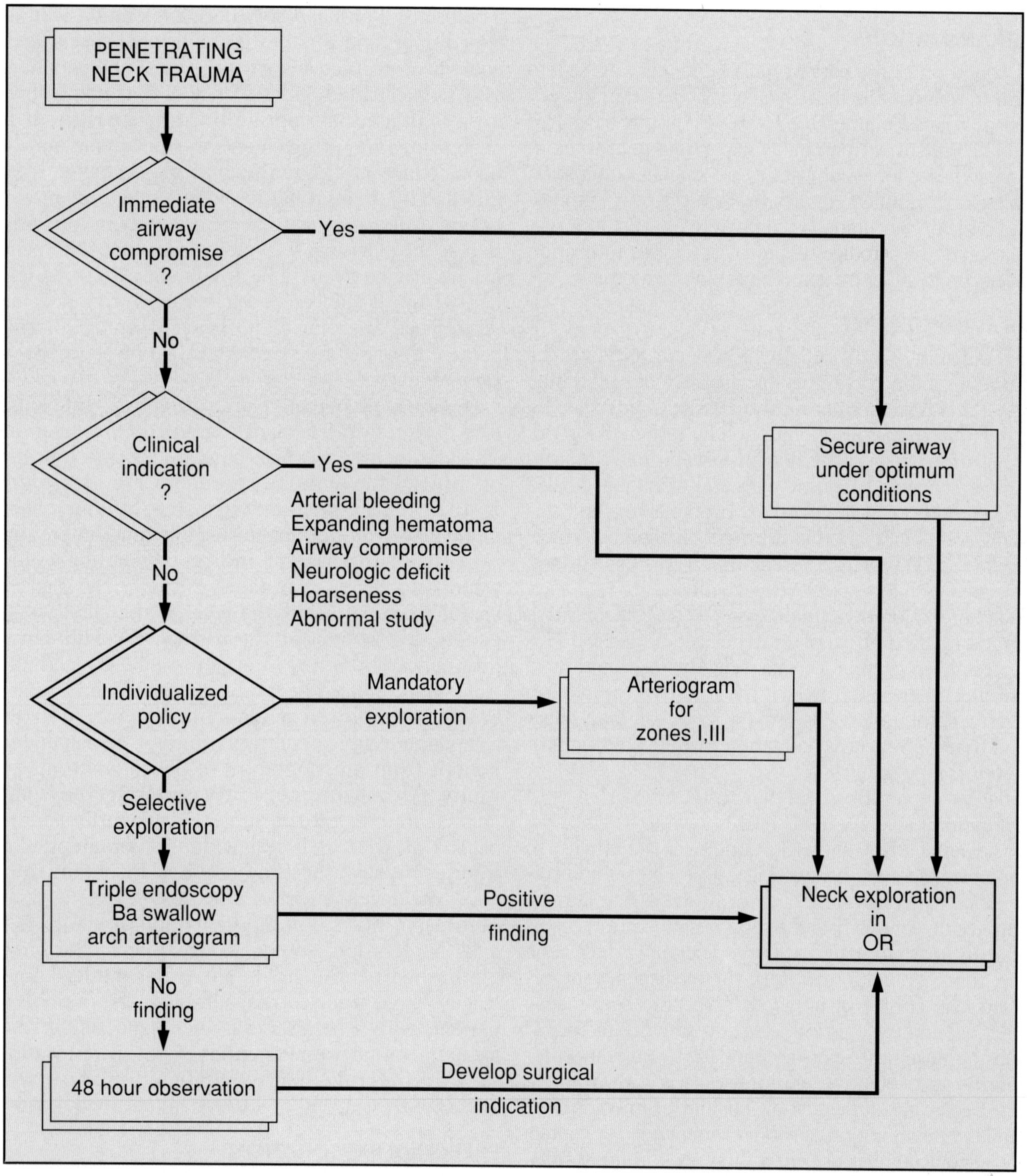

FIGURE 15.12 Suggested protocol for the management of penetrating neck trauma. To date, policies of selective and mandatory exploration have both been justified, with no clearly demonstrated advantage of one over the other.

This evaluation includes arch arteriography, contrast swallow, and triple endoscopy. Any positive finding in these studies mandates surgical exploration. Such a selective program can reduce, but not totally eliminate, negative explorations. Negative results from diagnostic evaluation–selective exploration average 10% to 25%.[6,10,11]

Biplane arteriography, now generally done by the transfemoral route, can identify transected vessels, pseudoaneurysms, intimal flaps, traumatic arteriovenous fistulas, and major venous injuries. A positive arteriogram is shown in Fig. 15.14. Arteriography is associated with very low morbidity, especially if selective injections are not needed. The remainder of the diagnostic studies are not necessary if an arteriographic abnormality is identified. If the arteriogram is normal, it is followed with contrast studies of the esophagus. A water-soluble swallow is typically followed by barium for better mucosal coating, and finally a barium-soaked cotton ball is swallowed, since some tiny tears may require a swallowed bolus for visualization. This study is followed by triple endoscopy including laryngoscopy, esophagoscopy, and bronchoscopy. While modern flexible fiberoptic endoscopes can be used without general anesthesia in cooperative patients, it should be kept in mind that the combined morbidity of the complete diagnostic evaluation equals that of a negative neck exploration.[6,10]

SURGICAL EXPLORATION

Several surgical approaches can be taken for exploration of the neck for penetrating wounds, but the patient should always be positioned, prepared, and draped to allow for access to both sides of the neck, base of the skull, supraclavicular regions, and both

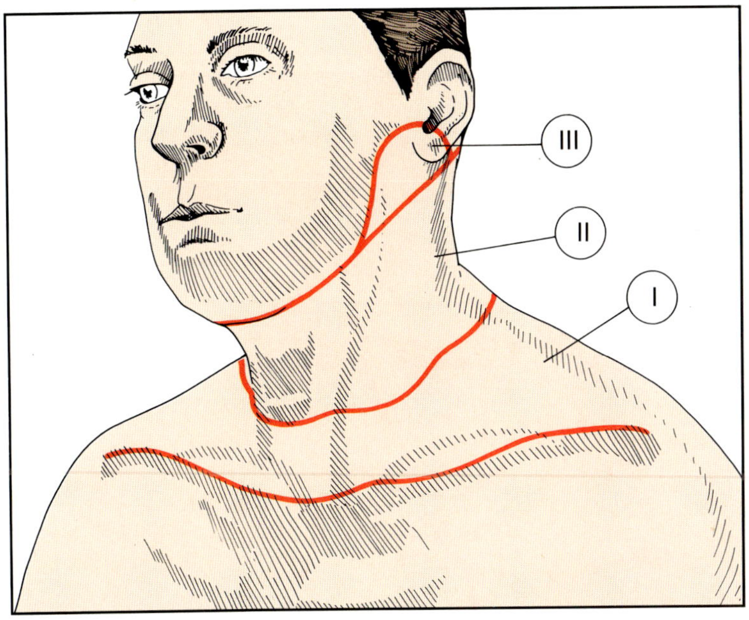

FIGURE 15.13 Topographic zones for classification of penetrating neck trauma.

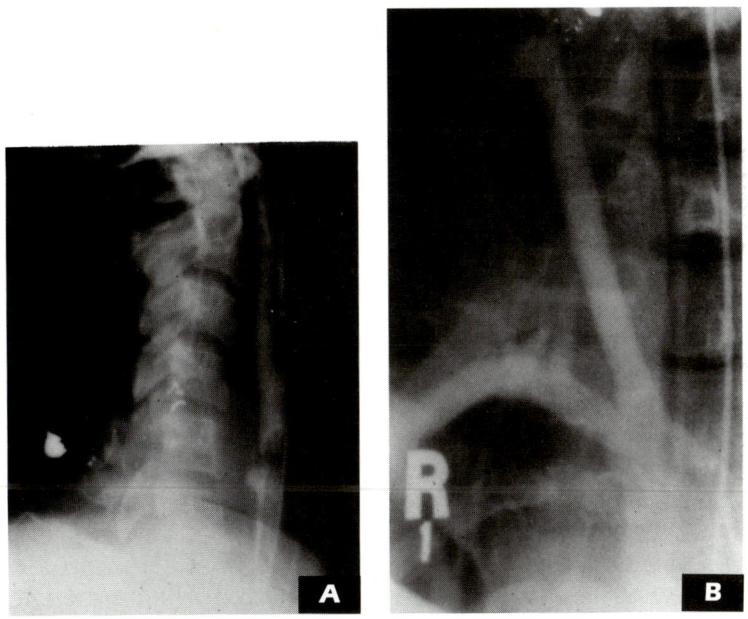

FIGURE 15.14 Arteriogram obtained for an asymptomatic patient with a small-caliber gunshot wound to the neck. Complete transection of the common carotid artery and concomitant occlusion of the right vertebral artery are identified. Under a policy of mandatory exploration, preoperative arteriography is not necessary for zone II injuries.

sides of the chest. Several incisions are available for such an exploration, and these are illustrated in Fig. 15.15. The choice of incision depends on known structural injuries, the results of special studies, and individual preference.

The *anterior sternocleidomastoid carotid incision* is the classic approach for exploring the visceral compartment of the neck with a unilateral injury. It provides good exposure of the esophagus and hypopharynx, and can be readily extended to facilitate vascular exposure. The right carotid incision extended into the suprasternal notch can usually expose the innominate artery bifurcation. Zone I injuries with known or suspected perforations of the innominate artery itself may require extension of this incision, by means of an *upper median sternotomy* to the fourth interspace. Such an extension provides excellent proximal control of the innominate artery. A separate infraclavicular approach to the axillary artery may be required to complete the distal control of such an innominate injury.

Complete exposure of the subclavian artery for trauma is most easily accomplished with a *fourth interspace anterior thoracotomy* on the appropriate side. The anterior sternocleidomastoid incision, upper median sternotomy, and thoracotomy can be well combined in an "open-book" incision with excellent exposure of all of the arch great vessels.[7]

Known or suspected bilateral neck trauma may be explored through either *bilateral carotid incisions* or a *transverse "thyroid" incision*. The transverse incision produces the most cosmetic result and is also quite flexible. Lateral extension of the transverse incision, with division of the strap muscles if necessary, produces excellent exposure of the visceral compartment. It can also be extended superiorly toward the mastoid to enhance distal vasculature control. The transverse incision is probably the most appropriate for approaching a known isolated injury of the upper airway.

A neck exploration for trauma should proceed in an orderly fashion with direct visualization of all structures in the visceral and vascular compartments. The larynx, trachea, thyroid gland, hypopharynx, and esophagus must all be visually inspected. Low-energy penetrating trauma that clearly does not penetrate the carotid sheath does not mandate exploration of the vascular compartment, although high-energy missiles and complex blunt or penetrating mechanisms can produce a carotid intimal flap or pseudoaneurysm despite apparent nonpenetration of the carotid sheath. If there is penetration of the carotid sheath, with or without an obvious hematoma, proximal and distal arterial control should be established prior to exposure of the area of injury. Once the carotid sheath is open, the common, internal, and external carotid arteries, internal jugular vein, and vagus nerve should be visually inspected for integrity, bleeding, or intramural hematoma.

In the absence of any injury, the incision should be irrigated and closed without drainage. Direct perforations of the aerodigestive tract should be repaired primarily. A small, flat, closed suction drain is placed alongside esophageal repairs by most surgeons. A temporary distal tracheostomy is employed with laryngeal or upper tracheal repairs by many surgeons. Gunshot or stab wounds that penetrate very close to the hypopharynx or esophagus are probably best managed with closed suction drainage until an oral diet is begun, even if no violation of the visceral integrity can be demonstrated.

Injuries to the carotid artery are treated following the general principles of vascular trauma. Low-energy lateral lacerations can be debrided and primarily repaired with fine nonabsorbable monofilament suture. High-energy carotid trauma or injuries involving soft tissue destruction require extensive debridement and usually interposition grafting. PTFE (polytetrafluroethylene) synthetic grafts have been used with success,[8] but autologous saphenous vein remains the arterial substitute of choice for traumatic wounds.

Injuries to the common or internal carotid artery that will require complex repair or interposition grafting may employ a wire-wound Silastic internal shunt for intraoperative preservation of carotid blood flow. The criteria for using such internal shunts remain controversial. However, the use of such temporizing shunting has been shown to substantially reduce

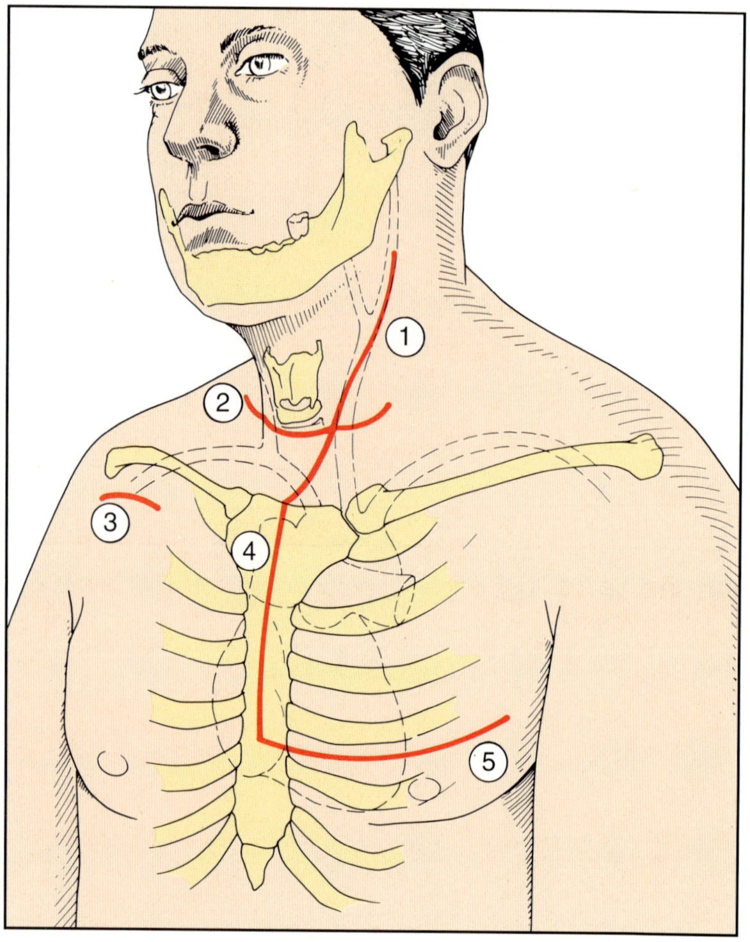

FIGURE 15.15 Incisions for exploration of penetrating neck trauma: (1) anterior sternocleidomastoid "carotid" incision, (2) transverse "thyroid" incision, (3) infraclavicular "axillary artery" incision, (4) upper median sternotomy, (5) fourth interspace thoracotomy. 1, 4, and 5 can be combined as an "open-book" incision for exposure of proximal control of arch vessels.

ischemic time in complex wounds. Cerebral perfusion can be promptly restored while the vessel is inspected, debrided, and grafted as necessary. Interposition grafting with either autologous saphenous vein or synthetic material can be accomplished by placing the conduit over the internal shunt with only momentary interruption of cerebral blood flow. The entire first suture line and almost all of the second suture line can then be completed with the shunt in place, reducing the ischemic time to the few minutes necessary to complete the final few stitches. Carotid internal shunting should be employed by surgeons familiar with its use to avoid intimal injury, elevation of atherosclerotic plaques, or air embolism, which can result from the improper use of the shunt.

Low-energy lateral lacerations of the internal jugular vein, in an otherwise clean wound, should be repaired if it can be accomplished with simple lateral venorraphy. Transected or otherwise badly damaged veins are usually simply ligated. Simultaneous acute ligation of both internal jugular veins should be avoided, if at all possible, because of the increased incidence of postoperative cerebral edema with bilateral internal jugular vein occlusion.

REFERENCES

1. American College of Surgeons Committee on Trauma: Advanced Trauma Life Support. Chicago, American College of Surgeons, 1984.
2. Berquist TH et al: Diagnostic Imaging of the Acutely Injured Patient. Baltimore, Urban & Schwarzenberg, 1985.
3. Bishara RA, Pasch AR, Douglas DD et al: The necessity of mandatory exploration of penetrating zone II neck injuries. Surgery 100:655–660, 1986.
4. Blahd WH, Iserson KV, Bjelland JC: Efficacy of the posttraumatic cross table lateral view of the cervical spine. J Emerg Med 2:243–249, 1985.
5. Doris PE, Wilson RA: The next logical step in the emergency radiographic evaluation of cervical spine trauma: The five-view trauma series. J Emerg Med 3:371–385, 1985.
6. Elerding SC, Manart FD, Moore EE: A reappraisal of penetrating neck injury management. J Trauma 20:695–697, 1980.
7. Flint LM, Snyder WH, Perry MO, Shires GT: Management of major vascular injuries in the base of the neck. Arch Surg 106:407–413, 1973.
8. Graham JM, Mattox KL, Feliciano DV, DeBakey ME: Vascular injuries of the axilla. Ann Surg 195:232–238, 1982.
9. Lewis VL Jr, Manson PN, Morgan RF et al: Facial injuries associated with cervical fractures: Recognition, patterns, and management. J Trauma 25:90–93, 1985.
10. Noyes LD, McSwain NE, Markowitz IP: Panendoscopy with arteriography versus mandatory exploration of penetrating wounds of the neck. Ann Surg 204:21–31, 1986.
11. Rakaschandra MR, Bhatti FK, Guadino E et al: Penetrating injuries of the neck: Criteria for exploration. J Trauma 23:47–49, 1983.
12. Saletta JD, Lowe RJ, Lim LT et al: Penetrating trauma of the neck. J Trauma 16:579–587, 1976.
13. Shaffer MA, Doris PE: Limitation of the cross table lateral view in detecting cervical spine injuries: A retrospective analysis. Ann Emerg Med 10:508–513, 1981.
14. Streitwieser DR, Knopp R, Wales LR et al: Accuracy of standard radiographic views in detecting cervical spine fractures. Ann Emerg Med 12:538–542, 1983.
15. Swan KG, Swan RC: The neck. In Gunshot Wounds: Pathophysiology and Management, pp 57–79 Littleton, MA, PSG Publishing, 1980
16. Unger SW, Tucker WS, Mrdeza MA et al: Carotid arterial trauma. Surgery 87:477–487, 1980.
17. Vines FS: The significance of occult fractures of the cervical spine. Radiology 107:493–504, 1969.
18. Williams CF, Bernstein TW, Jeleko: Essentiality of the lateral cervical spine radiograph. Ann Emerg Med 10:198–204, 1981.

principles of antibiotic use in trauma

Glenn D. Warden
Jeffrey R. Saffle

1 2 3 4 5 6 7 8 9 10 11 12 13 14 15 **16** 17 18 19 20

In the past 40 years, improvements in trauma care have greatly affected associated morbidity and mortality. Improvements in patient transport, triage, and resuscitation have reduced the frequency of early death from shock and hemorrhage. Technological advances in such areas as respiratory care, blood transfusion, and nutritional support have also reduced mortality from traumatic injuries.

In the face of this progress, infection remains the most common serious complication of penetrating trauma and the most frequent cause of death in trauma patients who survive the first 48 hours of care.[3,4,25] In addition, the economic consequences of infection in trauma patients are great. Even greater than the *direct* costs of infection (cultures, antibiotics, surgery) may be the *indirect* costs of prolonged hospitalization, disability, and time lost from work. In a study of penetrating trauma by Gentry and colleagues, the development of intraperitoneal infection was associated with a *threefold* to *fourfold* increase in hospital stay, much of the cost of which was "unrecoverable" under prospective payment schedules.[7] When these figures are multiplied by the ubiquitous frequency of penetrating trauma in America today, the potential expense is vast.

During World War II, the mortality associated with penetrating wounds of the colon was reduced from over 60% to under 30%.[27] The reasons for the decrease are multiple, but include the widespread use of colostomy, the decreased time from injury to operation, and the increased use of antibiotics, primarily sulfa drugs and penicillin.[25] Since then, the use of increasingly effective antibiotics has continued to reduce the mortality and complication rate of traumatic injuries. This chapter will review the principles of antibiotic administration in trauma patients and present guidelines for their use.

FACTORS INFLUENCING WOUND INFECTION

The likelihood of infection following any injury is influenced by a variety of factors. The most important and obvious of these is the degree of bacterial contamination that occurs with injury. The risk of infection arising in a wound can be correlated directly with the number of bacteria present in a tissue sample of the wound, as initially shown by Teplitz and others in burn wounds[14,24] and confirmed in abdominal wounds as well.[18] This principle was used by the National Academy of Science in 1964 to develop the following classification system for surgical wounds, based on the likelihood of significant bacterial contamination.[13] This system is extremely useful for the surgeon as a guide for making rational decisions about antibiotic administration.

Clean wounds occur under ideal operating room conditions. They include incisions made in surgically prepared skin, without entry into the gastrointestinal, respiratory, or genitourinary tracts. Such wounds are usually closed primarily. Wound infection rates under these circumstances should be less than 5% in the absence of other factors, and without the use of antibiotics.[2,13] This classification is usually reserved for elective surgical procedures and cannot be applied to penetrating traumatic wounds of any kind.

Clean-contaminated wounds include elective procedures that enter the gastrointestinal, respiratory, or genitourinary systems, or clean procedures in which a break in technique occurs. Examples include elective gastrectomy, pulmonary lobectomy, or transurethral prostatic surgery. Wound infection rates of approximately 10% are observed.

Contaminated wounds include fresh traumatic wounds, operations with major breaks in sterile technique, and procedures in which acute, nonpurulent inflammation is encountered. Examples include fresh penetrating abdominal wounds and acute perforations of the gastrointestinal tract. Infection rates are approximately 20%.

Dirty wounds are those involving old (greater than 4 hours) perforations of viscera, or established infections. Wounds that contain devitalized tissue or foreign bodies are also considered dirty. Infection rates in excess of 30% are observed.

In addition to bacterial contamination itself, a host of other factors also influence wound infection rates. Patient-related conditions such as preexisting diabetes mellitus, uremia, or malnutrition increase the likelihood of infection developing at any level of bacterial contamination. The same is true of various trauma-related factors such as shock, major hemorrhage, or multiple organ injury, all of which also increase the incidence of infectious complications.[4,14,17] Studies that evaluate the effect of therapeutic manipulations on infection rates should attempt to control for these factors. In all of these settings, the decision to use antibiotics in a particular patient must be individualized.

PROPHYLACTIC ANTIBIOTICS

The initial work of Miles and Burke demonstrated the increased effectiveness of antibiotics when given prior to the occurrence of bacterial contamination within wounds.[1,11] Using a guinea pig model, they found that the subcutaneous injection of staphylococci reliably produced an abscess. Various manipulations performed on the wound (injection of blood products, for example, or production of shock) affected the size of the infection, but only if performed within about 3 hours of inoculation. The administration of antibiotics (penicillin or streptomycin) *before* bacterial injection produced lesions which were no different in size from those that resulted from injection of killed bacteria. Antibiotic administration at the time of contamination was less effective in controlling abscess formation, while antibiotics given at various times following contamination were less and less effective. Antibiotics given more than 3 hours after bacterial injection had no apparent effect on subsequent abscess formation.

This research suggested that antibiotics given prior to the occurrence of bacterial contamination might reduce the incidence of infection more effectively than intraoperative or postoperative antibiotics. This led to trials of "prophylactic" regimens of antibiotic administration. Polk and Lopez-Mayor[18] gave intramuscular cephaloridine to patients undergoing elective gastrointestinal surgery and continued the drug for only two doses postoperatively. These patients had a markedly decreased incidence of both wound and intra-abdominal infections when compared to control patients randomized to receive placebo injections.

Since this study, an overwhelming body of evidence has accumulated in support of prophylactic antibiotics in a variety of surgical settings, including general, thoracic, and gynecologic surgery. They have been the subject of several recent reviews,[5,25] and as supportive evidence for their use grows, the indications for such "prophylactic" administration have become clearer and more restrictive. Perioperative prophylactic antibiotics are usually limited to clean-contaminated and contaminated procedures. Antibiotics are usually not used in clean procedures, since the chance of infection is usually too low to justify the expense and risk of antibiotic administration. Exceptions to this, however, are clean cases in which the development of infection would be disastrous to the patient, such as the placement of vascular grafts and orthopedic hardware, and open-heart procedures. In the opposite extreme, dirty cases essentially represent established infections that are unlikely to respond sufficiently to a limited course of prophylactic antibiotics. Such infections usually require formal courses of therapeutic antibiotic administration.

PROPHYLACTIC ANTIBIOTICS IN TRAUMA

In penetrating abdominal injuries, antibiotics can never be strictly "prophylactic," since contamination of both the traumatic wound and the peritoneal cavity has already occurred. The data of Burke and Miles, however, suggest that the prompt administration of antibiotics, even after contamination has occurred, could reduce the magnitude of infectious complications. In addition, antibiotics given prior to surgery in trauma patients should produce the same reduction in incisional infections as prophylactic antibiotics given in the setting of elective surgical procedures. Because most traumatic injuries are either contaminated or frankly dirty, the term "prophylactic antibiotics" is misleading—antibiotics are intended to control infection, not prevent it. We prefer to think of antibiotic use in this setting as *empiric* antibiotic therapy, which suggests that antibiotics are administered before the precise location of injury and its bacteriology are known. However, because the term prophylactic antibiotics is widely used to denote a specific method of antibiotic administration that includes the timing and duration of antibiotic use, we will continue to use it here.

A number of studies of prophylactic antibiotic use in penetrating trauma have been performed, some of which are reviewed in Figure 16.1. Studies were selected for review that (1) had comparable patients in each treatment group, (2) stated the incidence of significant intra-abdominal injuries in each treatment group, (3) reported infections according to their site of origin, and (4) did not include other antibiotic usage (such as peritoneal irrigation). The following studies illustrate a number of valid principles about the use of such antibiotics.

Antibiotics should be given as soon as possible following injury. This is a key principle in the empiric use of antibiotics. As Miles and Burke initially showed, after 3 hours from the time of bacterial contamination, antibiotics probably do not affect the development of infection. After this period, infection should be considered established; the wound is classified as dirty rather than contaminated. Antibiotics given in these circumstances should be given as a therapeutic course lasting several days.

Antibiotics should be given prior to surgery. They have been shown to reduce subsequent infection rates less effectively when given intraoperatively or postoperatively, as shown by Fullen and co-workers.[6] This effect appears to be additive to the absolute time following injury that antibiotics are administered. In addition, antibiotics given perioperatively act in a truly prophylactic manner in decreasing infection in the surgical wound.

The course of antibiotic use should be short. Stone and colleagues initially demonstrated that if antibiotics are begun promptly after injury, no more than one or two doses are needed to produce maximum reduction in the wound infection rate.[20] In two subsequent studies, Dellinger and associates and Oreskovich and co-workers demonstrated similar findings.[3,17] Giving prophylactic regimens for longer periods may increase the possibility of superinfection with resistant strains, or of complications related to the antibiotics themselves. In addition, the cost savings of prophylactic antibiotics may be negated by prolonged antibiotic use.

Antibiotics should be effective against the presumed target organisms. This principle is probably the most controversial, as well as the hardest to control, in trials of prophylactic antibiotic usage in trauma. Initial trials of empiric antibiotic therapy used penicillin, which is quite effective against streptococci and most staphylococci, but relatively ineffective against coliforms.[6] First-generation cephalosporins such as cephalothin have also been used in penetrating trauma[20,22] despite their limited activity against many enteric organisms. Trials that used aminoglycosides provided relatively good coverage against coliform bacteria, but gave poor anaerobic coverage. Despite their shortcomings, however, such regimens did reduce the incidence of infections, except of course those caused by organisms resistant to the antibiotics used.[23]

In fact, the significance of anaerobes in the etiology of surgical infections has been realized only within about the past 10 years. Stone and co-workers[22] recovered anaerobic bacteria from 47.7% of abdominal cultures taken from patients with penetrating trauma; up to nine anaerobic species were recovered from individual patients, and these authors observed that anaerobes were recovered almost uniformly in cases of abdominal trauma. Onderdonk and colleagues demonstrated that infections that follow peritoneal contamination from bowel contents have a polymicrobial, synergistic etiology involving both aerobic coliforms and anaerobic organisms.[16] They demonstrated in a rat model of peritoneal contamination that facultative aerobic organisms such as *E. coli*, when injected alone, produce peritonitis and early mortality. Injection of isolated colonies of

FIGURE 16.1
REVIEW OF PROPHYLACTIC ANTIBIOTIC USAGE IN TRAUMA

AUTHOR	PATIENTS	PT. GROUP	SAMPLE SIZE	ANTIBIOTIC ADMINISTRATION
Time of Administration				
Fullen et al 1972[6]	Penetrating abdominal injuries. Analyzed retrospectively over a 13-year period.	A	116	Penicillin and either tetracycline or chloramphenicol given before surgery.
		B	98	Same regimen given intraoperatively.
		C	81	Same regimen started postoperatively.
Length of Administration				
Stone et al 1979[20]	Patients with trauma randomized prospectively.	A	213	Cephalothin begun preop; continued for 4 doses.
		B	238	Cephalothin begun preop; continued 5–7 days.
Oreskovich et al 1982[17]	Penetrating abdominal trauma; prospectively randomized.	A	42	Penicillin and doxycycline begun preop; continued 12 hours.
		B	40	Same antibiotics; continued 5 days.
Dellinger et al 1986[3]	Penetrating abdominal injuries with bowel perforation confirmed; randomized initially to penicillin and doxycycline; later switched to cefoxitin.	A	31	Penicillin and doxycycline begun preop; continued 12 hours.
		B	30	Cefoxitin begun preop; continued 12 hours
		C	25	Penicillin and doxycycline begun preop; continued 5 days.
		D	28	Cefoxitin begun preop; continued 5 days.
Specific Antibiotics				
Thadepalli et al 1973[26]	Penetrating injuries of the GI tract randomized.	A	52	Cephalothin and kanamycin begun preop intraop; continued 7 days.
		B	48	Clindamycin and kanamycin begun preop intraop; continued 7 days.
O'Donnell et al 1978[15]	Penetrating injuries of the abdomen; randomized.	A	66	Clindamycin and gentamicin begun preop; continued 4–6 days.
		B	60	Carbenicillin begun preop; continued 4–6 days.
Hofstetter et al 1984[8]	Penetrating and blunt trauma; randomized.	A	69	Cefoxitin begun preop; continued 24 hours.
		B	50	Gentamicin, clindamycin and ampicillin begun preop; continued 24 hours.
Nichols et al 1984[13]	Patients with abdominal trauma; hollow viscous injury confirmed. Randomized.	A	70	Cefoxitin begun preop; continued 5 days.
		B	75	Clindamycin and gentamicin begun preop; continued 5 days.
Gentry et al 1984[7]	Patients with abdominal trauma and hollow viscous injury confirmed. Randomized.	A	51	Cefamandole begun preop; continued 48 hours.
		B	50	Cefoxitin begun preop; continued 48 hours.
		C	51	Ticarcillin and tobramycin begun preop; continued 48 hours.
Rowlands et al 1984[19]	Patients with penetrating injuries randomized to two separate studies.	1A	51	Cefamandole begun preop; continued 3 days.
		1B	54	Cefoxitin begun preop; continued 3 days.
		1C	46	Clindamycin and tobramycin begun preop; continued 3 days.
		2A	47	Moxalactam begun preop; continued 5 days.
		2B	45	Clindamycin and tobramycin begun preop continued 5 days.
Jones et al 1985[9]	Patients with penetrating trauma. Randomized.	A	85	Clindamycin and tobramycin begun preop; continued 48 hours.
		B	78	Cefamandole begun preopl continued 48 hours.
		C	94	Cefoxitin begun preop; continued 48 hours.

FIGURE 16.1
REVIEW OF PROPHYLACTIC ANTIBIOTIC USAGE IN TRAUMA (CONTINUED)

INFECTIONS: ABDOMINAL	INFECTIONS: WOUND	TOTAL	P-VALUE	COMMENTS
4%	7%			
25%	33%		ND*	Retrospective review of a heterogeneous patient group. However, when analyzed according to a degree of injury, colon injuries only, or year of injury, this relationship remains true.
19%	30%			
3.8%	9.8%	10.3%	NS†	Heterogenous patients. However, this relationship held true for all subgroups. The extra cost of 5 days of therapy was $100 per patient in 1979 (about $1000 now).
4.6%	13.1%	15.1%	NS	
4.7%	4.7%	9.5%	NS	No difference in infection rates when colon injuries analyzed separately.
2.5%	5%	7.5%	NS	
		26%	NS	Five days of therapy costs seven times as much as 12 hours.
		21%		
		27%	ND[1]	This early study showed that (1) anaerobes are cultured very frequently when bowel injuries are found; (2) anaerobes were cultured from 43% of group A, 3% group B patients. Anaerobic infections were much more common in group A; (3) prophylactic regimens should include anaerobic coverage.
		10%		
		7.5%	NS	Almost half of these patients had no visceral injury at surgery. Carbenicillin was chosen because of good activity against anaerobes and Enterobacteriaceae.
		10%		
4.3%	7.2%	14.5%	NS	Groups equivalent with respect to site and severity of injury. Hollow viscous injury present in only about half of patients.
8%	2%	18%		
9%	11%	20%	NS	Well done study limited to high-risk patients. Hospitalization 14 days if infection develops, 7 days otherwise.
9%	13%	23%		
11.8%	5.8%			The likelihood of an uneventful recovery was lower with cefamandole (80.3%) vs. cefoxitin or ticarcillin and tobramycin (94% and 90% respectively, $p > 0.05$). Wound infection doubles; abscess triples length of hospital stay.
6%	0%		NS	
5.8%	3.9%			
10%	10%	20%		In study 1, wound infections were significantly more common with cefoxitin compared to clindamycin and tobramycin; infection rates were significantly lower with clindamycin and tobramycin in study 1 in patients with gunshot wounds or high injury severity scores.
7%	13%	20%	NS	
9%	2%	11%		
2%	0%	2%	NS	
4%	4%	9%		
14%		20%		The significantly higher infection rate with cefamandole was increased in colon injuries. Bacteroides infections were more common with cefamandole.
26%		29%	≤0.05	
10%		13%		

* No statistical analysis performed.
† Nonsignificant difference.

anaerobes such as *Bacteroides fragilis* produced relatively little effect, while intraperitoneal abscesses were produced only when aerobic and anaerobic bacteria were injected together. This suggested that antibiotics which interrupt any part of this synergistic relationship might be effective in preventing abscess formation, and helped explain the success of early trials of antibiotics that lacked anaerobic coverage.

The efficacy of any regimen of antimicrobial prophylaxis depends largely on the bacteria encountered. Various abdominal organs have characteristic resident flora that differ greatly in number as well as type. In elective surgical procedures, prophylactic antibiotics can be chosen that are effective against the organisms which are likely to be encountered, as demonstrated in Polk and Lopez-Mayor's original study.[18] For example, the biliary tree is frequently sterile, but when contaminated, it usually contains coliform bacteria. In traumatic injuries, however, it is usually impossible to match "the bug and the drug," since the surgeon rarely knows what organ, if any, is injured until the abdomen is opened. The colon clearly represents the "dirtiest" of abdominal viscera, with as many as 10^{11} bacteria per gram of contents. It is not surprising that colon injury is invariably identified as a major predictor of infection following abdominal injury.[3,4,9,19]

In order to be widely useful and effective, any antibiotic prophylactic regimen must be effective in the setting of colon injury, yet in reviews of penetrating trauma, colon injury may be present in as little as 20% of injuries.[15,17] While the incidence of "negative laparotomy" in both blunt and penetrating trauma has been reduced by the development of selective approaches to these injuries, it remains true that many operations for trauma find no injury to abdominal viscera, or injuries limited to solid organs. The most powerful and broadest-spectrum antibiotic regimens are complicated, expensive, relatively risky, and usually unnecessary. A simpler regimen, however, may provide inadequate coverage for a severe injury, which is precisely the one in which antibiotic prophylaxis may be needed the most.

As mentioned previously, a prophylactic antibiotic need not be effective against all organisms encountered in order to be efficacious in trauma. Antibiotics should be selected that are effective against at least the major groups of bacteria anticipated, as abundant evidence suggests. In an important early study of patients with documented penetrating trauma to the gastrointestinal tract, Thadepalli and colleagues demonstrated that a regimen of cephalothin and kanamycin, with limited anaerobic activity, was inferior to a regimen of clindamycin and kanamycin in preventing infections.[26] Based on this and similar studies,[10] and on parallel studies in elective surgery, the most widely utilized prophylactic regimens consist of multiple drugs with activity against both anaerobes (usually clindamycin) and aerobic coliforms (usually an aminoglycoside). Such two-drug regimens (sometimes expanded to three drugs to cover enterococcus) have become the accepted standard for a variety of prophylactic situations, including trauma. These regimens have distinct disadvantages, however. Aminoglycosides have a relatively high frequency of complications. Optimum dosage for each of two or three drugs is usually decided individually and must be given separately. Both these facts complicate administration of antibiotics, and greatly increase the possibility that the antibiotics will not be administered as quickly as possible following injury. The cost of these multiple drug regimens is great and compounded by the appreciable cost of preparing separate IV doses for administration.

In an effort to avoid these difficulties, numerous trials of single-drug prophylaxis in trauma have been conducted. The best results have been obtained using antibiotics with effective gram-negative and anaerobic coverage, including carbenicillin,[15] cefoxitin,[7,9,14,19] or moxalactam.[19] O'Donnell and co-workers found that carbenicillin used alone was as effective in reducing the incidence of infections in trauma patients as a standard two-drug regimen.[15] Several studies have demonstrated that cefoxitin given preoperatively and continued for short periods postoperatively produces infection rates that are equivalent to those associated with effective doses of aminoglycosides and clindamycin.[7,9,14] Another third-generation cephalosporin, cefamandole, is somewhat less effective against *B. fragilis* than either cefoxitin or to aminoglycoside-clindamycin, and may have a slightly higher infection rate than either regimen, as demonstrated by Jones and colleagues,[9] arguing for the improved efficacy of regimens with powerful anaerobic coverage. However, other studies show no disadvantage of cefamandole compared to other antibiotic regimens.[7,19] Recently, Rowlands and associates demonstrated another third-generation cephalosporin, moxalactam, to be efficacious in the setting of acute trauma prophylaxis.[19]

Empiric antibiotics should be used only in appropriate candidates. Based on the classification of wounds reviewed previously, empiric antibiotics are best used in the setting of clean-contaminated or contaminated wounds. "Clean" traumatic wounds do not occur, but "clean" procedures are sometimes performed in trauma patients. Such procedures (splenorrhapy, closed reduction of a fracture) do not require antibiotic administration if no other open wounds are present. The most frequent of these "clean" procedures, however, is probably the negative laparotomy in the patient with blunt injury. This is technically clean, but usually cannot be so classified until the abdomen is opened. Hollow viscous injury is uncommon in blunt abdominal trauma, but certainly occurs. In addition, the high infection rate associated with solid organ injury (particularly the pancreas) in the presence of shock or hemorrhage argues strongly for a perioperative course of empiric antibiotics.

LIMITATIONS OF ANTIBIOTIC USE IN TRAUMA

It is equally important to recognize the limitations of empiric antibiotic administration in trauma. Two situations frequently render wounds dirty: first, if more than 4 hours have elapsed from injury to operation in contaminated wounds, empiric antibiotics are unlikely to be effective. Antibiotics should certainly be started, but they should probably be continued for longer periods postoperatively, and altered according to culture results. The other common "dirty" procedure is one in which contamination cannot be controlled completely. Crush injuries, open pelvic fractures, and other situations in which complete debridement may be impossible mandate continued antibiotic use beyond a short course of empiric therapy.

In this chapter we have intentionally avoided recommending antibiotics for various situations. As this review illustrates, a variety of drugs have demonstrated efficacy in trauma prophylaxis. Widely different regimens are used successfully at various institutions. In addition, the development of new antibiotics is proceeding rapidly, as the ongoing proliferation of cephalosporins illustrates. Improvements will continue to be made in the effectiveness, cost, and safety of antibiotics, and new drugs will continue to be tested. Instead we have reviewed the principles of antibiotic usage, adherence to which will result in the continued rational use of antibiotics in the initial management of the trauma patient.

REFERENCES

1. Burke JF: The effective period of preventive antibiotic action in experimental incisions and dermal lesions. Surgery 50:161–169, 1961.
2. Cruse PJ, Foord R: Five-year prospective study of 23,649 surgical wounds. Arch Surg 107:286, 1973.
3. Dellinger EP, Oreskovich MR, Wertz MJ et al: Risk of infection following laparotomy for penetrating abdominal injury. Arch Surg 119:20–27, 1984.
4. Dellinger EP, Wertz MJ, Lennard ES, Oreskovich MR: Efficacy of short-course prophylaxis after penetrating intestinal injury. Arch Surg 121:23–30, 1986.
5. DiPiro J, Bivins BA, Record KE et al: The prophylactic use of antimicrobials in surgery. Curr Probl Surg 20:71–132, 1983.
6. Fullen WD, Hunt J, Altmeier WA: Prophylactic antibiotics in penetrating wounds of the abdomen. J Trauma 12:282–289, 1972.
7. Gentry LO, Filiciano DV, Lea AS et al: Perioperative antibiotic therapy for penetrating injuries of the abdomen. Ann Surg 200:561–566, 1984.
8. Hofstetter SR, Pachter HL, Bailey AA, Coppa GF: A prospective comparison of two regimens of prophylactic antibiotics in abdominal trauma: Cefoxitin vs. triple drug. J Trauma 24:307–310, 1984.
9. Jones RC, Thal ER, Johnson NA, Gollihar LN: Evaluation of antibiotic therapy following penetrating abdominal trauma. Ann Surg 201:576–583, 1985.
10. Martinez OV, Lester JL, Arango A, Malinin TI: Antibiotic prophylaxis in penetrating colorectal injuries: The comparative effectiveness of clindamycin and cephalothin in combination with an aminoglycoside. Ann Surg 179:378–383, 1979.
11. Miles AA, Miles EM, Burke J: The value and duration of defence reactions of the skin to the primary lodgement of bacteria. Br J Exp Pathol 38:29–96, 1957.
12. Moncrief JA, Teplitz C: Changing concepts in burn sepsis. J Trauma 4:233, 1964.
13. National Academy of Sciences–National Research Council: Postoperative wound infections: Influence of ultraviolet irradiation of operating room and/or various other factors. Ann Surg (Suppl) 160:1, 1964.
14. Nichols RL, Smith JW, Klein DB et al: Risk of infection after penetrating abdominal trauma. N Eng J Med 311:1065–1070, 1984.
15. O'Donnell V, Mandel AK, Lou MA, Thadepalli H: Evaluation of carbenicillin and comparison of clindamycin and gentamicin combined therapy in penetrating abdominal trauma. Surg Gynecol Obstet 147:525–528, 1978.
16. Onderdonk AB, Bartlett JG, Louie T et al: Microbial synergy in experimental intra-abdominal abscess. Infect Immun 13:22–26, 1976.
17. Oreskovich MR, Dellinger EP, Lennard ES et al: Duration of preventive antibiotic administration for penetrating abdominal trauma. Arch Surg 117:200–205, 1982.
18. Polk HC, Lopez-Mayor JF: Postoperative wound infection: A prospective study of determinant factors and prevention. Surgery 66:97–103, 1969.
19. Rowlands BJ, Ericsson CD: Comparative studies of antibiotic therapy after penetrating abdominal trauma. Am J Surg 148:791–795, 1984.
20. Stone HH, Haney BB, Kolb LD et al: Prophylactic and preventive antibiotic therapy. Ann Surg 189:691–698, 1979.
21. Stone HH, Hester TR: Incisional and peritoneal infection after emergency celiotomy. Ann Surg 177:669–678, 1973.
22. Stone HH, Kolb LD, Geheber CE: Incidence and significance of intraperitoneal anaerobic bacteria. Ann Surg 181:705–715, 1975.
23. Stone HH, Kolb LD, Geheber CE, Dawkins EJ: Use of aminoglycosides in surgical infections. Ann Surg 183:660–666, 1976.
24. Teplitz C, Davis D, Mason AD Jr, Moncrief JA: Pseudomonas burn wound sepsis. I. Pathogenesis of experimental pseudomonas burn wound sepsis. J Surg Res 4:200, 1964.
25. Thadepalli H: Principles and practice of antibiotic therapy for post-traumatic abdominal injuries. Surg Gynecol Obstet 148:937–951, 1979.
26. Thadepalli H, Gorbach SL, Broido PW et al: Abdominal trauma, anaerobes, and antibiotics. Surg Gynecol Obstet 137:270–276, 1973.
27. Tucker JW, Fey WP: The management of perforating injuries of the colon and rectum in civilian practice. Surgery 35:213, 1954.

burn injury

Joseph A. Moylan

Burn injuries, including thermal, chemical, and electrical burns, are among the most challenging injuries treated by physicians. These injuries, experienced by over 2 million people each year in the United States, result not only in surface damage, but major metabolic, cardiovascular, and organ dysfunction. The purpose of this chapter will be to discuss each of these types of burn injuries in reference to initial care provided prehospital and in the emergency room, pathophysiology of the injury itself, and in-depth care by the surgical staff.

THERMAL INJURY

Thermal damage to the skin can result from contact with flame, liquids, or heated objects such as irons or electric stoves, or current. The majority of these injuries can be treated in outpatient facilities.[14] However, each year approximately 20% to 30% of the total burn injuries in the United States require hospitalization.

Surface injuries can be categorized as major, moderate, or minor (Fig. 17.1). Minor second-degree burns are those involving less than 15% of the total body surface, in children, less than 10%. Minor third-degree burns cover less than 2% to 3% of the body surface and do not involve any vital structures such as the eyes, hands, feet, or perineum.

Moderate-size burns are defined as second-degree burns of 15% to 25% of the body surface, slightly smaller areas in children, and third-degree burns of less than 10% of the total body surface excluding burns that involve vital structures. Patients with moderate-size burns can usually be treated effectively in a community hospital if resources and personnel with burn care experience are available.

Major burn injuries are defined as second-degree burns of more than 25% of the total body surface, and all third-degree burns of 10% of the body or more. In addition, all burns involving vital areas such as the hands, face, feet, eyes, ears, and perineum, as well as burns with inhalation injuries, electrical burns, and burns with other associated trauma are classified as major burns. Patients with major burns are usually stabilized and then transferred to a regional burn and trauma center.

Pathophysiology of the Burn Injury

While the burn causes primarily skin and subcutaneous damage, it has adverse effects on many other organ systems including the cardiovascular, pulmonary, and metabolic systems (Fig. 17.2). The extent and depth of the burn injury depend upon the temperature of the heat source and the duration of exposure. It is estimated that approximately 160°F heat applied at the skin surface for as little as 1 to 2 seconds can cause a full-thickness injury. Factors modifying the depth of skin damage include the insulating effect of clothes and the air, and the distance of the heat surface from the skin. The adverse effects of the burn injury and other organ dysfunction are also related to the extent of burn injury. However, mortality for burns has changed drastically over recent years with improved resuscitation, control of infection, and nutritional support.

Pathophysiologic changes can be divided into early, intermediate, and late. The earliest effects seen following a major burn injury involve primarily the cardiovascular and pulmonary systems.[3] Increased capillary permeability following the burn injury results in loss of fluids and protein from the intervascular to the extravascular compartment. This is secondary to cell disruption as well as the liberation of vasoactive materials. Edema may develop in both the unburned and burned areas secondary to these two mechanisms. In major burns there can be significant volume shifts proportional to the size of the burn. Cardiac output falls in the immediate postburn period and it continues to fall even after resuscitation has been begun. This is primarily due to a decrease in plasma volume as well as increased peripheral resistance. While a myocardial depressant factor has been suggested as the cause, multiple studies have failed to demonstrate its existence.

The effects of decreased cardiac output and inadequate plasma volumes are evident by signs of shock, including decreased urine output, confusion, and hypoxia. Decreased plasma volume persisting over the first 12 to 18 hours despite adequate resuscitation may well be due to arteriovenous shunting.[24]

Up to 8% to 10% of the red cell mass may be destroyed directly, depending upon the size of the burn injury, with subsequent sequestration. There may be alterations in the coagulation following burn injury, including depression in platelet and fibrinogen levels, but these are rapidly self-corrected and have little significance during the early resuscitation phase. Later in the burn period there may be disseminated intravascular coagulation secondary to sepsis, a common sequela of major burn injuries.

The immune system is also significantly affected, depending on the size of the injury. Burns have a higher incidence of infection than other kinds of trauma, due to not only destruction of the skin barrier, but also alterations in the immunoglobulins.

FIGURE 17.1
BURN CLASSIFICATION AND DISPOSITION

	SIZE AND DEPTH	TREATMENT MODE
Minor	2nd degree, less than 15% TBS* 3rd degree, less than 3%	Outpatient
Moderate	2nd degree, 15%–25% TBS* 3rd degree, less than 10%	Inpatient Community hospital
Major	2nd degree, over 25% TBS* 3rd degree, over 10% Burns involving face, hands, feet Inhalation injuries Burns plus multisystem injury	Inpatient Trauma/burn center

*TBS, total body surface.

Humoral factors are depressed in the early postburn period, but they rapidly respond and surpass original levels. These factors, however, may be significantly depressed when a secondary infection develops. Cellular components of infection response, including the lymphocyte and neutrophil functions, are also impaired following a burn injury.[2]

Alterations in pulmonary functions, including increased pulmonary vascular resistance, occur in the immediate postburn period. With the exception of patients with previously compromised right-sided heart function, these changes appear to have little clinical significance. However, patients with inhalation injuries and circumferential thoracic burns may experience significant alteration in their pulmonary function. These patients show either mechanical restriction in the presence of circumferential chest burn injuries or airway and parenchymal damage resulting in diffusion and breathing difficulties. These complications may require either chest escharotomy or intubation and mechanical support, or both. It is not uncommon for burn patients to demonstrate hyperpnea due to postinjury hypermetabolism, usually 24 hours after injury; however, it should not be confused with those changes in respiration produced by the initial injury itself. Delayed pulmonary complications include hypoxia and hypoventilation, and are usually secondary to sepsis either locally in the lung or systemically.

Metabolic changes are secondary to hormonal and chemical alterations, including elevated glucagon, cortisol and catechol levels, as well as depressed insulin and thyroxine levels.[27] These responses increase as the size of the burn increases. Patients remain hypermetabolic until the burn wound is healed. Alterations in endocrine function, as in other trauma, are influenced by sepsis or other complications.

Gastric and duodenal mucosal changes occurring in the early postburn period are due to low cardiac output. It is not uncommon to see guaiac-positive nasogastric aspirates during the early phase following injury. These are usually self-limiting, and when oral feedings and positive nitrogen balance are achieved they usually cause no difficulty. Sepsis, however, can result in additional mucosal ischemia, producing gastrointestinal bleeding, a frequent complication and indication of generalized sepsis.

FIGURE 17.2
PATHOPHYSIOLOGY OF BURN INJURY

LOCAL

1) Factors Influencing Depth and Extent
   a) Intensity of heat
   b) Length of exposure
   c) Area of exposure
   d) Mechanism of injury

SYSTEMIC EFFECTS

1) Cardiovascular
   a) Increased capillary permeability
   b) Decreased plasma volume
   c) Decreased cardiac output
   d) Red cell destruction
   e) Coagulopathies

2) Pulmonary
   a) Airway damage in upper and major airways
   b) Parenchymal damage in capillary pulmonary membrane
   c) Ventilatory insult by chest wall restriction

3) Immune
   a) Alteration in cellular and humoral response
   b) Sepsis

4) Metabolic
   a) Increased metabolic rate

5) Gastrointestinal
   a) Stress ulceration

6) Renal
   a) Acute failure

Prehospital and Emergency Care

Initial first aid provided at the scene of the burn accident includes extinguishing and removing any burning clothes. Burn accidents involving significant amounts of smoke may result in high carbon monoxide levels, producing cardiopulmonary arrest. Mouth-to-mouth resuscitation in the unconscious or poorly breathing patient may be lifesaving. The patient should be kept covered and warm prior to and during transport to the nearest medical facility to prevent any significant drop in body temperature and cardiac dysrhythmias, especially in colder climates. However, minor burns (i.e., those partial-thickness burns that are less than 15% of the body surface) may be treated with application of ice or cold-water soaks to decrease the pain. Cold applications should not be used in larger size burns, since they may result in an acute drop in body temperature and cardiac dysrhythmias, particularly in the elderly patient.

Transport should be as expeditious as possible, and start-up of an intravenous line should not be delayed, particularly if the nearest medical facility is less than 30 minutes away.[13] The burned extremity should be elevated during transport to minimize edema formation. Since carbon monoxide intoxication is a frequent sequela of most injuries, oxygen should be provided by mask for all patients incurring major- and moderate-size burns. Endotracheal or esophageal airways should be limited to those patients with apnea who cannot be adequately ventilated with an Ambu and an oral airway.

Initial care in the emergency department should include a complete primary and secondary physical survey. It is not unusual for patients in major fire accidents to have incurred other injuries that may not be obvious. Once the history and the physical assessment are rapidly completed, one or two large-caliber intravenous lines should be secured. Depending upon the size of the injury, it is preferable to place these intravenous accesses in nonburned areas. The patient should be weighed and then the size and depth of the burn injury calculated using the "rule of nines" to estimate the size (Fig. 17.3), and the appearance of the burn evaluated to determine partial- or full-thickness skin damage (Fig. 17.4). The amount of fluid required depends upon the size of the burn injury and the weight of the patient. In moderate or major burns, a Foley catheter should be inserted into the bladder to measure polyurine output. An initial ECG is indicated in patients over 45, patients with preexisting cardiovascular disease, or patients with other associated injuries in addition to thermal injury.

The presence of a severe inhalation injury, apnea, or significant carbon monoxide poisoning are indications for endotracheal intubation and possible mechanical ventilatory assistance. Patients with moderate and major burn injuries who do not require endotracheal intubation may benefit from oxygen administration during the resuscitative phase.

Having determined the disposition of the patient based on size and depth of the injury, (i.e., outpatient for minor burns, admission to the community hospital for moderate burns, or transfer to regional burn centers for major burns), all patients other than those requiring transfer to a regional burn center should have their burn areas treated. If transfer is indicated, it should be done as soon as cardiorespiratory stabilization has been achieved. The burned area should be cleaned gently using a mild soap not containing alcohol. Frequently this procedure is painful and administration of intravenous analgesia is beneficial. Bullae should be gently excised, particularly larger bullae which may become infected. Some physicians favor debridement of bullae less than 2 cm in diameter; others do not. Burns treated on an outpatient basis are by definition at minimal risk to infection and can therefore be treated without a topical antimicrobial agent. These are best treated in a closed fashion by dressing them with a nonadherent fine mesh gauze and then wrapped in a bulky dressing to prevent soaking through the dressing. Open or exposure treatment of these wounds is possible, since a more protective crust will form over the burn injury. However, this technique is certainly more painful and requires higher levels of analgesia, and thus the closed technique is preferred.

The patient should be seen frequently in the initial postburn period, at least every 48 hours, at which time the dressings are removed and the wound inspected, and if any evidence of infection is noted, the patient should be admitted to the hospital and treated with topical antimicrobial agents. It should be emphasized that minor burns are at minimal risk to infection and do not require either oral or topical antibacterial treatment.

Patients treated as outpatients should be warned of the potential complications of infection or ileus with vomiting in younger children. They should be advised to return to the emergency department immediately if fever, chills, or repeated vomiting occurs. An adequate supply of analgesia is an important aspect of outpatient care to assure the comfort of the patient. Frequently, severe pruritus requiring antihistamines may occur, particularly in cases of severe sunburn and other outpatient partial-thickness injuries.

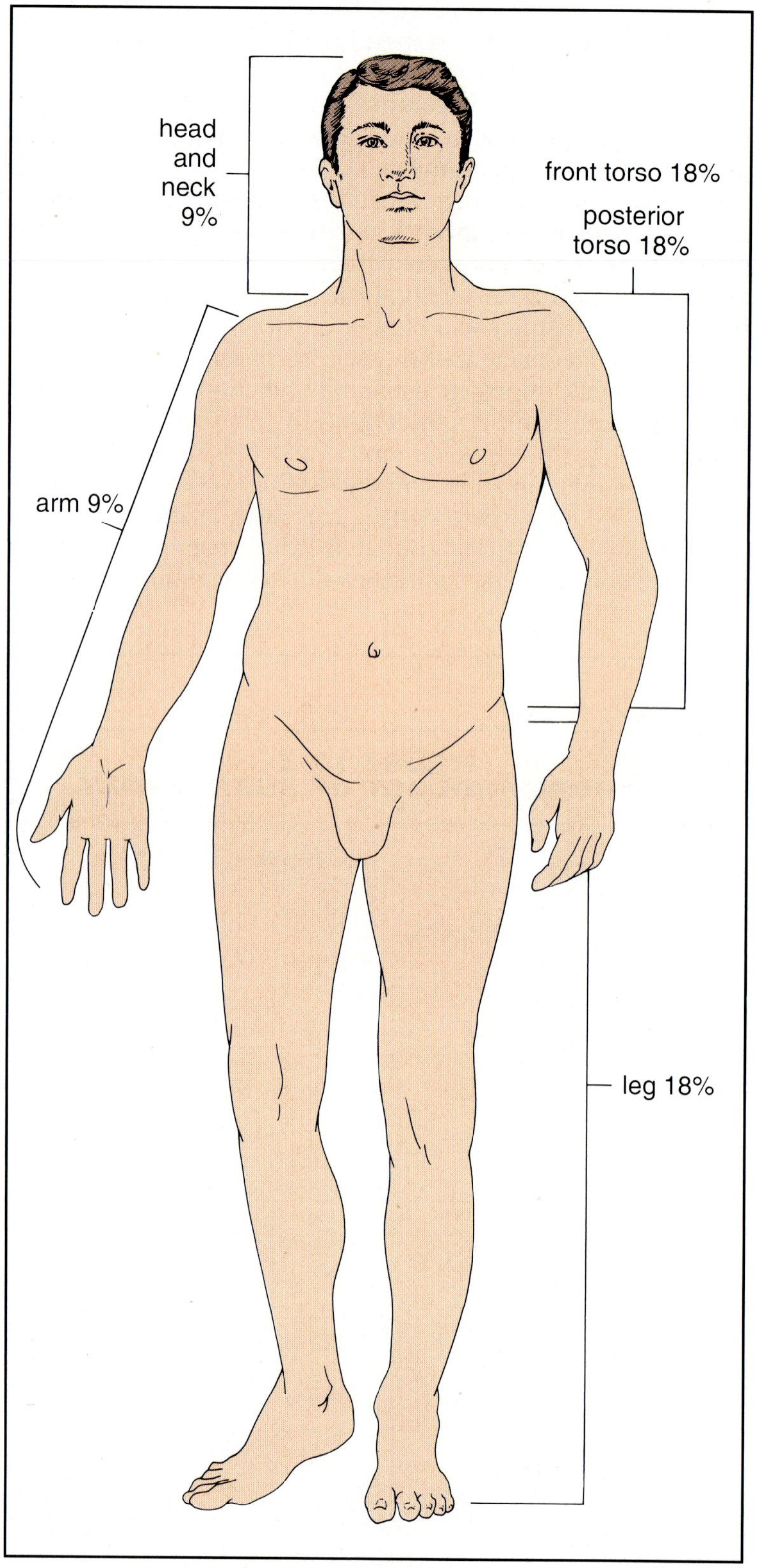

FIGURE 17.3 "Rule of nines" used in assessing areas of burn involvement.

Treatment

FLUID RESUSCITATION

Historically, many formulas have been suggested for burn shock resuscitation, including the Moore formula, the Evans formula, and the Brooke formula. In modern-day practice, however, the use of colloid in the first 24 hours is not common. Current approaches focus on the electrolyte solutions, which provide either slightly hypotonic, isotonic, or hypertonic resuscitation. All patients with burns over more than 15% of the body surface and requiring hospitalization should receive intravenous resuscitation. These patients are at risk for ileus, vomiting, and complications of inadequate perfusion. The amount of fluid required is determined by the size of the burn injury and the initial weight of the patient. The goal of burn resuscitation is to reverse burn shock and prevent organ dysfunction, especially in the renal, gastric, pulmonary, cerebral, and cardiac systems. Experimental studies have shown that return of cardiac output (CO) can be expressed in the formula,

$$CO = K, Na + H_2O$$

Resuscitation, within limits, can be accomplished by large quantities of water and small amounts of sodium, equal amounts of sodium and water, or larger amounts of sodium and lesser volumes of water. Experimental evidence reveals that 1 mEq of sodium has a resuscitative effect in this equation equal to 13 mEq of water. The complication and safety factors with various formulas are proportional to the ratios of sodium and water.

The most commonly used electrolyte solution for burn resuscitation is lactated Ringer's (Fig. 17.5). It is administered at 2 ml to 4 ml/kg/% burn. The Parkland approach, which provides 4 ml/kg/% burn is an effective resuscitation formula providing a wide margin of safety.[5] In a hypotonic resuscitative program such as the Parkland, the amount of water is greater, and therefore the incidence of tissue edema, particularly pulmonary, is higher. It is not unusual for major burn resuscitation patients given the Parkland formula to gain approximately 20% of their preburn weight at the end of the resuscitative period. This formula, however, has a high margin of safety and the incidence of renal failure is extremely low.

Isotonic resuscitation, which administers fluids which contain 150 to 160 mEq of sodium per liter, is the formula used at Duke University.[15] The solution is prepared by adding one half ampule of sodium bicarbonate to each liter of Ringer's lactate, which

FIGURE 17.4
FACTORS OF BURN DEPTH

	SECOND-DEGREE BURN	THIRD-DEGREE BURN
Etiologies	Hot liquid, explosion	Hot liquid (prolonged exposure), flame, electricity, chemical
Appearance	Erythematous, mottled	Ischemic, white-charred
Wound surface	Moist vesicles	Dry
Sensation	Present	Absent

FIGURE 17.5
ELECTROLYTE SOLUTIONS FOR BURN SHOCK RESUSCITATION

SOLUTION	SODIUM COMPOSITION	RATE OF ADMINISTRATION (1ST 24 HOURS)	COLLOID	ADVANTAGES	COMPLICATION
Hypotonic: Lactate Ringer's	130 mEq Na/liter	2–4 ml/kg/% (4 ml most common)	Yes	Safe, effective	Fluid overload, excessive edema
Isotonic: Lactate Ringer's plus 1/2 ampule $NaCO_3$ per liter	150 mEq Na/liter	3 ml/kg/%	Only if serum albumin <2g/dl after 24 hrs	Safe, effective	Formula may not give enough fluid for burns <25% total body surface
Hypertonic: Evaluated with sodium chloride and sodium Ringer's lactate	225–250 mEq Na/liter	2 ml/kg/% (approximate)	No	Limits amount of fluid	Under-resuscitation, hypernatremis, late renal failure

yields 150 mEq of sodium per liter. While the primary purpose of the sodium bicarbonate is to achieve an isotonic sodium load, the bicarbonate is theoretically beneficial during the initial resuscitation when the patient frequently has a base deficit. This formula is administered at approximately 3 ml/kg/% burn. The value of this resuscitative formula is that a major burn requires less total volume during the initial 24 hours, as evidenced by a gain of only 10% of the patient's preburn weight. The incidence of pulmonary edema, ileus, and cerebral edema is less with this resuscitative program than with a hypotonic resuscitative program. Extensive use of this formula over the past 10 years has shown that it is as safe as the hypotonic solution formula.

Hypertonic sodium resuscitation had been suggested over the past 15 years using a solution containing 225 mEq to 250 mEq of sodium per liter.[19] While a formula for instituting the resuscitative program has not been established, this program is frequently administered at approximately 2 ml to 2½ ml/kg/% burn, and increased to maintain an hourly urine output of 30 ml to 50 ml per hour. Proponents of this resuscitative technique suggest that less total fluid is used because the hypertonic solution recruits water from the intracellular and extravascular spaces into the intravascular space. Experience with this formula has shown that patients frequently gain somewhere between 7% to 9% of their preburn weight. However, because of the use of endogenous fluids to fill intravascular volume, the margin of safety with this formula is less. Also it appears that the incidence of delayed organ dysfunction may be higher with this formula; therefore, either isotonic or hypotonic resuscitation is recommended.

Colloid is not employed routinely in the first 24 hours in any of these formulas, but is reserved for that time when capillary permeability appears less (i.e., 24 hours postinjury). During the second 24-hour period, colloid is administered in the Parkland formula, with the hypotonic fluid continued at approximately 4 ml per liter and decreased as urine output increases. The Parkland formula also administers for approximately 20% to 60% of the calculated plasma volume as a colloid. This may be either plasma, plasmanate, or diluted salt-poor albumin. With the isotonic and hypertonic formulas, colloid is not usually employed during the second 24 hours unless the serum albumin falls below 2.5 g/dl. Then salt-poor albumin is administered to increase the osmotic pressure by raising the serum albumin level to 3 g/dl.

It should be emphasized that all formulas should be employed only as guides to initiating resuscitation. Careful monitoring of vital signs, overall general condition, and specifically hourly urine outputs of 30 ml to 50 ml in adults and 1 ml/kg in children less than 30 kg should be employed. If urine outputs of less than these parameters should occur during the first 48 hours, the volume of infused electrolyte solution should be increased. Oliguria during this time commonly indicates inadequate volume replacement. It is rare to have acute renal failure as the cause of early low urine output. Diuretics are rarely indicated in thermal injuries during the first 48 hours unless the patient has a documented history of congestive heart failure in the past or a very high filling pressure by Swan-Ganz catheter. Urine output in excess of 75 ml/hr in the adult and 2 ml/kg/hr in the child indicate over-resuscitation, unless glucosuria is to blame. Excessive resuscitation results in significant, unnecessary edema. If glucosuria is not present, the volume of resuscitative fluid should be reduced to compensate for excessive urine output. During the second postburn day, the amount of electrolyte infusion should be reduced if adequate urine output occurs. The hourly infusion rates can be arbitrarily reduced by 25% and, if stable urine output occurs over the next 24 hours, reduced again in a stepwise manner. If glucosuria is the cause of high urine output, it can be corrected by providing a sugar-free electrolyte solution. Adults tolerate dextrose-free electrolyte solutions for up to 24 hours without significant complications. However, children, particularly infants, if deprived of glucose infusion for longer than 12 hours, can incur significant metabolic disruption. In infants, once the urinalysis shows negative for sugar for a period of 4 hours, glucose should be added back to the resuscitative regimen. It is almost never necessary to provide exogenous insulin to control glucosuria during the resuscitative period, except in patients with preexistent diabetes.

CARDIOPULMONARY MONITORING

Standard monitoring of a major burn includes checking vital signs, hourly urine output, and daily weight, and assessing the general condition, especially mental response. Daily chest x-rays provide evidence of pulmonary complications common during the resuscitative phase, as well as of any infectious complications that could develop. Laboratory tests include serum electrolytes and blood gases at the time of admission. Serial blood gases including *p*H and oxygen saturation also provide vital parameters in major burn care. It should be pointed out that while serial hematocrit has been suggested as a good indicator of resuscitation, it has been found to be highly misleading. It is not uncommon to have the patient hemoconcentrate up to a hematocrit of 55 in spite of adequate resuscitation. An acute fall in hematocrit during the first 24 hours, however, is indicative of either hemolysis or bleeding from an underlying, unsuspected injury and should be carefully investigated.

Invasive central monitoring using a central venous pressure (CVP) or Swan-Ganz catheter is rarely indicated in major burn patients, since the risk of infection as well as endothelial damage is extremely high when these instruments are employed. CVP catheters may not provide true assessments of the intravascular volume during the phase of increased capillary permeability. Use of these invasive monitoring devices should be reserved for patients who, despite receiving large volumes of resuscitative fluid, fail to have the expected cardiac response—that is, patients who are on ventilators and patients with a history of congestive heart failure on cardiotonic and other types of cardiac medications.

EXTREMITY AND RESPIRATORY MONITORING

Full-thickness burns involving an extremity or chest wall may produce either circulatory or respiratory compromise. As edema forms, it increases interstitial pressure, which may produce compromise to venous and arterial flow as well as respiratory excursion. Initially, as pressure builds under an inelastic eschar in an extremity, venous return decreases and peripheral edema increases. As interstitial pressure equals or exceeds arterial pressure, inflow may cease. Similarly on the chest wall, as edema develops under a tight eschar, respiratory excursion of the chest wall is checked, resulting in decreased tidal volume, hyperpnea, and hypoxia.

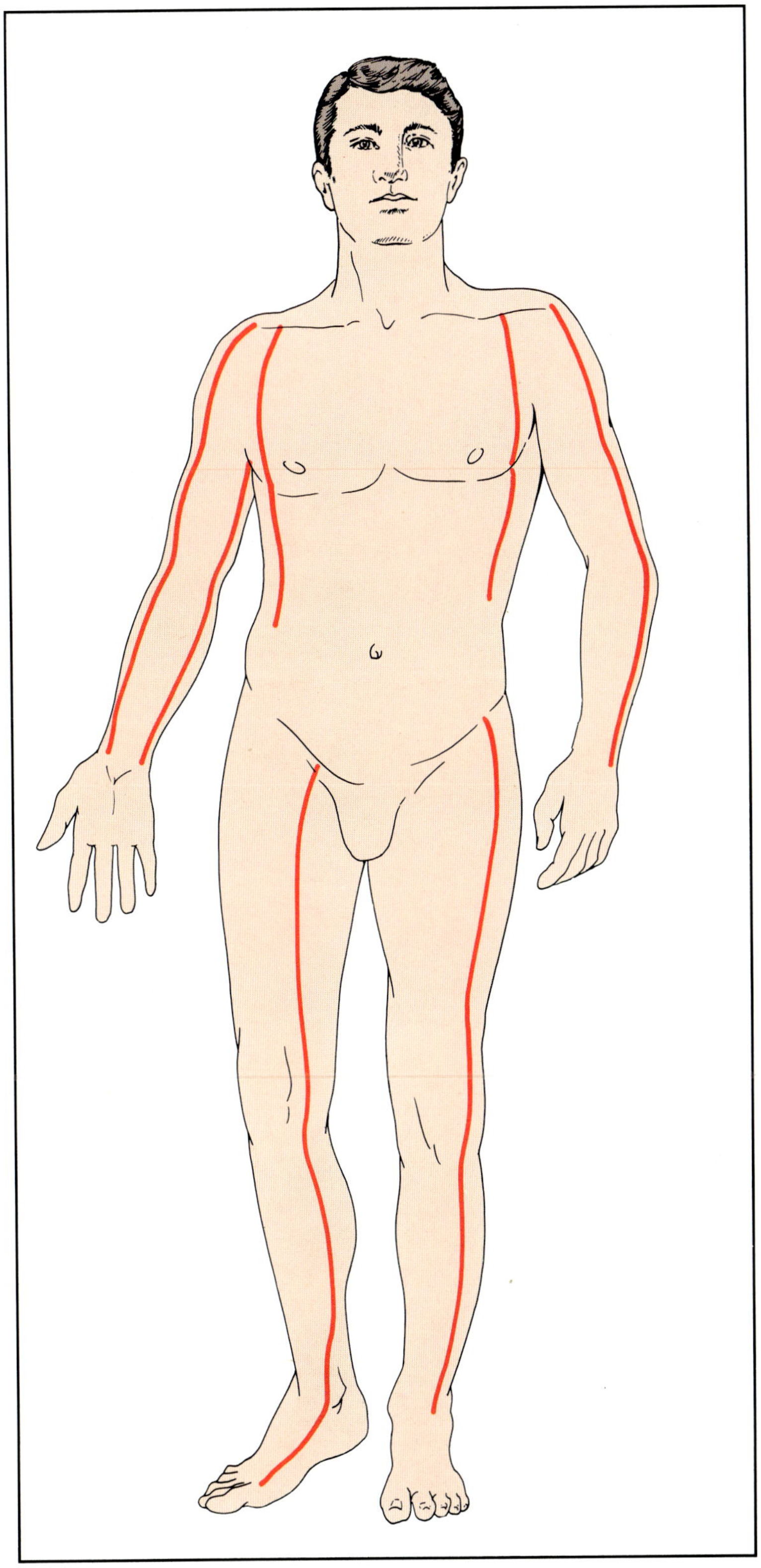

FIGURE 17.6 Location of incisions used for limb or chest escharotomies through full-thickness circumferential burns.

Preventive therapy is indicated in all patients with circumferential extremity and thoracic burns. The extremity should be elevated early in the treatment phase above the heart level: a sling system may be used for upper extremity burns or the lower end of the bed raised for lower extremity burns. In addition, active motion is indicated to augment the muscular pumping action for venous return. Active exercise of the upper or lower extremity for periods of two to three minutes should be carried out every 2 hours during the first 24 hours of postburn injury. If the chest wall is burned circumferentially, the head of the bed should be elevated to minimize upper body edema.

Careful monitoring of upper extremity blood flow is mandatory in all patients with circumferential limb burn. Clinical signs of decreasing distal flow include cyanosis, prolonged capillary refilling, change in normal sensation, paresthesia, or deep tissue pain. An objective measurement of flow may be made with the ultrasonic flowmeter.[18] This instrument is placed over the distal palmar arch for the upper limb or posterior tibial artery in the lower limb. If the presence of flow cannot be determined by using this instrument, an escharotomy is indicated. The adequacy of chest wall excursion can be determined by careful monitoring of the respiratory rate. If tachypnea develops associated with decreasing tidal volume, a chest wall escharotomy is indicated.

Escharotomy should be performed at the bedside, and the incisions should be carried out only through areas of full-thickness injury. Anesthesia is not required. For extremities the incisions are made on the medial and lateral aspects of the limb, extending over the entire length of the full-thickness burned areas (Fig. 17.6). The incision is carried down through the depth of the full-thickness injury to the subcutaneous level (Fig. 17.7). Extension of this incision through the fascia is not necessary in thermal injuries. If blood flow does not return to the palmar arch and digits after bilateral upper limb escharotomy and full-thickness burn is present over the digits, escharotomies of the

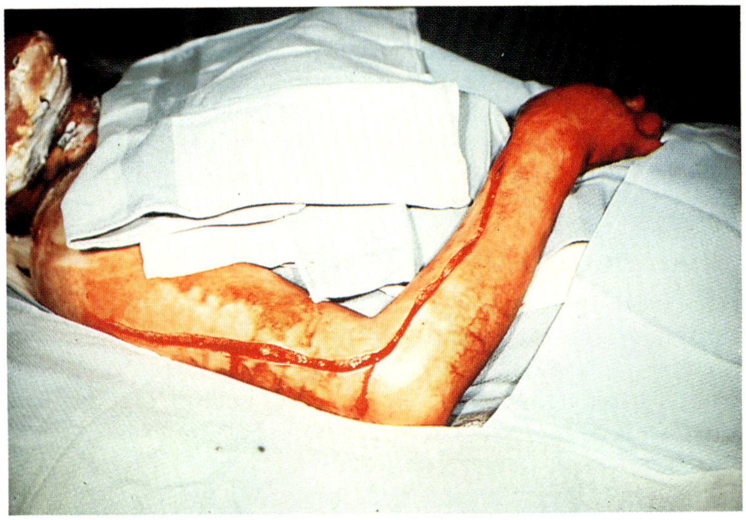

FIGURE 17.7 Lateral component of the escharotomy incision in the upper limb, third-degree burn.

medial and lateral aspect of the digits may be required. A chest escharotomy is usually carried out on the anterior thorax in a shield-like manner: the vertical limbs of the shield are at the anterior axillary line and the transverse or horizontal limb across the costochondral margin. Again, this escharotomy should be carried down only into the subcutaneous tissue. Bleeding is usually minimal and can be controlled by electrocautery or direct pressure. Since limb and chest escharotomies expose unburned, deep subcutaneous tissue, a topical antibiotic agent should be applied following this procedure and maintained until the time of healing or skin graft.

GENERAL SUPPORTIVE MEASURES

Adequate pain medication is required in patients with major burns, particularly partial-thickness injury. The analgesia program should be adjusted for each patient, since both the proportion of partial-thickness to full-thickness injuries and the individual's tolerance to pain will vary. Subcutaneous or intramuscular narcotics may be ineffective for pain during the early resuscitative period. Adequate analgesia is particularly important during the initial washing and debriding of the burn wound because this procedure may be very painful. Analgesia should be given intravenously during the first 24 hours.

Intravenous antibiotics have been shown not to be beneficial in the early care of burn patients. Use of prophylactic antibiotics, particularly penicillin, has been shown to result in the development of penicillin-resistant organisms and therefore should not be used. However, all patients should receive adequate tetanus prophylaxis. Patients who have undergone a previously effective active immunization and have received a toxoid booster within a year of the time of injury require no prophylaxis. Patients who received their most recent booster more than one year prior to injury should receive an additional booster dose of toxoid. Those who have not been adequately immunized or have associated injuries that are tetanus-prone should receive 250 to 500 units of human antitetanus globulin in addition to a toxoid booster. Those without any prior immunization should receive a similar program, as well as a complete immunization using toxoid in the usual routine dose schedule.

Ileus is not an uncommon occurrence following burn injury, particularly in burns in excess of 20% total body surface. A nasogastric tube may prevent aspiration and should be instilled immediately after adequate resuscitation has been started. It is not unusual for the ileus to last 2 to 3 days post injury, and therefore the nasogastric tube should be maintained during this period.

INHALATION INJURY

Inhalation injury continues to be one of the major factors in early mortality following burn injury.[17] This complication of thermal injury is actually a chemical burn of the airway caused by the inhalation of incomplete products of combustion. Inhalation injury has been reported in as much as 30% of patients involved in major burn accidents.

Inhalation injury has been anatomically divided into three areas: upper airway (i.e., inhalation injuries involving the pharynx and larynx down to the level of the vocal cord), major airway (those burns involving the tracheobronchial tree), and parenchyma (those involving the alveolar and capillary pul-

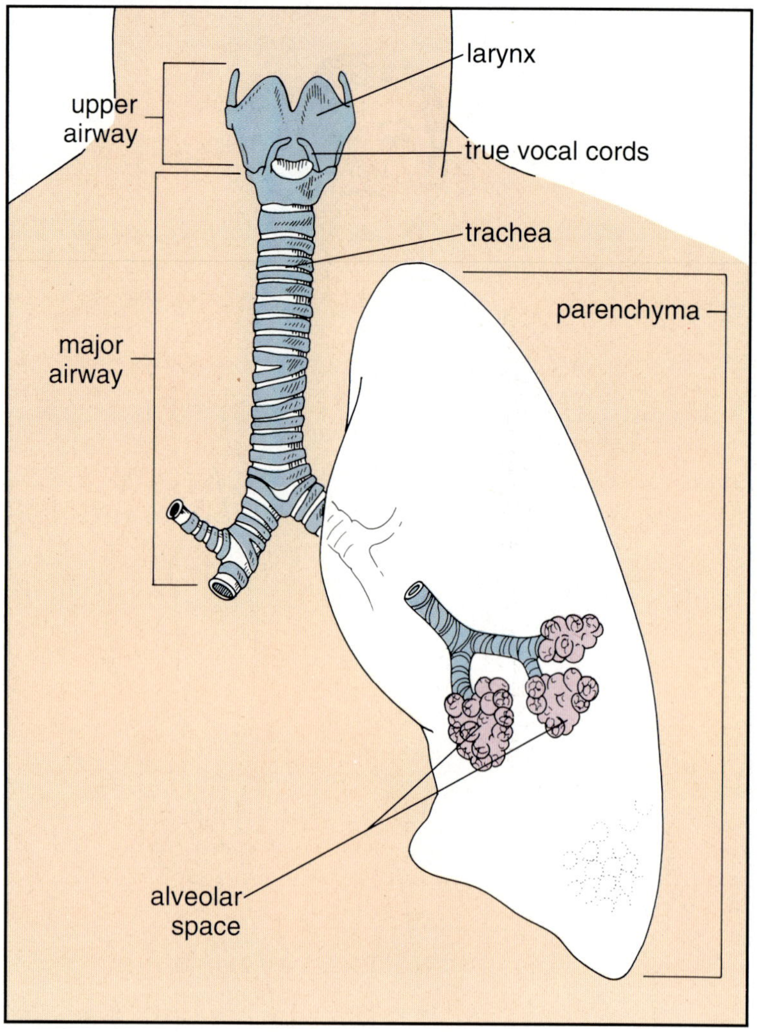

FIGURE 17.8 Levels of inhalation injury.

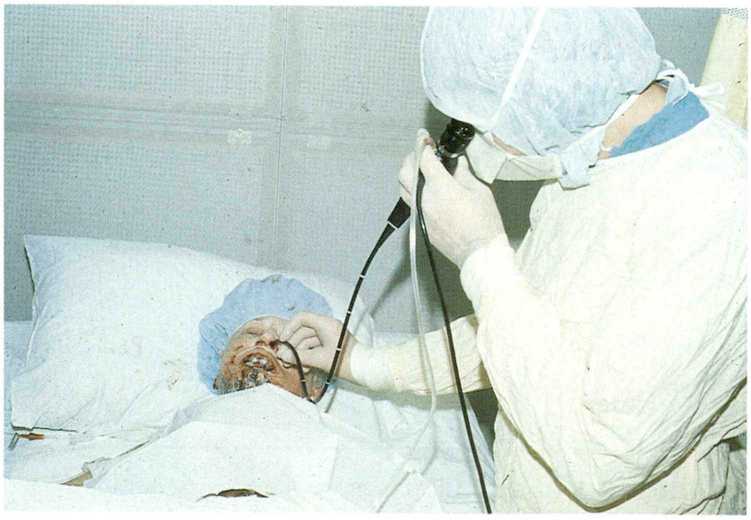

FIGURE 17.9 Bedside bronchoscopy under topical anesthesia.

monary membrane) (Fig. 17.8). Commonly, inhalation injuries produce mucosal damage, progressive swelling, possible upper airway occlusion, tracheobronchitis, mucosal plugs, and pneumonia. Rarely will inhalation injuries result in immediate hypoxia due to damage of the alveolar membrane.

All patients involved in a major thermal accident should be suspected of having an inhalation injury. The usual clinical signs such as head and neck burns, singeing of the nasal vibrissae, production of sooty sputum on cough, hoarseness, wheezing, and bronchorrhea may or may not be present in the early postburn period. Their appearance may be delayed until the patient is in dire respiratory stress.

Three common techniques have been used for the diagnosis of inhalation injury: fiberoptic bronchoscopy, xenon lung scans, and pulmonary function tests. The most commonly used approach is direct examination of the airway by *fiberoptic bronchoscopy*[16] (Figs. 17.9 and 17.10). This procedure can be accomplished at the bedside. The patient should be adequately oxygenated with 100% oxygen for a period of three minutes prior to the examination. The nasal mucosa is anesthetized with a topical anesthetic. Since upper airway edema may produce occlusion in the early postburn period, it is helpful to place a number 7 or 8 nasotracheal tube over the bronchoscope prior to beginning the diagnostic examination. The examination is begun by carefully observing the superglottic airway for evidence of inflammation and mucosal damage. The bronchoscope is then passed down to the level of the vocal cord, again looking for swelling, soot, or mucosal damage. If airway compromise is anticipated, the nasotracheal tube can be inserted at this time. Further examination is made of the major airway including the right and left main stem bronchus. Ulceration, deposition of carbon particles, and mucosal erythema are all indicators of inhalation injury. This technique provides a high level of accuracy. False-negative results occur only in those few patients with isolated parenchymal injuries due to incomplete combustion of aldehydes and other plastic derivatives.

Xenon-133 lung scan[20] involves the intravenous injection of an insoluble gas in the peripheral vein and clearance by the lung site. Areas of injury show retained radioactive isotope over serial scans. Failure to clear the gas within 90 seconds post injection is considered indicative of an inhalation injury. This test is also accurate, although false-negative results can occur due to hyperventilation and preexisting bronchitis.

Pulmonary function testing has also been used to diagnose inhalation injury. However, this testing is often difficult to perform in the early postburn period. It requires a moderate level of expertise and its sensitivity has been questioned.

The treatment of inhalation injury follows a graduated protocol based on the intensity or severity of the disease process. The patient should be carefully observed for progressive hypoxia and upper airway occlusion. Development of either of these complications should result in the insertion of a nasotracheal tube. Initially, patients with mild disease should be started on warm, humidified, oxygen-rich air and should be placed on an incentive spirometer to assist in clearing increased and insipid secretions of the airway. Repeat bronchoscopy may be necessary to help remove airway plugs. Progressive hypoxemia requires the use of mechanical ventilation including positive end-expiratory pressure. The use of prophylactic steroids has been shown to be hazardous, since these patients are already at risk of increased infection from their burn injury. Prophylactic antibiotics also have been shown to be unhelpful and to result in superinfections with resistant organisms.

Pulmonary infections, especially pneumonia, are common sequelae of inhalation injury.[23] Patients with the diagnosis of inhalation injuries require serial daily chest x-rays during the early postburn period. If a pulmonary infiltrate is present, endobronchial cultures should be made and the appropriate systemic antibiotic given. A variety of organisms have been cultured from patients with pneumonia following inhalation injury, most commonly staphylococci, pseudomonae, and other gram-negative bacteria.

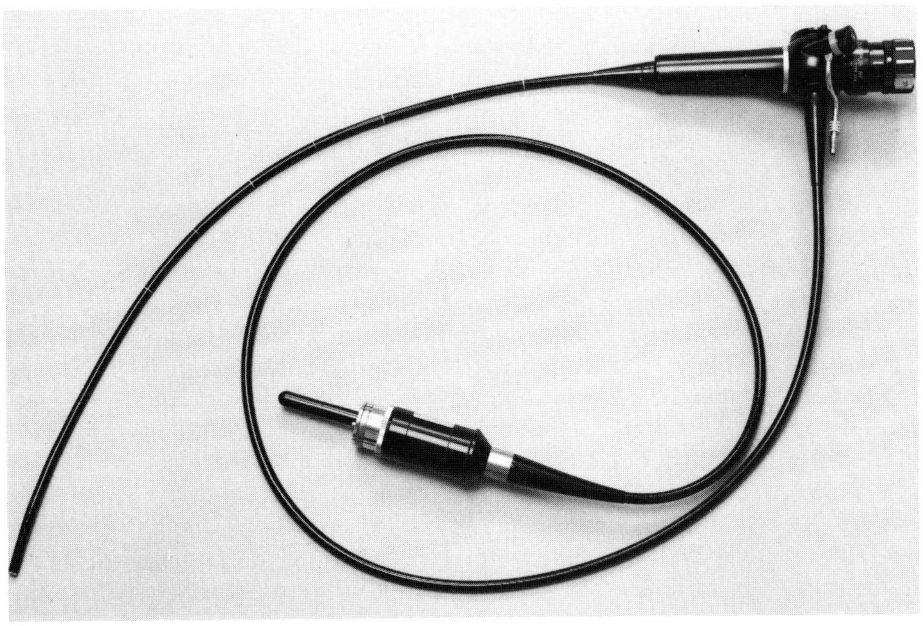

FIGURE 17.10 Flexible bronchoscope.

Careful regulation of fluid resuscitation in patients with inhalation injuries is important, because excessive hydration may result in increased pulmonary edema due to the altered capillary permeability. Patients requiring early intubation and mechanical ventilation because of extreme hypoxemia may benefit from central volume monitoring with a Swan-Ganz catheter to minimize excess fluid administration.

The presence of an inhalation injury markedly increases the mortality rate. While data are hard to acquire, it appears that it may cause a twofold increase. However, in patients with major burns mortality rates of more than 60% can be anticipated, and the effect of inhalation injury is obscure. Careful attention to treatment of inhalation injury and its complications will have a beneficial effect not only on the mortality rate, but also on the morbidity rate and length of hospitalization.

Care of the Burn Wound

After establishing ventilatory and hemodynamic stability, the key focus of burn care is the burn wound. Cleaning is accomplished by using a nonalcoholic surgical soap and gently debriding loose, nonviable tissue and shaving hair around the burned areas. Since this process may be painful, particularly in secondary burn areas, adequate intravenous analgesia should be provided prior to beginning the process. Two key principles in burn wound care should be kept in mind: antibacterial agents do not sterilize the burn wound, and mortality and morbidity are minimized by conversion of the burn wound from an open dirty wound to a closed healed wound as rapidly as possible. A combination of techniques have been employed to accomplish both these goals.

Topical and parenteral antibacterial agents do not sterilize the burn wound for a variety of factors. The burn tissue, which is rich in protein and moisture, secondary to edema and transeschar movement of fluid and serum, provides an excellent microbial culture medium. The avascular nature of the burn wound secondary to thrombosis of vessels limits the endogenous immune response as well as the penetration of a parenterally administered antibiotics. As granulation tissue develops and the eschar separates, exposed granulation tissue may become desiccated, resulting in secondary eschar formation. In addition to the local adverse circulatory phenomenon, a generalized condition (hypovolemia, resistant cardiac disease, and complications of septicemia) minimizes endogenous immune response and the delivery of systemically administered antibiotics.

Microbial factors also influence the burn wound interphase between the eschar and underlying viable tissue where the bacteria resides. These factors include the density of the bacteria, (i.e., the number of organisms per gram of tissue) and specific bacterial characteristics (i.e., the ability to produce both endotoxins and exotoxins, the presence of enzymes such as protease or elastase, and bacterial motility). Certain species of bacteria such as certain pseudomonae are more virulent and aggressive in converting a partial-thickness to a full-thickness injury as well as in invading otherwise healthy tissue. Wound microbial factors, combined with a depressed immune response mechanism, are responsible for the development of burn wound sepsis, that is, bacterial invasion of otherwise healthy or partially injured tissue, converting it to a full-thickness injury. As noted before, a variety of alterations occur in lymphocytic as well as opsonic proteins.[1] In the burned victim, T cell function is abnormal, but there is little evidence that it is related to bacterial infection. However, the development of fungal infections, particularly from *Candida,* may be influenced by this phenomenon. B-lymphocytes synthesize immunoglobins and antibodies in response to specific antigens following the burn injury. B-lymphocytes have an abnormal response to antigenic stimuli with depressed antibody function. Granulocytes and monocytes have abnormal ingestion of nonopsonized bacteria. The abnormality in the phagocytic function is directly related to the incidence and severity of burn wound invasion and septicemia. Opsonins are important substances that promote ingestion and intercellular killing by phagocytic cells within a few hours of burn injury. There is a progressive fall in a variety of opsonic proteins when malnutrition occurs in burn injury. These immunoproteins remain at low levels.

TOPICAL AGENTS

Since clinically effective topical antibiotic agents were first developed in the mid-1960s, three topical agents have emerged as the most common therapy for control of subeschar bacteria in burn wound sepsis: Sulfamylon cream, 0.5% silver nitrate soaks, and Silvadene burn cream (Fig. 17.11). Sulfamylon burn cream is a 10% suspension of mafenide acetate developed by Moncrief and associates, which is bacteriostatic, water soluble, and readily diffused through the eschar.[12] This water-base cream is applied twice a day usually without dressing and is removed for daily bathing and debridement of the wound, usually in a Hubbard tank, sometimes in the shower. This agent establishes an effective concentration at the interphase between eschar and viable tissue and has the broadest spectrum of activity against a variety of gram-negative organisms, especially pseudomonae. Its actual mechanism of action is unknown. It is locally nontoxic, is rapidly broken down in the blood to form an inactive form of the acid salt, and is excreted in the urine. While this agent has the broadest spectrum of coverage and is not inactivated by local substances, it has certain limitations related to its biochemical changes.[11] It is a carbonic anhydrase inhibitor, which results in bicarbonate excretion with secondary hyperventilation and carbon dioxide retention. In addition, application frequently results in surface pain of varying intensity. It has provoked allergic topical sensitivity in approximately 5% of patients.

Silvadene burn cream is a 1% suspension of silver sulfadiazine, which is a bacteriostatic agent.[6] Silvadene penetrates the eschar less effectively than Sulfamylon cream; however, it covers a broad spectrum of the usual burn bacteria. The agent is administered twice a day and is nontoxic. Besides its antibacterial effectiveness, its principal advantages are that it is pain-free, does not produce any respiratory or electrolyte abnormalities as Sulfamylon does, and has a low allergic topical sensitivity.[21]

The other agent commonly used is 0.5% silver nitrate solution.[10] This agent is applied in multilayered dressings. There is no pain associated with its application; however it may frequently adhere to the burn surface and can be painful upon removal. Because of the bulky nature of the dressing, this treatment limits joint motion. Since this agent does not penetrate the eschar, it is less effective as an antibacterial agent when applied late in the course of burn care. Other principal limitations include leaching of sodium, potassium, chloride, and calcium from the wound and the systemic absorption of the aqueous vehicle, which may result in alkalosis, mineral deficits, and water load. Silver ions are precipitated upon contact, causing proteinaceous material discoloration of the burn wound, the environment, and the skin of personnel in contact with the patient.

While many units use a single agent consistently, recent experience has shown that rotation of agents quarterly, semiannually, or annually may prevent the development of resistant organisms within a burn unit, as has occurred in the past with use of a single agent over several years. Silvadene cream and Sulfamylon still remain the two primary agents used in topical burn care, with 0.5% silver nitrate solution being used in those patients allergic to sulfa drugs.

INFECTIOUS COMPLICATIONS

The goal of burn wound care is removal of the eschar and rapid epithelialization of the partial-thickness injury, or the development of adequate beds for skin grafting when full-thickness injury is present. Daily wound observation and care are mandatory and must include inspection of the wound to note any changes indicating progression of infection at the interphase. A variety of approaches have been suggested to ensure safety of the process, to shorten the time to wound healing, and to improve cosmetic and functional results. These techniques include combinations of topical agents, use of biologic dressings, and early excision of the eschar followed by immediate autologous grafting or coverage with other types of biologic dressings. For the surgeon who treats an occasional major burn, the use of a single approach develops experience and confidence and assures optimal patient outcome.

Since infectious complications remain one of the most important factors affecting morbidity and mortality following burn injury, and the burn wound is a potential source of bacteria for these types of complications, daily inspection of the wound is mandatory until complete healing has taken place. Burn wound infection can occur at any time during the course of burn care. Although it is most common in the first 3 weeks, it must be carefully looked for during the entire healing period. Conversion of an area of partial-thickness burn to full-thickness necrosis and the presence of black or dark hemorrhagic discoloration are the most common findings indicative of burn wound sepsis. Other clinical signs that should alert the burn surgeon of changes in burn wound status are formation of "neoeschar," rapid eschar separation, bleeding into the subeschar fat, erythema and edema at the edge of the burn wound, and embolic hemorrhagic lesions in unburned tissue. In addition to bacterial wound sepsis, viral or fungal burn wound sepsis can also be present. The development of vesicular lesions on healed or healing second-degree burns is characteristic of viral infections.

Many have suggested serial, quantitative cultures of the burn wound surface to monitor burn wound status.[22] There is a general correlation between the results of one of these cultures and the presence of burn wound infection, but they are frequently difficult to perform from a microbiological point of view. Counts may be falsely low due to culturing an area with residual topical antibacterial agent on the wound or culturing the wound in an almost healed area. In addition, high counts may be caused by culturing pooled secretions or an area beneath the eschar at the time of separation. Both contact plates and swabs are time-consuming and expensive techniques.

The best technique for diagnosing burn wound invasion is the use of a lenticular-shaped, 500-mg biopsy that includes the eschar and the underlying, unburned tissue. This biopsy should be carried out when any of the clinical signs suggesting burn wound sepsis is present. One half of the specimen is sent for quantitative culture, the other half is examined under the microscope, where, by frozen section technique, the microorganisms can be seen to invade unburned, viable tissue. While this technique is not error free, it yields a high degree of accuracy in the early diagnosis of this major complication.

FIGURE 17.11
TOPICAL AGENTS

	BACTERIAL ACTIVITY	SIDE-EFFECTS	ADVANTAGES	DISADVANTAGES
Silvadene 1% silver sulfadiazine complex	Bacteriostatic, broad spectrum	Allergic reaction	Good antibacterial coverage No metabolic side-effects Pain-free	Sulfa hyperactivity
Mafenide 10% methylated sulfonamide cream	Bacteriostatic, broad spectrum	Painful Allergic reaction	Good antibacterial coverage Little bacterial resistance	Carbonic anhydrous inhibitor Sulfa hypersensitivity
Silver Nitrate 0.5% inorganic silver salt solution	Bacteriostatic, broad spectrum	Hypernatremia Hypochloremia	No allergic reaction Little bacterial resistance	Poor penetration Limits physical therapy Discolors environment

Burn wound sepsis treatment depends upon the location, extent, and depth of the invasive process. If Silvadene or silver nitrate soaks are being employed, changing to a topical Sulfamylon cream is indicated. Parenteral antibacterial therapy should be instituted based on the sensitivity of the microflora within the burn wound. At the time of instituting systemic therapy, new cultures of the burn wound and blood should be done so that systemic microbic therapy can be adjusted as new culture material becomes available. The infusion of an antibiotic solution such as carbenicillin directly into the infected tissue has been suggested. This process, called subeschar infusion, is particularly effective if the process is focal; it can be repeated every 12 hours beneath the eschar area using a long spinal needle to minimize the number of injection sites.

Excision of the area of burn wound sepsis should be performed if the burn extends into the subcutaneous tissue. Frequently in a wound extending over an extremity, amputation may be necessary, although every attempt should be made to control the process with localized excision, even if it involves fascia and muscle. An adequate level of parenteral antimicrobial agent should be administered both preoperatively and continuously during the excision to minimize hematogenous spread. Since widespread burn wound sepsis is associated with high mortality, every effort should be made to diagnose this complication early while it is still localized and can be treated with an adequate combination therapy as outlined above.

DEBRIDEMENT

Debridement of the wound is accomplished daily by sharp excision using scissors or scalpel as the eschar begins to separate. It is important that this process be carried out after separation begins, since exposure of fat or deeper tissues not covered by granulation will develop a neoeschar and will promote burn wound sepsis. Using topical antibacterial agents, separation usually begins around 12 to 21 days post burn, depending upon the type and density of the bacteria. In addition to sharp debridement, dressings can be used to debride the wound after large areas of eschar have been removed and only small residual necrotic debris is left. These dressings soaked in antimicrobial solutions can be applied several times each day to create a clean wound.

BIOLOGIC DRESSING

A variety of biologic dressings are now available to protect the underlying granulation tissue once nonviable tissue has separated.[26] The goal of biologic dressing is to allow granulation tissue to progress such that 100% of skin grafting or epithelialization of a deep second-degree wound is ensured, when the process may be slowed by desiccation, exposure, and evaporative water loss. A variety of biologic dressings are available, including cutaneous allograft and cutaneous xenograft. A variety of cutaneous allografts have been used, including viable allograft, in which the skin is harvested in the operating room using sterile technique from cadavers free of infection, viral diseases, cutaneous malignancies, and jaundice. This graft can be stored in the refrigerator for up to 2 weeks and facilitates wound healing by promoting the growth of granulation tissue, eliminating bacterial proliferation, and preventing desiccation of the wound by minimizing evaporative water loss and heat. In addition it decreases wound pain and thus makes physical therapy and joint movement more effective. This dressing can be left in place for 3 to 5 days depending upon the degree of separation beneath it. The allograft should be removed before it starts to adhere, since it may result in significant bleeding at the time of removal or even undergo rejection.

In addition to viable allograft, freeze-dried allograft skin is also available. Freeze-dried skin has an indefinite shelf life. However, it is in limited supply. It adheres less well to the wound than viable skin allograft, and is expensive to use.

Cutaneous xenograft is harvested primarily from pig and is commercially available. This agent is less effective than cutaneous allograft as a physiologic dressing. Since the xenograft is less effective in controlling bacterial proliferation, careful observation is mandatory because suppuration may develop when this agent is used early as eschar begins separation.

A variety of synthetic membranes have been attempted, but none are able to control suppuration when small segments of eschar remain on the wound. Alternatives to allograft or xenograft lack good drapability and conformity to the burn wound, and thus permit submembrane suppuration. Their use should be limited to those circumstances in which allograft or xenograft is not available and the wound base is almost totally free of nonviable tissue. Continued research in this area is directed toward the development of a bilaminated membrane with a collagen base, made of dermal and a tissue-cultured-derived sheets of autogenous epithelium.[7] While this membrane appears promising it is not yet available for general use.

Careful wound observation for the signs of systemic sepsis is particularly important after the application of biologic dressing. During the initial use of biologic dressing on any wound, especially the 24 hours following the first application, there may be extensive bacterial growth. The membrane should be removed at this time, the wound cleaned, and either a new biologic dressing applied or topical antimicrobial therapy reinstated. It is better to err on the side of the topical antibacterial agent, since destruction of granulation tissue at this point seriously sets back the goal of early wound coverage. As suppuration decreases and graft adherence increases, biologic dressings need not be changed as frequently. While some have suggested that allograft can be left in place up to 7 days, it is probably better to change it every 5 days to avoid the hazards of rejection or the need to excise the allograft at the time of skin grafting.

EXCISION

Excision of the burn wound, or surgical removal of the burn eschar, and immediate closure of the wound have been suggested to shorten the hospital stay, reduce the risk of burn wound invasion, and minimize metabolic demands. Proponents of this technique have suggested a variety of approaches including scalpel excision of extensive burn wounds to the level of the fascia, with either immediate skin grafting or the use of cutaneous allograft followed by delayed skin grafting. While this technique meets the principle of conversion of an open wound to a closed wound, it has been associated with extensive blood loss, limiting the amount of excision that can be carried out during a single procedure. Use of a tourniquet on the extremity has minimized blood loss but has created some other undesirable complications. The development of laser technology has minimized the blood loss but has increased the anesthetic time and made this an expensive procedure.

Others have suggested tangential excision, that is, stripping away of successive thin layers of burned tissue using a dermatome or guarded skin knife until nonviable tissue has been excised, as indicated by capillary bleeding from the entire bed. The resultant wound can have a xenograft of a biologic dressing or skin substitute, or can be immediately autografted if donor sites are available. The blood loss associated with tangential excision is less than with scalpel excision and is controlled by application of sponges soaked in topical agents to produce clotting. The advantage of tangential excision is that it can be repeated several times, since the metabolic insult is less than that of total and sharp excision. However, it does require a general anesthetic.

Current use of excision has evolved into a combination of scalpel excision and tangential excision. Scalpel excision to or below the fascial level is usually used in small full-thickness burns and for excision of the area of burn wound infection. Tangential excision is used in deep partial excision of burns covering less than 20% of the body surface. In larger burns it is used in procedures allowing serial coverage of full-thickness burns. Initial enthusiasm for both of these procedures has been moderated by randomized, controlled studies that have shown no significant difference in mortality rate or incidence of severe infection in patients with and without excision if their burn is in excess of 15% of the body surface. In another study of patients with burns of 20% to 40%, there was a smaller incidence of burn wound infection, but no reduction in the mortality rate. In full-thickness burns of less than 15% of the body surface, studies have indicated a shorter hospital stay for those who were treated by early excision with immediate skin grafting.

Burn Injury Complications

METABOLIC STRESS

Following a burn injury, metabolic stress is significant and results in increased hypermetabolism, producing increased oxygen consumption, elevated cardiac output, increased core temperature, and significant catabolism. The supermetabolic state appears to be secondary to an increase in catechol production and excretion, with a reciprocal relation between the thyroid hormone and catechol excretion such that the initial depression in the thyroid hormone is followed by a gradual return to normal as catechol levels decrease. There is a significant breakdown in muscle protein throughout the whole healing period until the wound is closed, resulting in major muscle breakdown using the gluconeogenetic pathway to produce energy.

Careful attention must be paid to nutritional support, since this hypermetabolic response continues until the wound is healed. Although pharmacologic agents such as beta blockers significantly decrease this response, a pharmacologic manipulation appears physiologically unwise and does not prevent complications.

A variety of nomograms have been proposed to estimate the amount of carbohydrate and protein required.[25] Estimates of protein replacement and caloric needs can be based on preburn weight and the size of the burn injury, as shown in Figures 17.12 and 17.13.

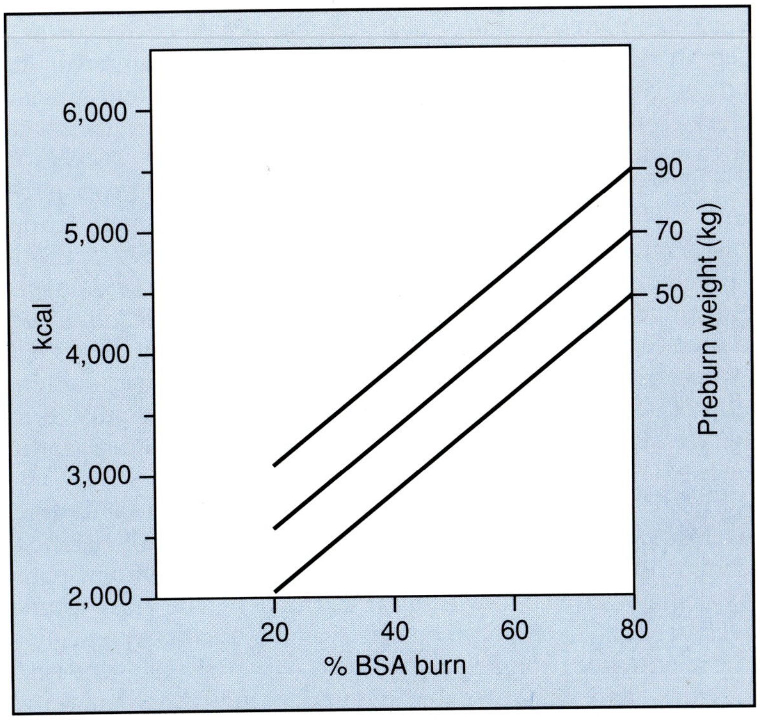

FIGURE 17.12 Daily caloric requirements based on weight of patient and magnitude of burn. BSA, body surface area.

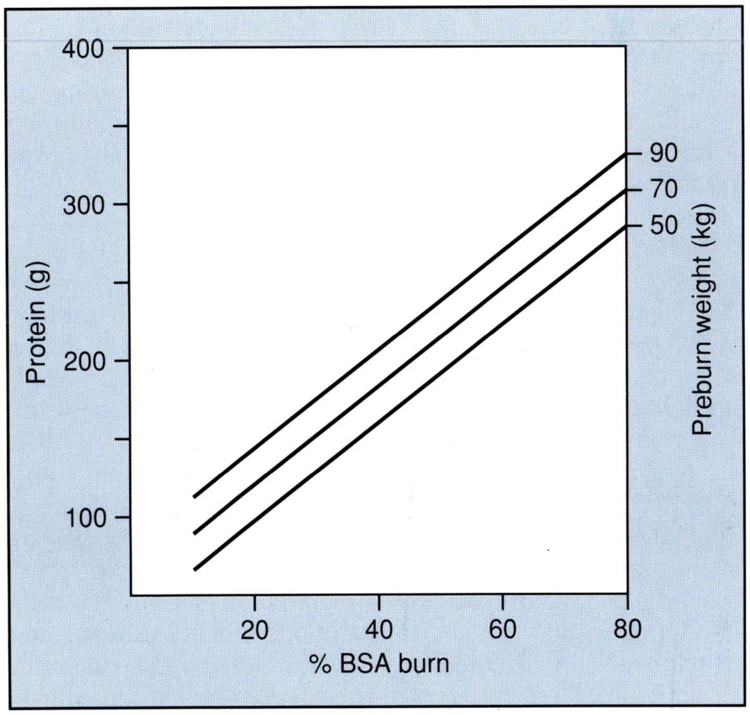

FIGURE 17.13 Daily protein requirement based on burn size and weight. BSA, body surface area.

A major challenge is providing adequate nutrition, and frequently a feeding tube must be used, since chronic pain and depression make it difficult for the patient to use ordinary dietary approaches. The goal of the nutritional program should be to prevent loss of 10% of the preburn weight. Infectious complications are very significant and can lead to death; every effort should be made to avoid the use of intravenous parenteral nutrition, since catheter-related sepsis is very high in patients with major burns. Diarrhea following tube feeding can be controlled with the use of oral antimotility agents such as paregoric. Since cold stress also affects the metabolic rate, every effort should be made to prevent chills and to keep the ambient temperature above 32°C.

GASTROINTESTINAL COMPLICATIONS

Gastrointestinal complications in the burn patient are similar to those of other patients with major trauma and include stress ulceration, acalculous cholecystitis, and bleeding. Gastric and duodenal ulceration can be prevented with the use of antacids and early feeding. While histamine-2 receptor antagonists decrease gastric acidity, they are found to be no more effective than early feeding and use of an antacid program.

SEPTIC COMPLICATIONS

The most common infection in burn patients other than involvement of the wound itself is pneumonia. Depressed immune response following the burn injury makes the burn patient a high risk for bronchial pneumonia, particularly in the presence of an inhalation injury that destroys the normal cilia. Most commonly, gram-negative bacteria are the cause of pneumonia in the burn patient. Since these are found on the burn surface itself, the pulmonary status of burn patients requires close monitoring, including daily chest x-rays during the early phase of burn care and careful daily physical assessment to note any evidence of increased pulmonary secretions, atelectasis, or other evidence of an infiltrate beginning. Rapid culturing and specific antimicrobial therapy is important, since broad-spectrum antibiotic coverage leads to the development of a resistant organism.

Hematogenous pneumonia is an unusual type of pneumonia found in the burn injury. This complication results from the hematogenous spread of microorganisms from distant septic foci, such as the burn wound itself and infected suppurative thrombophlebitis or gastrointestinal tract. This type of pneumonia is virulent and requires not only the treatment of pneumonia itself, but eradication of the primary source; otherwise, repeated bouts may occur.

SUPPURATIVE THROMBOPHLEBITIS

Thrombophlebitis is a complication resulting from direct infection of a vein secondary to the use of continuous intravenous supports, particularly during the early phase of care. The presence of induration over a vein and purulent drainage at the time of removal of a catheter are clinical evidence of suppurative thrombophlebitis. Frequently these symptoms are associated with gram-negative organisms, and hematogenous pneumonia may be the first indication of a distant site of such an infection. Unlike other infectious complications, thrombophlebitis usually fails to respond to systemic antibiotics alone and requires total excision of the involved vein segment.

BACTEREMIA AND SEPTICEMIA

Since direct invasion of the burn wound involves hematogenous seeding, bloodstream infection is a common phenomenon. This complication may occur particularly during the evolving phase of the burn wound when the eschar is separating and the burn wound is undergoing daily debridement.

Any signs of infection, including hypothermia, hyperthermia, tachycardia, or sepsis, should be regarded as suspect and identified by blood cultures. Septic shock demands immediate therapy, since mortality rates in immune-compromised patients are high. Therefore, initial broad-spectrum antibiotics should be given for both gram-negative and gram-positive organisms. However, availability of specific culture data should result in appropriate antibiotic regulation. It is not unusual for inappropriate use of antibiotics in a burn setting to result in resistant organisms. Therefore, prophylactic antibiotics should not be used in burn treatment except during the perioperative period when the patient is undergoing surgical debridement and skin grafting.

ELECTRICAL INJURY

Electrical injury presents a significant challenge in terms of diagnosis and management since the extent of underlying damage beneath the skin may not be apparent for up to 72 hours post accident. The type of circuit and voltage when electrical contact is made have a profound effect upon the resulting injury. Electrical accidents can result in immediate death, cardiopulmonary arrest, cerebral damage resulting in disruption of the cardiorespiratory center, or negligible damage other than painful sensation when contact with low amperage is encountered. An amperage above 15 milliamperes of alternating current flowing through the body when electrical contact is made is associated with significant damage.

The pathway of current through the body is also important. It may pass through vital organs such as the heart or brain resulting in immediate death. The longer the duration of contact with the electrical current, the greater the amount of damage. Resistance to the electrical current in tissue varies and may influence the course of the current through the body from point of entrance to exit. Resistance is greatest in bone, fat, and tendon and is less in skin and muscle; the least resistance is in nerve. Moisture at the point of contact and at exit also influences the amount of surface damage seen.

Electrical accidents produce three types of wound injury (Fig. 17.14).[9] Actual electrical injury caused by passage of electrical current to the skin characteristically produces an entrance and exit cutaneous wound with local destruction. The entry wound is charred and depressed. The exit wound is usually dry and gives the appearance of an actual explosion of the current at the time of exit. There may be extensive underlying tissue damage as indicated by immediate swelling. While the electrical path is not exactly known, it appears to travel along nerves and blood vessels, producing significant intimal destruction with progressive thrombosis. While a limb may initially appear viable following an electrical accident, thrombosis and spasm of arteries with progressive necrosis may result in ischemia and ultimate necrosis of an entire limb including the subcutaneous and muscular tissue. The second type of injury seen with electrical accident is the arc burn produced when the current temporarily courses external to the body across a joint. High-tension currents are commonly involved and produce severe, deep damage because the electrical arc temperatures are in excess of 2500°C. Arc injuries can also occur between the high-voltage line itself and the patient. The third type of injury is flame and is associated with ignition of clothing by electrical sparks or arcing. These burns are very similar to the usual thermal burns; however, full-thickness injury will frequently occur because of the prolonged exposure to the high temperatures.

Physiologic Effects

CARDIORESPIRATORY EFFECTS

Acute anoxia and ventricular fibrillation form a severe sequela resulting in immediate death. In addition, there can be significant myocardial damage similar to that produced by coronary artery disease. The current may also produce pulmonary parenchymal and pleural damage resulting in effusion and lobular contusion.

RENAL DAMAGE

Renal damage is secondary to both major muscle protein breakdown releasing myoglobin and hemolysis releasing hemoglobin. Initial severe shock may also contribute to the renal dysfunction, as in a crush injury. The goal of the initial fluid therapy, which will be described below, is to ensure adequate urine to prevent tubular cast formation.

NEUROMUSCULAR DAMAGE

Electrical injury to points near the brain results in significant cerebral dysfunction and respiratory center depression. Spinal cord injuries are more frequent than is generally recognized; they include spastic paresis and little or no sensory deficit. It is not unusual to find no neurologic deficit at the time of the accident and for signs and symptoms of spinal cord dysfunction to develop in a delayed manner. These are usually permanent. Electrical current can produce severe contraction of the muscles, resulting in fractures and dislocations.

FIGURE 17.14
ELECTRICAL INJURY

TYPES OF DAMAGE	CHARACTERISTICS
Direct Current Injury	Entrance and exit wounds Organs damaged dependent upon course through body and type of current and voltage Delayed necrosis due to ischemia
Arc Injury	Current temporarily courses external to body across a joint
Surface Thermal Injury	Ignition of clothing

GASTROINTESTINAL DAMAGE

The electrical current may also traverse the gastrointestinal tract, producing mucosal and submucosal injuries resulting in hemorrhagic necrosis of the small bowel or colon. Frequently, these symptoms may not be evident until after 48 hours postinjury. Careful assessment of the abdominal cavity is important over the first 3 to 4 days postinjury.

VASCULAR DAMAGE

As noted above, the electrical current may course along the intimal layer of the vessels, producing intimal disruption, thrombosis, or even hemorrhage. Delayed rupture of blood vessels has been reported, and careful monitoring of the adequacy of peripheral blood flow is imperative.

Treatment

The treatment of electrical burns is broken down into two phases, prehospital and hospital care. Since major cardiac and cerebral complications are related to continuous contact with the current source, the victim should be freed from the electrical current as soon as possible, while rescuers must take care to avoid being injured by the electrical source. The current could be switched off and the wire pushed away from the victim with a nonconductive instrument. Since cardiac and respiratory arrest are common sequelae, rapid assessment of the vital functions should be made and cardiopulmonary resuscitation (CPR) instituted immediately. Ventricular fibrillation is also a common sequelae and CPR maneuvers are begun with a chest thump if defibrillation is not immediately available.

If intravenous skills by an emergency medical technician are available, a large-bore needle should be inserted in a noninjured extremity and lactated Ringer's solution administered. Since large volumes of fluid may be required in the early resuscitation, contact with the responsible medical physician should be sought by radio so that the proper rate can be instituted based on the prehospital resuscitation protocols for electrical injuries.

The electrical accident results in significant fluid loss from the intravascular space into the damaged areas, as well as disruption of the muscle cells, causing release of myoglobin into the circulation. Large volumes of fluid may be required in the early phase of resuscitation, since major electrical accidents cause damage to the skin and subcutaneous tissue as well as muscle. Frequently, the external injury does not indicate the amount of underlying damage. This is particularly true of muscle, hollow viscus such as the gastrointestinal tract, or lung injuries. No true resuscitation formula exists for calculating the amount of fluid required by individuals with electrical burns. The key to monitoring resuscitation following electrical injury is urine output. The goal of therapy is to keep the urine output in excess of 100 ml an hour and to prevent acute renal failure. The initial appearance of the urine can give an indication of the amount of myoglobinuria as well as hemochromogens. If the urine appears a port-wine color or reddish black, it indicates significant muscle disruption and the need for osmotic diuretics in addition to isotonic resuscitation. Mannitol can be administered in a bolus dose with 25 g/dl in a continuous mannitol infusion. A diuretic may be necessary to augment urine output at the rate of 100 ml per hour or greater.

Severe acidosis is associated with myoglobin cast precipitation, and sodium bicarbonate administration should be considered. Systemic acidosis is frequently reversed by adequate fluid replacement; however, persistent aciduria is associated with a higher incidence of acute renal failure, and sodium bicarbonate should be used to ensure alkalinization of the urine. Careful attention to the urine *p*H to keep it in excess of 6 is valuable in preventing renal complications.

If a massive amount of dead muscle is apparent during the initial evaluation, consideration should be given to surgical amputation or excision of the dead tissue, which contributes significantly to myoglobin formation and renal failure.

Wound Management

The three types of electrical injuries require three different treatments. An electrical injury may result in minimal skin damage when the source of the current is of low voltage. Common sites include contact points of the hands, feet, and lips in children. These small areas of damage are best treated with topical antibacterial agents such as Silvadene and allowed to slough and heal. After conservative therapy, reconstruction may be necessary at a later date. However, if the low-voltage wound is in an area that is full thickness and total excision is technically and cosmetically possible, this may be accomplished in the early postburn period.

High-voltage contact produces a significant injury with underlying muscle damage. The physician needs to ascertain the underlying damage by making small incisions to directly visualize the muscle. When the injury involves an extremity, these incisions should be placed such that a fasciotomy can be performed if there is underlying significant muscle injury. In the presence of muscle damage, the patient should be taken to the operating room after being stabilized, where all dead skin, subcutaneous tissue, and dead muscle should be excised. It should be remembered that the electrical injury produces progressive vascular damage over 48 to 72 hours, and repeated inspection of the wound is necessary. Multiple debridements are often required and it is important to remember that what appears to be viable muscle immediately following an accident may undergo necrosis due to arterial thrombosis. These wounds should be kept open initially and dressed with an antibiotic-impregnated dressing, since sepsis with closed wounds is common.

Every effort should be made to preserve an extremity although amputation may be necessary to protect life. Small wounds of the hands and feet can be tolerated with nonexcisional therapy, but extensive injuries involving a distal or proximal extremity may require amputation. Repeat dressing changes and debridement require general anesthesia; they may be extremely painful.

When initial evaluation reveals no underlying muscle damage, management should include treatment of the entry and exit wounds with topical agents and debridement of loose devitalized tissue. Frequently these wounds, properly located, may be excised and closed with autogenous grafting after the first week.

Arc burns should be treated as full-thickness injuries and excised with either primary or delayed skin grafting when possible. Thermal burns secondary to a flash or explosion in an electrical accident should be treated as other thermal burns. Extensively burned areas should be treated with local topical agents such as silver sulfadiazine, debrided, and grafted as the granulating bed develops. Smaller full-thickness injuries can be excised and grafted to minimize the length of hospitalization.

CHEMICAL BURNS

Chemical burns are a common occurrence in industry, agriculture, research, and in the home. While the number of accidents occurring each year is not clearly defined, they are frequent enough that the trauma physician should be well acquainted with the specialized diagnostic, therapeutic, and prognostic considerations of chemical injuries. Many household, industrial, and laboratory products are capable of producing a chemical burn. The use of lye and acid in industry, home cleaning, manufacturing, and agricultural preparations is widespread. Phenols are used in sanitizers and disinfectants, and acids are components in common household cleaning preparations.

While most chemical accidents result in minimal tissue damage owing to the brief and limited exposure to the agent, chemical burns may result in significant morbidity, particularly those burns involving the face and eyes. Mortality rates for chemical burns (oxalic and hydrofluoric) have been reported for both massive skin exposure and the systemic effects of absorbed agents, such as hypocalcemia. Other effects include hepatic necrosis or nephrotoxicity following formic acid, picric acid, and phosphorus burn exposure. Creosol (Lysol) has produced methemoglobinemia and massive hemolysis, resulting in acute anemia and hemoglobinuria. Ingestion or inhalation of agents such as chromic acid or other strong acids like ammonia may result in a significant inhalation injury.

The pathophysiology of the tissue damage from a chemical agent is dependent upon the strength and concentration of the agent, the quantity of the agent, the duration of skin contact, the penetration into the tissue, and the mechanism of its action.[8] There are a variety of mechanisms in which a chemical agent produces damage, most importantly oxidation of tissue, protein denaturation, dessication of tissue, and increased capillary permeability with edema (Fig. 17.15). Oxydizing agents such as chromic acid and sodium hypochlorite (Clorox) produce extensive protein coagulation. Corrosives produce extensive protein denaturation. Some chemical agents denature protein by forming salts or by binding ions such as calcium which are necessary for cell viability. Other agents such as sulfuric acid and muriatic acid are desiccants that produce severe cellular dehydration and tissue disruption. Some agents cause massive blistering, which results in local tissue anoxia due to liberation of tissue amines.

Treatment

Initial evaluation of chemical burns may be misleading because these skin injuries frequently appear superficial at first, but result in full-thickness demarcation after 24 to 48 hours. It is not unusual to underestimate the extent and depth of injury; therefore, repeated evaluation is necessary, and hospitalization is occasionally required to ensure optimal outcome. The treatment of chemical burns consists of initial dilution, neutralization, and debridement of the wound. In addition, since some agents have systemic effects, the agent must be detoxified. The victim's garments are rapidly removed and massive amounts of water or physiologic saline are given intravenously, thus decreasing the concentration and the duration of contact and therefore minimizing the amount of skin damage. Multiple studies have shown that rapid irrigation with water is more effective in minimizing skin damage than delaying therapy while seeking a specific neutralizing agent. It must be emphasized that the amount of damage is related to the concentration and the duration of exposure to the chemical agent and therefore copious water irrigation should be started immediately. Specific agents can be provided as they become available.

Since fluoridine and hydrochloric acid penetrate the soft tissue rapidly and cause liquefaction and decalcification of the bone, subcutaneous injections of calcium gluconate following water dilution have been shown valuable in binding fluoride to prevent further damage and in decreasing pain.

Chemical Burn Complications

TRACHEOBRONCHIAL INJURY

Exposure to chemical gases such as ammonia may produce a significant inhalation injury, evidenced by tachypnea, hypoxia, and bronchospasm. Patients may require ventilatory support; a bronchoscopy should be performed to define the extent of injury. Delayed complications of chemical burns have been reported, so that a long-term follow-up with pulmonary function studies and radiographs is mandatory. While steroids may be contraindicated in thermal injury, in isolated chemical burns of the airway without skin damage, there may be some potential benefit.

EYE DAMAGE

Significant morbidity is associated with ocular burns.[4] Rapid emergency treatment consists of copious irrigation with water, preferably started at the time of the accident and continued during transport to a medical facility. Initial physical findings include blepharospasm, tearing, conjunctivitis, and uncontrolled rubbing of the eyes. Initial evaluation with a slit lamp reveals corneal swelling, potential clouding of the anterior chamber, and foreign bodies in the anterior chamber. Damage to the iris may occur despite massive continuing irrigation and may not be avoidable depending upon the characteristics of the chemical agent; a specific ophthalmologic consultation should be secured as soon as possible. Late sequelae of a chemical burn of the eye include ulceration and scarring of the cornea. Topical antibiotics should be provided to minimize corneal complications. Failure to control bacterial infection may result in corneal or scleral perforation. Frequently, conjunctival flap or grafting may be required. The sequelae of ocular burns include cataract formation or secondary glaucoma. Use of cycloplegics may be indicated if iritis occurs. Monitoring of the potential glaucoma with daily measurements of intraocular pressure is frequently required. Early referral for ophthalmologic evaluation and follow-up is indicated once initial emergency treatment is completed.

FIGURE 17.15
MECHANISMS OF CHEMICAL INJURY

Oxidation of tissue
Protein denaturation
Desiccation of tissue
Increased capillary permeability and edema

REFERENCES

1. Alexander JW: The body's response to infection. In Artz CP, Moncrief JA, Pruitt Jr BA (eds): Burns—A Team Approach, pp 107–119. Philadelphia, WB Saunders, 1979.
2. Alexander JW, Ogle CK, Stinnett JD, MacMillan BG: Sequential prospective analysis of immunologic abnormalities and infection following severe thermal injury. Ann Surg 188:809, 1978.
3. Asch MJ et al: Systemic and pulmonary hemodynamic changes accompanying thermal injury. Ann Surg 178:218, 1973.
4. Asch MJ, Moylan JA, Bruck HM, Pruitt BA Jr: Ocular complications associated with burns: Review of a five year experience including 104 patients. J Trauma 11:857–861, 1971.
5. Baxter CR: Crystalloid resuscitation of burn shock. In Stone H, Polk HA (eds): Contemporary Burn Management. Boston, Little, Brown & Co, 1971.
6. Baxter CR: Topical use of 1.0% silver sulfadiazine. In Polk HC, Stone HH (eds): Contemporary Burn Management. Boston, Little, Brown & Co, 1971.
7. Burke JF, Yannas IV, Quinby WC Jr et al: Successful use of a physiologically acceptable artificial skin in the treatment of extensive burn injury. Ann Surg, 194:413, 1981.
8. Curreri PW: Chemical burns. In Burns—A Team Approach, pp 363–369. Philadelphia, WB Saunders, 1979.
9. Hunt JL, Sato RM, Baxter CR: Acute electric burns. Current diagnostic and therapeutic approaches to management. Arch Surg 115:434, 1980.
10. Monafo WW: The management of burns: The silver nitrate method. Curr Probl Surg, Feb 1969, pp 53–56.

11. Moncrief JA: Topical antibacterial therapy of the burn wound. Clin Plast Surg 1:563, 1974.
12. Moncrief JA, Lindberg RB, Switzer WE, Pruitt BA Jr: Use of topical antibacterial therapy in the treatment of the burn wound. Arch Surg 92:558, 1966.
13. Moylan JA: First aid and transportation of burned patients. In Artz CP, Moncrief JA, Pruitt BA (eds): Burns—A Team Approach, p 151. Philadelphia, WB Saunders, 1979.
14. Moylan JA: Outpatient treatment of burns. Postgrad Med 73:235, 1983.
15. Moylan JA: Resuscitation and early management of the acutely burned child. In Serafin D, Georgiade N (eds): Pediatric Plastic Surgery, p 112. Philadelphia, WB Saunders, 1984.
16. Moylan JA, Birnbaum M, Adib K: Fiberoptic bronchoscopy following thermal injury. Surg Gynecol Obstet 140:541, 1975.
17. Moylan JA, Chan CK: Inhalation injury—an increasing problem. Ann Surg 188:34, 1978.
18. Moylan JA, Inge WW Jr, Pruitt BA Jr: Circulatory changes following circumferential extremity burns evaluated by the ultrasonic flowmeter: An analysis of 60 thermally injured limbs. J Trauma 11:763, 1971.
19. Moylan JA, Rickler JA, Mason AD: Resuscitation with hypertonic lactate saline in thermal injury. Am J Surg 125:580, 1973.
20. Moylan JA, Wilmore DW, Mounton DE, Pruitt BA Jr: Early diagnosis of inhalation injury using Xenon 133 lung scan. Ann Surg 176:477, 1972.
21. Ollstein R, Symonds FC, Crikelair GF, Belle L: Alternate case study of topical sulfamylon and silver sulfadiazine in burns. Plast Reconstr Surg 48:311, 1971.
22. Pruitt BA Jr: The burn wound. In Cameron JL (ed): Current Surgical Therapy, pp 513–524. Philadelphia, BC Decker, 1984.
23. Pruitt BA Jr, Erickson DR, Morris A: Progressive pulmonary insufficiency and other pulmonary complications of thermal injury. J Trauma, 15:369–379, 1975.
24. Pruitt BA Jr, Moylan JA: Current management of thermal burns. Adv Surg 6:237–288, 1972.
25. Schenk WG III, Moylan JA: Nutritional aspects of burn care. In Practical Approaches to Burn Management, p 42. Dearfield, IL, Flint Laboratories, 1977.
26. Shuck JM: Biologic dressings. In Artz CP, Moncrief JA, Pruitt BA Jr (eds): Burns—A Team Approach, pp 211–223. Philadelphia, WB Saunders, 1979.
27. Wilmore DW, Long JM, Mason AD Jr et al: Catecholamines: Mediator of the hypermetabolic response to thermal injury. Ann Surg 180:653, 1974.

hand trauma

William C. Pederson
Donald Serafin

1

2 6

3 7 11

4 8 12 16

5 9 13 17

10 14 18

15 19

20

The appropriate management of the traumatized hand follows many of the tenets of the basic approach to any trauma, yet there are certain points of evaluation and treatment that are specific for the hand.

PRIMARY EXAMINATION

Proper diagnosis of hand injury begins with a thorough examination of the injured hand based on an understanding of anatomic and functional relationships.

Patient History

As with any trauma patient, a knowledge of past medical history including allergies, immunizations (particularly tetanus), other systemic medical problems, current medications, and prior operations is important. Additional pertinent details are sought in patients with traumatic hand injuries.

The patient is questioned as to handedness and the state of hand function prior to injury. Patients with hand trauma will often have sustained prior injuries, and knowledge of these can bear on assessment of severity of injury and therapeutic approach. The patient's occupation should be considered in the selection of therapeutic alternatives as related to eventual hand function. The fact that the patient suffered injury on the job is relevant to treatment in the future and to eventual disability evaluations.

The position of the hand and what the patient was doing at the time of injury should be ascertained. Tendon injuries often occur with the fingers bent, necessitating a modified operative approach because of the increased distance between the ends of the severed tendons and the skin wound. Wounds occurring on the job can be contaminated with various tissue toxins, which demand proper management. Severe underlying injuries can occur in mill workers whose hands are caught in heated presses. All open injuries from farm or lawn machinery are considered contaminated and should be treated accordingly. Similarly, lacerations over the metacarpophalangeal joints of the fingers incurred in a fistfight are considered human bites and treated accordingly.

Certain diagnostic tests can add further to the initial assessment of hand injury.

PHYSICAL EVALUATION

The hand has many specialized structures related to its function and a thorough knowledge of its anatomy is essential to performing a proper physical examination. While a detailed review of hand anatomy is beyond the scope of this chapter, certain points of importance in the traumatized hand will be discussed. The reader is referred to monographs and texts on the subject for further study.[26,49,54]

It is important to use proper anatomic terminology in describing hand injuries. While some parts of the hand may be described adequately by several different terms, consistency is important. The hand is generally divided into palmar and dorsal areas (in the AP plane), and radial and ulnar areas (in the sagittal plane). The palm may be further divided into hypothenar (the ulnar aspect over the fifth metacarpal), thenar (the radical aspect overlying the thumb base), and mid-palmar areas. The digits may be further described in terms of their flexor and extensor surfaces.

The digits are properly designated as thumb, index, middle (or long), ring, and little. Numbering of the digits, although often used, is confusing and best avoided when describing traumatic injuries. The metacarpophalangeal (MCP) joints of the fingers are located at the level of the distal palmar crease. The joint between the first and second phalanges is the proximal interphalangeal (PIP) joint, and the joint between the second and third phalanges is the distal interphalangeal (DIP) joint. The thumb has an MCP joint and only two phalanges, with a single interphalangeal (IP) joint (Fig. 18.1).

The skin of the hand serves as a specialized covering to allow proper functioning of the underlying structures. The palmar skin (glabrous) is hairless and intimately attached to the underlying palmar fascia by many fibrous bands in order to allow tight grasping of objects. The dorsal skin lies very loosely over the dorsal fascia to allow motion of the joints and extensor tendons. The majority of the lymphatic drainage of the hand is in the loose dorsal areolar tissue and thus swelling in the hand is usually found dorsally. Abscess or inflammation in the palmar area may thus present as swelling on the dorsum due to these differences in skin coverage.

Examination of the skin of the injured hand may reveal functional abnormalities of proximal or underlying structures. Assessment of circulation in the digits is done by checking for adequate capillary refill. Interruption of sensory innervation to the digits results in cessation of sweating and this may facilitate diagnosis in patients unable to cooperate for a sensory examination.

The fingernail is a specialized skin appendage present on each digit. In patients with pigmented skin or with staining of the surrounding skin, the nail bed may be the only area available for examination of capillary refill. The presence of a subungual hematoma should alert the examiner to the possibility of nail bed laceration and distal phalanx fracture.

The hand is innervated by three major nerves: the median, the ulnar, and the radial. The median and ulnar nerves supply both motor and sensory functions while the radial is purely sensory. Sensory innervation of the tactile surfaces of the digits is through the ulnar and median nerves (Fig. 18.2). The median nerve supplies the thumb, the index and middle fingers, and the radial surface of the ring and the little fingers. While touch and pinprick afford a gross assessment of sensory function in the digits, proper evaluation of sensibility is done with two-point discrimination testing, using a paper clip bent so that the two ends are parallel and 5 mm to 10 mm apart. The patient is asked to discriminate between a one- and two-point light touch in the pulp skin of each digit, beginning with the clip ends 4 mm to 5 mm apart. If unable to do so, the ends of the clip are moved apart until two points are felt, and that distance is then recorded for each digit. Normal sensibility ranges from 4 mm to 6 mm in the pulp skin, increasing as one proceeds proximally in the hand. In the case of a totally severed nerve, the digit may be totally anesthetic to even a pinprick, and this data should be recorded as well.

The skin of the dorsum is innervated by the radial, median, and ulnar nerves (Fig. 18.2). The dorsal sensory branch of the ulnar nerve innervates the ulnar side of the dorsum (generally from the dorsal wrist crease to the ulnar aspect of the ring finger). The radial nerve innervates the remainder of the dorsum, except for an area from the tips of the index, middle and radial ring fingers to the mid-portion of the middle phalanges, which are innervated by the median nerve. Sensation to the dorsum is tested by examining for light touch and pinprick sensation. It is important to note that there can be variations in the above innervation patterns.

Motor function to the hand is supplied by extrinsic and intrinsic muscle groups. The extinsic muscles act to flex and extend the wrist, flex the fingers and thumb, and extend the MCP joints. The intrinsic muscles abduct and abduct the digits, extend the IP joints, and abduct and oppose the thumb.

Each finger is supplied with two extrinsic flexor tendons, the flexor digitorum profundus (FDP) and the flexor digitorum superficialis (FDS). These two muscle groups originate on the volar forearm and their tendons run through the carpal tunnel on their way to the fingers. The superficialis muscle is entirely median innervated, while the profundus muscle has median innervation to the radial two digits and ulnar innervation to the ulnar two digits. When passing through the carpal tunnel, the profundus tendons lie in series dorsal to the superficialis tendons. The superficialis tendons are layered with the tendons to the middle and ring fingers on top of the tendons to the index and little fingers. At the level of the metacarpal head to each digit, the two tendons enter a fibro-osseous canal called the tendon sheath. The FDS tendon lies superficial to the FDP tendon in the sheath until its decussation over the proximal phalanx. At this point the two slips of the FDS go around the FDP and

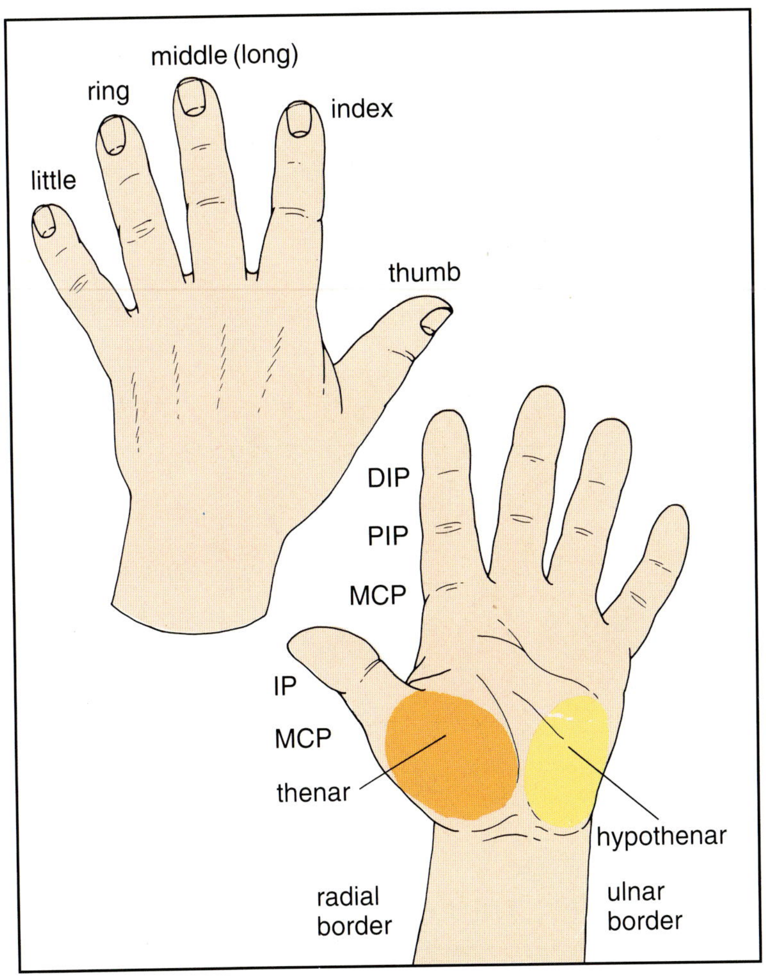

FIGURE 18.1 External hand anatomy.

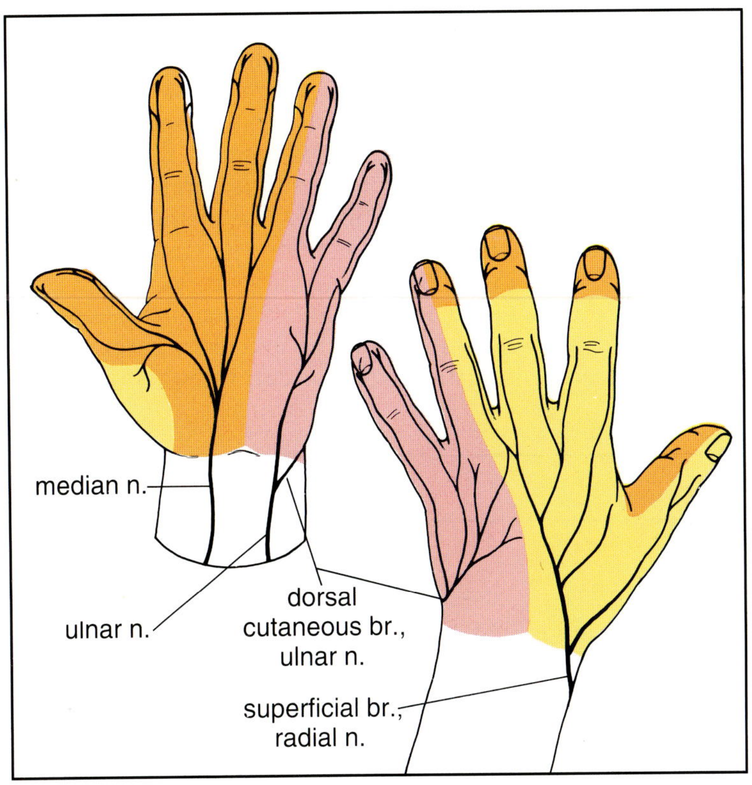

FIGURE 18.2 Sensory innervation of the hand.

insert behind it on the proximal portion of the middle phalanx (Fig. 18.3). The FDP proceeds to its insertion on the distal phalanx. Based on this anatomy, an intact FDS tendon will flex the MCP and PIP joints (with the other digits blocked in extension), and an intact FDP tendon will flex the DIP joint (with the other joints blocked in extension).

The flexor pollicis longus muscle is the single extrinsic flexor to the thumb and is median innervated. Its tendon runs radial to the finger flexors in the carpal tunnel out to the distal phalanx of the thumb. It acts to flex the IP joint of the thumb and, secondarily, the MCP joint of the thumb.

There are two extrinsic wrist flexors acting on opposite sides of the wrist. The flexor carpi ulnaris (FCU) is ulnarly innervated and inserts outside the carpal tunnel on the pisiform bone. The flexor carpi radialis (FCR) is median innervated and inserts on the volar second metacarpal. These two tendons are examined by having the patient flex the wrist. They may be palpated under the skin on their respective sides of the wrist and forearm. The palmaris longus is median innervated and inserts into the palmar fascia. It may be seen on examination lying just ulnar to the FCR tendon. However, it is entirely absent in 10% to 15% of people and thus may not be seen at all.

The extrinsic extensors originate in the dorsum of the forearm and are innervated entirely by the radial nerve. They pass over the dorsum of the wrist to the hand through a series of six tendon compartments. Tendons from the common extensor muscle serve each of the four fingers, with the thumb, index, and little fingers having their own separate additional extensors. The extrinsic finger extensors insert in the dorsal hood at the MCP joints and act to extend the digits at this level. Due to their dual extrinsic extensors, the index and little fingers may show no extension deficit if only one of their respective extensor tendons is injured. In addition, juncturae tendinum (tendinous bands) join adjacent tendons again, making diagnosis difficult even when a tendon has been completely severed. There are three wrist extensors, the extensors carpi radialis longus and brevis and the extensor carpi ulnaris. They are examined by having the patient extend the wrist and by palpating the tightened tendon under the skin.

The intrinsic muscles of the hand are innervated by the ulnar nerve, with the exception of the radial two lumbrical muscles, the opponens pollicis, the abductor pollicis, and the short flexor of the thumb, which are median innervated. The interosseous muscles and lumbricales act to extend the fingers at the IP joints, flex the MCP joints, and abduct and adduct the fingers to the central axis of the hand. The thenar muscles act to oppose, flex, abduct, and adduct the thumb. A good test of motor function for the ulnar nerve at the wrist is to feel for contraction of the first dorsal interosseous muscle in the first web space with index finger abduction.[45] The underlying bony structure of the hand is composed of the carpal bones and metacarpals (Fig. 18.4). The structural and functional interrelationships of the carpus are complex and knowledge of these is required for proper management of wrist trauma.[27] The carpometacarpal joints and metacarpal heads are stabilized by systems of ligaments. Diagnosis of instabilities in these structures is often based on radiologic examination.

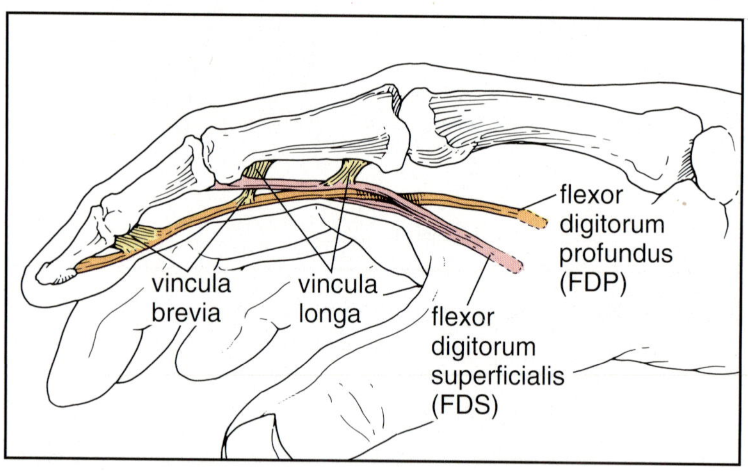

FIGURE 18.3 Anatomy of flexor system in the digit.

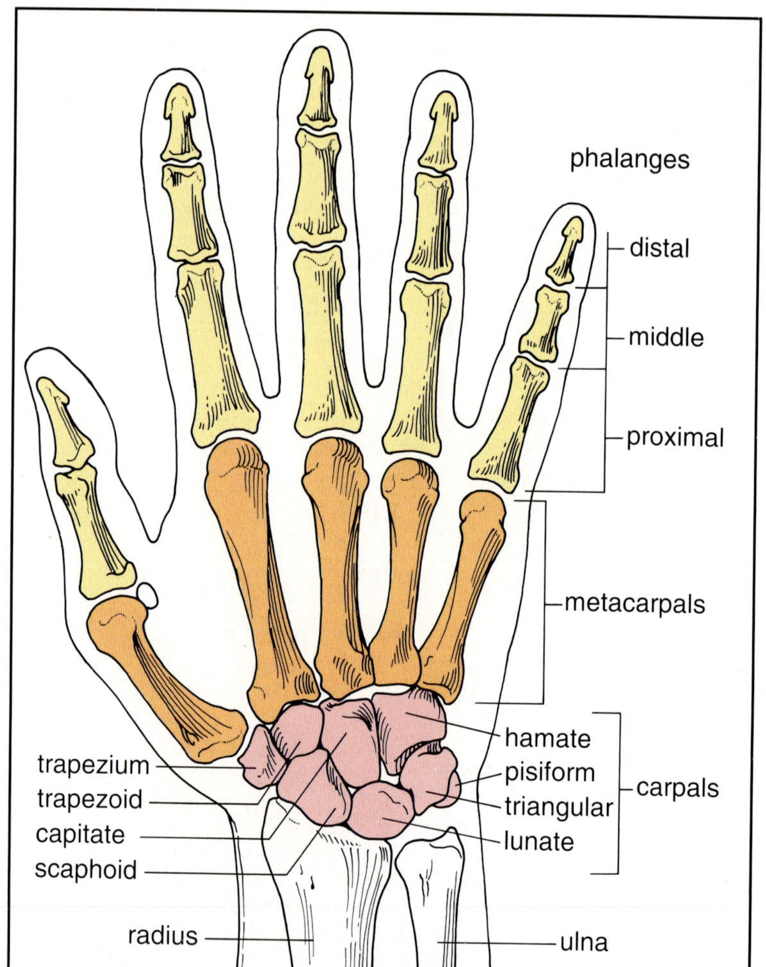

FIGURE 18.4 Bony anatomy of the hand.

RADIOLOGIC EVALUATION

X-ray examination of the injured hand plays an important role in diagnosis and planning of therapy. In most cases plain films in the standard views will suffice; however, certain specific studies may be required.

An adequate radiologic examination of the hand usually consists of plain films in the AP, lateral, and oblique views (Fig. 18.5). These should include the hand from the distal radius and ulna to the tips of the fingers. With any question of wrist injury, a forearm series should be included to evaluate the radius and ulna completely.

Closed injuries with areas of tenderness on palpation deserve close review of local radiologic findings to rule out fracture. This is particularly true in the patient with tenderness to palpation in the anatomist's snuff-box, which may be indicative of a scaphoid fracture. When no fracture is visible on routine series, a "scaphoid view" with the hand in an oblique position is obtained (Fig. 18.6, B). Sometimes a fracture is not apparent

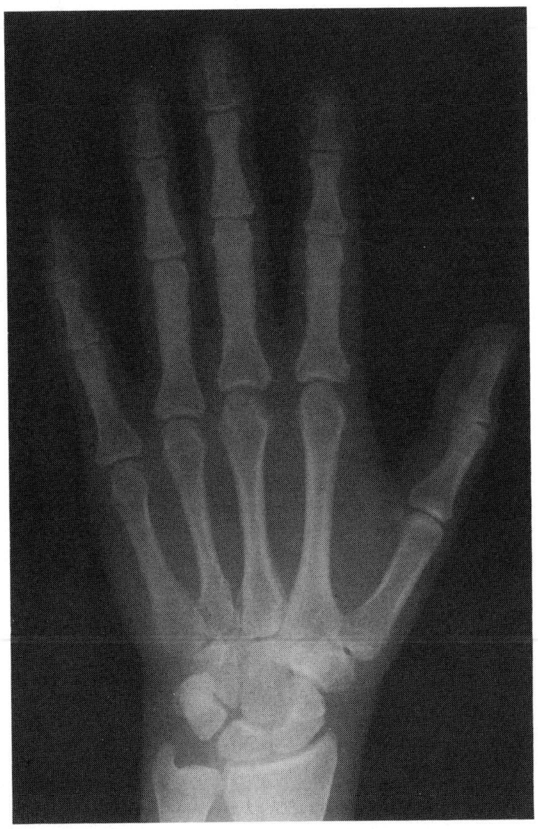

FIGURE 18.5 Normal AP hand x-ray.

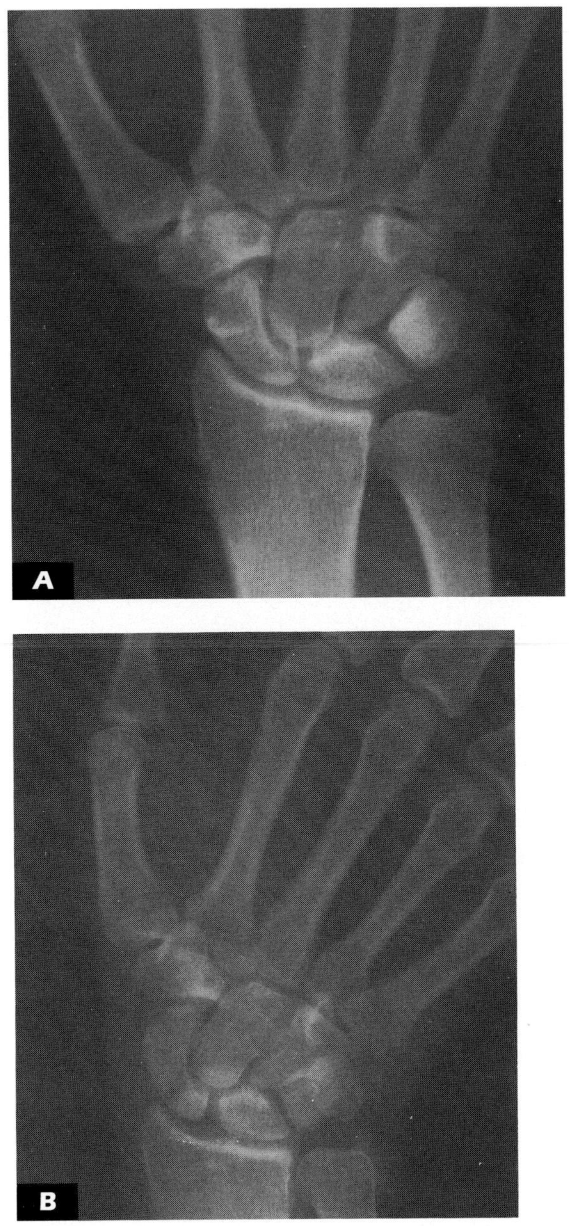

FIGURE 18.6 A Scaphoid fracture, routine AP wrist view. **B** "Scaphoid view," showing the fracture line of the scaphoid.

radiographically for two weeks. Patients with possible ligamentous injuries, particularly of the IP joint of the thumb, may require stress films of the involved joint to evaluate stability. The films often cannot be taken until a nerve block has been performed, however, to allow manipulation of the joint without undue pain.

Minor lacerations usually do not merit x-ray studies, except if incurred with power tools or with the possibility of injury from foreign bodies. Electrical or gas-driven tools can often cause bony injury which is unsuspected on external examination. These tools can cause deep deposition of foreign material such as metallic fragments, leaded paint (Fig. 18.7), and certain types of glass (coated or lead glass). X-rays will often reveal the location of embedded particles, but pinpointing them in three-dimensional space can be difficult; radiopaque markers on the skin at the entrance site may be required. Operative use of fluoroscopy or image intensification equipment may be required for particle removal.

Evaluation of the soft tissues on x-ray examination can reveal information about the extent of damage to these tissues and to underlying bony structures. Infections can lead to air in the soft tissues and tendon sheath. The tracks of puncture wounds can often be delineated by air bubbles as well. Particular attention should be paid to fat-plane swelling in the hand, which correlates well with underlying fractures, particularly in the thenar, scaphoid, and radial areas.[8]

In the case of strong clinical suspicion of fracture in the presence of normal plain films, polytomography may be necessary. This technique is particularly useful for carpal bone injuries. While useful for unusual wrist pathology, computed tomographic scanning is of little use in the acutely traumatized hand. And due to their lack of specificity, bone scans similarly are of little use in acute trauma.

Arteriography of the forearm and hand is generally not done in the acute setting. Open injuries are usually explored, the nature of vascular injury is ascertained, and repair is carried out

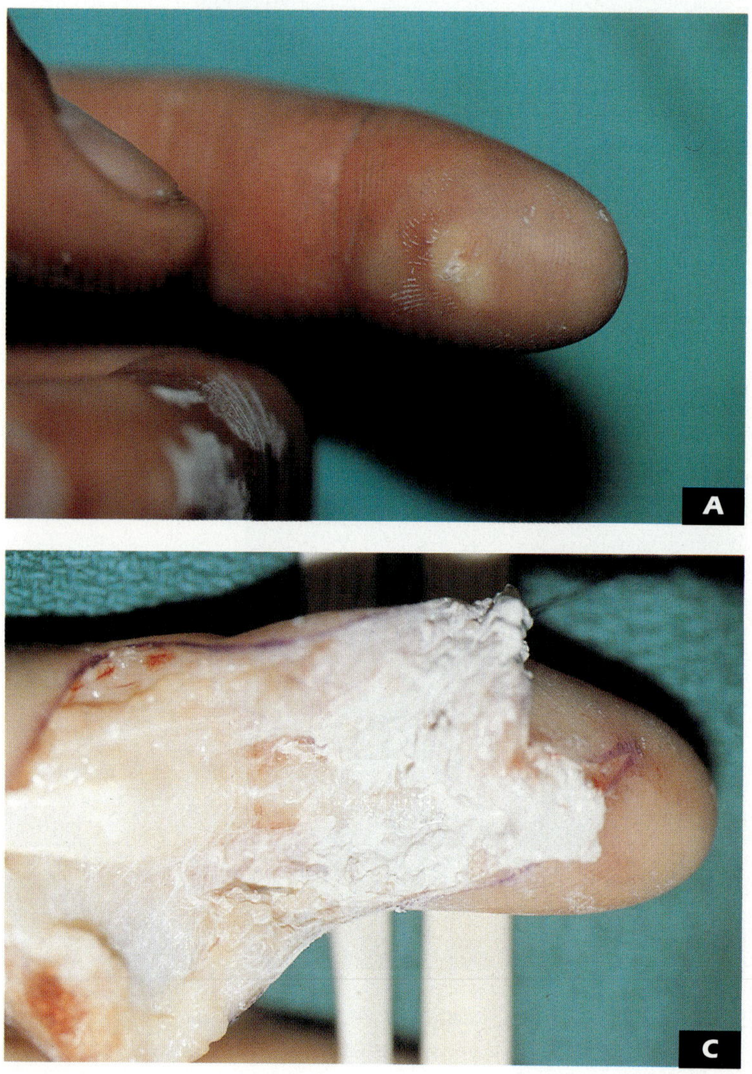

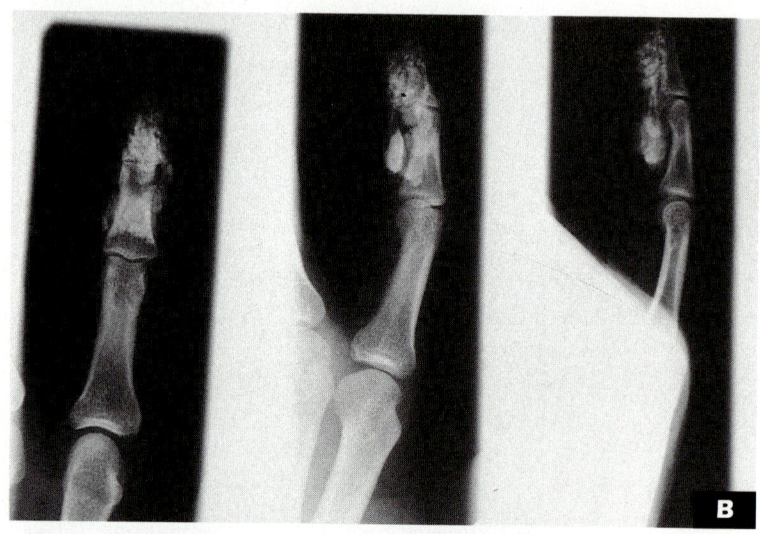

FIGURE 18.7 A Patient's finger after sustaining paint sprayer injury. Note minimal signs of paint injection. **B** X-ray of digit showing paint (lead-based) in distal digit. **C** View of finger at operative exploration.

at this time. Obvious exceptions occur in cases of a closed fracture with a question of vascular compromise or of suspected vascular anomalies. In any case, exploration of any hand with potential nonviability due to vascular injury should not be unreasonably delayed to obtain vascular radiography.

TREATMENT

While the aims of treatment of traumatic injuries in other parts of the body primarily stress wound healing, long-term results in injuries to the hand are assessed in terms of function. The hand is a sophisticated tool with which we make contact and manipulate our environment. Hand function has a direct bearing on employment for the majority of persons in our society, and the goal of treatment should be to return the injured hand to a functional state as rapidly as possible. Treatment decisions made early in the management of the injured hand have a direct bearing on the final result.

Most patients presenting with minor hand injuries can have treatment directed to the specific injury incurred. Those patients with more extensive injuries merit close examination of the entire involved extremity, including shoulder and possibly neck and thorax. Severe mutilating trauma to the hand can cause proximal injury to neural, vascular, and muscular structures and this possibility should be carefully explored on history and physical examination.

In the patient with multiple traumatic injuries including hand injury, priorities of treatment are important. The evaluation and treatment of a hand injury never takes precedence over other, potentially life-threatening injuries. Definitive repair of injured nerves and tendons may be done several days after injury in a clean wound with reasonable results. In the patient with ongoing systemic problems, the skin wound should be managed appropriately and repair of underlying structures carried out on a delayed basis. The hand should be splinted and elevated to obviate swelling and potential extension of underlying damage while awaiting definitive repair.

Minor closed soft tissue injuries and simple closed fractures may often be managed in the emergency room without compromising function. Small, obviously superficial injuries with negative physical findings may similarly be treated in the emergency room. Complex injuries or those with possible or suspected injury to deeper structures are properly managed only under the controlled conditions of the operating room. Attempts to treat these injuries should not be made with marginal anesthesia, improper lighting, poor instruments, or untrained help. Probing of wounds and attempts at exploration in the emergency room by untrained personnel are hazardous and often lead to improper treatment or injury to undamaged structures. After a brief examination of the surface wound and an inventory of hand function, a dry sterile dressing should be applied and the hand elevated. Simple prefabricated splints may be used to avoid further motion and trauma. Final examination and treatment is reserved for the operating room.

All hand injuries explored in the operating room should be managed with loupe magnification to aid in structure identification and with tourniquet control of bleeding. Most hand surgeons prefer magnification in the 23 to 4.53 range for routine work. The microscope is used for microsurgical repair of nerves and vessels.

Repair of digital injuries may be done with a digital tourniquet made from a Penrose drain or a rolled-up glove finger. If a 1/4-inch Penrose drain is used, the digit is first exsanguinated by wrapping it with a moist gauze sponge, and then the drain is carefully placed around the proximal digit. In order to avoid undue pressure on the digital nerves and vessels, two marks are made on the drain 2 cm apart and these two marks approximated with a small hemostat (Fig. 18.8). When using a glove finger, the tip is cut out and the rubber rolled proximally, effectively exsanguinating the finger and achieving hemostasis. Care must be taken to remember to remove the tourniquet after surgery to avoid necrosis of the digit. In forearm or wrist injuries, a standard arm tourniquet is used. The arm is exsanguinated with an Ace or Martin's bandage and the tourniquet is inflated to 75 to 100 mm Hg over systolic arterial pressure. This pressure may be maintained safely in the upper arm for up to two hours.[53] No exsanguination is used, however, in the presence of infection.

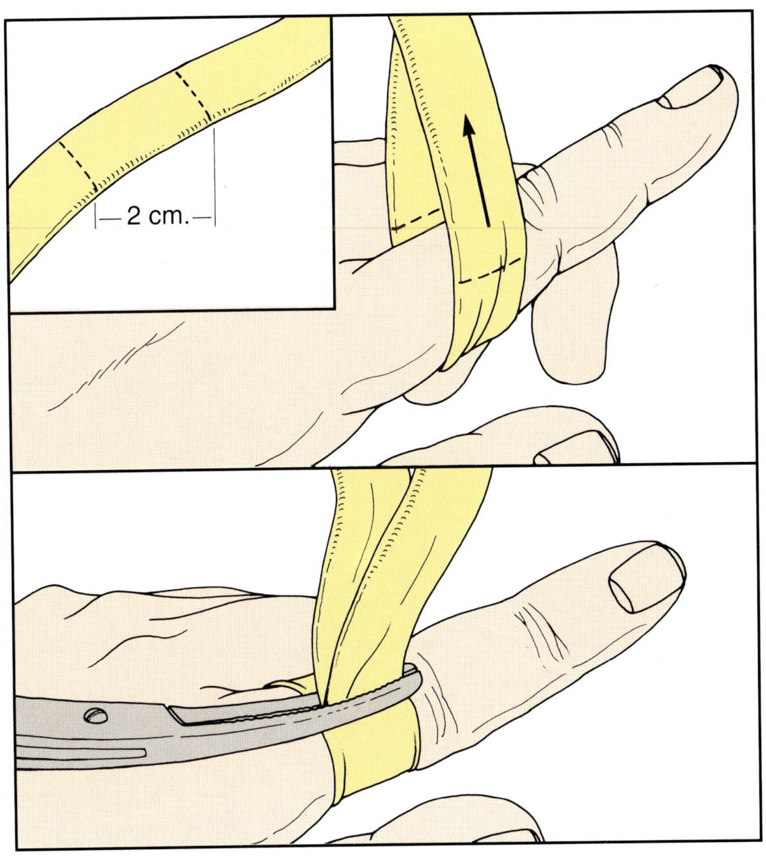

FIGURE 18.8 Digital tourniquet application.

Anesthesia

Nearly all injuries of the hand may be managed with local or regional anesthesia. Patients with complex injuries involving bone or flexor tendons should all have some type of block which affords forearm muscle relaxation (axillary or more proximal block).[20] If total relaxation is not required, an intravenous regional (Bier) block is often useful.[1] Children, patients with bilateral injury, and those requiring prolonged operative procedures should be given general anesthesia.

As a general rule, local infiltration anesthesia is reserved for superficial hand wounds on the dorsum. Lacerations in the palm and digits are difficult to anesthetize well without incurring a great deal of pain with infiltration and often a poor level of anesthesia will result. The subcutaneous skin of the palmar aspect of the hand has many fibrous septae, which impede diffusion of the anesthetic. Similarly there is little room for infiltration in the digits. These two areas should be treated with proximal nerve block with an appropriate local anesthetic.

Nerve block of the palm is accomplished by block of the median or ulnar nerve at the wrist level. The needle is inserted in the proximity of the nerve at the wrist level and anesthetic is injected. Care is taken to avoid injection into the nerve trunk, which can result in permanent damage. Paresthesiae in the distal distribution of the nerve caused by insertion of the needle are evidence that the needle is intraneural. The needle is withdrawn and repositioned until no paresthesiae are encountered. Only at this point is the anesthetic agent injected.

Digital nerve block is done by injection at the base of the involved digit in the vicinity of the digital nerves on the palmar surface (Fig. 18.9). It is important to use an agent without epinephrine, which can cause vasoconstriction of the digital vessels with subsequent necrosis of the distal digit. Complete anesthesia is obtained after dorsal infiltration to block the sensory branches of the radial nerve. Further descriptions of anesthetic techniques and agents may be found in texts on hand surgery and anesthesia.[40]

Closed Injuries

Closed injuries to the hand are usually the result of blunt trauma or abnormal stress placed on joints, ligaments, or tendons. Closed fractures are most often the result of a blow to the hand and may result in significant soft tissue injury. Dislocations and ligamentous damage arise from either a blow or momentary strain on the joints of the hand. This type of trauma can also cause avulsions of tendons with or without a portion of their bony insertions. An approach to the more common types of injuries will be discussed.

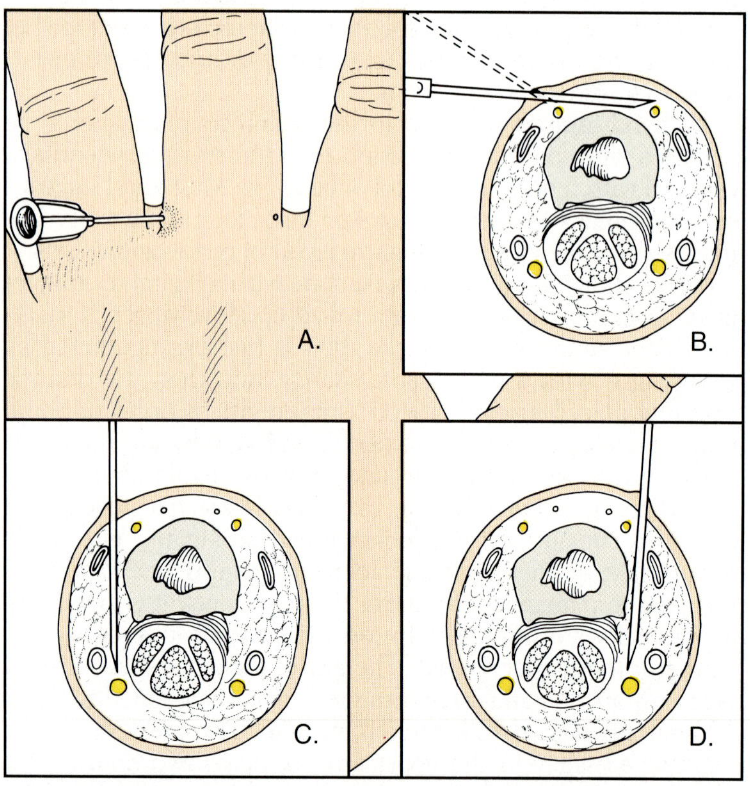

FIGURE 18.9 Digital block. **A** Dorsal insertion of the needle at the web space. **B** Dorsal infiltration of the radial sensory branches. **C** and **D** Injection surrounding the volar proper digital nerves.

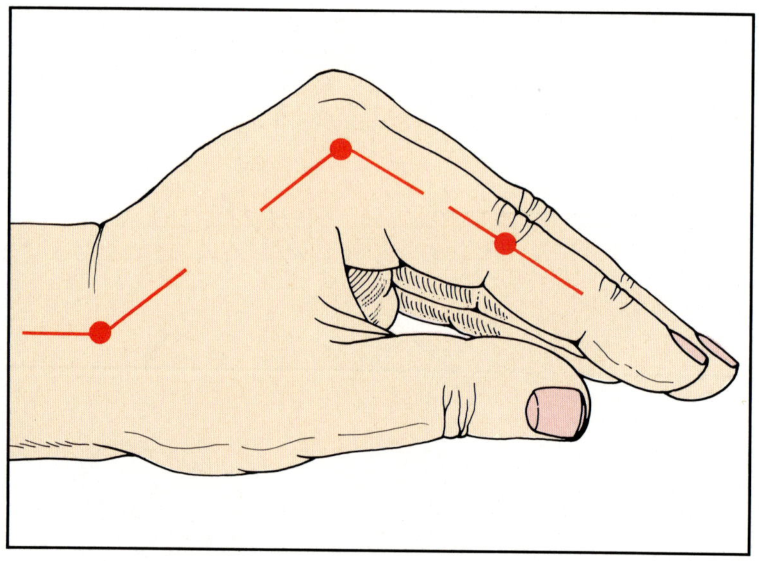

FIGURE 18.10 The "safe position."

Significant closed trauma to the hand will always result in tissue damage and swelling. One of the primary goals of treatment in hand trauma is to limit this swelling as much as possible. Swelling causes decreased motility in the hand by decreasing elasticity of the overlying skin and available space for motion of the digits. Marked swelling in the closed osseofascial compartments of the hand or forearm leads to a compartment syndrome which can have disastrous sequelae if left untreated.

The hand with closed trauma should first be elevated. This is important whether or not there is underlying fracture. The hand should also be splinted in the so-called "safe position," with the wrist in moderate extension (25° to 35°), the MCP joints flexed 90°, and the IP joints in extension, or 20° flexion (Fig. 18.10). Care is taken to avoid wrapping the splint so tight as to further compromise circulation.

COMPARTMENT SYNDROME

With increasing edema, resultant pressure in the closed spaces of the hand compromises circulation to muscles and nerves, leading to a compartment syndrome. The edema may be due to proximal vascular injury, closed fractures, snake bites, burns, or crush injuries. If the pressure is not relieved in an expeditious fashion, irreparable damage to these structures may occur, which can progress to frank necrosis. The long-term result is fibrosis of the involved structures, or Volkmann's contracture. The diagnosis of a compartment syndrome is made on a clinical basis, and thus, close and frequent examination of the involved part is necessary.

The hallmark of increased compartmental pressure is pain in the involved compartment which is not relieved by immobilization and elevation. Examination of the hand may reveal tense, painful swelling on the dorsum or over involved muscles of the forearm. Passive extension of involved muscles increases the pain while ischemia of the involved sensory nerves leads to decreased sensibility distally. A decrease in or loss of distal circulation is a late sign and may become evident only after irreversible damage has occurred to muscular and neural structures.

Direct measurement of compartmental pressures may be done with a catheter placed percutaneously in the involved osseofascial space and attached to a mercury or water manometer. Depending on the technique used in measurement, an intracompartmental pressure of greater than 30 to 45 mm Hg dictates the necessity of compartment release.[35,12] While direct measurements are useful for observing a patient with potential compartment syndrome, a high clinical index of suspicion is necessary to avoid tissue necrosis. Release of the involved compartment should not be delayed in the patient exhibiting classic signs in order to obtain pressure documentation.

Decompression of the interosseous compartment of the hand is accomplished with two incisions on the dorsum: one between the second and third metacarpal, and a second between the fourth and fifth metacarpal, thus avoiding tendon exposure when possible (Fig. 18.11, A). By these two skin incisions, the fascia over the four intrametacarpal spaces is released. Care is taken to avoid the overlying extensor tendons and sensory branches of the radial nerve. If necessary, the thenar and hypothenar compartments can be opened through mid-medial and mid-lateral incisions over these spaces. Digital fasciotomies are performed in the midaxial-lateral position of the nondominant side of the finger (Fig. 18.11, B). The fascia of the volar forearm is released with a curvilinear incision running from the base of the thenar eminence in the palm to the antecubital fossa. After release, the skin edges are left apart and a moist dressing applied over the exposed muscles. The hand is splinted and elevated, with wound closure accomplished by skin approximation or skin grafting in five to ten days.

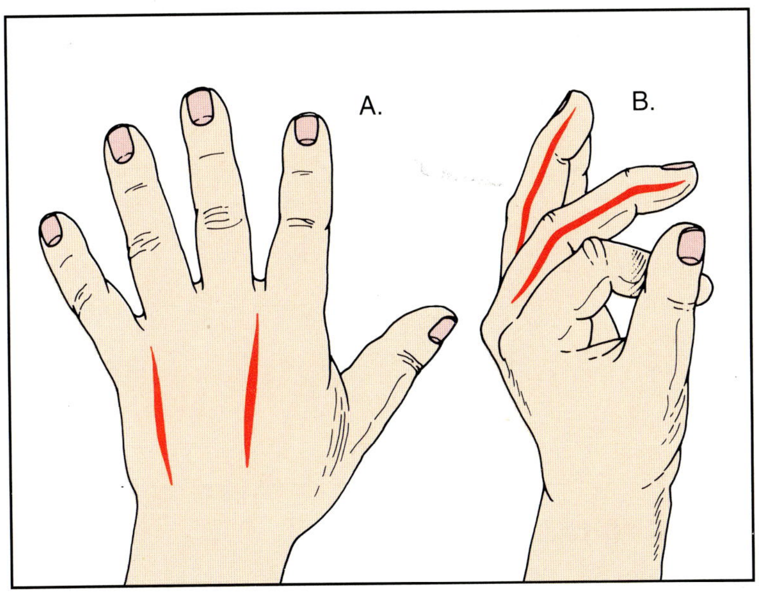

FIGURE 18.11 A Incisions for hand fasciotomies. **B** Incisions for digital fasciotomies or escharotomies.

FRACTURES

Closed fractures of the hand result in external deformities from swelling and angulation at the fracture site, due to both the mechanism of injury and the forces on the bone by surrounding musculotendinous units. The primary goals of treatment in hand fractures are stable and accurate reduction with early motion. Although many fractures will heal well with little or no treatment, improper treatment can result in significant functional impairment. An important step in management is recognition of those hand fractures requiring specific treatment and referring them to a specialist.[3]

Simple nondisplaced fractures of the phalanges can be treated with "buddy taping" and early motion. Those fractures of the shaft with displacement may be treated with closed reduction and splinting with an aluminum splint outrigger on a forearm cast. The MCP and IP joints are placed in moderate flexion and the digit taped to the splint. If postreduction x-rays reveal nonanatomic positioning of fragments or angulation, percutaneous pinning or open reduction should be considered.[17] Oblique fractures or those involving joint surfaces should all be treated with some form of internal fixation.

The majority of metacarpal fractures are satisfactorily managed with closed reduction and plaster splinting. After closed reduction of the fracture, the hand is placed in an ulnar or radial gutter splint with the adjacent metacarpal included and the MCP joint in 60° of flexion. For proper reduction, this parameter must be followed closely; any rotation after reduction is unacceptable. With the metacarpal in proper alignment, the flexed digits should all converge towards the scaphoid in the palm (Fig. 8.12). Open reduction is reserved for oblique fractures, those with unstable rotatory forces, and multiple displaced fractures.[37] The fractured hand is left immobilized for approximately four weeks, at which time the splint is removed and a program of progressive motion is begun. X-ray evidence of healing may be more prolonged than clinical healing and thus the patient with a stable and nontender fracture site should be considered to have bony union.

A direct blow to the metacarpal head results in a transverse impacted fracture of the head. When this occurs in the fourth and fifth metacarpals it is known as a *boxer's fracture* (Fig. 18.13). These fractures are usually adequately treated with closed reduction and immobilization for three to five weeks in an ulnar gutter splint.

Closed injuries to the carpus are usually the result of extraordinary stresses placed on the wrist. Fractures and dislocations with resulting ligamentous instability may occur in concert, and for this reason most carpal fractures should be managed by a competent orthopedist or hand specialist.

The most common fracture of the wrist is of the scaphoid and results from a sudden stress on the dorsiflexed wrist. Any patient presenting with a history of such an injury and tenderness to palpation in the anatomist's snuff-box should be considered to have a scaphoid fracture until it is ruled out with certainty. X-ray studies of the wrist including a scaphoid view should be taken (see Fig. 18.6). Lateral films may reveal instability patterns associated with scaphoid fractures.[27] The symptomatic patient without radiographic evidence of fracture should be treated with appropriate immobilization and follow-up films in two to three weeks. These later studies will outline fractures more readily due to bone resorption at the fracture line. Nondisplaced scaphoid fractures should be immobilized in a short arm–thumb spica cast with the wrist in flexion and radial deviation and the thumb in abduction for six to 12 weeks. Adequate initial treatment of these fractures should result in union in 90% to 95% of cases. Those fractures with displacement, wrist instability, or evidence of nonunion after appropriate immobilization will require open treatment by a trained specialist.[7]

TENDINOUS INJURIES

The two most common closed injuries to tendons involve avulsion of the end of the flexor or extensor tendon from its insertion on the distal phalanx. The extensor tendon is avulsed when a blow is delivered to the extended digit. The resulting deformity is called a *mallet finger* due to loss of extension of the DIP joint. Tendon avulsion may or may not be associated with avulsion of a small portion of the dorsal distal phalanx (Fig. 18.14). Acute injuries without bony involvement or small dorsal chips (less than 30% of the articular surface) are treated with mild hyperextension with a dorsal or volar splint. The patient is instructed to avoid any flexion of the joint for a period of four to six weeks and splinting should be continued for at least six to eight weeks total. The PIP joint is left free for motion during this period. With large bony fragments or an unsuccessful closed treatment, open reduction with K-pin or wire fixation of the tendon and fragment is required. Avulsion of the FDP tendon from the distal phalanx occurs with forced hyperextension of the digit or strong force applied to the flexed DIP joint, such as that exerted by a football player when grabbing an opponent's jersey. The patient presents with volar pain and swelling with no active flexion of the DIP joint. There may be an avulsed bone fragment, occasionally quite proximal, in the tendon sheath. Treatment is by open reinsertion of the tendon or bone fragment into the distal phalanx with routine postoperative treatment for flexor tendon injury. Both of these injuries are common in athletes and awareness of their occurrence aids in diagnosis and proper treatment.[43]

LIGAMENTOUS INJURIES

Closed ligamentous injuries in the hand without concomitant bony injury most often occur with dislocation of the interphalangeal joints, most commonly the PIP joint. If the joint is easily reducible and is stable to active and passive motion post reduction, immobilization is required for only two to three weeks. Active motion is begun at this point with the involved digit buddy-taped to an adjacent finger. The patient should be advised that swelling may persist for many months. Open repair is advo-

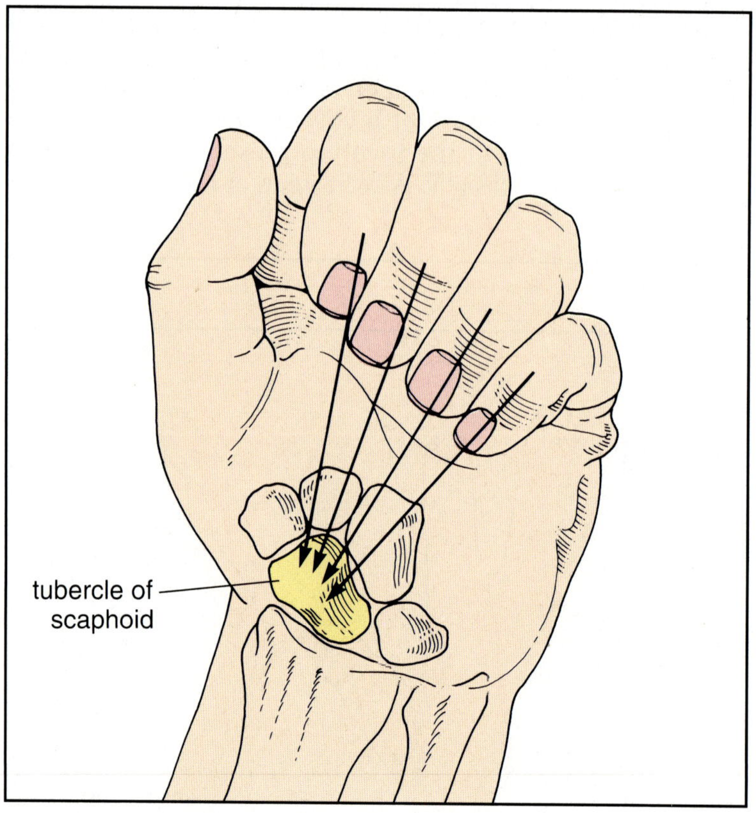

FIGURE 18.12 Tubercle of scaphoid.

cated for instability from the volar plate or a collateral ligament tear, which may be presumed when a large fracture fragment of the distal volar proximal phalanx is apparent on x-ray.[59]

Another common ligamentous injury is that to the ulnar collateral ligaments of the MCP joint of the thumb. This is common in skiers and baseball players and is known as a *gamekeeper's thumb*. About one third of these injuries will have an associated bony avulsion. Full evaluation of instability may require local block anesthesia and subsequent x-ray films with appropriate stress on the joint. Patients with no gross instability can be treated in a thumb spica cast for four to six weeks. Those with instability on initial evaluation, bony fragments, or ongoing complaints after closed treatment should have operative repair of the involved ligament.[46]

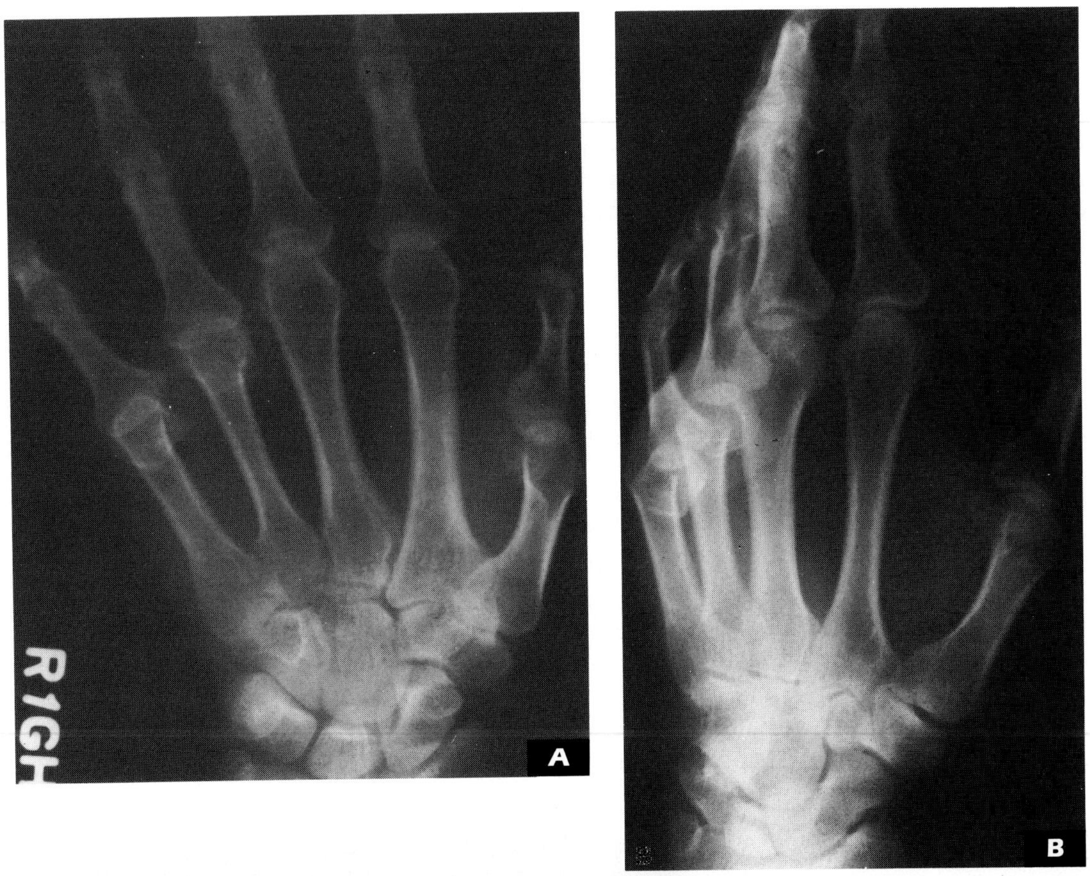

FIGURE 18.13 Boxer's fracture. **A** AP view shows the fracture at the heads of the 4th and 5th metacarpals. **B** Lateral view.

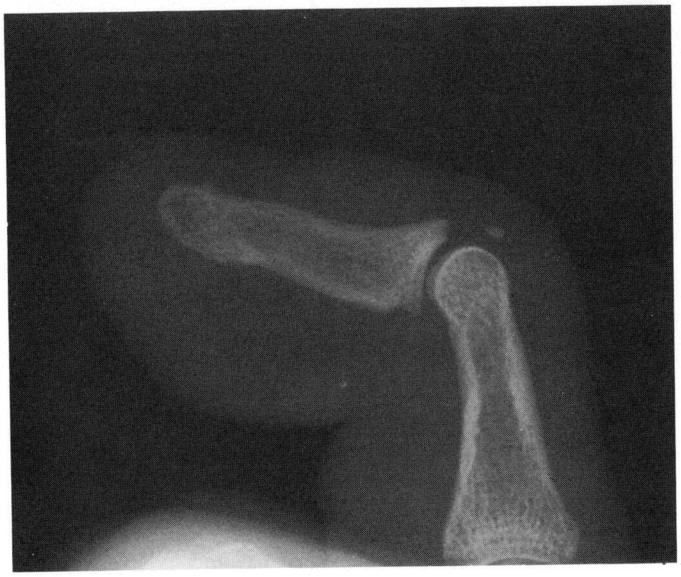

FIGURE 18.14 Traumatic closed mallet finger with a dorsal chip avulsion.

In some cases, the avulsed ulnar collateral ligament can become trapped behind the adductor aponeurosis (Fig. 18.15). This can only occur with a complete avulsion of the ligament such that the phalangeal attachment lies outside the adductor aponeurosis. In this situation, the ligament cannot properly heal to its normal insertion to the base of the proximal phalanx, and thus must be operatively repaired. This situation is known as a Stener Lesion 50.

Open Injuries

MINOR LACERATIONS

A great majority of patients with hand injuries will present with minor lacerations. In the patient with an unremarkable physical examination (no evidence of significant vascular, neurologic or tendinous injury), skin lacerations may be closed in the emergency room without untoward sequelae. Any patient with potential injury to deeper structures should be taken to the operating room for exploration.

An adequate level of anesthesia is obtained with either local infiltration or block as outlined earlier. The skin and wound edges are prepared with a surgical disinfectant (povidone-iodine solution or another agent, but not soap); deeper wound cleansing is deferred until exploration. Irrigation with a balanced saline or antibiotic solution may also be done at this time. While soaking of hand wounds is often performed in the emergency room, it is contraindicated because it does little to disinfect the skin and leads to maceration of skin and wound edges. Sterile drapes are applied and the wound is explored. Even with a normal physical examination, injury to underlying tendons, nerves, or vascular structures is occasionally discovered upon emergency room exploration. When this is the case, a sterile dressing is placed over the wound and the patient is taken to the operating room for final exploration and repair.

Assuming that inspection in the emergency room reveals only superficial injury, the wound edges are debrided of only that tissue that is obviously contaminated or nonviable. Careful closure is then accomplished with a suitable synthetic suture (monofilament nylon or polypropylene). Dermal or subcutaneous sutures are not done to avoid future suture abscesses or extrusion. Depending on the nature of injury, the hand is splinted and a sterile dressing is applied. Skin sutures are removed in two weeks on nonstressed surfaces and in three weeks on areas exposed to stresses of joint motion. While somewhat controversial, postinjury antibiotics are often useful to avoid infection in potentially contaminated injuries.

One area of injury commonly seen in the emergency room involves the fingertip and nail bed. Crush injuries to the fingertip often result in a subungual hematoma. Simple release of the hematoma through a hole made in the nail will diminish the pain, but may leave untreated significant injury to the underlying nail bed, leading to problems of nail growth and adherence.[24,60] In the case of all fingertip crush injuries with any more than a minimal subungual hematoma, the nail should be carefully removed and the nail bed repaired with interrupted 6-0 plain gut suture and loupe magnification. After repair of the nail bed, the cleansed nail should be replaced underneath the cuticle to prevent adherence of the cuticle to the bed. If the nail has been lost or damaged, a piece of nonadherent gauze is placed under the cuticle. Fractures of the tuft of the distal phalanx should be splinted for two to three weeks, allowing motion of the interphalangeal joints.

While most contaminated hand wounds can be safely closed without difficulty, some wounds are better treated openly. When appropriate, primary closure and healing are preferred to avoid

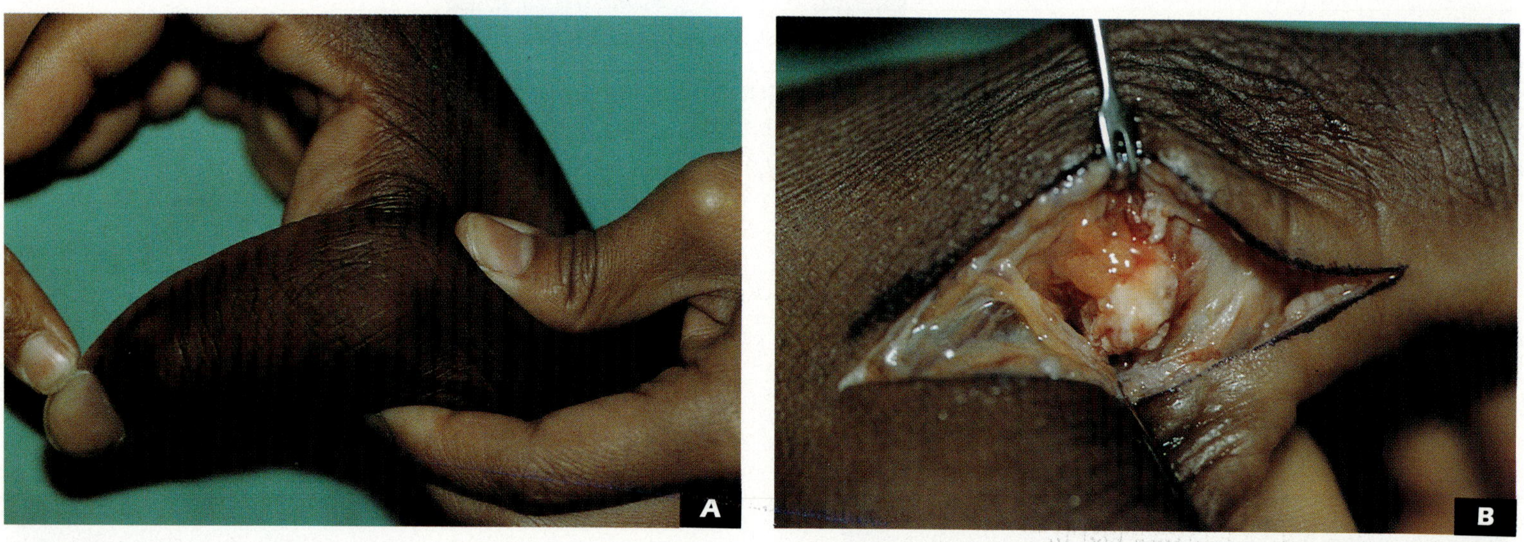

FIGURE 18.15 A Preoperative view of patient with acute disruption of the ulnar collateral ligament to the thumb. Note laxity under stress. **B** Intraoperative view of avulsed ulnar collateral ligament with Stener lesion. Note proximal end of ligament in a position outside of adductor aponeurosis, arrow pointing to ulnar collateral ligament.

prolonged pain, although they result in decreased motion and eventual function. Any bite wound, particularly of human origin, should be left open. Similarly, wounds incurred on the blades of lawn mowers or garden equipment are extremely prone to infection and should not be closed primarily unless debridement and cleansing is meticulous. These lacerations may be safely closed with skin tapes in three to five days if there is no evidence of soft tissue infection. Markedly contaminated wounds require thorough cleansing and debridement, which should only be carried out in the operating room.

SOFT TISSUE LOSS

In the case of significant soft tissue loss to the hand, coverage must be obtained. The type of coverage required depends on what is lost and what underlying structures are exposed. With simple skin loss, skin grafting with either split-thickness or full-thickness grafts will often suffice. On the other hand, if underlying tendons or neurovascular structures are exposed, they may require flap coverage. Injuries and infections on the dorsum of the hand frequently result in exposed extensor tendons, denuded of their peritenon, which will reject skin graft. Even if skin grafting is successful, these tendons are not likely to glide well underneath a skin graft.

The choice of flap coverage is dependent on the surgeon's particular experience and expertise, however several options exist. The pedicled groin flap offers an excellent option for hand coverage in most patients (Fig. 18.16). It can be designed to afford coverage of the entire surface of either the palm or dorsum of the hand. It does require keeping the patient's hand in a dependent position for about three weeks prior to pedicled division, which may not be desirable in older patients or those with other injuries. It may not be a good choice in patients with severe hand injuries, as it hinders early motion and the required positioning may compromise vascular flow, but it is probably the flap of choice for smaller dorsal tissue losses, particularly if the surgeon is unfamiliar with other techniques.

Another option for soft tissue coverage of the hand is the radial forearm flap. This flap may be based on a distal vascular pedi-

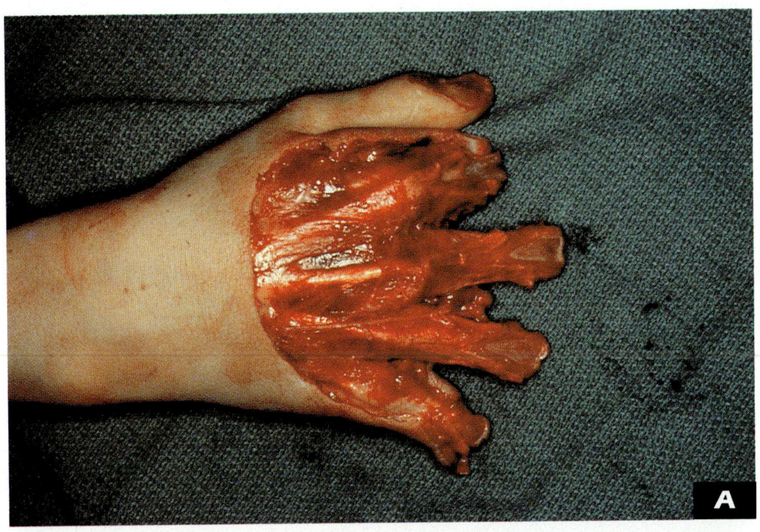

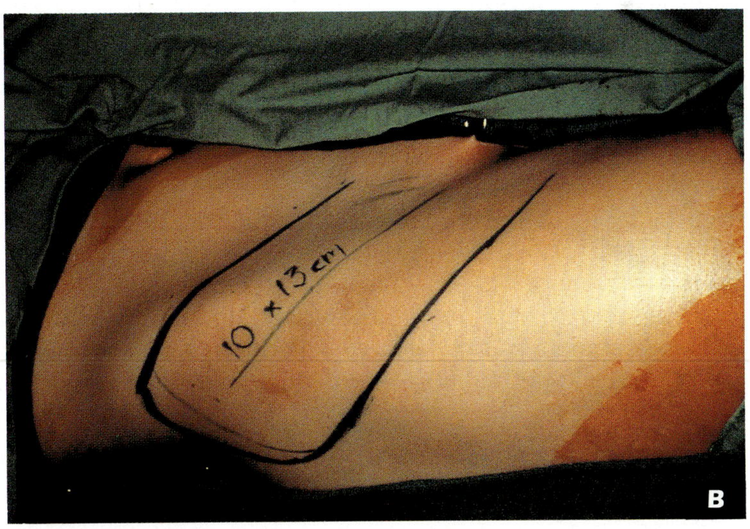

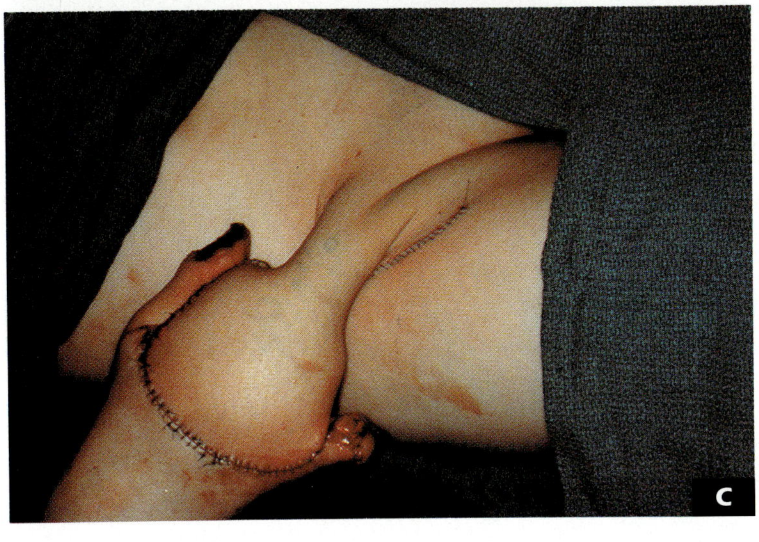

FIGURE 18.16 A Patient who sustained avulsion of the soft-tissues of the hand in farm equipment. **B** Markings for pedicled axial-pattern groin flap on right groin. **C** Intraoperative view after placement of groin flap on hand. Note tubing of proximal flap to allow some motion.

cle and rotated to cover almost any part of the hand (Fig. 18.17). It may not be indicated in patients with more proximal vascular injuries and in elderly patients with vascular disease, as it requires sacrifice of the radial artery.

Since the advent of microsurgical free tissue transfer, many soft tissue losses in the hand can be treated with a one-stage flap transfer. This technique imports well-vascularized tissue which may provide other tissues (i.e., tendon and/or nerve) required for definitive reconstruction (Fig. 18.18). There are many donor sites available for such transfer, and while a discussion of these is beyond the scope of this chapter, this technique may offer the best option for coverage in many cases of hand injury.

SOFT TISSUE: VASCULAR

Vascular injury in the hand is managed in a manner similar to vascular injury elsewhere in the body. Repair of the major vessels to the hand at the wrist level or proximally may be done in standard fashion with loupe magnification.[21] If division or injury to both ulnar and radial arteries has occurred, repair using microvascular techniques can result in excellent patency rates.[13] Some controversy exists as to the necessity for repair of an injured radial or ulnar artery at the wrist with an intact palmar arch, but repair should be attempted under reasonable circumstances. Brisk back-bleeding from the distal end of a severed radial or ulnar artery with decompression of the tourniquet indicates adequate flow from the remaining vessel. If repair is not done, both ends of the severed vessel should be ligated to avoid future false aneurysm formation.

Repair of the small vessels in the hand or digits should be done under the microscope by personnel trained in microvascular techniques. While adequate capillary refill of the distal digits is an indication of viability, compromised flow from digital vascular injury may result in significant late morbidity. Therefore, exploration and repair of damaged digital vessels is usually indicated, especially with injury to the dominant digital vessel.

SOFT TISSUE: NERVE

The proper approach to open injuries of the major nerves of the hand and forearm is of paramount importance in the management of hand trauma. Inappropriate care of nerve injuries, despite proper repair of other injured structures, can lead to a poorly functioning hand. Indeed, a sensate hand with other structural deformities is more useful than a mechanically sound hand with abnormal sensibility.

An understanding of the anatomy of peripheral nerves is necessary in order to carry out proper coaptation. Nerves consist of nerve fibers arranged in fascicles surrounded by connective tissue. Each fascicle is surrounded by perineurium, and groups of fascicles are surrounded by epineurium to form a complete peripheral nerve (Fig. 18.19). Within the connective tissue of nerves course vessels necessary for normal nutrition of the nerve fibers. Detailed studies of the internal topography of the nerves of the forearm and hand have been done which show that the fascicles do not follow a single straight course but tend to intermingle and rearrange themselves.[51] Knowledge of these interrelationships is very important.

The timing of nerve repair in peripheral injuries has been the subject of some controversy in the past, but current practice

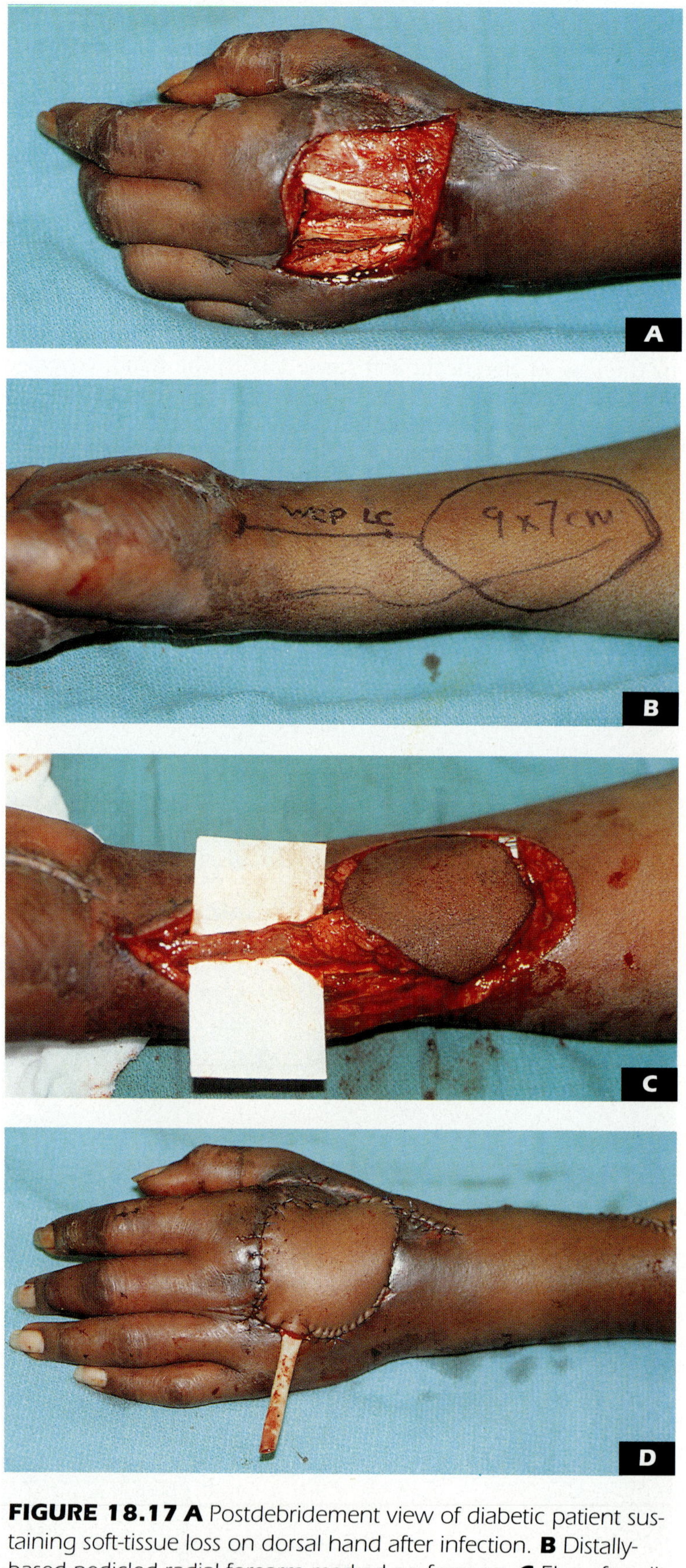

FIGURE 18.17 A Postdebridement view of diabetic patient sustaining soft-tissue loss on dorsal hand after infection. **B** Distally-based pedicled radial forearm marked on forearm. **C** Flap after dissection. Distal radial artery and venae comitans highlighted by background material. **D** Flap placed in defect after rotation and tunneling. Note that forearm was closed primarily.

divides repair into early (primary) and late (secondary). Primary repair is defined as repair of a lacerated nerve soon following injury and prior to final wound healing, whereas secondary repair is that which is done at a later date after wound healing is complete. Primary repair should be accomplished in injuries meeting the following criteria:

Injuries with sharply incised edges and without crush injury
Injuries with minimal contamination
Injuries without other injuries which compromise skeletal stability, circulation, or coverage
Injuries in patients in suitable condition for surgery[58]

Of course, repair should only be done by personnel trained in microvascular techniques with proper staff and instrumentation. Results of primary repair of both sensory and motor nerves show that it offers the best chance of normal return of function.[25]

Delayed repair is carried out after primary wound healing has taken place, in the range of three weeks or more after injury. Delayed repair with primary nerve suture can result in acceptable return of function if properly performed. Late repair of injuries with tissue loss or marked scarring may require nerve grafting and should only be performed by skilled, experienced personnel.

Sharply divided nerves are repaired by either an epineurial coaptation (suture of the surrounding epineurium) or a perineurial coaptation (suture of individual fascicles). A perineurial fascicular coaptation is most often indicated in a mixed motor and sensory nerve whose motor fascicles can be identified. This procedure, however, requires a thorough knowledge of interneurial anatomy and exacting technique.[52]

In most hands, epineurial repair of injured peripheral nerves is the method of choice.[39] The injured nerve ends are identified and freed from surrounding tissue, with care being taken to avoid further injury to the nerve or its sheath (epineurium). Lack of tension at the anastomosis is important for proper axonal bridging at the site of repair. Under direct vision, the fascicular bundles are arranged in apposition and fine monofilament sutures are placed in the epineurium (Fig. 18.20). In larger nerves, such as the median, orientation is often simplified by the presence of vessels on the nerve surface, which may be lined up. Manipulation of the free cut ends is kept to a minimum to

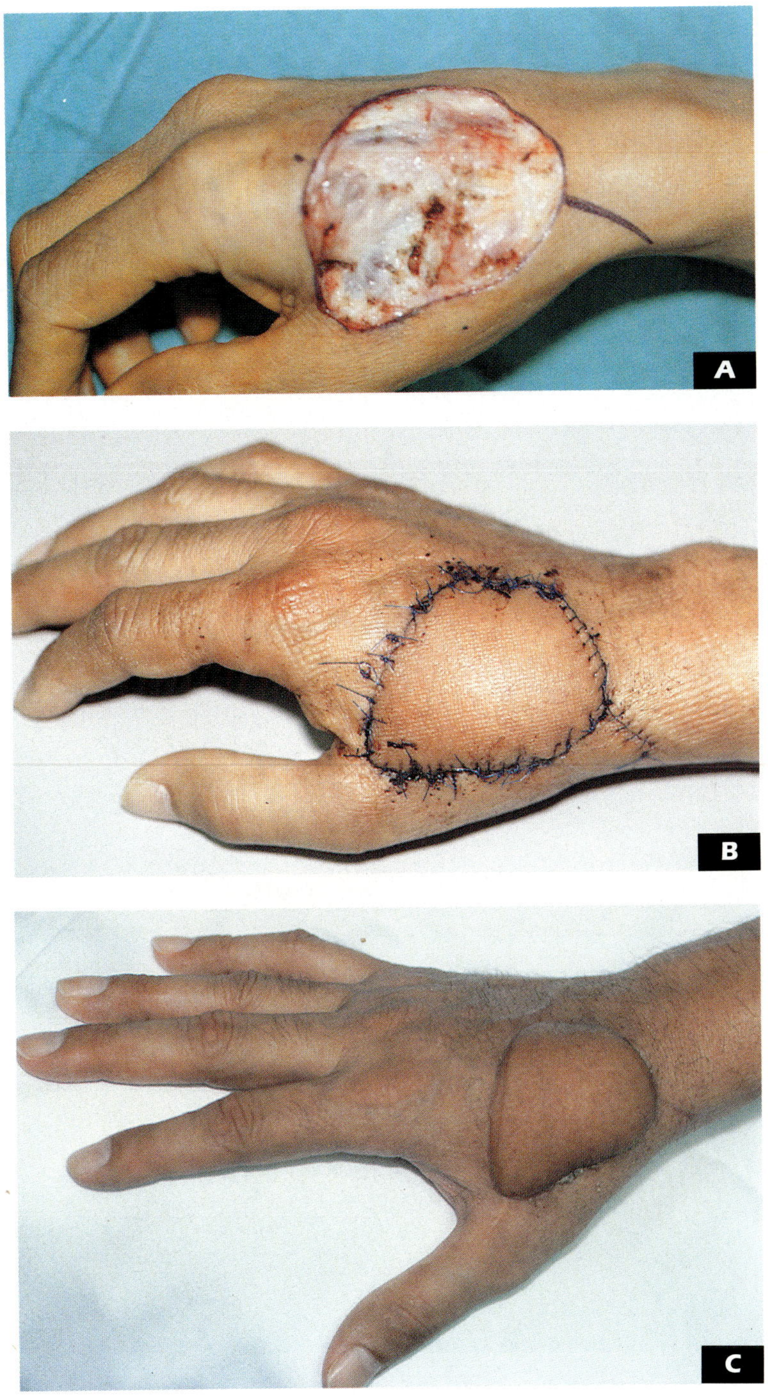

FIGURE 18.18 A Patient with unstable skin graft over dorsal hand after debridement of skin. **B** Showing area after placement of microvascular lateral arm cutaneous free flap. Anastomoses to radial artery and vein in snuffbox. **C** View at eight months after flap transfer.

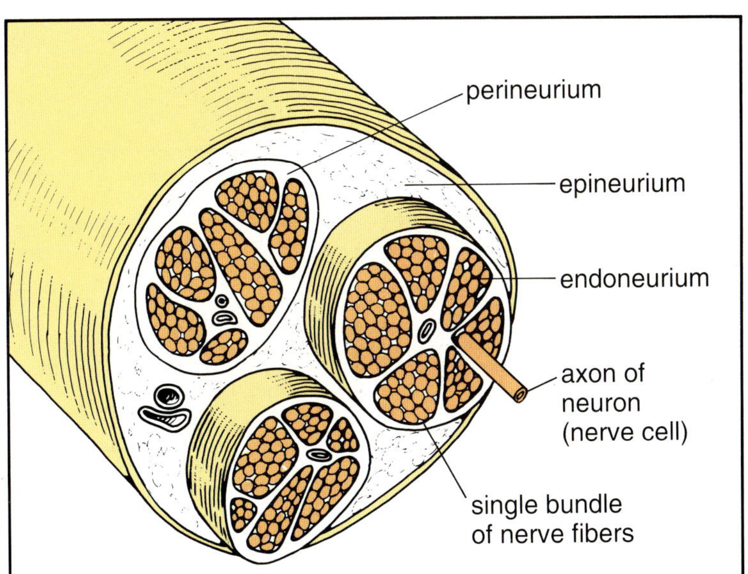

FIGURE 18.19 Internal neural anatomy.

decrease scar formation at the anastomosis. In the case of ragged edges, the ends may require careful trimming prior to suture placement. The smaller nerves in the hand and fingers are repaired in a similar manner, placing the minimum number of sutures needed for accurate approximation of the cut ends.

Postoperative nerve repair takes precedence over the desire for early motion. In general, the area of repair should be immobilized for three weeks following repair. After this period, motion is gradually begun, depending somewhat on the nature of other bony or tendinous injuries. Regeneration takes place at the rate of about a millimeter per day or an inch per month. The rate of regeneration is evaluated postoperatively by following the presence of an advancing Tinel's sign along the involved nerve trunk. There may be a delay of four to six weeks before the Tinel's sign becomes evident.[38] When there is no evidence of advancing regeneration, electrodiagnostic studies and subsequent reexploration may be required. The patient with sensory nerve injury should be cautioned as to proper care of the insensate portion of the hand while nerve regeneration is occurring (Fig. 18.21). A period of reeducation is often necessary to properly restore normal sensibility in reinnervated digits.

SOFT TISSUE: TENDONS

The approach to repair of open injuries to the tendons of the extrinsic muscles of the hand differs somewhat, depending on whether the extensor or flexor tendons are involved. The two systems have a number of anatomic and mechanical differences. The extrinsic flexor tendons pass from the forearm via the carpal tunnel into the palm of the hand where they enter their respective sheaths. Precise flexion of the digits is controlled by the smooth gliding of the flexor tendons in the canal over each other and through the pulley system (see Fig. 18.3). Damage to this system can result in binding of the tendons together and to the surrounding fibro-osseous canal, leading to decreased flexion of the involved digit. The extensor tendon system, in contrast, has no tendon sheaths or pulley system. The juncturae tend-

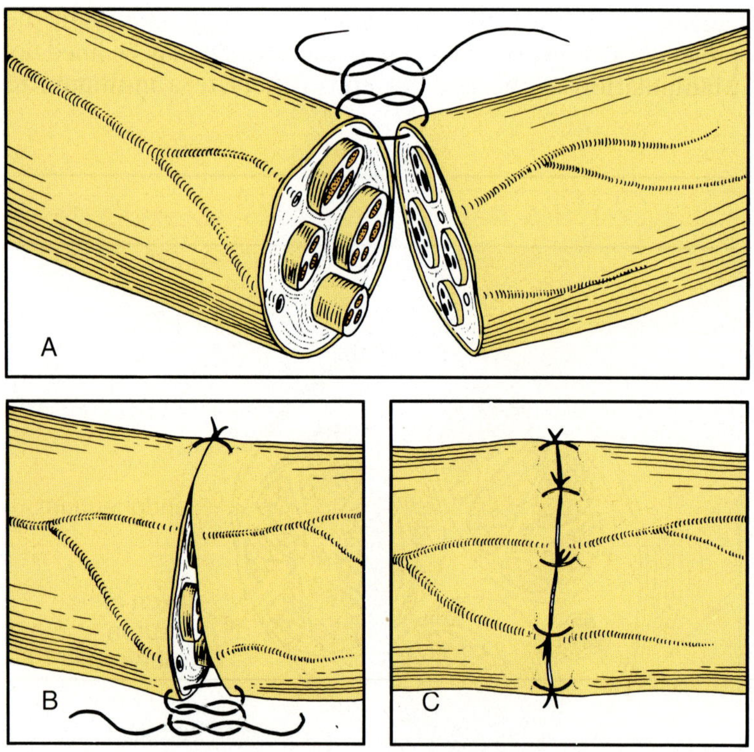

FIGURE 18.20 Technique of epineurial repair. **A** Placement of the epineurial sutures. **B** Alignment of the epineurium based on surface vessels. **C** Completed epineurial repair.

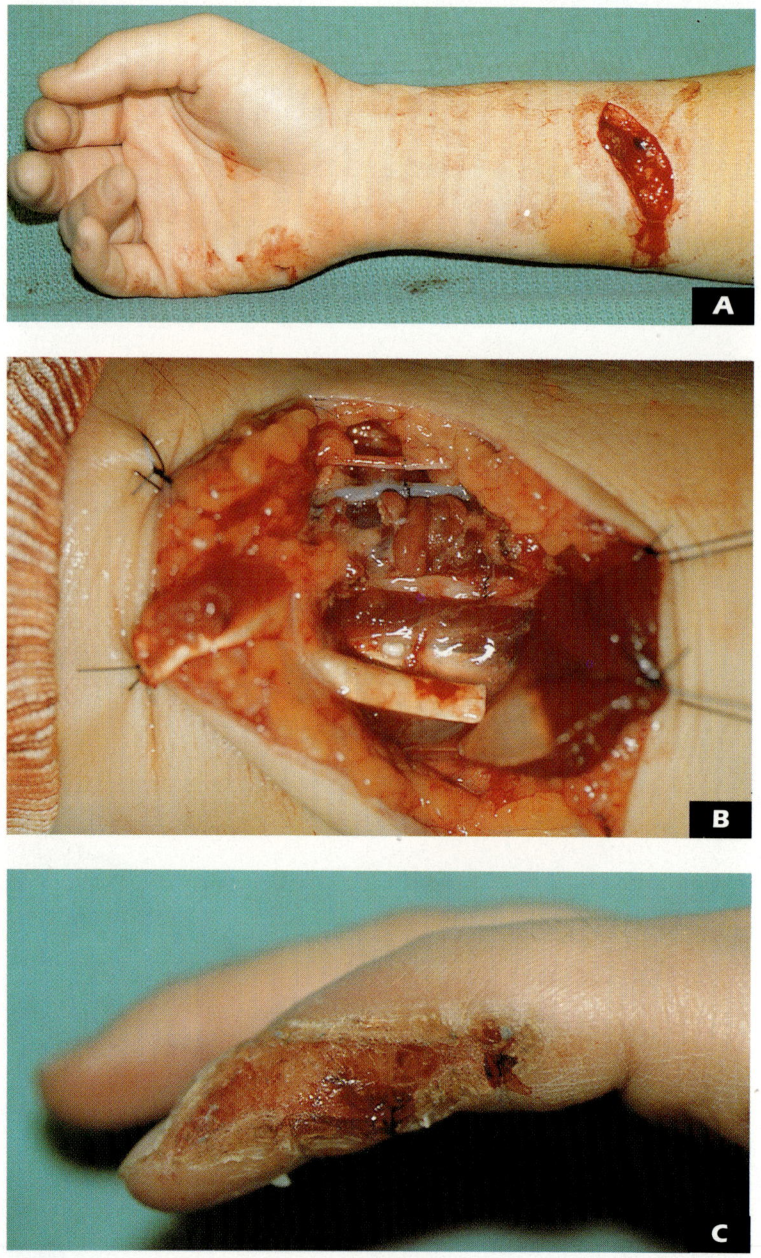

FIGURE 18.21 A Patient sustaining laceration to forearm from glass with division of radial artery, median nerve and tendons. **B** Intraoperative view of repairs of radial artery, median nerve and flexor tendons. **C** Burn sustained to index finger two months post-injury, secondary to lack of sensation.

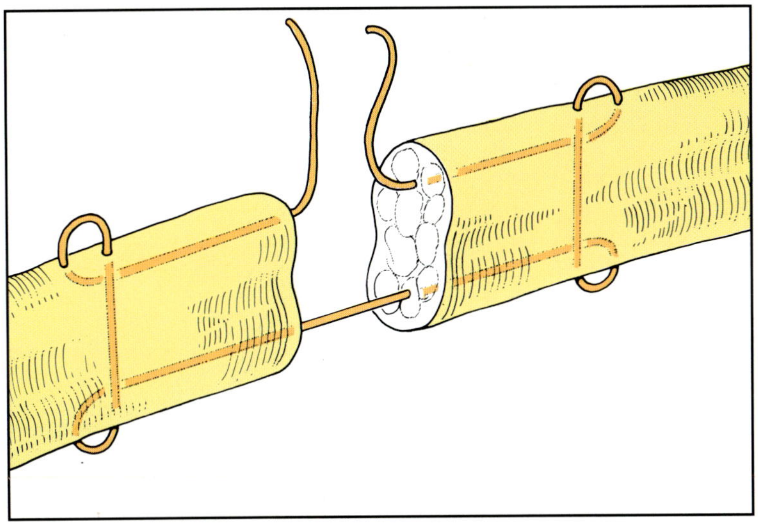

FIGURE 18.22 Kessler-Mason-Allen core tendon suture.

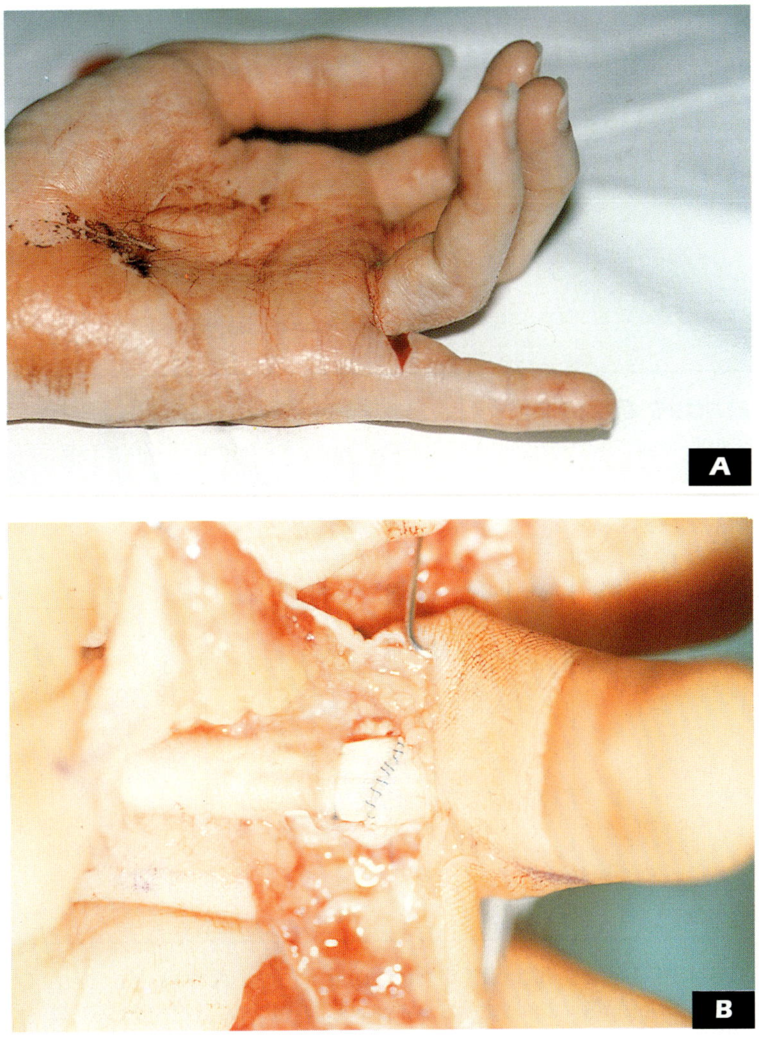

FIGURE 18.23 A Little finger with laceration of both flexors. Note lack at flexion due to total division of tendon. **B** Tendon after repair showing epitenon suture.

inum interconnect the various extrinsic extensors of the fingers, resulting in some mass motion in MCP joint extension. Because of these and other differences, the specifics of management of open injury to these two systems will be discussed separately.

Timing of tendon repair may be either primary or secondary. In general, tendon injuries are best managed at the time of primary wound management. While controversy existed in the past as to the wisdom of primary repair of flexor tendons, the so-called "no man's land," studies in large numbers of patients have shown excellent results with primary suture using proper techniques.[22] Primary suture of divided tendon ends may be done up to three to five days following injury without compromising results. In the presence of other life-threatening systemic problems contraindicating primary repair, delayed repair (possibly with tendon grafting) may be necessary.

The actual technique of repair varies with the type of tendon involved. The rounder flexor tendons should be repaired with some type of "core" suture. While many types of sutures have been proposed, all in use today use the principle of grasping tendon bundles for strength. We prefer the modified Kessler-Mason-Allen technique with the knot buried within the substance of the repair (Fig. 18.22). The extensor tendons are of a somewhat flatter configuration and are more easily repaired with a simple or figure-of-eight type of suture. Suture material in either type of repair should be a nonabsorbable synthetic to give strength to the repair during healing. Most authors prefer a braided suture for ease of handling, using 4-0 sutures for larger tendons and 5-0 for smaller ones.

Partial lacerations of tendons should only be sutured if greater than 30% of the diameter is involved. Lesser injuries are adequately treated with proper splinting and early controlled motion. With total division of a tendon, contraction of the corresponding muscle acts to retract the proximal end. This may occur at varying distances, from only a few millimeters to several centimeters. Mitigating factors are the presence of a nearby vincula (in the case of a flexor tendon) or a juncturae tendinum (in extensor tendons), which will decrease the distance of separation. If the proximal tendon is not easily located, the skin laceration should be extended proximally or a second counterincision made over the proximal course of the tendon. Once the tendon is located, it is advanced until the ends are in approximation and a Keith needle is passed through the tendon and surrounding skin proximally to hold it in position for repair. With the ends in approximation, the tendon is sutured with one of the above techniques. Care should be taken not to pull the suture too tight or it will bunch up at the repair site.

Approximation of cut tendon ends will suffice for repair in most areas. However, injuries to flexor tendons in the digits require special techniques. The flexor tendons are surrounded by the fibro-osseous canal from the distal palmar crease to the distal phalanx. Both careful handling and precise technique are required for proper return of function after repair in this area. The tendon sheath may be opened, but only in such a manner as to not damage the pulley system. The cut tendon ends are handled meticulously to minimize scarring; ideally, the tendon is grasped only by the cut surface. After placement of the core suture, the epitenon is carefully approximated with a fine (6-0) running monofilament suture (Fig. 18.23). This technique should decrease scarring around the repair and allow easier gliding of the repaired tendon within the sheath. The sheath is then repaired with fine monofilament suture, if feasible. Damaged pulleys over the proximal portion of the proximal phalanx and mid-portion of the middle phalanx should be repaired or reconstructed, as bowstringing of the tendons can result if either of these is not intact.

In the case of a tendon divided near the distal phalanx, reinsertion of the tendon may be required. If there is not enough distal tendon for core suturing, the proximal tendon is reinserted into the distal phalanx by notching the palmar surface of the distal phalanx and wiring the tendon to the bone. The wire is placed in the proximal tendon in the fashion of a core suture and brought either through or around the distal phalanx. It is then brought out through the distal digit or nail and tied over a button. The wire is removed after healing is adequate (usually in six to eight weeks).

When both the FDS and FDP tendons are lacerated in the sheath, both should generally be repaired. Full flexion of the digit can occur with the profundus only, however. Therefore, in elderly patients or those with other complicating factors, the FDS tendon by itself does not necessarily require repair for adequate function. In these cases, excision of the FDS tendon should be done to avoid tenodesis with the FDP tendon from scarring.

Repairs of the extensor tendon system in the digits require special consideration as well. Lacerations of the extensor tendons on the dorsum of the digits may be repaired by figure-of-eight sutures in standard fashion. Care is required to repair all involved structures on the dorsum and laterally, or late boutonnière or swan-neck deformities of the involved digits may result. With injuries over the PIP joint, immobilization in full extension should be employed for a period of five to six weeks. With an open injury at the DIP joint, the so-called mallet finger will result. The tendon is repaired and the joint splinted either externally or with a K-pin across the joint for three to four weeks. If the digit lacks full extension after this period, splinting should be continued for another two to three weeks.

Early controlled mobilization with passive motion of the flexor tendons has been shown to give excellent long-term results with repairs in the fibro-osseous canal.[29] At surgery, a suture is placed through the distal fingernail of the involved digit. The suture is then connected to a rubber band attached to the dressing at the wrist (Fig. 18.24). A dorsal splint is made with the wrist in moderate flexion, the MCP joints at approximately 20°, and the IP joints at 10°. The patient is then instructed to actively *extend* the digit against the pull of the rubber band as often as possible for the period of splinting, or about three weeks. At no time is the patient allowed to actively flex the digit during this time. After removal of the splint, the digit is reattached to an ace bandage at the wrist and active extension exercises are continued for another two weeks. At this point, the patient may gradually begin normal activities. Extensor tendon injuries in the wrist and hand should be splinted with the wrist in 45° extension and the MCP joints in 15° flexion for four weeks. In the case of obvious loss of motion after two to three months, operative tenolysis may be required.

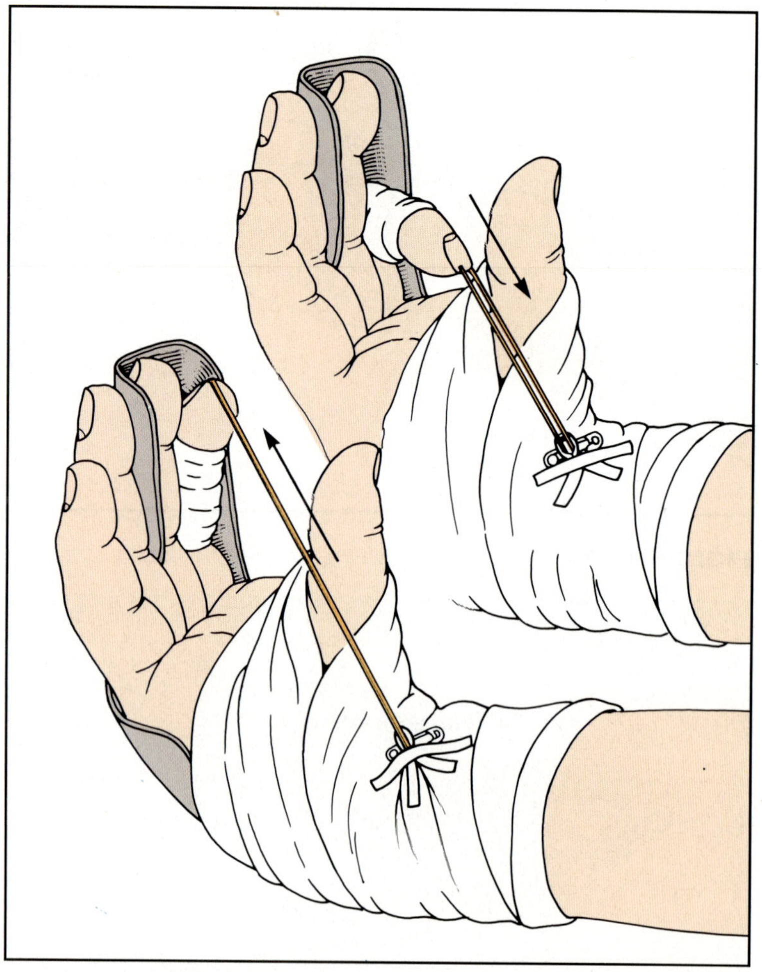

FIGURE 18.24 Rubber band traction to the nail with a dorsal splint for early controlled mobilization of a flexor tendon repair.

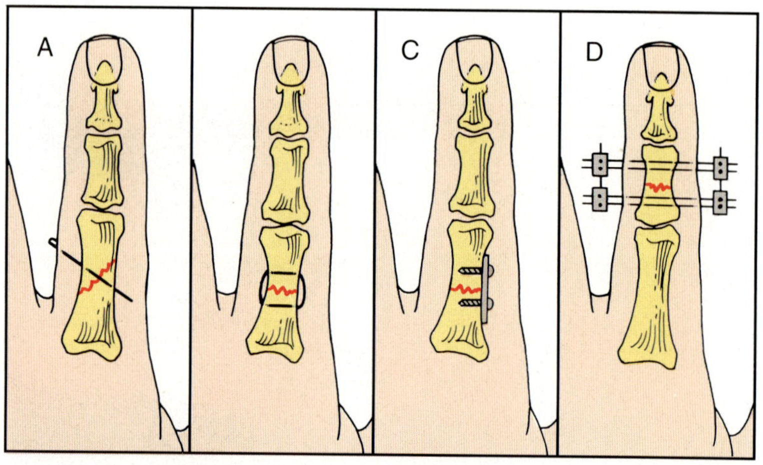

FIGURE 18.25 Types of fixation of fractures. **A** Kirschner wire (C wire, K wire). **B** Interosseous wiring. **C** Miniplate with screws. **D** External fixator.

BONE AND JOINT INJURIES

Open fractures are treated in a manner similar to closed fractures, with proper consideration given to adequate local cleansing of the fracture site and stabilization. After debridement of contaminated and nonviable tissues, the area of fracture is irrigated with an antibacterial/balanced saline solution. Stable fractures, as noted in the section on closed fractures, are treated after repair of soft tissue injuries and skin closure. Coverage of exposed bone is given primary consideration with the exception of grossly contaminated wounds. Unstable fractures are stabilized prior to wound closure by one of the accepted methods described in the following discussion.

Most simple fractures of the small bones of the hand may be managed by placement of transosseous Kirschner wires or interosseous wiring, or a combination of both (Fig. 18.25, A and B). Linear fractures are well stabilized by an interosseous wire placed through small holes drilled on either side of the fracture. Greater stability is obtained with two wires placed at 90° to each other across the fracture site. Relatively stable fractures and oblique fractures are well managed with small K-wires placed either through the wound or percutaneously across the fracture site. Care must be taken to avoid distraction of the fragments with inaccurate placement of K-wires, particularly when the crossed K-wire technique is used. Fixation is maintained for a period of six to eight weeks in most fractures, with a follow-up radiologic evaluation at appropriate intervals. Lack of tenderness and motion at the site of fracture indicates adequate clinical healing, while radiologic consolidation at the fracture site may lag behind for several months.

In the case of bone loss or marked comminution of fragments, an external fixator may be used (Fig. 18.25, D). Use of this type of fixation follows the basic principles of external fixation; nevertheless its proper application requires the skill of trained personnel.

Internal fixation of fractures of the hand with plates and screws has been used increasingly in recent years. However, its usefulness is limited by the requirements of wide tissue mobilization and periosteal stripping. Again, the method should be performed only by those trained in the techniques involved.

Open injuries to the joints and ligaments of the hand are managed with standard techniques of bony fixation and soft tissue repair. Loose pieces of joint cartilage should be debrided if not attached to larger bony fragments. After fixation of fracture fragments, repair of the ligamentous supporting structures of the joint is undertaken. Special attention must be given to the collateral ligaments and volar plates in the MCP and IP joints. These structures give lateral and volar support to the joint and their improper repair can lead to joint instability. After repair, the joint is immobilized for a period of up to six weeks, depending on the severity of injury. With severe injury to the joint surface or supporting structures, late reconstruction or joint fusion may be required for painless functioning.

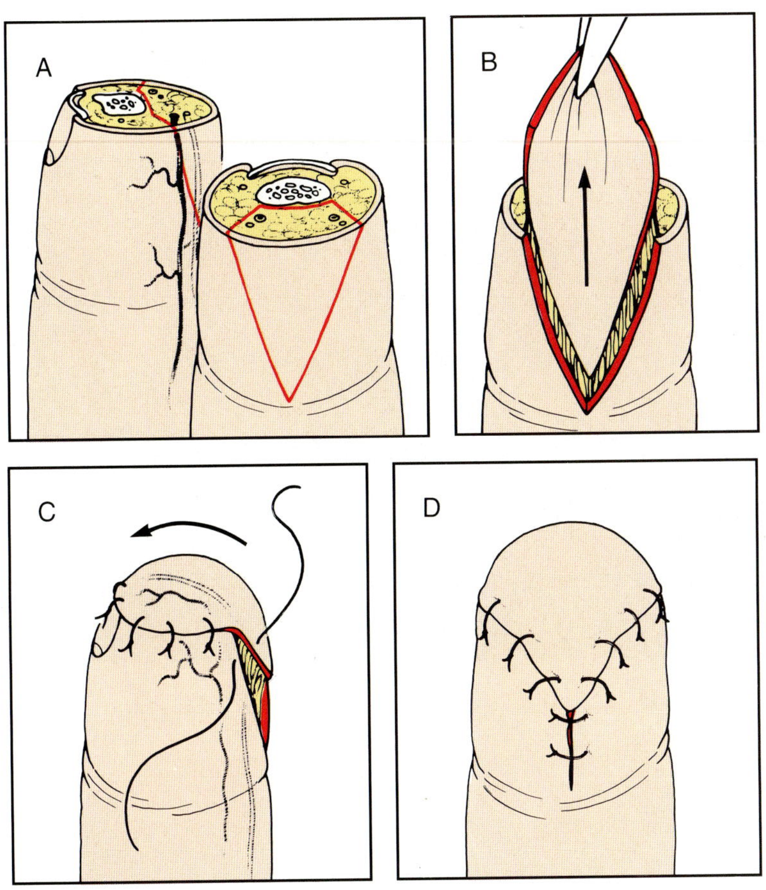

FIGURE 18.26 V-Y advancement flap for fingertip coverage.

AMPUTATION

Amputation of the tip of one of the digits is a commonly seen injury. The aims of proper management are to restore normal sensation without pain and to achieve stable coverage. In the case of a simple amputation of the tip of a finger without bony involvement, some controversy exists as to the necessity of coverage. If the portion amputated is available and has not been damaged by the injury, it may simply be replaced by careful suturing as a composite graft. This type of tip graft usually takes reasonably well, and even if the replaced portion of tissue fails to take, it acts as a biologic dressing while healing takes place underneath.

When the raw surface is less than 1 cm in diameter, the wound will reepithelialize from the periphery. While some authors have advocated skin grafting or flap coverage of tip amputations in the past, most today prefer allowing the injury to heal by secondary intention. The results are comparable, and while the wound may take up to six weeks to heal, the patient is off from work not significantly longer than the skin-grafted patient. Ultimate sensation is better than with grafts, as contraction of the wound acts to bring in pulp skin with normal sensation. Dressing of the fingertip while healing progresses is a matter of choice, as a number of satisfactory dressings have been used with success.

When a larger portion of the digital tip or pulp is amputated or there is exposed bone, coverage with a local flap should be considered. When there is more dorsal skin than volar skin lost, a V-Y advancement flap from the digital pulp may be used (Fig. 18.26). The flap is raised as a bipedicled island flap on the radial and ulnar digital bundles at the mid-distal phalanx level. It is then advanced over the digital tip and the defect closed as a "Y". This flap has reasonable sensation and gives good coverage to exposed bone at the tip.[2] When there is not enough volar skin for advancement, a cross-finger flap may work, particularly for the index finger and thumb. The flap is raised on the dorsum of an adjacent digit, usually over the middle phalanx. It may be based either proximally, distally, or laterally, with the latter being the most common approach. The flap is raised carefully off the paratenon of the extensor tendon under tourniquet control with magnification. The donor defect is covered at the time of the flap elevation with a full- or split-thickness skin graft. Good design is very important to avoid problems of inadequate flap size and tension on the pedicle. The flap is divided at two to three weeks and inset. The unused portion of the pedicle can be replaced on the donor site. Long-term studies have shown excellent return of sensibility, which improves with time (Fig. 18.27).[23]

Amputations occurring more proximally are treated by replantation. While the services of a replantation team are not available in every hospital, the patient and the amputated part can be safely transported to a properly staffed center. Proper preservation of the digits allows replantation to occur up to 24 hours after amputation with a reasonable chance for success. When performed by well-trained personnel in the proper setting, replantation today gives quite acceptable results to both the clinician and patient (Fig. 18.28).[34]

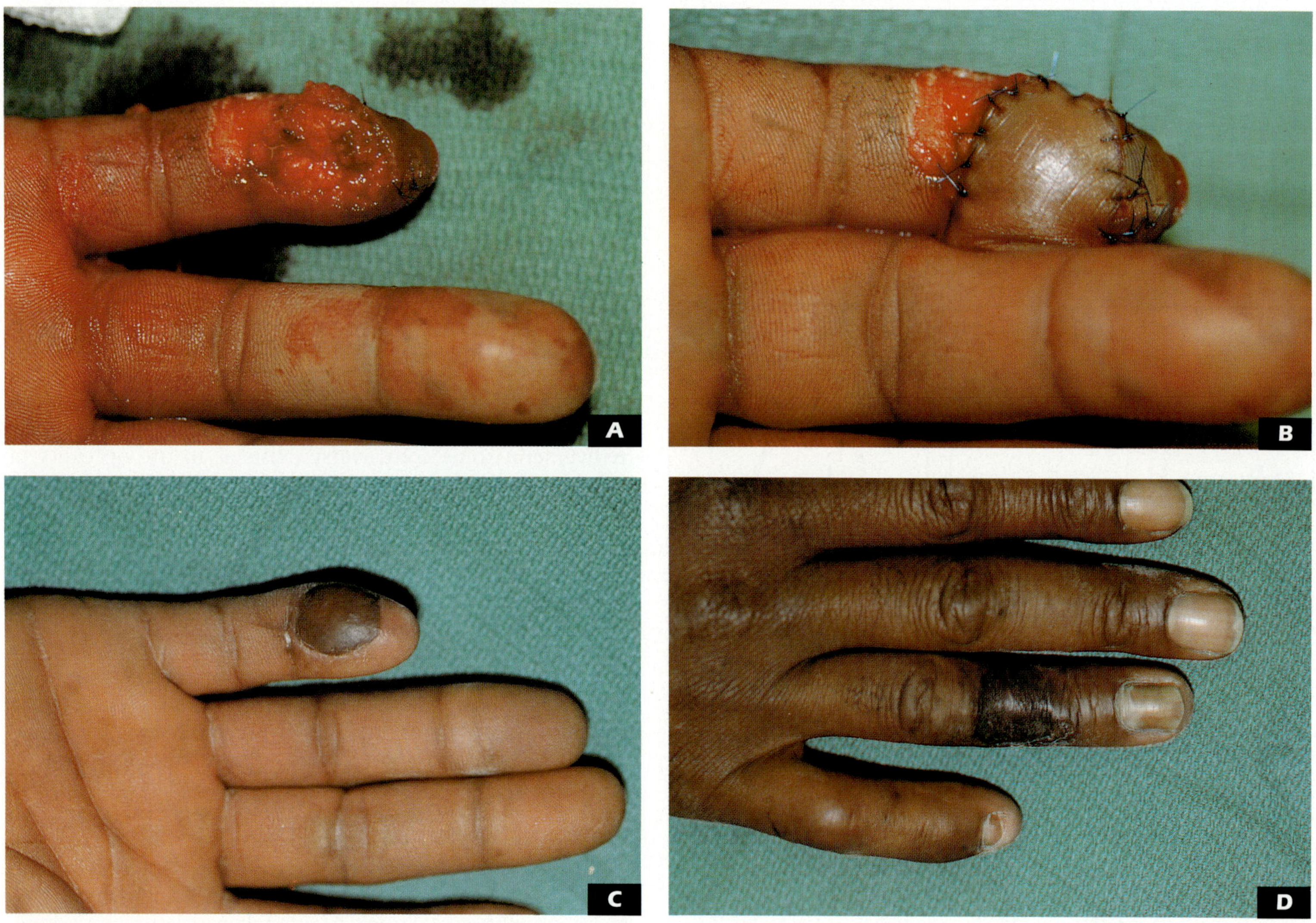

FIGURE 18.27 A Patient who sustained crush-avulsion injury to his little finger. **B** Post-debridement and placement of cross-finger flap from dorsum of ring finger. **C** Flap in situ three months after division. **D** Dorsum of ring finger covered with STSG at three months.

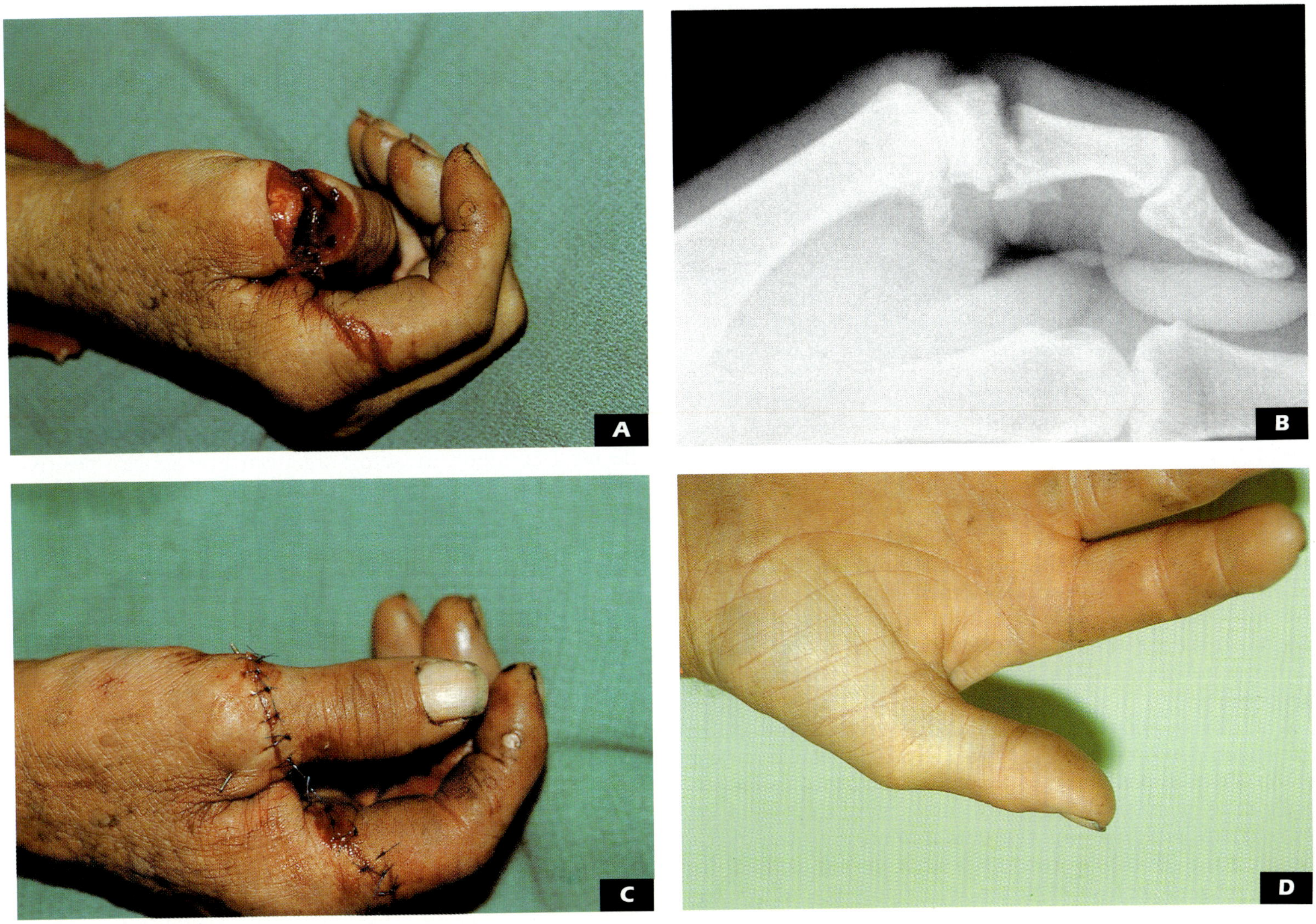

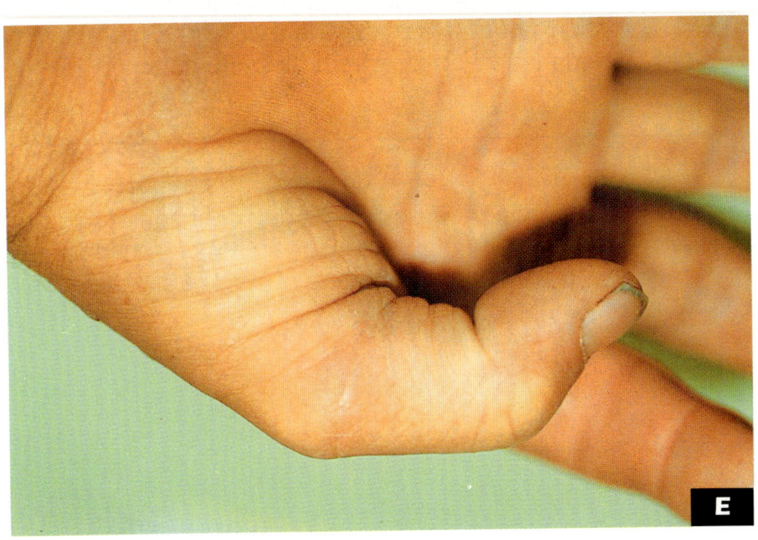

FIGURE 18.28 A Patient with near-amputation of right thumb. There was no vascular flow and only a small volar skin attachment was present. **B** X-ray showing level of division of proximal phalanx. **C** Immediate postoperative view after repair of digital vessels and nerves. **D** View at six months postop—extension. **E** View at 6 months postop—flexion.

The clinician should know the indications for replantation to avoid subjecting the patient to unnecessary expectations and delays in treatment. In general, the following amputations are considered favorable for replantation:

Thumb
Multiple digits
Partial hand (amputation at the level of the palm)
Almost any part in a child
Wrist or forearm
Elbow and above elbow (with sharp amputation or minimal tissue crush)
Individual digits distal to the flexor superficialis insertion

Those parts not considered favorable for replantation include severely crushed or mangled parts; amputations at multiple levels; amputations in patients with other serious injuries or diseases; amputations in patients with arteriosclerosis; those in patients with mental instability; and individual digital amputations in adults proximal to the FDS insertion.[55]

If the patient presents with one of the favorable indications and transportation to another hospital is necessary, the amputated part needs to be cleansed and sterilely dried. It is then placed dry in a sterile container, which is placed in ice; the part must not touch the ice or iced saline or maceration will occur. The patient is stabilized and transferred in the most expeditious manner possible.

When the patient is not a candidate for replantation or the amputated portion of the digit is not available, simple revision of the site of amputation is performed. In the digits, this is generally done by the development of simple dorsal and volar flaps. In order to avoid painful neuroma formation of the digital nerves at the site of amputation, the nerves to the digit are dissected proximally a short distance, divided, and allowed to retract proximally. Volar skin is generally preferable for distal tip coverage because of its better sensation. If preservation of length is important, a cross-finger flap may be necessary for tip coverage. Divided tendons are simply allowed to retract proximally, unless they can be reattached in a normal position to allow motion of joints just proximal to the site of amputation. The extensor and flexor tendons should not be sutured together, or a functional deformity may result. More proximal amputations of the hand and wrist are closed in standard fashion, allowing for as much length as possible.

HAND INFECTIONS

Cutaneous Infections

Acute infections of the hand are common but, if treated early and properly, can be managed primarily on an outpatient basis. The most common invading organism is coagulase-positive *Staphylococcus aureus* and is frequently associated with abscess formation. These abscesses can develop at varying levels. A subcuticular abscess lies directly beneath the epidermis. Abscesses may also be intracutaneous, subcutaneous, or subfascial. At times various levels may communicate with one another through a small opening, the so-called "collar button" abscess. Treatment consists of proper incision and drainage over the area of purulence, with care taken that all spaces are carefully decompressed and adequately drained. On the dorsum of the hand, particularly in hair-bearing areas, the abscess may be multiple and communicative, and is called a *carbuncle* or *Whitlow*.

Paronychia

Acute inflammation may be localized to anatomical compartments. The eponychium overlying the root of the nail may be involved. Inflammation or paronychia is quite common in this

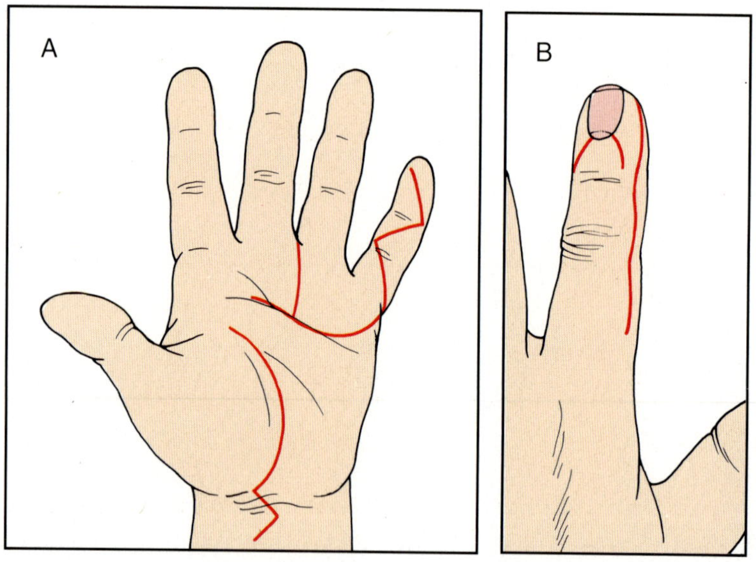

FIGURE 18.29 Incisions for exploration or drainage of hand infections. **A** Incisions on the palmar surface for digital and palmar abscesses. **B** Incisions for drainage of paronychia and digital infections.

location and is often the result of minor trauma; frequently, an intraepithelial abscess may be present. Treatment consists of hot soaks and adequate incision and drainage when purulence is noted (Fig. 18.29, B).

Apical Abscess

Inflammation localized to the very tip of the finger is termed an apical abscess. Fibrous septae attach the skin to the distal phalanx and divide the fingertip into multiple compartments. An abscess in this area may actually extend beneath the nail.

Volar Compartment Abscess

Digital creases divide the fingers into multiple volar pulp spaces. These creases are firmly attached to the underlying tendon sheath thus limiting inflammation to these compartments. The initial insult is frequently a small puncture wound.

Tendon Sheath Infections

Tendon sheath infections most likely result from a direct puncture wound frequently in the digital crease where the overlying skin is attached to the underlying tendon sheath with minimal subcutaneous tissue. Tenosynovitis is an inflammation that involves the tendon and its surrounding sheath. Kanavel's four signs of tenosynovitis include the following: (1) the affected digit is held in a slightly flexed position (2) the digit is red and swollen (3) there is pain on extension and (4) tenderness is present along the entire tendon sheath even outside the area of penetration into the tendon sheath.[19]

It is important to recognize that the little finger frequently communicates with the ulnar bursa and the thumb with the radial bursa, so that acute inflammation of the tendon sheath in either of these two digits will result in the extension of the inflammation to the wrist and forearm. Treatment consists of adequate incision and drainage. A controlled environment and operating conditions are mandatory[47]; this includes magnification, tourniquet control, and adequate anesthesia. Often regional anesthesia is contraindicated because of associated lymphangitis and cellulitis. Treatment should only be undertaken by an experienced hand surgeon knowledgeable of current techniques and anatomy, and especially skilled in postoperative management. Irrigation catheters are frequently employed postoperatively (Fig. 18.30). A balanced lactated Ringer's solution is selected as an irrigator with or without a bacteriocidal antibiotic (i.e., neomycin, bacitracin). Both the proximal and digital portions of the tendon sheath are exposed to permit adequate irrigation and drainage. After a period of immobilization, usually three to five days, limited progressive active motion is begun. Systemic antibiotics (cephalosporin type) are employed initially until the results of the cultures are available. Both aerobic and anaerobic cultures must be taken. If the history of the injured patient is out of the ordinary, as in a meat handler or a fisherman, then uncommon organisms must be considered and appropriate cultures obtained, for example, for *Mycobacterium* and *Erysipelothrix*.

Web Space Infections

Web space infections are common between the digits, often as a result of an innocuous scratch or fissure. Inflammation is usually confined to the area between the opposing digits. Swelling of the dorsum of the hand is also common. Abduction of the adjacent fingers at rest is pathognomonic of the site of infection.

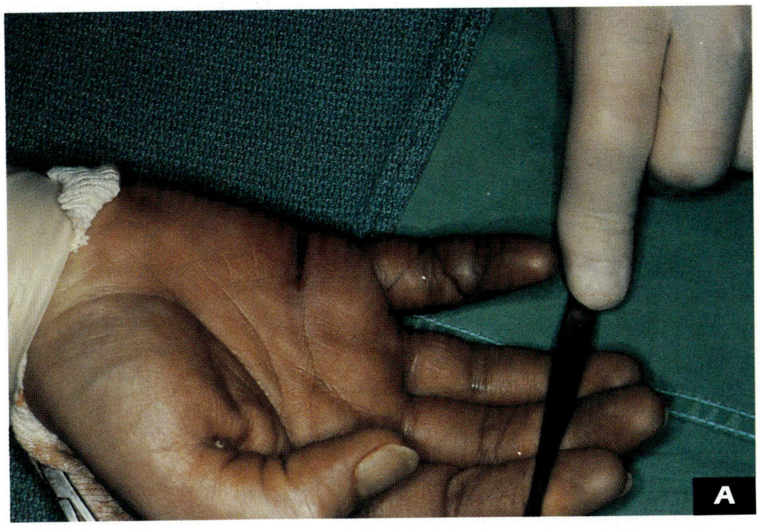

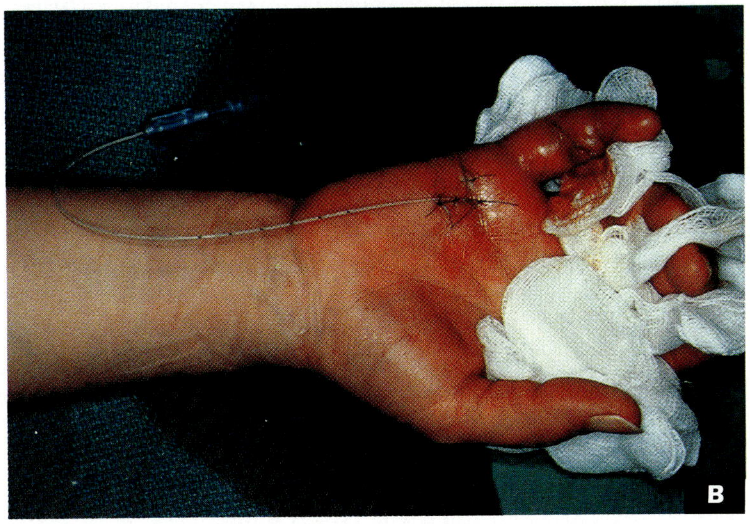

FIGURE 18.30 A Patient with tenosynovitis of little finger after dog bite. Note lines for incision in finger and palm. **B** Postop view showing placement of epidural catheter for continuous irrigation.

Deep Palmar Space Infections

Deep palmar space infection is frequently associated with a penetrating wound. The symptoms are inflammation beneath the palmar fascia, intense pain with obvious swelling on the volar aspect of the hand, and marked dorsal edema. The ability to move adjacent fingers differentiates a deep palmar infection from tenosynovitis. Treatment consists of expert surgical incision and drainage directly over the site of maximal tenderness (Fig. 18.29, A).

It should be recognized that not all inflammation is bacterial in origin, and therefore the history and physical findings are essential in establishing a correct diagnosis. Rheumatoid arthritis, gout, and gonorrhea must be considered in the differential diagnosis, particularly when the history is vague regarding trauma and is characterized by polyarthritis. The symptoms are of sudden onset (within 24 and 48 hours) combined with a prior history of trauma with intense pain and inflammation. Throbbing pain localized to a tendon sheath or space is pathognomonic of purulence within that space.[28] Surgical incision and drainage is mandatory.

SPECIAL INJURIES OF THE HAND

Human Bites

The largest percentage of human bites occur in the hand; mostly in males, and frequently as a result of an altercation.[15] In a recent review of hand infection requiring admission to the hospital, 21% were due to human bites.[4]

Diagnosis is established by inspection and careful history. Radiologic examination within the first week to ten days contributes little to the diagnosis, other than perhaps to document the presence of a fracture or the presence of air in the subcutaneous tissues and muscle indicating the possibility of a gas-forming organism. Radiologic changes indicating septic arthritis, tenosynovitis, and osteomyelitis are most reliably interpreted on the basis of clinical findings of pain on motion.

Treatment is dictated by the findings noted on physical examination and the amount of time following injury before the patient presents for evaluation. Generally, patients present either within the first 24 hours or later during the first week following injury. Although some controversy exists regarding the early treatment of human bites to the hand,[28] the following is recommended by most experienced hand surgeons. All injuries presenting during the first 24 hours are explored in a suitable environment, that is, with magnification and tourniquet control available. The wound is cultured prior to irrigation and debridement. When excising the wound edges at each tissue plane, the clinician must keep in mind that the puncture wound occurs usually when the fist is clenched and that the tract or penetration is changed when the digits are extended. The most common organism is *Eikenella corrodens,* which is sensitive to penicillin and cephalosporins.[28,33] Tetanus prophylaxis is given, as well as an initial dose of cephalosporin. Antibiotics are continued postoperatively, pending culture results. Wounds are left open and a soft dressing with a plaster splint is applied. Within 24 hours the wound is again examined, preferably by the same clinician administering primary care.

Patients presenting within the first 24 hours after injury with signs of cellulitis, lymphangitis, and possible joint penetration are treated in a similar fashion. The wound is debrided and irrigated and the joint explored. It is important that the examining physician be experienced in hand surgery; otherwise, improper exploration and debridement could result in the extension of the infection to adjacent, uninvolved structures. Patients with a suspected diagnosis of septic arthritis or tenosynovitis are admitted, following surgical care of the wounds, and observed for progression or diminution of symptoms and administered systemic antibiotics.

Patients presenting late (after 24 hours) with obvious signs of inflammation, tenosynovitis, or septic arthritis are treated similarly. These patients are all hospitalized.

In general, patients presenting with a human bite are frequently intoxicated and usually not reliable for follow-up. These patients should be observed in a holding area for 24 hours or admitted to the hospital.

Dog Bites

Unlike human bites, dog bites are common to both sexes and all ages. They can occur on any exposed location of skin, frequently the hand, face, and neck region. One can see a spectrum of injuries which varies from tissue loss and lacerations to isolated puncture wounds. Most patients seek treatment soon after injury.

Initial treatment consists of wound debridement and copious irrigation. Injuries to the hand are frequently left open, especially if they are puncture wounds and small lacerations. Patients with partially avulsed skin flaps, particularly with exposed neurotendinous structures, can be treated with primary wound closure as long as there are the following: an experienced hand surgeon to provide evaluation and treatment, an adequate surgical facility, and available magnification and tourniquet control. Injuries to the head and neck region frequently are debrided and closed primarily. All wounds require a strict follow-up in 24 hours and patients usually do not require admission. Tetanus prophylaxis is given and necessary radiographs and wound cultures are obtained. The organism most frequently cultured is *Pasteurella multocida.*[30]

Puncture wounds require special attention and follow-up. They may be deep, made by the large canine teeth in both dogs and cats, and involve either joint or tendon spaces. These wounds should be managed the same way as human bite injuries.

The following factors seem to increase the incidence of wound infection following dog bites:

Patients more than 50 years of age
Puncture wounds
Wounds involving the hand
Wounds that have been sutured

Prognostic stratification and sample size are not considered and full statistical comparison is lacking in most studies.[6] For this reason, there is disagreement over whether to administer prophylactic antibiotics following dog bite injuries to the hand. Most hand surgeons support the use of prophylactic antibiotics.

Snake Bites

Snake bite injuries to the hand are uncommon in the United States. Rattlesnake and water moccasin (Crotalidae) bites account for 96% to 98% of all snake bite envenomations,[48] and most bites are to the upper extremity. Prompt, early treatment minimizes morbidity significantly. Initial treatment should consist of wound suction and is most efficacious during the first three minutes following envenomation. The amount of venom removed by this technique drops off precipitously with time; after 30 minutes no significant benefit can be achieved.[32]

Significant controversy still exists as to the routine administration of antivenom to snake bite victims. Since most antivenoms are made of horse serum, the possibility of anaphylaxis and serum sickness must be weighed against the beneficial effects. Obviously, treatment with antivenom no longer manufactured from horse serum minimizes these complications. Most authors advocate the use of antivenoms as part of the initial treatment.[5,10,11,16,32,44,60] Antivenoms are administered intravenously in usual doses of four to five vials (10 ml per vial) for moderate envenomation, five to ten vials for more serious envenomation, and 15 or more vials when large doses of venom have been received and systemic manifestations are uncontrolled. The antivenom should be given over a 30- to 60-minute period with a large amount of crystalloids for volume replacement. Corticosteroids and cryotherapy have fallen into disrepute as primary treatment modalities.

In recent years, there have been many advocates of fasciotomies and debridement as the sole treatment modality in snake bite injuries of the hand.[14]

Surgical management consists of longitudinal fasciotomies of the fingers, with care to avoid injury to the dorsal and volar neurovascular structures. More proximal swelling may dictate decompression of the carpal tunnel and forearm compartments. Recent evidence[42] advocates the routine use of intracompartmental pressure monitoring in the management of pit viper envenomation as a way of preventing the disastrous sequelae of undiagnosed compartment syndromes.

Spider Bites

Loxosceles reclusa is native to the south and south central United States. Unlike the Black Widow spider, the venom of which is neurotoxic, the recluse spider's venom is cytotoxic. The bite may go unnoticed for six to eight hours because pain is not an early presenting symptom. Within 24 hours a central area of hemorrhage with induration is noted at the site, with a surrounding area of erythema. The zone of hemorrhage eventually becomes necrotic, turning dark with an eschar on the seventh day.

Early treatment consists of local injection of the antivenom, although it is not readily available.[41] Systemic symptoms that may accompany the bite may be treated early with either intralesional or systemic steroids, but their benefit and use remain questionable. Late treatment consists of ulcer excision and grafting when necessary.

BURN INJURIES

Thermal Injuries

In the emergency room the examining physician must first determine the exact location of the burn. Contact burns frequently occur on the palmar surface of the digits and hand, whereas flame burns occur more commonly on the dorsum. A diagram is made of the burn surface area and every attempt is made to indicate the depth of the burn. Burns are classified in terms of depth of injury as either first, second, third, or fourth degree. A first-degree burn is characterized by erythema and hyperesthesia. A second-degree burn is accompanied by more edema, blistering, and varying degrees of hyperesthesia and hypoesthesia. A third-degree burn is characterized by a hard, grayish-white anesthetic eschar. A fourth-degree burn is one that involves neurovascular or tendinous structures beneath the dermis as well as complete and irrevocable injury to the overlying skin.

The depth of the burn and its extent dictates the treatment.[9] First-degree and superficial second-degree burns with hyperesthesia or normal sensibility are best treated with topical antibiotics (Silvadine) and a loose-fitting polyethylene or rubber glove, which will minimize infection and the extension of the degree of tissue loss. Mobility of the joints is also maintained. The occlusive nature of the treatment significantly diminishes the pain that often accompanies such injury. Healing of the burn surface area is complete without hypertrophic scarring, changes in pigmentation, and limitation of motion, as frequently occurs with deeper burns.

Deeper second-degree and third-degree burns are best treated by early observation; splint immobilization with joint collateral ligaments in the maximally stretched position (MCP joints at 90° flexion, IP joints at 20° flexion, wrist at 25° to 35° flexion); application of a topical antibiotic; gentle compression to minimize edema; and frequent inspection and evaluation.[28] The burned hand must frequently be evaluated to rule out any possibility of vascular compromise as the result of direct endothelial injury and coagulation or progressive compartmental swelling. If vascular compromise has occurred, a fasciotomy or escharotomy is indicated. Whenever possible, incisions should be so planned as to avoid exposure of the deep structures and the deleterious effects of drying and secondary infection.

Treatment of deep second-degree burns and limited third-degree burns consists of excision of the eschar to viable tissue and grafting.[57] Excision is best performed during the early post-burn period when the wounds have demarcated and other systemic complications and injuries have been successfully treated or eliminated from consideration.[36]

Deep third- and fourth-degree burns require excision and flap coverage. Deeper structures such as tendons are best not debrided even though they appear nonviable, as late function may still result.

Special attention should be given to deep burns of the palmar surface of the hand. Evaluation of the exact mechanism of injury should consist of a good neurologic examination. Frequently deep palmar burns are associated with epilepsy, loss of consciousness, and prolonged contact to a hot object (infrequently noted in the alert, preinjury patient).

Palmar or volar skin is highly specialized in order to communicate with the environment. This glabrous skin contains a high concentration of mechanoreceptors and an increased number of myelinated nerve fibers and is also heavily keratinized and contains a thick, well-vascularized dermis. Again, thermal injuries to palmar skin are frequently not third-degree, thus treatment may consist of topical antibiotics and observation.

Burn wound contractures are less common in children than in the adult. Factors that contribute to contractures include protracted immobilization, extensive edema, and secondary bacterial invasion. As a result there is excessive collagen deposition, probably from myofibroblasts, which causes the undesirable late sequelae.[31] As indicated before, early excision and grafting for full-thickness and deep second-thickness injuries is most desirable, especially on the dorsum of the hand and fingers. Obviously, in patients with extensive burn injuries involving a significant total body surface area, treatment of hand injuries is secondary to resuscitative efforts and lifesaving procedures. During this time proper splint immobilization and antibiotic coverage is mandatory; following stabilization, treatment may proceed, based on the extent of burn injury.

Electrical Injuries

Electrical injuries are uncommon, accounting for only 3% of all burn wounds. They are frequently divided into low tension injuries (less than 500 volts) and high tension injuries (more than 500 volts). Burn injury is a direct consequence of heat and high voltage injuries may result in tissue temperatures of 5,000°C to 20,000°C.[18]

Low voltage injuries are confined to contact points, frequently involving the upper extremity in those areas containing glabrous skin. Contact may be prolonged because of tetanic muscle contraction precipitated by the alternating current. In addition to the time of contact, injury is related to the amount of heat or calories of the contacting object transmitted to the skin. This can be represented by the following formula:

$$\text{Calories: Amperage}^2 \times \text{Resistance}$$

High-voltage injuries are obviously more extensive, with often serious systemic manifestations. Cardiac dysrhythmias, myoglobinuria, convulsions, and falls from high places complicate the resuscitative effort. Wounds of entrance and exit are often of third and fourth degree and, because of the high resistance of bone and tendinous structures, excessive heat is generated with injury not only to these structures but also to the surrounding soft tissue. Arcing may occur across joint spaces or points of skin contact and cause a full-thickness thermal injury.

In extensive injuries amputation is common. However, recent reports indicate the usefulness of early excision of the involved tissue and vein grafting of major extremity arteries in order to provide distal perfusion through an area of third- or fourth-degree burn.[56] Aggressive surgical treatment follows treatment of the systemic manifestations and frequently includes escharotomies, fasciotomies, grafting, and flap coverage. Full-thickness excision and delayed wound coverage is thought to promote wound desiccation and accelerate necrosis from ischemic but viable tissue in the burn wound.

Chemical Burn Injuries

Chemical burn injuries to the hands are frequently associated with industrial injuries. Pain is a common accompanying symptom and its diminution with treatment often reflects the adequacy of the treatment provided. Initial treatment should consist of immediate, adequate irrigation. Then, the irrigating solution can be adjusted to a weak acid or alkali depending on the offending agent. With the advent of silicon wafers manufactured by the emerging computer industry, hydrofluoric acid burns have become increasingly more common. Treatment should consist of both a topical and intracutaneous injection of 10% calcium gluconate until the pain associated with the injury has been alleviated.[18]

REFERENCES

1. Adams JP, Dealy EJ, Kenmore PI: Intravenous regional anesthesia in hand surgery. J Bone Joint Surg 46A:811, 1964.
2. Atasoy E, Ioakimidis E, Kasdan ML et al: Reconstruction of the amputated fingertip with a triangular volar flap: A new surgical procedure. J Bone Joint Surg 52A:921, 1970.
3. Barton NJ: Fractures of the hand. J Bone Joint Surg 66B:159, 1984.
4. Bite N: Human bite injuries of the hand. Can J Surg 27:616, 1984.
5. Boyden TW: Snake venom poisoning: Diagnosis and treatment. Ariz Med 37:639, 1980.
6. Brown CG, Ashton JJ: Dog bites: The controversy continues. Am J Emergency Med 3:84, 1985.
7. Cooney WP, Dobyns JH, Linscheid RL: Fractures of the scaphoid: A rational approach to management. Clin Orthop 149:90, June 1980.
8. Curtis DJ, Downey EF, Barower AC et al: Importance of soft-tissue evaluation in hand and wrist trauma: Statistical evaluation. AJR 142:781–788, Apr 1984.
9. First W, Ackroyd F, Burke J, Bondoc C: Long-term functional results of selective treatment of hand burns. Am J Surg 149:516, 1985.
10. Garfin SR, Mubarak SJ, Davidson TML: Rattlesnake bites: Current concepts. Clin Orthop 140:50, 1979.
11. Garfin SR, Mubarak SJ: Treatment of rattlesnake bites—letter to the editor. J Hand Surg 5:619, 1980.
12. Gelberman RH, Garfin SR, Hewrgenroeder PT et al: Compartment syndromes of the forearm: Diagnosis and treatment. Clin Orthop 161:252, 1981.

13. Gelberman RH, Nunley JA, Koman LA et al: The results of radial and ulnar arterial repair in the forearm: Experience in three medical centers. J Bone Joint Surg 64A:383, 1982.
14. Glass TG Jr: Early debridement in pit viper bites. Surg Gynecol Obstet 136:774, 1973.
15. Glass KD: Factors related to the resolution of treated hand infections. J Hand Surg 7:388–94, 1982.
16. Grace TG, Omer GE: The management of upper extremity pit viper wounds. J Hand Surg 5:168, 1980.
17. Green DP, Anderson JR: Closed reduction and percutaneous pin fixation of fractured phalanges. J Bone Joint Surg 55A:1651, 1973.
18. Hentz VR: Burns of the hand: Thermal, chemical, electrical. Emergency Med Clin 3:391–403, 1985.
19. Kanaval AB: Infections of the Hand. Philadelphia, Lea & Febiger, 1925.
20. Kasdan ML, Kleinert HE, Kasdan AP, Kutz JE: Axillary block anesthesia for surgery of the hand. Plast Reconstr Surg 46:256, 1970.
21. Kleinert HE, Kasdan ML, Romero JL: Small blood-vessel anastomosis for salvage of severely injured upper extremity. J Bone Joint Surg 45A:788, 1963.
22. Kleinert HE, Kutz JE, Ashbell TS et al: Primary repair of lacerated flexor tendons in "No Man's Land." J Bone Joint Surg 49A:577, 1967.
23. Kleinert HE, McAlister CG, McDonald CJ, Kutz JE: A critical evaluation of cross-finger flaps. J Trauma 14:756, 1974.
24. Kleinert HE, Putcha SM, Ashbell TS, Kutz JE: The deformed fingernail, a frequent result of failure to repair nail bed injuries. J Trauma 7(2):177, 1967.
25. Kline DG, Hackett ER: Reappraisal of timing for exploration of civilian peripheral nerve injuries. Surgery 78(1):54, 1975.
26. Lampe EW: Surgical Anatomy of the Hand. Clinical Symposia 21(3). Summit, NJ; CIBA, 1969.
27. Linscheid RL, Dobyns JH, Beabout JW, Bryan RS: Traumatic instability of the wrist: Diagnosis, classification, and pathomechanics. J Bone Joint Surg 54A:1612, 1972.
28. Lister G: The Hand. 2nd ed. New York, Churchill Livingston, 1984.
29. Lister GD, Kleinert HE, Kutz JE, Atasoy E: Primary flexor tendon repair followed by immediate controlled mobilization. J Hand Surg 2(6):441, 1977.
30. Lucas GL, Bartlett DH: Pasteurella multocida infection in the hand. Plast Reconstr Surg 67:49, 1981.
31. Madden JW, Enna CD: The management of acute thermal injuries to the upper extremity. J Hand Surg 8:785–788, 1983.
32. McCollough NC, Gennaro JF Jr: Evaluation of venomous snake bite in the southern United States from parallel clinical and laboratory investigations. J Fla Med Assoc 49:956, 1963.
33. McDonald I: Eikenella corrodens infection of the hand. Hand 11:224, 1979.
34. Morrison WA, O'Brien BM, MacLeod A: Digital replantation and revascularization: A long term review of one hundred cases. Hand 10:125, 1978.
35. Mubarak SJ, Owen CA, Hargens AR et al: Acute compartment syndromes: Diagnosis and treatment with the aid of the wick catheter. J Bone Joint Surg 60A:1091, 1978.
36. Nielsen AB, Sommer J: Surgical treatment of the deeply burned hand. Burns 9:214–217, 1983.
37. O'Brien ET: Fractures of the metacarpals and phalanges. In Green DP (ed): Operative Hand Surgery. New York, Churchill Livingstone, 1982.
38. Omer GE: Report of the committee for evaluation of the clinical result in peripheral nerve injury. J Hand Surg 8(5):754, 1983.
39. Orgel MG: Epineurial versus perineurial repair of peripheral nerves. Symposium on Peripheral Nerve Microsurgery. Clin Plast Surg 11(1):101, 1984.
40. Ramamurthy S: Anesthesia. In Green DP (ed): Hand Surgery, p 23. New York, Churchill Livingston, 1982.
41. Reese R, Shack RB, Withers E et al: Management of the brown recluse spider bite. J Plast Reconstr Surg 68:769, 1981.
42. Roberts RS, Csencsitz TA, Heard CW Jr: Upper extremity compartment syndromes following pit viper envenomation. Clin Orthop 193:181, 1985.
43. Ruby LK: Common hand injuries in the athlete. Clin Sports Med 2(3):609, Nov 1983.
44. Russel FE, Carlson RW, Wainschel J, Osborne AH: Snake venom poisoning in the United States. JAMA 233:341, 1975.
45. Smith RJ: Intrinsic muscles of the fingers: Function, dysfunction, and surgical reconstruction. Instruct Course Lect 24:200, 1975.
46. Smith RJ: Post-traumatic instability of the metacarpophalangeal joint of the thumb. J Bone Joint Surg 59A:14, 1977.
47. Sneedon J: The Care of Hand Infections. Baltimore, Williams & Wilkins, 1970.
48. Sowder WT, Gehres GW: Snakebites in Florida. J Fla Med Assoc 49:973, 1963.
49. Spinner M: Kaplan's Functional and Surgical Anatomy of the Hand, 3rd ed. Philadelphia, J B Lippincott, 1984.
50. Stener, B: Displacement of the ruptured ulnar collateral ligament of the metacarpophalangeal joint of the thumb: A clinical and anatomical study. J Bone Joint Surg 44B:869, 1962.
51. Sunderland S: The interneural topography of the radial, median and ulnar nerves. Brain 68:243, 1945.
52. Sunderland S: The pros and cons of funicular nerve repair. J Hand Surg 4(3):201, 1979.
53. Tajima T: Considerations on the use of the tourniquet in surgery of the hand. J Hand Surg 8(5):799, Sept 1983.
54. Tubiana R: Examination of the Hand and Upper Limb. Philadelphia, WB Saunders, 1984.
55. Urbaniak JR: Replantation. In Green DP (ed): Operative Hand Surgery. New York, Churchill Livingston, 1982.
56. Wang XW, Lin HC, Sang HH et al: Early vascular grafting to prevent upper extremity necrosis after electrical burns: II. Experience with wound infection management. Burns 10:179–183, 1984.
57. Wang XW, Sun YH, Ahang ZM, Davies JWL: Tangential excision of eschar for deep burns of the hand: Analysis of 156 patients collected over 10 years. Burns 11:92–98, 1984.
58. Wilgis EFS: Nerve repair and grafting. In Green DP (ed): Operative Hand Surgery, p 915. New York, Churchill Livingstone, 1982.
59. Woods GL, Burton RI: Avoiding pitfalls in the diagnosis of the acutely injured proximal interphalangeal joint. Clin Plast Surg 8(1):95, Jan 1981.
60. Ya PM, Perry JF Jr: Experimental evaluation of methods for the early treatment of snake bite. Surgery 47:975, 1960.
61. Zook EG: The perionychium: Anatomy, physiology, and care of injuries. Clin Plast Surg 8(1):21, 1981.

nutrition in the trauma patient

John P. Grant

Since the introduction of intravenous parenteral nutrition by Dudrick and co-workers in 1968,[31] much has been learned about human nutrition, in particular, the metabolic requirements of the malnourished, hospitalized patient. The importance of providing essential fatty acids, various trace elements, vitamins, and proper proportions of the macronutrients protein, carbohydrate, fat, potassium, sodium, magnesium, and phosphorus, has all been stressed. The provision of parenteral and enteral nutrition to malnourished patients whose oral intake of nutrients is inadequate has become standard clinical practice in providing optimal care.

The extension of this highly effective medical therapy to the trauma patient in the critical care unit appears natural, for although many of these patients are not initially malnourished, they have heightened energy expenditures and nitrogen wasting, which lead to rapid nutritional deterioration if not adequately supported. Although the impact of aggressive nutritional support on clinical outcome of the trauma patient has been difficult to determine because of multiple other variables, including the severity of injury, there is no question as to its ability to provide safely necessary nutrients to fuel metabolic processes.

Intensive research has explored metabolic changes associated with trauma and evaluated the role of substrates in an attempt to develop the most effective formula for nutritional support. Although research is ongoing and much needs to be learned, complications induced by progressive starvation in patients who are otherwise salvageable are unacceptable with current technology. Quality care of all trauma patients must include an early evaluation of nutritional status and metabolic needs with institution of complete nutritional support. This chapter will deal with current concepts for the nutritional support of the trauma patient.

NORMAL METABOLIC RESPONSE TO STARVATION

Dietary intake is carefully modulated by complex neuroendocrine feedback mechanisms, so that caloric intake usually equals caloric expenditure and nitrogen intake equals nitrogen loss. A state of metabolic balance is established, which results in stable body weight and composition. When dietary intake is interrupted, the body adapts by cannibalizing body tissues to meet the metabolic needs of various organs.[19]

During the first two to three days of uncomplicated starvation, the body reacts by mobilizing body fat, glycogen, and protein. Certain tissues in the body, the central nervous system in particular, but also the renal medulla, red blood cells, and fibroblasts, require glucose as their energy substrate. The brain requires approximately 100 g to 120 g of glucose a day to meet its energy needs. This amount coupled with the needs of the renal medulla, red blood cells, fibroblasts, and other peripheral nerves brings the daily requirements of glucose to approximately 150 g. Glucose reserves in the body are quite limited, however, with only about 300 g to 400 g being present as glycogen in liver and muscle and as glucose in the intravascular space. The integrity of the central nervous system could not be maintained long without some mechanism for glucose production. A very efficient mechanism has evolved for glucose synthesis in starvation called *gluconeogenesis*. The process involves the breakdown of body protein and the full oxidation of the amino acid carbon skeleton to carbon dioxide and water or its use in subsequent synthetic pathways. The amino group from the amino acid is transaminated onto pyruvate, the anaerobic product of glucose metabolism, to form the amino acid alanine.[34,82] Alanine is subsequently transported to the liver where the amino group is split off with the formation of urea and the carbon skeleton channeled into pathways to synthesize glucose. The newly formed glucose is subsequently transported to peripheral tissues where it undergoes either complete oxidation to carbon dioxide and water or anaerobic metabolism to pyruvate, thus completing the cycle. It is estimated that for every 1800 calories used early in starvation, approximately 75 g of protein are broken down for gluconeogenesis and approximately 160 g of fat are metabolized.

As starvation continues, the body adapts by a gradual decrease in the basal metabolic rate associated with decreased activity, mild lethargy, decreased body core temperature, decreased cardiac rate and output, and decreased respiratory rate. The ability to reduce metabolic expenditure, however, is limited to 5% to 10% of the usual basal metabolic rate. Further reductions in energy expenditure are seldom recognized.

The hormonal response to prolonged starvation includes a decrease in circulating triiodothyronine (T_3) and an increase in reverse T_3, an inactive form.[87] Catecholamines and glucocorticoids slightly increase and growth hormone rises. The most significant change, however, is a fall in insulin and a rise in glucagon, causing a marked decrease in the molar insulin/glucagon ratio. As a result of the altered hormonal levels, or the increased alanine concentrations, or perhaps, some other process, the brain converts to using ketone bodies as an energy substrate and no longer requires glucose. This metabolic adaptation allows for a significant decrease in proteolysis and gluconeogenesis, with only 20 g to 25 g of protein turned over per day after five to seven days of starvation and a slight increase in lipid metabolism. The increase in lipolysis and oxidation of fat results in an increased production of ketone bodies and the development of starvation ketosis, reflecting a favorable metabolic response.

RESPONSE TO STARVATION IN THE TRAUMA PATIENT

Neuroendocrine Response to Trauma

The complex neuroendocrine response to stress has a marked impact on the metabolic response to trauma. The effects of the various hormones can be categorized as catabolic, anabolic, or modulating fluid and electrolyte balance.

CATABOLIC HORMONES

Glucocorticoids Injury causes a rapid increase in cortisol secretion for up to 24 to 48 hours. Even with minor injuries, two to five times the normal values of urinary hydrocorticoids can be detected for up to seven to ten days. In cases of severe or prolonged stress, urinary hydrocorticoids may be elevated for weeks to months and can eventually result in hypertrophy of the adrenal cortex. Cortisol, along with catecholamines, strongly stimulates lipolysis; inhibits protein synthesis in the periphery but stimulates protein synthesis in the liver; facilitates amino acid mobilization from muscle; induces the enzymes of gluconeogenesis; enhances secretion of glucagon while inhibiting insulin secretion; and stimulates conversion of lactic acid to glycogen.

Catecholamines The catecholamines, epinephrine and norepinephrine, can be detected in the bloodstream within seconds of injury. Although the biologic half-lives of both are short, they may be secreted for several days or longer in patients with severe stress, resulting in a prolonged metabolic effect. Epinephrine induces hepatic enzyme production, leading to glycogen breakdown, glycogenolysis, and gluconeogenesis; stimulates glucagon secretion; inhibits insulin secretion; stimulates lipolysis; enhances amino acid release from skeletal muscle; and inhibits the uptake of glucose by peripheral tissues. Epinephrine further leads to the secretion of pituitary adrenocorticotropic hormone (ACTH) and thus augments the release of glucocorticoids.

Glucagon Glucagon is a potent catabolic hormone secreted by the pancreas in response to trauma and is, in part, mediated by cortisol and cathecholamines as outlined above. Glucagon acts predominately on the hepatocyte, stimulating gluconeogenesis and glycogenolysis. In peripheral tissues it may enhance lipolysis and proteolysis, although these activities are less well documented.

ANABOLIC HORMONES

Insulin Insulin plays a central role in regulation of glucose metabolism. It inhibits gluconeogenesis and glycogenolysis in hepatic cells with the stimulation of glucokinase and uridine diphosphoglucose-glycosyl transferase, and the inhibition of pyruvate carboxylase and phosphorylase. Insulin further promotes glucose and potassium uptake by peripheral tissues, inhibits lipolysis, and favors amino acid uptake and protein synthesis in muscle. The stress reaction largely mediated by catecholamine release results in a marked depression in insulin production with increased glucagon production, lowering the molar ratio of insulin/glucagon and increasing gluconeogenesis and glycogenolysis. Although the sensitivity of adipose tissue to the effects of insulin following trauma change little, skeletal muscle has been shown to develop insulin resistance.[93]

Growth Hormone Stress is a strong stimulant of growth hormone secretion. Growth hormone stimulates nitrogen, phosphorus, and potassium retention, fatty acid oxidation, and ketogenesis. It also inhibits the action of insulin and promotes amino acid uptake with protein synthesis.

Androgens Testosterone, in addition to its other functions, acts as a potent anabolic hormone. It stimulates protein synthesis and decreases amino acid catabolism. During stress, catecholamines suppress testosterone production, and androgen concentrations are reduced.

FLUID AND ELECTROLYTE HORMONES

Antidiuretic Hormone Antidiuretic hormone is a powerful hormone responsible for maintaining a proper solute/solvent ratio in the serum. Hypovolemia and hypertonicity during stress stimulate antidiuretic hormone release from the posterior pituitary gland. The hormone's primary site of activity is the kidney, where it promotes water reabsorption.

Aldosterone This hormone promotes absorption of sodium bicarbonate and loss of potassium and hydrogen in the urine. Aldosterone secretion during stress is augmented by catecholamines and by hyponatremia. In addition, isotonic hypovolemia, by increasing renin production, leads to angiotensin release which in turn stimulates aldosterone secretion.

With the onset of trauma and associated pain and changes in intravascular volume, there is an increase in the central nervous system's sympathetic tone. This increase stimulates the pancreas to release increased amounts of glucagon and decreased amounts of insulin. The altered molar ratio of insulin/glucagon results in mobilization of peripheral muscle by proteolysis and the release of amino acids into the portal vein. The hypothalmus stimulates the anterior pituitary to secrete ACTH, which activates the adrenal gland to secrete catecholamines and cortisol. The hormonal response to trauma stimulates gluconeogenesis and glycolysis in the liver and results in an overall picture of glucose production and proteolysis. At the site of injury, afferent pain stimuli result in increased stimulation of the central nervous system, augmenting the neuroendocrine response. Bacterial growth in injured tissue produces various endotoxins that interfere with carbohydrate metabolism and can result in altered neurovascular tone and decreased organ perfusion and oxygenation. Inflammatory cells which migrate to the area of injury release a glycopeptide called interleukin I which induces fever, elicits granulocytopenia, increases amino acid release from muscle, and stimulates acute phase reactant protein synthesis by the liver.[7,22] In addition, interleukin I stimulates the pancreas to secrete both insulin and glucagon.

In uncomplicated trauma, the neuroendocrine response runs its course usually within four to seven days with eventual normalization of all values. In extensive trauma, particularly when complicated by repeated stress or the onset of sepsis, the neuroendocrine response can be sustained for weeks or months, converting an initial favorable response with respect to survival into a deleterious response leading to protein wasting, multiple organ system failure, and patient death.

Metabolic Response to Starvation During Trauma

Since the pioneering work of Cuthbertson in 1930,[28] it has been recognized that stress and trauma are associated with an increase in the basal metabolic rate. The degree and duration of this so-called catabolic response depends on the extent of injury and on the nutritional status of the patient. A patient who is nutritionally depleted tends to have a lower rate of catabolism and a poorer prognosis.[58] Body temperature is often elevated, probably by a temperature-regulator in the hypothalamus sensitive to catecholamines.[110] Cardiac and respiratory rates increase and the measured oxygen consumption increases to as high as twice the basal metabolic rate. There is a significant rise in protein synthesis, which accounts in large part for the increased metabolic rate. However, the rate of protein breakdown is even greater, resulting in a net nitrogen loss. As much as 120 g of protein per day can be broken down and used for gluconeogenesis. Increased glucose production along with a relative "insulin resistance" induced by catecholamine and cortisol release commonly results in hyperglycemia. Increased serum insulin concentrations blunt the effects of epinephrine on mobilization of fatty tissues for oxidation, resulting in only a mild increase in lipolysis for energy during starvation and stress (up to 160 g/day). Proteolysis occurs from different organs at different rates. Glucocorticoids stimulate immediate release of amino acids from skeletal muscle and skin accounting for most of the negative nitrogen balance.[36] Simultaneously, there is increased uptake of amino acids by the liver, both for gluconeogenesis and for acute-phase reactant of synthesis proteins, including fibrinogen, gamma globulin, haptoglobulin, ceruloplasmin, certain β-globulins, α_1-acid glycoprotein, α_1-antitrypsin, and the α_2-globulins.[40]

Consequences of Starvation During Trauma and Stress

Proteolysis during starvation and stress occurs in all protein-containing tissues with none spared, except perhaps the central nervous system. Seven-day fasting in rats produces a 30% body weight loss with a 30% to 40% decrease in mass of the liver, kidney, lung, gastrointestinal tract, and heart, with similar losses of organ protein content.[2,52] Similar data have been reported in man.[62] Associated with the loss of organ mass and protein content is impairment of organ function. Skeletal muscle function declines as starvation progresses. This was demonstrated in 1944[57] by the Minnesota experiment and again more recently by Lopes and colleagues.[69] Respiratory muscle function is also impaired in chronic malnutrition, as measured by pulmonary function tests.[6] Acute starvation decreases the maximal inspiratory vacuum and maximal expiratory pressure in hospitalized patients. Doekel and associates demonstrated that short periods of semistarvation in normal volunteers impaired the ventilatory response to hypoxia.[29] Likewise, Weissman and co-workers demonstrated loss of chemoreceptor sensitivity to hypercarbic gas mixtures following short periods of protein-free diets in normal volunteers.[109] Catabolism of the gastrointestinal tract leads to loss of villous height and absorptive surface with depletion of brush border enzymes and malabsorption.[103] Loss of normal gastric secretions is associated with bacterial overgrowth of the upper gastrointestinal tract contributing to diarrhea.[3] Delayed gastric emptying with small bowel hypermotility leads to nausea, vomiting, and diarrhea.[108] Hepatic function is markedly impaired in cases of undernutrition, with respect to both the mixed oxidative enzyme system and protein synthetic pathways.[85] In contrast, some enzyme systems, including the gluconeogenic series, increase in activity with progressive starvation. Changes in renal function during starvation include loss of concentrating ability with progressive diuresis in the face of dehydration and impaired ability to excrete acid leading to metabolic acidosis.[60,61] In children, clearance of aminoglycosides may be impaired because of altered glomerular and tubular function and severe protein depletion.[59] Cardiac contractility and output are depressed and tolerance to volume challenge limited.[1,63] Immune system function becomes impaired as starvation progresses, causing loss of chemotactic and phagocytic activity of the lymphocyte, anergy to common skin test antigens, and impairment of the humoral response.[64,74]

Due to these alterations in organ function, as well as other complex interactions, undernourished patients have an increased incidence of morbidity and mortality. Surveys of infectious complications in patients undergoing clean surgical procedures demonstrate that malnutrition (defined as weight loss and low serum albumin concentrations) is as important a factor in outcome as old age, obesity, diabetes, and infections in other parts of the body.[23,27] Relationships have been reported between morbidity and mortality and various nutritional parameters, including serum albumin and transferrin concentrations, delayed type hypersensitivity skin test reactions, percent weight loss from usual weight, and various combinations of these.[49,76] As a rule, patients admitted to critical care units for evaluation and treatment of major trauma should be receiving adequate nutritional support within the first 24 to 48 hours of admission after resuscitation. Optimal care must include drainage of septic foci, good surgical techniques, correction of metabolic abnormalities, and resuscitation from shock to avoid repeated stressful events leading to multiple organ failure.

NUTRITIONAL SUPPORT OF THE TRAUMA PATIENT

Substrate Requirements

FLUID REQUIREMENTS

Fluid requirements for patients receiving nutritional support are considerably higher than those required during 5% dextrose infusion. Formulas used to calculate fluid needs when 5% dextrose is infused are based either on weight (100 ml/kg for the first 10 kg, 50 ml/kg for the next 10 kg, and 20 ml/kg for each kilogram thereafter) or body surface area (1500 ml/square meter). Both formulas assume a catabolic state to be present with breakdown of body tissues for energy releasing 300 ml to 500 ml of water from intercellular spaces. With introduction of nutritional support, new body tissue is synthesized and, indeed, if therapy is effective, there is a net increase in lean body mass requiring new intercellular water. It is therefore necessary to provide from 300 ml to 500 ml fluid per day more than normal during adequate nutritional support. In addition, with fever there is an increased fluid loss via perspiration of approximately 360 ml/C per day which must be replaced. Third-space fluid losses due to trauma as well as measured external losses from fistulas, nasogastric drainage, and open wounds must also be replaced.

However, intubated patients receiving humidified air can absorb from 200 ml to 500 ml of fluid from the inhaled gas mixture. Often trauma patients are receiving multiple antibiotics and other drugs diluted in various volumes of intravenous solutions which may total a liter or more a day. The presence of renal failure and congestive heart failure limit fluid supplementation, while hemodialysis or peritoneal dialysis cause variable fluid losses. It is therefore necessary to monitor fluid needs of the trauma patient closely during nutritional support. Carefully kept records of input and output and daily weight are vital.

CARBOHYDRATE REQUIREMENTS

The neuroendocrine response and the heightened metabolic rate of trauma and stress prevent adaptation to starvation. The brain continues to require glucose as a fuel substrate and the overall caloric expenditure may be from 10% to 100% greater than the resting state, which requires from 35 to 45 kcal/kg/day. Patient studies using indirect calorimetry performed by Long and colleagues led to a modification of the original Harris-Benedict equation, which gave a better estimate of daily caloric expenditure (Fig. 19.1).[68] The modification includes an activity factor as well as an injury factor.

In early clinical experience with nutritional support, it was felt that the estimated caloric expenditure of traumatized and stressed patients should be met by providing an appropriate amount of glucose. Subsequent studies, however, have shown that in stress the maximal rate of glucose utilization is actually reduced because of the neuroendocrine response. Black and associates demonstrated the maximal rate of glucose utilization in stressed, critical-care patients to be 6.23 ± 0.87 mg/kg/min, while normal control subjects could use 9.46 ± 0.79 mg/kg/min.[9] Studies by Burke and colleagues demonstrated that as intravenous glucose infusion rates were increased, the percentage of carbon dioxide excreted from glucose oxidation rose progressively up to approximately 5 mg/kg/min glucose infusion, after which no further increase occurred, suggesting maximal utilization as an energy source.[17] Furthermore, when protein synthesis was measured during increasing glucose infusion, maximal protein synthesis was observed at 5 mg/kg/min glucose infusion. Thus, optimal carbohydrate support during stress is considered to be approximately 5 mg/kg/min. Attempts to improve glucose oxidation and nitrogen sparing with exogenous insulin has been of little value. Although blood glucose concentrations can be lowered by insulin injection, increased glucose oxidation and nitrogen sparing have not been documented. Potential adverse effects of insulin administration must also be considered. Insulin is known to stimulate the uptake of amino acids in the muscle and to block the release of amino acids from muscle protein, thus reducing the availability of amino acids in the vascular pool for protein synthesis in the liver. Furthermore, it has been proposed that the increased serum insulin and free fatty acids associated with the neuroendocrine response to stress may inhibit the activity of pyruvate dehydrogenase and therefore limit entry of glucose into the Krebs cycle for oxidative metabolism. Excessive glucose infusion leads to increased pyruvate concentration favoring fat synthesis pathways, which use up energy and produce carbon dioxide.

In general, it is suggested that carbohydrate support be provided to each patient's tolerance as indicated by an increase in blood sugar concentrations above 150 to 200 mg/dl or a rise in respiratory quotient above 1. In some patients with low levels of stress, all caloric requirements can be met by the infusion of glucose alone. As the stress level increases and glucose tolerance decreases, glucose infusion must be reduced as necessary to 5 mg/kg/min. Controversy exists as to whether to provide additional calories up to total calculated needs after glucose infusion is reduced, and whether the additional calories should be long-chain triglycerides, medium-chain triglycerides, standard crystalline amino acids, branched-chain amino acids, glucose, or other carbohydrates such as fructose or xylose.

In patients receiving peritoneal dialysis, it is important to recognize that up to 25 g glucose can be absorbed from the peritoneal cavity during the dialysis cycle. Patients receiving 4.25% dialysis solutions on hourly cycles may require no additional carbohydrate infusion intravenously.

FIGURE 19.1
ESTIMATION OF DAILY CALORIC EXPENDITURE

ACTIVITY FACTOR	USE	INJURY FACTOR	USE
Confined to bed	1.20	Minor operation	1.20
Out of bed	1.30	Skeletal trauma	1.35
		Major sepsis	1.60
		Severe thermal burn	2.10

Men: $(66.47 + 13.75W + 5.0H - 6.76A) \times$ (activity factor) $\times$ (injury factor) = kcal/day

Women: $(655.10 + 9.56W + 4.85H - 4.68A) \times$ (activity factor) $\times$ (injury factor) = kcal/day

W, weight in kg; H, height in cm; A, age in years.
Modified from Long CL, Schaffel N, Geiger JW et al: Metabolic response to injury and illness: Estimation of energy and protein needs from indirect calorimetry and nitrogen balance. JPEN 3:452–456, 1979.

FAT REQUIREMENTS

Three fatty acids cannot be synthesized by the human body and are therefore essential in the diet: linolenic, arachidonic, and linoleic acids. Although linolenic acid has no known metabolic function in the adult, it appears to be important in the development and maturation of the nervous system in the premature and newborn baby. Arachidonic acid can be synthesized in the presence of the third essential amino acid, linoleic acid. For this reason, in the adult, linoleic acid is considered the main essential fatty acid and, when provided, all symptoms of essential fatty acid deficiency can be avoided. Arachidonic acid is a precursor to the prostaglandin series, and as such plays a critical role in responses to stress and trauma. The body has ample amounts of essential fatty acids stored in fatty tissues. However, with infusion of dextrose solutions, insulin concentrations rise sufficiently to dampen mobilization of these fatty acid pools and numerous cases of essential fatty acid deficiency involving both the adult and infant populations have now been reported during total parenteral nutrition using carbohydrate as a caloric source.[39,84] To avoid essential fatty acid deficiency syndrome, exogenous essential fatty acids must be provided. The minimal amount of linoleic acid required daily is estimated to be between 1% and 2% of the total caloric support (the most commonly recommended safe amount is 4%). The provision, therefore, of 500 ml to 1000 ml of a 10% lipid emulsion given intravenously weekly can prevent essential fatty acid deficiency during total parenteral nutrition and should be the minimal amount infused.

Clinical symptoms of essential fatty acid deficiency may take weeks or months to become obvious. They include a dry, thick, desquamated skin, loss of muscle tone, fatty liver with hepatomegaly, thrombocytopenia, alopecia, and, in the infant population, growth retardation.[39,84] Biochemical evidence of essential fatty acid deficiency occurs when the enzyme system responsible for converting linoleic acid to arachidonic acid, in the absence of linoleic acid, generates 5,8,11-eicosatrienoic acid from oleic acid. A triene (5,8,11-eicosatrienoic acid) to tetraene (arachidonic acid) ratio greater than 0.4 in tissue and plasma phospholipids has been considered diagnostic of essential fatty acid deficiency.[50] Biochemical evidence of essential fatty acid deficiency has been detected as early as one to three weeks after the beginning of fat-free parenteral nutrition.

Lipid emulsions have also been proposed as a caloric source in the treatment of trauma patients, especially when intolerance prevents adequate caloric support from glucose infusions. Clinical studies have shown rapid clearance of lipid emulsions from the bloodstream in most patients. Theoretically, lipid catabolism should be enhanced by hormones released during stress: epinephrine, glucagon, and cortisol. Hormone-sensitive lipases hydrolyze triglycerides in the tissues, leading to an elevation of the level of nonesterified fatty acids in plasma and thus increasing their availability for oxidation. Indeed, several investigators have reported an increased rate of elimination of fat emulsions during stress.[46] Yet there appears to be a breakdown in the clearance mechanism as Lindholm and co-workers found significant impairment of lipid clearance in patients with multiple organ failure; most clinicians recommend that lipid infusions be greatly reduced in this clinical setting.[65]

Whenever lipids are used as a caloric source, it is assumed that the infused triglycerides will be taken up, as endogenous triglycerides are, by the lipocyte, hepatocyte, and peripheral tissues for oxidation, and that energy will be generated. Yet in a study by Goodenough and colleagues, only about 8% of infused lipids were immediately oxidized, with the remainder retained as neutral fats within the body and either stored or used later for energy production.[38] Further studies are needed to document both improved nitrogen sparing with increased caloric support using lipid emulsions and improved nitrogen flux. Fischer has stated that fat as a fuel drives hepatic tissue protein synthesis more efficiently than does carbohydrate and that hepatic gluconeogenesis is fueled by fat.[35] Whether infusion of lipid emulsions to provide the additional needed calories in excess of glucose tolerance is of actual clinical benefit in the trauma patient remains to be documented. Nonetheless, it is common clinical practice to infuse from 20% to 40% of caloric requirements in the form of lipid emulsions during stress and trauma without significant adverse clinical effects. Beneficial effects reported include a reduction in the respiratory quotient, decreased requirement for insulin, and lower blood sugar concentrations.

Some concerns have been raised about using long-chain fatty acids in total parenteral nutrition solutions. Lipid emulsions have a higher propensity to support bacterial growth than dextrose solutions or dextrose and amino acid solutions and there is some concern that 3-in-1 mixes may result in increased exposure to possible septic complications.[73] Furthermore, when the rate of lipid administration exceeds clearance by the lipolytic system, activation of the reticuloendothelial system may occur with phagocytosis of fat particles and impairment of the reticuloendothelial system's ability to phagocytose and kill invading organisms.[47] When this occurs, it may increase the risk of septicemia.

Lipid emulsions containing both long-chain fatty acids and medium-chain fatty acids (so-called *structured lipids*) are under investigation. An advantage of these products is that the medium-chain fatty acids may be more readily used as an energy source. Unlike long-chain fatty acids, medium-chain fatty acids do not require carnitine for entry into mitochondria for oxidation. Carnitine deficiency, although rare, may be seen in patients with abnormal renal function or liver, cardiac, or muscle disease; patients under metabolic stress or during hemodialysis; and patients with inadequate dietary intake of carnitine or its precursors.[12,104] Maiz and associates showed an improved nitrogen balance in rats with 25% full-thickness, scald skin burns when part of the caloric load was given as a structured lipid (60% medium-chain fatty acids and 40% long-chain fatty acids).[70] Hamaway and colleagues demonstrated better bactericidal capabilities of the reticuloendothelial system in injured and septic rats who were given the structured lipid product than those who received only long-chain fatty acids.[47] It might be preferable, therefore, to give lipid emulsions as a caloric source in the traumatized patient at no more than 40% of the nonprotein caloric input and preferable that they be given as a structured lipid formula. Structured lipid formulas are still under investigation. They may be marketed in the near future.

In conclusion, lipid emulsions should be provided to meet at least essential fatty acid requirements of all patients, and if tolerated, as a nonprotein caloric source in patients who are carbohydrate intolerant. Until further studies document effectiveness and safety, no more than 50% of the nonprotein calories should be supplied as a lipid emulsion. Care must be taken to ensure that the lipid emulsions are cleared from the bloodstream by monitoring either serum triglyceride levels (less than 350 mg/dl six hours following infusion in an adult) or free fatty acids, or by simple observation of plasma samples for turbidity. To avoid impairment of the reticuloendothelial system, it is suggested that the lipid emulsion not be given at a rate greater than 1 kcal/kg/hr.

Lipid infusion has not been adequately tested in patients with severe sepsis and multiple organ failure. To date, clinical experience in the very ill patient contraindicates intravenous lipid. Cerra and co-workers have claimed that in sepsis, lipid catabolism is decreased while glucose catabolism is increased.[21] In this setting, intravenous lipids would only have value if there were indeed a shortage of branched-chain amino acids and if their oxidation could be reduced by the increased oxidation of fatty acids. The presence of anoxia, or failure of the liver or kidneys, probably negates the usefulness of lipids. Further investigation is necessary.

Ketone Bodies Studies using conjugated ketone bodies as a caloric source are under way. These intermediates of fat metabolism enter the energy cycle more easily than either long-chain fatty acids or medium-chain fatty acids. Preliminary studies have demonstrated reasonable tolerance and some nitrogen-sparing capabilities; however, the product is far from being clinically available.[96]

NITROGEN NEEDS

The requirement for protein in a trauma patient is significantly greater than in a healthy individual. The minimal protein requirement to maintain neutral nitrogen balance in the well-nourished, unstressed individual has been estimated at 0.6 g/kg/day.[4] Hartley and Lee[48] found 1.5 g/kg/day of protein minimal for routine postoperative patients, while Bozzetti reported requirements of 1.5 g to 2.9 g/kg/day with stress.[13] Burn patients have been reported to require up to 12.9 g to 15.9 g of nitrogen per square meter per day during the acute catabolic phase.[102]

Requirements for protein and calories are interrelated. Studies of nitrogen balance during constant infusion of adequate protein have demonstrated a proportional relationship between nitrogen retention and the level of caloric support.[77] Similarly, with fixed adequate caloric intake, patients show improved nitrogen retention with increasing protein infusion.[102] Coexistence of increased nitrogen wastage requiring heightened nitrogen input due to stress, and the relationship between improved nitrogen balance with increased protein loading, has led to the common practice of infusing trauma patients with from 1.5 g to 2.5 g/kg/day of protein, depending upon the degree of stress. Documentation of optimal protein infusion can be obtained clinically by collecting 24-hour urine samples and assaying for total nitrogen excretion, and then combining that with any nitrogen lost through wounds or fistulas or from the gastrointestinal tract; the total output is compared with the infused nitrogen to determine nitrogen balance. In optimal states of metabolic support, a 3-g to 5-g positive nitrogen balance can be expected. Accumulations of greater than this are of unknown clinical significance. Negative nitrogen balances are indicative of a continued catabolic state. Infusion of 1.5 g to 2.5 g/kg/day of protein in the trauma patient is often associated with a rise in the blood urea nitrogen, but usually requires no attention unless the value exceeds 100 mg/dl.

With recent documentation of impaired glucose utilization in trauma patients, and with the questionable ability of lipid emulsions to improve nitrogen retention, research has been focused on the use of other fuel substrates during trauma and sepsis. Much attention recently has been given to branched-chain amino acid metabolism.[56] Unlike other amino acids, which are predominantly metabolized by the liver, leucine, isoleucine, and valine appear to be metabolized solely in muscle, heart, and kidney tissue, with the major site of oxidation in muscle. The process in skeletal muscle is characterized by transamination of the amino group (—NH_2) to form the gluconeogenic amino acids alanine and glutamine,[91] which are then transported to the gut, kidney, and liver as substrates for subsequent gluconeogenesis. The branched-chain amino acid carbon skeleton following transamination can be used in protein synthesis or can be oxidized to carbon dioxide and water in gut, muscle, heart, and kidney tissue to generate needed ATP for other metabolic processes. If the branched-chain amino acids are provided intravenously, they are oxidized directly and thus appear to reduce the amount of muscle degradation which might otherwise occur, thereby improving nitrogen balance. At the same time they can serve as an alternate donor of an amino group for alanine and glutamine synthesis to participate in gluconeogenesis.[10]

Freund and others have shown in animal models that branched-chain amino acids, in addition to providing nitrogen, have a nitrogen-sparing effect beyond the calculated balance.[37,71] Nitrogen flux studies suggest this nitrogen-sparing effect is due to a reduction in protein catabolism. Moyer and colleagues demonstrated improved nitrogen retention and survival rates using branched-chain amino acid infusion in patients with multiple organ failure,[75] and Cerra and co-workers[20] and Nuwer and associates[81] have shown improved immunocompetence. These studies have lead to the current recommendation for use of branched-chain amino acid enriched solutions during nutritional support in the traumatized and stressed patient. Optimal enrichment appears to range from the standard solutions of 15% to 25% branched-chain amino acids by weight to solutions containing from 45% to 50% branched-chain amino acids by weight. Studies have documented leucine to be the most important regulator of protein synthesis.[78] One clinical study has demonstrated a higher whole body catabolism rate in patients who received a 45% branched-chain amino acid solution low in leucine as compared with those who received the same solution containing high leucine concentrations.[11] Therefore it appears that optimal supplementation should have high leucine concentrations. It is suggested that these enriched solutions be given to provide between 1.5 g and 2.0 g/kg/day of protein supplemented by as much nonprotein caloric support as tolerated. This typically results in solution formulations with a nonprotein calorie/nitrogen ratio of 100:1 or 80:1, the lower ratio being required in late sepsis or during marked insulin resistance. In severe sepsis, protein loading can be increased to as high as 3 g/kg/day.

Three formulas of branched-chain amino acids for intravenous use are currently available: Aminosyn-HBC 7%, which is a 45% branched-chain amino acid solution containing molar ratios of isoleucine/leucine/valine of 1:2:1; BranchAmin 4%, which is a 100% branched-chain amino acid solution with a molar ratio of

1:1:1; and FreAmine HBC 6.9% with a molar ratio of 1:1.8:1.4. Several branched-chain enriched enteral feeding products are available and will be discussed in the next section.

Enteral Nutrition

Whenever possible, the gut should be used for nutritional support in trauma patients. The provision of nutrients enterally results in lower costs and lower risk of sepsis and maintains the integrity of the gut mucosa better than intravenous nutritional support. The latter point is very important in light of one postulate that suggests that the breakdown of the gut mucosal barrier with transport of intraluminal toxins into the portal blood is an initial step leading to multiple organ failure and death. Some preliminary data suggest the addition of glutamine to intravenous solutions preserves the gut histologically, but further studies are necessary to test whether glutamine protects the mucosal barrier and reduces the incidence of and mortality from multiple organ failure. One report suggests a lower incidence of upper gastrointestinal hemorrhage in stressed patients when a glutamine-containing solution is given enterally as compared to parenterally.[86]

ACCESS

Voluntary oral intake in the trauma patient is rarely adequate to meet daily nutrient requirements. The patient often has oropharyngeal injuries, obstruction of oral or nasal airways, and anorexia. When oral intake is possible, all efforts should be made to organize the patient's daily schedule to allow for pleasant eating conditions to encourage maximal intake. Calorie and protein intake records should be maintained to document the adequacy of the oral diet. When oral intake is impossible or inadequate, yet the gastrointestinal tract is capable of assimilating nutrients, some other access must be tried. If gastric emptying is adequate and there is minimal risk of aspiration, simple placement of a nasogastric tube or a gastrostomy is usually effective. In the presence of delayed gastric emptying or in patients with altered mental status in whom aspiration would represent a significant risk, enteral feeding accesses should be placed distal to the stomach and preferably in the proximal jejunum. If surgical exploration is undertaken, consideration should be given to placing a needle-tube jejunostomy.[105] More permanent access can be achieved by placing a larger bore Witzel jejunostomy. If it is expected that an oral diet will be resumed relatively quickly after an operative procedure, a nasojejunal tube can be placed during surgery with the assistance of anesthesia. As the tube is passed into the stomach, the surgeon can direct it around the duodenal sweep and draw it into the proximal jejunum.

If no surgical procedure is done, or if access is not established at the time of surgery, nasojejunal access can still be achieved by either passing an 8F or 10F feeding tube under fluoroscopic guidance[44] or by endoscopy.[30] The possible complications of pulmonary intubation must be recognized.[66]

SOLUTION ADMINISTRATION

Gastric tube feeding solutions can be either continuous infusion or bolus type. Continuous infusion should be begun at 50 ml/hr with full-strength feeding solution advanced at 25 ml/hr every six to eight hours until full support has been reached. Gastric residuals should be checked every four to six hours and if greater than 100 ml residuals are identified, 100 ml should be reinjected into the stomach and the remainder discarded and replaced by intravenous solutions. The feeding solution should be continued at the same rate. As tolerance improves, residuals will decrease to less than 100 ml.

Bolus feedings may be administered effectively in several ways. One satisfactory method begins with infusion of 50 ml of full-strength solution each hour and advancing it after eight to 12 hours to 100 ml/hr, and eight to 12 hours later to 200 ml every two hours. Thereafter, the amount infused and time between infusions is gradually increased until full support is obtained with six to nine feedings per day. No more than 500 ml of feeding solution should be bolused at one time and the rate of infusion should be over five minutes or more, since both high volume and rapid rate of infusion delay gastric emptying. Residuals should be checked before each feeding and handled in the manner described for continuous infusion. Feedings into the jejunum, whether by nasojejunal or jejunostomy tube, should be begun at 50 ml/hr using a diluted formula (one-half strength) to avoid hyperosmotic diarrhea. Every six to eight hours either the strength of the solution should be increased (by one quarter) or the rate of administration (by 25 ml/hr), depending on whether the patient has volume or osmotic intolerance. Within 48 to 72 hours, the patient should be advanced to full-strength solution at the appropriate rate to administer calculated needs. If intolerance is encountered, the feedings should be decreased to the previous rate and strength that were tolerated and then advanced more slowly.

AVAILABLE SOLUTIONS

Four basic groups of enteral feeding products are available commercially. The first group contains intact protein and complex carbohydrates along with various combinations of long- and medium-chain triglycerides. These products are isotonic or only slightly hypertonic, usually low residue (although some high-residue products are now available), lactose-free, and relatively inexpensive. They provide all known nutrients in adequate amounts to meet daily needs and are usually palatable for oral ingestion. Their consistency is such that they pass through nearly all feeding catheters including the small needle-tube jejunostomy catheters. However they require frequent flushing with boluses of water and still occasionally clog small-bore feeding tube systems.

The second group of products, called *chemically defined,* are also low residue and lactose-free, but contain partially hydrolized protein, which the package insert usually reports by percentage within specified molecular weight ranges. The carbohydrate is a polymer of glucose or a combination of simple and complex sugars; fat is present as medium- and long-chain triglycerides, although the total is less than in the first group of products. These solutions are less viscous and pass through small feeding tubes without difficulty. They provide all required nutrients when given in adequate amounts. They are mildly hypertonic, less palatable, and more expensive.

The third group of products are so-called *elemental* solutions and consist of crystalline amino acids, glucose, and minimal amounts of long-chain triglycerides. They are hypertonic, low residue, lactose-free, unpalatable, and expensive. In adequate amounts, they meet all daily requirements for vitamins and minerals; however, they are borderline to deficient in providing essential fatty acids.

The final group are specialized products intended to be used with failure of selected organs such as the kidneys, liver, and lungs. Also within this group are enteral products designed specifically for use during trauma and stress. These products contain partially hydrolized protein or crystalline amino acids modulated by the addition of branched-chain amino acids to comprise 23% to 44% of the total protein. The carbohydrate content is typically maltodextrins and sucrose; fat content is a combination of medium- and long-chain triglycerides providing 10% to 40% of the caloric load. They are generally concentrated solutions providing between 1.0 and 1.5 kcal/ml and have a calorie/nitrogen ratio of from 175:1 to 100:1 (Fig. 19.2).

Modular substrates are available for alteration of specific formulas. Fig. 19.3 lists some of the available products. Not all are compatible with enteral feeding products and testing should be performed prior to administration to assure compatibility.

FIGURE 19.2
EXAMPLES OF ENTERAL PRODUCTS FOR STRESS CONDITIONS

PRODUCT	KCAL/ML	CARBOHYDRATE	PROTEIN*	FAT*	OSM	NONPROTEIN CALORIES†	%BCAA
Traum-Acid HBC	1.0	166	56	12	640	102	50%
TraumaCal	1.5	95	55	45	550	90	23%
Stresstein	1.2	142	58	23	910	97	44%
Vivonex T.E.N.	1.0	206	38	2.8	630	149	33%

* Grams per 1000 kcal solution.
† Per gram of nitrogen.

FIGURE 19.3
EXAMPLES OF AVAILABLE MODULAR PRODUCTS

PRODUCT	CARBOHYDRATE*	PROTEIN*	FAT*	SODIUM†	POTASSIUM†	CHLORIDE†	MAGNESIUM†	PHOSPHATE‡
PROTEIN								
ProMod	24	179	21	20	59			758
Casec		238	5	18	1	1		2162
ProPac	15	190	20	25	32			
ProMix	15	208	12	28	59			
CARBOHYDRATE								
Polycose	250	0	0	12	1	14		
Moducal	250	0	0	8	0.3	13		
Sumacal	250	0	0	11		16		
FAT								
Microlipid	0	0	111	0	0	0		
MCT Oil	0	0	121	0	0	0		
Lipomul	0	0	111	0	0	0		

* Grams per 1000 kcal solution.
† mEq per 1000 kcal solution.

COMPLICATIONS OF ENTERAL FEEDING

Clogging of the enteral feeding tube is a frequent complication which can require replacement of the tube to reestablish flow. This is seldom a problem with the larger bore gastrostomy or nasogastric tubes, but with smaller nasoenteric and jejunostomy tubes the feeding solution can curdle and solidify under the influence of the gastric acidity or the alkalinity of the small bowel, causing blockage of the tube exit ports. Frequent irrigation with tap water or normal saline can assist in dislodging debris, but it will not always prevent clogging. Sometimes a change to a chemically defined or elemental product, or even to another brand within the same group of products can alleviate clogging. Gentle irrigation should be tried with a syringe no smaller than 50 ml; anything smaller can generate excessive pressure and result in rupture of the feeding tube. If this occurs in the nasopharyngeal area, aspiration can occur. Insertion of a guidewire to attempt to break up the blockage is always fruitless, fraught with danger of disruption of the catheter and perforation of the intestine, and should be avoided. If patency is not established with irrigation, the tube should be exchanged.

Diarrhea is the most common complication of enteric feedings. Diarrhea with enteral feeding is often appropriate because most enteral products have minimal residue, resulting in a semiliquid or liquid stool. The debilitation brought on by trauma and sickness often includes poor voluntary sphincter control and the patient's continual soilage of liquid stool can be misinterpreted as diarrhea. Instead of turning off the feeding solution when diarrhea is reported, a thorough evaluation should be performed. The first question to ask is whether diarrhea is really present. Unless 1000 ml or more of diarrhea occurs a day, the loss is probably clinically insignificant and requires no specific management. Normal stool water content ranges from 200 ml to 500 ml/day and significant losses of electrolytes and water rarely occur until over 1000 ml/day are lost. A simple measurement is the first procedure to do when diarrhea is suspected.

If significant diarrhea is indeed documented, it may be due to one of several causes. Too rapid an increase in rate or concentration is simply treated by returning to the previous rate or concentration tolerated and advancing more slowly. Bolus feeding administered without a pump or a catch-up attempt that is made when the infusion falls behind schedule is often met with a dumping–type syndrome and massive diarrhea. The rate of infusion should vary by no more than 20%. In particular, bolus administration in the jejunum will be followed by significant diarrhea. Bacterial overgrowth of the feeding solution can result in enteritis with diarrhea. None of the commercially available feeding solutions contain preservatives and if exposed to room temperature for over eight hours can acquire significant bacterial overgrowth.[5,94] Feeding bags should be filled with no more than enough solution for eight hours and care should be taken to maintain as much sterility as possible.

Steatorrhea is an uncommon complication of enteral feeding but may occur with solutions containing high concentrations of fat. A change to products containing combinations of long- and medium-chain triglycerides may help, or a change to products containing low fat may be necessary. The addition of lactose to the diet by ordering full-liquid oral diets may well result in diarrhea. Improper administration of hypertonic medications through the enteral feeding tube can also cause diarrhea by an osmotic load. A look at the osmolality of typical medications administered to trauma patients will reveal why administration of these products directly into the small bowel without dilution can cause an osmotic diarrhea (Fig. 19.4).[80] All drugs are best given parenterally or through the stomach, but when it is necessary to give medications through the small bowel, they should be appropriately diluted with feeding solution or tap water. Severe atrophy of the mucosal surface with loss of brush border enzymes associated with malnutrition can be another cause for tube feeding intolerance. In this case, continued administration of enteral feedings is important to stimulate mucosal regrowth and enzyme recovery, which cannot be accomplished with intravenous nutrition alone. Finally, less common causes of diarrhea include hypoalbuminemia, essential fatty acid deficiency, zinc deficiency, and laxative abuse.

Treatment of the cause of the diarrhea usually suffices to resolve the problem and the use of agents to slow bowel motility such as codeine, Lomotil, paregoric, or Imodium, is rarely necessary. When indicated, these medications can be added to the tube feeding solution so that they are infused slowly and continuously, or they can be given in divided doses.

Aspiration of feeding solutions is not uncommon, occurring most often when the solutions are administered into the stomach. Patients with altered mental states from stress or following head trauma are at highest risk for aspiration, with reports of up to 40% showing signs of aspiration pneumonitis clinically or at

FIGURE 19.4
OSMOLALITY OF VARIOUS DRUGS

DRUG	CONCENTRATION	MOSM/KG
Aldactone suspension	25 mg/ml	2245
Digoxin elixir	50 mg/ml	3000
E.E.S. suspension	200 mg/5 ml	4475
Keflex suspension	250 mg/5 ml	2445
KCl elixir 10% (sugar-free)		3000
KCl injection	2 mEq/ml	3600
K phosphate injection	3 mM P/ml	5450
Lasix Oral	10 mg/5 ml	3938
NaCl injection	4 mEq/ml	7090
Na phosphate injection	3 mM P/ml	4650
$NaHCO_3$ injection	1 mEq/ml	1730
Phenobarbitol elixir	400 mg/dl	3000
Tagamet liquid	300 mg/ml	4035
V-Cillin-K suspension	250 mg/5 ml	2995

autopsy.[83] Although it is recommended that the head of the bed be elevated 30° during gastric feedings, many trauma patients cannot tolerate elevation. Metoclopramide has occasionally improved gastric emptying, but its effects are unpredictable. Even passage of the feeding tube into the jejunum does not entirely eliminate risks of aspiration pneumonitis, gastric acid secretion will continue and may reflux, even though gastric feedings are not being administered. In addition, a few patients develop gastric hypersecretion in response to jejunal feedings with production of 3 to 4 liters of gastric juice per day. This response appears not to be abated by H_2 receptor antagonists and may require placement of a nasogastric tube for gastric decompression to protect the patient from aspiration.

An unusual but serious complication of enteral feeding is the development of transmural necrotizing enteritis. This complication occurs most commonly in the elderly, critically ill patient with low cardiac output and poor intestinal motility. Although the exact etiology is not clear, forced feeding into the jejunum may lead to pooling of the feeding solution in the lumen of the bowel with subsequent bacterial overgrowth. Bacterial toxins and intact bacteria may penetrate the wall leading to localized enteritis, ischemia, and transmural necrosis with microperforations of the intestine usually along the antimesenteric border. The development of necrotizing enteritis is indicated clinically by fever, tachycardia, abdominal cramps, bloating, and diarrhea which is occasionally bloody. Continuation of the enteral feedings may lead to gangrene and perforation. The histologic changes are most severe at the tip of the feeding catheter and decrease distally, suggesting that this is not a problem of vascular occlusion. Abdominal x-ray films initially show a mottled appearance of the intestines, followed by pneumatosis, and finally, free intraperitoneal air when perforation occurs. To avoid this complication of enteral feeding in the jejunum in patients in whom gastrointestinal motility may be compromised, water soluble contrast material should first be injected through the catheter and then gut motility evaluated fluoroscopically. If gut motility and gross anatomic appearance are normal, enteral feedings can be carefully initiated. If mild to moderate dilation of the bowel is observed with dysmotility characterized by a churning motion or retrograde peristalsis, it is best to avoid enteral feedings and give parenteral nutrition instead.

Drug-nutrient interactions can occur any time drugs are given during enteral feedings. The pharmacokinetics of most drugs have been studied following oral ingestion on an empty stomach. The simultaneous administration of medications with enteral feeding products raises questions of compatibility, with possible precipitation or gel formation, denaturation of either the feeding solution or the drug, and interference of one with the other's absorption. Of further concern is the administration of a drug at a site which may alter its properties, including absorbability and activity. Some drugs require acidification in the stomach, while others have not been studied with respect to direct administration into the small intestine. Some drugs exert their effect only at a specific site, such as antacids in the stomach. Timed-release properties of drug preparations can be destroyed if they are pulverized for administration through small tubes in the jejunum. Finally, the hypertonicity of drugs must be taken into consideration any time a drug is placed into the gastrointestinal tract through a tube for fear of inducing a dumping-type syndrome.

Parenteral Nutrition

When the gastrointestinal tract is unusable for nutritional support in the trauma patient, either due to ileus, enterocutaneous fistulas, or inability to gain access, there should be no hesitancy to turn to intravenous nutritional support. Although risks of electrolyte imbalance, substrate intolerance, and sepsis are higher and cost is significantly greater than with enteral nutrition, the greatest risk is of progressive malnutrition. Much has been written about the application of total parenteral nutrition to the hospitalized patient.[42,55] Only those issues which are unique to the trauma patient are discussed here.

ACCESS

Standard techniques may be used for placement of a subclavian catheter for vascular access in the trauma patient. At times, trauma of the head and neck area renders access through the subclavian or internal jugular vein impossible and occasionally the antecubital or femoral veins must be used. Use of these alternative routes is associated with a higher incidence of thrombophlebitis and sepsis and should be restricted. Recently, there has been increased use of right atrial Silastic catheters placed in the subclavian vein in critically ill patients. The single- or dual-lumen Silastic catheter does provide excellent vascular access for blood sampling and fluid administration and yet still allows total parenteral nutrition to progress with a minimal increase in infectious complications. However, polyvinyl chloride catheters used for multiple access have been repeatedly shown to be associated with an unacceptable increase (30% to 50%) in septic complications. There has been a recent trend to use triple-lumen polyvinyl chloride subclavian catheters in the trauma patient without ample documentation of their safety. Experience with multiple-access polyvinyl chloride catheters suggests that the rate of infectious complications would be unacceptable with triple-lumen catheters as well. Indeed, some studies have documented a tenfold increase in septic complications when triple-lumen catheters are left in place more than 48 to 72 hours.[72] Other studies have demonstrated acceptable infectious complication rates from prolonged use of triple-lumen catheters when sterile isolation techniques are practiced on each of the lumens and access is limited to only that mandated by clinical needs.[26] In general, it is suggested that the triple-lumen subclavian catheter be left in place for a maximum of 72 hours. This limits the usefulness of the triple-lumen catheter for total parenteral nutrition, but it serves to initiate therapy until an isolated subclavian catheter can be placed. Piggybacking into arteriovenous fistulas or shunts has been done on occasion. This technique has a slightly increased incidence of access thrombosis and the possibility of significant hemorrhage should the administration needle become detached.

Complications of vascular access are summarized in Figure 19.5 as a reminder of the importance of proper technique and experience. Review of the literature suggests that insertion complications are related to the experience of the physician and increase in emergency conditions. With an experienced physician placing the catheter electively in a cooperative patient, major complications should occur at an incidence of less than 1%. Trauma patients in the intensive care unit seldom present optimal conditions for catheterization because of the altered anatomy, difficulty with proper positioning, and poor patient cooperation. It is therefore important that subclavian vein catheter placement be done by the most accomplished and experienced individual available.

A recent report documents the problem of multiple central venous access catheters tangling *in situ*, making catheter removal difficult and central venous thrombosis more likely.[41] When superior vena caval access for total parenteral nutrition is established, therefore, an attempt should be made to remove all other unnecessary central venous access catheters. Further, care should be taken to perform cannulation on a side where no other catheters are passing through the subclavian vein or innominate vein. Occasionally, the other catheter is damaged during cannulation by the insertion needle, and even severed, resulting in catheter embolization.

ADMINISTRATION OF TOTAL PARENTERAL NUTRITION

Fifty percent to 75% of the calculated caloric and nitrogen requirement should be administered during the first 24 hours to allow determination of substrate tolerance and a clearer definition of electrolyte requirements. Laboratory values should be reviewed following 12 hours of nutrient infusion and the necessary adjustments made in formulation and the rate advanced to full support. Typically, patients can be started on 1500 ml to 2000 ml of nutrient solution and advanced 24 hours later to full support. Severe glucose intolerance can mandate changes in solution formulation, including adding more fat and reducing carbohydrate and perhaps using a branched–chain amino acid–enriched formula. All solutions should be administered using electronic control devices to assure steady infusion of nutrient solutions without the danger of interruption or runaway infusions. If solutions are prepared properly under sterile technique in the pharmacy, and no additives are placed in the bags after delivery to the ward, in-line millipore filters are unnecessary. Such filters cannot be used when albumin or lipid emulsions are added to the nutrient solution as both will rapidly clog the filters.

AVAILABLE SOLUTIONS

Multiple carbohydrate solutions are available which range in concentration from 5% to 70%. Selection of carbohydrate concentration is based upon needed fluid restriction. Many pharma-

FIGURE 19.5
COMPLICATIONS OF SUBCLAVIAN VASCULAR ACCESS

AUTHOR	DATE	#	THROMBOSIS	PNEUMOTHORAX	WRONG VEIN	UNSUCCESSFUL	ART INJURY	BRACHIAL PLEXUS INJURY
Newsome[79]	1984	137		4			4	
Jones[54]	1984	307		5	2	5		
Conces[24]	1984	500		7	160	20		
Lockwood[67]	1984	131		10				
Falcone[32]	1985	140		4	11	23	4	
Sitzman[100]	1985	200		6	10		10	
Fares[33]	1986	225		4	10	6	2	
Schug[95]	1986	210	1	5	9		6	
Grant	1989	3164	22	43	189	110	10	1
Total		5104	23	88	391	164	36	1

cies find that a 70% dextrose solution that can be diluted with sterile water as necessary to meet fluid requirements is less expensive overall and allows maximal flexibility with the least inventory.

There are five lipid products available in the United States: Intralipid, Liposyn, Liposyn II, Travamulsion, and Soyacal. Each is available as a 10% (1.1 kcal/ml) or a 20% (2 kcal/ml) emulsion. All contain glycerine for isotonicity and egg yolk phospholipids as emulsifier agents. Polyunsaturated fatty acid profiles vary between products due to their different fat sources: Travamulsion, Intralipid, and Soyacal contain soybean oil, while Liposyn contains safflower oil and Liposyn II contains equal amounts of safflower and soybean oil.

Although protein and fibrin hydrolysates were important during the development of nutritional support, they have no clinical use today. Amino acid products now available consist of synthetic crystalline amino acids. Depending upon the respective amino acid salts, various electrolytes are also present. The various solutions range in concentration from 3.5% to 11.4%. When one is compounding solution formulations, the electrolyte composition of the various solutions must be carefully considered. As noted earlier, three branched-chain enriched amino acid formulas are available, Aminosyn-HBC 7%, BranchAmin 4%, and FreAmine HBC 6.9%. Aminosyn-HBC 7% and FreAmine HBC 6.9% are intended to be used as a complete amino acid product to be added to dextrose and supplemented with fat to provide total parenteral nutrition. BranchAmin 4%, in contrast, is intended as an additive to enrich the branched-chain amino acid component of other amino acid solutions.

Following is a list of the electrolyte salts most commonly used for total parenteral nutrition. The sequence of mixing is quite important to reduce the incidence of precipitation:

1. Calcium salts
2. Multivitamin solution
3. Folic acid
4. Ascorbic acid
5. Sodium chloride
6. Sodium lactate and acetate
7. Potassium chloride and acetate
8. Magnesium sulfate
9. Potassium phosphate
10. Sodium phosphate
11. Heparin
12. Trace elements
13. Albumin
14. Regular insulin

Following each addition, the solution should be thoroughly mixed, and after all additives are mixed the solution should be carefully inspected for precipitants against both a light and dark

FIGURE 19.5
COMPLICATIONS OF SUBCLAVIAN VASCULAR ACCESS (CONTINUED)

AUTHOR	THORACIC DUCT INJURY	SKIN BLEED	HEMOTHORAX	HYDROTHORAX	SUBCUT EMPHYS	AIR EMBOL	CATH EMBOL	TOTAL COMPL	% COMPL
Newsome[79]		3						12	8.8
Jones[54]								13	4.2
Conces[24]								187	37.4
Lockwood[67]								10	7.6
Falcone[32]								45	32.1
Sitzman[100]								26	13.0
Fares[33]								22	9.8
Schug[95]								20	9.5
Grant	3	15	1	1	4	3	1	402	12.7
	3	18	1	1	4	3	1	737	14.4

background. After final inspection, the solution should be sent to the patient's floor and refrigerated until used. An expiration date of 48 hours should be placed on each unit once additives have been injected. Compatibility of various electrolytes with the amino acid and carbohydrate solutions will allow complete support to be established in most cases through the central access catheter. On occasion, however, calcium, phosphorus, and magnesium requirements may be so great that precipitation will occur when all are added to the same intravenous formulation. In these instances, additional mineral support should be given through a peripheral intravenous catheter. In my experience, 1 liter of standard nutrition solution, when mixed appropriately, will tolerate any concentration of sodium, potassium, and chloride, up to 15 mEq calcium, 30 mEq magnesium, and 30 mM of phosphate.

Insulin can be added in any concentration and is completely compatible. Monocomponent insulin, preferably recombinant DNA synthetic human insulin, should be used to reduce allergic reactions. Albumin, steroids, cimetidine and ranitidine appear to be compatible in all concentrations. Hydrochloric acid can be added directly to the nutrient solution without adverse effects, except possibly on vitamins and trace elements. If other central accesses are available, it is recommended that hydrochloric acid be administered through those lines. It is generally recommended that antibiotics be administered through separate peripheral intravenous lines rather than piggyback into the central catheter along with the nutrient solution. Studies, however, have suggested that many antibiotics and various drugs are compatible with the nutrient solution (Fig. 19.6) and may be given piggyback if sterile technique is observed.

COMMON ELECTROLYTE ADDITIVES IN TOTAL PARENTERAL NUTRITION

- Sodium
  - acetate
  - chloride
  - lactate
  - phosphate
  - iodide
- Potassium
  - acetate
  - chloride
  - phosphate
- Calcium
  - gluconate
  - gluceptate
- Magnesium
  - sulfate
- Chronic chloride
- Manganese sulfate
- Cupric sulfate
- Selenous acid
- Zinc sulfate chloride
- Ammonium
  - molybdate
  - tetrahydrate

FIGURE 19.6
COMPATIBILITY OF VARIOUS DRUGS WITH TOTAL PARENTERAL NUTRITION SOLUTIONS

DRUG	COMMENTS
* Albumin	Soluble
* Aminophylline	500 mg/L
+ Ampicillin	1 g/L, decays rapidly
+ Carbenicillin	8 g/L, decays with time
+ Cefamandole	
+ Cefazolin	1 g/L
+ Cefoxitin	
+ Cephalothin	2 g/L, impaired by vitamins, stable
+ Cephapirin	
+ Cephadine	
O Chloramphenicol	700 mg/L
* Cimetidine	300 mg/L, stable
+ Clindamycin	600 mg/L
* Cyanocobalamin	1 mg/L, degraded by vitamin C
* Cyclophosphamide	500 mg/L
* Cytarabine	100 mg/L
+ Dobutamine	
* Dopamine	400 mg/L
+ Erythromycin	1 g/L
* Fluorouracil	1000 mg/L, stable up to 48 hr
* Furosemide	40 mg/L
+ Gentamincin	80 mg/L, impaired by vitamins, stable
* Heparin	Soluble
* Hydrochloric acid	0 1 N
* Hydrocortisone	Soluble
* Insulin	Soluble
* Iron dextran	100 mg/L, stable
* Isoproterenol	2 mg/L
+ Kanamycin	500 mg/L, impaired by vitamins, decays with time
* Levarterenol	4 mg/L
* Lidocaine	1 g/L
* Metaraminol	100 mg/L
+ Methicillin	1.5 g/L, stable
* Methotrexate	50 mg/L
* Methyldopate	500 mg/L
* Methylprednisolone	250 mg/L
* Metoclopramide	3 g/L
+ Oxacillin	500 mg/L
+ Penicillin G	5 million units, intramuscularly preferred, limited stability
O Phytonadione	10 mg/L, intramuscularly preferred
* Polymyxin B	40 mg/L, stable over 24 hr
+ Tetracycline	500 mg/L
+ Tobramycin	80 mg/L

* Mixable; + best to piggyback only; O uncertain compatibility.
Note: Stability and availability depend on amino acid solution, pH, electrolyte additives, temperature, and storage time. Risk of formation of immunogenic and allergenic breakdown products with time must be considered. Multiple additive compatibility unknown. Read all references before using. Never mix unless necessary. Piggyback when possible.
Reprinted from Ref. 55, p 140, by courtesy of Marcel Dekker, Inc.

Complications of Total Parenteral Nutrition

SUBCLAVIAN VEIN THROMBOSIS

Subclavian vein thrombosis may occur in 5% to 20% of patients who receive total parenteral nutrition.[14] Often the thrombosis is not recognized clinically because collateral vessels form rapidly. When symptoms are recognized, unilateral swelling of the arm, shoulder, neck, or head may occur, or even bilateral swelling may be observed. Occasionally headaches and blurred vision are reported. Thrombosis may occur as early as 24 to 48 hours following insertion of the catheter, but more commonly occurs after one to two weeks. Studies have noted the rapid formation of a fibrin sleeve on the outside of the subclavian catheter and have suggested that continual deposition of platelets and fibrin results in gradual occlusion of the subclavian vein.[51] These patients commonly demonstrate some or all of Virchow's triad of factors conducive to venous thrombosis: local vessel trauma, a hypercoagulable state, and reduced blood flow. Bern and coworkers have suggested that a fall in antithrombin III is associated with thrombosis in selected patients and have recommended prophylactic administration of low-dose Coumadin when the antithrombin III level is abnormal.[8] Use of heparin-bonded catheters, Silastic catheters, and catheters coated with water-activated lubricants and the addition of 1000 to 2000 units of heparin per liter of parenteral nutrition solution have all reduced the incidence of subclavian catheter thrombosis.

Treatment of subclavian vein thrombosis is dictated by clinical symptoms. If no symptoms are observed, no treatment can be given. If arm swelling and edema is observed, the catheter should be removed and the extremity elevated. Heparinization is recommended with conversion to Coumadin with anticoagulant therapy continued for four to six weeks. If total parenteral nutrition is still needed, a new catheter can be placed by way of the opposite subclavian vein. Occasionally, the thrombosed vein will recannulate, but usually it fibroses to a thin cord and is no longer useful for catheterization. Early infusion of streptokinase or urokinase to dissolve subclavian vein thrombosis should be highly effective and will obviate removal of the catheter and avoid fibrosis of the vein, but experience with this technique is minimal and long-term results are unknown.[101] Although rare, it is possible for the patient to suffer a pulmonary embolis from subclavian vein thrombosis.

CATHETER-RELATED SEPSIS

The actual incidence of catheter-related septic complications when a standard protocol is followed for catheter insertion, dressing care, and catheter utilization is less than 1% in noninfected patients and less than 3% in patients harboring infections elsewhere in the body.[42] Achievement of such safety requires meticulous care of the catheter exit site and isolation of the catheter infusion system to prevent contamination. Nutrient solutions must be prepared under laminar flow hood conditions and no additives should be injected after initial preparation.

When the fever of catheter-related sepsis does occur, it is often difficult to recognize in trauma and critically ill patients because there are other known causes of fever. Sometimes, however, a change in the febrile pattern, an elevation in white blood count, or clinical signs of sepsis will dictate concern. When sepsis is suspected, all other intravenous catheters should be removed. A thorough physical examination should be performed and appropriate laboratory and radiographic studies ordered to define the source of sepsis. If a source of sepsis is identified, appropriate therapy should be given and total parenteral nutrition continued through the same catheter. If no septic source is identified, a culture should be drawn through the subclavian catheter with a simultaneous peripheral blood culture also drawn. The catheter should be removed and the tip of the catheter sent for culture. If the catheter tip culture is positive, or if the differential colony count shows a 100-fold increase in the blood from the catheter, a primary catheter infection can be assumed to be present. After 24 to 48 hours of appropriate antibiotics, a new subclavian catheter can be inserted for continued parenteral nutrition. It should be stressed that all *Candida* infections should be treated with therapeutic doses of amphotericin to avoid systemic candidiasis and endophthalmitis. Some clinicians have proposed exchange of the subclavian catheter over a guidewire with culture of the removed catheter as an alternative to removal of the catheter.[15] This technique carries the potential risk of introducing skin contaminants into the bloodstream during catheter exchange and is to be discouraged.

ELEVATION OF LIVER ENZYMES

Elevation of the serum liver enzymes SGOT, SGPT, and occasionally LDH and bilirubin may occur between the seventh and eighth day of nutritional support in 60% to 90% of patients, with a second elevation after 20 days in 20% to 40% of patients receiving carbohydrate-based total parenteral nutrition.[43] Typically, SGPT and SGOT are elevated, with LDH and serum bilirubin elevations less frequently observed. Physical examination may demonstrate an enlarged, tender liver, but liver failure is usually absent. This clinical syndrome appears to be unique to total parenteral nutrition and is not observed during enteral nutrition.

Etiology of elevated liver enzymes is probably multifactorial. It has been variously attributed to toxic effects of a product of tryptophane breakdown, to essential fatty acid deficiency, to fatty acid surplus, and to biliary stasis. The most commonly proposed mechanism, however, is steatosis secondary to carbohydrate overload. Hall and colleagues used an intravenously fed rat model to demonstrate that hepatic steatosis occurred during intravenous nutrition because of abnormalities in all four possible mechanisms for fat deposition in the liver.[45] There was increased hepatic lipogenesis, decreased fat oxidation, increased mobilization of fat from peripheral tissues with uptake in the liver, and decreased mobilization of fat from the liver to the peripheral tissues. Provision of an isocaloric and isonitrogenous nutrition solution that had 30% of the glucose caloric load replaced with lipid emulsion resulted in a marked decrease in lipid deposition and decreased elevation of liver enzymes.[90] Although long-term effects of hepatic steatosis secondary to total parenteral nutrition remain to be identified, concern has been raised that progressive liver failure and cirrhosis may occur. Injury to the rat hepatic microsomal enzyme system has been documented with both decreased absolute concentrations and depression of antipyrine clearance.[89] These effects might have a serious impact on the trauma patient as many drugs used in the intensive care unit are cleared similarly through the hepatic microsomal enzyme system (Fig. 19.7).[16]

ALLERGIC REACTIONS

Allergic reactions to B-complex vitamin additives and lipid emulsions have occasionally been reported during total parenteral nutrition. Reaction to vitamins is characterized by a rash with perhaps some increased fever and tachycardia. Allergic reaction to lipid emulsions may take one of two forms. The first occurs rapidly during infusion and is characterized by fever, chills, vomiting, and pain in the chest or back. The second type of reaction is generalized pruritic urticaria and occurs later, often several hours after infusion. Other associated symptoms may include palpations, tachypnea, nausea, wheezing, headache, and occasionally an oily taste in the mouth. Following prolonged lipid administration, the patient may exhibit hepatomegaly, jaundice with centrilobular cholestasis, thrombocytopenia, eosinophilia, leukopenia, and occasionally splenomegaly. Rarely, a fat overload syndrome occurs, characterized by hyperlipidemia, acute fever, focal seizures, leukocytosis, hepatosplenomegaly, shock, and spontaneous bleeding due to platelet dysfunction. This syndrome appears to be dose-related, occurring usually when doses exceed 4 g/kg/day.

Complications of Refeeding

REFEEDING SYNDROME

Occasionally, the initiation of enteral or parenteral nutritional support is associated with an idiosyncratic reaction referred to as the "refeeding syndrome." The patient will experience severe intermittent headaches, usually felt to be due to carbohydrate loading, progressive lethargy which may result in a semicomatose state and, on occasion, loss of bladder and bowel control. These symptoms usually resolve with no alteration in feeding. Occasionally a hypermetabolic response is observed, characterized by a progressive rise in cardiac and respiratory rate, a rise in body core temperature, and an increase in oxygen consumption. This response is best treated by reduction in caloric support followed by a very gradual increase and careful monitoring. The greater the degree of malnutrition, in particular cardiac wasting, the more the patient is intolerant to fluid loading and is susceptible to heart failure or pulmonary edema. Concomitant administration of diuretics and careful fluid management is usually required. Finally, rapid onset of hypophosphatemia with paresthesia, mental obtundity, and even coma may be seen during refeeding, especially during administration of high glucose loads.[99] Glucose mobilizes phosphorus intracellularly and chemically binds it. Interruption in the glucose load results in rapid restoration of serum phosphorus. The syndrome can be avoided by providing adequate phosphorus supplementation. Monitoring of serum phosphorus is necessary to identify this complication and the treatment is to administer supplemental intravenous phosphate using sodium or potassium salts.

ELECTROLYTE DEFICIENCIES

The requirements for sodium and chloride, extracellular electrolytes, are little different during nutritional support than during routine 5% dextrose infusion. However, requirements for electrolytes concentrated within the cells—potassium, phosphorus, and magnesium—differ significantly during nutritional support. If starvation has led to body wasting, total body content of potassium, phosphorus, and magnesium may be significantly depleted, even though serum concentrations are relatively normal. With refeeding, these electrolytes are carried by the flux of carbohydrate and water into intracellular spaces, resulting in a rapid fall in serum concentrations, which may lead to clinically detectable deficiency syndromes. In addition to the need to

FIGURE 19.7
DRUGS CLEARED BY THE HEPATIC MICROSOMAL ENZYME SYSTEM

DRUG METABOLISM	ENZYME
Oxidation of Aliphatic and Aromatic Groups	Cytochrome P-450
Barbiturates	
Diazepoxides	
Phenothiazines	
Meprobamate	
Phenytoin	
Antihistamines	
Antipyrine	
Acetophenetidin	
Aminopyrine	
Some synthetic steroids	
Reduction of Azo- and Nitro- Groups	Flavin enzymes
Choramphenicol	
Propylthiouracil	
Hydrolases of Esters and Amides	Esterases
Procaine	
Lidocaine	
Atropine	
Meperidine	
Conjugations with Glucuronic Acid	Transferases
Alcohols	(UDP-GT)*
Phenols	
Acetaminophen	

*UDP-GT, uridine diphosphate-glucose transferase.
Brodie BB, Gillette JR, LaDu BN: Enzymatic metabolism of drugs and other foreign compounds. Annu Rev Biochem 27:427-452, 1958 and Remmer H: The role of the liver in drug metabolism. Am J Med 49:617–629, 1970.

replace total body deficits, establishment of an anabolic state is associated with new cell formation and a need for new intracellular water, which contains high concentrations of these three electrolytes. Daily requirements for potassium during anabolism range from 60 to 150 mEq, phosphorus 20 to 60 mM, and magnesium between 15 and 20 mEq.

Potassium depletion is characterized by alterations in the electrocardiogram with sagging ST segments, low voltage, flat or inverted T-waves, and prolongation of the QT intervals. Clinically, it is identified by cardiac arrythmias with ectopic atrial impulses, hyporeflexia, muscle weakness, general malaise, paresthesias, gastrointestinal ileus, metabolic alkalosis, and pseudodiabetic glucosuria. Clinical symptoms of phosphate depletion occur usually when the inorganic phosphate concentration falls below 1.0 mg/dl. Symptoms include paresthesia; absent knee tendon reflexes; weakness of the muscles of the extremities, neck, mastication, and respiration; hyperventilation; mental obtundity; rhabdomyolysis, and an abnormal electromyogram.[99] Hypophosphatemia may also lead to depletion of ATP, with associated conformational changes of red blood cell membranes leading to rigid spherocytosis. The oxyhemoglobin curve is shifted to the left with impaired oxygen delivery to peripheral tissues and a decrease in red blood cell and platelet survival time.[106] Impaired white blood cell chemotaxis and phagocytosis has also been reported.[25] Clinical symptoms of hypomagnesemia are seldom seen unless serum magnesium falls below 1.0 mEq/liter. Symptoms mimic those of hypocalcemia and to differentiate them it is often necessary to obtain serum values. Typically confusion, hyperactive deep tendon reflexes, convulsions, tetany, positive Chvostek's and Trousseau's signs, tremor, clonus, nystagmus, paresthesias, weakness, and muscle fasciculations are observed.[97,107] Marked hypomagnesemia may also lead to severe potassium wasting in the urine. The importance of proper electrolyte supplementation was stressed by Rudman and associates when they demonstrated optimal nitrogen repletion required adequate supplementation of all electrolytes in addition to nitrogen and calories.[92] Depletion of any individual electrolyte was associated with an impaired nitrogen repletion rate.

TRACE ELEMENT DEFICIENCIES

In addition to the well known signs of iodine and iron deficiencies, clinical deficiency syndromes have now been identified for zinc, copper, chromium, manganese, and selenium. Total parenteral nutrition solutions contain minimal amounts of trace elements and enteral solutions contain a highly variable amount. Careful monitoring and supplementation are necessary during nutritional support to avoid clinical deficiency states. Abnormal losses of trace elements are not infrequent in the trauma patient; zinc, for example, is lost in fluid from fistulas or stomas with up to 17 mg/kg lost from the distal small bowel and 12.2 mg/kg lost nasogastrically. Copper and manganese are excreted in the bile and depletion can occur when biliary diversion is present or increased serum concentrations can occur with biliary obstruction. Chromium is excreted in increased amounts during stress through the kidneys and can lead to chromium deficiency.

Clinical settings where zinc deficiency is commonly observed include chronic liver disease as with cirrhosis, long-term corticosteroid therapy, after major surgery or trauma, malabsorption syndromes, and zinc-deficient total parenteral nutrition or oral diet. Clinical symptoms of zinc deficiency include diarrhea; mental depression; paranasal, paraoral, scrotal, and generalized dermatitis; alopecia; poor wound healing; decreased taste and smell acuity; and a distorted sense of taste and smell with anorexia and weight loss. Copper deficiency is associated with a hypochromic normocytic anemia, depressed reticulocyte count, and neutropenia, which is marked by a severe decrease in the percentage of polymorphonuclear cells. Occasionally, hypoproteinemia with periorbital or presacral edema is present. In animals, hair loss and skin discoloration due to depression of tyrosinase has been reported. Chromium deficiency results in decreased glucose tolerance due to altered sensitivity of peripheral tissues to insulin. Manganese deficiency has been infrequently observed but has been reported to be associated with weight loss, slow growth, a transient dermatitis, occasional nausea and vomiting, and hypocholesterolemia. In experimental animals, a diabetic-like glucose intolerance has been observed. Selenium was declared an essential trace element in humans relatively recently; lack of it causes muscle tenderness, and perhaps red blood cell rigidity and white blood cell dysfunction.

NUTRITIONAL SUPPORT IN PATIENTS WITH SELECTED ORGAN FAILURE

Acute and Chronic Renal Failure

Depressed renal function, associated with variable degrees of fluid and nitrogen retention, presents problems primarily of waste elimination. Basic metabolic processes remain mostly unchanged. This is not to say that there are no metabolic abnormalities during renal failure; but these are usually secondary to the clinical condition causing the renal failure rather than to renal failure itself, for example, sepsis, hemodynamic instability, drug toxicity, and severe liver disease. It follows, therefore, that nutritional support should be tailored to fit the altered metabolic status due to the primary disease and rarely should changes be made due to just renal failure.

It is preferable to provide optimal nutritional support and use hemodialysis or peritoneal dialysis as a substitute for the kidney in clearing metabolic waste products. If effective dialysis can be established, nitrogen retention is rarely a problem and full support can be provided. If dialysis is inadequate, however, fluid restriction may be necessary and can be accomplished by using concentrated solutions of dextrose, amino acids, and lipid emulsions. Nitrogen restriction is unnecessary until blood urea nitrogen reaches a level of clinical concern, usually at or above 100 mg/dl. Levels of blood urea nitrogen exceeding 100 mg/dl increase the risk of platelet dysfunction and may alter mental function, thus compromising patient cooperation. If this is encountered, the amount of protein infused should be progressively reduced until a satisfactory concentration is obtained. However, less than 50 g/day may result in inadequate delivery of essential amino acids and possibly amino acid deficiency syndromes. It is therefore recommended that infusions of less than 50 g/day be supplemented with essential amino acids. For enteral infusions, products available include Amin-Aid and Travasorb Renal. Products available for intravenous infusion include Nephramine and Aminosyn R.F. These products rarely need to be given as the sole source of nutrition as neither the enteral nor intravenous products contain trace elements, vitamins, or minerals. To check that total supplementation is adequate, the amount of each essential amino acid in the standard amino acid product should be added to the amounts in the supplemental product.

In a few trauma patients, hemodialysis or peritoneal dialysis is not possible and severe restrictions in fluid and protein are required. In this clinical setting, the essential amino acid solutions with concentrated dextrose and lipids for calories with no electrolyte, mineral, or vitamin components can be used, which will allow continued limited metabolic support—a preferable alternative to complete withdrawal. By infusing this very high biologic value protein diet with adequate caloric support, in the presence of adequate liver function, urea nitrogen can be reused in the synthesis of nonessential amino acids and subsequent protein. Low nitrogen input coupled with use of endogenous urea nitrogen can result in a reduction of blood urea nitrogen with stabilization usually under 100 mg/dl, depending upon the degree of trauma and catabolism. Whether the liver retains the capability to synthesize all other necessary nonessential amino acids remains unproven, and use of this highly specialized diet should be limited to for very specific clinical indications.

Effective metabolic support in patients with renal failure will often significantly reduce mobilization of cellular electrolytes and may initiate lean body mass synthesis. Careful monitoring of potassium, phosphorus and magnesium is therefore necessary and at times supplementation may be required to avoid deficiencies. Trace element and vitamin supplementation may be necessary to avoid deficiency syndromes.

Cardiac Failure

Two types of cardiac failure must be distinguished as they mandate different metabolic support. One type is secondary to primary myocardial disease, such as atherosclerosis with subsequent myocardial infarction and dysfunction, valvular disease, constrictive pericarditis, and various myocardiopathies. The second type is due to malnutrition with wasting of myocardial mass, depression of contractility, and loss of volume tolerance.

In primary diseases of the myocardium, the nutritional status is limited by cardiac output. Any increase in lean body mass or metabolic demand can aggravate cardiac failure. The goals of nutritional support should solely be to maintain current nutritional status, matching input as nearly as possible to daily metabolic needs and making no attempt to increase lean body mass. Attempts to improve the nutritional status can only be undertaken if the primary myocardial disease is corrected, such as following coronary artery bypass grafting or replacement of a defective cardiac valve. No special nutritional solutions are mandated, except as indicated by volume restriction and other organ dysfunction. Enteral nutritional support may not be possible because of poor gastrointestinal motility if cardiac output is severely compromised.

Nutritional support in patients who suffer severe cardiac wasting with cardiac dysfunction due to starvation presents an entirely different clinical problem. In this setting, the goal is to gradually rehabilitate the nutritional status allowing time for recovery of cardiac mass and function. It is this patient population, however, that poorly tolerates volume and caloric loading and that frequently experiences the refeeding syndrome. Nutritional support should be instituted gradually, with careful monitoring for signs of a hypermetabolic state or volume overload. Diuretics may be necessary early in the treatment program for several days to a week to achieve full nutritional support. Caloric and nitrogen requirements should initially be based on the patient's current weight, and then advanced to reflect the patient's usual or ideal body weight. So far, no special substrate formulation profiles have been identified, and some controversy exists as to whether nonprotein calories are best given as carbohydrate or in combination with fat.

Pulmonary Failure

It is also important to recognize two etiologies of pulmonary failure, since they mandate different programs of metabolic support. The first mechanism occurs after parenchymal disease with alteration in gas exchange, lymphatic drainage, alveolar ventilation, and perfusion. The clinical conditions of pulmonary edema, adult respiratory distress syndrome, chronic obstructive pulmonary disease, and congestive heart failure characterize this population. The second mechanism of pulmonary failure follows wasting of the intercostal and diaphragmatic respiratory muscles along with a depression of ventilatory drive, all secondary to severe malnutrition.

In the first setting, appropriate nutritional support mandates nonprotein caloric support formulations least conducive to generation of carbon dioxide. Excessive infusions of carbohydrate, as discussed previously, will result in a gradual elevation of the respiratory quotient to more than 1, as carbohydrate is converted into storage molecules of fat. With the increase in carbon dioxide production associated with some increased requirements for oxygen to support fat synthesis, the capacity of the lung can be exceeded resulting in progressive hypercarbia, respiratory acidosis, and increasing respirator dependency. Optimal feeding formulations substitute lipid for some carbohydrate with 30% to 40% of nonprotein calories derived from fat. With this formulation, the respiratory quotient will usually fall below 1, providing optimal metabolic support without compromising pulmonary function further. Pulmocare is marketed as an enteral product with these characteristics; parenteral products simply increase lipid and decrease carbohydrate content.

Patients who suffer from malnutrition, loss of pulmonary muscles, and a depressed ventilatory drive usually have no compromise of gas exchange, yet simply do not move enough air to achieve normal blood gases. Many times these patients require intubation and respirator support which further reduce muscle activity and contribute to continued disuse atrophy. Optimal respiratory care in this setting is intermittent ventilation, which allows the patient to continue some ventilatory effort to maintain respiratory muscle exercise. There is no need to alter the carbohydrate lipid composition to reduce carbon dioxide production. Instead optimal substrate support is needed for rehabilitation of respiratory muscle mass and function. This substrate profile remains to be determined, but from experience with athletic training programs, high carbohydrate and high protein diets would appear optimal. Further data supporting this concept come from body compositional studies by Shizgal and colleagues[98] of isonitrogenous, isocaloric diets with respect to their ability to replenish lean body mass over time. Carbohydrate-based formulas produced optimal gain in lean body mass, while fat-based formulas were the least efficient. Intermediate replenishment resulted from mixed-fuel formulations. Studies by Weissman and co-workers demonstrated that patients recover from depression of ventilatory drive during malnutrition when treated with refeeding of protein alone.[109] Optimal support would therefore appear to be high protein, glucose-based formulations with at least enough lipid support to provide essential fatty acids. Additional studies are necessary to further clarify optimal substrate support.

Liver Failure

The onset of liver dysfunction is often very difficult to determine clinically during care of the trauma patient. Reliance on elevation of liver enzymes such as SGOT, SGPT, LDH, and serum bilirubin can be misleading as they reflect cellular injury rather than alteration in hepatic metabolism. Elevations in serum bilirubin often reflect hemoglobin breakdown or altered hepatic secretion and not necessarily hepatic function. Elevations in serum ammonia are perhaps more useful, since with normal hepatic function, the liver can clear even elevated production of ammonia while normal serum concentrations are maintained. However, determination of true liver function requires more involved clinical testing, such as clearance of sulfobromophthalein, antipyrine, or barbiturate. Measurement of serum amino acid profiles can also be of help as elevated levels of the straight-chain amino acids which are usually cleared by the liver indicate liver dysfunction. Such tests unfortunately require expensive laboratory equipment and a significant amount of time. Clinically, altered liver function is often characterized by progressive mental dysfunction, starting as confusion and then progressing to lethargy and eventually coma, a syndrome termed *hepatic encephalopathy*.

In the early stages of liver dysfunction, feeding formulations require few alterations. Even with moderate hepatic dysfunction, restrictions are seldom necessary. In severe liver dysfunction, however, gluconeogenesis as well as lipid clearance may be depressed. Changes in protein supplementation also become necessary because of the increasing elevations of the straight-chain amino acids, which are metabolized by the liver, and the decreasing levels of branched-chain amino acids, which are metabolized by muscle. In severe hepatic dysfunction, formulation modification should include adequate glucose loading to avoid hypoglycemia, restriction of lipid infusion based on monitoring of lipid clearance to avoid hypertriglyceridemia or lipemic serum, and modification of the amino acid infusion to provide higher concentrations of branched-chain amino acids and restricted amounts of the straight-chain amino acids.[53] Specialized enteral formulas which meet these specifications include Hepatic-Aid II and Travasorb Hepatic. If should be noted that these formulations do not include electrolyte, mineral, or vitamin supplementation, hence these need to be provided separately. The one available specialized parenteral formulation is Hepatamine. Use of these specialized protein formulations should be restricted to patients in whom abnormal serum amino acid profiles have been documented by aminoacidograms. If the profile is not abnormal, routine amino acid formulations are recommended. Specialized products are significantly more expensive and are only effective in normalizing the serum amino acid profile. Even when abnormal amino acid profiles are documented, use of these specialized amino acid formulations does not necessarily improve patient survival, although it does allow high protein support without aggravation of hepatic encephalopathy.

Multiple Organ System Failure

The clinical syndrome of multiple organ failure resulting from continued prolonged stress and often complicated by repeated insults such as gastrointestinal bleeding, surgical interventions, severe local infections, and generalized sepsis with disseminated intravascular coagulation, presents the most difficult metabolic challenge for nutritional support. The extensive substrate modifications required by the failure of two or more organs usually result in such severe restrictions that adequate nutritional support can no longer be maintained. The goal of nutritional support becomes, therefore, to provide optimal support within the restrictions, with the hope that improvement in organ function will allow adequate nutritional support before the onset of starvation or other complications. As long as support is indicated, the clinician must continue to strive to provide the most effective nutrient formulation possible based on careful monitoring and clinical judgment.

As discussed earlier, with the onset of multiple organ failure, lipid clearance dramatically deteriorates and the use of lipid emulsions for nonprotein caloric support must be abandoned in favor of glucose-based solutions that use lipid emulsions for essential fatty acids only. This change in support is mandated by the identification of lipemic serum or of elevated serum triglycerides, confirming poor clearance. In this setting, however, glucose utilization also decreases because of the neuroendocrine response and the presence of an insulin postreceptor abnormality. Glucose infusion is often limited to less than 5 mg/kg/hr, sometimes to as little as 2 mg/kg/hr. Alternative fuel substrates may well be indicated, such as branched-chain amino acids and medium-chain triglycerides. Moyer and co-workers[75] and Cerra and colleagues[20] have found improved nitrogen retention and survival in patients with multiple organ failure when branched-chain amino acids comprise 45% to 50% of infused amino acids by weight. In spite of metabolic substrate modulation, mortality in this group of patients remains greater than 50%, generally because of the multiple other problems present in addition to the major breakdown in the metabolic processes.

REFERENCES

1. Abel RM, Alonso DR, Grimes J et al: Biochemical, ultrastructural, and hemodynamic changes in chronic protein-calorie malnutrition in dogs. Circulation (Suppl II) 56:205, 1977.
2. Addis T, Poo LJ, Lew W: The quantities of protein lost by the various organs and tissues of the body during a fast. J Biol Chem 115:111–116, 1936.
3. Adesola AO: The influence of severe protein deficiency on gastric acid secretion in Nigerian children. Br J Surg 55:866, 1968.
4. Anderson GH, Patel DG, Jeejeebhoy KN: Design and evaluation by nitrogen balance and blood aminograms of an amino acid mixture for total parenteral nutrition of adults with gastrointestinal disease. J Clin Invest 53:904–912, 1974.
5. Anderson KR, Norris DJ, Godfrey LB et al: Bacterial contamination of tube-feeding formulas. JPEN 8:673–678, 1984.
6. Arora NS, Rochester DF: Respiratory muscle strength and maximal voluntary ventilation in undernourished patients. Am Rev Respir Dis 126:5–8, 1982.
7. Beisel WR: Mediators of fever and muscle proteolysis. N Engl J Med 308:586–588, 1983.
8. Bern MM, Bothe A Jr, Bistrian B et al: Prophylaxis against central vein thrombosis with low-dosed warfarin. Surgery 99:216–220, 1986.
9. Black PR, Brooks DC, Bessey PQ et al: Mechanisms of insulin resistance following injury. Ann Surg 196:420–435, 1982.
10. Blackburn GL, Moldawer LL, Usui S et al: Branched chain amino acid administration and metabolism during starvation, injury and infection. Surgery 86:307–315, 1979.
11. Bonau RA, Ang SD, Jeevanandam M et al: High-branched chain amino acid solutions: Relationship of composition to efficacy. JPEN 8:622–627, 1984.
12. Borum PR: Role of carnitine supplementation in clinical nutrition. Adv Clin Nutr 315–324, 1983.
13. Bozzetti F: Parenteral nutrition in surgical patients. Surg Gynecol Obstet 142:16–20, 1976.
14. Bozzetti F, Scarpa D, Terno G et al: Subclavian venous thrombosis due to indwelling catheters: A prospective study on 52 patients. JPEN 7:560–562, 1983.
15. Bozzetti F, Terno G, Bonfanti G, et al: Prevention and treatment of central venous catheter sepsis by exchange via a guidewire. A prospective controlled trial. Ann Surg 198:48–52, 1983.
16. Brodie BB, Gillette JR, LaDu BN: Enzymatic metabolism of drugs and other foreign compounds. Annu Rev Biochem 27:427–454, 1958.
17. Burke JF, Wolfe RR, Mullany CJ et al: Glucose requirements following burn injury. Ann Surg 190:274–285, 1979.
18. Burri C, Krischak G: Techniques and complications of administration of total parenteral nutrition. In Manni C, Magalini SI, Scrascia E (eds): TPN, pp 306–315. New York, American Elsevier Scientific Publishing, 1976.
19. Cahill GF Jr: Starvation in man. N Engl J Med 282:668–675, 1970.
20. Cerra FB, Mazuski JE, Chute E et al: Branched chain metabolic support. A prospective, randomized, double-blind trial in surgical stress. Ann Surg 199:286–291, 1984.
21. Cerra FB, Siegel JH, Border JR et al: The hepatic failure of sepsis: Cellular versus substrate. Surgery 86:409–422, 1979.
22. Clowes GHA, George BC, Villel CA Jr et al: Muscle proteolysis induced by a circulating peptide in patients with sepsis or trauma. N Engl J Med 308:545–552, 1983.
23. Committee on Trauma, National Academy of Sciences–National Research Council: Postoperative wound infections: The influence of ultraviolet irradiation of the operating room and of various other factors. Ann Surg (Suppl) 160:1–192, 1964.
24. Conces DJ, Holden RW: Aberrant locations and complications in initial placement of subclavin vein catheters. Arch Surg 119:293, 1984.
25. Craddock PR, Yawata Y, VanSanten L et al: Acquired phagocyte dysfunction. A complication of the hypophosphatemia of hyperalimentation. N Engl J Med 290:1043–1047, 1974.
26. Crocker KS, Pine RW, Steffee WP: The triple lumen central venous catheter. Nutrition in Clinical Practice 1:90–96, 1986.
27. Cruse PJE, Foord R: A five-year prospective study of 23,649 surgical wounds. Arch Surg 107:206–210, 1973.
28. Cuthbertson DP: The disturbance of metabolism produced by bony and non-bony injury, with notes on certain abnormal conditions of bone. Biochem J 24:1224–1263, 1930.
29. Doekel RC Jr, Zwillich CW, Scoggin CH et al: Clinical semi-starvation: Depression of hypoxic ventilatory response. N Engl J Med 295:358–361, 1976.
30. Douglas DD, Morrissey JF: A new technique for rapid endoscopic-assisted intubation of the small intestine. Arch Surg 113:196–198, 1978.
31. Dudrick SJ, Wilmore DW, Vars HM et al: Long-term total parenteral nutrition with growth, development and positive nitrogen balance. Surgery 64:134–142, 1968.
32. Falcone RE, Hickman DM, Rophie R: The complication rate of elective subclavian vein puncture by the novice. JPEN 9:379, 1985.
33. Fares LG, II, Block PH, Feldman SD: Improved house staff results with subclavian cannulation. Am Surg 52:108, 1986.
34. Felig P: The glucose-alanine cycle. Metabolism 22:179–207, 1973.
35. Fischer JE: Amino acid metabolism in sepsis. In Fischer JE, Alexander JW (eds): Relevance of Nutrition to Sepsis, pp 54–59. Columbus, Ross Labs, 1981.
36. Fleck A, Munro HN: Protein metabolism after injury. Metabolism 12:783–789, 1963.
37. Freund HR, James JH, Fischer JE: Nitrogen-sparing mechanisms of singly administered branched-chain amino acids in the injured rat. Surgery 90:237–243, 1981.
38. Goodenough RD, Wolfe RR: Effect of total parenteral nutrition on free fatty acid metabolism in burned patients. JPEN 8:357–360, 1984.
39. Goodgame J, Lowry S, Brennan M et al: Essential fatty acid deficiency in total parenteral nutrition: Time course of development and suggestions for therapy. Surgery 84:271–276, 1978.
40. Gordon AH: Effects of trauma and partial hepatectomy on the rates of synthesis of plasma proteins by the liver. In Rothschild, MA, Waldmann T (eds): Plasma Protein Metabolism. Regulation of Synthesis, Distribution, and Degradation, pp 351–369. New York, Academic Press, 1970.
41. Graff J, Gong R, Byron R et al: Knotting and entanglement of multiple central venous catheters. JPEN 10:319–321, 1986.
42. Grant JP: Handbook of Total Parenteral Nutrition, a, pp 47–69; b, pp 124–129. Philadelphia, WB Saunders, 1980.
43. Grant JP, Cox CE, Kleinman LM et al: Serum hepatic enzyme and bilirubin elevations during parenteral nutrition. Surg Gynecol Obstet 145:573–580, 1977.
44. Grant JP, Curtas MS, Kelvin FM: Fluoroscopic placement of nasojejunal feeding tubes with immediate feeding using a nonelemental diet. JPEN 7:299–303, 1983.
45. Hall RI, Grant JP, Ross LH et al: Pathogenesis of hepatic steatosis in the parenterally fed rat. J Clin Invest 74:1658–1668, 1984.
46. Hallberg D: Studies on the elimination of exogenous lipids from the bloodstream. The effect of fasting and surgical trauma in man on the elimination rate of a fat emulsion injected intravenously. Acta Physiol Scand 65:151–163, 1965.
47. Hamaway KJ, Moldawer LL, Georgieff M et al: The effect of lipid emulsions on reticuloendothelial system function in the injured animal. JPEN 9:559–565, 1985.
48. Hartley TF, Lee HA: Investigations into the optimal nitrogen and caloric requirements and comparative nutritive value of three intravenous amino acid solutions in the postoperative period. Nutr Metabol 19:201–211, 1975.
49. Harvey KB, Moldawer LL, Bistrian BR et al: Biological measures for the formulation of a hospital prognostic index. Am J Clin Nutr 34:2013–2022, 1981.
50. Holman RT: The ratio of the trienoic:tetraenoic acid in tissue lipids as a measure of essential fatty acid requirements. J Nutr 70:405–410, 1960
51. Hoshal VL Jr, Ause RG, Hoskins PA: Fibrin sleeve formation on indwelling subclavian central venous catheters. Arch Surg 102:353–358, 1971.

52. Jackson CM: Effects of acute and chronic inanition upon the relative weight of the various organs and systems of adult albino rats. Am J Anat 18:75–116, 1915.
53. James JH, Jeppsson B, Ziparo V et al: Hyperammonaemia, plasma amino acid imbalance, and blood-brain amino acid transport: A unified theory of portal-systemic encephalopathy. Lancet 2:772–775, 1979.
54. Jones KW, Seltzer MH, Slocum BA, et al: Parenteral nutrition complications of percutaneous subclavian catheters. JPEN 8:385, 1984.
55. Kaminski MV: Hyperalimentation: A Guide for Clinicians. New York, Marcel Dekker, Inc., 1985.
56. Kern KA, Bower RH, Atamian S et al: The effect of a new branched chain–enriched amino acid solution on postoperative catabolism. Surgery 92:780–785, 1982.
57. Keys A, Brozek J, Henschel A et al: The Biology of Human Starvation. Minneapolis, University of Minnesota Press, 1950.
58. Kinney JM: Calories-nitrogen-disease and injury relationships. In Symposium on Total Parenteral Nutrition, pp 35–45. Chicago, American Medical Association, 1972.
59. Klahr S, Alleyne GAO: Effects of chronic protein-calorie malnutrition on the kidney. Kidney Int 3:129–141, 1973.
60. Klahr S, Tripathy K, Garcia FT et al: On the nature of the renal concentrating defect in malnutrition. Am J Med 43:84–96, 1967.
61. Klahr S, Tripathy K, Lotero H: Renal regulation of acid-base balance in malnourished man. Am J Med 48:325–331, 1970.
62. Krieger M: Ueber die Atrophie der menschlichen Organe bei Inanition. Z. angew. Anat Knostitutional 7:87–134, 1921.
63. Kyger ER, Block WJ, Roach G et al: Adverse effects of protein malnutrition on myocardial function. Surgery 84:147–156, 1978.
64. Law DK, Dudrick SJ, Abdou NI: Immunocompetence of patients with protein-calorie malnutrition: The effects of nutritional repletion. Ann Intern Med 79:545–550, 1973.
65. Lindholm M, Rossner S: Rate of elimination of the intralipid fat emulsion from the circulation in ICU patients. Crit Care Med 10:740–746, 1982.
66. Lipman TQ, Kessler T, Arabian A: Nasopulmonary intubation with feeding tubes: Case reports and review of the literature. JPEN 9:618–620, 1985.
67. Lockwood AH: Percutaneous subclavian vein catherization. Arch Intern Med 144:1407, 1984.
68. Long CL, Schaffel N, Geiger JW et al: Metabolic response to injury and illness: Estimation of energy and protein needs from indirect calorimetry and nitrogen balance. JPEN 3:452–456, 1979.
69. Lopes J, Russell D, Whitwell J et al: Skeletal muscle function in malnutrition. Am J Clin Nutr 36:602–610, 1982.
70. Maiz A, Yamazaki K, Sobrado J et al: Protein metabolism during total parenteral nutrition in injured rats using medium-chain triglycerides. Metabolism 33:901–909, 1984.
71. Maksoud JG, Tannuri U: Effect of branched-chain amino acids and insulin on postinjury protein catabolism in growing animals. JPEN 8:416–420, 1984.
72. McCarthy MC, Shives J, Robinson RJ et al: Prospective evaluation of triple and single lumen catheters in total parenteral nutrition. JPEN (Suppl) 10:6S, 1976.
73. Melly MA, Meng HC, Schaffner W: Microbial growth in lipid emulsions used in parenteral nutrition. Ann Surg 110:1479–1481, 1975.
74. Miller CL: Immunological assays as measurements of nutritional status: A review. JPEN 2:554–566, 1978.
75. Moyer ED, Border JR, Cerra FB et al: Multiple systems organ failure: IV. Imbalances in plasma amino acids associated with exogenous albumin in the trauma-septic patient. J Trauma 21:543–547, 1981.
76. Mullen JL: Consequences of malnutrition in the surgical patient. Surg Clin North Am 61:465–488, 1981.
77. Munro HN: General aspects of the regulation of protein metabolism by diet and hormones. In Munro HN, Allison JB (eds): Mammalian Protein Metabolism, vol 1, pp 267–319. New York, Academic Press, 1964.
78. Nachbauer CA, James JH, Edwards LL et al: Infusion of branched chain-enriched amino acid solutions in sepsis. Am J Surg 147:743–752, 1984.
79. Newsome HH, Jr, Armstrong CW, Mayhall GC, et al: Mechanical complications from insertion of subclavian venous feeding catheters: Comparison of de novo percutaneous venipuncture to change of catheter over guidewire. JPEN 8:560, 1984.
80. Niemiec PW Jr, Vanderveen TW, Morrison JI et al: Gastrointestinal disorders caused by medication and electrolyte solution osmolality during enteral nutrition. JPEN 7:387–389, 1983
81. Nuwer N, Cerra FB, Shronts EP et al: Does modified amino acid total parenteral nutrition alter immune response in high level surgical stress? JPEN 7:521–524, 1983
82. Odessey R, Khairallah EA, Goldberg AL: Origin of possible significance of alanine production by skeletal muscle. J Biol Chem 249:7623–7629, 1974.
83. Olivares L, Segovia A, Revuelta R: Tube feeding and lethal aspiration in neurological patients. A review of 720 autopsy cases. Stroke 5:654–657, 1974.
84. O'Neill JA Jr, Caldwell MD, Meng HC: Essential fatty acid deficiency in surgical patients. Ann Surg 185:535–542, 1977.
85. Onicescu D, Radu A: Histochemical researches on the hepatocyte under experimental starvation conditions. On the activity of some oxido-reducing enzymes. Acta Histochem 32:418–424, 1969.
86. Pingleton SK, Hadzima SK: Enteral alimentation and gastrointestinal bleeding in mechanically ventilated patients. Crit Care Med 11:13–16, 1983.
87. Portnay GI, O'Brian JT, Bush J et al: The effect of starvation on the concentration and binding of thyroxine and triiodothyroine in serum and on the response to TRH. J Clin Endocrinol Metabol 39:191–194, 1974.
88. Remmer H: The role of the liver in drug metabolism. Am J Med 49:617–629, 1970.
89. Ross LH, Griffeth L, Hall RI et al: Hepatotoxic effects of parenteral nutrition upon the in vivo pharmacokinetics of antipyrine. Surg Forum 34:34–36, 1983.
90. Ross LH, Griffeth L, Hall RI et al: Elimination of hepatotoxicity of total parenteral nutrition using fat-carbohydrate mixture. Surg Forum 35:97–99, 1984.
91. Ruderman NB, Berger M: The formation of glutamine and alanine in skeletal muscle. J Biol Chem 249:5500–5506, 1974.
92. Rudman D, Millikan WJ, Richardson TJ et al: Elemental balances during intravenous hyperalimentation of underweight adult subjects. J Clin Invest 55:94–104, 1975.
93. Ryan NT, Blackburn GL, Clowes HA Jr: Differential tissue sensitivity to elevated endogenous insulin levels during experimental peritonitis in rats. Metabolism 23:1081–1089, 1974.
94. Schroeder P, Fisher D, Volz M et al: Microbial contamination of enteral feeding solutions in a community hospital. JPEN 7:364–368, 1983.
95. Schug CB, Culhane DE, Knopp RK: Subclavian vein catheterization in the emergency department: a comparison of guidewire and nonguidewire technique. Ann Emer Med 15:769, 1986.
96. Sherwin RS, Hendler RG, Felig P: Effect of ketone infusions on amino acid and nitrogen metabolism. J Clin Invest 55:1382–1390, 1975.
97. Shils ME: Experimental human magnesium depletion. Medicine 48:61–85, 1969.
98. Shizgal HM, Forse RA: Protein and calorie requirements with total parenteral nutrition. Ann Surg 192:562–569, 1980.
99. Silvis SE, Paragas PD Jr: Paresthesias, weakness, seizures, and hypophosphatemia in patients receiving hyperalimentation. Gastroenterology 62:513–520, 1972.
100. Sitzmann JV, Townsend TR, Siler MC, Bartlett JG: Septic and technical complications of central venous catheterization. A prospective study of 200 consecutive patients. Ann Surg 202:766, 1985.
101. Smith NL, Ravo B, Soroff HS et al: Successful fibrinolytic therapy for superior vena cava thrombosis secondary to long-term total perenteral nutrition. JPEN 9:55–57, 1985.
102. Soroff HS, Pearson E, Artz CP: An estimation of the nitrogen requirements for equilibrium in burned patients. Surg Gynecol Obstet 112:877–883, 1971.
103. Tejada C, Restrepo C: Effect of malnutrition on the gastrointestinal tract and on the pancreas. Proceedings of the 8th Pan American Congress of Gastroenterology, New York, 1962.

104. Toa RC, Yoshimura NN: Carnitine metabolism and its application in parenteral nutrition. JPEN 4:469–486, 1980.
105. Torosian MH, Rombeau JL: Feeding by tube enterostomy. Surg Gynecol Obstet 150:918–927, 1980.
106. Travis SF, Sugerman HJ, Ruberg RL et al: Alterations of red-cell glycolytic intermediates and oxygen transport as a consequence of hypophosphatemia in patients receiving intravenous hyperalimentation. N Engl J Med 285:763–768, 1971.
107. Vallee BL, Wacker WEC, Ulmer DD: The magnesium-deficiency tetany syndrome in man. N Engl J Med 262:155–161, 1960.
108. Viteri FE, Schneider RE: Gastrointestinal alterations in protein-calorie malnutrition. Med Clin North Am 58:1487–1505, 1974.
109. Weissman C, Askanazi J, Rosenbaum S et al: Amino acids and respiration. Ann Intern Med 98:41–44, 1983.
110. Wilmore DW: The Metabolic Management of the Critically Ill, p 197. New York, Plenum Press, 1977.
111. Wilmore DW: Energy production, metabolism of fat and glucose. In Fischer JE, Alexander JW (eds): Relevance of Nutrition to Sepsis, pp 51–54. Columbus, Ross Labs, 1981.

critical care management for trauma

Anthony A. Meyer

20

Critical care is a relatively recent addition to medicine, although the concept has been evolving for over a century. The development of critical care is closely linked to trauma management. During the Crimean War, the most seriously injured patients were kept close together after surgery to make better use of the limited nursing personnel. Preoperative resuscitation areas were established in North Africa during World War II to improve the early treatment of the most seriously injured. As general anesthesia became routine, recovery rooms were used to manage postoperative patients during the unstable period of emergence from anesthesia. As techniques and equipment for treating the critically injured improved, the rationale developed for consolidating these resources and the personnel trained to treat respiratory failure.[85] Since then, patients requiring specialized personnel or equipment developed into what we presently know as the intensive care unit (ICU).

The ICU is integral to the management of severely injured patients. Whether patients come to the ICU after surgery or directly from the emergency room, their acute, evolving problems must be managed appropriately to achieve the best outcome. The types of ICUs in which trauma patients may be managed vary greatly. Recently, an NIH Consensus Conference established guidelines for classification of ICUs (Fig. 20.1).[23] Such identification may be useful in assessing the capabilities of any unit in managing specific patients or problems. Type I units are capable of managing patients with any problems; the physicians in the ICU have no other responsibilities. Type II units are frequently specialty service ICUs, such as cardiothoracic surgery, or neurosurgery, and have covering physicians who are in the hospital, but with other responsibilities. Type III units have limited monitoring capability and may be covered by physicians not familiar with the patients. Type IV units are not critical care units and provide only increased nursing observation. Understanding this system of classification aids in the identification of the type of ICU necessary for hospitals treating severely injured patients. Major trauma centers should have at least a type I and possibly a type II unit. Patients with severe multiple-system injuries should be managed in a type I unit.

Although there has been some recent reduction, trauma accounts for 150,000 deaths and 400,000 disabling injuries each year.[113] The majority of these deaths occur within an hour of injury, frequently before the victim receives medical attention, but there are still a significant number of deaths that occur days and weeks after injury. It is this group of eventual fatalities and the larger number of seriously injured survivors that receive treatment in ICUs. Trauma patients may be brought to ICUs for any of several reasons, but generally because they require the use of the supportive devices restricted to ICUs, monitoring of unstable physiologic status, or constant nursing and physician care.

As a very important part of trauma care, critical care must be an integral part of any major trauma center.[68,73,114,117] In some institutions, critical care is provided by a separate service, and management of any patient entering the ICU must be transferred to that service. This interruption in the continuity of patient care is not in the best interest of the patient or of medical education.[50,73] However, few trauma services have sufficient personnel to assign one member solely to the ICU. This dilemma can best be solved by developing a critical care service that actively participates in the management of all ICU patients and functions as an integral part of each service, while the patients remain on the primary service. Such a system requires excellent communication between the services, which can be accomplished by performing joint rounds.

The educational requirements for surgical residents in the areas of trauma and critical care have been expanded.[50,107] Both the qualifying and certifying exams of the American Board of Surgery dedicate a large segment to these areas. Furthermore, the American Board of Surgery began issuing Certificates of Added Qualification in Critical Care in 1987.

The goals in the management of critically ill trauma victims are not really different from those of all medical care: to provide optimal care for the patient, including limitation of injury, and to prevent complications. Although the patients have already suffered an injury, attention to care can limit further injury by preventing unnecessary blood loss and promptly restoring perfusion. Complications that can arise include sepsis and iatrogenic complications.

Fulfillment of these management goals requires an understanding of both trauma and critical care. Patients who have suffered severe injury have profound physiologic response. Physicians treating these patients must be familiar with the pathophysiology of injury and the body's response to that injury. Appropriate treatment of the injury in the ICU will be the result, whether the treatment is the primary means of managing the injury or secondary, as in supportive care after operative management of

FIGURE 20.1
NIH CONSENSUS CONFERENCE CLASSIFICATION OF CRITICAL CARE UNITS

TYPE OF UNIT	PHYSICIAN COVERAGE	NURSE:PATIENT RATIO	MONITORING CAPABILITIES
I	Present in ICU	1:1 or 1:2	All invasive monitoring
II	Present in hospital	1:1 or 1:2	All invasive monitoring
III	Covering physician in hospital with resuscitation skills	1:3 to 1:4	Limited invasive monitoring
IV	Physician on call, not always in hospital	1:3 to 1:5	No invasive monitoring

the injury. Monitoring is important in the optimal treatment of trauma, but selection of monitoring techniques must be done with serious consideration. Trauma patients need frequent reassessment, since change in status is common. Also, complications that occur more often after severe injury must be prevented or treated promptly and appropriately.

This chapter will discuss the general topics of pathophysiology, treatment, supportive care, monitoring, and preventive management of complications; then these topics will be applied to a review of the major organ systems. It is hoped this will serve as a successful format in the critical care treatment of not only the severely injured, but all surgical patients.

Pathophysiology of and Response to Injury

Trauma occurs when there is transmission of energy to the victim. The severity of the injury depends on the amount and concentration of the energy, the tissues which sustain the injury, and the degree to which normal physiology is disturbed by either blood loss or contamination. Both penetrating and blunt trauma transmit energy. The injury will be severe if a great deal of energy is transmitted, as in a high-speed vehicular accident or a 50-foot fall, or if less energy is concentrated to a small area such as the head, or if even less energy results in severe hemorrhage and shock, as in a stab wound to a great vessel.

All these mechanisms produce some cell injury and death. Prostaglandin synthesis is increased after injury, with further chemical alteration to such vasoconstrictors as thromboxane, and vasodilators such as prostacyclin.[19,49,61,87] Furthermore, leukotrienes, another arachidonic acid metabolite group, are increased and act as a chemotactant and greatly increase vascular permeability.[30,87,104] The local cell injury also leads to coagulation and the activation of the complement cascade. Platelet aggregation in the thrombotic mechanisms also release thromboxane. Some of the intermediate components of the complement cascade and their by-products also increase vascular permeability and have chemotactic activity.

Injury also produces several other systemic effects on the victim. Adrenergic stimulation leads to release of catecholamines. Epinephrine and norepinephrine produce vasoconstriction, increase cardiac contractility and heart rate, and decrease blood flow to some tissues. Aldosterone and antidiuretic hormone (ADH) secretion are increased, which leads to increased sodium and water reabsorption. Cortisol, insulin, and growth hormone are also released in higher amounts after injury.

The extent of both the local and systemic responses to injury are to some extent proportional to the amount of energy transmitted or the amount of blood loss or contamination. If any of these are significant, there will be generalized fluid sequestration, an increase in metabolic rate, and a rise in myocardial demand. Major injuries may require many liters of fluid resuscitation as long as the patient has low intravascular pressures. Epinephrine increases lipolysis and blocks the anabolic effects of insulin. The normal host defenses are adversely affected, with suppression of hormonal and cellular, specific and nonspecific components of the immune system.

These local and systemic reaction to injury cause a net effect called the physiologic response to injury. An appreciation of these individual effects makes it easier to understand the variability in the net response, and permits a more rational pharmacologic support of the patient. It also provides a basis for understanding the research being done to alter the response of arachidonic acid metabolites, with the goal of controlling the response to injury.

ICU Treatment of Traumatic Injuries

The management of injuries in the ICU can generally be classified as primary and secondary treatment and the management of complications. The use of these classifications permits more defined goals and methods of treatment. An example of primary treatment is a patient with blunt trauma and severe pulmonary contusion who requires mechanical ventilation as the sole means of managing that injury. In another example, a victim of blunt trauma may need an emergency laparotomy to repair a severe liver injury. Postoperatively the patient may need mechanical ventilation because of limited ability to breathe after prolonged anesthesia and massive transfusion. In this situation, the need for ventilatory treatment is secondary to surgery and resuscitation, not to the injury. A last example is the patient who, several days after severe injury, becomes septic from an abdominal abscess and develops respiratory failure. In this case, the ventilation is part of the management of the complication. The expected time course and potential outcome are frequently different for these three types of management.

Supportive Care

Many physiologic effects of injury and ensuing complications are limited; however, some can lead to significant organ dysfunction, and even to organ-system failure. In some instances, there may be failure of multiple systems and organs, frequently related. In these situations, supportive care is needed to sustain the patient until that organ or system returns to a level of function sufficient to sustain life. Much of what is described as curing a patient in the ICU is merely providing supportive care until the patient cures him- or herself.

Generally, it is wise to begin supportive care early to avoid further deterioration of the patient or systems. It is also necessary to reassess supportive care frequently.

Monitoring

Although we usually associate monitoring with invasive catheters and electronic displays of a physiologic parameter, monitoring includes all methods of evaluating a patient over time. Monitoring evaluates not only the status of the patient, but also the effectiveness of any treatment he is receiving. Monitoring in the ICU can be divided into three general groups: physiologic, clinical, and laboratory techniques.[72]

The physiologic monitoring methods are the ones most often associated with critical care. They permit continuous measurement and immediate availability of data. Examples of these are catheters measuring intravascular pressure in the pulmonary artery, central veins, and peripheral arteries, as well as intracranial pressure. A very simple but extremely useful physiologic method of monitoring is of urine output.

Monitoring techniques require varied amounts of time and expertise to institute. They are all associated with some level of risk. Before selecting any monitoring technique, it is important to assess the usefulness of the information to be obtained as well as all the risks.[46,72] Some of the more common methods of physiologic monitoring are listed in Figure 20.2, along with the more common complications. Monitoring must be used selectively on an individual basis and reevaluated at least daily.

Clinical methods of monitoring are subjective. Frequently the value of the clinical observation is influenced by other factors such as low temperature, decreasing skin perfusion, or alcohol or sedative drugs impairing mental status. Still, clinical monitoring of any body system can be very useful if done by an experienced observer. Organ-system dysfunction is often apparent to an attentive clinician long before it is confirmed by physiologic or laboratory information.

Laboratory results can also serve as a means for monitoring. These results provide evidence for evolving changes that may only be suggested by other methods of monitoring. Hematocrit levels parallel blood loss, and elevated creatinine implies deteriorating renal function. One important limitation to these tests is that they do require some time for completion.

Physiologic, clinical, and laboratory monitoring provide different information about the patient. The most crucial role of the physician in managing the critically ill patient is to review this information and assess the patient. This must be done often, depending upon the instability of the patient, for without such frequent reassessment, the information available is of little use. Too often, more effort is placed in the gathering of information than in consideration of what is available. It must be remembered that the information may be incorrect because of technical problems, or its interpretation may be wrong. In situations where information appears contradictory or misleading, a general reassessment should precede another battery of tests.

These assessments can conveniently be done by system review. First the physiologic status, support treatment, and possible complications of each system are reviewed using available information. A treatment plan is considered, including how much information will be necessary for future assessments. The plans for all the systems are then integrated to provide optimal care for the patient. This is the culmination of monitoring critically ill patients. It is important to remember, however, that the patient is an individual, not just an amalgamation of interrelated systems.

Prevention and Management of Complications

Patients with severe injury are at increased risk of complications. Complications may be secondary to the injury and the course of disease, or to iatrogenic intervention. The goal of patient care is to prevent them from occurring or, if they have developed, limit them and provide appropriate treatment.

There are simple accepted prophylactic measures to prevent complications, such as antacids to prevent stress gastritis, skin care and the use of padding and special beds to prevent pressure sores, and sterile technique in placing and dressing indwelling venous catheters to prevent septic thrombophlebitis. Close medical and nursing attention to these measures will prevent many complications.

FIGURE 20.2
RISKS AND BENEFITS OF VARIOUS MONITORING METHODS

METHOD	RISKS	BENEFITS
Arterial line	Thrombosis, ischemia, limb loss, distal and proximal embolization infection	Continuous reading of systemic pressure
Central venous catheter (jugular or subclavian)	Thrombosis, hemorrhage, arterial injury, pneumothorax, hydrothorax, infection, arrhythmias	Continuous measurement of right heart filling pressure
Pulmonary artery catheter (Swan-Ganz)	Thrombosis, hemorrhage, arterial injury, pneumothorax, arrhythmias, infection, endocarditis, pulmonary artery rupture, air emboli	Continuous measurement of right and left heart filling pressures; cardiac output determination
Urinary catheter	Bladder colonization, urethral injury	Continuous measure of renal perfusion
Intracranial pressure catheter (intraventricular)	Bleeding, neurologic deficit, infection	Continuous measure of intracranial pressure and potential drainage route to decrease pressure

Frequent reassessment of the injury will aid in the early diagnosis of any complication, and its expeditious treatment will limit the consequences. Frequent review of the patient's problems, organ-system function, and therapies will identify such problems as compartment syndrome, pneumothorax while on mechanical ventilation, and deteriorating renal function in a patient on aminoglycoside antibiotics. Attention to these complications will limit their number and significantly improve the critical care management of these patients.

SYSTEM INJURIES AND MANAGEMENT

Treatment, supportive care, monitoring, and prevention and management of complications are the methods used in providing critical care. The severely injured patient has many problems common to all critically ill patients, as well as some problems unique to his or her injury. These common and unique problems are presented in a system-review fashion, as they would be encountered when assessing a patient. The treatment of these problems, along with the supportive care, monitoring, and complications frequently associated with injury, are discussed for each system. When evaluating and considering treatment, it is crucial to remember that these systems and problems are interrelated, and any management plan must be comprehensive enough to take them all into account.

Cardiovascular System

The cardiovascular system is affected by many of the problems and complications of injury. In turn, because it determines perfusion and thus ultimate survival of all other systems, the adequate function of the cardiovascular system is essential for patient survival.

There are few injuries that cause direct damage to the heart which require treatment. Myocardial contusion is the most commonly encountered of these injuries. Despite radionuclide scan evidence of significant dysfunction in up to 55% of patients with severe contusion,[108] clinically significant problems are rare.[86,109] Patients with new arrhythmias, changes in ECG, chest pain, or high clinical suspicion of injury should be monitored for approximately 24 hours with telemetry. If hemodynamic instability is present, an ICU setting may be appropriate. Prophylactic lidocaine is not indicated.

Monitoring of the cardiovascular system is highly developed and has many options. Arterial blood pressure, central venous pressure, and pulmonary artery wedge pressure are all available in type I or type II ICUs. Cardiac output and vascular resistance, calculated by thermodilution techniques available with the pulmonary artery catheters, can be very useful information in the critically ill but incur significant risk. Pneumothorax, bleeding, and arrhythmias are associated with central line placement.[58,77] Arterial catheters can produce arterial thrombosis with subsequent limb loss in upper extremity as well as lower extremity sites. Central venous catheters can cause occlusion or septic thrombophlebitis.[81] The latter is a surgical emergency requiring excision of the vein. Pulmonary artery catheters have an incidence of endocardial injury of over 50% and of infective endocarditis in as many as 7% of cases.[91] New, less invasive methods of monitoring the cardiovascular system are being used in some clinical situations, including transesophageal echocardiography and pulse aximetry.[52] These methods may provide more useful information with less risk to the patient.

Although these cardiovascular monitoring techniques are very useful, they only measure pressure, not perfusion. Moreover, the calculated cardiac output has many sources of potential error, frequently as much as 25%. One other method of monitoring cardiovascular status is following urine output. This is a direct measure of organ perfusion and, in patients with normal renal function, it is probably as useful as any pressure measurement. Clinical assessment of perfusion can also be very useful. A patient with cool, mottled extremities is obviously poorly perfused, no matter what the blood pressure reads.

Supportive care of the cardiovascular system centers around improving perfusion. The determinants of perfusion are preload, heart rate, contractility, and afterload.[47] It is important to remember that the goal is good perfusion, not an arbitrary blood pressure. Blood pressure is only one parameter of perfusion, determined by cardiac output and systemic vascular resistance. A patient can have a normal or high blood pressure and be inadequately perfused. Insufficient perfusion will lead to lactic acidosis, detectable on arterial blood gas measurement. Patients may also have low blood pressure and be well perfused, as in a patient with spinal cord injury and neurogenic shock from sympathetic interruption.

Injured patients with poor perfusion are almost always improved by increasing preload through a bolus infusion of isotonic salt solution or blood. Whether reduced preload is due to bleeding, fluid sequestration associated with injury, or sepsis, a volume challenge is the first response to decreased perfusion.

Although arrhythmias are not a common cause of impaired perfusion after injury, they do occur and can be a chronic problem requiring treatment. The management is the same as with arrhythmias of any cause, and has been extensively reviewed.[97] Supraventricular tachycardia may develop and lead to impaired cardiac output, because of the poor ventricular filling with heart rates over 140/min. The usual treatment is small doses of verapamil (5 mg) given intravenously, or beta blockers such as Inderal. Atrial fibrillation is associated with thoracic injuries and procedures. Treatment consists of rate control with digoxin. If the patient is in acute distress verapamil may be useful, and in extreme situations cardioversion may be necessary.

Impaired myocardial contractility after injury or sepsis has been described by several investigators,[28,64,75,98,123] but the nature of this impairment and its cause remain unclear. Nevertheless, there are several situations in which support of myocardial contractility is necessary. When a patient has inadequate perfusion not due to low preload or high afterload, contractility is likely to be the problem. Too often, however, patients with inadequate preload are treated with ionotropic agents to increase contractility in an attempt to avoid fluid resuscitation. Such attempts will be unsuccessful and may lead to further decrease in perfusion and deterioration of the patient. Furthermore, prolonged treatment with catecholamines leads to myocardial injury.[3,21,92]

Afterload is the vascular resistance the heart must work against during systole. It determines blood pressure in conjunction with cardiac output. Afterload is increased by the vasoconstrictor effect of circulating catechols after injury or hypovolemia. Afterload is often reduced during sepsis, possibly as a result of false neurotransmitters produced by protein catabolism and altered amino acid breakdown.[102] Sepsis also leads to pulmonary hypertension, which will cause right ventricular dilation and impair left ventricle function by limiting the interventricular system.[28,44,100,125]

There are several drugs frequently used to support the cardiovascular system. Dopamine is useful in improving contractility and selectively increasing renal perfusion at low doses where its beta effects prevail. At high doses, its alpha effects are more prominent, leading to increased afterload and significant tachycardia. Dobutamine has the positive ionotropic effects without the chronotropic or alpha effects of dopamine at high doses. It is useful in patients who are already tachycardic.

Sodium nitroprusside is effective in reducing systemic vascular resistance by causing vasodilation.[20] It will result in a significant drop in filling pressure and perfusion when used in hypovolemic patients who have compensated by vasoconstriction. In such patients, volume infusion must precede and continue during nitroprusside infusion. Its effectiveness in improving cardiac output in septic patients with a low-output state and high systemic vascular resistance has not been consistently noted.[17,101]

It remains essential to remember that the goal of supportive care of the cardiovascular system is perfusion and oxygen delivery, not arterial blood pressure, central venous pressure, or pulmonary capillary wedge pressure.[99] For that reason, clinical assessment of perfusion, as well as determination of lactic acidosis, is useful following treatment. Patients are too often treated with alpha-adrenergic agents, such as Levophed, or alpha-effect levels of dopamine, to produce an artificially elevated blood pressure. This is typical with patients with sepsis who may have a normal or high cardiac output, a very low vascular resistance, and as a result, a systolic pressure of 70 to 80 torr. As long as the patient is adequately perfused, with sufficient urine output, the cardiovascular system needs no support. Infusion of agents that produce an alpha-adrenergic effect will raise the blood pressure, but also may decrease perfusion and increase myocardial work and oxygen consumption because of the increased afterload.

Complications of the cardiovascular system are usually limited to arrhythmias, myocardial infarctions, or problems associated with monitoring techniques, such as those just described. Arrhythmias can often be prevented by maintenance of normal electrolyte balance and drug dosages. Complications due to monitoring devices or cannulas can cause death or severe morbidity.[43,88] Proper supervision and technique in placement and maintenance of these monitors is essential. The number of complications is closely associated with the length of time an indwelling device is in place.[32] A reassessment of the risk versus the benefit of each catheter should be made at least daily to avoid prolonged, unjustified use. Routine catheter change and care has been found to reduce these complications. Alternatives to invasive cardiovascular monitoring such as pulse oximeters can be used, and provide adequate information in many patients.

Respiratory System

Thoracic injury occurs in 25% of trauma victims and includes several specific injuries which are treated primarily in the ICU. Soft tissue injuries of the face and neck, generalized edema, and impaired ability to protect the airway may lead to loss of the airway. Blunt chest trauma can cause rib fractures, flail chest, and pulmonary contusion, all of which can lead to respiratory failure. Treatment of these injuries centers on maintenance of the airway, preventing respiratory failure, and providing support if it develops.

Airway impairment is best treated by prompt endotracheal intubation, either through an oral or a nasal route, although nasal tubes are much better tolerated for prolonged intubation. Patients with unstable neck fractures or severe maxillofacial injuries may require cricothyroidotomy or tracheostomy to establish an airway acutely.[118]

Treatment of rib fractures requires pain control to permit adequate lung expansion and clearance of secretion. Oral or parenteral opiates can be used. However, patients with multiple, comminuted fractures or limited pulmonary reserves are at greater risk of developing respiratory failure or pneumonia. More effective pain control can often be achieved by multiple intercostal nerve blocks of the injured ribs. Epidural morphine has also been used successfully to provide relief of pain. Aggressive pulmonary toilet is an integral part of this and all other treatment plans for chest injury.[6]

Flail chest injuries result in paradoxical motion of a segment of the chest wall. Respiratory failure will result if the segment or motion is large enough to prevent adequate ventilation, or if other thoracic injuries have occurred. Many patients have limited paradox and do not develop respiratory failure. Treatment of severe flail chest injuries requiring ventilation consists of stabilizing the chest wall by preventing negative intrathoracic pressure and reducing the paradoxical motion.[22,56,63] Assist/control volume ventilation is given in order to limit the amount of negative intrathoracic pressure and therefore the paradoxical motion. The chest wall muscles and eventually the bony callus will stabilize the chest wall and return to spontaneous ventilation. Occasionally, operative stabilization of flail chest injuries is required.[111]

Pulmonary contusion produces direct injury to the lung parenchyma with hemorrhage, atelectasis, and significant shunting. These patients develop hypoxia which may be severe enough to require intubation and ventilation. Treatment of severe pulmonary contusion requires ventilation with end-expiratory pressure. The amount of positive end-expiratory pressure (PEEP) required will vary between patients, but will frequently be 10 cm to 15 cm H_2O before oxygenation improves.

Monitoring of respiratory function also entails physiologic, clinical, and laboratory methods. Simple pulmonary mechanics measure the ability to ventilate, and more complete flow-loop curves provide information on the compliance of the lung and chest wall. Clinical assessment of the respiratory system identifies system failure earlier than other means of monitoring. Early recognition of respiratory distress does require an appreciation of normal and abnormal ventilatory efforts. Laboratory monitoring of the respiratory system is usually confined to arterial blood gas determination. In general, PCO_2 determines the adequacy of ventilation, PO_2 the adequacy of gas exchange, and *p*H the adequacy of oxygen delivery and CO_2 clearance. More specialized monitors of the respiratory function, such as mass spectroscopy or capnometers, measure end-tidal CO_2. Pulse oximeters measure arterial oxygen saturation and provide a noninvasive, continuous method of following oxygen delivery. Pediatric patients are frequently monitored with transcutaneous oxygen monitors which provide measures of tissue oxygenation.

Ventilatory support is the most common reason why patients are admitted to the ICU. While respiratory failure may be the direct result of a thoracic injury requiring specific treatment, more often it develops during the treatment of multiple injuries or subsequent complications. In these situations, support of the respiratory system must be provided while the primary problem is treated and respiration improves.

Airway management has already been mentioned. Intubation of critically ill patients can be simple, but is frequently difficult and occasionally a major problem. Usually, these intubations should be performed or supervised by someone very skilled in airway management, or an attending anesthesiologist. Awake nasal intubations work well in many patients. If the patient is *in extremis*, oral intubation should be performed to minimize delay; conversion to a nasal tube can be made at a later time. Muscle relaxants should be used by those experienced with them and capable of mask ventilation if intubation proves impossible. Depolarizing muscle relaxants, such as succinylcholine, should not be used after severe injury because of the risk of hyperkalemic cardiac arrest. The endotracheal tubes used should have the high-volume low-pressure cuffs, such as those on Lance tubes, as they greatly reduce the incidence of tracheal stenosis and tracheoesophageal fistula in patients requiring intubation for several weeks.

Mechanical ventilators vary greatly and provide several different methods of ventilatory support. These instruments are usually described as either time-, pressure-, or volume-cycled instruments. Most ventilators used today on adults are time- or volume-cycled ventilators which deliver a fixed tidal volume over a predetermined period and have pressure-release mechanisms to prevent inadvertent generation of too high a pressure.

Choice of the ventilatory mode depends on the patient and goal of therapy. Controlled ventilation delivers only the minute volume set on the instrument and does not permit additional breathing. Assist/control ventilation also delivers a set minute volume but in addition, will deliver a preset volume breath with very limited respiratory effort, usually a negative intrathoracic pressure of 3 to 5 cm H_2O. Intermittent mandatory ventilation (IMV) permits the patient to breathe in addition to the preset minute volume. This can be synchronized (SIMV) to prevent the instrument from delivering a preset breath on top of a spontaneous breath. A recently added ventilator feature is the use of pressure support. Most systems have significant impedance to flow, making spontaneous ventilation more difficult with the tubes and ventilators than without them. Pressure support delivers gas at a preset pressure during spontaneous ventilation to offset some of this difficulty. The pressure support can be set arbitrarily at some pressure above baseline, or increased while monitoring tidal volume to achieve the volume desired. High-frequency jet ventilators and oscillating ventilators are being used extensively in some ICUs.[14,59] Presently there is no evidence that they are any improvement over standard ventilatory management, except in patients with bronchopleural fistulas and in neonates with lung immaturity.[43,115]

Another consideration in providing ventilatory support is the use of end-expiratory pressure, as either PEEP with mechanical ventilation or continuous positive airway pressure (CPAP) with spontaneous ventilation. The effect of end-expiratory pressure is to increase the functional residual capacity (FRC).[95,96,121] The relationship of FRC to other pulmonary volumes is seen in Figure 20.3. The FRC maintains the resting volume of the lung above the closing volume, the level at which the terminal airways begin to collapse. Loss of surfactant or inflammatory processes of the lung, such as with ARDS, causes the closing volume to exceed the FRC. If the FRC falls below the closing volume, atelectasis develops with perfusion of the nonventilated lung, an increase in the shunt fraction, and resultant hypoxia. Increasing inspiratory pressure will only overinflate the already patent areas of the lung and not significantly affect collapsed areas. The addition of PEEP or CPAP will begin to reexpand those collapsed areas when the FRC rises above the closing volume.[29,96,116] A low level (3 cm–5 cm H_2O) of end-expiratory pressure is recommended for all intubated patients unless contraindicated. Although PEEP is part of the treatment for ARDS, there is conflicting evidence that early use of PEEP will prevent ARDS.[78,119] Patients with severe chronic obstructive pulmonary disease (COPD) may develop trapped gas with PEEP. An elevated intracranial pressure (ICP) may increase when PEEP is added

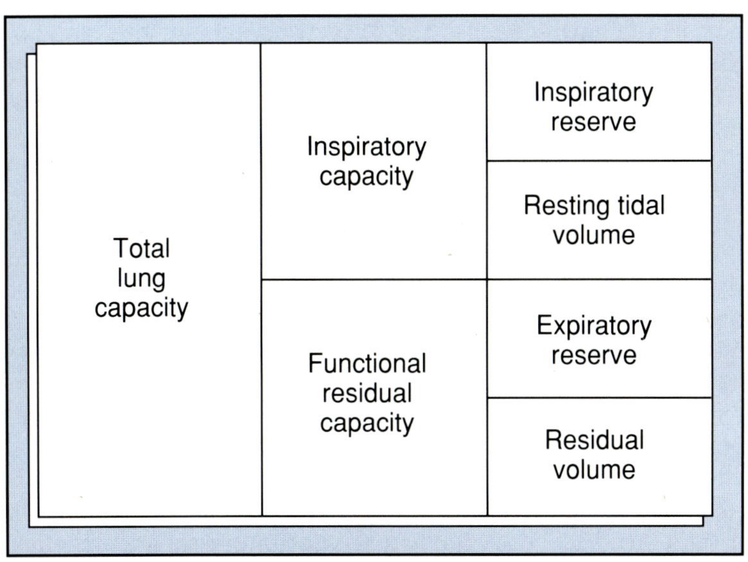

FIGURE 20.3 Relative lung volumes.

or increased. Cardiac filling has been found to decrease, adversely affecting cardiac output, but only to a significant degree at a PEEP above 10 cm H_2O.[11,16,55,67,82] The choice of the amount of PEEP to use is somewhat arbitrary. Maximum compliance and minimal shunt fraction are two variables that have been used to select the correct level of PEEP.[108] End-expiratory pressure can also be delivered in a nonintubated patient using mask CPAP.[84] This is not, however, an alternative for the patient in respiratory distress.

The choice of the mode of ventilation depends on the status of the patient. Assist/control and SIMV are standard modes for continued ventilatory support. Patients with a nonrespiratory drive to breathe will frequently develop significant respiratory alkalosis from overventilation on assist/control. This increased drive can often be blunted by sedation, but if sedation is unsuccessful, an IMV mode may be more effective. However, patients should not be permitted to spontaneously ventilate at low-rate IMV when they exhibit the signs of respiratory distress: the use of accessory muscles and high ventilatory rates. For example, a patient who is on an IMV of 6 with a delivered volume of 1 liter may have a minute volume requirement of 10 liters. The spontaneous tidal volume is only 200 cc, the patient must breathe 20 times per minute over the IMV rate to achieve the 10-liter minute volume. Such a patient on assist/control would only have to breathe four times over the preset rate of six to receive the 10-liter minute volume. If the patient develops respiratory alkalosis from significant hyperventilation on this mode, sedation will usually decrease the respiratory drive. Those patients who fail to slow their overbreathing with sedation may need to be changed to SIMV with pressure support.

Oxygen therapy is an important part of support of the respiratory system. Many patients develop hypoxia as part of their respiratory failure. This may be due to poor gas diffusion or increased shunting and perfusion of the nonventilated lung. Oxygen therapy is more likely to help in the patients with decreased perfusion, since transport is directly proportional to alveolar oxygen content. Patients with shunting, however, already have near-maximal saturation of the blood from the ventilated and perfused lung, and increased alveolar oxygen will not significantly increase the oxygen content in the blood.[57] Since the increased alveolar oxygen does not interface with blood in the perfused but not ventilated lung, there is no increase in oxygen in the blood from that part of the lung. Thus oxygen therapy will be most useful in patients with hypoxia from poor diffusion, but of limited benefit in those with shunting, which responds best to end-expiratory pressure.

When applying oxygen therapy, it is crucial to pay attention to the period of time the patient is receiving a high fraction of inspired oxygen (F_IO_2).[93,124] An F_IO_2 of greater than 0.6 for more than 48 hours will increase pulmonary fibrosis and the surfactant, produces type II alveolar cells.[26,39,40] The F_IO_2 should be reduced to the lowest level that produces acceptable oxygen saturation, usually above 95%.

Returning patients to spontaneous, unassisted ventilation remains a recurrent problem in all of critical care. Most patients do not need to be weaned from ventilatory support. If they required short-term ventilation, had good premorbid pulmonary function, and are awake and alert, they can simply be placed on spontaneous ventilation after they have the plan explained to them. Once they demonstrate the ability to ventilate adequately, they can be extubated. Patients will have less postextubation hypoxia if they are extubated from a T-piece with zero end-expiratory pressure (ZEEP).[89]

Those patients with premorbid pulmonary disease, prolonged intubation, or some evidence of ARDS with ensuing pulmonary fibrosis, do require weaning from ventilatory support but not until the underlying problem, whether it is COPD, pneumonia, or sepsis, is adequately treated. Patients with CO_2 retention who are receiving nutritional support should have their CO_2 production measured. A decrease in carbohydrate intake will also decrease their CO_2 production and make weaning easier.[4,5]

There are many techniques for weaning, but none have been proven superior. Once the patient is stable and has acceptable blood gases on an F_IO_2 of 0.4 or less and 5 cm of PEEP, he or she is more likely to tolerate weaning and be able to be extubated.[94] One effective technique of weaning is to decrease the IMV stepwise to a level of two to four breaths/min. Then the patient can be placed on progressively longer periods of CPAP, until he or she tolerates several hours on this mode without respiratory distress. The use of pressure support has significantly improved the effectiveness of this technique during the IMV and CPAP phases. Once extubated, the patient will require close respiratory monitoring for evidence of worsening respiratory distress. If the patient begins to have increased ventilatory effort, it is more prudent to reintubate early rather than late. This limits some of the rebound respiratory failure that the patient may develop.

Complications of treatment and supportive care of the respiratory system are most often related to the injury or the effects of injury. Pneumonia develops frequently in the severely injured because of direct pulmonary injury, immobility, immune suppression, and ARDS. Pneumonia in these patients is treated identically to pneumonia in other patients: with appropriate antibiotics, chest physical therapy, and general supportive care.

Endotracheal tubes, pediatric tubes especially, can become plugged more easily than might be expected. The routine use of humidified gas and suctioning decreases this problem. If it does occur, the tube should be removed immediately and replaced, rather than try to remove the obstruction.

Barotrauma is a relatively frequent complication of mechanical ventilation, occurring as often as 8% in some studies.[24,80] Barotrauma, usually pneumothorax, pneumomediastinum, or subcutaneous air, is often seen in patients on higher levels of PEEP (more than 10 cm H_2O). It is related to the peak pressures needed to ventilate the patient, rather than PEEP.[62] The patients on high levels of PEEP usually have very noncompliant lungs and need that level of peak pressure to ventilate them. The treatment of pneumothorax is tube thoracostomy. Pneumomediastinum and subcutaneous air do not require treatment, but the patient should be closely monitored for other forms of barotrauma.

Neurologic System

The incidence of head injury varies between regions and institutions, but it remains the most common cause of death in patients who survive resuscitation and initial management after injury. Although there is no direct treatment of head injury in the ICU, ICU management does include monitoring ICP, which rises after severe brain injury.[69] Monitoring of patients with impaired neurologic function depends a great deal on the extent of the impairment.

As in other systems, monitoring in patients with neurologic dysfunction after trauma includes physiologic, clinical, and laboratory methods. Physiologic monitors are limited because of access to the brain. Presently ICP monitoring constitutes the principal method of physiologic brain monitoring.[10,37,90] The most accurate measurements are obtained with intraventricular catheters. Subdural catheters, although very useful, occasionally yield misleading information. When one is monitoring ICP, it is important to have a simultaneous measurement of mean arterial pressure. The difference between the two equals the cerebral perfusion pressure, which is a reasonable index of brain perfusion.

Clinical monitoring of brain function of critically injured patients consists primarily in assessing the mental status and gross motor changes. The Glasgow coma scale remains the standard system used to clinically evaluate head injury patients.[110] Medications and metabolic effects often prevent an in-depth neurologic exam, but simple changes in pupillary size and reactivity, response to stimuli, and symmetry of motor and sensory exams may indicate an acute change in the neurologic status.

Laboratory methods of monitoring neurologic injury and dysfunction are advancing rapidly. The computed tomography scan permits evaluation of anatomy, but not function. As continual video display printouts of limited EEG readings become available, this type of monitoring will be reclassified as a physiologic method.

Supportive care of the dysfunctional neurologic system is relatively limited to control of ICP and maintenance of cerebral perfusion pressure (CPP). There is a balance between keeping the ICP low enough and the arterial pressure high enough to maintain good blood flow to the brain.[70]

Mannitol is an effective oncotic agent that causes a decrease in ICP, probably by several mechanisms, including net diffusion of fluid from the brain into the vascular space. Reduction of CO_2 by hyperventilation will raise blood *p*H relative to the *p*H of cerebrospinal fluid (CSF), leading to vasoconstriction and lowering of ICP.[33,48,79,83] This effect is blunted in 24 to 48 hours, when the blood and CSF *p*H have equilibrated. Other measures to lower ICP include a decrease in temperature or the use of muscle relaxants in agitated patients.[41]

Adrenergic agents that raise the blood pressure will increase the mean arterial pressure measured at the brain level. This is thought to increase the brain blood flow, including the site of injury. Ionotropic drugs and those with adrenergic activity have been used to raise the mean arterial pressure. These manipulations permit maintenance of adequate CPP despite abnormally high ICP. This is probably an effective means of managing the limited elevations of ICP. When the ICP remains higher than 40 to 50 cc H_2O, there is probably some neurologic damage from pressure, despite an adequate CPP. There may also be significant cardiovascular effects of this artificial elevation of blood pressure, which may adversely affect other organs. The goal of neurologic system support is to maintain perfusion of the brain, not ICP or CPP, although these variables are related to brain perfusion. Dehydration to lower ICP and excess alpha-adrenergic stimulation to raise blood pressure by vasoconstriction may actually decrease blood flow to the brain. It remains essential that treatment be focused on the goal of optimal brain perfusion.[9,41]

Complications associated with the neurologic system are limited in number. Critically ill patients frequently have reversible mental status changes, many of which are not associated with a focal brain injury or deficit. This nonspecific encephalopathy commonly resolves when the patient recovers. Intracranial hemorrhage may develop as a late complication in some cases, requiring surgical control.

There are two fluid and electrolyte problems associated with head injury: inappropriate ADH (SIADH) and diabetes insipidus. SIADH is characterized by hyponatremia with rising urine sodium, and urine osmolality greater than serum osmolality. This problem usually resolves spontaneously and is frequently not treated, or treated with water restriction. Diabetes insipidus is most often the result of brain injury with decreased release of ADH. The result is a loss of large volumes of very dilute urine. Treatment usually consists of replacing the lost fluid with an IV of a hypotonic solution, such as D5W saline. If the problem persists, vasopressin (Pitressin, plain, or in oil) can be administered.[83]

Infection is uncommon, but ventriculitis is associated with ICP monitors and carries a high mortality. Brainstem herniation is usually not a complication of ICU treatment, but represents the eventual course of some very severe brain injuries. Since head injuries are the most common cause of late trauma deaths, advances in the critical care management of these patients may significantly improve the outcome.

Urinary System

Although hematuria is common with blunt trauma, severe damage to the kidneys, ureters, and bladder occurs in less than 5% of major injuries. In those patients with urinary system injury, there is no direct treatment in the ICU other than maintenance of urine output and, rarely, bladder irrigation for clearance of clots.

Monitoring of the urinary system is simple and relatively easy in most cases and consists in measurement of urine output. This requires a Foley catheter or, in cases of lower urinary injury or urethral obstruction, a suprapubic catheter. Urine output greater than 0.5 ml/kg/hr in an adult and 1/mg/kg/hr in a child younger than two years indicates adequate perfusion of the kidneys and patent tubules. Urine output below this level may be from a prerenal cause, hypovolemia, a renal cause such as tubular necrosis, or a postrenal cause such as obstructive uropathy.[66]

Further assessment of renal function requires laboratory testing. Serum creatinine is a good measure of renal function. Specific tubular function can be better assessed by measuring urinary electrolytes, or calculating the fractional excretion of sodium (FEN):

$$\text{FEN} = \frac{\text{Urinary sodium}}{\text{Urinary creatinine}} \times \frac{\text{Plasma creatinin}}{\text{Urinary sodium}} \times 100$$

If the FEN is less than 1, the likelihood of severe tubular dysfunction is small; any oliguria is probably due to nontubular causes.[34]

Supportive care of the urinary system is the maintenance of adequate urine output. This is accomplished by providing adequate perfusion of the kidneys and a patent collecting system. Further intervention is rarely needed. Occasionally, dopamine may be needed to increase renal perfusion and urine output.[76] If renal failure does develop, dialysis may be required. Early dialysis after injury and renal failure is associated with better survival[112] and can be accomplished either by peritoneal dialysis or hemodialysis. Some patients only require removal of fluid without dialysis, and this can be accomplished by plasma ultrafiltration.

Complication of the urinary function develops in severely ill trauma victims for several major reasons. Diminished perfusion after injury may lead to renal dysfunction and possibly failure.[65] Sepsis is another potential cause of decreased renal perfusion and subsequent renal failure. Renal function is also impaired by circulating myoglobin and hemoglobin. Since Bywaters first described this problem both clinically and experimentally, increased attention has been paid to avoiding renal failure after crush injuries, limb ischemia, and hemolysis.[12,13,51,54] Again, the most important treatment is prevention by maintenance of adequate urine output, usually over 100 ml/hr until the urine clears. Sodium bicarbonate can be added to make the urine alkaline and prevent precipitation of the pigment in the tubules; mannitol has been used as an osmotic diuretic to maintain urine output. However, the addition of these two measures has never proven to be superior to maintaining adequate urine output.

Renal toxicity from medicines and other agents such as IV radiograph contrast continue to occur. Prevention is usually possible by monitoring drug levels and adequate hydration during radiology procedures whenever contrast is used.

The mortality of renal failure after injury remains high.[103] As in all other systems, prevention of urinary dysfunction is the best method of treatment.

Gastrointestinal System

Injuries to the gastrointestinal (GI) system are usually produced by penetrating trauma, although blunt injuries of the liver and spleen can also occur. Treatment is usually surgical repair, except for some very selective injuries of the liver and spleen, which are managed nonoperatively with close monitoring, preferably in an ICU. Such nonoperative management should be undertaken only in a major trauma center with the personnel and resources for immediate surgical intervention if it is needed.

Monitoring of the GI system is done to look for complications, rather than as a treatment follow-up. The passage of gas and stool is a good indicator of general bowel function and indicates obstruction is absent. Nasogastric tube output and stool can be tested for blood to detect occult or clinically obvious bleeding. The physical exam and right or left decubitus films of the abdomen are the best indicators of perforation or infection.

Complications of the gastrointestinal system can be summarized as bleeding, obstruction, and perforation. Bleeding may develop in the colon from diverticula or vascular malformations. This problem is uncommon in the ICU and has no apparent preventive measures. Significant upper GI bleeding does develop after injury, especially when complicated by sepsis. Prevention has significantly reduced the incidence of stress gastritis with bleeding. The most effective technique of preventing stress gastritis with bleeding is antacids. Antacids titrated to maintain gastric *p*H of or greater than 5 have been documented to be effective. Cimetidine and other H_2 blockers have been used to reduce gastric acid and limit bleeding.[106] Sucralfate, a coating agent that covers ulcers, is another option. Endoscopy is indicated if significant bleeding occurs. Nonoperative techniques of control are appropriate, though if the bleeding isn't stopped surgery may be indicated.

Obstruction of the bowel occurs occasionally during ICU management of the severely injured. This problem is most often seen after abdominal exploration, but may be related to other metabolic effects, including sepsis. Most acute obstructions will resolve with appropriate decompression. If the obstruction persists after 4 to 7 days, reexploration is often indicated.

Perforation with infection can develop in several organs of the gastrointestinal system. The gallbladder most often develops infection associated with acalculous cholecystitis.[45] This infection is associated with decreased perfusion of the gallbladder and often with overdistention. Enteral feeding with fat has not been proven to prevent this problem. The most common sites of perforation of the bowel are the duodenum, from ulcer disease, and the cecum, from colon obstruction. Perforation can also develop in other portions of the gut, however. Preventive treatment for colonic perforation is to monitor cecal size by KUB films and early cecostomy if it becomes distended more than 13 cm. In patients whose condition is deteriorating, occult gastrointestinal perforation and infection have to be considered.

Metabolic System

Other than direct injury to an endocrine organ, trauma does not injure the metabolic system. Trauma does, however, have dramatic effects on the metabolic system, producing an increased release of catecholamines and hormones, as presented in the review of pathophysiology.[31,122] Monitoring of these effects requires the complex measurement of circulating mediators. Indirect monitoring of the effects of hormones on end-organs is inaccurate because of the many other factors that affect those organs.

Metabolic support of the severely injured ICU patient can be broadly interpreted to include radiant warming to maintain temperature and thyroid replacement in hypothyroid patients. Much of metabolic support is nutrition, and this is a major factor in the treatment of these critically injured patients.[16,36,60] Recovery from acute renal failure can be improved with early metabolic support.[1] That is why it is crucial for the clinician to have a clear understanding of the metabolic and nutritional system, its support, and its potential complications in caring for the critically ill.

Hematologic System

Trauma can disturb the hematologic system by blood loss or injury to blood-producing (bone marrow) or blood-processing (liver and spleen) organs. Ther is no specific ICU treatment for this disturbance. Massive transfusion (the replacement of one and one half total body blood volumes) has associated problems that require treatment and monitoring to prevent complications. These problems are compounded by the fact that massively transfused patients have been in shock.

Monitoring of patients who are receiving massive transfusions is done by physiologic and laboratory means. Physiologic monitoring includes temperature and urine output to ensure perfusion. Hypothermia is a common problem after infusion of room temperature crystalloid and refrigerated blood products. Laboratory monitoring of massively transfused patients includes hematocrit, platelet count, and coagulation parameters. Increased bleeding after massive transfusion is due to general factors including dilutional thrombocytopenia and hypothermia.

Supportive care of the massively transfused patient requires maintenance of perfusion and delivery of oxygen. Once the source of blood loss is controlled, reestablishment of the normal homeostasis can begin. Transfusion requirements will continue as transfused blood is typed and cleared at an accelerated rate and hematopoesis is limited by the severity of the injury.

Massive transfusion causes both immediate complications of hypothermia and coagulopathy as well as later problems. A transfusion reaction can be immediate or delayed and may be limited to a febrile reaction or massive hemolysis. The hematologic system is very interrelated with other systems and prevention of complications is best handled by scrupulous attention to blood transfusion in the ICU. If a transfusion reaction is suspected, the infusion must be stopped and tests ordered for transfusion reaction. Another later complication of transfusion is infection. The incidence of infection with non-A—non-B hepatitis after transfusion of a single unit remains well over 5%. Cytomegalovirus occurs in over 5% of donors; other viruses are less commonly found. Units of blood are presently screened for human immunodeficiency virus and type B hepatitis, so that infection with those agents should be uncommon.

Musculoskeletal System

Injuries to the musculoskeletal system occur commonly in most forms of injury. The severity of the injuries varies greatly. Although critical care is not usually associated with the treatment of these injuries, many complex musculoskeletal injuries are managed in ICUs.

Patients with multiple fractures and other problems requiring critical care need traction to limit their injury and prevent complications. This treatment is limited and often followed by definitive operative fixation. Traction and splints should be examined frequently to ensure that they are fulfilling their purpose.

Monitoring of the musculoskeletal system is largely limited to following perfusion and, in some injuries, compartment pressures. Doppler measurement of arterial and venous flow is useful in those situations in which edema or depth of the vessel limits palpation of arterial inflow. Clinical assessment of the limb perfusion is also very useful. Measurement of compartment pressures is more standardized now with the use of the slit-catheter technique.

Complications of the musculoskeletal system may be preventable by close attention to the patient's complaints at physical examination. Occasionally, musculoskeletal problems are overlooked during the management of more unstable life-threatening injuries with other systems. Compulsive attention to detail, however, may prevent or limit significant disability which becomes apparent when the patient is more stable.

Immune System

The immune system is the sum of the body's defense mechanisms to infection. Of the patients who survive the first 48 hours after injury and subsequently die, 80% of those deaths which are not the result of head injury are due to sepsis.[123] Injury suppresses all of the measurable components of immune response and increases susceptibility to infection.[2,71,104] Patients who are severely injured and require critical care measures are at extremely high risk of death from infection. The most common infection is pneumonia, but other infections occur, especially at sites of injury.

Treatment of problems of the immune system is essentially the treatment of infection. Location of the site of infection is frequently difficult in critically ill patients. Routine portable films, especially chest x-rays, identify a large number of infectious problems. Bedside ultrasound has proved very useful in the unstable patient. CT scans or other tests may identify and locate a source of infection. There continue to be cases that require surgical exploration to determine if infection is present.

The fundamental rules of management of infection are no different in the critically ill trauma patient. These are:

Appropriate antibiotics
Drainage of debridement of infection
Adjunctive measures

High-dose corticosteroids have been used with varied results, but a recent randomized study noted no increased survival from sepsis with dexamethasone or methylprednisolone.[105]

Antibiotics are chosen to cover suspected organisms and adjusted when cultures are available. Loculated infection must be drained, and recent advances in percutaneous techniques have made this an effective option for many types of abscess. Infected, devitalized tissue must be debrided to aid percutaneous drainage.

Adjunctive measures are very important, for example chest physiotherapy for pneumonia or elevation of infected limbs.

Monitoring requirements of patients with infection and sepsis vary according to their stability and the presence of other organ-system dysfunction. Patients who are hemodynamically stable and have adequate respiratory function require no extensive monitoring. Patients who are hypotensive but well perfused generally only need arterial lines. Pulmonary artery catheters in such patients will only confirm what is known clinically, that cardiac output is high and systemic vascular resistance and filling pressures are low. Pulmonary artery catheters should be used in patients with poor peripheral perfusion or severe respiratory failure, but it is not known if they improve survival. Urine output remains the most reliable measure of perfusion in sepsis in the absence of deteriorating renal function.

Supportive care for infected and septic patients also varies tremendously. Stable patients being treated for their infection will require little supportive care unless there is other system dysfunction. Sepsis, like injury, leads to increased release of local mediators and a rise in circulating catecholamines, aldosterone, ADH, insulin, and glucagon.[15] However, some patients with profound sepsis may require hemodynamic and pulmonary support. Circulating myocardial depressants have been noted in clinical and experimental sepsis.[120] Hemodynamic support should be directed at improving perfusion, not achieving an arbitrary blood pressure. Dobutamine and beta-adrenergic doses of dopamine frequently provide this effect. Myocardial depression will usually resolve with appropriate treatment of the infection.

Sepsis may produce dramatic changes in the respiratory system and is the most common cause of ARDS.[27] Supportive care for respiratory failure is as described in the section on the respiratory system. Despite some early studies, the use of steroids to treat ARDS has not been shown to be beneficial.[74] Sepsis has extensive effects on all other systems.[7,8,15,42] Patients develop increased metabolic demands, while the mechanism to respond to those demands is impaired.[25,53] Hepatic protein synthesis and bile metabolism are impaired with sepsis.[18,35,38] Renal failure can develop as a consequence of sepsis.[65] Some coagulopathy is common, but severe bleeding diatheses are rare. Supportive care of this multiple-system dysfunction is designed to maintain the patient until he or she responds to the treatment of the underlying infection. The mortality rate for sepsis with multiple-system failure remains at 80% to 90%.

Complications develop as a result of infection and are much more frequent if the patient has systemic sepsis. Acutely, patients may have dysfunction of several other body systems, which may lead to permanent organ failure. The ARDS associated with sepsis will often result in significant impairment of pulmonary function if the patient survives. Sepsis can lead to other localized infection, spread by circulating bacteria. There are no apparent means of preventing these complications other than prompt treatment of any infection.

REFERENCES

1. Abel RM, Beck CH Jr, Abbot WM et al: Improved survival from acute renal failure after treatment with intravenous essential L-amino acids and glucose. N Engl J Med 288:695–699, 1973.
2. Abraham E: Immunologic mechanisms underlying sepsis in the critically ill surgical patient. Surg Clin North Am 65:991–1003, 1985.
3. Archer LT, Black MR, Hinshaw MB: Myocardial failure with altered response to adrenaline in endotoxin shock. Br J Pharmacol 54:145–154, 1975.
4. Askanazi J, Rosenbaum SH, Hyman AI et al: Respiratory changes induced by the large glucose loads of total parenteral nutrition. JAMA 243:1444–1447, 1980.
5. Askanazi J, Weisman C, Rosenbaum SH et al: Nutrition and the respiratory system. Crit Care Med 10:163–172, 1982.
6. Bartlett RH: Postoperative pulmonary prophylaxis. Chest 81:1–9, 1982.
7. Barzotta AP, Polk HC Jr: Multiple system organ failure. Surg Clin North Am 63:315–336, 1983.
8. Baue AE, Chaudry IH: Prevention of multiple systems failure. Surg Clin North Am 60:1167–1181, 1980.
9. Becker DP, Miller JD, Hard JD et al: The outcome from severe head injury with early diagnosis and intensive management. J Neurosurg 47:491–502, 1977.
10. Borel C, Hanley D: Neurologic intensive care unit monitoring. Crit Care Clin 1:223–237, 1985.
11. Buda AJ, Pinsky MR, Engels NB: Effect of intrathoracic pressure on left ventricular performance. N Engl J Med 301:453–459, 1979.
12. Bywaters EGL, Beall O: Crush injuries with impairment of renal function. Br Med J 1:427–430, 1941.
13. Bywaters EGL, Stead JK: The production of renal failure following injection of solutions containing myoglobin. Q J Exp Physiol 33:53–60, 1944.
14. Carlon GC, Kahn RC, Howland WS et al: Clinical experience with high frequency jet ventilation. Crit Care Med 9:1–6, 1981.
15. Cerra FB: The systemic septic response: Multiple systems organ failure. Crit Care Clin 1:591–607, 1985.
16. Cerra FB: The role of nutrition in the management of metabolic stress. Crit Care Clin (in press).
17. Cerra FB, Hassett J, Siegel JH: Vasodilator therapy in clinical sepsis with low output syndrome. J Surg Res 25:180–188, 1978.
18. Cerra FB, Siegel JH, Border JR et al: The hepatic failure of sepsis: Cellular versus substrate. Surgery 86:409–422, 1979.
19. Chandry IH: Cellular mechanisms in shock and ischemia and their correction. Am J Physiol 245:R117–R134, 1983.
20. Chatterjee K, Parmley WW: The role of vasodilator therapy in heart failure. Prog Cardiovasc Dis 19:301–355, 1977.
21. Chernow B, Rainey TG, Lake R: Endogenous and exogenous catecholamines in critical care medicine. Crit Care Med 10:409–416, 1982.
22. Clemmer TP, Fairfax WR: Chest injury: Critical care management. Crit Care Clin (in press).
23. Critical care medicine. NIH Consensus Conference. JAMA 250:798–804, 1983.
24. Cullen DJ, Caldera DL: The incidence of ventilator-induced pulmonary barotrauma in critically ill patients. Anesthesiology 50:185–191, 1979.
25. Curnow RT, Rayfield EJ, George DT et al: Altered hepatic glycogen metabolism and glucoregulatory hormones during sepsis. Am J Physiol 230:1296–1301, 1976.
26. Davis WB, Rennard ST, Bitterman PB et al: Pulmonary oxygen toxicity: Early reversible changes in human alveolar structures induced by hyperoxia. N Engl J Med 309:878–882, 1983.
27. Demling RH: The pathogenesis of respiratory failure after trauma and sepsis. Surg Clin North Am 60:1373–1390, 1981.
28. Demling RH: The cardiopulmonary effects of sepsis on the trauma patient. Crit Care Clin (in press).

29. Demling RH, Nerlich M: Acute respiratory failure. Surg Clin North Am 63:337–355, 1983.
30. Denzliger C, Rapp S, Hagmann W et al: Leukotrienes as mediators in tissue trauma. Science 230:330–332, 1985.
31. Egdahl RH, Meguid MM, Aun F: The importance of the endocrine and metabolic responses to shock and trauma. Crit Care Med 5:257–263, 1977.
32. Elliott CG, Zimmerman GA, Clemmer TA: Complications of pulmonary artery catheterization in the care of critically ill patients: A prospective study. Chest 76:647–652, 1979.
33. Enevoldsen EM, Jensen FT: Autoregulation and CO[cf15]2 responses of cerebral blood flow in patients with acute severe head injury. J Neurosurg 48:689–703, 1978.
34. Espinel CH, Gregory AW: Differential diagnosis of acute renal failure. Clin Nephrol 13:73–88, 1980.
35. Fahrlander H, Huber F, Gloor F: Intrahepatic retention of bile in severe bacterial infections. Gastroenterology 46:590–599, 1964.
36. Fischer JE: Nutritional support in the seriously ill patient. Curr Probl Surg 17:469–531, 1980.
37. Fleischer AS, Payne NS, Tindall GT: Continuous monitoring of intracranial pressure in severe closed head injury without mass lesions. Surg Neurol 6:31–40, 1976.
38. Flint LM: Liver failure. Surg Clin North Am 62:157–165, 1982.
39. Frank L, Bucher JR, Roberts RJ: Oxygen toxicity in neonatal and adult animals of various species. J Appl Physiol 45:699–704, 1978.
40. Frank L, Massaro D: Oxygen toxicity. Am J Med 69:117–127, 1980.
41. Frost EAM: The intensive care of the neurosurgical patient. Semin Anesth 1:340–353, 1982.
42. Fry DE: Multiple organ system failure: The role of uncontrolled infection. Arch Surg 115:136–141, 1980.
43. Gardner RM, Schwartz R, Wong HC et al: Percutaneous indwelling radial artery catheters for monitoring cardiovascular function: Prospective study of the risk of thrombosis and infection. N Engl J Med 290:1227–1231, 1974.
44. Glantz SA, Hisbach GY, Moores WY et al: The pericardium substantially affects the left ventricular diastolic pressure-volume relationship in the dog. Circ Res 42:433–441, 1978.
45. Glenn F, Berker AG: Acute acalculous cholecystitis. Ann Surg 195:131–138, 1982.
46. Goldenheim PD, Kazenu H: Cardiopulmonary monitoring of critically ill patients. N Engl J Med 311:717–720, 776–780, 1984.
47. Gorlin R: Practical cardiac hemodynamics. N Engl J Med 296:203–205, 1977.
48. Greenberg JH, Alavi A, Reivich M et al: Local cerebral blood volume response to carbon dioxide in man. Circ Res 43:324, 1978.
49. Hechtman HB, Huval WV, Mathieson MA: Prostaglandin and thromboxane mediation of cardiopulmonary failure. Surg Clin North Am 63:263–283, 1983.
50. Holcroft JW: Responsibility for care of the critically ill surgical patient. J Surg Res 38:315–318, 1985.
51. Honda N: Acute renal failure and rhabdomyolysis. Kidney Int 23:888–898, 1983.
52. Horton JW, Coln D, Mitchell JH: Left ventricular volumes and contractility during hemorrhagic hypertension: Dimensional analysis and biplane cineflourography. Circ Shock 11:73, 1983.
53. Houtchens BA, Westenskow DR: Oxygen consumption in septic shock: Collective review. Circ Shock 13:361–384, 1984.
54. Iaina A, Reisin E, Eliahou H: Acute renal failure in combat injuries. J Trauma 15:281–289, 1975.
55. Jardin F, Fracot J, Boisante L et al: Influence of positive end-expiratory pressure on left ventricular performance. N Engl J Med 304:387–392, 1981.
56. Jones KW: Thoracic trauma. Surg Clin North Am 60:957–981, 1980.
57. Katz JA, Zinn SE, Ozanne GM et al: Pulmonary, chest wall, and lung-thorax elastances in acute respiratory failure. Chest 80:304–311, 1981.
58. Kaye W: Invasive monitoring techniques: Arterial cannulation, bedside pulmonary artery catheterization, and arterial puncture. Heart Lung 12:395–427, 1983.
59. Klain M, Keszler H: High-frequency jet ventilation. Surg Clin North Am 65:917–930, 1985.
60. Kudsk KA, Stone JM, Sheldon GF: Nutrition in trauma and burns. Surg Clin North Am 62:183–192, 1982.
61. Kuehl FA Jr, Egan RW: Prostaglandins, arachidonic acid, and inflammation. Science 210:978–984, 1980.
62. Kumar A, Pontoppidan H, Falke KJ et al: Pulmonary barotrauma during mechanical ventilation. Crit Care Med 1:181–189, 1973.
63. Lewis FR: Thoracic trauma. Surg Clin North Am 62:97–104, 1982.
64. Lovett WM, Wangensteen SL, Gleen TM et al: Presence of a myocardial depressant factor in patients with circulatory shock. Surgery 70:223–230, 1981.
65. Lucas CE: The renal response to acute injury and sepsis. Surg Clin North Am 56:953–970, 1976.
66. Lucas CE: Renal considerations in the injured patient. Surg Clin North Am 62:133–148, 1982.
67. Luce JM: The cardiovascular effects of mechanical ventilation and positive end-expiratory pressure. JAMA 252:807–811, 1984.
68. Machiedo GW, Blackwood JM, Rush BF Jr: Practice of critical care in academic surgical centers. J Surg Res 30:223–228, 1981.
69. Marsh ML, Marshall LF, Shapiro HM: Neurosurgical intensive care. Anesthesiology 47:149–158, 1977.
70. Marshall LF, Smith RW, Shapiro HM: The outcome with aggressive treatment in severe head injuries. Part I. The significance of intracranial pressure monitoring. J Neurosurg 50:20–32, 1979.
71. McIrvine AJ, Mannick JA: Lymphocyte function in the critically ill surgical patient. Surg Clin North Am 63:245–261, 1983.
72. Meyer AA, Lewis FR: Hemodynamic monitoring in the trauma patient. Semin Anesth 3:143–154, 1984.
73. Meyer AA, Trunkey DD: Critical care as an integral part of trauma care. Crit Care Clin (in press).
74. Nicholson DP: Corticosteroids in the treatment of septic shock and the adult respiratory distress syndrome. Med Clin North Am 67:717–724, 1983.
75. Parker MM, Shelhamer JH, Bacharach SL et al: Profound but reversible myocardial depression in patients with septic shock. Ann Intern Med 100:483–491, 1984.
76. Parker S, Carlon GC, Issacs M et al: Dopamine administration in oliguria and oliguric renal failure. Crit Care Med 9:630–631, 1981.
77. Parsa MH, Tabora F: Establishment of intravenous lines for long-term intravenous therapy and monitoring. Surg Clin North Am 65:835–865, 1985.
78. Pepe PE, Hudson LD, Carrico CJ: Early application of positive end-expiratory pressure in patients at risk for the adult respiratory distress syndrome. N Engl J Med 311:281–286, 1984.
79. Perini S, Beltramella A, Pasut ML et al: CNS trauma: Head injuries. Crit Care Clin 1:241–265, 1985.
80. Peterson GW, Baier H: Incidence of pulmonary barotrauma in a medical ICU. Crit Care Med 11:67–69, 1983.
81. Pinilla JC, Ross DF, Martin T et al: Study of the incidence of intravascular catheter infection and associated septicemia in critically ill patients. Crit Care Med 11:21–25, 1983.
82. Pinsky MR: The influence of positive-pressure ventilation on cardiovascular function in the critically ill. Crit Care Clin 1:699–717, 1985.
83. Pitts LH, Martin N: Head injuries. Surg Clin North Am 62:47–60, 1982.
84. Pontoppidan H: Mechanical aids to lung expansion in non-intubated surgical patients. Am Rev Respir Dis 122:109–119, 1980.
85. Pontoppidan H, Wilson RS, Rie MA et al: Respiratory intensive care. Anesthesiology 47:96–116, 1977.
86. Potkin RT, Werner JA, Trobaugh GB et al: Evaluation of noninvasive tests of cardiac damage in suspected cardiac contusion. Circulation 66:627–631, 1982.

INDEX

Note: Numbers in **boldface** refer to Figure or Table numbers.

B